DATE DUE			

PARASITES OF LABORATORY ANIMALS

PARASITES OF LABORATORY ANIMALS

Robert J. Flynn, D.V.M.

DIVISION OF BIOLOGICAL AND MEDICAL RESEARCH
ARGONNE NATIONAL LABORATORY
ARGONNE, ILLINOIS

THE IOWA STATE UNIVERSITY PRESS | AMES

THIS WORK was supported by the U.S. Atomic Energy Commission and the Air Force Office of Scientific Research.

ROBERT J. FLYNN is a veterinarian who has been professionally concerned with the production and maintenance of research animals since 1948. He is a certified specialist in laboratory animal medicine and co-founder of both the American Association for Laboratory Animal Science and the American College of Laboratory Animal Medicine. His professional activities have been devoted to advancing medical and biological science by improving the quality of the animals used in biomedical research. In recognition of his achievements, he has been awarded the Griffin Award, the highest honor of the American Association for Laboratory Animal Science.

Library of Congress Cataloging in Publication Data

Flynn, Robert J   1923–
    Parasites of laboratory animals.
    Includes bibliographies.
    1. Parasites—Laboratory animals.   2. Laboratory
animals—Diseases.   I. Title.

SF810.A3F6   636.08′85   77—171165

ISBN 0—8138—0470—1

Composed and printed by
The Iowa State University Press

First edition, 1973

COLLABORATORS

FLIES

E. PAUL CATTS
University of Delaware
Newark, Delaware

LICE

KARY C. EMERSON
Arlington, Virginia

PENTASTOMIDS

ALEX FAIN
Institute de Médecine Tropicale
Prince Léopold
Antwerp, Belgium

NEMATODES, ACANTHOCEPHALANS,
LEECHES

DONALD HEYNEMAN
University of California
San Francisco, California

PARASITES OF FISHES

GLENN L. HOFFMAN
Eastern Fish Disease Laboratory
Leetown, West Virginia

TICKS

HARRY HOOGSTRAAL
U.S. Naval Medical Research Unit
No. 3
Cairo, U.A.R.

PARASITES OF AMPHIBIANS
AND REPTILES

HAROLD M. KAPLAN
Southern Illinois University
Carbondale, Illinois

LICE

KE CHUNG KIM
Pennsylvania State University
University Park, Pennsylvania

PROTOZOANS

NORMAN D. LEVINE
University of Illinois
Urbana, Illinois

FLEAS

ROBERT E. LEWIS
Iowa State University
Ames, Iowa

LICE

ROGER D. PRICE
University of Minnesota
St. Paul, Minnesota

BUGS

RAYMOND E. RYCKMAN
Loma Linda University
Loma Linda, California

TREMATODES, CESTODES

MARIETTA VOGE
University of California
Los Angeles, California

MITES

CONRAD YUNKER
Rocky Mountain Laboratory
Hamilton, Montana

TO MY WIFE AND FAMILY
*in partial restitution for the time taken from them
for this book*

CONTENTS

ix

PREFACE

ALTHOUGH much is known about the parasites of laboratory animals, information is often lacking and what is available is scattered. It is the purpose of this book to gather what is known in this field so that it is readily accessible to those who need it, and to point out what is not known.

Some of the stated deficiencies in our knowledge are probably incorrect in that the information is available but either has been overlooked or has not been published. It is hoped that these incorrect statements will stimulate persons with contrary information to point out the error or to divulge previously unpublished data.

It is also recognized that in a work of this sort, other errors are likely. It would be appreciated if these are pointed out so that they can be corrected in future editions, should the reception of this book warrant future revisions.

Many people helped write this book. The principal contributors are listed in the front. They are called "collaborators" rather than authors, not in any way to detract from their contributions but to prevent their being criticized for errors which are mine. A draft of each chapter was first prepared by the appropriate collaborator and then rewritten by me. The rewriting was done primarily to emphasize laboratory animals and secondarily to provide uniformity of style. The rewritten chapter was then reviewed by the collaborator and, in some cases, by others. Thus, each chapter in the book represents a joint effort of at least two people and, in some cases, of several.

Many people, besides the listed collaborators, assisted in the preparation of this volume. These include persons who reviewed chapters or parts of chapters, furnished illustrations, made literature searches and helped or advised in various ways. These people are listed under Acknowledgments. Although great effort was made to make the listing complete, it is recognized that the contributions of some may have been inadvertently omitted. For this, I apologize and I assure these people that the omissions were unintentional.

The parasites described are those that occur spontaneously. Experimentally induced conditions are mentioned only if they are of special significance. No attempt is made to include the parasites of all domestic and wild animals. As a general rule, those of the common laboratory animals (mouse, rat, hamster, guinea pig, rabbit, dog, cat, rhesus monkey, chicken) are all included, but for the less common species (such as other rodents, other primates, reptiles, amphibians, fishes), only the commonest parasites of the animal species most likely to be used in the laboratory are described. Agents that occur only in domestic animals of agricultural importance are not described, even though these animals are sometimes used in the laboratory, as this information is readily available elsewhere.

The common and proper names of animals included are given in the Appendix. Except for a few rare or uncommon animals, the common name only is used in the text. Although this may appear unscientific, the repeated use, for example, of *Mesocricetus auratus,* when one means the usual laboratory hamster, and *Oryctolagus cuniculus,* when one means the laboratory rabbit, is undesirable. Also, scientific names sometimes change, but common names tend to remain the same. Great care was taken to ensure that the scientific name is given for every common name that appears in the text, and that the common name is specific. Authorities used to determine the appropriate names are cited.

It is my sincere hope that the usefulness of this book will justify the efforts of all who helped prepare it.

ROBERT J. FLYNN

ACKNOWLEDGMENTS

THE preparation of this book required the assistance and cooperation of many people. The principal contributors are those listed in the front of the book as "Collaborators." Special recognition is also due to the following Argonne personnel who gave unselfishly of their time and talents:

L. J. Roder and Eve Albertson: For editorial assistance without which this book would never have been completed.

Susan J. Clegg: For a variety of tasks, including typing and retyping the entire manuscript several times.

Doris J. Flynn: For patiently and uncomplainingly verifying every reference in the book.

N. P. Zaichick: For searching exhaustively for hard-to-find reference articles and for other bibliographic assistance.

Jane K. Glaser: For photographic assistance, including the mounting of every illustration in the book.

Others who reviewed chapters, who made literature searches, who prepared chapters which were subsequently deleted from this book, or who advised or assisted in a variety of other ways include:

C. H. Andrewes, Salisbury, England
L. M. Ashley, Western Fish Nutrition Laboratory
W. A. Austin, Detroit Zoological Park
T. Balazs, Smith, Kline and French
Aeleta Barber, Louisiana State University
S. Barker, University of Adelaide
J. E. Beach, Fisons Pharmaceuticals Limited
B. N. Berg, Columbia University
N. R. Brewer, University of Chicago
B. A. Briody, New Jersey College of Medicine and Dentistry
A. O. Broome, University of Texas
D. G. Brown, University of Tennessee
W. L. Bullock, University of New Hampshire
L. K. Bustad, University of California, Davis
J. H. Calaby, Commonwealth (Australian) Scientific and Industrial Research Organization
B. W. Calnek, Cornell University
R. W. Camden, Argonne National Laboratory
J. Camin, University of Kansas
L. E. Carmichael, Cornell University
Helen E. Cesvet, W. Alton Jones Cell Science Center
L. R. Christensen, University of Toronto
J. J. Christian, Albert Einstein Medical Center
T. B. Clarkson, Wake Forest University
G. R. Clements, Armour Pharmaceutical Company
J. M. Clinton, Cherry Hill, New Jersey
R. A. Crandell, University of Illinois
C. N. W. Cumming, Carworth
Edith Cumming, Carworth
Gretchen M. Dayton, Argonne National Laboratory
F. Deinhardt, Presbyterian-St. Luke's Hospital
L. S. Diamond, U.S. Public Health Service
W. H. Dieterich, Animal Resources
E. Dougherty, Cornell University
J. D. Douglas, Holloman Air Force Base
G. Dryden, University of Missouri
G. A. Elliott, Upjohn Company
R. D. Estep, National Institutes of Health

Sylvia L. Eubanks, Chattanooga, Tennessee

J. S. Evans, Upjohn Company

E. S. Feenstra, Upjohn Company

J. F. Ferrell, Hazleton Laboratories

M. H. Fisher, Argonne National Laboratory

M. B. Flack, St. Mary's Hospital Medical School

H. L. Foster, Charles River Breeding Laboratories

Theresa Fox, Carshalton, England

J. K. Frenkel, University of Kansas Medical Center

M. H. Friedman, Sloan-Kettering Institute

C. E. Fuller, U.S. Air Force

D. P. Furman, University of California, Berkeley

Mildred M. Galton (deceased)

J. R. Ganaway, U.S. Public Health Service

Lucille K. Georg, National Communicable Disease Center

J. P. Gibson, Wm. S. Merrell Company

J. H. Gillespie, Cornell University

R. C. Good, National Center for Primate Biology

J. R. Gorham, Washington State University

J. W. Gowen (deceased)

W. R. Graham, Upjohn Company

J. E. Gray, Upjohn Company

M. L. Gray (deceased)

E. T. Greenstein, Bristol Laboratories

Melissa R. Gregory, Argonne National Laboratory

R. A. Griesemer, National Center for Primate Biology

K. W. Hagen, Jr., Washington State University

Patricia O. Halloran, Staten Island Zoo

J. E. Halver, Western Fish Nutrition Laboratory

Janet W. Hartley, National Institutes of Health

J. M. Heinen, Hinsdale, Illinois

W. L. Henning, Bryan College

W. R. Hinshaw, Frederick, Maryland

D. D. Holmes, Veterans Administration Hospital, Oklahoma City

B. M. Honigberg, University of Massachusetts

W. R. Horsfall, University of Illinois

J. R. M. Innes, Bionetics Research Laboratories

R. T. Jordan, Bio-Medical Research Laboratories

D. W. Jolly, Huntingdon Research Centre

L. D. Jones, Fitzsimons General Hospital

T. C. Jones, Harvard Medical School

L. H. Karstad, Ontario Veterinary College

Elaine B. Katz, Highland Park, Illinois

C. F. Kauffeld, Staten Island Zoo

W. O. Kester, Golden, Colorado

L. Kilham, Dartmouth Medical School

R. F. Kinard, U.S. Public Health Service

G. M. Kohls, Rocky Mountain Laboratory

Lisbeth M. Kraft, Goshen, New York

J. H. Krupp, University of Colorado

T. J. Lafeber, Niles, Illinois

W. Lane-Petter, Huntingdon Research Centre

E. J. Larson, National Drug Company

A. M. Leash, Case Western Reserve University

J. H. Litchfield, Battelle Memorial Institute

J. K. Loosli, Cornell University

Sally Lust, Washington State University

K. T. Maddy, National Institutes of Health

W. L. Margard, Battelle Memorial Institute

R. O. McClellan, Lovelace Foundation

S. J. McConnell, Texas A & M University

E. Meerovitch, McGill University

R. W. Menges (deceased)

D. B. Meyer, Michigan Department of Health

K. F. Meyer, University of California, San Francisco

M. C. Meyer, University of Maine

F. E. Mitchell, University of Georgia

J. B. Moloney, National Institutes of Health

D. H. Moore, Institute for Medical Research

J. A. Moore, National Institutes of Health

W. W. Moss, Academy of Natural Sciences

G. W. Nace, University of Michigan

M. K. Nadel, Xerox Corporation

J. B. Nelson, Rockefeller University

J. W. Newberne, Wm. S. Merrell Company

E. V. Orsi, Seton Hall University

L. A. Page, National Animal Disease Laboratory

T. W. Penfold, University of Washington

A. C. Peters, Battelle Memorial Institute

J. E. Prier, Pennsylvania Department of Health

H. E. Rhoades, University of Illinois

V. T. Riley, Pacific Northwest Research Foundation

Jane F. Robens, Hoffman-LaRoche

Lynne Roder, Wheaton, Illinois
Norma Rothman, Philadelphia
W. P. Rowe, National Institutes of Health
R. A. Runnells, Kalamazoo
G. A. Sacher, Argonne National Laboratory
Mary Sasso, Argonne National Laboratory
H. E. Savely, Air Force Office of Scientific Research
L. H. Saxe, West Virginia University
F. W. Scott, Cornell University
L. A. Selby, University of Missouri
G. B. Sharman, Commonwealth (Australian) Scientific and Industrial Research Organization
R. C. Simkins, Argonne National Laboratory
S. K. Sinha, Central Wisconsin Colony and Training School
B. H. Skold, Iowa State University
R. L. Smiley, U.S. Department of Agriculture
J. M. B. Smith, Massey University of Manawatu
L. DS. Smith, Virginia Polytechnic Institute
Rebecca F. Smith, Argonne National Laboratory
C. H. Snider, U.S. Air Force
S. F. Snieszko, Eastern Fish Disease Laboratory
V. Sprague, University of Maryland
W. T. S. Thorp, University of Minnesota
R. Ellen Thro, Downers Grove, Illinois
D. V. Tolle, Argonne National Laboratory
B. F. Trum, Harvard Medical School
D. C. Tudor, Rutgers University
A. A. Tuffery, University of Western Australia
E. P. Walker (deceased)
T. G. Ward, Microbiological Associates
H. D. Webster, Upjohn Company
J. A. Weir, University of Kansas
E. Weiss, Naval Medical Research Institute
G. W. Wharton, Ohio State University
L. F. Whitney, Orange, Connecticut
R. E. Wilsnack, Huntington Research Center
K. E. Wolf, Eastern Fish Disease Laboratory
J. M. Woodward, University of Tennessee
A. N. Worden, Huntingdon Research Centre

J. T. Yoder, Veterans Administration Center, Des Moines
A. Zervins, Westinghouse

Persons who generously furnished illustrations for this book are:

S. H. Abadie, Louisiana State University Medical Center
A. M. Allen, U.S. Public Health Service
H. D. Anthony, Kansas State University
N. Ashton, University of London
W. S. Bailey, Auburn University
K. P. Baker, University of Dublin
F. Bloom, Flushing, New York
R. E. Bostrom, Edgewood Arsenal
B. C. Bullock, Wake Forest University
W. L. Bullock, University of New Hampshire
G. R. Burch, Pitman-Moore
R. B. Burrows, Burroughs Wellcome and Company
E. H. Coles, Kansas State University
P. B. Conran, Dow Chemical Company
G. E. Cosgrove, Oak Ridge National Laboratory
M. Dorothy Cox, Loma Linda University
L. S. Diamond, U.S. Public Health Service
C. van Duijn, Zeist, Netherlands
E. E. Elkan, London
R. R. Estes, School of Aerospace Medicine
S. A. Ewing, Oklahoma State University
R. K. Farrell, Washington State University
J. F. Ferrell, Hazleton Laboratories
M. J. Forstner, University of Munich
J. K. Frenkel, University of Kansas Medical Center
T. E. Fritz, Argonne National Laboratory
K. Fujiwara, University of Tokyo
M. Fukui, Chugai Pharmaceutical Company
S. M. Gaafar, Purdue University
P. Ghittino, Fish Disease Laboratory, Torino
G. L. Graham, University of Pennsylvania
J. H. Greve, Iowa State University
A. H. Groth, Auburn University
R. T. Habermann, U.S. Public Health Service
K. W. Hagen, Jr., Washington State University
A. H. Handler, Rutgers Medical School
J. L. Hansen, Armed Forces Institute of Pathology

G. R. Healy, National Communicable Disease Center

L. H. Herman, Edgewood Arsenal

J. R. M. Innes, Bionetics Research Laboratories

R. F. Jackson, St. Augustine

Helen Jarvis, Walter Reed Army Medical Center

T. C. Jones, Harvard Medical School

W. Klemm, School of Veterinary Medicine, Cluj, Romania

G. M. Kohls, Rocky Mountain Laboratory

J. R. Lindsey, University of Alabama, Birmingham

R. D. Manwell, State University of New York, Syracuse

B. Matanic, State University of New York, Brooklyn

A. Meshorer, Weizmann Institute of Science

J. H. L. Mills, University of Saskatchewan

T. Møller, Royal Veterinary and Agricultural College (Denmark)

Betty J. Myers, Southwest Foundation for Research and Education

Dawn G. Owen, Laboratory Animals Centre

C. M. Poole, Argonne National Laboratory

W. H. Pryor, School of Aerospace Medicine

H. Reichenbach-Klinke, Munich

W. M. Reid, University of Georgia

Bonny Rininger, Bionetics Research Laboratories

W. A. Rogers, Auburn University

T. C. Ruch, University of Washington

E. H. Sadun, Walter Reed Army Medical Center

H. F. Smetana, Tulane University

Alma D. Smith, Rocky Mountain Laboratory

E. J. L. Soulsby, University of Pennsylvania

E. F. Staffeldt, Argonne National Laboratory

W. B. Stone, State University of New York, Syracuse

R. K. Strickland, U.S. Department of Agriculture

W. H. Taliaferro, Argonne National Laboratory

H. Tanaka, University of Tokyo

J. M. Tufts, Ralston Purina Company

E. W. Van Stee, Ohio State University

J. H. Vickers, Lederle Laboratories

R. A. Whitney, Edgewood Arsenal

M. J. Worms, National Institute for Medical Research

W. T. Yasutake, Western Fish Disease Laboratory

PART 1

Parasites of Endothermal Laboratory Animals

Chapter 1

FLAGELLATES

ANY flagellates occur in endothermal laboratory animals. Although most are nonpathogenic, some are distinctly pathogenic and others are of unknown pathogenicity. To assess the possible role of a flagellate as a disease agent, it is first necessary to identify it. This chapter therefore contains descriptions of both pathogenic and nonpathogenic flagellates.

HEMOFLAGELLATES

Several species of *Trypanosoma* and *Leishmania* affect endothermal laboratory species.

The trypanosomes are parasites of the circulatory system and tissue fluids; a few sometimes invade cells. Almost all are transmitted by bloodsucking invertebrates in which they may or may not undergo cyclic development, depending on the species of trypanosome. Some are pathogenic while others are not. They have an elongate, leaflike body with a central nucleus, a posterior basophilic kinetoplast, and a flagellum. The flagellum arises from a basal granule just anterior to the kinetoplast and extends forward along the side of the body to form an undulating membrane; it may or may not extend beyond the body as a free anterior flagellum (Fig. 1.1). Four stages occur in the life

Tables are placed at the ends of the chapters.

cycle: amastigote (leishmanial) (Fig. 1.1*A*), promastigote (leptomonad) (Fig. 1.1*B*), epimastigote (crithidial) (Fig. 1.1*C*), and trypomastigote (trypanosomal) (Fig. 1.1*D*) (Hoare and Wallace 1966). Usually only the trypomastigote stages occur in the vertebrate host, except for *Trypanosoma cruzi* in which the amastigote form also occurs.

Members of the genus *Leishmania* are found in the macrophages and other cells of the reticuloendothelial system where they multiply by binary fission. Some 22 different specific and subspecific names have been given to mammalian leishmanias. Different strains are associated with different types of disease, different hosts, or different epidemiologic features. Most strains are euryxenous, with a wide host range, but a few are stenoxenous, infecting only a single host under natural conditions. All species are morphologically similar but sometimes differ in size.

The hemoflagellates which occur in endothermal laboratory animals are listed in Table 1.1. The most important species are discussed below.

Trypanosoma lewisi

This relatively nonpathogenic species is common in the wild Norway rat, black rat, and other rats throughout the world (Bonfante, Faust, and Giraldo 1961; Eyles 1952). It is not usually transmissible to mice. Because fleas are the vectors of this

3

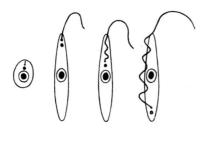

A   B   C   D

FIG. 1.1. Types of trypanosomatid flagellates. *(A)* Amastigote (leishmanial). *(B)* Promastigote (leptomonad). *(C)* Epimastigote (crithidial). *(D)* Trypomastigote (trypanosomal). (From Levine 1961. Courtesy of N. D. Levine, University of Illinois.)

parasite, it can occur only in laboratory rodents obtained from their natural environment or in colonies infested with fleas.

MORPHOLOGY

This flagellate is 26 to 34 μ long and has a pointed posterior end with a medium-sized nonterminal kinetoplast, a well-defined undulating membrane, and a free anterior flagellum (Fig. 1.2) (Levine 1961).

LIFE CYCLE

The vectors, the northern rat flea *(Nosopsyllus fasciatus)* and possibly the

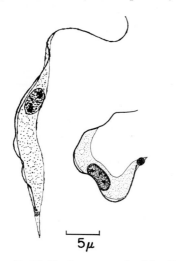

5μ

FIG. 1.2. *(Left) Trypanosoma lewisi. (Right) Trypanosoma cruzi.* (From Levine 1961. Courtesy of N. D. Levine, University of Illinois.)

oriental rat flea *(Xenopsylla cheopis),* become infected by ingesting blood (Minchin and Thomson 1915). The trypanosomes penetrate the gastric epithelial cells of the flea and produce long, free transitional forms by multiple fission. After several intracellular multiplications, the epithelial cells are destroyed, and the transitional forms pass to the rectum. Here the epimastigote form develops, attaches to the wall of the rectum, and multiplies for the life of the flea. About 5 days after infection, some epimastigote stages transform into small, metacyclic, infective trypanosomes which cannot reproduce in the flea and which pass out in the feces. Rats become infected by the ingestion of fleas or moist flea feces, but are not infected by the bite of the flea. The trypanosomes appear in the rat blood 5 to 7 days after infection, multiply for about a week, and disappear.

PATHOLOGIC EFFECTS

Trypanosoma lewisi is usually non-pathogenic although it sometimes produces anemia in a host experimentally inoculated simultaneously with the parasite and a corticosteroid (Sherman and Ruble 1967).

A spontaneous arthritis in the laboratory rat associated with a trypanosome, presumably *T. lewisi,* has been reported (Fujiwara and Suzuki 1967). It occurs in 4- to 5-week-old rats and is characterized by erythema and edema of the pedal extremities. The rear paws are most frequently involved and the tibiotarsal articulation is the most severely affected (Fig. 1.3*A*). Exudate from articular lesions contains many trypanosomes but no bacteria (Fig. 1.3*B*). Microscopic lesions are those of a purulent arthritis, with inflammation of the adjacent subcutaneous and muscular tissues (Fig. 1.3*C, D*). The condition has been experimentally reproduced by inoculating young rats subcutaneously in the foot with affected tissue materials.

DIAGNOSIS

Diagnosis is made by identifying the organism in blood or organ smears or in tissue sections.

CONTROL

The elimination of fleas will eliminate *T. lewisi* infection from a colony. Many

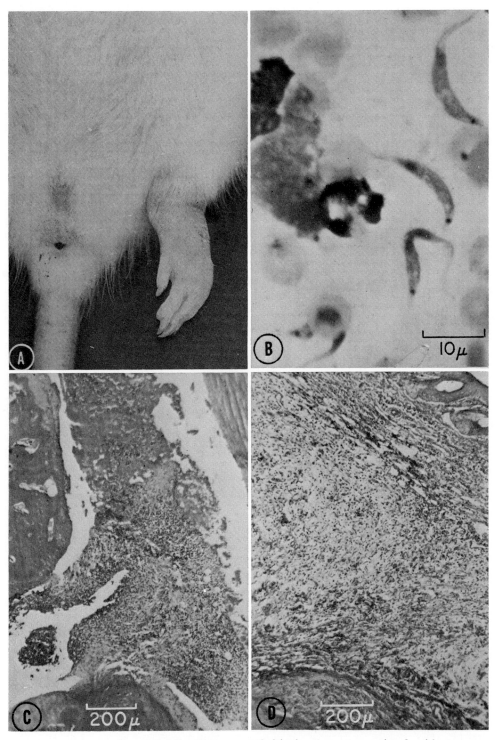

FIG. 1.3. Spontaneous arthritis in the rat associated with trypanosomes. *(A)* Edema of tibiotarsal joint. *(B)* Trypanosomes in exudate
from affected joint. *(C)* Purulent arthritis. *(D)* Edema and inflammatory
cell infiltration of adjacent subcutaneous tissue. (From Fujiwara and
Suzuki 1967. Courtesy of Japan Experimental Animal Research Association.)

drugs have been tried against this trypanosome without success (Levine 1961).

There is no definite evidence that this flagellate is a public health problem although a trypanosome indistinguishable from *T. lewisi* occurred in a Malayan infant in close contact with rats and rat fleas (Johnson 1933). The child had anemia and fever which lasted 2 weeks, and many trypanosomes were present in the blood. Recovery was spontaneous.

Trypanosoma duttoni

This usually nonpathogenic species occurs in the house mouse and other wild mice throughout the world (Levine 1961). Although morphologically indistinguishable from *T. lewisi,* it is not usually transmissible to rats. Its vector is the northern rat flea, *Nosopsyllus fasciatus,* and its life cycle is the same as that of *T. lewisi.*

Although *T. duttoni* is ordinarily considered nonpathogenic, it is harmful to mice under conditions of stress caused by inadequate nutrition and reduced temperature (Sheppe and Adams 1957). Extensive gastric and intestinal hemorrhages are produced. Even under normal conditions, weight gains are significantly reduced in infected mice.

This parasite cannot occur in laboratory colonies in the absence of fleas.

Trypanosoma conorhini

This nonpathogenic flagellate has been found in wild Norway and black rats or in its insect vector, a reduviid bug, *Triatoma rubrofasciata,* in Hawaii, Brazil, India, Taiwan, and Indonesia (Dias and Campos Seabra 1943; Morishita 1935; Wood 1946). Natural infection has not been reported in laboratory animals but could possibly occur in specimens obtained from their natural habitat or in those maintained in facilities infested with the insect vector. The laboratory mouse, rat, and monkey have been infected experimentally. The trypomastigote form is 27 to 54 μ long, including a free flagellum. It has a long, pointed posterior end and a prominent undulating membrane. The kinetoplast is of medium size. It lies some distance from

the posterior end and has a pot-shaped structure anterior to it.

Trypanosoma nabiasi

This nonpathogenic flagellate has been found in wild rabbits in Europe and Turkey (Króo 1936). *Trypanosoma nabiasi* is 24 to 36 μ long, including a free flagellum 4 to 10 μ long, and has a sharply pointed posterior end, a very large kinetoplast near the posterior end, and a prominent undulating membrane. It is extremely rare in laboratory rabbits and is not likely to occur unless they are infested with the insect vector, the rabbit flea *(Spilopsyllus cuniculi)* (Grewal 1956).

Trypanosoma cruzi

This species is an important pathogen of man. It has been found in many wild and domestic animals, including the house mouse, wood rats, other rodents, dog, cat, other carnivores, armadillo, opossum, and bats in southern United States and Mexico and in marmosets, capuchins, squirrel monkeys, spider monkeys, and other simian primates in Central and South America (Belding 1965; Dunn, Lambrecht, and du Plessis 1963; Levine 1961). The Norway rat can be infected experimentally, but natural infections in laboratory colonies have not been reported. Natural *Trypanosoma cruzi* infection has been reported from laboratory squirrel monkeys and capuchins (Bullock, Wolf, and Clarkson 1967; Eastin and Roeckel 1968). It is important in these species because it can interfere with experimental results and also because it is a potential hazard to man. Although it is generally considered that *T. cruzi* is confined to the Western Hemisphere, there are reports of a similar trypanosome in laboratory monkeys obtained from Asia (Kabat, Wolf, and Bezer 1952; Seneca and Wolf 1955). The Asian form has been found in rhesus monkeys in the United States after the monkeys were inoculated with corticosteroids.

Two forms of *T. cruzi* are found in mammals (Levine 1961). The trypomastigote form (Fig. 1.2) occurs in the blood. It is 16 to 20 μ long and has a pointed posterior end, a curved, stumpy body, a large subterminal kinetoplast, a narrow undulating membrane, and a moderately long free flagellum. The amastigote form occurs in groups in the cells of skeletal muscle, the myocardium, the reticuloendothelial system, and other tissues. It is 1.5 to 4.0 μ in diameter.

LIFE CYCLE

The trypanosomes enter the bloodstream, invade the cells of the reticuloendothelial system and striated muscle, especially the myocardium, and turn into amastigote forms. These multiply by binary fission, destroy the tissue cells, and form nests of parasites. The amastigote forms become trypomastigote forms and return to the blood. Vectors are the kissing or cone-nosed bugs, the most important being *Panstrongylus megistus* and *Triatoma infestans*.

In the insect vector, the trypanosomes turn into amastigote forms. These multiply by binary fission, change into metacyclic trypomastigote forms, and are excreted in the feces. This cycle takes 6 to 15 days or more. Animals become infected either by active penetration of the parasite through the skin or mucous membranes or by the ingestion of infected bugs, bug feces, or rodents. Intrauterine infection also occurs.

PATHOLOGIC EFFECTS

Trypanosoma cruzi causes either an acute or a chronic disease in laboratory animals, depending upon the strain of the parasite and the age and species of the host (Belding 1965; Levine 1961). Young animals are the most susceptible. Signs are usually nonspecific. Generalized edema without necrosis or hemorrhage is common. Anemia, splenomegaly, hepatomegaly, and lymphadenitis also occur. The commonest lesion is myocarditis. Muscle cell fibers, particularly those of the heart, are often destroyed (Fig. 1.4).

DIAGNOSIS

Diagnosis is made by identifying the organism in blood or organ smears or in tissue sections (Fig. 1.5). Another technique, known as xenodiagnosis, is to examine reduviid bugs for trypanosomes after they have fed on suspected hosts.

CONTROL

Elimination of the insect vectors will eliminate *T. cruzi* infections. There is no effective treatment (Faust, Beaver, and Jung 1968).

PUBLIC HEALTH CONSIDERATIONS

Trypanosoma cruzi causes Chagas' disease in man and is a serious pathogen (Levine 1961). Care should be taken to avoid exposure either by accidental inoculation with trypanosomes or by contamination of mucous membranes or skin with infected material.

Trypanosoma sanmartini

This species, of unknown pathogenicity, was described from squirrel monkeys in Colombia (Garnham and Gonzales-Mugaburu 1962). It greatly resembles *T. cruzi* and may be an aberrant strain or subspecies (Dunn, Lambrecht, and du Plessis 1963). It is curved, often S-shaped, with a large ovoid kinetoplast at its posterior tip and a moderately developed undulating mem-

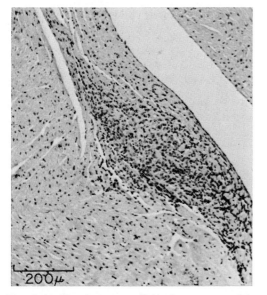

FIG. 1.4. Focal myocarditis in a capuchin caused by *Trypanosoma cruzi*. (From Bullock, Wolf, and Clarkson 1967. Courtesy of American Veterinary Medical Association.)

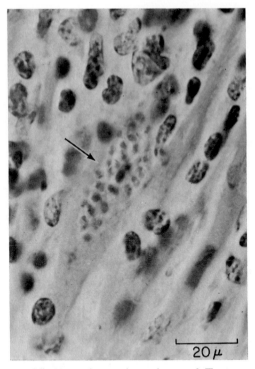

Fig. 1.5. Nest of amastigote forms of *Trypanosoma cruzi* in cardiac muscle fiber in a capuchin. (From Bullock, Wolf, and Clarkson 1967. Courtesy of American Veterinary Medical Association.)

brane. It is 17 to 24 μ long, including a free flagellum 4 to 9 μ long, and is 2 to 3 μ wide. It is unlikely to occur in the laboratory except in squirrel monkeys obtained from endemic areas.

Trypanosoma minasense
(Syn. *Trypanosoma mycetae, T. devei, T. escomeli, T. florestali, T. manguinhense, T. brimonti, T. advieri*)

This apparently nonpathogenic flagellate occurs in marmosets, capuchins, squirrel monkeys, spider monkeys, howler monkeys, night monkeys, woolly monkeys, and man in Central and South America (Dunn, Lambrecht, and du Plessis 1963). The trypomastigote form in the blood is sinuous and 29 to 46 μ long; the nucleus is usually at, or just anterior to, the middle of the body. The kinetoplast is small and well anterior to the posterior end. The undulating membrane is fairly well developed, and the free flagellum is usually one-sixth to one-third of the body length.

Trypanosoma minasense does not appear to be pathogenic for vertebrates and therefore must be distinguished from the pathogenic *T. cruzi* with which it is sometimes found in mixed infection. It is unlikely to occur in the laboratory except in primates obtained from endemic areas.

Trypanosoma rangeli
(Syn. *Trypanosoma ariarii, T. cebus, T. guatemalense*)

This apparently nonpathogenic flagellate occurs in the dog, cat, opossum, capuchins, and man in Central and South America (Dunn, Lambrecht, and du Plessis 1963; Groot 1951; Groot, Renjifo, and Uribe 1951; Levine 1961). It is common in the dog, cat, and man in certain areas of Venezuela, Colombia, and Guatemala. Young mice, rats, and rhesus monkeys can be infected experimentally. It is unlikely to occur in the laboratory except in animals obtained from endemic areas.

The trypomastigote form in the blood is about 26 to 36 μ long and has a pointed posterior end, a small, subterminal kinetoplast, and a rippled undulating membrane with a free flagellum (Levine 1961). The commonest vector is the reduviid bug *Rhodnius prolixus*, but *Triatoma dimidiata* and other reduviids have also been found infected. Infection of the vertebrate host is either by bite or by fecal contamination.

Trypanosoma rangeli does not appear to be pathogenic for animals and man (Levine 1961). However, it must be distinguished from pathogenic trypanosomes, and especially from *T. cruzi*, with which it is sometimes found in mixed infection. *Trypanosoma rangeli* is larger than *T. cruzi* and has a much smaller kinetoplast.

Trypanosoma saimirii, Trypanosoma diasi

These two biologically and morphologically similar species may be identical (Dunn, Lambrecht, and du Plessis 1963). Both are apparently nonpathogenic, and neither is likely to occur in the laboratory except in primates obtained from endemic areas.

Trypanosoma saimirii has been reported from squirrel monkeys in Brazil (Deane and Damasceno 1961; Rodhain 1941). It resembles *T. minasense* morphologically. It is 19 to 29 μ long, with a free flagellum extending 6 to 9 μ beyond the body, and is 3 μ wide. The kinetoplast is relatively small and is located 5 μ from the elongate, slender, pointed posterior end.

Trypanosoma diasi has been reported from capuchins in Brazil (Deane and Damasceno 1961; Deane and Martins 1952). It is 33 to 36 μ long and 3 to 4 μ wide, with a free flagellum extending 7 to 9 μ beyond the body.

Trypanosoma primatum

This apparently nonpathogenic flagellate has been reported in guenons, the chimpanzee, and gorilla in western Africa (Reichenow 1917). It is apparently common in the chimpanzee and gorilla in west central Africa, but it has not been found in these species in the laboratory. It resembles *T. lewisi*, having a long, pointed posterior end with the kinetoplast well back from it, a prominent undulating membrane, and a free flagellum, but its kinetoplast is larger, constricted in the middle, and shaped like a figure 8.

Leishmania

Leishmania has been found in many parts of the tropics and subtropics where it is an important parasite of the dog, certain wild rodents, and man. Several species of endothermal laboratory animals have been infected experimentally, but only the dog and guinea pig are subject to natural infections, and even these infections do not occur in the temperate zone (Levine 1961). It is unlikely to occur in the laboratory except in dogs obtained from pounds or in wild rodents obtained from their natural habitat in endemic areas.

MORPHOLOGY

All species of *Leishmania* are ovoid, usually measure 2.5 to 5.0 μ by 1.5 to 2.0 μ, and contain a nucleus, a small kinetoplast, and a trace of an internal filament representing the flagellum (Fig. 1.1*A*) (Levine 1961). In culture and in the invertebrate vectors, they assume the promastigote (leptomonad) form (Fig. 1.1*B*), are 14 to 20 μ by 1.5 to 3.5 μ, and have a kinetoplast anterior to the nucleus, a flagellum, and no undulating membrane.

LIFE CYCLE

Leishmania is transmitted by sand flies of the genus *Phlebotomus*, either by bite or by being crushed on the skin. It multiplies by binary fission in the promastigote form in the sand fly gut.

PATHOLOGIC EFFECTS

In the mammalian host, *Leishmania* occurs in the macrophages and other cells of the reticuloendothelial system, and in the skin, spleen, liver, bone marrow, lymph nodes, and mucosa (Levine 1961). Various strains are associated with different signs, lesions, hosts, and epidemiologic features. *Leishmania donovani* causes visceral leishmaniosis in the dog, cat, and man. *Leishmania tropica* causes cutaneous leishmaniosis in the dog, cat, wild rodents, and man. In visceral leishmaniosis, the spleen is greatly enlarged, congested, and purple or brown. The liver and sometimes the lymph nodes are also enlarged. The reticuloendothelial cells are increased in number and invaded by the parasites. In cutaneous leishmaniosis, there may be abundant scurfy desquamation of the skin and, in some dogs, numerous cutaneous ulcers. *Leishmania enriettii* causes ulcers of the skin of the guinea pig, especially of the paws, ears, and nose (Muniz and Medina 1948a, b).

DIAGNOSIS

Diagnosis is by demonstration of the organism. Blood or bone marrow is used for the visceral type, and material from skin lesions is used for the cutaneous type (Levine 1961).

CONTROL

Because of the need for a sand fly intermediate host, the life cycle cannot be completed in the laboratory, and no special control procedures are required.

PUBLIC HEALTH CONSIDERATIONS

Both visceral leishmaniosis, or kala azar, and cutaneous leishmaniosis are important zoonoses in endemic areas (Faust,

Beaver, and Jung 1968). The visceral form can be transmitted only by an infected sand fly and is therefore of little public health importance in the laboratory, but the cutaneous form can be transmitted mechanically by the stable fly *(Stomoxys)*, and for this reason, infected laboratory animals should be destroyed.

ENTERIC FLAGELLATES

The most important enteric flagellates in endothermal laboratory animals are the trichomonads and *Giardia*.

The five genera of trichomonads affecting endothermal laboratory animals are similar (Honigberg 1963). *Tritrichomonas* has three anterior flagella and no pelta (a crescent-shaped, silver-stained structure anterior to the axostyle). The other four genera all have a pelta. *Trichomitus* has three anterior flagella, *Trichomonas* and *Tetratrichomonas* have four, and *Pentatrichomonas* has five. In *Tritrichomonas*, *Trichomitus*, *Tetratrichomonas*, and *Pentatrichomonas*, the posterior flagellum extends free beyond the body; in *Trichomonas* it does not. With the curious exception of the rabbit and other lagomorphs, species of trichomonads have been found in the intestinal tract, especially in the cecum, of practically every species of mammal or bird, many lower vertebrates, and even some invertebrates. They are common in laboratory animals throughout the world.

Members of the genus *Giardia* have been found in all classes of vertebrates but mainly in mammals. It has generally been assumed that most species are host-specific; consequently, different names have been given to the forms from different hosts. However, because of the lack of morphologic differences, it has been suggested that there are actually only two species in mammals, each with a number of races: *G. muris* in the mouse, rat, and hamster, and *G. duodenalis* in the rat, ground squirrels, deer mice, pocket mice, guinea pig, chinchilla, rabbit, dog, cat, cattle, other animals, and man (Filice 1952). The essential difference between these two forms is that the median bodies of *G. muris* are small and rounded while those of *G. duodenalis* are long and shaped like the claws of a hammer. Further research is needed to determine if this view is correct. In this chapter,

the various species-specific names are used.

The enteric flagellates which occur in endothermal laboratory species are listed in Table 1.2. Some of the more important species are discussed below.

Tritrichomonas muris

This nonpathogenic flagellate is common in the cecum, colon, and small intestine of the house mouse, Norway rat, black rat, and other wild rodents throughout the world (Andrews and White 1936; Bonfante, Faust, and Giraldo 1961). It is also common in the conventional laboratory mouse, rat, and hamster (Heston 1941; Wantland 1955; Wenrich 1949), but it does not occur in cesarean-derived, barrier sustained rodent colonies (Foster 1963; Owen 1968).

MORPHOLOGY

Tritrichomonas muris measures 16 to 26 μ by 10 to 14 μ (Fig. 1.6*A*) (Levine 1961). It has an anterior vesicular nucleus. Anterior to this is a blepharoplast from which arise the anterior flagella, a posterior flagellum, a fibrillar costa, a stiff rodlike axostyle, and a parabasal body and filament.

LIFE CYCLE

Reproduction is by simple binary fission (Levine 1961). No cysts are formed, and transmission is by ingestion of trophozoites passed in the feces. Cross infection between the mouse, rat, and hamster has been accomplished experimentally (Saxe 1954a).

PATHOLOGIC EFFECTS

Tritrichomonas muris is nonpathogenic (Levine 1961).

DIAGNOSIS

This flagellate is often found in abundance in the feces of animals with diarrhea, but this is only because fluid or semifluid intestinal contents provide a favorable habitat for its growth and multiplication. Thus it must not be diagnosed as a cause of enteric disease.

CONTROL

Because it is nonpathogenic, no control measures are necessary. The organism

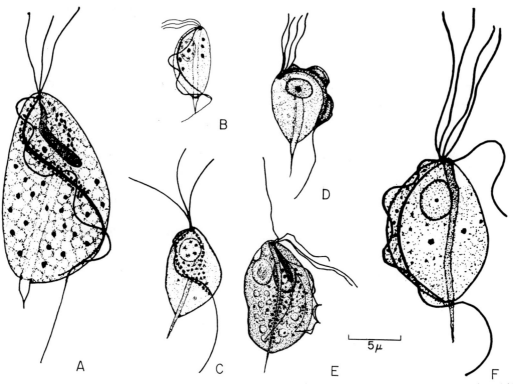

Fig. 1.6. Trichomonads affecting endothermal laboratory species. *(A) Tritrichomonas muris. (B) Tritrichomonas minuta. (C) Trichomitus wenyoni. (D) Tetratrichomonas microti. (E) Trichomonas gallinae. (F) Pentatrichomonas hominis.* (From Wenrich 1930; Wenrich and Saxe 1950. Courtesy of American Society of Parasitologists.)

can be eliminated from a colony by cesarean section (Foster 1963).

PUBLIC HEALTH CONSIDERATIONS

Tritrichomonas muris is not a public health problem.

Tritrichomonas minuta, Trichomitus wenyoni

These nonpathogenic trichomonads occur in the cecum and colon of the mouse, rat, and hamster (Levine 1961). *Trichomitus wenyoni* also occurs in the rhesus monkey and baboons. *Tritrichomonas minuta* measures 4 to 9 μ by 2 to 5 μ (Fig. 1.6B) (Wenrich 1924). *Trichomitus wenyoni* measures 4 to 16 μ by 2.5 to 6.0 μ (Fig. 1.6C) (Wenrich and Nie 1949). These flagellates are common in some colonies, but absent in others (Foster 1963; Owen 1968).

Tritrichomonas caviae, Tritrichomonas sp., Tritrichomonas criceti

Tritrichomonas caviae is common in the cecum and colon of the guinea pig throughout the world (Nie 1950). It measures 10 to 22 μ by 6 to 11 μ. A smaller, unnamed species has also been reported in the guinea pig in the United States (Nie 1950). It measures 6 to 13 μ by 4.5 to 6.5 μ. *Tritrichomonas criceti* occurs in the cecum and colon of the hamster in North America (Wantland 1956). It measures 12 to 25 μ by 5 to 10 μ. The incidence of these species in laboratory colonies is unknown; *T. caviae* is probably common. None of these species is pathogenic.

Tetratrichomonas microti

This nonpathogenic flagellate is common in the cecum of the mouse, rat, hamster, voles, and other wild rodents in North America and has been experimentally transmitted from the hamster to the rat (Levine 1961; Saxe 1954a). It is 4 to 9 μ long (Fig. 1.6*D*) (Wenrich and Saxe 1950). Its incidence in laboratory colonies is unknown. It is probably common in specimens obtained from their natural environment.

Tetratrichomonas macacovaginae

Tetratrichomonas macacovaginae has been found in the vagina of the rhesus monkey in North America (Hegner and Ratcliffe 1927). It measures 8 to 16 μ by 3 to 6 μ and has a free posterior flagellum which differentiates it from *T. vaginalis*, a common parasite of man. Nothing is known of its pathogenicity or incidence.

Trichomonas tenax

This nonpathogenic trichomonad is common in the mouth, especially between the gums and teeth, of the rhesus monkey, cynomolgus monkey, baboons, and man throughout the world (Hegner and Chu 1930; Wenrich 1947). It measures 4 to 16 μ by 2 to 15μ (Honigberg and Lee 1959; Wenrich 1947). Its incidence in laboratory colonies is unknown. It is probably common in primates obtained from their natural environment.

Trichomonas gallinae

This frequently pathogenic flagellate occurs in the mouth, sinuses, pharynx, esophagus, crop, proventriculus, orbital sinuses, and liver of the chicken, pigeon, and other birds throughout the world (Levine 1961). It is common in the pigeon, but rare in the chicken. There are no specific reports of its occurrence in laboratory birds; it is probably rare.

MORPHOLOGY

Trophozoites are piriform, 6 to 19 μ long and 2 to 9 μ wide, with four anterior flagella and an axostyle (Fig. 1.6*E*) (Levine 1961). There are no cysts.

LIFE CYCLE

Reproduction is by binary fission, and transmission is by ingestion. In pigeons, transmission is usually from adult to offspring in pigeon milk.

PATHOLOGIC EFFECTS

Trichomonas gallinae causes trichomonosis of the upper digestive tract (Levine 1961). The disease is often rapidly fatal in the pigeon. Caseous, necrotic nodules or ulcers occur in affected organs, especially in the crop, esophagus, and pharynx.

DIAGNOSIS

Diagnosis is made by identifying the organism in smears or tissue sections of typical lesions.

CONTROL

Control depends on elimination of the parasite from adults (Levine 1961). Oral treatment with 2-amino-5-nitrothiazole (Enheptin), 28 to 45 mg per kg of body weight daily for 7 days or 0.16% in the drinking water for 7 to 14 days, is effective.

PUBLIC HEALTH CONSIDERATIONS

This trichomonad is of no public health importance.

Pentatrichomonas hominis

This nonpathogenic flagellate is a common inhabitant of the cecum and colon of the mouse, rat, hamster, dog, cat, rhesus monkey, cynomolgus monkey, chimpanzee, orangutan, and other primates, including man, throughout the world (Andrews and White 1936; Burrows and Lillis 1967; Hegner 1934; Hegner and Chu 1930; Poindexter 1942). It usually has five anterior flagella, but some organisms have only four and a few only three (Levine 1961). It is piriform and measures 8 to 20 μ by 3 to 14 μ (Fig. 1.6*F*). The incidence of this flagellate in laboratory primates is unknown. It is probably common in specimens obtained from their natural habitat. It is common in laboratory dogs obtained from pounds (Burrows and Lillis 1967).

Monocercomonas

This nonpathogenic flagellate resembles *Tritrichomonas* but lacks an undulating membrane and a costa (Levine 1961). It is piriform and has an anterior nucleus, three anterior flagella, a trailing flagellum, a pelta, a parabasal body, and a projecting

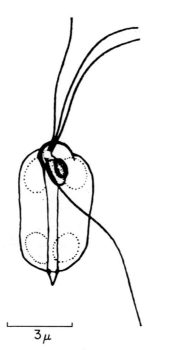

FIG. 1.7. *Monocercomonas caviae*. (From Nie 1950. Journal of Morphology 86:415, Fig. 7*A*.)

axostyle. It reproduces by binary fission; there are no cysts.

Monocercomonas caviae, M. pistillum, and *M. minuta* are common in the cecum of the guinea pig (Nie 1950). *Monocercomonas caviae* occurs throughout the world; it is 4 to 9 μ long and 2 to 4 μ wide (Fig. 1.7). *Monocercomonas pistillum* and *M. minuta* have been reported from North America. *Monocercomonas pistillum* is 4 to 7 μ long by 3 to 4 μ wide; *M. minuta* is 3 to 6 μ long by 2 to 3 μ wide.

Monocercomonas cuniculi occurs in the cecum of the rabbit throughout the world (Tanabe 1926). It is 5 to 14 μ long. Its incidence is unknown; it is probably common.

Hexamastix

This nonpathogenic flagellate has a piriform body with an anterior nucleus and cytostome, a pelta, a conspicuous axostyle, a prominent parabasal body, five anterior flagella, and a trailing flagellum (Levine 1961). Reproduction is by binary fission; there are apparently no cysts.

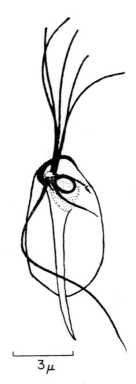

FIG. 1.8. *Hexamastix caviae*. (From Nie 1950. Journal of Morphology 86:421, Fig. 8*A*.)

Hexamastix caviae (Fig. 1.8) and *H. robustus* are common in the cecum of the guinea pig (Nie 1950). *Hexamastix caviae* occurs throughout the world; it is 4 to 10 μ long and 3 to 5 μ wide. *Hexamastix robustus* has been reported from North America; it is 7 to 14 μ by 3 to 8 μ. *Hexamastix muris* (Fig. 1.9) occurs in the cecum of the rat, hamster, and other rodents throughout the world (Kirby and Honigberg 1949; Wenrich 1946); it is 5 to 12 μ long. Its incidence is unknown; it is probably common.

Chilomitus

This nonpathogenic flagellate has an elongate body with a convex aboral surface, a well-developed pellicle, a cuplike cytostome near the anterior end from which four flagella emerge, an anterior nucleus, a parabasal body, and an axostyle which is often rudimentary (Levine 1961). Cysts sometimes occur.

Chilomitus caviae (Fig. 1.10) is com-

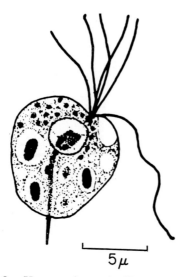

FIG. 1.9. *Hexamastix muris.* (Courtesy of N. D. Levine, University of Illinois.)

mon in the cecum of the guinea pig throughout the world; it is 6 to 14 μ long and 3 to 5 μ wide. *Chilomitus conexus* has been reported from North America. It also occurs in the cecum of the guinea pig but is uncommon. It is 4 to 7 μ by 1 to 2 μ (Nie 1950).

Enteromonas

This nonpathogenic flagellate has been reported from many mammals, but the number of species of this genus is uncertain since adequate cross-transmission experiments have not been carried out. The trophozoite is spherical or piriform, with three short anterior flagella, one of which is sometimes difficult to see; a fourth long flagellum runs along the flattened body surface and extends freely at the posterior end. It also has an anterior nucleus and a strand-like funis which extends posteriorly from the blepharoplast along the body surface (Levine 1961). There is no cytostome. The cysts are ovoid and contain four nuclei when mature.

Enteromonas hominis (syn. *Tricercomonas intestinalis, Octomitus hominis, Enteromonas bengalensis*) occurs in the cecum of the rat, hamster, rhesus monkey, other macaques, and man throughout the world (Levine 1961; Reardon and Rininger 1968). It is not common. The trophozoites are 4

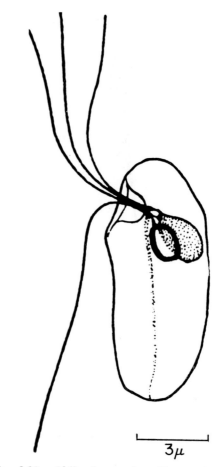

FIG. 1.10. *Chilomitus caviae.* (From Nie 1950. Journal of Morphology 86:408, Fig. 6A.)

to 10 μ long by 3 to 6 μ wide and have many food vacuoles containing bacteria.

Enteromonas caviae (syn. *E. fonsecai*) (Fig. 1.11) is common in the cecum of the guinea pig throughout the world (Nie 1950). It is 3 to 5 μ long by 2 to 4 μ wide. *Enteromonas* sp. occurs in the cecum of the rabbit throughout the world (Harkema 1936). Its incidence is unknown.

Retortamonas

The trophozoites of this nonpathogenic flagellate are piriform or fusiform and are drawn out posteriorly, with an anterior nucleus, a large anterior cytostome, an anterior flagellum, a posteriorly directed trailing flagellum which emerges from the cytostomal groove, and a cytostomal fibril

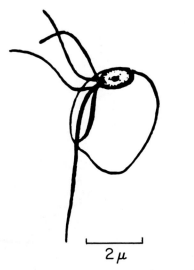

FIG. 1.11. *Enteromonas caviae*. (From Nie 1950. Journal of Morphology 86:392, Fig. 4.)

around the anterior end and sides of the cytostome (Fig. 1.12) (Ansari 1955, 1956). The cysts are piriform or ovoid and have one or two nuclei.

Retortamonas intestinalis (syn. *Embadomonas intestinalis*) occurs in the cecum of man and probably also of the rhesus monkey, chimpanzee, and other simian primates throughout the world (Levine 1961). The trophozoites are 4 to 9 μ long by 3 to

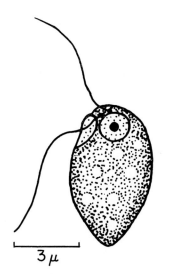

FIG. 1.12. *Retortamonas*. (Courtesy of N. D. Levine, University of Illinois.)

4 μ wide, and the cysts are 4 to 7 μ long by 3 to 5 μ wide. Its incidence is unknown.

Retortamonas caviae is common in the cecum of the guinea pig throughout the world (Nie 1950). Its trophozoites are 4 to 8 μ long by 4 μ wide, and its cysts are 4 to 6 μ long by 3 to 4 μ wide.

Retortamonas cuniculi is sometimes found in the cecum of the rabbit throughout the world (Collier and Boeck 1926). Its trophozoites are 7 to 13 μ long by 5 to 10 μ wide, and its cysts are 5 to 7 μ long by 3 to 4 μ wide. Its incidence in laboratory colonies is unknown.

Retortamonas sp. was found in the cecum of 1.7% of 2,515 wild Norway rats in eastern United States (Andrews and White 1936). Its incidence in laboratory colonies is unknown.

Chilomastix

The trophozoites of this nonpathogenic flagellate are piriform, with an anterior nucleus, a large cytostomal groove near the anterior end, three anterior flagella, a short fourth flagellum which undulates within the cytostomal groove, and a cytoplasmic fibril along the anterior end and sides of the cytostomal groove (Levine 1961). The cysts are usually lemon shaped and contain one nucleus and the organelles of the trophozoite.

Chilomastix mesnili (syn. *C. hominis*, *C. suis*) is common in the cecum and colon of the rhesus monkey, cynomolgus monkey, other macaques, green monkey, other guenons, baboons, capuchins, orangutan, chimpanzee, pig, and man (Hegner 1934; Hegner and Chu 1930; Myers and Kuntz 1965; Poindexter 1942; Reardon and Rininger 1968). Its trophozoites are 6 to 24 μ long by 3 to 10 μ wide, and its cysts are 6.5 to 10.0 μ long. Its incidence in laboratory colonies is unknown; it is probably common in primates obtained from their natural environment.

Chilomastix cuniculi is common in the cecum of the rabbit throughout the world (Levine 1961). Its trophozoites are ordinarily 10 to 15 μ long but may range from 3 to 20 μ.

Chilomastix intestinalis and *C. wenrichi* occur in the cecum of the guinea pig (Levine 1961). The trophozoites of *C. intestinalis* are 9 to 28 μ by 7 to 11 μ, and its

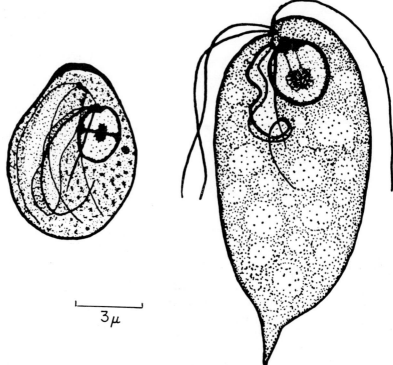

FIG. 1.13.   *Chilomastix
bettencourti. (Left)* Cyst.
(Right) Trophozoite.
(From Wenrich 1930.)

3μ

cysts are 9 to 11 μ by 7 to 10 μ (Nie 1950).
The trophozoites of *C. wenrichi* are 7.5 to
12.0 μ by 4 to 5 μ (Nie 1950). *Chilomastix
intestinalis* is common throughout the
world. *Chilomastix wenrichi* has been reported from North America; its incidence
is unknown.

Chilomastix bettencourti (Fig. 1.13) occurs in the cecum of the mouse, Norway
rat, black rat, and hamster (Levine 1961).
It is structurally identical to *C. mesnili*
(Wenyon 1926). It has been found in 2 to
78% of wild Norway rats, in up to 88%
of wild black rats, and in up to 80% of
wild house mice in various surveys throughout the world (Andrews and White 1936;
Bonfante, Faust, and Giraldo 1961). It has
also been found in 9.2% of 412 hamsters
in the United States (Wantland 1955). Its
incidence in laboratory rats and mice is
unknown; it is probably common in conventional colonies.

Chilomastix gallinarum occurs in the
ceca of the chicken and other birds
throughout the world (Levine 1961). It has
been found in 40% of a large number of

chickens surveyed in eastern United States.
The body is 11 to 20 μ long by 5 to 12 μ
wide. Its incidence in laboratory chickens
is unknown; it is probably common.

Selenomonas palpitans

This nonpathogenic flagellate occurs
in the cecum and colon of the guinea pig
throughout the world (Levine 1961). It is
7 to 9 μ long and 2 μ wide, kidney or crescent shaped with blunt ends, and has a
tuft of flagella emerging from the middle
of the concave side. The nucleus is highly
refractile and lies on the concave side near
the base of the flagella. Reproduction is by
transverse binary fission through the flagellar region. The incidence of *Selenomonas
palpitans* is unknown.

Monocercomonoides

Species of this nonpathogenic genus
have an anterior nucleus, two pairs of anterior flagella, a pelta, an axostyle which is
usually filamentous, and one to four strand-
like funises which extend backward just
beneath the body surface (Levine 1961).

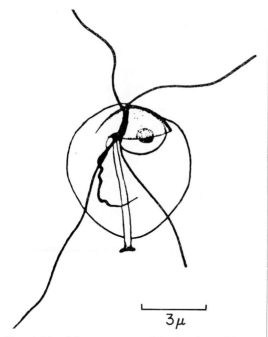

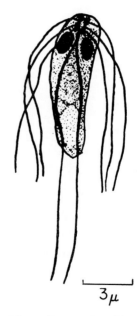

FIG. 1.14. *Monocercomonoides caviae.* (From Nie 1950. Journal of Morphology 86:396, Fig. 5*A*.)

FIG. 1.15. *Hexamita muris.* (From Wenrich 1930.)

Monocercomonoides caviae (Fig. 1.14), *M. quadrifunilis, M. wenrichi,* and *M. exilis* occur in the cecum of the guinea pig (Levine 1961). *Monocercomonoides wenrichi* is the commonest species. *Monocercomonoides caviae* and *M. quadrifunilis* are also common; the incidence of *M. exilis* is unknown. *Monocercomonoides caviae* occurs throughout the world; it is 4 to 8 μ long and 3 to 7 μ wide and has three funises. *Monocercomonoides quadrifunilis, M. wenrichi,* and *M. exilis* have been reported from North America. *Monocercomonoides quadrifunilis* is 4 to 13 μ by 3 to 11 μ and has four funises; *M. wenrichi* is 3 to 12 μ by 3 to 8 μ and has a single, thick sinuous funis; and *M. exilis* is 4 to 9 μ by 3 to 6 μ and has a single, short funis (Nie 1950).

Monocercomonoides sp. has been reported in the cecum of the rat and hamster in North America (Saxe 1954a). Its incidence is unknown.

Hexamita

Some members of this genus are free-living while others have been found in the digestive tract of insects, other invertebrates, and all classes of vertebrates. Some species cause enteritis in birds, but little is known of the pathogenicity of those which occur in mammals (Levine 1961). The trophozoites are piriform and bilaterally symmetrical, with two anterior nuclei, six anterior flagella, two posterior flagella, and two separate axostyles (which may possibly be hollow tubes rather than rods). Some species form cysts.

Hexamita muris (syn. *Octomitus muris, Syndyomita muris*) (Fig. 1.15) is 7 to 9 μ long and 2 to 3 μ wide. It occurs in the small intestine and cecum of the mouse, rat, hamster, and various wild rodents throughout the world (Levine 1961); it is common in some colonies (Bonfante, Faust, and Giraldo 1961; Heston 1941; Tsuchiya and Rector 1936) and absent in others (Foster 1963; Owen 1968). Enteritis in the laboratory mouse has been associated with this flagellate (Meshorer 1969; A. Meshorer, personal communication). Although the disease was reported from Israel, the affected mice were obtained from a North American commercial breeder. Young animals develop an acute form of the disease; older animals usually develop a chronic form. Signs

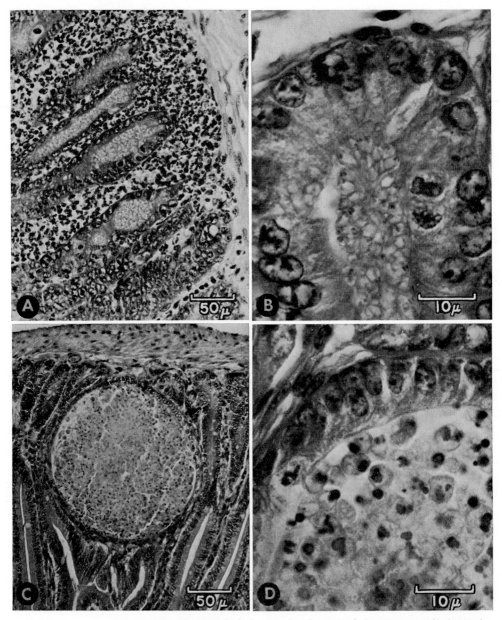

Fig. 1.16. Hexamitiosis in the duodenum of the mouse. *(A)* Acute infection. Note cellular infiltration and organisms in crypts. *(B)* Higher magnification of organisms in crypt. *(C)* Chronic infection. Note pseudocyst in intestinal wall. *(D)* Higher magnification of portion of pseudocyst. (Courtesy of A. Meshorer, Weizmann Institute of Science.)

of the acute form are diarrhea, rapid loss of weight, and sometimes death. The primary signs of the chronic form are weight loss and listlessness; diarrhea is uncommon and death is rare. The lesions are restricted to the anterior part of the small intestine and consist of a duodenitis. The duodenal crypts are filled with *H. muris* and the walls appear to contain cysts (pseudocysts) (Fig. 1.16). Treatment with dimetridazole, nitrofurantoin, or oxytetracycline is apparently ineffective.

Hexamita pitheci has been reported in the cecum and colon of the rhesus monkey in South America (da Cunha and Muniz 1929). Its incidence is unknown; it is 2.5 to 3.0 μ long and 1.5 to 2.0 μ wide. A similar and perhaps identical species of *Hexamita* has been found in feces of the rhesus monkey and the chimpanzee in North America (Hegner 1934; Wenrich 1933). It is 4 to 6 μ long and 2 to 4 μ wide. Its incidence is unknown.

Octomitus

The trophozoite of this nonpathogenic flagellate is bilaterally symmetrical and has a piriform body, two anterior nuclei, six anterior flagella, and two posterior flagella (Levine 1961). There are two axostyles which originate at the anterior end; these come together and fuse as they pass posteriorly, emerging from the body as a single central rod. The fusion of the axostyles differentiates this genus from *Hexamita* (Gabel 1954).

Octomitus pulcher (syn. *Hexamita pulcher, Octomitus intestinalis*) (Fig. 1.17) occurs in the cecum of the mouse, rat, hamster, ground squirrels, and other wild rodents throughout the world (Levine 1961). It is 6 to 10 μ long and 3 to 7 μ wide. Its incidence is unknown.

Giardia lamblia

(Syn. *Lamblia intestinalis, Megastoma entericum*)

Giardia lamblia, the cause of giardiosis, is common in the duodenum, jejunum, and upper ileum of man, the rhesus monkey, cynomolgus monkey, chimpanzee, other primates, and the pig (Levine 1961; Ruch 1959). It is found throughout the world. It has been reported in the laboratory rhesus monkey (Reardon and Rininger

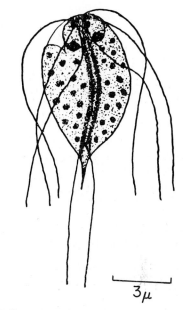

Fig. 1.17. *Octomitus pulcher.* (From Wenrich 1930.)

1968), and it is probably common in specimens obtained from their natural habitat.

MORPHOLOGY

The trophozoites are bilaterally symmetrical and measure 9 to 21 μ long, 5 to 15 μ wide, and 2 to 4 μ thick (Levine 1961). They have a piriform body with a broadly rounded anterior end, an extended posterior end, and a large sucking disc on the anterior ventral side. There are two anterior nuclei, two slender axostyles, eight flagella which emerge at different locations, and a pair of darkly staining median bodies which are curved bars shaped like the claws of a claw hammer. Cysts are ovoid, measure 8 to 12 μ by 7 to 10 μ, and contain four nuclei.

LIFE CYCLE

Reproduction is by binary longitudinal fission. Transmission is by ingestion of the organism in contaminated feces.

PATHOLOGIC EFFECTS

Giardia lamblia has been reported to cause diarrhea in monkeys, but controlled studies have not been conducted (Ruch 1959).

DIAGNOSIS

Tentative diagnosis is made by identifying the organism in the feces or intestine in association with diarrhea. Since the pathogenicity of *G. lamblia* is uncertain, it is important that other possible causes be considered before ascribing the diarrhea to this organism.

CONTROL

Quinacrine, chloroquine, and amodiaquine are effective in man, but there are no reports of treatment in lower primates (Lamadrid-Montemayor 1954). Rigid sanitation is important for control. Cysts are resistant, but 2 to 5% phenol or cresol will destroy them (Červa 1955).

PUBLIC HEALTH CONSIDERATIONS

Giardia lamblia sometimes causes diarrhea in man. For this reason, infected animals should be handled with caution.

Giardia muris

This possibly pathogenic flagellate occurs in the anterior small intestine of the mouse, Norway rat, hamster, black rat, and other wild rodents throughout the world (Andrews and White 1936; Bonfante, Faust, and Giraldo 1961). It is common in wild specimens and in conventional laboratory colonies (Bemrick 1961; Heston 1941) but does not occur in cesarean-derived, barrier-sustained colonies (Foster 1963; Owen 1968).

MORPHOLOGY

Trophozoites are 7 to 13 μ long by 5 to 10 μ wide, and the median bodies are small and round (Fig. 1.18) (Levine 1961). Other characteristics are similar to those of *G. lamblia*.

LIFE CYCLE

The life cycle is similar to that of *G. lamblia*.

PATHOLOGIC EFFECTS

Although controlled studies of the organism's pathogenicity have not been conducted, *G. muris* has reportedly caused chronic enteritis, especially in young mice (Kofoid and Christiansen 1915).

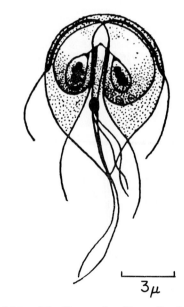

FIG. 1.18. *Giardia muris*. (From Lavier 1924.)

DIAGNOSIS

Diagnosis is made by identifying the organism in association with enteric lesions. Since the pathogenicity of *G. muris* is uncertain, other possible causes must be considered before ascribing the lesions to this organism.

CONTROL

Lead arsenate, given orally at the rate of 0.5% in the feed for 1 to 3 days, eliminates *G. muris* from mice, but it is toxic (Bemrick 1962). Metronidazole, given at 0.5% in the drinking water for 11 days, and quinacrine hydrochloride, given orally at a rate of 0.25 mg per g of body weight, are effective (Bemrick 1963; Mandoul, Dargelos, and Millan 1961).

PUBLIC HEALTH CONSIDERATIONS

Giardia muris is of no known public health importance.

Giardia simoni

Giardia simoni occurs in the anterior small intestine of the rat, hamster, and various wild rodents throughout the world; it is common in some laboratory colonies (Levine 1961; Saxe 1954a) and absent in others (Foster 1963; Owen 1968). Attempts to in-

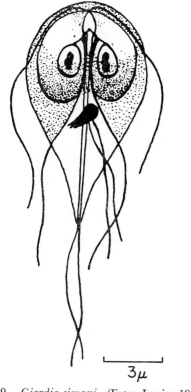

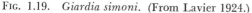

3μ

FIG. 1.19. *Giardia simoni.* (From Lavier 1924.)

fect mice experimentally have been unsuccessful (Bemrick 1962). The trophozoites (Fig. 1.19) are 11 to 19 μ by 5 to 11 μ, and the median bodies are curved bars similar to those of *G. lamblia*. A mild jejunal tympanites has been associated with this infection in the rat, but controlled pathogenicity studies have not been conducted (Boeck 1919).

Giardia caviae

This apparently nonpathogenic flagellate occurs in the anterior small intestine of the guinea pig throughout the world (Hegner 1923; Levine 1961; Nie 1950). It is apparently rare. Its trophozoites are 8 to 15 μ by 6 to 10 μ, and its median bodies are curved bars similar to those of *G. lamblia*.

Giardia duodenalis

This apparently nonpathogenic flagellate is common in the anterior small intestine of the rabbit throughout the world (Levine 1961). It also occurs in a South American porcupine (*Coendou villosus*). Its trophozoites are 13 to 19 μ by 8 to 11 μ and have median bodies similar to those of *G. lamblia*.

Giardia canis

This possibly pathogenic flagellate occurs in the anterior small intestine of the dog throughout the world (Levine 1961). It is common in laboratory dogs obtained from pounds, but its incidence in those raised in kennels is unknown (Burrows and Lillis 1967).

MORPHOLOGY

Trophozoites are 12 to 17 μ long and 7 to 10 μ wide, with median bodies which are curved bars like those of *G. lamblia* (Levine 1961). The cysts are 9 to 13 μ long and 7 to 9 μ wide. Other characteristics are the same as those of *G. lamblia*.

LIFE CYCLE

The life cycle is similar to that of *G. lamblia*.

PATHOLOGIC EFFECTS

The pathogenicity of *G. canis* is uncertain. It has been reported as causing diarrhea in young dogs, but the conditions under which it is pathogenic are unknown (Levine 1961).

DIAGNOSIS

Diagnosis is made by identifying the organism in the feces or intestine in association with diarrhea. Since the pathogenicity of *G. canis* is uncertain, other possible causes of the diarrhea should be considered.

CONTROL

Sanitation will prevent transmission of the infection. Quinacrine hydrochloride, given orally (50 to 100 mg twice daily for 2 to 3 days, and repeated if necessary after 3 to 4 days), is an effective treatment (Levine 1961).

PUBLIC HEALTH CONSIDERATIONS

Giardia canis may be a form of *G. lamblia;* therefore, care should be taken to prevent contamination from dog feces.

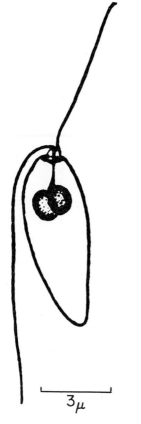

FIG. 1.20. *Proteromonas brevifilia.* (From Nie 1950. Journal of Morphology 86:389, Fig. 3.)

Giardia cati

This flagellate, which may be identical with *G. canis,* has been reported from the anterior small intestine of the cat in the United States and Europe (Levine 1961). Its incidence and pathogenicity are unknown. The trophozoites are 10 to 18 μ long and 5 to 9 μ wide. The median bodies are curved bars similar to those of *G. lamblia.* The cysts are 10.5 μ long and 7.0 μ wide.

Proteromonas brevifilia

Proteromonas brevifilia (Fig. 1.20), an apparently nonpathogenic flagellate, is common in the cecum of the guinea pig throughout the world (Alexieff 1946; Levine 1961; Nie 1950). It is 4 to 9 μ long and 2 to 4 μ wide. The body is spindle shaped, with an anterior and a free-trailing

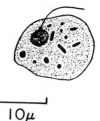

FIG. 1.21. *Histomonas meleagridis.* Trophozoite from cecum of chicken. (From Wenrich 1943. Journal of Morphology 72:295, Fig. 1.)

flagellum, an anterior nucleus, a rhizoplast running from the flagellar blepharoplast to the nuclear membrane, a perirhizoplastic ring which is thought to be a parabasal body, and a paranuclear body the same size as the nucleus.

Histomonas meleagridis

Histomonas meleagridis is common in the ceca and liver of the chicken, turkey, and other birds throughout the world (Levine 1961). Although it is a serious pathogen in the turkey, infection in the chicken is usually inapparent. Its incidence in the laboratory chicken is unknown; it is probably rare or absent.

MORPHOLOGY

This organism is pleomorphic (Levine 1961; Lund 1963; Tyzzer 1919). The form found in the cecal lumen is flagellated (Fig. 1.21). It ranges from about 6 to 18 μ and usually has a clear outer zone of cytoplasm with a granular inner zone. Bacteria and food particles are often present; the nucleus is variable. Typically one, but sometimes two, flagella arise from a basal granule near the nucleus.

The forms that occur in the cecal wall and liver are extracellular. A basal granule is located near the nucleus, but no discernible flagella are present. There are invasive, actively ameboid forms measuring 8 to 17 μ long, vegetative forms measuring 12 to 15 μ by 12 to 21 μ, and compact forms measuring 4 to 11 μ. The vegetative and compact forms usually occur in groups. There are no cysts.

LIFE CYCLE

Transmission is primarily by ingestion of the organism in eggs of the cecal worm

(*Heterakis gallinarum*). Ingestion of feces containing the parasite and mechanical transmission by insects also occur but are of minor importance.

PATHOLOGIC EFFECTS

Although the turkey is more commonly affected, serious disease sometimes occurs in the young chicken (Levine 1961). Clinical signs are listlessness, ruffled feathers, and yellow diarrhea. Ulcers and caseous inflammation are seen in the cecal mucosa, and depressed, yellow, necrotic foci measuring up to 1 cm in diameter occur in the liver. Parasites are easily seen in histologic sections of the cecal and hepatic lesions.

DIAGNOSIS

Diagnosis is based on the characteristic liver lesions and on the microscopic identification of the organism in histologic sections or in cecal scrapings.

CONTROL

Good management and sanitation, including elimination of the cecal worm, are important in preventing this disease (Levine 1961). The drug 2-amino-5-nitrothiazole (Enheptin), given in the feed at a level of 0.1 to 0.2%, is an effective treatment.

PUBLIC HEALTH CONSIDERATIONS

Histomonas meleagridis does not affect man.

Oikomonas termo

Most members of the genus *Oikomonas* are apparently nonpathogenic and free-living, but some occur in animals (Levine 1961). *Oikomonas termo* has been found in the feces and large intestine of the guinea pig throughout the world. Its trophozoites lack chromatophores, lorica, or test. It has a single flagellum and a nucleus near the center of the body and is about 10 to 11 μ long and 7 to 10 μ wide (Nie 1950). Its incidence is unknown.

Sphaeromonas communis

Not much is known about the genus *Sphaeromonas*. It is closely related to *Oikomonas* and may even be a synonym of that genus (Levine 1961). *Sphaeromonas communis* occurs in the cecum and colon of the guinea pig throughout the world (da Fonseca 1916; Yakimoff et al. 1921). Its body is spherical or ellipsoidal, with a somewhat central nucleus, a single long flagellum arising from a basal granule on the nuclear membrane, and a cytoplasm that contains many dark-staining granules; it is 3 to 14 μ in diameter. Its incidence is unknown.

Caviomonas mobilis

Caviomonas mobilis (Fig. 1.22), a nonpathogenic flagellate, has been reported in the cecum of the hamster and guinea pig in North America (Levine 1961; Saxe 1954b). It has been found in 11% of 56 guinea pigs in eastern United States (Nie 1950). The body is naked, with a vesicular nucleus at the anterior end, a single flagellum arising from the nuclear membrane, and a band-like peristyle arising from the nuclear membrane opposite to the origin of the flagellum and extending posteriorly along the periphery of the body surface. It is 2 to 7 μ long and 2 to 3 μ wide. There are no cysts.

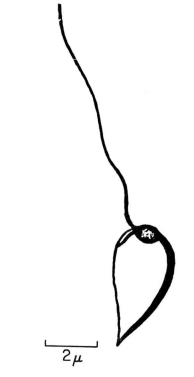

FIG. 1.22. *Caviomonas mobilis*. (From Nie 1950. Journal of Morphology 86:386, Fig. 1.)

TABLE 1.1. Hemoflagellates affecting endothermal laboratory animals

Parasite	Geographic Distribution	Endothermal Host	Location in Host	Method of Infection	Incidence		Pathologic Effects	Public Health Importance	Reference
					In nature	In laboratory			
*Trypanosoma lewisi**	Worldwide	Rat, black rat, other rats	Blood	Ingestion of flea vector or flea feces	Common	Absent; can occur only if fleas are present	Usually none; sometimes anemia; possibly arthritis of pedal extremities	Possibly causes anemia, fever	Bonfante et al. 1961; Eyles 1952; Fujiwara and Suzuki 1967; Levine 1961; Sherman and Ruble 1967
*Trypanosoma duttoni**	Worldwide	Mouse, other mice	Blood	Ingestion of flea vector or flea feces	Apparently uncommon	Absent; can occur only if fleas are present	Usually none; sometimes gastritis, enteritis	None known	Levine 1961; Sheppe and Adams 1957
*Trypanosoma conorhini**	Hawaii, Brazil, India, Taiwan, Indonesia	Rat, black rat	Blood	Ingestion of reduviid bug vector or wound contamination with bug feces	Apparently uncommon	Absent; can occur only if reduviid bugs are present	None	None	Dias and Campos Seabra 1943; Morishita 1935; Wood 1946
*Trypanosoma nabiasi**	Europe, Turkey	Rabbit	Blood	Ingestion of flea vector or flea feces	Common	Absent; can occur only if fleas are present	None	None	Grewal 1956; Kroó 1936
*Trypanosoma cruzi**	Southern United States, Mexico, Central America, South America, possibly Asia	Mouse, wood rats, other rodents, dog, cat, other carnivores, armadillo, opossum, bats, marmosets, capuchins, squirrel monkeys, spider monkeys, other simian primates, man	Blood, reticulo-endothelium, muscle, heart, other tissues	Ingestion of reduviid bug vector or wound contamination with bug feces	Common in some areas; uncommon in others	Occurs only in animals obtained from natural habitat in endemic areas	Edema, myocarditis, anemia, splenomegaly, hepatomegaly, lymphadenitis	Causes trypanosomosis (Chagas' disease)	Belding 1965; Dunn et al. 1963; Kabat et al. 1952; Levine 1961; Seneca and Wolf 1955
*Trypanosoma sanmartini**	Colombia	Squirrel monkeys	Blood	Wound contamination with feces of reduviid bug vector	Unknown	Unknown; likely to occur only in animals obtained from natural habitat in endemic areas	Unknown	Unknown	Dunn et al. 1963; Garnham and Gonzales-Mugaburu 1962

*Discussed in text.

TABLE 1.1 (continued)

Parasite	Geographic Distribution	Endothermal Host	Location in Host	Method of Infection	Incidence		Pathologic Effects	Public Health Importance	Reference
					In nature	In laboratory			
Trypanosoma minasense*	Central America, South America	Marmosets, capuchins, spider monkeys, howler monkeys, night monkeys, woolly monkeys, squirrel monkeys, man	Blood	Unknown; probably similar to T. sanmartini	Common in some areas; uncommon in others	Occurs only in animals obtained from natural habitat in endemic areas	Probably none	Infects man; probably non-pathogenic	Dunn et al. 1963
Trypanosoma rangeli*	Central America, South America	Dog, cat, opossum, capuchins, man	Blood	Reduviid bug bite or contamination with bug feces	Common in dog, cat	Occurs only in animals obtained from natural habitat in endemic areas	Probably none	Infects man; probably non-pathogenic	Dunn et al. 1963 Groot 1951 Groot et al. 1951 Levine 1961
Trypanosoma saimirii*	Brazil	Squirrel monkeys	Blood	Reduviid bug bite or contamination with bug feces	Unknown	Unknown; likely to occur only in animals obtained from natural habitat in endemic areas	None	None known	Deane and Damasceno 1961 Dunn et al. 1963 Rodhain 1941
Trypanosoma diasi*	Brazil	Capuchins	Blood	Wound contamination with feces from reduviid vector	Unknown	Unknown; likely to occur only in animals obtained from natural habitat in endemic areas	None	None known	Deane and Damasceno 1961 Deane and Martins 1952 Dunn et al. 1963
Trypanosoma primatum*	West Africa	Guenons, chimpanzee, gorilla	Blood	Unknown	Unknown; probably common	Unknown; likely to occur only in animals obtained from natural habitat in endemic areas	None	None known	Reichenow 1917

*Discussed in text.

25

TABLE 1.1 (continued)

Parasite	Geographic Distribution	Endothermal Host	Location in Host	Method of Infection	Incidence — In nature	Incidence — In laboratory	Pathologic Effects	Public Health Importance	Reference
Trypanosoma brucei	Africa	Dog, domestic animals, wild game animals	Blood, cerebro-spinal fluid	Tsetse fly bite	Common in domestic animals	Occurs only in animals obtained from natural habitat in endemic areas	Fever, anemia, edema, emaciation, muscular atrophy, incoordina-tion, paraly-sis, death	None	Levine 1961
Trypanosoma congolense	Africa	Dog, domestic animals, wild game animals	Blood, cerebro-spinal fluid	Tsetse fly bite	Common in domestic animals	Occurs only in animals obtained from natural habitat in endemic areas	Fever, anemia, edema, emaciation, muscular atrophy, incoordina-tion, paraly-sis, death	None	Levine 1961
Trypanosoma dimorphion	Africa	Dog, domestic animals	Blood, cerebro-spinal fluid	Tsetse fly bite	Uncommon	Occurs only in animals obtained from natural habitat in endemic areas	Fever, anemia, edema, emaciation, muscular atrophy, incoordina-tion, paraly-sis, death	None	Levine 1961
Trypanosoma evansi	Central America, South America, North Africa, Asia	Dog, domestic animals, wild game animals	Blood, cerebro-spinal fluid	Tabanid fly bite	Common	Occurs only in animals obtained from natural habitat in endemic areas	Fever, anemia, edema, emaciation, muscular atrophy, in-coordination, paralysis, death	None	Levine 1961
Trypanosoma avium	Worldwide	Chicken, pigeon, other birds	Blood	Black fly or mosquito bite	Common in wild birds	Unknown; probably rare or absent	None	None known	Bennett 1961
*Leishmania donovani**	Tropics, subtropics	Black rat, other wild rodents, dog, cat, man	Reticulo-endothelium	Sand fly bite; skin contamination with crushed flies or fly feces	Common	Occurs only in animals obtained from natural habitat in endemic areas	Splenomegaly; sometimes hepato-megaly, enlarged lymph nodes	Causes visceral leishmaniosis (kala azar)	Hoogstraal et al, 1963 Levine 1961
*Leishmania tropica**	Tropics, subtropics	Wild rodents, dog, cat, man	Reticulo-endothelium, skin, mucous membranes	Sand fly bite; skin contamination with crushed flies or fly feces	Common	Occurs only in animals obtained from natural habitat in endemic areas	Desquamation of skin, cutaneous ulcers	Causes cutaneous leishmaniosis	Levine 1961
*Leishmania enrietti**	Brazil	Guinea pig	Skin	Unknown	Unknown	Unknown	Cutaneous ulcers	None	Muniz and Medina 1948a, b

*Discussed in text.

TABLE 1.2. Enteric flagellates affecting endothermal laboratory animals

Parasite	Geographic Distribution	Endothermal Host	Location in Host	Method of Infection	Incidence In nature	Incidence In laboratory	Pathologic Effects	Public Health Importance	Reference
Tritrichomonas muris*	Worldwide	Mouse, rat, black rat, hamster, other wild rodents	Cecum, colon, small intestine	Ingestion of organism passed in feces	Common	Common in some colonies; absent in others	None	None	Andrews and White 1936 Bonfante et al. 1961 Levine 1961 Wantland 1955
Tritrichomonas minuta*	North America, Europe	Mouse, rat, hamster	Cecum, colon	Ingestion of organism passed in feces	Common	Common in some colonies; absent in others	None	None	Wenrich 1924
Tritrichomonas caviae*	Worldwide	Guinea pig	Cecum, colon	Ingestion of organism passed in feces	Unknown	Unknown; probably common	None	None	Nie 1950
Tritrichomonas sp.*	United States	Guinea pig	Cecum	Ingestion of organism passed in feces	Unknown	Unknown	None	None	Nie 1950
Tritrichomonas criceti*	North America	Hamster	Cecum, colon	Ingestion of organism passed in feces	Unknown	Unknown	None	None	Wantland 1956
Tritrichomonas eberthi	Worldwide	Chicken, other birds	Ceca	Ingestion of organism passed in feces	Common	Unknown	None	None	Levine 1961
Trichomitus wenyoni*	North America	Mouse, rat, hamster, rhesus monkey, baboons	Cecum, colon	Ingestion of organism passed in feces	Unknown	Common in some colonies; absent in others	None	None	Wenrich and Nie 1949
Tetratrichomonas microti*	North America	Mouse, rat, hamster, voles, other wild rodents	Cecum	Ingestion of organism passed in feces	Common	Unknown; probably common in animals obtained from natural habitat	None	None	Wenrich and Saxe 1950
Tetratrichomonas macacovaginae*	North America	Monkey	Vagina	Venereal contact	Unknown	Unknown	Unknown	Unknown	Hegner and Ratcliffe 1927
Tetratrichomonas gallinarum	Worldwide	Chicken, other birds	Ceca	Ingestion of organism in food or water	Common	Unknown; probably common	None	None	Levine 1961
Trichomonas tenax*	Worldwide	Rhesus monkey, cynomolgus monkey, baboons, man	Mouth	Oral contact	Common	Unknown; probably common in animals obtained from natural habitat	None	Infects man; probably non-pathogenic	Hegner and Chu 1930 Honigberg and Lee 1959 Wenrich 1947

*Discussed in text.

27

TABLE 1.2 (continued)

Parasite	Geographic Distribution	Endothermal Host	Location in Host	Method of Infection	Incidence — In nature	Incidence — In laboratory	Pathologic Effects	Public Health Importance	Reference
Trichomonas canistomae	United States, Europe	Dog	Mouth	Oral contact	Probably rare	Rare	None	None	Levine 1961
Trichomonas felistomae	United States	Cat	Mouth	Oral contact	Probably rare	Rare	None	None	Levine 1961
*Trichomonas gallinae**	Worldwide	Chicken, pigeon, other birds	Mouth, sinuses, pharynx, esophagus, crop, proventriculus, liver	Ingestion of organism in pigeon milk or in contaminated water	Common in pigeon; rare in chicken	Unknown; probably rare	Caseous nodules or ulcers of crop, esophagus, pharynx	None	Levine 1961
*Pentatrichomonas hominis**	Worldwide	Mouse, rat, hamster, dog, cat, rhesus monkey, cynomolgus monkey, chimpanzee, orangutan, other simian primates, man	Cecum, colon	Ingestion of organism passed in feces	Common in rat, dog, monkey, cynomolgus monkey, chimpanzee	Unknown; probably common in animals obtained from natural habitat	None	Infects man; probably non-pathogenic	Andrews and White 1936; Burrows and Lillis 1967; Hegner 1934; Hegner and Chu 1930; Poindexter 1942
Pentatrichomonas sp.	Probably worldwide	Chicken, other birds	Ceca, liver	Ingestion of organism passed in feces	Unknown	Unknown	Unknown	None known	Levine 1961
*Monocercomonas caviae**	Worldwide	Guinea pig	Cecum	Ingestion of organism passed in feces	Unknown	Common	None	None	Nie 1950
*Monocercomonas pistillum**	North America	Guinea pig	Cecum	Ingestion of organism passed in feces	Unknown	Common	None	None	Nie 1950
*Monocercomonas minuta**	North America	Guinea pig	Cecum	Ingestion of organism passed in feces	Unknown	Common	None	None	Nie 1950
*Monocercomonas cuniculi**	Worldwide	Rabbit	Cecum	Ingestion of organism passed in feces	Unknown	Unknown; probably common	None	None	Levine 1961; Tanabe 1926
*Hexamastix caviae**	Worldwide	Guinea pig	Cecum	Ingestion of organism passed in feces	Unknown	Common	None	None	Levine 1961; Nie 1950
*Hexamastix robustus**	North America	Guinea pig	Cecum	Ingestion of organism passed in feces	Unknown	Common	None	None	Levine 1961; Nie 1950

*Discussed in text.

TABLE 1.2 (continued)

Parasite	Geographic Distribution	Endothermal Host	Location in Host	Method of Infection	Incidence In nature	Incidence In laboratory	Pathologic Effects	Public Health Importance	Reference
Hexamastix muris*	Worldwide	Rat, hamster, other rodents	Cecum	Ingestion of organism passed in feces	Common	Unknown; probably common	None	None	Kirby and Honigberg 1949 Levine 1961 Wenrich 1946
Chilomitus caviae*	Worldwide	Guinea pig	Cecum	Ingestion of organism passed in feces	Unknown	Common	None	None	Levine 1961
Chilomitus conexus*	North America	Guinea pig	Cecum	Ingestion of organism passed in feces	Unknown	Uncommon	None	None	Levine 1961 Nie 1950
Enteromonas [hominis*	Worldwide	Rat, hamster, rhesus monkey, other macaques, man	Cecum	Ingestion of organism passed in feces	Uncommon	Unknown	None	Infects man; probably non-pathogenic	Levine 1961 Reardon and Rininger 1968
Enteromonas caviae*	Worldwide	Guinea pig	Cecum	Ingestion of organism passed in feces	Unknown	Common	None	None	Nie 1950
Enteromonas sp.*	Worldwide	Rabbit	Cecum	Ingestion of organism passed in feces	Unknown	Unknown	None	None	Harkema 1936
Retortamonas intestinalis*	Worldwide	Rhesus monkey, chimpanzee, other simian primates, man	Cecum	Ingestion of organism passed in feces	Unknown	Unknown	None	Infects man; probably non-pathogenic	Levine 1961
Retortamonas caviae*	Worldwide	Guinea pig	Cecum	Ingestion of organism passed in feces	Unknown	Common	None	None	Nie 1950
Retortamonas cuniculi*	Worldwide	Rabbit	Cecum	Ingestion of organism passed in feces	Unknown	Unknown	None	None	Collier and Boeck 1926 Levine 1961
Retortamonas sp.*	Eastern United States	Rat	Cecum	Ingestion of organism passed in feces	Uncommon	Unknown	None	None	Andrews and White 1936
Chilomastix mesnili*	Worldwide	Rhesus monkey, cynomolgus monkey, other macaques, green monkey, other guenons, baboons, capuchins, orangutan, chimpanzee, pig, man	Cecum, colon	Ingestion of organism passed in feces	Common	Common in animals obtained from natural habitat	None	Infects man; probably non-pathogenic	Hegner 1934 Hegner and Chu 1930 Levine 1961 Myers and Kuntz 1965 Poindexter 1942 Reardon and Rininger 1968

* Discussed in text.

TABLE 1.2 (continued)

Parasite	Geographic Distribution	Endothermal Host	Location in Host	Method of Infection	Incidence In nature	Incidence In laboratory	Pathologic Effects	Public Health Importance	Reference
Chilomastix cuniculi*	Worldwide	Rabbit	Cecum	Ingestion of organism passed in feces	Common	Common	None	None	Levine 1961
Chilomastix intestinalis*	Worldwide	Guinea pig	Cecum	Ingestion of organism passed in feces	Unknown	Common	None	None	Levine 1961 Nie 1950
Chilomastix wenrichi*	North America	Guinea pig	Cecum	Ingestion of organism passed in feces	Unknown	Unknown	None	None	Levine 1961 Nie 1950
Chilomastix bettencourti*	Worldwide	Mouse, rat, black rat, hamster	Cecum	Ingestion of organism passed in feces	Common	Unknown; probably common	None	None	Andrews and White 1936 Bonfante et al. 1961 Wantland 1955 Wenyon 1926
Chilomastix gallinarum*	Worldwide	Chicken, other birds	Ceca	Ingestion of organism passed in feces	Common	Unknown; probably common	None	None	Levine 1961
Selenomonas palpitans*	Worldwide	Guinea pig	Cecum, colon	Ingestion of organism passed in feces	Unknown	Unknown	None	None	Levine 1961
Monocercomonoides caviae*	Worldwide	Guinea pig	Cecum	Ingestion of organism passed in feces	Unknown	Common	None	None	Levine 1961 Nie 1950
Monocercomonoides quadrifunilis*	North America	Guinea pig	Cecum	Ingestion of organism passed in feces	Unknown	Common	None	None	Levine 1961 Nie 1950
Monocercomonoides wenrichi*	North America	Guinea pig	Cecum	Ingestion of organism passed in feces	Unknown	Common	None	None	Levine 1961 Nie 1950
Monocercomonoides exilis*	North America	Guinea pig	Cecum	Ingestion of organism passed in feces	Unknown	Unknown	None	None	Levine 1961 Nie 1950
Monocercomonoides sp.*	North America	Rat, hamster	Cecum	Ingestion of organism passed in feces	Unknown	Unknown	None	None	Levine 1961 Saxe 1954a
Hexamita muris*	Worldwide	Mouse, rat, hamster, wild rodents	Small intestine, cecum	Ingestion of organism passed in feces	Common	Common in some colonies; absent in others	Associated with duodenitis in mouse	None	Bonfante et al. 1961 Heston 1941 Levine 1961 Meshorer 1969 Tsuchiya and Rector 1936
Hexamita pitheci*	South America	Rhesus monkey	Cecum, colon	Ingestion of organism passed in feces	Unknown	Unknown	None	None	da Cunha and Muniz 1929

*Discussed in text.

TABLE 1.2 (continued)

Parasite	Geographic Distribution	Endothermal Host	Location in Host	Method of Infection	Incidence In nature	Incidence In laboratory	Pathologic Effects	Public Health Importance	Reference
Hexamita sp.*	North America	Rhesus monkey, chimpanzee	Cecum	Ingestion of organism passed in feces	Unknown	Unknown	None	None	Hegner 1934 Wenrich 1933
*Octomitus pulcher**	Worldwide	Mouse, rat, hamster, ground squirrels, other rodents	Cecum	Ingestion of organism passed in feces	Unknown	Unknown	None	None	Gabel 1954 Levine 1961
*Giardia lamblia**	Worldwide	Rhesus monkey, cynomolgus monkey, chimpanzee, other simian primates, pig, man	Anterior small intestine	Ingestion of organism passed in feces	Common	Unknown; probably common in animals obtained from natural habitat	Possibly enteritis in monkey	Causes enteritis	Levine 1961 Ruch 1959
*Giardia muris**	Worldwide	Mouse, rat, hamster, black rat, other wild rodents	Anterior small intestine	Ingestion of organism passed in feces	Common	Common in some colonies; absent in others	Possibly enteritis in mouse	None	Andrews and White 1936 Bemrick 1961 Bonfante et al. 1961 Heston 1941 Kofoid and Christiansen 1915 Levine 1961 Mandoul et al. 1961 Owen 1968
*Giardia simoni**	Worldwide	Rat, hamster, wild rodents	Anterior small intestine	Ingestion of organism passed in feces	Common	Common in some colonies; absent in others	Associated with tympanites in rat	None known	Bemrick 1962 Boeck 1919 Levine 1961 Saxe 1954a
*Giardia caviae**	Worldwide	Guinea pig	Anterior small intestine	Ingestion of organism passed in feces	Unknown	Unknown; apparently rare	None	None known	Hegner 1923 Levine 1961 Nie 1950
*Giardia duodenalis**	Worldwide	Rabbit, South American porcupine (*Coendou villosus*)	Anterior small intestine	Ingestion of organism passed in feces	Unknown	Common	None	None known	Levine 1961
*Giardia canis**	Worldwide	Dog	Anterior small intestine	Ingestion of organism passed in feces	Unknown	Common in dogs obtained from pounds	Uncertain; probably diarrhea	Unknown; possibly causes enteritis	Burrows and Lillis 1967 Levine 1961

*Discussed in text.

TABLE 1.2 (continued)

Parasite	Geographic Distribution	Endothermal Host	Location in Host	Method of Infection	Incidence		Pathologic Effects	Public Health Importance	Reference
					In nature	In laboratory			
Giardia cati*	United States, Europe	Cat	Anterior small intestine	Ingestion of organism passed in feces	Unknown	Unknown	Unknown	Unknown	Levine 1961
Proteromonas brevifilia*	Worldwide	Guinea pig	Cecum	Ingestion of organism passed in feces	Unknown	Common	None	None	Alexieff 1946 Levine 1961 Nie 1950
Histomonas meleagridis*	Worldwide	Chicken, other birds	Ceca, liver	Ingestion of organism in Heterakis eggs or in feces	Common	Unknown; probably rare or absent	Mild to severe entero-hepatitis	None	Levine 1961 Lund 1963 Tyzzer 1919
Oikomonas termo*	Worldwide	Guinea pig	Large intestine	Ingestion of organism passed in feces	Unknown	Unknown	None	None	Levine 1961 Nie 1950
Sphaeromonas communis*	Worldwide	Guinea pig	Cecum, colon	Ingestion of organism passed in feces	Unknown	Unknown	None	None	da Fonseca 1916 Levine 1961 Yakimoff et al. 1921
Caviomonas mobilis*	North America	Hamster, guinea pig	Cecum	Ingestion of organism passed in feces	Unknown	Common	None	None	Levine 1961 Nie 1950 Saxe 1954b

*Discussed in text.

REFERENCES

Alexieff, A. 1946. Notes protistologiques. Arch. Zool. Exp. Genet. 84:150–54.

Andrews, J., and H. F. White. 1936. An epidemiological study of protozoa parasitic in wild rats in Baltimore, with special reference to *Endamoeba histolytica*. Am. J. Hyg. 24:184–206.

Ansari, M. A. R. 1955. The genus *Retortamonas* Grassi (Mastigophora: Retortamonidae) Biologia 1:40–69.

———. 1956. The genus *Retortamonas* Grassi, its cultivation and development. Pakistan J. Health 5:189–95.

Belding, D. L. 1965. Textbook of parasitology. 3d ed. Appleton-Century-Crofts, New York. 1374 pp.

Bemrick, W. J. 1961. A note on the incidence of three species of *Giardia* in Minnesota. J. Parasitol. 47:87–89.

———. 1962. The host specificity of *Giardia* from laboratory strains of *Mus musculus* and *Rattus norvegicus*. J. Parasitol. 48:287–90.

———. 1963. A comparison of seven compounds for giardiacidal activity in *Mus musculus*. J. Parasitol. 49:819–23.

Bennett, G. F. 1961. On the specificity and transmission of some avian trypanosomes. Can. J. Zool. 39:17–33.

Boeck, W. C. 1919. Studies on *Giardia microti*. Univ. Calif. (Berkeley) Publ. Zool. 19:85–134.

Bonfante, R., E. C. Faust, and L. E. Giraldo. 1961. Parasitologic surveys in Cali, Departmento del Valle, Colombia: IX. Endoparasites of rodents and cockroaches in Ward Siloe, Cali, Colombia. J. Parasitol. 47:843–46.

Bullock, B. C., R. H. Wolf, and T. B. Clarkson. 1967. Myocarditis associated with trypanosomiasis in a Cebus monkey *(Cebus albifrons)*. J. Am. Vet. Med. Assoc. 151:920–22.

Burrows, R. B., and W. G. Lillis. 1967. Intestinal protozoan infections in dogs. J. Am. Vet. Med. Assoc. 150:880–83.

Červa, L. 1955. Resistence cyst Lamblia intestinalis vuči zevnim faktorum. Cesk. Parasitol. 2:17–21.

Collier, Jane, and W. C. Boeck. 1926. The morphology and cultivation of *Embadomonas cuniculi* n. sp. J. Parasitol. 12:131–40.

Cunha, A. da, and J. Muniz. 1929. Nota sobre os parasitas intestinaes do *Macacus rhesus* com a descripcao de uma nova especie de Octomitus. Mem. Inst. Oswaldo Cruz (Supp.) 5:34–35.

Deane, L. M., and R. G. Damasceno. 1961. Tripanosomídeos de mamíferos de regiano Amazonica: II. Tripanosomas de macacos de zona do Salgado, estado do Pará. Rev. Inst. Med. Trop. Sao Paulo 3:61–70.

Deane, L. M., and Regina Martins. 1952. Sobre um tripansoma encontrado em macaco da Amazonia e que evolui em triatomineos. Rev. Brasil. Malariol. Doencas Trop. Publ. Avulsas 4:47–61.

Dias, E., and C. A. Campos Seabra. 1943. Sobre o *Trypanosoma conorrhini*, hemoparasito do rato transmitido pelo *Triatoma rubrofasciata*. Presenca do vector infectado na cidade do Rio de Janeiro. Mem. Inst. Oswaldo Cruz 39:301–30.

Dunn, F. L., F. L. Lambrecht, and R. du Plessis. 1963. Trypanosomes of South American monkeys and marmosets. Am. J. Trop. Med. Hyg. 12:524–34.

Eastin, C. E., and Irene Roeckel. 1968. *Trypanosoma cruzi* complicating *Prosthenorchis* infestation in the squirrel monkey *(Saimiri sciureus)*. Abstr. 52. 19th Ann. Meeting Am. Assoc. Lab. Animal Sci., Las Vegas.

Eyles, D. E. 1952. Incidence of *Trypanosoma lewisi* and *Hepatozoon muris* in Norway rats. J. Parasitol. 38:222–25.

Faust, E. C., P. C. Beaver, and R. C. Jung. 1968. Animal agents and vectors of human disease. 3d ed. Lea and Febiger, Philadelphia. 461 pp.

Filice, F. P. 1952. Studies on the cytology and life history of a *Giardia* from the laboratory rat. Univ. Calif. (Berkeley) Publ. Zool. 57:53–145.

Fonseca, O. da. 1916. Estudos sobre os flajelados parasitos dos mamiferos do Brazil. Mem. Inst. Oswaldo Cruz 8:5–40.

Foster, H. L. 1963. Specific pathogen-free animals, pp. 109–38. *In* W. Lane-Petter, ed. Animals for research: Principles of breeding and management. Academic Press, New York.

Fujiwara, K., and Y. Suzuki. 1967. Spontaneous arthritis in laboratory rats associated with trypanosomal infection (in Japanese). Bull. Exp. Animals 16:103–5.

Gabel, J. R. 1954. The morphology and taxonomy of the intestinal protozoa of the American woodchuck, *Marmota monax* Linnaeus. J. Morphol. 94:473–549.

Garnham, P. C. C., and L. Gonzales-Mugaburu. 1962. A new trypanosome in *Saimiri* monkeys from Colombia. Rev. Inst. Med. Trop. Sao Paulo 4:79–84.

Grewal, M. S. 1956. Life cycle of the rabbit trypanosome, *Trypanosoma nabiasi* Railliet, 1895. Trans. Roy. Soc. Trop. Med. Hyg. 50:2–3.

Groot, H. 1951. Nuevo foco de trypanosomiasis humana en Colombia. Anales Soc. Biol. Bogota 4:220–21.

Groot, H., S. Renjifo, and C. Uribe. 1951. *Trypanosoma ariarii*, n. sp., from man, found in Colombia. Am. J. Trop. Med. 31:673–91.

Harkema, R. 1936. The parasites of some North Carolina rodents. Ecol. Monographs 6:151–232.

Hegner, R. W. 1923. Giardias from wild rats and mice and *Giardia caviae* sp. n. from the guinea pig. Am. J. Hyg. 3:345–49.

———. 1934. Intestinal protozoa of chimpanzees. Am. J. Hyg. 19:480–501.

Hegner, R. W., and H. J. Chu. 1930. A survey of protozoa parasitic in plants and animals of the Philippine Islands. Philippine J. Sci. 43:451–82.

Hegner, R. W., and H. Ratcliffe. 1927. Trichomonads from the vagina of the monkey, from the mouth of the cat and man, and from the intestine of the monkey, opossum and prairie-dog. J. Parasitol. 14:27–35.

Heston, W. E. 1941. Parasites, pp. 349–79. *In* G. D. Snell, ed. Biology of the laboratory mouse. Blakiston, Philadelphia.

Hoare, C. H., and F. G. Wallace. 1966. Development stages of trypanosomatid flagellates: A new terminology. Nature 212:1385–86.

Honigberg, B. M. 1963. Evolutionary and systemic relationships in the flagellate order Trichomonadida Kirby. J. Protozool. 10:20–63.

Honigberg, B. M., and J. J. Lee. 1959. Structure and division of *Trichomonas tenax* (O. F. Müller). Am. J. Hyg. 69:177–201.

Hoogstraal, H., P. F. D. Van Peenen, T. P. Reid, and D. R. Dietlein. 1963. Leishmaniasis in the Sudan Republic: 10. Natural infections in rodents. Am. J. Trop. Med. Hyg. 12:175–78.

Johnson, P. D. 1933. A case of infection by *Trypanosoma lewisi* in a child. Trans. Roy. Soc. Trop. Med. Hyg. 26:467–68.

Kabat, E. A., A. Wolfe, and Ada E. Bezer. 1952. Studies on acute disseminated encephalomyelitis produced experimentally in rhesus monkeys: VII. The effect of cortisone. J. Immunol. 68:265–75.

Kirby, H., and B. Honigberg. 1949. Flagellates of the caecum of ground squirrels. Univ. Calif. (Berkeley) Publ. Zool. 53:315–65.

Kofoid, C. A., and Elizabeth B. Christiansen. 1915. On binary and multiple fission in *Giardia muris* (Grassi). Univ. Calif. (Berkeley) Publ. Zool. 16:30–54.

Kroó, H. 1936. Die spontane, apathogene Trypanosomeninfektion der Kaninchen. Z. Immunitaetsforsch. 88:117–28.

Lamadrid-Montemayor, F. 1954. Comparative study of chloroquine and amodiaquin in the treatment of giardiasis. Am. J. Trop. Med. Hyg. 3:709–11.

Lavier, G. 1924. Deux espèces de *Giardia* du rat d'égout parisien *(Epimys norvegicus)*. Ann. Parasitol. 2:161–68.

Levine, N. D. 1961. Protozoan parasites of domestic animals and of man. Burgess, Minneapolis. 412 pp.

Lund, E. E. 1963. *Histomonas wenrichi* n. sp. (Mastigophora: Mastigamoebidae), a nonpathogenic parasite of gallinaceous birds. J. Protozool. 10:401–4.

Mandoul, R., R. Dargelos, and J. Millan. 1961. Destruction des protozoaires intestinaux de la souris par un dérivé nitré de l'imidazole. Bull. Soc. Pathol. Exotique 54:12–16.

Meshorer, A. 1969. Hexamitiasis in laboratory mice. Lab. Animal Care 19:33–37.

Minchin, E. A., and J. D. Thomson. 1915. The rat-trypanosome, *Trypanosoma lewisi*, in its relation to the rat flea, *Ceratophyllus fasciatus*. Quart. J. Microscop. Sci. 60:463–692.

Morishita, K. 1935. An experimental study on the life history and biology of *Trypanosoma conorhini* (Donovan), occurring in the alimentary tract of *Triatoma rubrofasciata* (de Geer) in Formosa. Japan. J. Zool. 6:459–546.

Muniz, J., and H. Medina. 1948a. Leishmaniose tegumentar do cobaio: *Leishmania enriettii* n. sp. Arquiv. Biol. Tecnol. Inst. Biol. Pesquisas Tecnol. 3:13–30.

———. 1948b. Leishmaniose tegumentar do cobaio: *Leishmania enriettii* n. sp. Hospital (Rio de Janeiro) 33:7–25.

Myers, Betty J., and R. E. Kuntz. 1965. A checklist of parasites reported for the baboon. Primates 6:137–94.

Nie, D. 1950. Morphology and taxonomy of the intestinal protozoa of the guinea-pig, *Cavia porcella*. J. Morphol. 86:381–493.

Owen, Dawn. 1968. Investigations: B. Parasitological studies. Lab. Animals Centre News Letter 35:7–9.

Poindexter, H. A. 1942. A study of the intestinal parasites of the monkeys of the Santiago Island primate colony. Puerto Rico J. Public Health Trop. Med. 18:175–91.

Reardon, Lucy V., and Bonny F. Rininger. 1968. A survey of parasites in laboratory primates. Lab. Animal Care 18:577–80.

Reichenow, E. 1917. Parásitos de la sangre y del intestino de los monos antropomorfos africanos. Bol. Real Soc. Espan. Hist. Nat. Secc. Biol. 17:312–32.

Rodhain, J. 1941. Notes sur Trypanosoma minasense Chagas: Identité spécifique du trypanosome du saimiri: *Chrysothrix sciureus*. Acta Biol. Belg. 1:187–93.

Ruch, T. C. 1959. Diseases of laboratory primates. W. B. Saunders, Philadelphia. 600 pp.

Saxe, L. H. 1954a. Transfaunation studies on the host specificity of the enteric protozoa of rodents. J. Protozool. 1:220–30.

———. 1954b. The enteric protozoa of the laboratory golden hamster. Abstr. J. Parasitol. 40(Supp.):20.

Seneca, H., and A. Wolf. 1955. *Trypanosoma cruzi* infection in the Indian monkey. Am. J. Trop. Med. Hyg. 4:1009–14.

Sheppe, W. A., and J. R. Adams. 1957. The pathogenic effect of *Trypanosoma duttoni* in hosts under stress conditions. J. Parasitol. 43:55–59.

Sherman, I. W., and Judith A. Ruble. 1967. Virulent *Trypanosoma lewisi* infections in cortisone-treated rats. J. Parasitol. 55:258–62.

Tanabe, M. 1926. Morphological studies on *Trichomonas*. J. Parasitol. 12:120–30.

Tsuchiya, H., and L. E. Rector. 1936. Studies on intestinal parasites among wild rats caught in Saint Louis. Am. J. Trop. Med. 16:705–14.

Tyzzer, E. E. 1919. Developmental phases of the protozoon of "Blackhead" in turkeys. J. Med. Res. 40:1–30.

Wantland, W. W. 1955. Parasitic fauna of the golden hamster. J. Dental Res. 34:631–49.

———. 1956. Trichomonads in the golden hamster. Trans. Illinois State Acad. Sci. 48:197–201.

Wenrich, D. H. 1924. Trichomonad flagellates in the caecum of rats and mice. Anat. Record 29:118.

———. 1930. Intestinal flagellates of rats, pp. 124–42. *In* R. Hegner and J. Andrews, eds. Problems and methods of research in protozoology. Macmillan, New York.

———. 1933. A species of *Hexamita* (Protozoa, Flagellata) from the intestine of a monkey *(Macacus rhesus)*. J. Parasitol. 19:225–29.

———. 1943. Observations on the morphology of Histomonas (Protozoa, Mastigophora) from pheasants and chickens. J. Morphol. 72:279–303.

———. 1946. Culture experiments on intestinal flagellates: I. Trichomonad and other flagellates obtained from man and certain rodents. J. Parasitol. 32:4053.

———. 1947. The species of *Trichomonas* in man. J. Parasitol. 33:177–88.

———. 1949. Protozoan parasites of the rat, pp. 486–501. *In* E. J. Farris and J. Q. Griffith, eds. The rat in laboratory investigation. J. B. Lippincott, Philadelphia.

Wenrich, D. H., and D. Nie. 1949. The morphology of *Trichomonas wenyoni* (Protozoa, Mastigophora). J. Morphol. 85:519–31.

Wenrich, D. H., and L. H. Saxe. 1950. *Trichomonas microti*, n. sp. (Protozoa; Mastigophora). J. Parasitol. 36:261–69.

Wenyon, C. M. 1926. Protozoology: A manual for medical men, veterinarians and zoologists. 2 vol. Baillière, Tindall, and Cox, London.

Wood, S. F. 1946. The occurrence of *Trypanosoma conorhini* Donovan in the reduviid bug *Triatoma rubrofasciata* (Degeer) from Oahu, T. H. Proc. Hawaiian Entomol. Soc. 12:651.

Yakimoff, W. L., W. J. Wassilewsky, M. T. Korniloff, and N. A. Zwietkoff. 1921. Flagellés de l'intestin des animaux de laboratoire. Bull. Soc. Pathol. Exotique 14:558–64.

Chapter 2

SARCODINES

THE sarcodines which occur in endothermal laboratory animals, the amebas, are parasites of the digestive tract (Levine 1961). Most are nonpathogenic, a few are pathogenic, and the role of others is uncertain. For purposes of differential diagnosis, all amebas that occur in endothermal laboratory animals are listed in Table 2.2. The most important are discussed below.

Entamoeba histolytica
(SYN. Entamoeba caudata)

This pathogenic ameba occurs in the cecum and colon of the rat, dog, cat, pig, and most primates, including man, throughout the world (Levine 1961). It has been reported in the rhesus monkey, cynomolgus monkey, pigtail monkey, bonnet monkey, green monkey, baboons, langurs, capuchins, spider monkeys, howler monkeys, woolly monkeys, marmosets, gibbons, orangutan, and chimpanzee (Benson, Fremming, and Young 1955; Bond et al. 1946; Bourova 1946; Dunn 1968; Hegner 1934; Johnson 1941; Kessel 1928; Kuntz and Myers 1966; Kuntz, Myers, and Vice 1967; Miller and Bray 1966; Reardon and Rininger 1968; Ruch 1959; Van Riper et al. 1966; Young et al. 1957). This organism is apparently common in Old World monkeys but uncommon or rare in New World monkeys obtained from their natural habitat (Ruch 1959; Vickers 1969). Although the infection rate in nature is often low, in the laboratory it can increase rapidly and persist for an extended period (Miller and Bray 1966).

Entamoeba histolytica is occasionally found in the dog in southern and eastern United States and in many other parts of the world and is likely to be present in laboratory dogs obtained from pounds in these regions (Burrows and Lillis 1967; Levine 1961). It is rare in the cat.

This ameba has often been reported in wild Norway rats throughout the world (Andrews and White 1936; Bonfante, Faust, and Giraldo 1961; Levine 1961). There are no specific reports of it in laboratory rodents. It is probably rare in conventional colonies and is completely absent from cesarean-derived, barrier-sustained colonies (Foster 1963).

The mouse, guinea pig, and rabbit have been infected experimentally.

MORPHOLOGY

Entamoeba histolytica is divided into a nonpathogenic race with trophozoites 12 to 15 μ in diameter and a pathogenic race with trophozoites 20 to 30 μ in diameter (Fig. 2.1) (Hoare 1958, 1961; Levine 1961). In both races, the nucleus is vesicular and contains a small, central endosome with a ring of small, peripheral granules (Levine 1961). Cysts are 10 to 20 μ in diameter and have four nuclei when mature. Rodlike chromatoid bodies with rounded ends are often present.

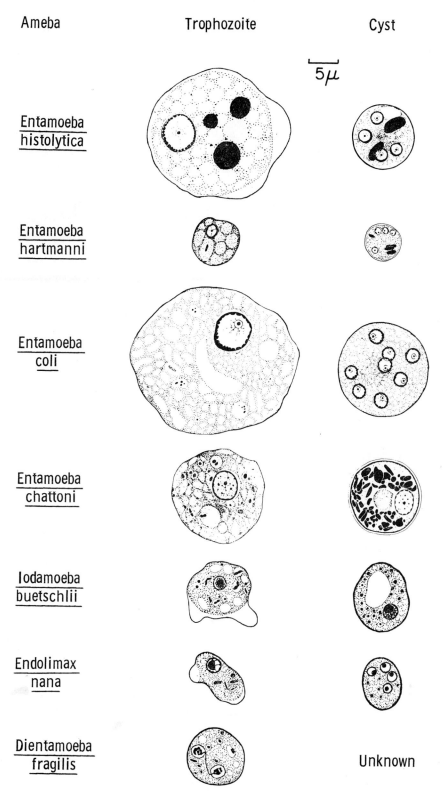

| Ameba | Trophozoite | Cyst |

5μ

Entamoeba
histolytica

Entamoeba
hartmanni

Entamoeba
coli

Entamoeba
chattoni

Iodamoeba
buetschlii

Endolimax
nana

Dientamoeba
fragilis

Unknown

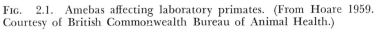

FIG. 2.1. Amebas affecting laboratory primates. (From Hoare 1959.
Courtesy of British Commonwealth Bureau of Animal Health.)

LIFE CYCLE

Reproduction is by binary fission (Levine 1961). Before encysting, the ameba becomes round and small. It produces a cyst wall, and the nucleus divides twice, producing four small nuclei. These nuclei emerge from the cyst and divide, and the organism separates into eight minute amebas. Each of these grows into a trophozoite.

Transmission is by ingestion of cysts which are passed in the feces of chronic carriers. Hosts with dysentery pass trophozoites only and are not important sources of infection.

PATHOLOGIC EFFECTS

In most cases, *E. histolytica* causes mild signs or none at all; however, different strains vary in virulence. The species and nutritional status of the host, environmental factors, and the enteric bacterial flora also affect pathogenicity. New World monkeys are more susceptible than Old World monkeys (Ruch 1959; Vickers 1969). Varying degrees of diarrhea, sometimes hemorrhagic, have been reported in the dog and in subhuman primates (Eichhorn and Gallagher 1916; Herman and Schroeder 1939; Hill 1953; Levine 1961; Miller and Bray 1966; Patten 1939; von Prowazek 1912; Ratcliffe 1931; Suldey 1924; Vickers 1968, 1969; Weidman 1923).

Chronic, mild colitis, characterized by congestion, petechial hemorrhages, and ulcers, sometimes occurs in simian primates (Bond et al. 1946; Bostrom, Ferrell, and Martin 1968; Fremming et al. 1955; Miller and Bray 1966; Vickers 1969). The amebas first invade the mucosa and form small colonies. These colonies then extend into the submucosa and occasionally the muscularis. They produce typical bottle- or flask-shaped ulcers (Fig. 2.2) that range in size from a few millimeters to large confluent lesions involving wide areas of the colon. Ameboid trophozoites are present in and adjacent to the ulcers (Fig. 2.3), but tissue reaction is minimal in the absence of secondary bacterial invasion. Amebas sometimes enter the lymphatics but are generally filtered out in the lymph nodes. Occasionally they enter the mesenteric venules and are carried to the liver, lungs, brain, and other organs where they cause abscesses ranging up to several centimeters in diameter.

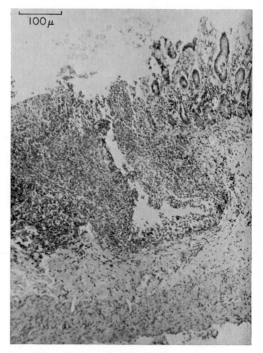

FIG. 2.2. *Entamoeba histolytica* infection in a capuchin. Typical bottle- or flask-shaped intestinal ulcer. (From Vickers 1969. Courtesy of New York Academy of Sciences.)

DIAGNOSIS

Diagnosis is made by microscopic identification of the organism in the feces or lesions (Levine 1961). Since *E. histolytica* is common and often nonpathogenic, other possible causes of enteritis must be eliminated before a definitive diagnosis of amebic dysentery is made. Bacillary dysentery sometimes coexists with amebic dysentery in simians (Bisseru 1967). It is also important to differentiate *E. histolytica* from nonpathogenic amebas (Table 2.1).

CONTROL

Sanitation is important in the prevention of amebiasis. Trophozoites are readily destroyed with common disinfectants, but cysts are more resistant, and hot water or steam is required to kill them (Beaver and Deschamps 1949; Chang 1955; Halpern and Dolkart 1954; Jones and Newton 1950; Simitch, Petrovitch, and Chibalitch 1954).

Since *E. histolytica* is common in primates, all animals in a colony should be ex-

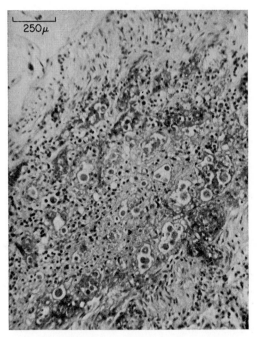

FIG. 2.3. *Entamoeba histolytica* infection in a capuchin. Trophozoites in and adjacent to intestinal ulcers. (Courtesy of J. H. Vickers, Lederle Laboratories.)

amined periodically. New animals should be quarantined for at least 2 months, and during this period they should be examined several times (Britz et al. 1961; Ratcliffe 1954; Whitney, Johnson, and Cole 1967). Infected animals should be treated whether or not they show signs of disease.

Effective treatments for the monkey include fumagillin given orally, 20 mg twice a day for 14 days; carbarsone given orally, 250 mg daily for 10 days; and diiodohydroxyquin given orally, 650 mg daily for 7 to 20 days (Cass 1952; Whitney, Johnson, and Cole 1967; Young et al. 1957). Effective treatments for the chimpanzee include fumagillin given orally, 20 to 30 mg twice a day for 10 days; carbarsone given orally, 500 mg daily for 10 days; and diiodohydroxyquin given orally, 2 g daily for 20 days (Benson, Fremming, and Young 1955; Cass 1952; Ruch 1959; Van Riper et al. 1966). An effective treatment for the dog is iodochlorhydroxyquin given orally, 250 mg three times a day for 7 to 14 days (Seneviratna 1963).

As *E. histolytica* is common in man and most cases of amebiasis in dogs are of human origin, all caretakers, especially those handling primates and dogs, should be examined routinely (Geiman 1964; Hoare 1959; Levine 1961).

PUBLIC HEALTH CONSIDERATIONS

This parasite causes amebic dysentery, a serious disease of man. Because of the high incidence of *E. histolytica* in nonhuman primates, all these animals should be considered infected and handled with care. Man has acquired amebic dysentery from laboratory primates, and animal technicians and caretakers who work with primates obtained from their natural environment are at great risk of infection (Bisseru 1967; Geiman 1964). This is especially true among individuals who practice poor personal hygiene or who are unaware of the hazard involved. Training courses for such personnel are recommended.

Entamoeba hartmanni

Entamoeba hartmanni closely resembles *E. histolytica* but is nonpathogenic (Levine 1961). It is differentiated essentially on the basis of its smaller size (Table 2.1; Fig. 2.1). The incidence and distribution of *E. hartmanni* in laboratory animals are unknown because in the past it has been confused with *E. histolytica*. It has been reported in the cecum and colon of the dog, rhesus monkey, and man in North America and probably occurs throughout the world. In one study of naturally infected monkeys, two types of *Entamoeba* with tetranucleate cysts were seen (Bond et al. 1946). The smaller race was undoubtedly *E. hartmanni*. In a survey of 660 stray dogs in eastern United States, only 1 dog was found infected with *E. hartmanni* (Burrows and Lillis 1967).

Entamoeba coli

This nonpathogenic ameba is the commonest species in man and probably in other primates (Kuntz and Myers 1966; Kuntz, Myers, and Vice 1967; Levine 1961). It occurs in the cecum and colon of the rhesus monkey, cynomolgus monkey, other macaques, the green monkey, baboons, gibbons, orangutan, chimpanzee, gorilla, other nonhuman primates, and the pig throughout the world. It is common in laboratory primates obtained from their natural habitat (Poindexter 1942; Reardon and Rininger 1968; Rowland and Vandenbergh 1965; Van Riper et al. 1966). *Entamoeba coli* reproduces by binary fission and is generally transmitted by ingestion of cysts. Its structure is described in Table 2.1 and illustrated in Figure 2.1.

Entamoeba chattoni

(SYN. *Entamoeba polecki*)

This species occurs in the cecum and colon of the monkey and other primates, including man (Levine 1961). *Entamoeba chattoni* is probably commoner in monkeys than *E. histolytica,* but most workers have failed to recognize it. It has been reported from laboratory monkeys in the United States and Germany and probably occurs throughout the world (Kessel and Johnstone 1949; Kessel and Kaplan 1949; Mudrow-Reichenow 1956). It has been associated with diarrhea in man (Burrows and Klink 1955), but its pathogenicity for laboratory primates is unknown. The structural characteristics of *E. chattoni* are described in Table 2.1 and illustrated in Figure 2.1.

Entamoeba gingivalis

This nonpathogenic species occurs in the mouth of the dog, cat, rhesus monkey, cynomolgus monkey, baboons, chimpanzee, and man throughout the world (Levine 1961). It is found between the teeth, under the edge of the gums, and in the tartar. *Entamoeba gingivalis* thrives on diseased gums and was once thought to cause pyorrhea in man. The distinguishing characteristics of its trophozoites are given in Table 2.1. They feed on leucocytes, epithelial cells, sometimes bacteria, and rarely erythrocytes. There are no cysts, and transmission is generally by oral contact. It is common in primates (Ruch 1959) but uncommon in the dog and cat (Levine 1961). It is usually associated with diseased gums.

Entamoeba muris

This nonpathogenic species is common in the cecum and colon of the house mouse and wild rats and occurs in high incidence in conventional laboratory mouse, rat, and hamster colonies throughout the world (Bonfante, Faust, and Giraldo 1961; Ful-

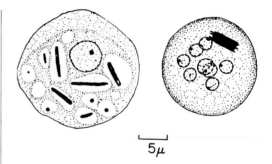

FIG. 2.4. *Entamoeba muris. (Left)* Trophozoite. *(Right)* Cyst. (From Hoare 1959. Courtesy of British Commonwealth Bureau of Animal Health.)

ton and Joyner 1948; Levine 1961; Mudrow-Reichenow 1956; Wantland 1955). It does not occur in cesarean-derived, barrier-sustained colonies (Foster 1963). The structure of *Entamoeba muris* is similar to that of *E. coli* (Levine 1961). Its trophozoites are 8 to 30 μ long; its cysts are 9 to 20 μ in diameter and contain eight nuclei when mature (Fig. 2.4).

Entamoeba caviae

Entamoeba caviae is common in the cecum of the laboratory guinea pig throughout the world (Mudrow-Reichenow 1956; Nie 1950). It resembles *E. coli* (Levine 1961). Its trophozoites are 10 to 20 μ in diameter; its cysts are 11 to 17μ in diameter and contain eight nuclei when mature. *Entamoeba caviae* is nonpathogenic, but it must be differentiated from other amebas in experimentally infected animals.

Entamoeba cuniculi

This nonpathogenic species occurs in the cecum and colon of the rabbit (Levine 1961). It is apparently common and worldwide in distribution but is seldom reported. It has been found in 25% of the domestic rabbits in the USSR (Kheisin 1938). Its trophozoites are 12 to 30 μ long, its cysts are 7 to 21 μ in diameter and have eight nuclei when mature.

Iodamoeba buetschlii

This nonpathogenic ameba is common in the cecum and colon of the rhesus monkey, cynomolgus monkey, other macaques, green monkey, other guenons, mangabeys, mandrills, baboons, capuchins, chimpanzee, gorilla, and man throughout the world (Dunn 1968; Hegner 1934; Hegner and Chu 1930; Kuntz, Myers, and Vice 1967; Levine 1961; Mackinnon and Dibb 1938; Poindexter 1942; Reardon and Rininger 1968; Wenrich 1937). It is frequently found in laboratory primates obtained from their natural habitat. The structure and distinguishing characteristics of *Iodamoeba buetschlii* are given in Table 2.1 and are illustrated in Figure 2.1.

Endolimax nana

Endolimax nana is nonpathogenic. It is common in the cecum and colon of the rhesus monkey, cynomolgus monkey, other macaques, patas monkeys, guenons, mangabeys, baboons, capuchins, chimpanzee, gorilla, pig, and man throughout the world (Dunn 1968; Hegner 1934; Hegner and Chu 1930; Kuntz, Myers, and Vice 1967; Levine 1961; Mackinnon and Dibb 1938; Poindexter 1942; Reardon and Rininger 1968; Rowland and Vandenbergh 1965). It is common in laboratory primates obtained from their natural habitat. The structure and distinguishing characteristics of this ameba are given in Table 2.1 and are illustrated in Figure 2.1.

Endolimax ratti

Endolimax ratti may be a synonym of *E. nana;* the two organisms are structurally identical (Levine 1961). It is nonpathogenic and occurs occasionally in the cecum and colon of the wild Norway rat and conventional laboratory rat throughout the world (Andrews and White 1936; Baldassari 1935; Cable and Headlee 1936).

Dientamoeba fragilis

Dientamoeba fragilis sometimes causes a mucous diarrhea in man, but its pathogenicity for lower primates is unknown (Levine 1961). It occurs in the cecum and colon of the rhesus and cynomolgus monkeys in Asia and in man throughout the world (Hegner and Chu 1930; Knowles and Das Gupta 1936; Levine 1961). Although it has not been observed in baboons in nature, an 8% incidence has been noted in these animals in captivity in south central United States (Kuntz and Myers 1967). The structure and distinguishing characteristics of *D. fragilis* are given in Table 2.1 and illustrated in Figure 2.1.

TABLE 2.1. Structural characteristics of amebas affecting laboratory primates

Ameba	Trophozoite			Cyst		
	Size	Usual number of nuclei	Nuclear characteristics	Size	Usual number of nuclei	Other Characteristics
Entamoeba histolytica	12 to 15 μ (small race) 20 to 30 μ (large race)	1	Small central endosome surrounded by ring of small peripheral granules	10 to 20 μ	4	Rod-shaped chromatoid bodies with rounded ends; large glycogen vacuole sometimes present
Entamoeba hartmanni	3 to 10.5 μ	1	Small central endosome; peripheral granules variable in arrangement	4 to 8 μ	4	Rod-shaped chromatoid bodies with rounded ends; large glycogen vacuole sometimes present
Entamoeba coli	15 to 50μ (usually 20 to 30 μ)	1	Large eccentric endosome surrounded by ring of large peripheral granules	10 to 33 μ	8	Splinter-shaped chromatoid bodies; usually few to many small glycogen vacuoles
Entamoeba chattoni	9 to 25 μ	1	Variable: endosome large or small, central or eccentric, compact or diffuse; peripheral granules fine or coarse, uniform, irregular or diffuse	6 to 18 μ	1	Variable chromatoid bodies, usually irregular and small but also oval, spherical or rod shaped with rounded or pointed ends; glycogen vacuole sometimes present
Entamoeba gingivalis	5 to 35 μ (usually 10 to 20 μ)	1	Small central endosome surrounded by ring of small peripheral granules			Cysts not formed
Iodamoeba buetschlii	4 to 20 μ (usually 9 to 14 μ)	1	Large central endosome surrounded by lightly staining globules; peripheral granules usually not present	5 to 14 μ (usually 8 to 10 μ)	1	No chromatoid bodies; large compact glycogen body present, which stains darkly with iodine
Endolimax nana	6 to 15 μ	1	Large irregular endosome connected to nuclear membrane by achromatic strands; peripheral granules usually not present	5 to 14 μ	4	Oval, irregular, thin walled; no chromatoid bodies; poorly defined glycogen bodies sometimes present
Dientamoeba fragilis	3 to 22 μ (usually 6 to 12 μ)	2 (connected by filament)	Endosome consists of several chromatin granules; fine strands connect endosome to nuclear membrane; peripheral granules not present			Cysts unknown

TABLE 2.2. Sarcodines affecting endothermal laboratory animals

Parasite	Geographic Distribution	Endothermal Host	Location in Host	Method of Infection	Incidence — In nature	Incidence — In laboratory	Pathologic Effects	Public Health Importance	Reference
Entamoeba histolytica＊	Worldwide	Rat, dog, cat, rhesus monkey, cynomolgus monkey, pigtail monkey, bonnet monkey, green monkey, baboons, langurs, capuchins, spider monkeys, howler monkeys, woolly monkeys, marmosets, gibbons, orangutan, chimpanzee, pig, man	Cecum, colon	Ingestion of cysts passed in feces	Common in rat, dog, Old World primates; rare in cat, New World primates	Common in animals obtained from natural habitat	Diarrhea, sometimes hemorrhagic; colitis, sometimes ulcerative; occasionally abscesses in liver, lungs, brain, other organs	Causes amebic dysentery	Benson et al. 1955, Bourova 1946, Dunn 1968, Kuntz and Myers 1966, Kuntz et al. 1967, Levine 1961, Miller and Bray 1966, Reardon and Rininger 1968, Ruch 1959, Van Riper et al. 1966, Vickers 1968, 1969, Young et al. 1957
Entamoeba hartmanni＊	North America, probably worldwide	Dog, rhesus monkey, man	Cecum, colon	Ingestion of of cysts passed in feces	Unknown	Unknown	None	None	Bond et al. 1946, Burrows and Lillis 1967, Levine 1961
Entamoeba coli＊	Worldwide	Rhesus monkey, cynomolgus monkey, other macaques, green monkey, baboons, gibbons, orangutan, chimpanzee, gorilla, other simian primates, pig, man	Cecum, colon	Ingestion of cysts passed in feces	Common	Common in animals obtained from natural habitat	None	None	Kuntz and Myers 1966, Kuntz et al. 1967, Levine 1961, Poindexter 1942, Reardon and Rininger 1968, Rowland and Vandenbergh 1965, Van Riper et al. 1966
Entamoeba chattoni＊	United States, Germany, probably worldwide	Rhesus monkey, other simian primates, man	Cecum, colon	Ingestion of cysts passed in feces	Unknown	Unknown	Unknown	Associated with diarrhea	Burrows and Klink 1955, Kessel and Johnstone 1949, Kessel and Kaplan 1949, Levine 1961, Mudrow-Reichenow 1956

＊Discussed in text.

43

TABLE 2.2 (continued)

Parasite	Geographic Distribution	Endothermal Host	Location in Host	Method of Infection	Incidence — In nature	Incidence — In laboratory	Pathologic Effects	Public Health Importance	Reference
Entamoeba gingivalis*	Worldwide	Dog, cat, rhesus monkey, cynomolgus monkey, baboons, chimpanzee, man	Mouth	Oral contact	Common in primates; uncommon in dog, cat	Unknown; probably common in primates; uncommon in dog, cat	Associated with diseased gums, but non-pathogenic	Associated with diseased gums, but non-pathogenic	Levine 1961 Ruch 1959
Entamoeba muris*	Worldwide	Mouse, rat, black rat, hamster	Cecum, colon	Ingestion of cysts passed in feces	Common	Common	None	None	Bonfante et al. 1961 Fulton and Joyner 1948 Levine 1961 Mudrow-Reichenow 1956 Wantland 1955
Entamoeba caviae*	Worldwide	Guinea pig	Cecum	Ingestion of cysts passed in feces	Unknown	Common	None	None	Levine 1961 Mudrow-Reichenow 1956 Nie 1950
Entamoeba cuniculi*	Apparently worldwide	Rabbit	Cecum, colon	Ingestion of cysts passed in feces	Apparently common	Apparently common	None	None	Kheisin 1938 Levine 1961
Entamoeba gallinarum	Worldwide	Chicken, other birds	Ceca	Ingestion of cysts passed in feces	Common	Common	None	None	Levine 1961
Iodamoeba buetschlii*	Worldwide	Rhesus monkey, cynomolgus monkey, other macaques, green monkey, other guenons, mangabeys, baboons, mandrills, capuchins, chimpanzee, gorilla, man	Cecum, colon	Ingestion of cysts passed in feces	Common	Common in animals obtained from natural habitat	None	None	Dunn 1968 Hegner 1934 Hegner and Chu 1930 Kuntz et al. 1967 Levine 1961 Mackinnon and Dibb 1938 Poindexter 1942 Reardon and Rininger 1968 Wenrich 1937

* Discussed in text.

44

TABLE 2.2 (continued)

Parasite	Geographic Distribution	Endothermal Host	Location in Host	Method of Infection	Incidence — In nature	Incidence — In laboratory	Pathologic Effects	Public Health Importance	Reference
Endolimax nana*	Worldwide	Rhesus monkey, cynomolgus monkey, other macaques, patas monkeys, guenons, mangabeys, baboons, capuchins, chimpanzee, gorilla, pig, man	Cecum, colon	Ingestion of cysts passed in feces	Common	Common in animals obtained from natural habitat	None	None	Dunn 1968, Hegner 1934, Hegner and Chu 1930, Kuntz et al. 1967, Levine 1961, Mackinnon and Dibb 1938, Poindexter 1942, Reardon and Rininger 1968, Rowland and Vandenbergh 1965
Endolimax ratti*	Worldwide	Rat	Cecum, colon	Ingestion of cysts passed in feces	Uncommon	Unknown	None	None	Andrews and White 1936, Baldassari 1935, Cable and Headlee 1936, Levine 1961
Endolimax gregariniformis	Worldwide	Chicken, other birds	Ceca	Ingestion of cysts passed in feces	Common	Unknown	None	None	Levine 1961
Dientamoeba fragilis*	Worldwide	Rhesus monkey, cynomolgus monkey, baboons, man	Cecum, colon	Unknown	Unknown	Unknown	Unknown	Causes mucous diarrhea	Hegner and Chu 1930, Knowles and Das Gupta 1936, Kuntz and Myers 1967, Levine 1961

*Discussed in text.

45

REFERENCES

Andrews, J., and H. F. White. 1936. An epidemiological study of protozoa parasitic in wild rats in Baltimore, with special reference to *Endamoeba histolytica*. Am. J. Hyg. 24:184–206.

Baldassari, M. T. 1935. Le parasitisme des rats à Toulon. Marseille Med. 1:716–18.

Beaver, P. C., and G. Deschamps. 1949. The viability of *E. histolytica* cysts in soil. Am. J. Trop. Med. 29:189–91.

Benson, R. E., B. D. Fremming, and R. J. Young. 1955. Care and management of chimpanzees at the Radiobiological Laboratory of the University of Texas and the United States Air Force. School Aviation Med., U.S. Air Force Rept. 55–48. 7 pp.

Bisseru, B. 1967. Diseases of man acquired from his pets. William Heinemann Medical Books, London. 482 pp.

Bond, V. P., W. Bostick, E. L. Hansen, and H. H. Anderson. 1946. Pathologic study of natural amebic infection in macaques. Am. J. Trop. Med. 26:625–29.

Bonfante, R., E. C. Faust, and L. E. Giraldo. 1961. Parasitologic surveys in Cali, Departmento del Valle, Colombia: IX. Endoparasites of rodents and cockroaches in Ward Siloe, Cali, Colombia. J. Parasitol. 47:843–46.

Bostrom, R. E., J. F. Ferrell, and J. E. Martin. 1968. Simian amebiasis with lesions simulating human amebic dysentery. Abstr. 51. 19th Ann. Meeting Am. Assoc. Lab. Animal Sci., Las Vegas.

Bourova, L.-F. 1946. Étude expérimentale des amibes du type *histolytica* chez les singes inférieurs. Ann. Parasitol. Humaine Comparee 21:97–118.

Britz, W. E., J. Fineg, J. E. Cook, and E. D. Miksch. 1961. Restraint and treatment of young chimpanzees. J. Am. Vet. Med. Assoc. 138:653–58.

Burrows, R. B., and G. E. Klink. 1955. *Endamoeba polecki* infections in man. Am. J. Hyg. 62:156–67.

Burrows, R. B., and W. G. Lillis. 1967. Intestinal protozoan infections in dogs. J. Am. Vet. Med. Assoc. 150:880–83.

Cable, R. M., and W. H. Headlee. 1936. The incidence of animal parasites of the brown rat *(Rattus norvegicus)* in Tippecanoe County, Indiana. Proc. Indiana Acad. Sci. 46:217–19.

Cass, J. S. 1952. Enteric infections in monkeys. Proc. Animal Care Panel 3:14–22.

Chang, S. L. 1955. Survival of cysts of *Endamoeba histolytica* in human feces under low-temperature conditions. Am. J. Hyg. 61:103–20.

Dunn, F. L. 1968. The parasites of *Saimiri:* in the context of platyrrhine parasitism, pp. 31–68. *In* L. A. Rosenblum and R. W. Cooper, eds. The squirrel monkey. Academic Press, New York.

Eichhorn, A., and B. Gallagher. 1916. Spontaneous amebic dysentery in monkeys. J. Infect. Diseases 19:395–407.

Foster, H. L. 1963. Specific pathogen-free animals, pp. 110–38. *In* W. Lane-Petter, ed. Animals for research: Principles of breeding and management. Academic Press, New York.

Fremming, B. D., F. S. Vogel, R. E. Benson, and R. J. Young. 1955. A fatal case of amebiasis with liver abscesses and ulcerative colitis in a chimpanzee. J. Am. Vet. Med. Assoc. 126:406–7.

Fulton, J. D., and L. P. Joyner. 1948. Natural amoebic infections in laboratory rodents. Nature 161:66–68.

Geiman, Q. M. 1964. Shigellosis, amebiasis and simian malaria. Lab. Animal Care 14:441–54.

Halpern, B., and R. E. Dolkart. 1954. The effect of cold temperatures on the viability of cysts of *Endamoeba histolytica*. Am. J. Trop. Med. Hyg. 3:276–82.

Hegner, R. W. 1934. Intestinal protozoa of chimpanzees. Am. J. Hyg. 19:480–501.

Hegner, R. W., and H. J. Chu. 1930. A survey of protozoa parasitic in plants and animals of the Philippine Islands. Philippine J. Sci. 43:451–82.

Herman, C. M., and C. R. Schroeder. 1939. Treatment of amoebic dysentery in an orang-utan. Zoologica 24:339.

Hill, W. C. O. 1953. Report of the Society's prosector for the year 1952. Proc. Zool. Soc. London 123:227–51.

Hoare, C. A. 1958. The enigma of host-parasite relations in amebiasis. Rice Inst. Pamphlet 45:23–35.

———. 1959. Amoebic infections in animals. Vet. Rev. Annotations 5:91–102.

———. 1961. Considérations sur l'étiologie de l'ambiase d'aprés la rapport hôte-parasite. Bull. Soc. Pathol. Exotique 54:429–41.

Johnson, C. M. 1941. Observations on natural infections of *Endamoeba histolytica* in Ateles and rhesus monkeys. Am. J. Trop. Med. 21:49–61.

Jones, Myrna F., and W. L. Newton. 1950. The survival of cysts of *Endamoeba histolytica* in water at temperatures between 45° C. and 55° C. Am. J. Trop. Med. 30:53–58.

Kessel, J. F. 1928. Intestinal protozoa of monkeys. Univ. Calif. (Berkeley) Publ. Zool. 31:275–306.

Kessel, J. F., and H. G. Johnstone. 1949. The occurrence of *Endamoeba polecki* Prowazek, 1912, in *Macaca mulatta* and in man. Am. J. Trop. Med. 29:311–17.

Kessel, J. F., and Fay Kaplan. 1949. The effect of certain arsenicals on natural infections of *Endamoeba histolytica* and of *Endamoeba polecki* in *Macaca mulatta*. Am. J. Trop. Med. 29:319–22.

Kheisin, E. M. 1938. Observations on the morphology of *Entamoeba coli* var. *cuniculi* Brug from the rabbit intestine (in Russian). Vestn. Mikrobiol. Epidemiol. Parasitol. 17:384–90.

Knowles, R., and B. M. Das Gupta. 1936. Some observations on the intestinal protozoa of macaques. Indian J. Med. Res. 24:547–56.

Kuntz, R. E., and Betty J. Myers. 1966. Parasites of baboons *(Papio doguera* Pucheran, 1856) captured in Kenya and Tanzania, East Africa. Primates 7:27–32.

———. 1967. Microbiological parameters of the baboon *(Papio* sp.): Parasitology, pp. 741–55. *In* H. Vagtborg, ed. The baboon in medical research. Vol. 2. Univ. of Texas Press, Austin.

Kuntz, R. E., Betty J. Myers, and T. E. Vice. 1967. Intestinal protozoans and parasites of the gelada baboon *(Theropithecus gelada* Rüppel, 1835). Proc. Helminthol. Soc. Wash. D.C. 34:65–66.

Levine, N. D. 1961. Protozoan parasites of domestic animals and of man. Burgess, Minneapolis. 412 pp.

Mackinnon, D. L., and M. J. Dibb. 1938. Report on intestinal protozoa of some mammals in the Zoological Gardens at Regent's Park. Proc. Zool. Soc. London Ser. B. 108:323–45.

Miller, M. J., and R. S. Bray. 1966. *Entamoeba histolytica* infections in the chimpanzee *(Pan satyrus)*. J. Parasitol. 52:386–88.

Mudrow-Reichenow, Lilly. 1956. Spontanes vorkommen von Amöben und Ciliaten bei Laboratoriumstieren. Z. Tropenmed. Parasitol. 7:198–211.

Nie, D. 1950. Morphology and taxonomy of the intestinal protozoa of the guinea-pig, *Cavia porcella*. J. Morphol. 86:381–493.

Patten, R. A. 1939. Amoebic dysentery in orang-utans *(Simia satyrus)*. Australian Vet. J. 15:68–71.

Poindexter, H. A. 1942. A study of the intestinal parasites of the monkeys of the Santiago Island primate colony. Puerto Rico J. Public Health Trop. Med. 18:175–91.

Prowazek, S. von. 1912. Weiterer Beitrag zur Kenntnis der Entamöben. Arch. Protistenk. 26:241–49.

Ratcliffe, H. L. 1931. A comparative study of amebiasis in man, monkeys and cats, with special reference to the formation of the early lesions. Am. J. Hyg. 14:337–52.

———. 1954. Disease control and colony management of infra-human primates at the Philadelphia Zoological Garden. Proc. Animal Care Panel 5:8–15.

Reardon, Lucy V., and Bonny F. Rininger. 1968. A survey of parasites in laboratory primates. Lab. Animal Care 18:577–80.

Rowland, Eloise, and J. G. Vandenbergh. 1965. A survey of intestinal parasites in a new colony of rhesus monkeys. J. Parasitol. 51:294–95.

Ruch, T. C. 1959. Diseases of laboratory primates. W. B. Saunders, Philadelphia. 600 pp.

Seneviratna, P. 1963. Amoebic dysentery in dogs in Ceylon. Ceylon Vet. J. 11:130–31.

Simitch, T., Z. Petrovitch, and D. Chibalitch. 1954. La vitalité des kystes de Entamoeba dysenteriae en dehors de l'organisme de l'hôte. Arch. Inst. Pasteur Algerie 32:223–31.

Suldey, E. W. 1924. Dysenterie amibienne spontanée chez le chimpanze *(Troglodytes niger)*. Bull. Soc. Pathol. Exotique 17:771–73.

Van Riper, O. C., J. W. Day, J. Fineg, and J. R. Prine. 1966. Intestinal parasites of recently imported chimpanzees. Lab. Animal Care 16:360–63.

Vickers, J. H. 1968. Gastrointestinal diseases of primates, pp. 393–96. *In* R. W. Kirk, ed. Current veterinary therapy: III. Small animal practice. W. B. Saunders, Philadelphia.

———. 1969. Diseases of primates affecting the choice of species for toxicologic studies. Ann. N.Y. Acad. Sci. 162:659–72.

Wantland, W. W. 1955. Parasitic fauna of the golden hamster. J. Dental Res. 34:631–49.

Weidman, F. D. 1923. The animal parasites, their incidence and significance, pp. 614–59. *In* H. Fox, ed. Disease in captive wild mammals and birds: Incidence, description, comparison. J. B. Lippincott, Philadelphia.

Wenrich, D. H. 1937. Studies on *Iodamoeba bütschlii* (Protozoa) with special reference to nuclear structure. Proc. Am. Phil. Soc. 77:183–205.

Whitney, R. A., D. J. Johnson, and W. C. Cole. 1967. The subhuman primate: A guide for the veterinarian. EASP 100-26. Edgewood Arsenal, Maryland.

Young, R. J., B. D. Fremming, R. E. Benson, and M. D. Harris. 1957. Care and management of a *Macaca mulatta* monkey colony. Proc. Animal Care Panel 7:67–82.

Chapter 3

SPOROZOANS and NEOSPORANS

THESE groups contain a wide variety of pathogens, including the coccidian and malarial parasites, the toxoplasmasids, and the piroplasmasids.

Of the coccidian parasites affecting endothermal laboratory animals, *Eimeria, Isospora,* and *Cryptosporidium* are enteric parasites; *Klossiella* primarily affects the kidneys; and *Hepatozoon* and *Haemogregarina* occur in the circulatory system.

The malarial parasites found in endothermal laboratory animals are *Plasmodium,* which occurs in primates and rodents; *Hepatocystis* and *Sergentella,* which occur in lower primates; and *Haemoproteus* and *Leucocytozoon,* which are avian parasites. The only species of significance in laboratory animals are those which occur in lower primates obtained from their natural habitat.

The toxoplasmasids, *Sarcocystis, Toxoplasma,* and *Besnoitia,* are usually not important pathogens in endothermal laboratory animals.

The piroplasmasids are blood parasites. *Babesia, Aegyptianella, Entopolypoides,* and *Theileria* are the genera which occur in endothermal laboratory animals; *Babesia* is the most important.

Only one neosporan, *Nosema cuniculi,* occurs in endothermal laboratory animals.

COCCIDIAN PARASITES

The coccidia proper are those sporozoans that belong to the suborder Eimeriorina. *Eimeria, Isospora,* and *Cryptosporidium,* the members of this group which affect endothermal laboratory animals, are all monoxenous; that is, they involve a single type of host. The gametes develop independently, the microgametocyte typically producing many small microgametes. The zygote becomes a thick-walled, resistant oocyst containing many sporozoites enclosed in secondary cysts known as sporocysts.

The coccidian genus *Klossiella* belongs to the suborder Adeleorina. A typical oocyst is not formed, but a number of sporocysts, each containing many sporozoites, develop within a membrane which is perhaps laid down by the host cell. Each microgametocyte forms two to four nonflagellated microgametes which develop in syzygy with, that is, lying up against, the macrogametes. The life cycle involves a single host, with gametogony and schizogony occurring in different locations.

The genera *Hepatozoon* and *Haemogregarina* also belong to the suborder Adeleorina, but to different families than *Klossiella.* The life cycle of *Hepatozoon* involves two hosts, one of which is a bloodsucking invertebrate. The parasites are found in the cells of the circulatory system of the endothermal vertebrate host and in the digestive system of the invertebrate host. The vertebrate host becomes infected by ingesting the invertebrate host. The life cycle of the one species of *Haemogregarina* that occurs in endothermal laboratory animals is unknown.

The coccidian parasites which occur in endothermal laboratory animals are listed in Table 3.1. The most important are discussed below.

Eimeria nieschulzi
(Syn. *Eimeria halli*)

Eimeria nieschulzi is common in the small intestine of the wild Norway and black rats throughout the world, but it is uncommon in the laboratory rat (Levine and Ivens 1965a). It does not occur in cesarean-derived, barrier-sustained colonies (Foster 1963). Reports of disease associated with *E. nieschulzi* are rare, but it has been a serious problem in at least one colony, causing diarrhea and death in young animals (Becker 1934; Pérard 1926). It is not transmissible from the rat to the mouse (Marquardt 1966).

MORPHOLOGY

A mature oocyst characteristic of the genus *Eimeria* is shown in Figure 3.1. The oocyst of *E. nieschulzi* is ellipsoidal to ovoid, is tapered at both ends, and has a smooth, colorless-to-yellow wall (Fig. 3.2*A*) (Roudabush 1937). It measures 16 to 26 μ by 13 to 21 μ and has one polar granule. No oocyst residuum or micropyle is present. Sporocysts are elongate ovoid and have a small Stieda body and a residuum. Sporozoites are 10 to 12 μ long and contain a central nucleus with an eosinophilic globule at each end. These globules are not present in the merozoites. The four generations of merozoites are 7 to 10 μ, 13 to 16 μ, 17 to 22 μ, and 4 to 7 μ long, respectively.

LIFE CYCLE

Oocysts containing a single cell, or sporont, are passed in the feces (Dieben 1924; Roudabush 1937). In the presence of oxygen, sporulation occurs after about 3 days. Four sporocysts are formed, each containing two sporozoites. The rat is infected by ingestion of sporulated oocysts. Sporozoites *(1)* (Fig. 3.3) escape from the oocysts and enter the intestinal epithelium *(2)* to become first-generation schizonts *(3)*. Schizogony occurs after 1.5 days, and 20 to 36 first-generation merozoites *(4)* are formed. The epithelial cells rupture and release the merozoites *(5)*, which then enter other cells *(6)*. These develop and produce 10 to 14 second-generation merozoites *(7, 8)* on the 2nd day after infection. Schizogony occurs two more times, producing third-generation *(9, 10, 11)* and fourth-generation *(12, 13)*

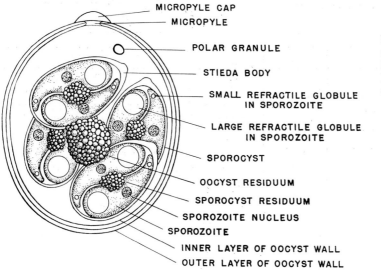

MICROPYLE CAP
MICROPYLE
POLAR GRANULE
STIEDA BODY
SMALL REFRACTILE GLOBULE IN SPOROZOITE
LARGE REFRACTILE GLOBULE IN SPOROZOITE
SPOROCYST
OOCYST RESIDUUM
SPOROCYST RESIDUUM
SPOROZOITE NUCLEUS
SPOROZOITE
INNER LAYER OF OOCYST WALL
OUTER LAYER OF OOCYST WALL

Fig. 3.1. *Eimeria,* typical sporulated oocyst. (From Levine 1961a. Courtesy of N. D. Levine, University of Illinois.)

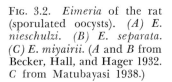

Fig. 3.2. *Eimeria* of the rat (sporulated oocysts). *(A) E. nieschulzi. (B) E. separata. (C) E. miyairii. (A* and *B* from Becker, Hall, and Hager 1932. *C* from Matubayasi 1938.)

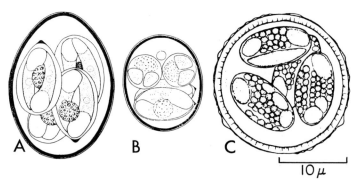

merozoites on the 3rd and 4th days after infection. Fourth-generation merozoites *(14)* enter epithelial cells and form microgametocytes *(15, 16, 17)* and macrogametes *(19).* The microgametocytes produce a large number of flagellated microgametes *(18)* by multiple fission. The macrogametes enlarge *(20)* and, after fertilization by a microgamete, form a wall and become oocysts *(21).* These oocysts enter the intestinal lumen from the epithelial cells and pass out in the feces *(22, 23).* The prepatent period, the period of time from infection to the appearance of oocysts in the feces, is 7 days. Oocysts continue to be discharged for 4 to 5 days. Unless reinfection occurs, the infection is self-limiting since asexual reproduction (schizogony) continues for only four generations.

PATHOLOGIC EFFECTS

Eimeria nieschulzi primarily affects young animals and causes diarrhea, weakness, and emaciation (Pérard 1926). The severity of the disease depends on the size of the infecting dose of oocysts (Becker 1934). Animals which recover are relatively immune, but the disease sometimes recurs in adults under stress.

DIAGNOSIS

Tentative diagnosis is based on the presence of oocysts in the feces, but accurate identification is sometimes difficult. Also, oocysts can occur in the absence of disease. A positive diagnosis can be made only at necropsy by finding lesions containing coccidia in association with signs of disease.

CONTROL

Infection with *E. nieschulzi* is self-limiting both in the individual and the colony. Control depends primarily on good sanitation. There are several coccidiostatic drugs, but none has been reported effective in the rat. Deriving a new colony by cesarean section will eliminate the infection (Foster 1963).

PUBLIC HEALTH CONSIDERATIONS

Eimeria nieschulzi is not transmissible to man.

Eimeria separata

This slightly pathogenic species is apparently common in the cecum and colon of the wild Norway rat and other rats throughout the world (Levine and Ivens 1965a). Its incidence in the conventional laboratory rat is unknown; it does not occur in cesarean-derived, barrier-sustained colonies (Foster 1963).

MORPHOLOGY

The oocyst is usually ellipsoidal, with a smooth, colorless, or pale yellow wall (Fig. 3.2B). It measures 10 to 19 μ by 10 to 17 μ and contains one to three polar granules but no residuum or micropyle. The sporocysts are ellipsoidal and have a small Stieda body and a residuum.

LIFE CYCLE

The life cycle is similar to that of *E. nieschulzi* (Roudabush 1937).

PATHOLOGIC EFFECTS

Eimeria separata does not usually cause clinical signs even when large infective doses are administered, but a mild

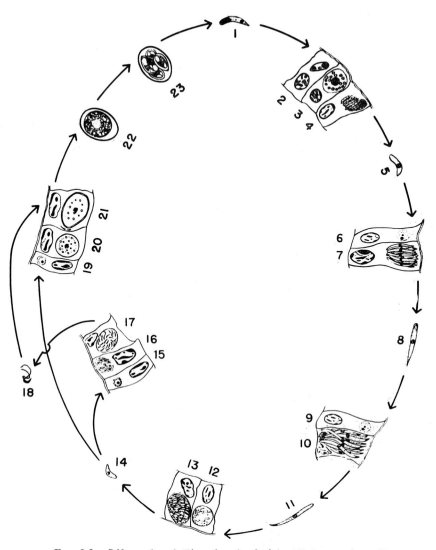

Fig. 3.3. Life cycle of *Eimeria nieschulzi*. *(1)* Sporozoite. *(2)* Sporozoite after entering host intestinal cell. *(3)* First-generation schizont in host cell (merozoites shown in cross section; note refractile globule). *(4)* First-generation merozoites in host cell. *(5)* First-generation merozoite. *(6)* Second-generation schizont in host cell. *(7)* Second-generation merozoites in host cell. *(8)* Second-generation merozoite. *(9)* Third-generation schizont in host cell. *(10)* Third-generation merozoites in host cell. *(11)* Third-generation merozoite. *(12)* Fourth-generation schizont in host cell. *(13)* Fourth-generation merozoites in host cell. *(14)* Fourth-generation merozoite. *(15)* Young microgametocyte in host cell. *(16)* Older microgametocyte in host cell. *(17)* Mature microgametocyte in host cell (surface view). *(18)* Microgamete. *(19)* Young macrogamete in host cell. *(20)* Developing macrogamete in host cell (note plastic granules inside macrogamete). *(21)* Young oocyst (zygote) in host cell. *(22)* Unsporulated oocyst in feces. *(23)* Sporulated oocyst in feces. (From Levine 1957. Courtesy of N. D. Levine, University of Illinois.)

hyperemia of the cecum and colon has been reported in rats examined 6 days after infection (Becker 1934).

DIAGNOSIS

Diagnosis is based on identification of oocysts in the feces in association with enteric lesions.

CONTROL

Control is similar to that described for *E. nieschulzi.*

PUBLIC HEALTH CONSIDERATIONS

Eimeria separata is not transmissible to man.

Eimeria miyairii

This coccidium occurs in the small intestine of the wild Norway rat and possibly the black rat throughout the world (Levine and Ivens 1965a). It is not common, and nothing is known of its pathogenicity. Its incidence in conventional laboratory rat colonies is unknown; it does not occur in cesarean-derived, barrier-sustained colonies (Foster 1963). The oocyst is spherical to subspherical, with a thick, rough, yellow-brown, radially striated wall (Fig. 3.2C). It measures 17 to 29 μ by 16 to 26 μ, with a mean of 24 by 22 μ. Micropyle, oocyst polar granule, and oocyst residuum are absent. A sporocyst residuum is present.

Eimeria falciformis

This somewhat pathogenic coccidium occurs in the small and large intestine of the mouse throughout the world (Levine and Ivens 1965a). It is common in Europe, and in one survey of conventional laboratory mice in the British Isles, it was found in 8 of 13 colonies (Owen 1968). It does not occur in cesarean-derived, barrier-sustained colonies (Foster 1963).

MORPHOLOGY

The oocyst is oval or spherical, with a smooth, colorless wall (Fig. 3.4A) (Levine and Ivens 1965a). It measures 14 to 26 μ by 11 to 24 μ. Polar granules are sometimes present, but there is no micropyle or residuum. Sporocysts are ovoid and have a small Stieda body and a residuum.

LIFE CYCLE

The life cycle is similar to that of *E. nieschulzi.*

PATHOLOGIC EFFECTS

Mild infections have little effect, but severe ones cause anorexia, diarrhea, and sometimes death (Breza and Jurasek 1959; Cordero del Campillo 1959; Nieschulz and Bos 1931; Owen 1968). Catarrhal enteritis, hemorrhages, and epithelial sloughing occur in the small intestine.

DIAGNOSIS

Diagnosis is based on identification of oocysts in the feces in association with clinical signs and enteric lesions.

CONTROL

Control depends primarily on sanitation. Infection can be eliminated by deriving a new colony by cesarean section (Foster 1963).

PUBLIC HEALTH CONSIDERATIONS

Eimeria falciformis is not a public health hazard.

Other Species of Eimeria in the Mouse

Several other species of *Eimeria* affect the mouse (Levine and Ivens 1965a). These include *E. ferrisi* (Fig. 3.4B), *E. hansonorum* (3.4C), *E. hindlei* (Fig. 3.4D), *E. keilini* (Fig. 3.4E), *E. krijgsmanni* (Fig. 3.4F), *E. musculi* (Fig. 3.4G), and *E. schueffneri* (Fig. 3.4H). Nothing is known of their pathogenicity, and none has been reported in the laboratory mouse.

Eimeria caviae

This usually nonpathogenic species is common in the large intestine of the guinea pig throughout the world and has been reported from the wild guinea pig, *Cavia aperea,* in Brazil (Levine and Ivens 1965a). In one survey in the British Isles it was found in 4 of 20 laboratory colonies (Owen 1968). It does not occur in cesarean-derived colonies (Calhoon and Matthews 1964).

MORPHOLOGY

Oocysts are oval, ellipsoidal, or subspherical, smooth, and usually brown (Fig.

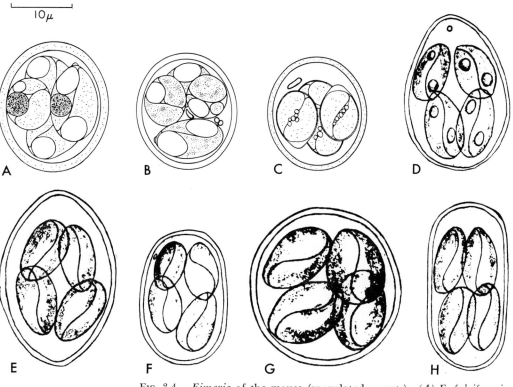

FIG. 3.4. *Eimeria* of the mouse (sporulated oocysts). *(A) E. falciformis.
(B) E. ferrisi. (C) E. hansonorum. (D) E. hindlei. (E) E. keilini. (F)
E. krijgsmanni. (G) E. musculi. (H) E. schueffneri. (A, B, C from
Levine and Ivens 1965a; courtesy of University of Illinois Press.
D, E, F, G, H from Yakimoff and Gousseff 1938.)*

3.5) (Henry 1932; Lapage 1940). They measure 13 to 26 μ by 12 to 23 μ, but have no
micropyle or polar granule. Both the oocyst
and sporocysts contain a residuum.

LIFE CYCLE

The life cycle is similar to that of *E.
nieschulzi.*

PATHOLOGIC EFFECTS

Eimeria caviae is usually nonpathogenic, but it sometimes causes diarrhea and
death. The lesions seen at necropsy occur
in the mucosa of the colon and consist of
small white or pale yellow plaques and petechial hemorrhages; sometimes the entire
mucosa is destroyed. Hepatomegaly and
yellow, necrotic, oocyst-containing areas in
the liver of the guinea pig have been attributed to infection with this coccidium,

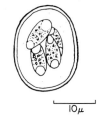

FIG. 3.5. *Eimeria ca-
viae* of the guinea
pig (sporulated oo-
cyst). (From Ryšavy
1954.)

but it is uncertain if the organism involved
was *E. caviae* (Kleeberg and Steenken 1963).

DIAGNOSIS

Diagnosis is based on identification of
oocysts in the feces in association with diarrhea and enteric lesions.

CONTROL

Sanitation plus treatment with succinylsulfathiazole, 0.1% in the drinking

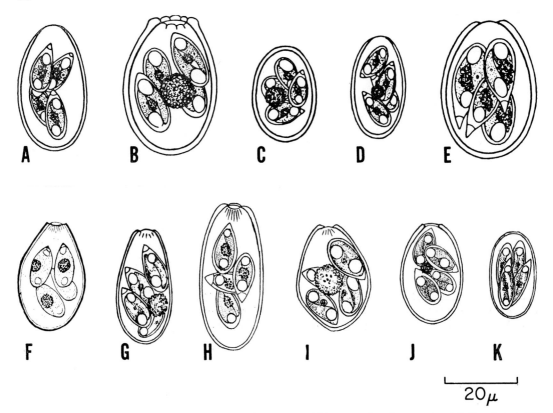

FIG. 3.6. *Eimeria* of the rabbit (sporulated oocysts). *(A) E. stiedai. (B) E. magna. (C) E. perforans. (D) E. media. (E) E. irresidua. (F) E. piriformis. (G) E. coecicola. (H) E. elongata. (I) E. intestinalis. (J) E. matsubayashii. (K) E. nagpurensis. (A, B, C, D, E from Carvalho 1942. F from Kheisin 1948. G, H, I, J, K from Gill and Ray 1960; courtesy of Zoological Society of Calcutta.)*

water, is reportedly effective (Kleeberg and Steenken 1963). Infection of a colony can be eliminated by deriving a new colony by cesarean section (Calhoon and Matthews 1964; Wills 1968).

PUBLIC HEALTH CONSIDERATIONS

Eimeria caviae is not transmissible to man.

Eimeria stiedai

Eimeria stiedai, an extremely pathogenic coccidium of the rabbit, is common in the laboratory rabbit throughout the world (Berson-Organiściak 1966; Niak 1967; Owen 1968; Poole et al. 1967; Seamer and Chesterman 1967; Sevim 1967). It has

also been reported from the cottontail rabbit and hares (Levine 1961a).

MORPHOLOGY

The oocyst is ovoid or ellipsoidal and is 28 to 40 μ by 16 to 25 μ (Fig. 3.6A) (Levine 1961a). It has a flat micropylar end, a smooth, salmon-colored wall, and a micropyle, but no polar granule or residuum. Sporocysts are ovoid and have a Stieda body and a residuum.

LIFE CYCLE

The rabbit is infected by ingestion of sporulated oocysts (Becker 1934; Horton 1967; Smetana 1933a, b). Sporozoites penetrate the mucosa of the small intestine and

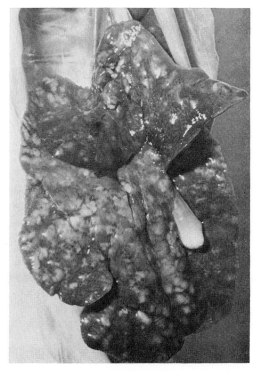

FIG. 3.7. *Eimeria stiedai* lesions in liver of a rabbit. Note white nodules (dilated bile ducts) throughout the liver. (Courtesy of K. Hagen, Washington State University.)

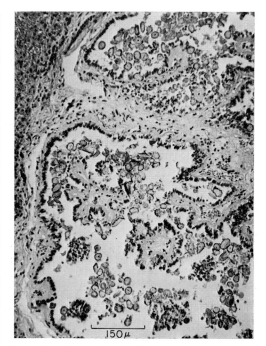

FIG. 3.8. Hepatic coccidiosis of the rabbit. Note proliferation of biliary epithelium and several developmental stages of *Eimeria stiedai*. (Courtesy of B. Matanic, State University of New York.)

pass via the mesenteric lymph nodes and hepatic portal system to the liver. In the liver, they enter the epithelial cells of the bile ducts and occasionally the liver parenchymal cells, where they become schizonts. The schizonts produce merozoites, but the number of asexual generations is unknown. Oocysts pass out with the bile and appear in the feces 18 days after infection. Sporulation occurs in 3 days.

PATHOLOGIC EFFECTS

Light infections are often inapparent; heavy infections are characterized by anorexia, a distended abdomen, and weight loss (Cook 1969; Levine 1961a; Ostler 1961). Diarrhea and icterus sometimes occur. The liver is enlarged. The bile ducts are dilated and appear on the surface of the liver as white nodules (Fig. 3.7). These nodules, when incised, are found to contain a green, creamy fluid packed with oocysts.

Microscopically, the bile ducts are hyperplastic. Developmental forms of the parasite are seen in the epithelium, and oocysts appear in the lumen (Fig. 3.8). (Ruebner, Lindsey, and Melby 1965). Hepatic cirrhosis is common in rabbits that have recovered from the clinical disease (Smetana 1933c).

Mortality is variable. *Eimeria stiedai* infection is one of the commonest causes of death in the rabbit; it is severest in the young rabbit.

DIAGNOSIS

Diagnosis is based on identification of oocysts and direct association of the organism with disease. Since several species of *Eimeria* with similar oocysts occur in the rabbit, accurate identification is essential. The presence of oocysts in the feces of a rabbit with anorexia, diarrhea, and weight loss does not necessarily mean that these signs are caused by the parasite. Conversely, coccidia sometimes cause severe disease early in their life cycle before oocysts are formed. Therefore, a definitive diagnosis of *E. stiedai* infection can be made only at necropsy and requires the recognition of the coccidium in the typical lesions.

CONTROL

Eimeria stiedai infection can be eliminated by proper management and sanitation (Lund 1949). The oocysts are extremely resistant but can be destroyed by bacterial action in the absence of oxygen or by ultraviolet light, heat, or desiccation (Farr and Wehr 1949; Hagen 1958; Koutz 1950; Pérard 1924; Warner 1933). Autoclaving and ammonia fumigation are also effective (Horton-Smith, Taylor, and Turtle 1940).

No drugs are known that will cure coccidiosis once signs of disease appear; all are prophylactic and must be given at the time of exposure or soon thereafter to be effective. Coccidiostats affect schizonts and merozoites only and prevent the completion of the life cycle. Since the stages which invade the tissues (sporozoites) are not affected, immunity develops (Horton-Smith

1947). Recommended coccidiostats include succinylsulfathiazole, sulfamerazine, or sulfamethazine, given orally at the rate of 0.5 to 1.0% in the feed (Gerundo 1948; Horton-Smith 1947, 1958), and sulfaquinoxaline or sulfamerazine, given orally at the rate of 0.02 to 0.10% in the drinking water (Hagen 1961; Horton-Smith 1958; Lund 1954). Sulfadiazine and sulfaquinoxaline are also effective when given subcutaneously in a 20% aqueous solution at the rate of 0.1 g per kg of body weight (Miklovich and Pellérdy 1960). Nitrofurazone and furacin are also reportedly effective (Boch 1957; Kamyszek 1963).

PUBLIC HEALTH CONSIDERATIONS

Eimeria stiedai infection is not transmissible to man.

Eimeria magna

Eimeria magna is one of the most pathogenic intestinal coccidia of the rabbit (Lund 1949; Ostler 1961). It occurs in the jejunum, ileum, and sometimes the cecum (Fig. 3.9*A*) of the rabbit throughout the

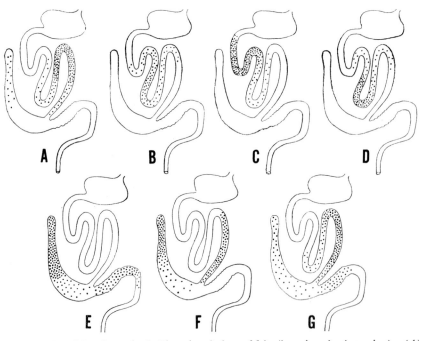

FIG. 3.9. Intestinal *Eimeria* of the rabbit (location in intestine). *(A)* *E. magna.* (B) *E. perforans.* (C) *E. media.* (D) *E. irresidua.* (E) *E. piriformis.* (F) *E. coecicola.* (G) *E. intestinalis.* (From Kheisin 1957.)

world and has been transmitted experimentally to the cottontail rabbit (Kheisin 1957; Levine 1961a; Sevim 1967). *Eimeria magna* has also been reported in hares, but its occurrence in these lagomorphs is uncertain (Pellérdy 1956). It is common in the laboratory rabbit (Niak 1967; Owen 1968; Poole et al. 1967; Seamer and Chesterman 1967).

The oocyst is ovoid or ellipsoidal, smooth, and orange-yellow or brown, and measures 27 to 41 μ by 17 to 29 μ (Fig. 3.6*B*) (Kheisin 1947b). There is a large micropyle surrounded by shoulders and an oocyst residuum, but there is no polar granule. Sporocysts are ovoid and have a Stieda body and a sporocyst residuum. The endogenous states are found below the epithelial cell nuclei of the villi and in the submucosa (Rutherford 1943). There are two asexual generations of merozoites. Oocysts appear in the feces 7 to 8 days after infection, and sporulation time is 2 to 3 days.

Eimeria magna infection is characterized by loss of weight, anorexia, mucous diarrhea, and death. Inflammation and sloughing of the intestinal mucosa are seen at necropsy.

Diagnosis, control, and treatment are similar to those described for *E. stiedai* except that the coccidiostatic drugs used for hepatic coccidiosis of the rabbit are less effective for intestinal coccidiosis (Cook 1969; Horton-Smith 1958; Ostler 1961). *Eimeria magna* is not transmissible to man.

Eimeria perforans

(SYN. *Eimeria exigua*)

This mildly pathogenic parasite occurs in the small intestine (Fig. 3.9*B*) of the rabbit throughout the world and has been transmitted experimentally to the cottontail rabbit (Kheisin 1957; Levine 1961a; Sevim 1967). It is common in the laboratory rabbit (Niak 1967; Owen 1968; Poole et al. 1967; Seamer and Chesterman 1967).

The oocyst is ovoid, smooth, and colorless to pink, and measures 24 to 30 μ by 14 to 20 μ (Fig. 3.6*C*). It has an oocyst residuum but no micropyle or polar granule. Sporocysts are ovoid and contain a Stieda body and a residuum. The endogenous stages are found above the nuclei of the intestinal epithelial cells (Rutherford 1943). There are two asexual generations

of merozoites. The prepatent period is 5 to 6 days, and the sporulation time is 2 days.

Eimeria perforans sometimes causes mild diarrhea. The duodenum appears white and edematous; petechiae and white spots and streaks are seen in the ileum and jejunum. Diagnosis, control, and treatment are similar to those described for *E. stiedai* (Horton-Smith 1958; Ostler 1961). Sanitation, elimination of infected animals, and prophylactic treatment with sulfaquinoxaline, given orally at the rate of 0.1% in the feed or drinking water, are effective (Horton-Smith 1958; McPherson et al. 1962). *Eimeria perforans* is not transmissible to man.

Eimeria media

Eimeria media, a moderately pathogenic coccidium, occurs in the small intestine (Fig. 3.9*C*) of the rabbit throughout the world (Kheisin 1957; Levine 1961a; Ostler 1961; Sevim 1967). It is also found in the cottontail rabbit. It is common in the laboratory rabbit (Niak 1967; Owen 1968; Poole et al. 1967; Seamer and Chesterman 1967).

The oocyst is ovoid, smooth, and 19 to 33 μ by 13 to 21 μ, and has a micropyle and residuum (Fig. 3.6*D*). There is no polar granule. Sporocysts are elongate ovoid and have a Stieda body and a residuum (Pellérdy and Babos 1953; Rutherford 1943). The endogenous stages are found above or below the epithelial cell nuclei of the intestinal villi and in the submucosa. There are two asexual generations of merozoites. The prepatent period is 5 to 6 days, and the oocyst sporulation time is 2 days.

Eimeria media sometimes causes a moderate enteritis and diarrhea (Pellérdy and Babos 1953). Edema and gray foci are seen in the intestine. Diagnosis, control, and treatment are similar to those described for *E. stiedai* (Ostler 1961). *Eimeria media* is not transmissible to man.

Eimeria irresidua

Eimeria irresidua is one of the more pathogenic coccidia that occurs in the small intestine (Fig. 3.9*D*) of the rabbit (Kheisin 1957; Levine 1961a; Ostler 1961). It is found throughout the world and is common in the laboratory rabbit (Niak 1967;

Owen 1968; Poole et al. 1967; Seamer and Chesterman 1967; Sevim 1967).

The oocyst is ovoid, smooth, and 38 by 26 μ, and has a prominent micropyle but no polar granule or residuum (Fig. 3.6E) (Rutherford 1943). Sporocysts are ovoid and contain a Stieda body and a residuum. The endogenous stages are found above or below the epithelial cell nuclei of the intestinal villi and in the submucosa. There are two asexual generations of merozoites. The prepatent period is 9 to 10 days, and the oocyst sporulation time is 2.0 to 2.5 days.

Eimeria irresidua causes a hemorrhagic diarrhea and inflammation and sloughing of the enteric epithelium. Diagnosis, control, and treatment are similar to those given for *E. stiedai* (Horton-Smith 1958; Ostler 1961). *Eimeria irresidua* is not transmissible to man.

Eimeria piriformis

Eimeria piriformis occurs in the cecum and colon (Fig. 3.9E) of the rabbit in Europe and the Near East; it is uncommon (Levine 1961a; Niak 1967). Its oocyst is piriform to ovoid, smooth, yellow-brown, and 26 to 32 μ by 17 to 21 μ, and has a micropyle but no polar granule or residuum (Fig. 3.6F). The sporocysts have a residuum. Endogenous stages occur above the nuclei of the intestinal epithelial cells (Kheisin 1957). The prepatent period is 9 days, and the oocyst sporulation time is 2 days. Its pathogenicity is unknown.

Eimeria coecicola

This slightly pathogenic species is common in the posterior ileum and cecum (Fig. 3.9F) of the wild rabbit in eastern Europe and India but rare in domestic specimens (Gill and Ray 1960; Levine 1961a).

The oocyst is ovoid, smooth, and yellow, measures 25 to 40 μ by 15 to 21 μ, and has a micropyle and a residuum, but no polar granule (Fig. 3.6G). The sporocysts have a residuum. Endogenous stages are found in the epithelial cells of the cecal villi, and the sexual stages are below the nuclei of the cecal crypt cells (Kheisin 1947a). The prepatent period is 9 days, and the oocyst sporulation time is 3 days.

Eimeria coecicola does not cause clinical signs, but small white foci of developing oocysts sometimes occur in the cecum.

Eimeria elongata, Eimeria neoleporis

Eimeria elongata, a species of unknown pathogenicity, occurs in the intestine of the rabbit in western Europe (Levine 1961a). *Eimeria neoleporis,* a slightly to markedly pathogenic species, has been isolated from the cottontail rabbit in North America, from the domestic rabbit in India, and from the laboratory rabbit in Iran (Carvalho 1942; Gill and Ray 1960; Niak 1967).

The oocyst of *E. elongata* is elongate and ellipsoidal, with almost straight sides (Fig. 3.6H). It is gray, measures 35 to 40 μ by 17 to 20 μ, and has a thin wall and a broad micropyle. A polar granule and residuum are not present. Sporocysts are elongate and have a residuum. The life cycle and pathogenicity are unknown.

The structure of the *E. neoleporis* oocyst is the same as that of *E. elongata*. *Eimeria neoleporis* causes a mild to severe enteritis in the cottontail rabbit.

Eimeria intestinalis

This somewhat pathogenic coccidium occurs in the ileum, cecum, and colon (Fig. 3.9G) of the rabbit in eastern Europe and India (Kheisin 1957; Levine 1961a). It is uncommon in the domestic rabbit; its incidence in the laboratory rabbit is unknown.

The oocyst is piriform, smooth, yellow, and 21 to 36 μ by 15 to 21 μ, and has a micropyle and residuum but no polar granule (Fig. 3.6I). Sporocysts are ovoid and have a residuum. The endogenous stages occur above and sometimes beside the nuclei of the epithelial cells (Pellérdy 1953). There are at least two asexual generations of merozoites. The prepatent period is 9 days, and the oocyst sporulation time is 1 to 2 days. Experimental infection in young rabbits causes severe catarrhal enteritis, diarrhea, and sometimes death (Pellérdy 1953, 1954).

Eimeria matsubayashii

This slightly to moderately pathogenic species occurs primarily in the ileum of the rabbit in Japan and India (Levine 1961a). Its prevalence and endogenous stages are unknown. The oocyst is broadly ovoid, measures 22 to 29 μ by 16 to 22 μ, and has a micropyle and a residuum (Fig.

3.6*J*) (Gill and Ray 1960). Sporocysts are ovoid and contain a residuum. Oocyst sporulation time is 1.5 to 2.0 days. *Eimeria matsubayashii* causes a fibrinonecrotic enteritis (Tsunoda 1952).

Eimeria nagpurensis

This species of unknown pathogenicity has been isolated from the domestic rabbit in India and from the laboratory rabbit in Iran (Gill and Ray 1960; Niak 1967). Its prevalence and endogenous stages are unknown. The oocyst is barrel shaped, with the long sides parallel in their middle third (Fig. 3.6*K*). It is colorless or yellow, measures 20 to 27 μ by 10 to 15 μ, and has a thin wall but no micropyle or residuum. Sporocysts are oat shaped; the anterior end

is sharply pointed and a residuum is present.

Eimeria tenella

This extremely pathogenic coccidium is common in the ceca (Fig. 3.10*A*) of the chicken throughout the world (Levine 1961a), but it is uncommon in the laboratory chicken raised on wire under good sanitation.

MORPHOLOGY

The oocyst is broadly ovoid, 14 to 31 μ by 9 to 25 μ, with a smooth wall and no micropyle (Fig. 3.11) (Levine 1961a). It is unsporulated and contains a single cell (sporont) when passed in the feces. In the presence of oxygen it sporulates in 1 day

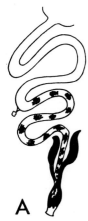
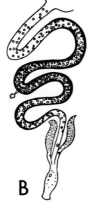
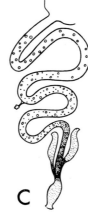

A   **B**   **C**

Fig. 3.10. *Eimeria* of the chicken (location in intestine). *(A) E. tenella. (B) E. necatrix. (C) E. brunetti. (D) E. acervulina. (E) E. maxima. (F) E. mitis.* (From Levine 1961a. Courtesy of N. D. Levine, University of Illinois.)

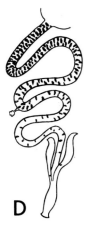
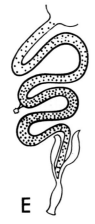
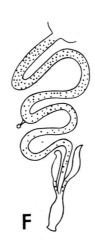

D   **E**   **F**

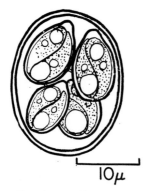

FIG. 3.11. *Eimeria tenella* (sporulated oocyst). (From Chandler and Read 1961. Courtesy of John Wiley & Sons.)

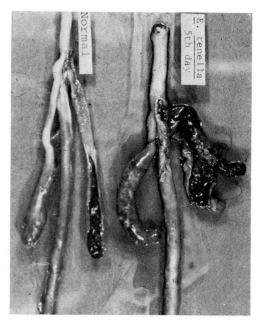

FIG. 3.12. Cecal coccidiosis (*Eimeria tenella* infection) in the chicken *(right)*. Note characteristic hemorrhage. (Courtesy of W. M. Reid, University of Georgia.)

or more and then contains four sporocysts, each with two sporozoites.

LIFE CYCLE

The chicken is infected by ingesting sporulated oocysts. Endogenous stages are similar to those of *E. nieschulzi;* they occur in the epithelial cells of the ceca. There are three generations of schizonts which produce merozoites. Third-generation merozoites produce macrogametes and microgametes which unite to form a zygote that secretes a wall around itself, becomes an oocyst, and passes out in the feces. The prepatent period is 7 days and the patent period is several days.

PATHOLOGIC EFFECTS

Eimeria tenella is the most pathogenic coccidium of the chicken (Levine 1961a). Depending on the age of the host and the size of the infective dose of oocysts, coccidiosis caused by this organism varies from inapparent infection to a severe, highly fatal disease. Young chickens about 4 weeks old are most susceptible, whereas those 1 to 2 weeks of age and birds 6 weeks and older are more resistant. Because adults frequently have partial immunity from prior exposure, they usually develop only inapparent infections.

Typical signs are listlessness, anorexia, and hemorrhagic diarrhea. Initially, the cecal mucosa is hemorrhagic and later, fibrinonecrotic; the wall is thickened and the lumen is filled with blood (Fig. 3.12).

Mortality varies with the age of the

host and the size of the infective dose. It usually ranges from 32 to 90% in young chickens.

DIAGNOSIS

A definitive diagnosis is made only when coccidia and lesions occur concurrently in the ceca. The presence of oocysts in the feces does not necessarily mean that coccidiosis is present, and conversely, clinical disease sometimes occurs before oocysts develop and appear in the feces.

CONTROL

The infection is self-limiting, but reinfection with less severe manifestations is common if proper sanitation and management are not practiced (Levine 1961a). Many drugs are used to treat coccidiosis in the chicken, but all are coccidiostatic and have no effect once clinical disease appears. Sulfaguanidine, at a level of 0.5% in the food, sulfamethazine and sulfamerazine, at a level of 0.10 to 0.25%, and sulfaquinoxaline, at a level of 0.025%, are effective against *E. tenella*. Sodium sulfamethazine, at a level of 0.2%, and sulfaquinoxaline, at a level of 0.04% in the drinking water, are also effective. Other recommended drugs, all administered in the feed, include nitrophenide, at a level of 250 to 500 ppm; bithionol, at a level of 500 ppm in combination with 100 ppm methiotriazamine; nitrofurazone alone, at a level of 110 ppm, or at a level of 55 ppm in combination with 8 ppm furazolidone; glycarbylamide, at a level of 30 ppm; nicarbazine, at a level of 100 to 125 ppm; and buquinolate, at a level of 83 to 110 ppm (Dunkley 1968; Edgar and Flanagan 1968; Levine 1961a).

PUBLIC HEALTH CONSIDERATIONS

Eimeria tenella is not transmissible to man.

Other Species of *Eimeria* in the Chicken

The chicken is host to eight other species of coccidia: *Eimeria necatrix,* which causes enteritis and thickening of the anterior and central small intestine (Fig. 3.10*B*); *E. brunetti,* which causes necrotic enteritis of the posterior small intestine and large intestine (Fig. 3.10*C*); *E. acervulina,* which sometimes causes inflammation of the anterior small intestine but is usually nonpathogenic (Fig. 3.10*D*); *E. maxima,* which occasionally causes slight to moderate enteritis of the small intestine (Fig. 3.10*E*); *E. mitis,* which is usually nonpathogenic in the small intestine (Fig. 3.10*F*); *E. praecox,* which is essentially nonpathogenic in the small intestine; *E. hagani,* which is slightly pathogenic in the anterior small intestine; and *E. mivati,* which causes mild enteritis in the upper and lower intestine (Edgar and Seibold 1964; Levine 1961a). Most are common in the chicken throughout the world, but all are uncommon in the laboratory chicken raised on wire under good sanitation.

The life cycles of all chicken coccidia are similar to that of *E. tenella* (Levine 1961a) except that the endogenous stages occur in the cells of the small and large intestine instead of the ceca. Except for *E. necatrix* and *E. brunetti,* none of these species is markedly pathogenic; all produce self-limiting infections. A relative immunity develops after infection, and adults usually become inapparent carriers. In general, most of the drugs which are effective against *E. tenella* are not effective against the intestinal coccidia; therefore, control depends primarily on sanitation. None of these coccidia is transmissible to man.

Isospora bigemina

This extremely pathogenic species is common in the small intestine of the dog, cat, and other carnivores throughout the world (Levine 1961a). It is frequently found in laboratory dogs obtained from pounds (Burrows and Lillis 1967) but is uncommon in those maintained in kennels that practice good sanitation and management (Johnson, Andersen, and Gee 1963) and is absent in cesarean-derived, barrier-maintained colonies (Sheffy, Baker, and Gillespie 1961).

MORPHOLOGY

The oocyst is broadly ellipsoidal, subspherical, or spherical (Fig. 3.13*A*) (Levine 1961a; Levine and Ivens 1965b). It measures 10 to 14 μ by 10 to 12 μ, has a smooth, colorless wall composed of a single layer, and is indistinguishable from the oocyst produced in cat feces by *Toxoplasma gondii* (Frenkel, Dubey, and Miller 1970; Overdulve 1970; Sheffield and Melton 1970; Siim, Hutchison, and Work 1969; Work and Hutchison 1969). There is no micropyle. Sporocysts are broadly ellipsoidal, measure 7 to 8 μ by 5 to 7 μ, and contain a sporocyst residuum and four sausage-shaped sporozoites but have no Stieda body.

LIFE CYCLE

Unsporulated oocysts are passed in the feces (Levine 1961a; Levine and Ivens 1965b). These sporulate in the presence of oxygen in a day or more. Two sporocysts are formed, each with four sporozoites. The dog and cat are infected by ingestion of the oocysts. Sporozoites are released and enter the epithelial cells of the small intestine and develop into schizonts containing 8 to 12 merozoites. After an unknown number of asexual generations, the merozoites produce sexual stages, macrogametes and microgametes, which unite to form a zygote. The zygote forms a wall, becomes an oocyst, and passes out in the feces.

PATHOLOGIC EFFECTS

This is probably the most pathogenic coccidium of the dog and cat (Levine

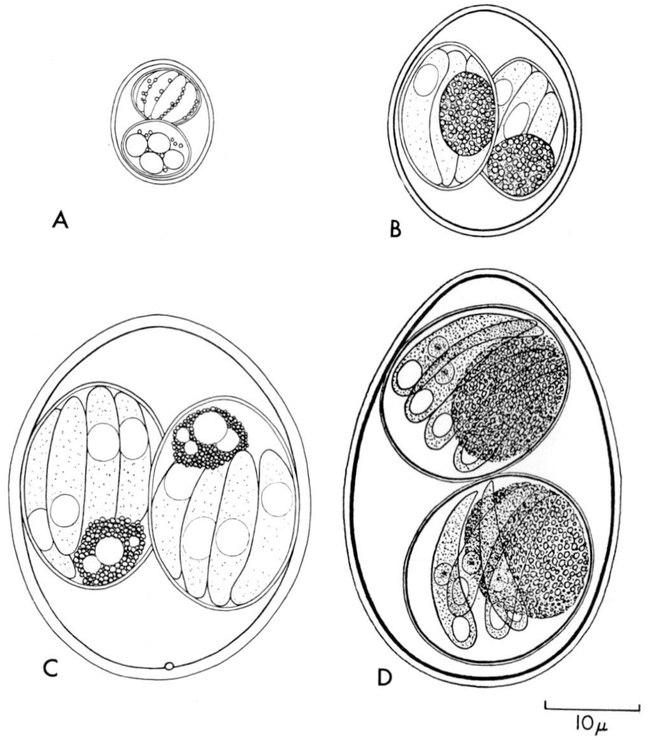

Fig. 3.13. *Isospora* of the dog and cat (sporulated oocysts). *(A) I. bigemina. (B) I. rivolta. (C) I. canis. (D) I. felis. (A, B, C from Levine and Ivens 1965b; courtesy of American Society of Parasitologists. D from Wenyon 1926.)*

1961a). Young animals are more seriously affected, whereas adults are usually inapparent carriers. Clinical signs appear 4 to 6 days after exposure; their severity depends on the number of oocysts ingested. They range from mild diarrhea to severe catarrhal or hemorrhagic diarrhea, and also include anorexia, listlessness, loss of weight, eosinophilia, anemia, and occasionally death. The small intestine, especially the ileum, is hemorrhagic and inflamed. The mucosa is thickened and ulceration and sloughing are common.

DIAGNOSIS

Diagnosis is based on recognition of oocysts in the feces in association with clinical signs and enteric lesions.

CONTROL

Sanitation and isolation will prevent the infection. There is no effective treatment once signs of the disease have appeared. Antibiotics, such as the tetracyclines, are sometimes used to control secondary bacterial infection. Supportive and symptomatic treatment is also recommended.

PUBLIC HEALTH CONSIDERATIONS

The oocysts of *Isospora bigemina* are morphologically indistinguishable from those of *I. hominis* of man, but no cross-transmission experiments have been carried out to determine whether they are the same (Levine 1961a). Since the oocysts of *Toxoplasma gondii*, produced in cat feces, are indistinguishable from those of *I. bigemina*, appropriate sanitary precautions should be taken in handling feces from infected cats.

Isospora rivolta

This apparently nonpathogenic species occurs in the posterior small intestine and sometimes in the cecum and colon of the dog, cat, and probably wild carnivores throughout the world (Levine 1961a; Mahrt 1966). It is common in the laboratory dog and cat obtained from pounds (Burrows and Lillis 1967; Scott 1967) but uncommon in those maintained in kennels that practice good sanitation and management (Johnson, Andersen, and Gee 1963) and absent in cesarean-derived, barrier-maintained colonies (Sheffy, Baker, and Gillespie 1961).

Its oocyst is ellipsoidal to ovoid, measures 20 to 27 μ by 15 to 24 μ, and resembles that of *Isospora bigemina* except for size (Fig. 3.13*B*). Sometimes sporocysts are found free in the feces; these have been called *Cryptosporidium* oocysts because they contain four naked sporozoites (Levine and Ivens 1965b). Dogs and cats are infected by ingestion of oocysts. Endogenous stages develop in the posterior small intestine and rarely in the cecum and colon. The prepatent period is 6 days, and the patent period 13 to 23 days (Mahrt 1967). Pathologic effects are unknown. Control measures effective against *I. bigemina* are also effective against this species. *Isospora rivolta* is apparently not transmissible to man.

Isospora canis

This presumably moderately pathogenic species is found in the small intestine of the dog throughout the world. It was formerly thought to be identical with *Isospora felis,* but it is now known to be a separate species (Levine and Ivens 1965b; Neméseri 1959). It is common in laboratory dogs obtained from pounds (Burrows and Lillis 1967) but uncommon in those maintained in kennels that practice good sanitation and management (Johnson, Andersen, and Gee 1963). Its oocyst is broadly ellipsoidal to slightly ovoid, measures 35 to 42 μ by 27 to 33 μ, and has a smooth wall composed of a single layer without a micropyle (Fig. 3.13*C*). The life cycle of *I. canis* is similar to that of *I. bigemina,* but it has not been studied in detail. Dogs become infected by the ingestion of sporulated oocysts; the parasite is thought to cause diarrhea. The same measures used to control *I. bigemina* are effective against this species. *Isospora canis* is not transmissible to man.

Isospora felis

This slightly to moderately pathogenic species occurs in the small intestine, sometimes the cecum, and occasionally the colon of the cat and other carnivores (Levine 1961a). It is common in the laboratory cat (Scott 1967). It resembles *I. canis* but differs in having an ovoid oocyst which measures 32 to 53 μ by 26 to 43 μ (Fig. 3.13*D*). Sporulation time ranges from 8 hours at 38 C and 40 hours at 20 C to several days at lower temperatures (Shah 1969). Endoge-

nous stages occur in the epithelial cells of the villi of the ileum and occasionally the duodenum and jejunum. There are two generations of schizonts and merozoites. The second generation merozoites give rise to gamonts, which in turn produce oocysts. The prepatent period is 7 to 8 days and the patent period, 10 to 11 days. The pathogenicity of *I. felis* is variable. It occasionally causes severe enteritis, emaciation, diarrhea, and death in young cats, but more often it has no apparent effect (Shah 1969). The same measures used to control *I. bigemina* are effective against this species. *Isospora felis* is not transmissible to man.

Isospora ratti

Isospora ratti was found in the intestinal contents of a wild Norway rat in central United States (Levine and Ivens 1965a). Its incidence, life cycle, pathogenicity, and public health importance are unknown. The oocyst is subspherical, smooth, and tan and measures 22 to 24 μ by 20 to 21 μ (Fig. 3.14). There is a polar granule but no micropyle or residuum. Within the oocyst are two ovoid sporocysts, each of which has a Stieda body, a residuum, and four sporozoites.

Cryptosporidium muris

This slightly pathogenic coccidium was reported once in the laboratory mouse in the United States early in the twentieth century but has not been reported with certainty since (Levine and Ivens 1965a; Tyzzer 1910). It occurs in the stomach, either in the lumen of the gastric glands or attached

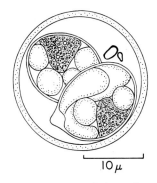

Fig. 3.14. *Isosopora ratti* (sporulated oocyst). (From Levine and Ivens 1965a. Courtesy of University of Illinois Press.)

to the epithelial surface, and sometimes causes dilation of the gastric glands and a slight increase in lymphoid cells. The oocyst is smooth, measures 7 by 5 μ, and contains four naked sporozoites and a residuum but no micropyle. Schizonts measure 7 by 6 μ and form eight merozoites. Schizonts, macrogametes, and oocysts have a knoblike attachment organ on their surface. Microgametes have no flagella.

Cryptosporidium parvum

This essentially nonpathogenic species has also been reported in the laboratory mouse in the United States, but it is rare (Hampton and Rosario 1966; Levine and Ivens 1965a; Tyzzer 1912). It occurs throughout the small intestine. The parasites are attached to the surface and either cause an indentation or are buried in the striated border of the epithelial cells of the villi. The oocyst is ovoid or spherical, 4 to 5 μ by 3 μ, and smooth; it has a residuum but no micropyle. Schizonts are 3 to 5 μ in diameter and form eight merozoites.

Cryptosporidium sp.

A slightly pathogenic species of Cryptosporidium has been observed in the small intestine of the guinea pig in eastern United States (Jervis, Merrill, and Sprinz 1966). The parasites are found embedded in the striated border of the epithelium of the intestinal villi (Fig. 3.15); they are round or ovoid, measure 1 to 4 μ in diameter, and resemble C. parvum. They do not produce overt clinical signs but cause a chronic enteritis characterized by shortening and thickening of the villi, infiltration of inflammatory cells in the lamina propria, and a decrease in the concentrations of a number of enzymes in the absorptive cells.

Klossiella muris

This ordinarily nonpathogenic coccidium is common in the kidneys of the conventional laboratory mouse throughout the world but has been reported only once in the wild house mouse (Levine and Ivens 1965a). It does not occur in cesarean-derived, barrier-sustained colonies (Foster 1963).

MORPHOLOGY

The sporocyst has a thin wall, measures 16 by 13 μ, and contains 25 to 34 ba-

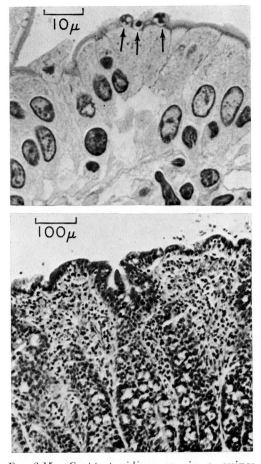

FIG. 3.15. *Cryptosporidium* sp. in a guinea pig. *(Top)* Organism *(arrows)* embedded in the striated border of the ileum. *(Bottom)* Ileal mucosa. Note infiltration of inflammatory cells. (From Jervis, Merrill, and Sprinz 1966. Courtesy of American Veterinary Medical Association.)

nana-shaped sporozoites (Levine and Ivens 1965a). Each merozoite is about 7 by 2 μ. The mature oocyst measures about 40 μ in diameter.

LIFE CYCLE

The mouse is infected by ingesting sporulated sporocysts (Levine and Ivens 1965a). Sporozoites pass into the bloodstream and enter the endothelial cells of the kidney glomeruli, where schizogony occurs (Fig. 3.16A). There are two types of schizonts: one forms 8 to 12 merozoites, the

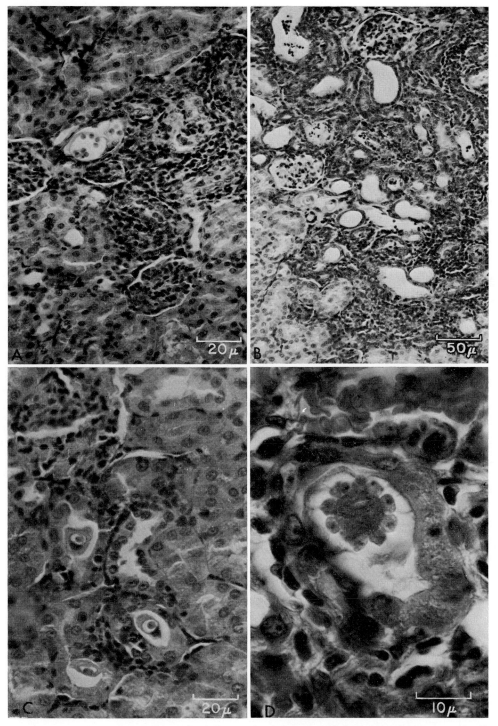

FIG. 3.16. *Klossiella muris* in mouse kidney. *(A)* Schizogony. *(B, C)* Early stage of sporogony. *(D)* Late stage of sporogony. (Courtesy of A. Meshorer, Weizmann Institute of Science.)

other 40 to 60 merozoites. Merozoites enter the epithelial cells of the convoluted tubules of the kidney, where they form gamonts which become macrogametes and microgametocytes. After fertilization, the zygote or oocyst grows and divides by sporogony (Fig. 3.16B, C, D) to form 12 to 16 sporoblasts, each of which becomes a sporocyst. The sporocysts rupture the host cell and pass out of the body in the urine.

PATHOLOGIC EFFECTS

Klossiella muris is usually nonpathogenic, but in heavy infections the kidneys are sometimes enlarged, and pale areas and small gray necrotic foci are seen on the surface (Smith and Johnson 1902; Yang and Grice 1964). Microscopically, organisms occur in the tubular epithelial cells, glomerular endothelium, and convoluted tubule lumens. The parasites are commoner in the cortex; they apparently cause little inflammation, although destruction of tubular epithelium has been reported. Foci of interstitial cellular infiltration are seen, but not in association with the organisms.

DIAGNOSIS

Diagnosis is based on the gross and microscopic lesions and on recognition of the organism in tissue sections. The presence of perivascular, follicular, lymphocytic infiltration in the outer zone of the medulla is said to be of diagnostic significance (Otto 1957).

CONTROL

Good sanitation is necessary for control of this parasite. No treatment has been reported.

PUBLIC HEALTH CONSIDERATIONS

Klossiella muris is not a public health problem.

Klossiella cobayae

This usually nonpathogenic coccidium is common in the kidneys and other organs of the conventional guinea pig throughout the world, but it does not occur in cesarean-derived colonies (Calhoon and Matthews 1964; Levine and Ivens 1965a). The first schizogony takes place in the capillary endothelial cells of the kidney and other organs. The last schizogony, along with gam-

etogony and sporogony, occurs in the endothelial cells of the kidney tubules. The mature zygote is 30 to 40 μ in diameter. It produces 30 or more sporocysts, each containing about 30 sporozoites. Although *Klossiella cobayae* is usually considered nonpathogenic, a chronic to subacute nephritis with degenerative lesions has been described (Bonciu et al. 1957; Cossel 1958). The parasite is often encountered in sections of the kidney, lungs, spleen, and other organs during routine histologic examination.

Hepatozoon muris

(SYN. *Hepatozoon perniciosum, Leucocytozoon muris, Leucocytozoon ratti, Leucocytogregarina innoxia*)

This usually nonpathogenic parasite is common in wild Norway and black rats throughout the world (Eyles 1952a; Laird 1959; Levine 1961a; Prakash 1954). It has also been reported from several other rodents, but these reports are of doubtful validity. *Hepatozoon muris* is rare in the laboratory rat (Miller 1908); it does not occur in cesarean-derived, barrier-sustained colonies (Foster 1963).

MORPHOLOGY

Schizonts, which are found in the liver, are 10 to 30 μ in diameter (Fig. 3.17A) (Kusama, Kasai, and Kobayashi 1919; Miller 1908). Gamonts, which occur in the lymphocytes, appear in stained blood smears as elongated oval or reniform bodies, 8 to

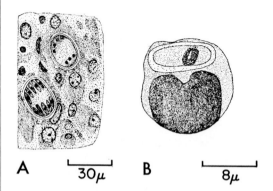

FIG. 3.17. *Hepatozoon muris* in the rat. (A) Schizonts in liver tissue. (B) Gamont in lymphocyte. (From Wenrich 1949. Courtesy of J. B. Lippincott Co.)

12 μ by 3 to 6 μ, with a light blue, non-granular cytoplasm and a pink central nucleus (Fig. 3.17B). No sexual differences can be seen. The cytoplasm of the lymphocyte around the parasite is unstained. Free forms of the parasite, which occur in the blood, are slender, curved or straight, and are often pointed at one end.

LIFE CYCLE

The rat becomes infected by ingesting the invertebrate vector, the spiny rat mite *Laelaps echidninus* (Kusama, Kasai, and Kobayashi 1919; Miller 1908). Sporozoites are released in the intestine, enter the hepatic portal system, and are transported to the liver. Schizogony takes place in the liver parenchymal cells. Merozoites enter the lymphocytes in the circulating blood and become gamonts. The gamonts are ingested by the mite; fertilization and sporogony occur in the arthropod vector.

PATHOLOGIC EFFECTS

Hepatozoon muris is usually considered nonpathogenic (Kusama, Kasai, and Kobayashi 1919). Anemia and emaciation, accompanied by splenomegaly and hepatic degeneration, have been reported in rats with severe infections, but these changes may have been caused by a concurrent, heavy infestation with the mite vector (Miller 1908).

DIAGNOSIS

Diagnosis is based on recognition of the parasite in blood smears and tissue sections in association with signs and lesions.

CONTROL

No effective drugs are known, but the elimination of mites will prevent transmission of the parasite. Recovered rats have some immunity (Kusama, Kasai, and Kobayashi 1919).

PUBLIC HEALTH CONSIDERATIONS

Hepatozoon muris is not known to occur in man.

Hepatozoon musculi, Hepatozoon microti

Hepatozoon musculi has been reported from the laboratory mouse in Great Britain (Porter 1908). *Hepatozoon microti*, found in the wild house mouse in central Europe,

is possibly the same organism (Erhardova 1955). *Hepatozoon musculi* differs from *H. muris* in that schizogony takes place only in the bone marrow. The incidence and pathologic effects of both species are unknown.

Hepatozoon cuniculi

This species has been reported from the rabbit in Italy (Sangiorgi 1914). Its gamonts are found in the leucocytes, and its schizonts in the spleen.

Hepatozoon canis

This usually nonpathogenic species occurs in the dog, cat, and several wild carnivores (Levine 1961a). Its incidence is unknown. Schizonts are found in the spleen, bone marrow, and to a lesser extent in the liver. Gamonts occur in the polymorphonuclear leucocytes. They are elongate and rectangular with rounded ends and measure about 8 to 12 μ by 3 to 6 μ. The dog and cat become infected by ingesting the vector, the brown dog tick (*Rhipicephalus sanguineus*). *Hepatozoon canis* usually causes no apparent signs, but fever, emaciation, anemia, splenomegaly, and death sometimes occur. No effective drugs are known, but elimination of the tick vector will prevent infection. *Hepatozoon canis* is not transmissible to man.

MALARIAL PARASITES

The malarial parasites belong to the suborder Haemospororina. They differ from the coccidian parasites (Eimeriorina and Adeleorina) in that microgametocytes produce a moderate number of microgametes, and sporozoites are naked. Gamonts are similar and develop independently; the zygote is motile. All species are heteroxenous; schizogony takes place in a vertebrate host and sporogony in an invertebrate host. If erythrocytes are invaded pigment is formed from the host cell hemoglobin.

There is a single family, Plasmodiidae. The most important genus is *Plasmodium*, which contains the malarial parasites of man and other vertebrates. Two other genera, *Hepatocystis* and *Sergentella*, occur in wild primates and some other mammals; and an additional two genera, *Leucocytozoon* and *Haemoproteus*, occur principally in wild birds.

The malarial parasites which occur in

endothermal laboratory animals are listed in Table 3.2. The most important species are discussed below.

Plasmodium cynomolgi

(Syn. *Plasmodium cyclopis*)

This mildly pathogenic species is common in the cynomolgus monkey, pigtail macaque, bonnet monkey, other macaques, and leaf monkeys in Asia (Eyles 1963; Eyles et al. 1962c). The rhesus monkey is frequently infected experimentally, but there is only one report of natural infection in this species (Schmidt et al. 1961b). A subspecies, *Plasmodium cynomolgi bastianellii,* occurs in the cynomolgus monkey of the Malay Peninsula (Bray 1963b; Eyles 1963; Garnham 1959).

Plasmodium cynomolgi is likely to be encountered in primates obtained from endemic areas. It is important because it is transmissible to man, because it is an excellent model for studies of human malaria, and because it can confuse research data (Conran 1967).

MORPHOLOGY

The structure of this parasite is illustrated in Figure 3.18 (Bray 1957a, 1963a; Eyles 1960b; Hawking, Perry, and Thurston 1948; Shortt 1948; Shortt and Garnham 1948). Schizonts (cryptozoites), which occur in the liver parenchymal cells *(1–9),* are 1.5 to 2.5 μ in diameter when young and about 40.0 μ in diameter when mature. When merozoites (metacryptozoites) occur in erythrocytes *(11, 16),* they occupy about one-third to one-half of the diameter of the cell. They have a large central vacuole and are called ring stages because they resemble a signet ring when stained with Romanovsky stain.

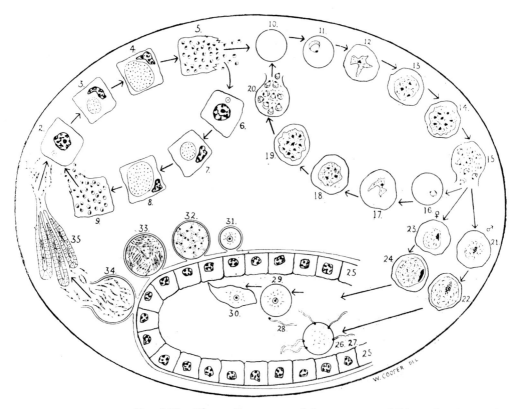

FIG. 3.18. *Plasmodium cynomolgi,* structure and life cycle. See explanation in text. (From Shortt 1948. Courtesy of Royal Society of Tropical Medicine and Hygiene.)

LIFE CYCLE

The life cycle of *P. cynomolgi* is typical of *Plasmodium* (Fig. 3.18) (Bray 1957a, 1963a; Eyles 1960b; Hawking, Perry, and Thurston 1948; Shortt 1948; Shortt and Garnham 1948). Sporozoites enter the blood through a mosquito bite *(1)*, invade the liver parenchymal cells *(2)*, and develop into schizonts (cryptozoites) *(3, 4)*. Rapid growth and nuclear division occur, and in 7 to 8 days, the cryptozoites contain a thousand or more nuclei. The parasite completely fills the host cell, but there is no tissue reaction. By the 8th day, merozoites (metacryptozoites) are formed in the cryptozoite; they are released from the host cell *(5)* at this time or later. A few enter another liver parenchymal cell and form a new generation of metacryptozoites *(6, 7, 8, 9)*. This exoerythrocytic cycle recurs every 8 to 11 days. It lasts indefinitely at a low level and provides a source of parasites for subsequent relapses.

Some first-generation metacryptozoites begin the erythrocytic phase of the life cycle. They enter the erythrocytes *(10)*, vacuolate *(11)*, enlarge, become schizonts (trophozoites) *(12)*, and undergo multiple fission (schizogony) *(13, 14)* to produce merozoites *(15)*. The erythrocytes rupture and the merozoites invade new erythrocytes. This asexual cycle takes 2 days and is repeated indefinitely *(16 to 20)*.

After an indeterminate number of asexual generations, some merozoites enter erythrocytes and form either microgametocytes *(21, 22)* or macrogametes *(23, 24)*. These remain unchanged until ingested by the proper species of mosquito. In the stomach of the mosquito *(25)*, the microgametocytes produce a moderate number of heavy, flagellumlike microgametes by exflagellation *(26, 27)*. A microgamete *(28)* fertilizes a macrogamete *(29)*, and the resultant zygote *(30)* migrates to the outer surface of the stomach wall to form an oocyst *(31)*. The oocyst grows, its nucleus divides *(32)*, and numerous sporoblasts are formed. Each sporoblast nucleus then divides until the oocyst contains several thousand slender, spindle-shaped sporozoites, each with a central nucleus *(33)*. These break out of the oocyst *(34)*, enter the body cavity, migrate to the salivary glands *(35)*, and are injected into a new host when the mosquito feeds *(1)*. The process of sporozoite development takes 10 to 20 days or longer.

Natural vectors are *Anopheles hackeri* and *A. balabacensis introlatus* (Warren and Wharton 1963). Experimental vectors are *A. maculipennis, A. maculatus, A. sundaicus, A. kochi, A. lesteri, A. philippinensis, A. quadrimaculatus,* and *A. freeborni* (Eyles, 1960a). Oocysts develop in *Mansonia uniformis,* but sporozoites rarely reach the salivary glands (Warren, Eyles, and Wharton 1962).

PATHOLOGIC EFFECTS

When the merozoites leave the erythrocytes, the toxic products of their metabolism sometimes cause a paroxysm of chills and fever. The schizogonous cycle of *P. cynomolgi* takes 2 days, thus causing paroxysms every other day. The clinical disease, tertian malaria, is characterized by anorexia, weakness, listlessness, fever, mild anemia, splenomegaly, and hepatic congestion. Thrombocytopenia lasting 2 to 6 days, mild leukopenia, progressive anemia, and reticulocytosis have been reported in experimental infection (Jeffery and Sodeman 1966). Pigment granules (hemozoin) sometimes occur in the spleen and other organs.

DIAGNOSIS

Diagnosis is based on the identification of the parasite in blood smears (Fig. 3.19). Schizonts are found in the liver parenchymal cells but must be differentiated from those of *Hepatocystis.* The presence of hemozoin indicates a *Plasmodium* infection.

CONTROL

Mosquito control will prevent transmission of the disease within a laboratory. A combination of chloroquine, given intramuscularly, 2.5 mg per kg of body weight daily for 7 days, and primaquine, given orally, 0.75 mg per kg of body weight daily for 14 days, is effective in suppressing the infection (Conran 1967; P. B. Conran, personal communication). Quinine and quinacrine are also used.

PUBLIC HEALTH CONSIDERATIONS

Accidental infection of man has occurred in the laboratory (Eyles, Coatney,

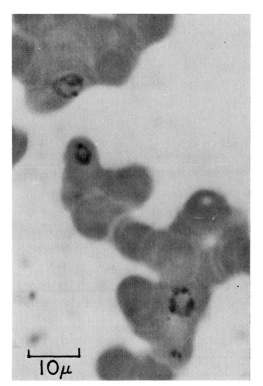

FIG. 3.19. *Plasmodium cynomolgi* in blood smear of a rhesus monkey. (Courtesy of P. B. Conran, Dow Chemical Co.)

and Getz 1960; Schmidt, Greenland, and Genther 1961a), and *P. cynomolgi* has been transmitted experimentally from macaques to man, using *Anopheles freeborni* and *A. quadrimaculatus* mosquitoes as vectors (Beye et al. 1961; Coatney et al. 1961; Contacos and Coatney 1963; Contacos et al. 1962; Eyles, Coatney, and Getz, 1960; Schmidt, Greenland, and Genther 1961a). Therefore, effective mosquito control is essential in laboratory facilities in which possibly infected nonhuman primates are housed (Gibson 1967).

Plasmodium knowlesi

Plasmodium knowlesi, a usually mild but sometimes severe pathogen, is common in the cynomolgus monkey and also occurs in the pigtail macaque, other macaques, leaf monkeys, and man (Chin et al. 1965; Eyles et al. 1962c; Lambrecht, Dunn, and Eyles 1961; Schmidt et al. 1961b). It is readily transmitted to the rhesus monkey

and several other lower primates (Bray 1963b; Eyles 1963). It occurs primarily in the Malay Peninsula but has also been found in the Philippine Islands and Taiwan (Lambrecht, Dunn, and Eyles 1961). A subspecies, *P. knowlesi edesoni*, has been isolated from the cynomolgus monkey in the Malay Peninsula (Garnham 1963a). *Plasmodium knowlesi* is likely to be encountered in laboratory primates obtained from endemic areas.

MORPHOLOGY

The structure of this parasite is similar to that of *P. cynomolgi* (Garnham, Lainson, and Cooper 1957). Ring stages are relatively small, about one-fourth the diameter of the host cell, and often have an accessory chromatin dot. Schizonts have dark brown pigment granules and are not markedly ameboid. Gamonts are round.

LIFE CYCLE

The life cycle of *P. knowlesi* is similar to but differs from all other species of *Plasmodium* in that its schizogonous cycle takes only 1 day (Garnham, Lainson, and Cooper 1957).

PATHOLOGIC EFFECTS

Because of its 1-day schizogonous cycle, this parasite produces a unique quotidian malaria. The disease is mild in the natural hosts, but it is acute and often fatal in experimentally infected rhesus, vervet, and patas monkeys and in baboons (Bray 1963b; Eyles 1963).

DIAGNOSIS

Diagnosis is based on demonstration of the parasite in blood smears. Host erythrocytes are not enlarged, are often pale, and sometimes contain fine stippling, depending on the staining method.

CONTROL

Mosquito control will prevent transmission of the disease in the laboratory.

PUBLIC HEALTH CONSIDERATIONS

Since *P. knowlesi* affects man, care should be taken to exclude mosquitoes from laboratory facilities housing primates which are possibly infected.

Plasmodium inui

(SYN. *Plasmodium osmaniae,*
Plasmodium shortti)

This mildly pathogenic species is common in the cynomolgus monkey, bonnet monkey, pigtail macaque, and other macaques in southern Asia, Indonesia, the Philippine Islands, and Taiwan (Eyles 1963; Eyles and Warren 1962; Howard and Cabrera 1961; Lambrecht, Dunn, and Eyles 1961; Sinton 1934). A subspecies, *Plasmodium inui shortti,* has been found in the bonnet monkey in India (Bray 1963b; Eyles 1963; Shortt et al. 1961). *Plasmodium inui* is readily transmitted to the rhesus monkey, but natural infection is uncommon (Mathis and Leger 1911; Schmidt et al. 1961b). Schizogony takes 3 days, and thus paroxysms of chills and fever occur every 3rd day. The resultant clinical disease is called quartan malaria (Sinton 1934). *Plasmodium inui* is likely to be encountered in primates obtained from endemic areas. It has been experimentally transmitted to man (Coatney et al. 1966).

Plasmodium coatneyi

Plasmodium coatneyi, a mildly pathogenic species, occurs in the cynomolgus monkey of the Malay Peninsula and the Philippine Islands (Eyles et al. 1962a; Warren and Wharton 1963). It has been transmitted experimentally to other macaques and leaf monkeys, and it causes a tertian malaria in the rhesus monkey (Eyles 1963). *Plasmodium coatneyi* may be encountered in primates obtained from endemic areas; its natural incidence is unknown.

Plasmodium gonderi

This mildly pathogenic malarial parasite is common in mangabeys and mandrills in west central Africa and is readily transmissible to the rhesus monkey (Bray 1959; Garnham, Lainson, and Cooper 1958; Rodhain and van den Berghe 1936). It causes a mild tertian malaria and is likely to be encountered in mangabeys and mandrills obtained from endemic areas.

Plasmodium malariae

(SYN. *Plasmodium rodhaini*)

Plasmodium malariae, an important pathogen of man, is also found in the chimpanzee in Africa, and cross transmission of the parasite between the two hosts has been reported (Bray 1959, 1960; Garnham, Lainson, and Gunders 1956; Rodhain 1948; Rodhain and Dellaert 1943). It causes quartan malaria in both man and the chimpanzee. *Plasmodium malariae* is common in nature and is likely to be encountered in chimpanzees obtained from endemic areas. Control of mosquitoes will prevent the transmission of the disease in the laboratory.

Plasmodium reichenowi

This mildly pathogenic species occurs in the chimpanzee and gorilla in Africa. It is structurally similar to *Plasmodium falciparum* of man, but attempts to transmit it to man have been unsuccessful (Bray 1956, 1963c; Garnham, Lainson, and Gunders 1956; Reichenow 1949–1953). *Plasmodium reichenowi* causes a mild tertian malaria in the chimpanzee (Bray 1957b), and it may be encountered in specimens obtained from endemic areas. Its natural incidence is unknown.

Plasmodium schwetzi

Plasmodium schwetzi, a mildly pathogenic species, occurs in the chimpanzee and gorilla in Africa and has been experimentally transmitted to man (Bray 1958, 1963b, c; Rodhain and Dellaert 1955). It causes a mild tertian malaria in the chimpanzee and man and may be found in chimpanzees obtained from endemic areas. Its natural incidence is unknown.

Plasmodium brasilianum

This sometimes markedly pathogenic species is the commonest malarial parasite of New World monkeys. It is frequently found in howler monkeys, spider monkeys, capuchins, squirrel monkeys, uakaris, and woolly monkeys in Central and South America (Aberle 1945; Clark 1930, 1931; Dunn and Lambrecht 1963; Gonder and von Berenberg-Gossler 1908; Hill 1936; Porter, Johnson, and De Sousa 1966; Taliaferro and Cannon 1936; Taliaferro and Taliaferro 1934). It has been transmitted experimentally to the night monkey, marmosets, and man. *Plasmodium brasilianum* causes quartan malaria (Taliaferro and Klüver 1940a, b). It is occasionally fatal in spider monkeys, howler monkeys, and capuchins but is more often fatal in experimentally infected night monkeys and marmosets. *Plasmodium brasilianum* is likely to be encountered in susceptible primates obtained from endemic areas. In man it produces a low level parasitemia with few or no clinical signs (Contacos et al. 1963). It is possible that this species is actually *P. malariae* introduced into the New World by early explorers and modified through numerous passages in wild monkeys (Dunn 1965).

Plasmodium simium

Plasmodium simium is common in the howler monkey in Brazil and has been reported in man (Deane, Deane, and Neto 1966; da Fonseca 1951; Garnham 1963b). It causes tertian malaria and is likely to be encountered in laboratory specimens obtained from the endemic area.

Plasmodium of Rodents

Four species of *Plasmodium* are maintained in laboratory rodents for research purposes.

Plasmodium berghei occurs naturally in the tree rat *(Thamnomys surdaster)* in central Africa (Vincke and Lips 1948). It is transmissible to the Norway rat, mouse, hamster, and various wild rodents, but not to the guinea pig or rabbit. A severe malaria is produced in the mouse and a mild form in the rat. It is used extensively in malarial research.

Plasmodium vinckei was obtained from a mosquito in central Africa (Rodhain 1952). It develops in certain African rats *(Thamnomys, Aethomys)* and the mouse and causes a severe type of malaria, probably quotidian, in the latter species. It is not transmissible to the Norway rat or hamster.

Plasmodium chabaudi, which may be a synonym for *P. vinckei,* was obtained from a tree rat *(Thamnomys rutilans)* in central Africa (Landau 1965). It can be transmitted to the mouse but not to the Norway rat. Mice simultaneously infected with *P. chabaudi* and *Eperythrozoon coccoides* develop a mild, chronic malaria which is seldom fatal; mice infected with *P. chabaudi* alone develop severe, fatal malaria (Ott and Stauber 1967).

Plasmodium inopinatum was obtained from a wild rat in Belgium (Resseler 1956). It develops in the mouse, rat, hamster, tree rat *(Thamnomys surdaster),* and fat mouse *(Steatomys).*

Hepatocystis kochi
(Syn. *Plasmodium kochi, Hepatocystis joyeuxi, H. cercopitheci, H. bouilliezi, H. simiae)*

Hepatocystis kochi is the commonest malarial parasite of the green monkey, other guenons, mangabeys, and baboons in central Africa, and it occurs in practically all monkeys of that region (Aberle 1945; Garnham 1947; Garnham, Heisch, and Minter 1961; Kuntz and Myers 1967). It is common in laboratory specimens acquired from endemic areas. Incidences of 42 to 56% have been reported in primates obtained from west central Africa (Bray 1959; Lefrou and Martignoles 1955), and 40 to 75% in specimens from east central Africa (Miller 1959; Pietrzyk and Umiński 1967; Strong, Miller, and McGill 1965; Vickers 1966). Although *H. kochi* rarely causes clinical disease, it can interfere with toxicologic tests and confuse research data (Vickers 1966).

MORPHOLOGY

The structure of this parasite is similar to that of *Plasmodium cynomolgi* (Garnham 1947, 1948). Macrogametes stain blue with Giemsa stain and have a two-part nucleus consisting of a pale pink area and dense central chromatin. Microgametocytes contain a large, oval, pale pink, two-part nucleus which is sometimes one-half the size of the parasite.

LIFE CYCLE

Schizonts in the liver parenchymal cells form large cysts (Garnham 1947, 1948; Garnham and Pick 1952; Miller 1959). The nuclei multiply and each cyst enlarges and forms cytomeres. These coalesce and become a merocyst or megaloschizont which measures up to 2 mm in diameter in guenons and 4 mm in diameter in baboons and contains a packed mass of merozoites. The merocyst bursts and releases merozoites which invade the erythrocytes. Ring stages develop into gamonts in 4 to 5 days. There are no schizonts in the blood.

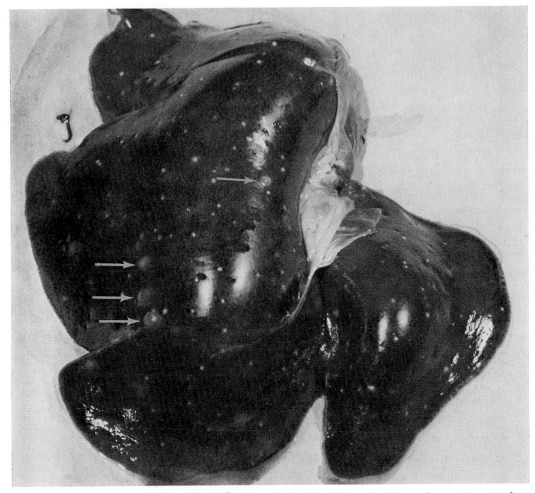

FIG. 3.20. *Hepatocystis kochi* lesions in liver of a green monkey. Note mature merocysts *(arrows)* and numerous white foci representing scars of old lesions. (From Vickers 1966. Courtesy of American Veterinary Medical Association.)

The vector of *H. kochi* is a midge *(Culicoides)* (Garnham, Heisch, and Minter 1961). Sporogony in the midge lasts 5 to 6 days. Oocysts develop in the hemocele and in 5 days are over 30 μ in diameter. Sporozoites are 13 μ long and have a subcentral nucleus. They break out of the oocysts, migrate to the salivary glands, and enter the host when the midge feeds.

PATHOLOGIC EFFECTS

Mature merocysts appear on the surface of the liver as grayish white, translucent foci; healed lesions appear as fibrotic spots (Fig. 3.20) (Vickers 1966). In histologic sections, enormous numbers of merozoites are seen in the merocysts (Fig. 3.21). Otherwise, *H. kochi* causes no lesions or signs of disease. Reports to the contrary are possibly the result of concurrent infection with *P. gonderi*.

DIAGNOSIS

Diagnosis is based on identification of the parasite in thick blood smears from the living animal (Fig. 3.22) (Pietrzyk and Umiński 1967) or in histologic sections of the liver at necropsy (Vickers 1966). Host

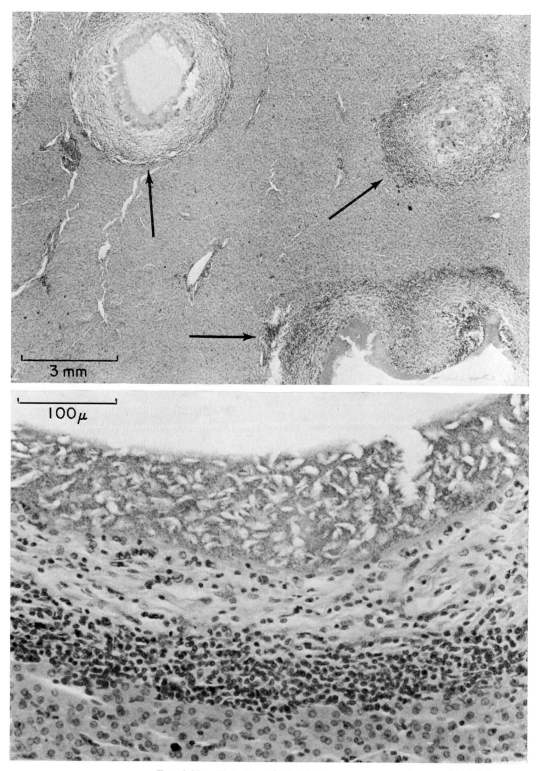

Fig. 3.21. *Hepatocystis kochi* in a green monkey. *(Top)* Merocysts *(arrows)* in histologic section of liver. *(Bottom)* Section through edge of merocyst. Note inner rim *(top)* containing innumerable merozoites. (From Vickers 1966. Courtesy of American Veterinary Medical Association.)

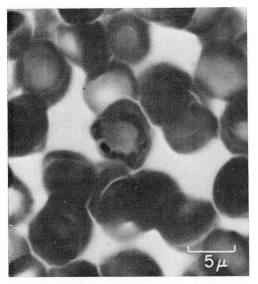

FIG. 3.22. *Hepatocystis kochi* in blood smear of a baboon. (Courtesy of Betty June Myers, Southwest Foundation for Research and Education.)

erythrocytes are not enlarged and contain no stippling; pigment granules are small.

CONTROL

In laboratory primates, *H. kochi* infection can be prevented by selecting specimens from areas of Africa relatively free of the parasite (Vickers 1966). Natural transmission does not occur in the laboratory in the absence of the insect vector. Treatment with antimalarial drugs is not effective (Miller 1959; Ruch 1959).

PUBLIC HEALTH CONSIDERATIONS

Hepatocystis kochi does not infect man.

TOXOPLASMASIDS

All toxoplasmasids are monoxenous parasites. Although their taxonomic position has been uncertain, electron microscopic evidence now indicates that they are definitely sporozoans (Levine 1961b). They have no spores. Cysts or pseudocysts containing many naked trophozoites are produced by binary fission or, perhaps sometimes, by schizogony. Pseudopods, flagella, and cilia are absent; locomotion is by body flexion or gliding. There are two families, Sarcocystidae and Toxoplasmatidae.

The family Sarcocystidae has but one genus, *Sarcocystis*. Its cysts occur in skeletal, cardiac, esophageal, and diaphragmatic muscles and are usually divided into compartments by internal septa. It is common in many animal species.

The family Toxoplasmatidae has two genera, *Toxoplasma* and *Besnoitia*. In the genus *Toxoplasma*, either pseudocysts (in which a thin "cyst" wall is formed by the host and not by the parasite) or cysts are formed. Trophozoites reproduce by binary fission or endodyogeny (in which two daughter cells form in a mother cell and then destroy it and escape), and possibly by schizogony in young pseudocysts. A single, euryxenous species, *Toxoplasma gondii*, is recognized. It occurs in a wide variety of mammals and in a few birds.

In the genus *Besnoitia*, the pseudocysts are present in the subcutaneous and connective tissues, serosal membranes, and elsewhere. They have a heavy wall containing nuclei and are not compartmented. Trophozoites are banana shaped, crescentic, or elongate and oval and are slightly pointed at one end. *Besnoitia* is rare in laboratory animals.

The toxoplasmasids which occur in endothermal laboratory animals are listed in Table 3.3. The most important are discussed below.

Sarcocystis

This relatively nonpathogenic parasite occurs in many animals throughout the world (Eisenstein and Innes 1956; Levine 1961a; Sahasrabudhe and Shah 1966). Numerous species have been named, but their validity is uncertain. Differentiation is based on the host, the structure of the cyst wall, and the size of trophozoites, but cross infection occurs, and the appearance of the parasite varies with the host.

Sarcocystis muris occurs in the wild Norway rat and, less commonly, in the black rat and house mouse throughout the world (Bonciu, Dincolesco, and Petrovici 1958; Calero 1952; Krampitz 1957; Liddo and Sangiorgi 1941; Tsuchiya and Rector 1936). It was once common in conventional laboratory rodents but is now rare (Deschiens, Levaditi, and Lamy 1957; Garner, Innes, and Nelson 1967; Levine 1961a). It has not been found in cesarean-derived, barrier-sustained colonies (Foster 1963).

Sarcocystis cuniculi occurs in rabbits throughout the world. It is common in the cottontail rabbit in the United States, but apparently uncommon in the domestic rabbit (Deschiens, Levaditi, and Lamy 1957; Erickson 1946; Morgan and Waller 1940).

Sarcocystis of undetermined species has been reported from the dog, cat, and other domestic animals sometimes used in the laboratory (Eisenstein and Innes 1956). It is common in the cat but rare in the dog.

Sarcocystis kortei and *S. nesbitti* occur in the rhesus monkey but are apparently uncommon (Dubin and Wilcox 1947; Hartman 1961; de Korté 1905; Mandour 1969; Offutt and Telford 1945). Other unnamed species have been reported from baboons (Strong, Miller, and McGill 1965), woolly monkeys (Henderson and Bullock 1968), squirrel monkeys, spider monkeys, tamarins *(Saguinus)*, and marmosets *(Callimico, Cal-*

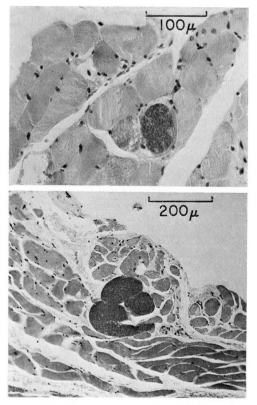

FIG. 3.23. *Sarcocystis* cysts in skeletal muscle of a tamarin *(Saguinus)*. (Courtesy of G. E. Cosgrove, Oak Ridge National Laboratory.)

lithrix) (Nelson, Cosgrove, and Gengozian 1966). An incidence of 16% has been reported in laboratory tamarins and 1% in laboratory rhesus monkeys (Habermann and Williams 1957; Nelson, Cosgrove, and Gengozian 1966).

MORPHOLOGY

The cysts, or Miescher's tubes, of *Sarcocystis* occur in the skeletal and cardiac muscles (Fig. 3.23) (Levine 1961a). They are cylindrical, spindle shaped, ellipsoidal, or irregular in structure and lie lengthwise in the muscles. Trophozoites, or Rainey's corpuscles, are banana shaped when mature; the anterior end is slightly pointed, and the posterior end is rounded. They vary in size with the species (Ludvík 1958b, 1960). Cysts of *S. muris* have smooth walls, are several millimeters long, and are not compartmented. Trophozoites measure 9 to 15 μ by 2.5 to 3.0 μ. Cysts of *S. cuniculi* are up to 5 mm long, are compartmented, and have a layer of radial villi, or cytophaneres, on the outer wall. Trophozoites are 4 to 5 μ in width and 6 to 16 μ, usually 12 to 13 μ, in length. Cysts of *S. kortei* are 0.3 to 0.8 mm long by 80 to 150 μ wide (Dubin and Wilcox 1947; Hartman 1961; Mandour 1969). Trophozoites are 3 to 14 μ long. Cysts of *S. nesbitti* occur only in skeletal muscle (Mandour 1969). They are 0.1 to 1.1 mm long by 165 μ wide. Trophozoites are 7 to 9 μ by 2 to 3 μ.

LIFE CYCLE

Sarcocystis has no sexual stages or intermediate hosts (Levine 1961b; Scott 1943). Animals become infected by ingesting trophozoites encysted in the muscle tissue or those free in the feces of other animals. The trophozoites presumably pass through the intestinal wall, enter the bloodstream, and are carried to the striated muscles, where they enter the muscle cells. They divide by binary fission or perhaps by schizogony into a number of rounded cells or trophoblasts surrounded by a cyst wall. These continue to reproduce by binary fission and later change into banana-shaped trophozoites. As multiplication proceeds, the cyst grows and is sometimes divided by septa into chambers or compartments. New trophozoites continue to be formed at the periphery. Trophozoites also reproduce by binary

fission. As the cyst becomes older, the trophozoites in its center degenerate and disappear. After it becomes mature, the wall dis-
integrates and the trophozoites are released.
They reach the digestive tract by way of
the bloodstream and pass out in the feces.

PATHOLOGIC EFFECTS

Sarcocystis usually does not cause clinical disease (Eisenstein and Innes 1956;
Garner, Innes, and Nelson 1967). The sar-
cocyst occurs in skeletal muscle and, less
commonly, in cardiac, esophageal, and diaphragmatic muscle. It destroys the portion of the muscle fiber which it occupies
and sometimes causes pressure atrophy of
adjacent cells. Cellular reaction around the
cyst is rare. The cyst contains an endotoxin,
sarcocystin, which is highly toxic for the
rabbit and mouse, but only mildly toxic
for the rat (Levine 1961a). There is no
evidence that it is important in natural infections.

DIAGNOSIS

Diagnosis is made by microscopic
identification of the characteristic cysts.
Sometimes they are seen macroscopically at
necropsy.

CONTROL

Infection is avoided through sanitation
and the prevention of cannibalism. There
is no effective treatment.

PUBLIC HEALTH CONSIDERATIONS

Sarcocystis occurs in man but it is rare.
However, because it is possible that the
species that occur in laboratory animals
are transmissible to man, feces from animals
likely to be infected should be handled
with caution.

Toxoplasma gondii

Toxoplasma gondii infection is common, but the disease it causes, toxoplasmosis, is uncommon, and its predisposing
causes are poorly understood (Levine
1961a). The organism occurs in various
tissues of the mouse, rat, black rat, guinea
pig, other rodents, rabbit, hares, dog, cat,
other carnivores, squirrel monkeys, capuchins, marmosets, lemurs, woolly monkeys,
baboons, the chimpanzee, other primates,
the chicken, other birds, most domestic

animals, and man (Dubey 1968a; Frenkel
1956; Galuzo 1966; Galuzo and Zasukhin
1963; Jacobs 1956; Levine 1961a, b; Møller 1968; Siim 1960; Stolz 1962; van Thiel
1964). *T. gondii* is common in the dog and
cat, particularly those obtained from
pounds, throughout the world (Levine
1961a). Reported incidences in the dog in
the United States range from 16 to 67%,
and in Europe from 8 to 87% (Work 1969).
Incidences in the cat in the United States
range from 5 to 83%, and in Europe from
39 to 63%. It has not been encountered in
cesarean-derived, barrier-sustained dogs
(Griesemer and Gibson 1963).

Toxoplasma gondii is less common in
laboratory primates, rodents, and lagomorphs. It has been found in New World
laboratory primates in the United States
(McKissick, Ratcliffe, and Koestner 1968);
in the laboratory rabbit in the United
States, Europe, and central Africa (Lainson
1955; Miller and Feldman 1953; Orio et al.
1959; Perrin 1943a; Szemerédi 1968); in the
guinea pig in the United States, Mexico,
Central America, southern Europe, and
central Africa (Makstenieks and Verlinde
1957; Mariani 1940; Miller and Feldman
1953; Orio et al. 1959; Rodaniche and Pinzon 1949; Varela, Martínez Rodríguez, and
Trevino 1953) in the wild Norway rat in
the United States and British Isles (Eyles
1952b; Lainson 1957); and in both the
house mouse and laboratory mouse in the
United States and Europe (Gibson and
Eyles 1957; Mooser 1950; Nicolau and Balmus 1934). The organism is frequently encountered in some conventional rodent colonies but is absent in others; it has not been
observed in cesarean-derived, barrier-sustained colonies (Calhoon and Matthews
1964; Foster 1963).

MORPHOLOGY

Trophozoites are crescent or banana
shaped and measure 4 to 8 μ by 2 to 4 μ
(Levine 1961a). One end is pointed and the
other rounded, and there is a central nucleus. They have an anterior conoid and
polar ring, 5 to 18 cylindrical or club-
shaped structures (toxonemes) extending
posteriorly from the anterior region, and
several subpellicular fibrils (Kikkawa and
Gueft 1964; Ludvík 1958a). The trophozoites occur in various tissue cells through-

out the host and also extracellularly in the blood and peritoneal fluid. Initially they occupy vacuoles in the host cells but, as they multiply, a cyst or pseudocyst forms around them. Oocysts, which have so far been observed only in the intestinal epithelial cells and feces of infected cats, are indistinguishable from those of *Isospora bigemina* (Frenkel, Dubey, and Miller 1970; Overdulve 1970; Sheffield and Melton 1970; Siim, Hutchison, and Work 1969; Work and Hutchison 1969).

LIFE CYCLE

Toxoplasma gondii reproduces sexually in the intestinal epithelium of the cat and by binary fission or endodyogeny in other tissues of the cat and other animals (Frenkel, Dubey, and Miller 1970). The usual natural mode of infection is unknown, but congenital toxoplasmosis occurs and it is postulated that most mammals and birds are infected by ingestion of oocysts in cat feces and that the cat is infected either by ingesting oocysts in feces or trophozoites or cysts in other animals. Experimental infections have been produced by inoculation of mucous membranes or scarified skin, and also by feeding flesh or feces of infected animals, oocysts, or trophozoites (Beverley 1959; Frenkel, Dubey, and Miller 1969, 1970; Galuzo 1966; Levine 1961a; Sheffield and Melton 1969; Siim, Hutchison, and Work 1969; Work and Hutchison 1969). At one time it was thought that *T. gondii* was carried in the egg of the cat ascarid, *Toxocara mystax* (Dubey 1968a; Hutchison 1965); however, it is now known that the nematode egg is not necessary for transmission (Dubey 1968b; Frenkel, Dubey, and Miller 1969; Hutchison, Dunachie, and Work 1968; Sheffield and Melton 1969), and it appears that the transmitting stage in cat feces is an oocyst indistinguishable from that of *Isospora bigemina* (see above).

PATHOLOGIC EFFECTS

Toxoplasmosis varies from an inapparent infection to an acutely fatal disease. Inapparent infection is commoner and is the form usually seen in adult animals; neonates are more frequently affected with clinical disease. In the dog, the disease is most commonly found in conjunction with canine distemper (Roberts 1966). The signs are variable. In the larger endothermal laboratory animals, such as the rabbit, dog, cat, and monkeys, they include fever, cough, anorexia, weakness, depression, ocular and nasal discharges, pale mucous membranes, leukopenia, dyspnea, vomiting, diarrhea, incoordination, convulsions, premature birth, abortion, and death (Conroy 1964; Frenkel 1956; McKissick, Ratcliffe, and Koestner 1968; Meier, Holzworth, and Griffiths 1957; Møller 1968; Smith and Jones 1966; Stolz 1962; Szemerédi 1968; van Thiel 1964). In the smaller endothermal laboratory animals, such as the mouse, the signs, as determined by experimental infection, range from a shortened life-span and decreased reproduction to acute, fulminating disease characterized by death (Beverley 1959; Bjotvedt 1964). Lesions include encephalitis, pneumonitis, myocarditis, nephritis, lymphadenitis, and chorioretinitis. Cellular and interstitial necrosis in the brain and necrotic foci in the liver, lungs, lymph nodes, and other organs sometimes occur (Fig. 3.24). *Toxoplasma*, either singly and in pairs or in pseudocysts containing numerous organisms, is usually associated with these lesions (McKissick et al. 1968).

DIAGNOSIS

Diagnosis in laboratory animals is based on finding the organism in smear preparations or in histologic sections, or by animal inoculation (Levine 1961a; Møller 1968). The Sabin-Feldman dye test is often used to survey a colony, but false positives frequently occur. A hemagglutination test is also used (Chordi, Walls, and Kagan 1964). Isolation of the organism itself is more reliable but is time-consuming and expensive. The presence of oocysts indistinguishable from those of *I. bigemina* in cat feces is not conclusive evidence of *T. gondii* infection.

CONTROL

Because the usual natural mode of transmission is unknown, specific preventive measures cannot be recommended. Routine sanitation should be employed, wild animal reservoirs controlled, and the ingestion of dog and cat feces prevented. No effective treatment is known.

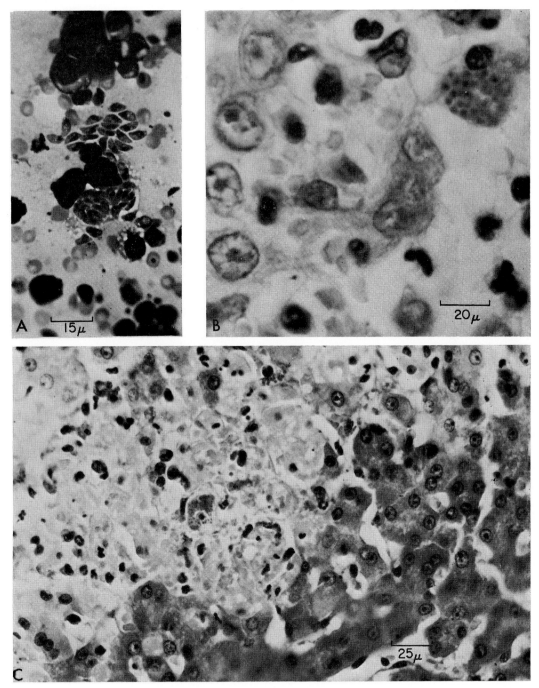

FIG. 3.24. Toxoplasmosis. *(A) Toxoplasma* in impression smear from lung of a mouse. *(B) T. gondii* in the lung of a cat. Note proliferation and cuboid shape of alveolar cells (AFIP neg. no. 56–11752). *(C) T. gondii* in the liver of a dog. Note sharply demarcated necrotic lesions (AFIP neg. no. 101348). (*A* from Frenkel 1956; courtesy of New York Academy of Sciences. *B* from Smith and Jones 1966; courtesy of Lea and Febiger and Armed Forces Institute of Pathology. *C* courtesy of Armed Forces Institute of Pathology.)

PUBLIC HEALTH CONSIDERATIONS

Toxoplasmosis occurs in man but is usually uncommon. Nevertheless, because it is a zoonosis, care should be taken to avoid infection. Persons working with potentially infected animals should be instructed in proper personal hygiene. Dog and cat feces should be handled with caution.

Besnoitia jellisoni

This parasite has been found in the subcutis, other connective tissues, serosal membranes, and venous sinuses of the dura mater of the deer mouse, kangaroo rat, and opossum in the United States (Ernst et al. 1968; Frenkel 1953; Stabler and Welch 1961). It causes either a chronic illness or an acute, fatal disease characterized by yellow-gray masses in the dural venous sinuses of the dura mater. The organism has been transmitted by parenteral inoculation to the mouse, rat, hamster, vole, and ground squirrel, but it does not occur naturally in these species. Its natural incidence in the deer mouse, kangaroo rat, and opossum are unknown. It is probably rare and is not likely to be encountered in laboratory specimens.

PIROPLASMASIDS

Piroplasmasids are blood parasites whose taxonomic position has long been uncertain (Levine 1961a). By electron microscopy they appear to belong with the sporozoans (Friedhoff and Scholtyseck 1968; Simpson, Kirkham, and Kling 1967). For this reason they are included here. Reproduction is by binary fission or schizogony; the existence of sexual reproduction is doubtful. All species are parasitic and heteroxenous, and all known vectors are ticks. *Babesia*, *Aegyptianella*, *Entopolypoides*, and *Theileria* are the genera which occur in endothermal laboratory animals; the genus *Babesia* is by far the most important.

All piroplasmasids known to occur in endothermal laboratory animals are listed in Table 3.4. The most important are discussed below.

Babesia decumani
(Syn. Nuttalia decumani)

This possibly pathogenic piroplasmasid is common in erythrocytes of wild Norway and black rats in Africa and southern Asia (Capponi, Sureau, and Deschiens 1955; Macfie 1915; Prakash 1954; Sureau and Capponi 1955). The mouse has been infected experimentally, but natural infection of laboratory rodents has not been reported.

MORPHOLOGY

Babesia decumani may be ameboid, ring shaped, circular, ovoid, or sausage shaped. Cytoplasmic processes are sometimes present. The parasite varies in size from a tiny ring to a body over half the diameter of the host erythrocyte and contains one or more vacuoles. The host cell is not enlarged. Dividing forms, consisting of four lanceolate parasites in the shape of a cross, sometimes occur.

LIFE CYCLE

The life cycle and specific vector of *B. decumani* are unknown, but it is presumably tick-borne.

PATHOLOGIC EFFECTS

Hemoglobinuria and death sometimes occur in experimentally infected wild Norway rats (Sureau and Capponi 1955). Degenerative changes are produced in the convoluted tubules of the kidneys, and large amounts of hematin are deposited in the kidneys and liver.

DIAGNOSIS

Diagnosis is based on the signs and lesions and identification of the parasite in erythrocytes.

CONTROL

There is no information on control; however, elimination of possible arthropod vectors should prevent transmission.

PUBLIC HEALTH CONSIDERATIONS

Babesia decumani is of no public health importance.

Babesia rodhaini

This piroplasmasid was isolated from erythrocytes of a tree rat (*Thamnomys sur-*

daster) in Africa (van den Berghe et al. 1950). The mouse, cotton rat, and hamster have been experimentally infected, but natural infection of laboratory rodents has not been reported (van den Berghe et al. 1950; Rodhain 1950). This parasite is maintained in mice in several laboratories for teaching and research purposes.

MORPHOLOGY

Babesia rodhaini resembles *B. decumani* structurally. It is 2 to 4 μ long and 2 to 3 μ wide. Its multiplication stages have four trophozoites, 2 by 1 μ, arranged in a cruciform pattern. Trophozoites ingest host cell cytoplasm by phagotrophy as do those of *Plasmodium,* but hemoglobin is digested more completely and no hemozoin is formed (Rudzinska and Trager 1962).

LIFE CYCLE

The life cycle is unknown; transmission is presumably by a tick.

PATHOLOGIC EFFECTS

Experimentally infected mice develop a severe hemolytic anemia, reticuloendothelial hyperplasia, focal liver necrosis, and hematuria (Paget, Alcock, and Ryley 1962). The incubation period is 3 to 10 days, and the infection reaches a peak in 6 to 13 days (Rodhain 1950).

DIAGNOSIS

Diagnosis is based on identification of the parasite in erythrocytes.

CONTROL

Natural infection does not occur in laboratory rodents, and no specific control measures other than elimination of possible arthropod vectors are required.

PUBLIC HEALTH CONSIDERATIONS

This parasite is of no public health importance.

Babesia canis

Babesia canis, the cause of canine babesiosis, occurs in the erythrocytes of the dog and other canids (Levine 1961a; Riek 1968; Rokey 1968). It has been reported from southern and southwestern United States, southern Europe, Central America, South America, Asia, Africa, and northern Australia. It is common in the tropics, but uncommon in temperate regions. It is rare in laboratory dogs and would be expected to occur only in animals obtained from pounds or from those maintained in tick-infested kennels in endemic areas. Research dogs given repeated blood transfusions from donors from endemic areas have an increased opportunity to acquire this infection. One epizootic in a research colony in California has been reported (Hirsh et al. 1969).

MORPHOLOGY

The trophozoites of *B. canis* are large, piriform, and 4 to 5 μ long, or round or ameboid and 2 to 4 μ in diameter (Fig. 3.25) (Levine 1961a). They generally contain a vacuole.

LIFE CYCLE

The life cycle requires a tick vector; the brown dog tick *(Rhipicephalus san-*

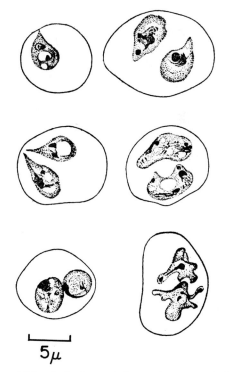

5μ

FIG. 3.25. *Babesia canis* in erythrocytes of the dog. (From Wenyon 1926.)

guineus) is probably the most important (Levine 1961a). When a tick ingests the parasites, most of them die in its intestine, but some become vermiform and enter the intestinal cells. Here they grow into large ameboid forms, multiply by a series of binary fissions, and produce over 1,000 individuals in 2 to 3 days. These become vermiform and pass into the body cavity; they are about 16 μ long. They enter the ovary, penetrate the eggs, become spherical, and divide a few times. They do not develop further in the larval tick that hatches from the egg, but when it molts to the nymphal stage, the parasites enter the salivary glands, multiply by a series of binary fissions, and fill each host cell with thousands of minute parasites. These become vermiform, break out of the host cell, enter the lumen of the salivary gland, and are injected into the vertebrate host by the nymph or adult tick while it feeds. The parasites enter the erythrocytes of the vertebrate host, divide by binary fission, and

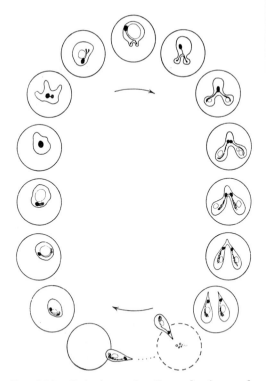

FIG. 3.26. *Babesia canis*. Reproductive cycle in circulating erythrocyte of the dog. (From Nuttall and Graham-Smith 1908.)

eventually destroy affected blood cells (Fig. 3.26). There are no sexual stages.

PATHOLOGIC EFFECTS

Different strains of *B. canis* vary in pathogenicity and in the disease manifestations each produces (Levine 1961a). The incubation period is 3 to 8 days (Dorner 1969). Clinical signs include pyrexia, anemia, icterus, inappetence, thirst, weakness, hemoglobinuria, prostration, and often death (Dorner 1969; Hirsh et al. 1969; Rokey and Russell 1961; Seibold and Bailey 1957). The spleen is enlarged and dark red and has prominent splenic corpuscles. The liver is enlarged and yellow, the heart and skeletal muscles are pale yellow, and the kidneys, fat, and mucous membranes are sometimes yellow.

DIAGNOSIS

Diagnosis is based on the clinical signs and identification of the parasite in erythrocytes (Hirsh et al. 1969). The latter is done effectively by centrifuging a blood sample collected in a microhematocrit tube containing an anticoagulant (EDTA). A thin smear is then made from the erythrocytes located just below the buffy coat and stained with Giemsa stain. The chances of finding the parasites can be further increased by staining the smear with acridine orange and then using fluorescent microscopy (Winter 1969).

CONTROL

Elimination of ticks will prevent infection. Effective treatments include a 1% solution of trypan blue given intravenously, 4 to 5 ml for a 15-kg dog; a 0.5% solution of acaprin given subcutaneously, 0.05 ml per kg of body weight; a 5% solution of phenamidine given subcutaneously, 0.2 ml per kg of body weight (Levine 1961a); and pyrimethamine given orally, 1.5 mg per kg of body weight (Hirsh et al. 1969).

PUBLIC HEALTH CONSIDERATIONS

This parasite is not transmissible to man.

Babesia pitheci

This usually nonpathogenic piroplasmasid has been found in erythrocytes of macaques, guenons, mangabeys, and ba-

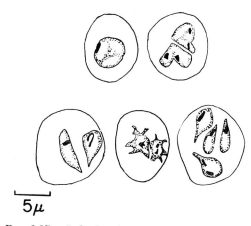

5μ

FIG. 3.27. *Babesia pitheci* in erythrocytes of a guenon. (From Garnham 1950. Courtesy of Cambridge University Press.)

boons in Africa and in European zoos (Garnham 1950; Hill 1953, 1954; Kikuth 1927; Ross 1905; Tanguy 1937). Its incidence in nature is unknown, and it has not been reported in the laboratory. The parasite could be encountered in nonhuman primates obtained from Africa.

MORPHOLOGY

Babesia pitheci is relatively large, 2 to 6 μ long, and may be round, oval, elliptical, piriform, lanceolate, or ameboid (Fig. 3.27) (Garnham 1950).

LIFE CYCLE

Reproduction is by binary fission. Although this parasite is presumably tick-borne, the specific vector is unknown.

PATHOLOGIC EFFECTS

This piroplasmasid is usually nonpathogenic, but it can be fatal after splenectomy (Tanguy 1937). In splenectomized animals, it causes an anemia accompanied by anisocytosis and poikilocytosis. From one to six, usually two, organisms are present in an erythrocyte, but macrocytosis does not occur.

DIAGNOSIS

Diagnosis is based on the clinical signs and on identification of the parasite in erythrocytes.

CONTROL

Elimination of possible arthropod vectors will prevent the spread of the infection. Treatment with 1% trypan blue solution intravenously, 1 ml per kg of body weight per day for 2 days in combination with a single injection of 0.5% acriflavine solution, 0.2 ml per kg of body weight, is helpful but will not eliminate the parasite (Tanguy 1937).

PUBLIC HEALTH CONSIDERATIONS

Babesia pitheci is of no known public health importance.

Entopolypoides macaci

(SYN. *Babesia macaci*)

This slightly pathogenic piroplasmasid has been reported in erythrocytes of cynomolgus monkeys from Indonesia and green monkeys from Africa (Fairbairn 1948; Mayer 1933, 1934). Cynomolgus and rhesus monkeys have been experimentally infected by intravenous or subcutaneous injection of infected blood (Mayer 1934). Its incidence in nature is unknown. Although there are no specific reports of this parasite in laboratory primates, it could be encountered in specimens obtained from endemic areas.

MORPHOLOGY

This parasite lacks true piriform stages. Its trophozoites are actively ameboid, with long, threadlike, branching pseudopods resembling polyp arms. The youngest stages in the erythrocytes are tiny ring forms or are small and disc shaped, one-third to one-half as large as the smallest *Plasmodium* rings. These grow into the larger branching forms characteristic of the genus. Parasitized erythrocytes are not enlarged, and pigment is not formed.

LIFE CYCLE

The life cycle is unknown, but it presumably involves a tick.

PATHOLOGIC EFFECTS

Entopolypoides macaci sometimes causes monocytosis and anemia (Mayer 1934).

DIAGNOSIS

Diagnosis is based on identification of the parasite in erythrocytes.

CONTROL

No control or treatment has been reported; however, the elimination of possible arthropod vectors should prevent the spread of the infection.

PUBLIC HEALTH CONSIDERATIONS

Entopolypoides macaci has not been reported in man.

NEOSPORANS

The neosporans (cnidosporans) contain forms which have an ameboid sporoplasm. Most are parasites of fishes and invertebrates, but a few occur in higher animals. Only one species, *Nosema cuniculi* (Table 3.5), occurs in endothermal laboratory animals.

Nosema cuniculi

(SYN. *Encephalitozoon cuniculi*)

Nosema cuniculi occurs throughout the world in the brain, kidneys, and other tissues of the mouse, rat, hamster, multimammate mouse, guinea pig, rabbit, cottontail rabbit, and dog and has been reported once in man (Frenkel 1956; Innes et al. 1962; Lainson 1954; Levine 1961a; Malherbe and Munday 1958; Møller 1968). It usually causes an inapparent infection that is seen during routine histologic examination, but acute disease sometimes occurs, particularly in the rabbit. It is common in some conventional rodent and rabbit colonies in some areas, but is rare or absent in others (Koller 1969; Malherbe and Munday 1958; Tuffery and Innes 1963). Infection has occurred in a cesarean-derived, barrier-sustained mouse colony (Innes et al. 1962).

Several other species of *Nosema* have been described, and the name has also been erroneously given to the Negri bodies of rabies (Innes et al. 1962; Levine 1961a; Nelson 1962; Weiser 1965). However, because of the transmissibility of the organism from one host to another, only a single species is recognized (Levine 1961a).

Although this parasite usually causes only inapparent infection, it is important because it can confuse research data, especially in studies involving the central nervous system (Innes et al. 1962).

MORPHOLOGY

The structure of *N. cuniculi* has been determined from histologic preparations of brain, kidneys, peritoneal exudate, liver, spleen, and other organs (Levine 1961a). Trophozoites are straight to slightly curved rods measuring 2 to 4 μ by 1.2 to 2.5 μ. They have an eccentric nucleus about one-fourth to one-third the size of the parasite. Pseudocysts containing 100 or more trophozoites occur in the nerve cells, macrophages, and other tissue cells. Spores have a polar capsule and filament which everts as it emerges and through which the sporoplasm enters a new host (Weiser 1965).

LIFE CYCLE

Multiplication is by schizogony (Weiser 1965). Little is known about the meth-

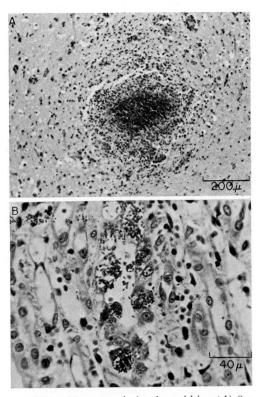

FIG. 3.28. Nosematosis in the rabbit. *(A)* Section of cerebrum with typical granuloma. *(B)* Section of kidney with organisms in cells and free in tubule. (From Møller 1968.)

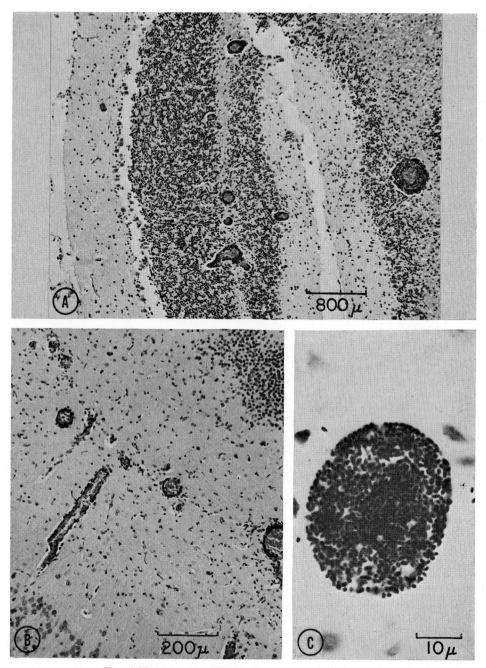

FIG. 3.29. Nosematosis in the mouse. *(A)* Cerebellum. Note several vessels with marked perivascular cuffing. *(B)* Hippocampus. Note perivascular cuffing. *(C)* Pseudocyst in brain. Note absence of wall. (From Innes et al. 1962. Courtesy of Journal of Neuropathology and Experimental Neurology.)

od of transmission. Congenital infection occurs in the mouse and probably in the rat, rabbit, and dog (Innes et al. 1962; Levine 1961a; Perrin 1943a). The organism is excreted in the urine and can be transmitted experimentally by parenteral inoculation of infected tissues (Perrin 1943a). Transmission by cannibalism of infected animals has also been suggested (Weiser 1965).

PATHOLOGIC EFFECTS

Nosema cuniculi usually does not cause a clinical disease, but encephalitis and nephritis sometimes occur in the rabbit and rarely in the young dog (Innes and Saunders 1962; Møller 1968; Tuffery and Innes 1963; Yost 1958). Signs in the rabbit, when they occur, are circling, paralysis, and death. Signs in the mouse and rat are absent in natural infections, but abdominal enlargement and ascites occur in experimental infection (Innes et al. 1962).

Gross lesions are rare and have been reported only in the acute disease in the rabbit. They consist of renal enlargement with gray streaks in the cortex and medulla (Møller 1968).

Microscopic lesions occur in all susceptible species. In the rabbit, they consist of focal granulomas and microglial nodules of the cerebrum, cerebellum, midbrain, and pons (Fig. 3.28*A*) (Innes and Saunders 1962; Innes et al. 1962; Møller 1968). Perivascular cuffing, focal infiltrations, and mild meningitis sometimes occur, but diffuse brain lesions are uncommon. Granulomas and lymphocytic infiltrations are also seen in the heart and kidneys (Fig. 3.28*B*), and sometimes a severe focal interstitial nephritis occurs.

Microscopic lesions in the dog are similar to those of the rabbit and consist of encephalitis or meningoencephalomyelitis and interstitial or tubular nephritis (Plowright 1952; Plowright and Yeoman 1952).

Microscopic lesions in the mouse consist of a chronic, diffuse meningoencephalitis (Fig. 3.29) (Innes et al. 1962). Perivascular infiltration and microglial nodules are common, but granulomas are rare.

These lesions occur in over 50% of the mice in affected colonies. Similar lesions also occur in the lungs, kidneys, adrenal glands, and other tissues. Mortality is usually extremely low.

DIAGNOSIS

Diagnosis is made by identifying the lesions and pseudocysts. Intraperitoneal inoculation of mice is also useful and typically produces abdominal enlargement and ascites. *Nosema cuniculi* is differentiated from *Toxoplasma gondii* on the basis of structural and staining characteristics (Frenkel 1956; Innes et al. 1962; Lainson 1954; Perrin 1943a). Trophozoites of *N. cuniculi* are rod shaped and smaller than those of *T. gondii*. They stain poorly with hematoxylin and eosin; those of *T. gondii* stain moderately well. *Nosema cuniculi* trophozoites stain dark red with carbol fuchsin-methylene blue, purple with carbol fuchsin, and blue with Giemsa-colophonium; those of *T. gondii* stain blue with carbol fuchsin-methylene blue, but do not stain with carbol fuchsin or Giemsa-colophonium. Pseudocysts of *N. cuniculi* are irregular in form and do not have a cyst wall; those of *T. gondii* are spherical with a well-defined cyst wall.

CONTROL

No treatment is reported. Because of the uncertainty of the method of transmission, definitive control measures cannot be recommended. Good sanitation and elimination of infected breeding stock should be helpful. The incidence of infection in the rabbit can be reduced and possibly eliminated by retaining only offspring from females free of the typical neural lesions (Howell and Edington 1968).

PUBLIC HEALTH CONSIDERATIONS

Although *N. cuniculi* has been reported only once from man, care should be taken to avoid infection. Individuals working with laboratory animals should be instructed in proper personal hygiene, and excreta from animals should be handled with caution.

TABLE 3.1. Coccidian parasites affecting endothermal laboratory animals

Parasite	Geographic Distribution	Endothermal Host	Location in Host	Method of Infection	Incidence		Pathologic Effects	Public Health Importance	Reference
					In nature	In laboratory			
Eimeria nieschulzi*	Worldwide	Rat, black rat	Small intestine	Ingestion of oocyst passed in feces	Common	Uncommon or absent	Diarrhea, weakness, emaciation, death	None	Becker 1934; Levine and Ivens 1965a; Pérard 1926
Eimeria separata*	Worldwide	Rat, wild rats	Cecum, colon	Ingestion of oocyst passed in feces	Common	Unknown	Slight enteritis	None	Becker 1934; Levine and Ivens 1965a
Eimeria miyairii*	Worldwide	Rat, possibly black rat	Small intestine	Ingestion of oocyst passed in feces	Uncommon	Unknown	Unknown	None known	Levine and Ivens 1965a
Eimeria falciformis*	Worldwide	Mouse	Intestine	Ingestion of oocyst passed in feces	Common, especially in Europe	Common in some colonies; absent in others	Anorexia, diarrhea, catarrhal enteritis, sometimes death	None	Breza and Jurasek 1959; Cordero del Campillo 1959; Levine and Ivens 1965a; Nieschulz and Bos 1931; Owen 1968
Eimeria ferrisi*	United States	Mouse	Cecum	Ingestion of oocyst passed in feces	Unknown	Unknown	Unknown	None known	Levine and Ivens 1965a
Eimeria hansonorum*	United States	Mouse	Intestine	Ingestion of oocyst passed in feces	Unknown	Unknown	Unknown	None known	Levine and Ivens 1965a
Eimeria hindlei*	USSR	Mouse	Intestine	Ingestion of oocyst passed in feces	Unknown	Unknown	Unknown	None known	Levine and Ivens 1965a
Eimeria keilini*	USSR	Mouse	Intestine	Ingestion of oocyst passed in feces	Unknown	Unknown	Unknown	None known	Levine and Ivens 1965a
Eimeria krijgsmanni*	USSR	Mouse	Intestine	Ingestion of oocyst passed in feces	Unknown	Unknown	Unknown	None known	Levine and Ivens 1965a
Eimeria musculi*	USSR	Mouse	Intestine	Ingestion of oocyst passed in feces	Unknown	Unknown	Unknown	None known	Levine and Ivens 1965a
Eimeria schueffneri*	USSR	Mouse	Intestine	Ingestion of oocyst passed in feces	Unknown	Unknown	Unknown	None known	Levine and Ivens 1965a
Eimeria caviae*	Worldwide	Guinea pig, wild guinea pig (Cavia aperea)	Large intestine	Ingestion of oocyst passed in feces	Unknown	Common in some colonies; absent in others	Usually none; sometimes diarrhea, hemorrhagic enteritis, death	None	Kleeberg and Steenken 1963; Levine and Ivens 1965a; Owen 1968

*Discussed in text.

TABLE 3.1 *(continued)*

Parasite	Geographic Distribution	Endothermal Host	Location in Host	Method of Infection	Incidence In nature	Incidence In laboratory	Pathologic Effects	Public Health Importance	Reference
Eimeria stiedai*	Worldwide	Rabbit, cottontail rabbits, hares	Liver	Ingestion of oocyst passed in feces	Common	Common	Anorexia, weight loss, distended abdomen, hepatomegaly, cirrhosis of liver, hyperplasia of bile duct; sometimes diarrhea, icterus, death	None	Berson-Organisciak 1966 Cook 1969 Levine 1961a Niak 1967 Ostler 1961 Owen 1968 Poole et al. 1967 Ruebner et al. 1965 Seamer and Chesterman 1967 Sevim 1967 Smetana, 1933a, b, c
Eimeria magna*	Worldwide	Rabbit	Jejunum, ileum, sometimes cecum	Ingestion of oocyst passed in feces	Common	Common	Anorexia, weight loss, mucous diarrhea, severe enteritis, sometimes death	None	Horton-Smith 1958 Kheisin 1957 Levine 1961a Lund 1949 Niak 1967 Ostler 1961 Owen 1968 Poole et al. 1967 Seamer and Chesterman 1967 Sevim 1967
Eimeria perforans*	Worldwide	Rabbit	Small intestine	Ingestion of oocyst passed in feces	Common	Common	Mild diarrhea, slight enteritis	None	Horton-Smith 1958 Kheisin 1957 Levine 1961a McPherson et al. 1962 Niak 1967 Ostler 1961 Owen 1968 Poole et al. 1967 Seamer and Chesterman 1967 Sevim 1967
Eimeria media*	Worldwide	Rabbit, cottontail rabbits	Small intestine	Ingestion of oocyst passed in feces	Common	Common	Moderate diarrhea, enteritis	None	Kheisin 1957 Levine 1961a Niak 1967 Ostler 1961 Owen 1968 Pellérdy and Babos 1953 Poole et al. 1967 Seamer and Chesterman 1967 Sevim 1967

* Discussed in text.

TABLE 3.1 *(continued)*

Parasite	Geographic Distribution	Endothermal Host	Location in Host	Method of Infection	Incidence In nature	Incidence In laboratory	Pathologic Effects	Public Health Importance	Reference
*Eimeria irresidua**	Worldwide	Rabbit	Small intestine	Ingestion of oocyst passed in feces	Common	Common	Hemorrhagic diarrhea, severe enteritis	None	Horton-Smith 1958 Kheisin 1957 Levine 1961a Niak 1967 Ostler 1961 Owen 1968 Poole et al. 1967 Seamer and Chesterman 1967 Sevim 1967
*Eimeria piriformis**	Europe, Iran	Rabbit	Cecum, colon	Ingestion of oocyst passed in feces	Uncommon	Uncommon	Unknown	None known	Kheisin 1957 Levine 1961a Niak 1967
*Eimeria coecicola**	Eastern Europe, India	Rabbit	Posterior ileum, cecum	Ingestion of oocyst passed in feces	Common	Rare	Occasional slight enteritis	None known	Gill and Ray 1960 Kheisin 1947a, 1957 Levine 1961a
*Eimeria elongata**	Western Europe	Rabbit	Intestine	Unknown; presumably by ingestion of oocyst passed in feces	Unknown	Unknown	Unknown	None known	Levine 1961a
*Eimeria neoleporis**	North America, India, Iran	Rabbit, cottontail rabbits	Intestine	Unknown; presumably by ingestion of oocyst passed in feces	Unknown	Uncommon	Mild to severe enteritis in cotton-tail rabbits	None known	Carvalho 1942 Gill and Ray 1960 Niak 1967
*Eimeria intestinalis**	Eastern Europe, India	Rabbit	Ileum, cecum, colon	Ingestion of oocyst passed in feces	Uncommon	Unknown	Diarrhea, severe catarrhal enteritis, sometimes death	None known	Kheisin 1957 Levine 1961a Pellérdy 1953, 1954
*Eimeria matsubayashii**	Japan, India	Rabbit	Ileum	Ingestion of oocyst passed in feces	Unknown	Unknown	Fibrino-necrotic enteritis	None known	Gill and Ray 1960 Levine 1961a Tsunoda 1952
*Eimeria nagpurensis**	India, Iran	Rabbit	Intestine	Unknown; presumably by ingestion of oocyst passed in feces	Unknown	Unknown	Unknown	None known	Gill and Ray 1960 Niak 1967
Eimeria canis	North America, Europe, Australia	Dog, cat	Intestine	Ingestion of oocyst passed in feces	Unknown	Unknown	Unknown	None	Levine 1961a

*Discussed in text.

TABLE 3.1 *(continued)*

Parasite	Geographic Distribution	Endothermal Host	Location in Host	Method of Infection	Incidence — In nature	Incidence — In laboratory	Pathologic Effects	Public Health Importance	Reference
Eimeria cati	USSR	Dog, cat	Intestine	Ingestion of oocyst passed in feces	Rare	Unknown	Unknown	None	Levine 1961a
Eimeria felina	Europe	Cat, other felids	Unknown	Ingestion of oocyst passed in feces	Rare	Unknown	Unknown	None	Levine 1961a
Eimeria galago	Africa	Galago	Intestine	Unknown; presumably by ingestion of oocyst passed in feces	Rare	Rare or absent	Unknown	None known	Poelma 1966
Eimeria lemuris	Africa	Galago	Intestine	Unknown; presumably by ingestion of oocyst passed in feces	Rare	Rare or absent	Unknown	None known	Poelma 1966
Eimeria otolicni	Africa	Galago	Intestine	Unknown; presumably by ingestion of oocyst passed in feces	Rare	Rare or absent	Unknown	None know	Poelma 1966
*Eimeria tenella**	Worldwide	Chicken	Ceca	Ingestion of oocyst passed in feces	Common	Uncommon	Severe hemorrhagic diarrhea, listlessness, anorexia, fibrinonecrotic enteritis, death	None	Levine 1961a
*Eimeria necatrix**	Worldwide	Chicken	Small intestine, ceca	Ingestion of oocyst passed in feces	Common	Uncommon	Diarrhea, enteritis	None	Levine 1961a
*Eimeria brunetti**	Worldwide	Chicken	Lower small intestine, colon	Ingestion of oocyst passed in feces	Uncommon	Uncommon	Necrotic enteritis	None	Levine 1961a
*Eimeria acervulina**	Worldwide	Chicken	Small intestine	Ingestion of oocyst passed in feces	Common	Uncommon	Slight enteritis	None	Levine 1961a
*Eimeria maxima**	Worldwide	Chicken	Small intestine	Ingestion of oocyst passed in feces	Common	Uncommon	Slight to moderate enteritis	None	Levine 1961a
*Eimeria mitis**	Worldwide	Chicken	Small intestine	Ingestion of oocyst passed in feces	Common	Uncommon	Sometimes slight enteritis	None	Levine 1961a

*Discussed in text.

TABLE 3.1 *(continued)*

Parasite	Geographic Distribution	Endothermal Host	Location in Host	Method of Infection	Incidence		Pathologic Effects	Public Health Importance	Reference
					In nature	In laboratory			
*Eimeria praecox**	Worldwide	Chicken	Small intestine	Ingestion of oocyst passed in feces	Common	Uncommon	None	None	Levine 1961a
*Eimeria hagani**	Worldwide	Chicken	Small intestine	Ingestion of oocyst passed in feces	Uncommon	Uncommon	Slight enteritis	None	Levine 1961a
*Eimeria mivati**	Worldwide	Chicken	Intestine	Ingestion of oocyst passed in feces	Common	Uncommon	Mild enteritis, sometimes death	None	Edgar and Seibold 1964
Eimeria labbeana	Worldwide	Pigeon	Intestine	Ingestion of oocyst passed in feces	Common	Rare or absent	Enteritis, sometimes death	None	Levine 1961a
*Isospora bigemina**	Worldwide	Dog, cat, other carnivores	Small intestine	Ingestion of oocyst passed in feces	Common	Common in dogs obtained from pounds; uncommon in dogs obtained from some kennels	Mild to severe enteritis, diarrhea, anorexia, listlessness, weight loss, sometimes death	None known	Burrows and Lillis 1967 Johnson et al. 1963 Levine 1961a
*Isospora rivolta**	Worldwide	Dog, cat, other carnivores	Small intestine, sometimes cecum, colon	Ingestion of oocyst passed in feces	Common	Common in dogs obtained from pounds; uncommon in dogs obtained from some kennels	None known	None known	Burrows and Lillis 1967 Levine 1961a Mahrt 1966, 1967 Scott 1967
*Isospora canis**	Worldwide	Dog	Small intestine	Ingestion of oocyst passed in feces	Common	Common	Unknown; possibly diarrhea	None	Burrows and Lillis 1967 Levine and Ivens 1965b Neméséri 1959
*Isospora felis**	Worldwide	Cat, other carnivores	Small intestine, sometimes cecum, colon	Ingestion of oocyst passed in feces	Common	Common	Usually none; sometimes severe enteritis, diarrhea, emaciation, death	None	Levine 1961a Shah 1969
*Isospora ratti**	Central United States	Rat	Intestine	Unknown; presumably by ingestion of oocyst passed in feces	Unknown	Unknown	Unknown	Unknown	Levine and Ivens 1965a

*Discussed in text,

TABLE 3.1 (continued)

Parasite	Geographic Distribution	Endothermal Host	Location in Host	Method of Infection	Incidence In nature	Incidence In laboratory	Pathologic Effects	Public Health Importance	Reference
Isospora arctopitheci*	South America	Marmosets	Intestine	Ingestion of oocyst passed in feces	Rare	Rare or absent	Unknown	None known	Rodhain 1933
Isospora sp.	Africa	Galago	Intestine	Unknown; presumably by ingestion of oocyst passed in feces	Rare	Rare or absent	Unknown	None known	Poelma 1966
Cryptosporidium muris*	United States	Mouse	Stomach	Unknown; presumably by ingestion of oocyst passed in feces	Unknown	Rare	Slight gastritis	None known	Levine and Ivens 1965a Tyzzer 1910
Cryptosporidium parvum*	United States	Mouse	Small intestine	Unknown; presumably by ingestion of oocyst passed in feces	Unknown	Rare	Insignificant	None known	Hampton and Rosario 1966 Levine and Ivens 1965a Tyzzer 1912
Cryptosporidium sp.*	Eastern United States	Guinea pig	Small intestine	Unknown; presumably by ingestion of oocyst passed in feces	Unknown	Rare	Slight enteritis	None known	Jervis et al. 1966
Klossiella muris*	Worldwide	Mouse	Kidneys	Ingestion of sporocysts passed in urine	Rare	Common in some colonies; absent in others	Usually none; sometimes necrotic foci in kidneys, enlargement of kidneys	None known	Levine and Ivens 1965a Otto 1957 Smith and Johnson 1902 Yang and Grice 1964

*Discussed in text.

92

TABLE 3.1 *(continued)*

Parasite	Geographic Distribution	Endothermal Host	Location in Host	Method of Infection	Incidence In nature	Incidence In laboratory	Pathologic Effects	Public Health Importance	Reference
Klossiella cobayae*	Worldwide	Guinea pig	Kidneys, lungs, spleen, other organs	Ingestion of sporocysts passed in urine	Rare	Common in some colonies; absent in others	Usually none; sometimes nephritis	None	Bonciu et al. 1957 Cossel 1958 Levine and Ivens 1965a
Hepatozoon muris*	Worldwide	Rat, black rat	Lymphocytes, liver parenchyma	Ingestion of mite vector	Common	Rare	Usually none; possibly anemia, emaciation	None	Eyles 1952 Kusama et al. 1919 Laird 1959 Levine 1961a Miller 1908 Prakash 1954
Hepatozoon musculi*	Great Britain	Mouse	Lymphocytes, bone marrow	Unknown	Unknown	Unknown	Unknown	None known	Porter 1908
Hepatozoon microti*	Central Europe	Mouse	Unknown	Unknown	Unknown	Unknown	Unknown	None known	Erhardova 1955
Hepatozoon cuniculi*	Italy	Rabbit	Leucocytes, spleen	Unknown	Unknown	Unknown	Unknown	None known	Sangiorgi 1914
Hepatozoon canis*	Southern Europe, Asia, Africa	Dog, cat, wild carnivores	Leucocytes, spleen, bone marrow, liver	Ingestion of tick vector	Unknown	Unknown	Usually none; sometimes fever, anemia, emaciation, spleno-megaly, death	None	Levine 1961a
Haemogregarina cynomolgi	Central Africa	Rhesus monkey, baboons	Blood	Unknown	Unknown	Unknown	Unknown	Unknown	Blanchard and Langeron 1913 Langeron 1920 Leger and Bédier 1922 Wenyon 1926

* Discussed in text.

TABLE 3.2. Malarial parasites of endothermal laboratory animals

Parasite	Geographic Distribution	Endothermal Host	Location in Host	Method of Infection	Incidence		Pathologic Effects	Public Health Importance	Reference
					In nature	In laboratory			
*Plasmodium cynomolgi**	Asia	Cynomolgus monkey, pigtail macaque, bonnet monkey, other macaques, leaf monkeys, man	Erythrocytes	Mosquito bite	Common	Common in monkeys obtained from endemic areas	Mild to moderate tertian malaria; anorexia, weakness, listlessness, fever, splenomegaly, hepatic congestion	Causes tertian malaria; accidental laboratory infection reported	Bray 1963b Conran 1967 Eyles 1963 Eyles et al. 1960, 1962c Garnham 1959 Schmidt et al. 1961a, b
*Plasmodium knowlesi**	Malay Peninsula, Philippine Islands, Taiwan	Cynomolgus monkeys, pigtail macaque, other macaques, leaf monkeys, man	Erythrocytes	Mosquito bite	Common in cynomolgus monkey; uncommon in other monkeys	Unknown; probably common in cynomolgus monkeys obtained from endemic areas; uncommon in other monkeys	Quotidian malaria	Causes quotidian malaria; natural infection reported	Chin et al. 1965 Eyles et al. 1962c Garnham 1963a Lambrecht et al. 1961 Schmidt et al. 1961b
*Plasmodium inui**	Southern Asia, Indonesia, Philippine Islands, Taiwan	Cynomolgus monkey, bonnet monkey, pigtail macaque, other macaques, man	Erythrocytes	Mosquito bite	Common	Unknown; probably common in monkeys obtained from endemic areas	Quartan malaria	Causes quartan malaria; experimentally transmissible to man	Bray 1963b Eyles 1963 Eyles and Warren 1962 Howard and Cabrera 1961 Lambrecht et al. 1961 Shortt et al. 1961 Sinton 1934
*Plasmodium coatneyi**	Malay Peninsula	Macques	Erythrocytes	Mosquito bite	Unknown	Unknown	Tertian malaria	None known	Eyles 1963 Eyles et al. 1962a Warren and Wharton 1963
Plasmodium fieldi	Malay Peninsula	Pigtail macaque	Erythrocytes	Mosquito bite	Unknown	Unknown	Mild tertian malaria	None known	Eyles 1963 Eyles et al. 1962b Held et al. 1967
Plasmodium sp.	India	Macaques	Erythrocytes	Unknown; presumably mosquito bite	Unknown	Unknown	Unknown	None known	Eyles 1963
Plasmodium pitheci	Indonesia	Orangutan	Erythrocytes	Unknown; presumably mosquito bite	Unknown	Unknown	Tertian malaria	None known	Halberstädter and von Prowazek 1907

*Discussed in text.

94

TABLE 3.2 *(continued)*

Parasite	Geographic Distribution	Endothermal Host	Location in Host	Method of Infection	Incidence — In nature	Incidence — In laboratory	Pathologic Effects	Public Health Importance	Reference
Plasmodium hylobati	Indonesia	Gibbon	Erythrocytes	Unknown; presumably mosquito bite	Unknown	Unknown	Quartan malaria	None known	Bray 1963c; Rodhain 1941
Plasmodium jefferyi	Malay Peninsula	Gibbon	Erythrocytes	Mosquito bite	Unknown	Unknown	Mild to moderate tertian malaria	None known	Warren et al. 1966
Plasmodium youngi	Malay Peninsula	Gibbon	Erythrocytes	Mosquito bite	Unknown	Unknown	Severe tertian malaria	None known	Eyles et al. 1964
Plasmodium eylesi	Malay Peninsula	Gibbon	Erythrocytes	Mosquito bite	Unknown	Unknown	Mild to moderate tertian malaria	None known	Warren et al. 1965
*Plasmodium gonderi**	West central Africa	Mangabeys, mandrills	Erythrocytes	Mosquito bite	Common	Unknown; probably common in monkeys obtained from endemic area	Mild tertian malaria	None known	Bray 1959; Garnham et al. 1958; Rodhain and van den Berghe 1936
*Plasmodium malariae**	Africa	Chimpanzee, man	Erythrocytes	Mosquito bite	Common	Unknown; probably common in chimpanzees obtained from endemic area	Quartan malaria	Causes quartan malaria; cross transmission between chimpanzee and man demonstrated	Bray 1959, 1960; Garnham et al. 1956; Rodhain 1948; Rodhain and Dellaert 1943
*Plasmodium reichenowi**	Africa	Chimpanzee, gorilla	Erythrocytes	Mosquito bite	Unknown	Unknown	Mild tertian malaria	Probably none	Bray 1956, 1957b, 1963c; Garnham et al. 1956; Reichenow 1949–1953
*Plasmodium schwetzi**	Africa	Chimpanzee, gorilla	Erythrocytes	Mosquito bite	Unknown	Unknown	Mild tertian malaria	Experimentally transmissible to man; causes tertian malaria	Bray 1958, 1963b; Rodhain and Dellaert 1955
Plasmodium girardi	Madagascar	Lemurs	Erythrocytes	Unknown; presumably mosquito bite	Unknown	Unknown	Mild quartan malaria	None known	Bück et al. 1952

*Discussed in text.

TABLE 3.2 *(continued)*

Parasite	Geographic Distribution	Endothermal Host	Location in Host	Method of Infection	Incidence In nature	Incidence In laboratory	Pathologic Effects	Public Health Importance	Reference
Plasmodium lemuris	Madagascar	Lemurs	Erythrocytes	Unknown; presumably mosquito bite	Unknown	Unknown	Unknown	None known	Huff and Hoogstraal 1963
Plasmodium fragile	India, Ceylon	Stumptailed macaque, toque monkey (*Macaca sinica*)	Erythrocytes	Unknown; presumably mosquito bite	Unknown	Unknown	Tertian malaria	None known	Dissanaike et al. 1965
Plasmodium simiovale	Ceylon	Toque monkey (*Macaca sinica*)	Erythrocytes	Mosquito bite	Unknown	Unknown	Tertian malaria	None known	Dissanaike et al. 1965
Plasmodium brasilianum*	Mexico, Central America, South America	Howler monkeys, spider monkeys, capuchins, squirrel monkeys, uakaris, woolly monkeys	Erythrocytes	Mosquito bite	Common	Common in monkeys obtained from endemic areas	Mild to severe quartan malaria	Experimentally transmissible to man; causes mild parasitemia	Dunn 1965 Dunn and Lambrecht 1963 Porter et al. 1966 Taliaferro and Taliaferro 1934
Plasmodium simium*	Brazil	Howler monkeys, man	Erythrocytes	Mosquito bite	Common	Common in monkeys obtained from endemic areas	Tertian malaria	Causes tertian malaria; reported once	Deane et al. 1966 da Fonseca 1951 Garnham 1963b
Plasmodium berghei*	Central Africa	Tree rat (*Thamnomys surdaster*)	Erythrocytes	Mosquito bite	Unknown	Experimental only	Severe malaria in mouse; mild malaria in rat	None	Vincke and Lips 1948
Plasmodium vinckei*	Central Africa	Unknown	Erythrocytes	Mosquito bite	Unknown	Experimental only	Severe malaria in mouse	None	Rodhain 1952
Plasmodium chabaudi*	Central Africa	Tree rat (*Thamnomys rutilans*)	Erythrocytes	Mosquito bite	Unknown	Experimental only	Malaria in mouse	None	Landau 1965 Ott and Stauber 1967
Plasmodium inopinatum*	Belgium	Rat	Erythrocytes	Mosquito bite	Unknown	Experimental only	Malaria in mouse, rat, hamster	None	Resseler 1956
Plasmodium gallinaceum	Asia	Chicken	Erythrocytes	Mosquito bite	Unknown	Unknown	Anemia, high mortality	None	Levine 1961a

*Discussed in text.

96

TABLE 3.2 (continued)

Parasite	Geographic Distribution	Endothermal Host	Location in Host	Method of Infection	Incidence — In nature	Incidence — In laboratory	Pathologic Effects	Public Health Importance	Reference
Plasmodium juxtanucleare	Mexico, South America, Japan, Philippine Islands	Chicken	Erythrocytes	Mosquito bite	Unknown	Unknown	Anemia, high mortality	None	Itagaki and Tsubokura, 1968a, b; Levine 1961a; Manuel 1967
Hepatocystis kochi*	Central Africa	Green monkey, other guenons, mangabeys, baboons	Erythrocytes	Bite of midge	Common in endemic areas	Common in specimens obtained from endemic areas	Foci in liver; no clinical signs	None	Aberle 1945; Bray 1959; Garnham 1947, 1948; Garnham et al. 1961; Kuntz and Myers 1967; Lefrou and Martignoles 1955; Miller 1959; Pietrzyk and Uminski 1967; Strong et al. 1965; Vickers 1966
Hepatocystis semnopitheci	Southeastern Asia, Indonesia	Cynomolgus monkey, pigtail macaque, other macaques, leaf monkeys	Erythrocytes	Unknown	Unknown	Unknown	Unknown	None	Eyles and Warren 1962, 1963; Knowles 1919; Poisson 1953; Reichenow 1949–1953
Hepatocystis taiwanensis	Taiwan	Macaques	Erythrocytes	Unknown	Unknown	Unknown	Unknown	None	Bray 1963b
Hepatocystis foleyi	Madagascar	Lemurs	Erythrocytes	Unknown	Unknown	Unknown	Mild tertian malaria	None	Bray 1963b; Bück et al. 1952
Sergentella anthropopitheci	Western Africa	Chimpanzee	Blood	Unknown	Rare	Unknown	None	None	Deschiens et al. 1927
Leucocytozoon sabrazesi	Southeastern Asia, Indonesia	Chicken	Leucocytes, erythrocytes	Unknown; probably bite of midge	Unknown	Unknown	Anemia, fever, diarrhea	None	Levine 1961a
Leucocytozoon caulleryi	Eastern United States, southeastern Asia, Indonesia	Chicken	Leucocytes, erythrocytes	Unknown; probably bite of midge	Unknown	Unknown	Uncertain; perhaps anemia, fever, diarrhea	None	Levine 1961a
Haemoproteus columbae	Worldwide	Pigeon	Erythrocytes	Bite of pigeon ked (Pseudolynchia canariensis)	Common	Rare or absent	Generally inapparent; sometimes anorexia, anemia, splenomegaly	None	Baker 1967; Levine 1961a

*Discussed in text.

97

TABLE 3.3. Toxoplasmasids affecting endothermal laboratory animals

Parasite	Geographic Distribution	Endothermal Host	Location in Host	Method of Infection	Incidence — In nature	Incidence — In laboratory	Pathologic Effects	Public Health Importance	Reference
Sarcocystis muris[*]	Worldwide	Mouse, rat, black rat	Striated muscle, smooth muscle	Ingestion of trophozoites in muscle or passed in feces	Rare in mouse; common in rat	Rare in some colonies; absent in others	Cysts in muscle; usually no clinical signs	Unknown; sarcocystiasis occurs in man but is rare	Boncitu et al. 1958 Deschiens et al. 1957 Krampitz 1957 Levine 1961a
Sarcocystis cuniculi[*]	Worldwide	Rabbit, cottontail rabbit	Striated muscle, smooth muscle	Ingestion of trophozoites in muscle or passed in feces	Uncommon in rabbit; common in cottontail rabbit	Uncommon or rare in rabbit	Cysts in muscle; usually no clinical signs	Unknown; sarcocystiasis occurs in man but is rare	Deschiens et al. 1957 Erickson 1946 Levine 1961a Morgan and Waller 1940
Sarcocystis sp.[*]	Worldwide	Dog, cat, domestic animals	Striated muscle, smooth muscle	Ingestion of trophozoites in muscle or passed in feces	Common in cat; rare in dog	Common in cat; rare in dog	Cysts in muscle; usually no clinical signs	Unknown; sarcocystiasis occurs in man but is rare	Eisenstein and Innes 1956
Sarcocystis kortei[*]	Worldwide	Rhesus monkey	Striated muscle, smooth muscle	Ingestion of trophozoites in muscle or passed in feces	Uncommon	Uncommon	Cysts in muscle; usually no clinical signs	Unknown; sarcocystiasis occurs in man but is rare	Dubin and Wilcox 1947 Habermann and Williams 1957 Hartman 1961 de Korté 1905 Mandour 1969 Offutt and Telford 1945
Sarcocystis nesbitti[*]	India	Rhesus monkey	Striated muscle	Unknown; presumably by ingestion of trophozoites in muscle or passed in feces	Uncommon	Uncommon	Cysts in muscle; usually no clinical signs	Unknown; sarcocystiasis occurs in man but is rare	Mandour 1969
Sarcocystis sp.[*]	East central Africa	Baboons	Striated muscle	Unknown; presumably by ingestion of trophozoites in muscle or passed in feces	Uncommon	Uncommon	Cysts in muscle; usually no clinical signs	Unknown; sarcocystiasis occurs in man but is rare	Strong et al. 1965
Sarcocystis sp.[*]	South America	Woolly monkeys	Striated muscle	Unknown; presumably by ingestion of trophozoites in muscle or passed in feces	Uncommon	Uncommon	Cysts in muscle; usually no clinical signs	Unknown; sarcocystiasis occurs in man but is rare	Henderson and Bullock 1968

[*]Discussed in text.

98

TABLE 3.3 (continued)

Parasite	Geographic Distribution	Endothermal Host	Location in Host	Method of Infection	Incidence — In nature	Incidence — In laboratory	Pathologic Effects	Public Health Importance	Reference
Sarcocystis sp.*	South America	Squirrel monkeys, spider monkeys, tamarins, marmosets	Striated muscle, smooth muscle	Unknown; presumably by ingestion of trophozoites in muscle or passed in feces	Common	Common in monkeys obtained from endemic areas	Cysts in muscle; usually no clinical signs	Unknown; sarcocystiasis occurs in man but is rare	Nelson et al. 1966
Sarcocystis rileyi	Worldwide	Chicken, duck, wild birds	Striated muscle, smooth muscle	Ingestion of trophozoites in muscle or passed in feces	Uncommon in chicken	Uncommon or absent	Cysts in muscle; usually no clinical signs	Unknown; sarcocystiasis occurs in man but is rare	Levine 1961a
*Toxoplasma gondii**	Worldwide	Mouse, rat, black rat, guinea pig, other rodents, rabbit, hares, dog, cat, other carnivores, squirrel monkeys, capuchins, marmosets, other primates, chicken, other birds, domestic animals, man	Brain, lungs, liver, heart, kidneys, lymph nodes, blood, other tissues	Ingestion of trophozoites or oocysts in tissues, feces; transplacentally; usual method unknown	Common in dog; uncommon in rodents, lagomorphs, primates	Common in dog and cat; common in some rodent colonies; uncommon or absent in others	Inapparent to fatal disease with varied signs including fever, cough, anorexia, weakness, depression, ocular discharge, nasal discharge, leukopenia, dyspnea, vomiting, diarrhea, convulsions, death	Causes toxoplasmosis in man; uncommon	Bjotvedt 1964 Conroy 1964 Dubey 1968a Galuzo 1966 Galuzo and Zasukhin 1963 Gibson and Eyles 1957 Lainson 1955, 1957 Levine 1961a, b McKissick et al. 1968 Miller and Feldman 1953 Moller 1968 Orio et al. 1959 Stolz 1962 Szemeredi 1968 van Thiel 1964 Work 1969
*Besnoitia jellisoni**	United States	Deer mice, kangaroo rats, opossum	Subcutis, other connective tissues, serosal membranes, cranial dural venous sinuses	Unknown	Unknown; probably rare	Unknown; probably rare	Acute, fatal, or chronic disease	Unknown	Ernst et al. 1968 Frenkel 1953 Stabler and Welch 1961

*Discussed in text.

TABLE 3.4. Piroplasmasids affecting endothermal laboratory animals

Parasite	Geographic Distribution	Endothermal Host	Location in Host	Method of Infection	Incidence		Pathologic Effects	Public Health Importance	Reference
					In nature	In laboratory			
*Babesia decumani**	Africa, southern Asia	Rat, black rat	Erythrocytes	Unknown; presumably by tick bite	Common	Unknown; probably rare or absent	Renal degeneration, hemoglobinuria, sometimes death	None	Capponi et al. 1955 Macfie 1915 Prakash 1954 Sureau and Capponi 1955
Babesia muris	Great Britain	Rat	Erythrocytes	Unknown; presumably by tick bite	Unknown	Unknown; probably rare or absent	Unknown	None	Fantham 1905, 1906
*Babesia rodhaini**	Africa	Tree rat (*Thamnomys surdaster*)	Erythrocytes	Unknown; presumably by tick bite	Unknown	Experimental only	Hemolytic anemia, reticulo-endothelial hyperplasia, liver necrosis, hematuria	None	van den Berghe et al. 1950 Paget et al. 1962 Rodhain 1950 Rudzinska and Trager 1962
*Babesia canis**	Worldwide in tropics and subtropics	Dog, other canids	Erythrocytes	Tick bite	Common in tropics	Rare	Fever, anemia, icterus, anorexia, weakness, hemoglobinuria, splenomegaly, hepatomegaly, death	None	Dorner 1969 Hirsh et al. 1969 Levine 1961a Riek 1968 Rokey 1968 Rokey and Russell 1961 Seibold and Bailey 1957
Babesia vogeli	Southern Asia, northern Africa	Dog	Erythrocytes	Tick bite	Unknown	Unknown	Fever, listlessness, anemia, icterus	None	Levine 1961a Riek 1968

*Discussed in text.

TABLE 3.4 *(continued)*

Parasite	Geographic Distribution	Endothermal Host	Location in Host	Method of Infection	Incidence In nature	Incidence In laboratory	Pathologic Effects	Public Health Importance	Reference
Babesia gibsoni	Asia, northern Africa	Dog, other canids	Erythrocytes	Tick bite	Unknown	Unknown	Anemia, listlessness	None	Groves and Yap 1968 Levine 1961a Riek 1968
Babesia felis	Southern Africa, India	Cat, wild felids	Erythrocytes	Unknown; presumably by tick bite	Unknown	Unknown	Anemia, listlessness	None	Levine 1961a
*Babesia pitheci**	Europe, Africa	Macaques, guenons, mangabeys, baboons	Erythrocytes	Unknown; presumably by tick bite	Unknown	Unknown	Usually none; anemia after splenectomy	None known	Garnham 1950 Hill 1953, 1954 Kikuth 1927 Ross 1905 Tanguy 1937
Aegyptianella pullorum	Southeastern Europe, Asia, Africa	Chicken, other birds	Erythrocytes	Tick bite	Unknown	Unknown	Anemia, fever, icterus, diarrhea, anorexia	None	Ahmed and Soliman 1966 Levine 1961a
Aegyptianella moshkovski	Asia, northern Africa	Chicken, other birds	Erythrocytes	Unknown; presumably by tick bite	Unknown	Unknown	Unknown	None	Levine 1961a
*Entopolypoides macaci**	Africa, Indonesia	Cynomolgus monkey, green monkey	Erythrocytes	Unknown; presumably by tick bite	Unknown	Unknown	Sometimes anemia	None known	Fairbairn 1948 Mayer 1933, 1934
Theileria cellii	Ceylon	Macaques	Erythrocytes	Unknown; presumably by tick bite	Unknown	Unknown	Unknown	None known	Castellani and Chalmers 1910, 1913

*Discussed in text.

TABLE 3.5. Neosporans affecting endothermal laboratory animals

Parasite	Geographic Distribution	Endothermal Host	Location in Host	Method of Infection	Incidence		Pathologic Effects	Public Health Importance	Reference
					In nature	In laboratory			
*Nosema cuniculi**	Worldwide	Mouse, rat, hamster, multimammate mouse, guinea pig, rabbit, cottontail rabbits, dog, man	Brain, kidneys, heart, lungs, adrenals, other tissues	Transplacentally; otherwise unknown	Common in rabbit; uncommon in other species	Common in some rodent and rabbit colonies; uncommon in others	Usually inapparent; sometimes encephalitis, nephritis, death	Causes nosematosis; reported once	Frenkel 1956 Innes et al. 1962 Koller 1969 Lainson 1954 Levine 1961a Malherbe and Munday 1958 Moller 1968 Nelson 1962 Perrin 1943a, b Tuffery and Innes 1963 Weiser, 1965 Yost 1958

*Discussed in text.

REFERENCES

Aberle, Sophie D. 1945. Primate malaria. Natl. Acad. Sci.–Natl. Res. Council Publ., Wash., D.C. 171 pp.

Ahmed, A. A. S., and M. K. Soliman. 1966. Observations made during a natural outbreak of aegyptianellosis in chickens. Avian Diseases 10:390–93.

Baker, J. R. 1967. A review of the role played by the *Hippoboscidae* (Diptera) as vectors of endoparasites. J. Parasitol. 53:412–18.

Becker, E. R. 1934. Coccidia and coccidiosis of domesticated game and laboratory animals and of man. Collegiate Press, Ames, Ia. 147 pp.

Becker, E. R., Phoebe R. Hall, and Anna Hager. 1932. Quantitative, biometric and host-parasite studies on *Eimeria miyairii* and *Eimeria separata* in rats. Iowa State Coll. J. Sci. 6:299–316.

Berghe, L. van den, I. H. Vincke, M. Chardome, and M. van den Bulcke. 1950. *Babesia rodhaini* n. sp. d'un rongeur du Congo Belge transmissible à la souris blanche. Ann. Soc. Belge Med. Trop. 30:83–86.

Berson-Organiściak, Janina. 1966. Kokcydioza niektórych zwierzat laboratoryjnych i jej zwalczanie. Zwierzeta Lab. 2:215–21.

Beverley, J. K. A. 1959. Congenital transmission of toxoplasmosis through successive generations of mice. Nature 183:1348–49.

Beye, H. K., M. E. Getz, G. R. Coatney, H. A. Elder, and D. E. Eyles. 1961. Simian malaria in man. Am. J. Trop. Med. Hyg. 10:311–16.

Bjotvedt, G. 1964. The nature and variety of diseases of laboratory animals. Vet. Scope 9:14–24.

Blanchard, R., and M. Langeron. 1913. Le paludisme des macaques (*Plasmodium cynomolgi* Mayer, 1907). Arch. Parasitol. 15:529–42.

Boch, J. 1957. Versuche zur Behandlung der Kaninchenkokzidiose mit Nitrofurazon (Furacin-W). Muench. Tieraerztl. Wochschr. 70:264–67.

Bonciu, C., B. Clecner, A. Greceanu, and A. Margineanu. 1957. Contribution à l'étude de l'infection naturelle des cobayes avec des sporozoaires du genre Klossiella. Arch. Roumaines Pathol. Exp. Microbiol. 16:131–43.

Bonciu, C., M. Dincolesco, and Monica Petrovici. 1958. Contribution à l'étude de la maladie d'Armstrong chez la souris blanche. Arch. Roumaines Pathol. Exp. Microbiol. 17:455–70.

Bray, R. S. 1956. Studies on malaria in chimpanzees: I. The erythrocytic forms of *Plasmodium reichenowi*. J. Parasitol. 42:588–92.

———. 1957a. Additional notes on the tissue stages of *Plasmodium cynomolgi*. Trans. Roy. Soc. Trop. Med. Hyg. 51:248–52.

———. 1957b. Studies on malaria in chimpanzees: III. Gametogony of *Plasmodium reichenowi*. Ann. Soc. Belge Med. Trop. 37:169–74.

———. 1958. Studies on malaria in chimpanzees: V. The sporogonous cycle and mosquito transmission of *Plasmodium vivax schwetzi*. J. Parasitol. 44:46–51.

———. 1959. Pre-erythrocytic stages of human malaria parasites: *Plasmodium malariae*. Brit. Med. J. 1959-2:679–80.

———. 1960. Studies on malaria in chimpanzees: VIII. The experimental transmission and pre-erythrocytic phase of *Plasmodium malariae*, with a note on the host-range of the parasite. Am. J. Trop. Med. Hyg. 9:455–65.

———. 1963a. The exoerythrocytic phase of malaria parasites. Intern. Rev. Trop. Med. 2:41–74.

———. 1963b. Malaria infections in primates and their importance to man. Ergeb. Mikrobiol. Immunitätsfor. Exp. Therap. 36:168–213.

———. 1963c. The malaria parasites of anthropoid apes. J. Parasitol. 49:888–91.

Breza, M., and V. Jurasek. 1959. Prispevok k vyznamu kokidiozy ako pricine hynutia laboratornych mysi. Vet. Casopis 8:372–78.

Bück, G., J. Courdurier, and J. J. Quesnel. 1952. Sur deux nouveaux plasmodium observés chez un lémurien de Madagascar splénectomisé. Arch. Inst. Pasteur Algerie 30:240–43.

Burrows, R. B., and W. G. Lillis. 1967. Intestinal protozoan infections in dogs. J. Am. Vet. Med. Assoc. 150:880–83.

Calero, M. C. 1952. Incidence of *Trypanosoma lewisi*, *Sarcocystis muris*, species of *Spirochaeta* and mirofilarial larvae in rats in Panama City and suburbs. J. Parasitol. 38:369.

Calhoon, J. R., and P. J. Matthews. 1964. A method for initiating a colony of pathogen-free guinea pigs. Lab. Animal Care 14:388–94.

Capponi, M., P. Sureau, and R. Deschiens. 1955. Présentation d'un hématozoaire observé dans le sang de *Mus norvegicus* au centre Vietnam. Bull. Soc. Pathol. Exotique 48:649–51.

Carvalho, J. C. M. 1942. *Eimeria neoleporis* n. sp., occurring naturally in the cottontail and transmissible to the tame rabbit. Iowa State Coll. J. Sci. 16:409–10.

Castellani, A., and A. J. Chalmers. 1910. Manual of tropical medicine. Baillière, Tindall and Cox, London. 1265 pp.

———. 1913. Manual of tropical medicine. 2d ed. Baillière, Tindall and Cox, London. 1779 pp.

Chandler, A. C., and C. P. Read. 1961. Introduction to parasitology. 10th ed. John Wiley, New York. 822 pp.

Chin, W., P. G. Contacos, G. R. Coatney, and H. R. Kimball. 1965. A naturally acquired quotidian-type malaria in man transferable to monkeys. Science 149:865.

Chordi, A., K. W. Walls, and I. G. Kagan. 1964. Studies on the specificity of the indirect hemagglutination test for toxoplasmosis. J. Immunol. 93:1024–33.

Clark, H. C. 1930. A preliminary report on some parasites in the blood of wild monkeys of Panama. Am. J. Trop. Med. 10:25–41.

———. 1931. Progress in the survey for blood parasites of the wild monkeys of Panama. Am. J. Trop. Med. 11:11–20.

Coatney, G. R. W. Chin, P. G. Contacos, and H. K. King. 1966. Plasmodium inui, a quartan-type malaria parasite of Old World monkeys transmissible to man. J. Parasitol. 52:660–63.

Coatney, G. R., H. A. Elder, P. G. Contacos, M. E. Getz, R. Greenland, R. N. Rossan, and L. H. Schmidt. 1961. Transmission of the M strain of Plasmodium cynomolgi to man. Am. J. Trop. Med. Hyg. 10: 673–78.

Conran, P. B. 1967. Monkey malaria. Abstr. 38. 18th An. Meeting Am. Assoc. Lab. Animal Sci., Washington, D.C.

Conroy, J. D. 1964. Diseases of the skin, pp. 322–47. In E. J. Catcott, ed. Feline medicine and surgery. American Veterinary Publications, Santa Barbara, Calif.

Contacos, P. G., and G. R. Coatney. 1963. Experimental adaptation of simian malarias to abnormal hosts. J. Parasitol. 49:912–18.

Contacos, P. G., H. A. Elder, G. R. Coatney, and Clara Genther. 1962. Man to man transfer of two strains of Plasmodium cynomolgi by mosquito bite. Am. J. Trop. Med. Hyg. 11:186–93.

Contacos, P. G., J. S. Lunn, G. R. Coatney, J. W. Kilpatrick, and F. E. Jones. 1963. Quartan-type malaria parasite of New World monkeys transmissible to man. Science 142:676.

Cook, R. 1969. Common diseases of laboratory animals, pp. 160–215. In D. J. Short and Dorothy P. Woodnott, eds. The I.A.T.

manual of laboratory animal practice and techniques. 2d ed. Charles C Thomas, Springfield, Ill.

Cordero del Campillo, M. 1959. Estudios sobre Eimeria falciformis (Einer, 1870) parasito del raton: I. Observaciones sobre el período pre-patente, esporulación, morfología de los ooquistes y estudio biométrico de los mismos, producción de ooquistes y patogenicidad. Rev. Iberica Parasitol. 19:351–68.

Cossel, L. 1958. Nierenbefunde beim Meerschweinchen bei Klossiella-Infektion (Klossiella cobayae). Schweiz. Z. Allgem. Pathol. Bakteriol. 21:62–73.

Deane, L. M., Maria P. Deane, and J. F. Neto. 1966. Studies on transmission of simian malaria and on a natural infection of man with Plasmodium simium in Brazil. Bull. World Health Organ. 35:805–8.

Deschiens, R., J. C. Levaditi, and L. Lamy. 1957. Sur quelques aspects morphologiques de sarcosporidies de divers mammifères. Bull. Soc. Pathol. Exotique 50:225–28.

Deschiens, R., H. Limousin, and J. Troisic. 1927. Eléments présentant les caractères d'un protozoaire sanguicole observés chez le chimpanzé. Bull. Soc. Pathol. Exotique 20:597–600.

Dieben, C. P. A. 1924. Over de morphologie en biologie van het rattencoccidium Eimeria nieschulzi n. sp. en zijne verspreiding in Nederland (tevens vergelijkend onderzoek van de bekende coccidium-opsporingsmethoden). Thesis. 119 pp.

Dissanaike, A. S., P. Nelson, and P. C. C. Garnham. 1965. Two new malaria parasites, Plasmodium cynomolgi ceylonensis subsp. nov. and Plasmodium fragile sp. nov., from monkeys in Ceylon. Ceylon J. Med. Sci. 14:1–9.

Dorner, J. L. 1969. Clinical and pathologic features of canine babesiosis. J. Am. Vet. Med. Assoc. 154:648–52.

Dubey, J. P. 1968a. Toxoplasma infection in English cats. Vet. Record 82:377–79.

———. 1968b. Isolation of Toxoplasma gondii from the feces of a helminth free cat. J. Protozool. 15:773–75.

Dubin, I. N., and A. Wilcox. 1947. Sarcocystis in Macaca mulatta. J. Parasitol. 33:151–53.

Dunkley, M. J. W. 1968. Laboratory trials with buquinolate—a new broad-spectrum coccidiostat for poultry. Vet. Record 83:30–34.

Dunn, F. L. 1965. On the antiquity of malaria in the Western Hemisphere. Human Biol. 37:385–93.

Dunn, F. L., and F. L. Lambrecht. 1963. The

hosts of *Plasmodium brasilianum* Gonder and von Berenberg-Gossler, 1908. J. Parasitol. 49:316–19.

Edgar, S. A., and C. Flanagan. 1968. Coccidiostatic effects of buquinolate in poultry. Poultry Sci. 47:95–104.

Edgar, S. A., and C. T. Seibold. 1964. A new coccidium of chickens, *Eimeria mivati* sp. n. (Protozoa: Eimeriidae) with details of its life history. J. Parasitol. 50:193–204.

Eisenstein, R., and J. R. M. Innes. 1956. Sarcosporidiosis in man and animals. Vet. Rev. Annotations 2:61–78.

Erhardova, B. 1955. *Hepatozoon microti* Coles, 1914 bei unseren kleinen Säugetieren. Folia Biol. (Prague) 1:282–87.

Erickson, A. B. 1946. Incidence and transmission of *Sarcocystis* in cottontails. J. Wildlife Management 10:44–46.

Ernst, J. V., B. Chobotar, Emily C. Oaks, and D. M. Hammond. 1968. *Besnoitia jellisoni* (Sporozoa: Toxoplasmae) in rodents from Utah and California. J. Parasitol. 54:545–49.

Eyles, D. E. 1952a. Incidence of *Trypanosoma lewisi* and *Hepatozoon muris* in Norway rats. J. Parasitol. 38:222–25.

———. 1952b. *Toxoplasma* in the Norway rat. J. Parasitol. 38:226–29.

———. 1960a. *Anopheles freeborni* and *A. quadrimaculatus* as experimental vectors of *Plasmodium cynomolgi* and *P. inui*. J. Parasitol. 46:540.

———. 1960b. The exoerythrocytic cycle of *Plasmodium cynomolgi* and *P. cynomolgi bastianellii* in the rhesus monkey. Am. J. Trop. Med. Hyg. 9:543–55.

———. 1963. The species of simian malaria: Taxonomy, morphology, life cycle, and geographical distribution of the monkey species. J. Parasitol. 49:866–87.

Eyles, D. E., G. R. Coatney, and M. E. Getz. 1960. Vivax-type malaria parasite of macaques transmissible to man. Science 131:1812–13.

Eyles, D. E., Y. L. Fong, F. L. Dunn, Elizabeth Guinn, McW. Warren, and A. A. Sandosham. 1964. *Plasmodium youngi* n. sp., a malaria parasite of the Malayan gibbon, *Hylobates lar lar*. Am. J. Trop. Med. Hyg. 13:248–55.

Eyles, D. E., Y. L. Fong, McW. Warren, Elizabeth Guinn, A. A. Sandosham, and R. H. Wharton. 1962a. *Plasmodium coatneyi*, a new species of primate malaria from Malaya. Am. J. Trop. Med. Hyg. 11:597–604.

Eyles, D. E., A. B. G. Laing, and Y. L. Fong. 1962b. *Plasmodium fieldi* sp. nov., a new species of malaria parasite from the pig-tailed macaque in Malaya. Ann. Trop. Med. Parasitol. 56:242–47.

Eyles, D. E., and McW. Warren. 1962. *Plasmodium inui* in Sulawesi. J. Parasitol. 48:739.

———. 1963. *Hepatocystis* from *Macaca irus* in Java. J. Parasitol. 49:891.

Eyles, D. E., McW. Warren, Y. L. Fong, A. A. Sandosham, and F. L. Dunn. 1962c. A malaria parasite of Malayan gibbons. Med. J. Malaya 17:86.

Fairbairn, H. 1948. The occurrence of a piroplasm, *Entopolypoides macaci,* in East African monkeys. Ann. Trop. Med. Parasitol. 42:118.

Fantham, H. B. 1905. Microscopic preparations of a new Haemosporidian parasite belonging to the genus *Piroplasma*, from the blood of the white rat. Proc. Zool. Soc. London 2:491.

———. 1906. *Piroplasma muris*, Fant. from the blood of the white rat, with remarks on the genus *Piroplasma*. Quart. J. Microscop. Sci. 50:493–516.

Farr, Marion M., and E. E. Wehr. 1949. Survival of *Eimeria acervulina*, *E. tenella* and *E. maxima* oocysts on soil under various field conditions. Ann. N.Y. Acad. Sci. 52:468–72.

Fonseca, F. da. 1951. Plasmódio de primata do Brasil. Mem. Inst. Oswaldo Cruz. 49:543–53.

Foster, H. L. 1963. Specific pathogen-free animals, pp. 110–37. *In* W. Lane-Petter, ed. Animals for research: Principles of breeding and management. Academic Press, New York.

Frenkel, J. K. 1953. Infections with organisms resembling *Toxoplasma*. 6th Intern. Congr. Microbiol., Rome 2:556–57.

———. 1956. Pathogenesis of toxoplasmosis and of infections with organisms resembling *Toxoplasma*. Ann. N.Y. Acad. Sci. 64:215–51.

Frenkel, J. K., J. P. Dubey, and Nancy L. Miller. 1969. *Toxoplasma gondii*: Fecal forms separated from eggs of the nematode *Toxocara cati*. Science 164:432–33.

———. 1970. *Toxoplasma gondii* in cats: Fecal stages identified as coccidian oocysts. Science 167:893–96.

Friedhoff, K., and E. Scholtyseck. 1968. Feinstrukturen von *Babesia ovis* (Piroplasmidea) in *Rhipicephalus bursa* (Ixodoidea): Transformation sphäroider Formen zu Vermiculaformen. Z. Parasitenk. 30:347–59.

Galuzo, I. G. 1966. Toxoplasmosis of animals, pp. 204–6. *In* A. Corradetti, ed. Proc.

First Intern. Congr. Parasitol. Pergamon Press, New York.

Galuzo, I. G., and D. N. Zasukhin. 1963. Toxoplasmosis of man and animals (in Russian). Izv. Akad. Nauk. Kaz. SSR, Alma-Ata, Kazakhstan, USSR. 410 pp.

Garner, F. M., J. R. M. Innes, and D. H. Nelson. 1967. Murine neuropathology, pp. 295–348. In E. Cotchin and F. J. C. Roe, eds. Pathology of laboratory rats and mice. Blackwell Scientific Publ., Oxford.

Garnham, P. C. C. 1947. Exoerythrocytic schizogony in Plasmodium kochi Laveran: A preliminary note. Trans. Roy. Soc. Trop. Med. Hyg. 40:719–22.

———. 1948. The development cycle of Hepatocystis (Plasmodium) kochi in the monkey host. Trans. Roy. Soc. Trop. Med. Hyg. 41:601–16.

———. 1950. Blood parasites of East African vertebrates, with a brief description of exoerythrocytic schizogony in Plasmodium pitmani. Parasitology 40:328–37.

———. 1959. A new sub-species of Plasmodium cynomolgi, Riv. Parassitol. 20:273–78.

———. 1963a. A new sub-species of Plasmodium knowlesi in the long-tailed macaque. J. Trop. Med. Hyg. 66:156–58.

———. 1963b. Distribution of simian malaria parasites in various hosts. J. Parasitol. 49:905–11.

Garnham, P. C. C., R. B. Heisch, and D. M. Minter. 1961. The vector of Hepatocystis (Plasmodium) kochi; the successful conclusion of observations in many parts of tropical Africa. Trans. Roy. Soc. Trop. Med. Hyg. 55:497–502.

Garnham, P. C. C., R. Lainson, and W. Cooper. 1957. The tissue stages and sporogony of Plasmodium knowlesi. Trans. Roy. Soc. Trop. Med. Hyg. 51:384–96.

———. 1958. The complete life cycle of a new strain of Plasmodium gonderi from the drill (Mandrillus leucophaeus), including its sporogony in Anopheles aztecus and its pre-erythrocytic schizogony in the rhesus monkey. Trans. Roy. Soc. Trop. Med. Hyg. 52:509–17.

Garnham, P. C. C., R. Lainson, and A. E. Gunders 1956. Some observations on malaria parasites in a chimpanzee, with particular reference to the persistence of Plasmodium reichenowi and Plasmodium vivax. Ann. Soc. Belge Med. Trop. 36:811–22.

Garnham, P. C. C., and F. Pick. 1952. Unusual form of merocysts of Hepatocystis (= Plasmodium) kochi. Trans. Roy. Soc. Trop. Med. Hyg. 46:535–37.

Gerundo, M. 1948. Control of hepatic coccidiosis of rabbits with succinylsulfathiazole

U.S.P.: a study of the mode of action of the sulfonamides. Arch. Pathol. 46:128–31.

Gibson, C. L., and D. E. Eyles. 1957. Toxoplasma infections in animals associated with a case of human congenital toxoplasmosis. Am. J. Trop. Med. Hyg. 6:990–1000.

Gibson, T. E. 1967. Parasites of laboratory animals transmissible to man. Lab. Animals 1:17–24.

Gill, B. S., and H. N. Ray. 1960. The coccidia of domestic rabbit and the common field hare of India. Proc. Zool. Soc. Calcutta 13: 129–43.

Gonder, R., and H. von Berenberg-Gossler. 1908. Untersuchungen über Malaria plasmodien der Affen. Malaria (Leipzig) 1:47–56.

Griesemer, R. A., and J. P. Gibson. 1963. The gnotobiotic dog. Lab. Animal Care 13:643–49.

Groves, M. G., and L. F. Yap. 1968. Babesia gibsoni in a dog. J. Am. Vet. Med. Assoc. 153:689–94.

Habermann, R. T., and F. P. Williams, Jr. 1957. Diseases seen at necropsy of 708 Macaca mulatta (rhesus monkey) and Macaca philippinensis (cynomolgus monkey). Am. J. Vet. Res. 130:419–26.

Hagen, K. W., Jr. 1958. The effects of age and temperature on the survival of oocysts of Eimeria stiedae. Am. J. Vet Res. 19:1013–14.

———. 1961. Hepatic coccidiosis in domestic rabbits treated with 2 nitrofuran compounds and sulfaquinoxaline. J. Am. Vet. Med. Assoc. 138:99–100.

Halberstädter, L., and S. von Prowazek. 1907. Untersuchungen über die Malariaparisiten der Affen. Arb. Gesundh. Amt., Berlin 26:37–43.

Hampton, J. C., and B. Rosario. 1966. The attachment of protozoan parasites to intestinal epithelial cells of the mouse. J. Parasitol. 52:939–49.

Hartman, H. A. 1961. The intestinal fluke (Fasciolopsis buski) in a monkey. Am. J. Vet. Res. 22:1123–26.

Hawking, F., W. L. M. Perry, and June P. Thurston. 1948. Tissue forms of a malaria parasite, Plasmodium cynomolgi. Lancet 1:783–89.

Held, J. R., P. G. Contacos, and G. R. Coatney. 1967. Studies of the exoerythrocytic stages of simian malaria. I. Plasmodium fieldi. J. Parasitol. 53:225–32.

Henderson, J. D., and B. C. Bullock. 1968. A summary of lesions seen at necropsy in eight spontaneous woolly monkey (Lagothrix spp.) deaths. Abstr. 31. 19th Ann.

Meeting Am. Assoc. Lab. Animal Sci., Las Vegas.

Henry, Dora P. 1932. Coccidiosis of the guinea pig. Univ. Calif. (Berkeley) Publ. Zool. 37:211–68.

Hill, W. C. O. 1936. Notes on malaria and tetanus in monkeys. J. Comp. Pathol. Therap. 49:274–78.

———. 1953. Report of the Society's prosector for the year 1952. Proc. Zool. Soc. London 123:227–51.

———. 1954. Report of the Society's prosector for the year 1953. Proc. Zool. Soc. London. 124:303–11.

Hirsh, D. C., R. L. Hickman, C. R. Burkholder, and O. A. Soave. 1969. An epizootic of babesiosis in dogs used for medical research. Lab. Animal Care 19:205–8.

Horton, R. J. 1967. The route of migration of *Eimeria stiedae* (Lindemann, 1865) sporozoites between the duodenum and bile ducts of the rabbit. Parasitology 57:9–17.

Horton-Smith, C. 1947. The treatment of hepatic coccidiosis in rabbits. Vet. J. 103:207–13.

———. 1958. Coccidiosis in domestic mammals. Vet. Record 70:256–62.

Horton-Smith, C., E. L. Taylor, and E. E. Turtle. 1940. Ammonia fumigation for coccidial disinfection. Vet. Record 52:829–32.

Howard, L. M., and B. D. Cabrera. 1961. Simian malaria in the Philippines. Science 134:555–56.

Howell, J. McC., and N. Edington. 1968. The production of rabbits free from lesions associated with *Encephalitozoon cuniculi.* Lab. Animals 2:143–46.

Huff, C. G., and H. Hoogstraal. 1963. *Plasmodium lemuris* n. sp. from *Lemur collaris* E. Geoffroy. J. Infect. Diseases 112:233–36.

Hutchison, W. M. 1965. Experimental transmission of *Toxoplasma gondii.* Nature 206:961–62.

Hutchison, W. M., J. F. Dunachie, and K. Work. 1968. The faecal transmission of *Toxoplasma gondii.* Acta Pathol. Microbiol. Scand. 74:462–64.

Innes, J. R. M., and L. Z. Saunders. 1962. Comparative neuropathology. Academic Press, New York. 839 pp.

Innes, J. R. M., W. Zeman, J. K. Frenkel, and G. Borner. 1962. Occult endemic encephalitozoönosis of the central nervous system of mice (Swiss-Bagg-O'Grady strain). J. Neuropathol. Exp. Neurol. 21:519–33.

Itagaki, K., and M. Tsubokura. 1968a. Studies on avian malaria in Japan: I. Life cycle, with special reference to the exoerythrocytic growth of the parasite. Japan. J. Vet. Sci. 30:1–6.

———. 1968b. Studies on avian malaria in Japan: II. Pathogenicity of the parasite. Japan. J. Vet. Sci. 30:73–80.

Jacobs, L. 1956. Propagation, morphology, and biology of *Toxoplasma.* Ann. N.Y. Acad. Sci. 64:154–79.

Jeffery, G. M., and W. A. Sodeman, Jr. 1966. Pathological and physiological response of the host to simian malarias, pp. 246–47. *In* A. Corradetti, ed. Proc. First Intern. Congr. Parasitol. Pergamon Press, New York.

Jervis, Helen R., T. G. Merrill, and H. Sprinz. 1966. Coccidiosis in the guinea pig small intestine due to a *Cryptosporidium.* Am. J. Vet. Res. 27:408–14.

Johnson, R. M., A. C. Andersen, and W. Gee. 1963. Parasitism in an established dog kennel. Lab. Animal Care 13:731–36.

Kamyszek, F. 1963. Furacoccid w zwalczaniu kokcydiozy królików. Med. Weterynar (Poland). 19:564–66.

Kheisin, E. M. 1947a. A new species of rabbit coccidia *(Eimeria coecicola* n. sp.). Akad. Nauk SSSR, Compt. Rend. (Dokl.) Acad. URSS, Intern. ed. 55:177–79.

———. 1947b. Variability of the oocysts of *Eimeria magna* Perard (in Russian). Zool. Zh. 26:17–30.

———. 1948. Development of two intestinal coccidia of the rabbit *Eimeria piriformis* Kotlan and Pospesch and *Eimeria intestinalis* nom. nov. (in Russian). Uch. Zap. Karelo-finsk. Univ. 3:3.

———. 1957. Topologic differences in the species of coccidians associated with the domestic rabbit *(Oryctolagus cuniculus* L.) (in Russian). Tr. Leningr. Obshchestvo Estestvoispytatlis. 73:150–58.

Kikkawa, Y., and B. Gueft. 1964. Toxoplasma cysts in the human heart: An electron microscopic study. J. Parasitol. 50:217–25.

Kikuth, W. 1927. Piroplasmose bei Affen. Arch. Schiffs-Tropen-Hyg. 31:37–40.

Kleeberg, H. H., and W. Steenken, Jr. 1963. Severe coccidiosis in guinea-pigs. J. S. African Vet. Med. Assoc. 34:49–52.

Knowles, R. 1919. Notes on the monkey plasmodium and on some experiments in malaria. Indian J. Med. Res. 7:195–202.

Koller, L. D. 1969. Spontaneous *Nosema cuniculi* infection in laboratory rabbits. J. Am. Vet. Med. Assoc. 155:1108–14.

Korté, W. F. de. 1905. On the presence of a Sarcosporidium in the thigh muscles of *Macacus rhesus.* J. Hyg. 5:451–52.

Koutz, F. R. 1950. The survival of oocysts of avian coccidia in the soil. Speculum (Ohio State Univ.) 3(3):3, 28–29, 32–35.

Krampitz, H. E. 1957. Ricerche sugli emo-parassiti dei micromammiferi selvatici della Sicilia. Riv. Parassitol. 18:219–33.

Kuntz, R. E., and Betty J. Myers. 1967. Micro-biological parameters of the baboon (Papio sp.): Parasitology, pp. 741–55. In H. Vogt-borg, ed. The baboon in medical research. Vol. 2. Univ. Texas Press, Austin.

Kusama, S., K. Kasai, and R. Kobayashi. 1919. The leucocytogregarine of the wild rat, with special reference to its life-history. Kitasato Arch. Exp. Med. 3:103–22.

Lainson, R. 1954. Natural infection of En-cephalitozoon in the brains of laboratory rats. Trans. Roy. Soc. Trop. Med. Hyg. 48:5.

———. 1955. Toxoplasmosis in England: I. The rabbit (Oryctolagus cuniculus) as a host of Toxoplasma gondii. Ann. Trop. Med. Parasitol. 49:384–96.

———. 1957. The demonstration of Toxo-plasma in animals, with particular ref-erence to members of the Mustelidae. Trans. Roy. Soc. Trop. Med. Hyg. 51:111–17.

Laird, M. 1959. Malayan protozoa: 2. Hepa-tozoon Miller (Sporozoa: Coccidia), with an unusual host record for H. canis (James). J. Protozool. 6:316–19.

Lambrecht, F. L., F. L. Dunn, and D. E. Eyles. 1961. Isolation of Plasmodium knowlesi from Phillippine macaques. Nature 191:1117–18.

Landau, Irène. 1965. Description de Plas-modium chabaudi n. sp., parasite de ron-geurs africains. Compt. Rend. Acad. Sci. 260:3758–61.

Langeron, M. 1920. Note additionnelle sur une hémogrégarine d'un macaque. Bull. Soc. Pathol. Exotique 13:394.

Lapage, G. 1940. The study of coccidiosis (Eimeria caviae [Sheather 1924]) in the guinea pig. Vet. J. 96:144–54, 190–202, 242–54, 280–95.

Lefrou, G., and J. Martignoles. 1955. Contri-bution à l'étude de Plasmodium kochi. Plasmodium des singes africans. Bull. Soc. Pathol. Exotique 48:227–34.

Leger, M., and E. Bédier. 1922. Hémo-grégarine du cynocéphale, Papio sphinx E. Geoffrey. Compt. Rend. Soc. Biol. 87:933–34.

Levine, N. D. 1957. Protozoan diseases of lab-oratory animals. Proc. Animal Care Panel 7:98–126.

———. 1961a. Protozoan parasites of domestic animals and of man. Burgess, Minneapolis. 412 pp.

———. 1961b. Problems in the systematics of the "Sporozoa." J. Protozool. 8:442–51.

Levine, N. D., and Virginia Ivens. 1965a. The coccidian parasites (Protozoa; Sporozoa) of rodents. Illinois Biol. Monograph 33. Univ. Illinois Press, Urbana. 365 pp.

———. 1965b. Isospora species in the dog. J. Parasitol. 51:859–64.

Liddo, S., and M. Sangiorgi. 1941. Reperti parassitologici nei ratti di Terra di Bari. Riv. Parassitol. 5:241–45.

Ludvík, J. 1958a. Morphology of Toxoplasma gondii in electron microscope. Vestn. Cesk. Spolecnosti Zool. 22:130–36.

———. 1958b. Elektronenoptische Befunde zur Morphologie der Sarcosporidien (Sar-cocystis tenella Railliet 1886). Zentr. Bak-teriol. Parasitenk. Abt. I. Orig. 172:330–50.

———. 1960. The electron microscopy of Sarcocystis miescheriana Kuhn 1865. J. Protozool. 7:128–35.

Lund, E. E. 1949. Considerations in the prac-tical control of intestinal coccidiosis of domestic rabbits. Ann. N.Y. Acad. Sci. 52:611–20.

———. 1954. The effect of sulfaquinoxaline on the course of Eimeria stiedae infections in the domestic rabbit. Exp. Parasitol. 3:497–503.

Macfie, J. W. S. 1915. Babesiasis and tryp-anosomiasis at Accra, Gold Coast, West Africa. Ann. Trop. Med. Parasitol. 9:457–94.

Mahrt, J. L. 1966. Life cycle of Isospora rivol-ta (Grassi, 1879) Wenyon, 1923 in the dog. Thesis. Univ. Illinois, Urbana. 62 pp.

———. 1967. Endogenous stages of the life cycle of Isospora rivolta in the dog. J. Protozool. 14:754–59.

Makstenieks, O., and J. D. Verlinde. 1957. Toxoplasmosis in the Netherlands. Clini-cal interpretation of parasitological and serological examinations and epidemi-ological relationships between toxoplas-mosis in man and in animals. Doc. Med. Geograph. Trop. 9:213–24.

Malherbe, H., and V. Munday. 1958. En-cephalitozoon cuniculi infection of labo-ratory rabbits and mice in South Africa. J. S. African Vet. Med. Assoc. 29:241–46.

Mandour, A. M. 1969. Sarcocystis nesbitti n. sp. from the rhesus monkey. J. Protozool. 16:353–54.

Manuel, M. F. 1967. The presence of Plasmo-dium juxtanucleare Versiani and Gomes, 1941 in the domestic fowls in the Philip-pines. Ceylon Vet. J. 15:133–37.

Mariani, G. 1940. Toxoplasmosi spontanea delle cavie ad Addis Abeba. Riv. Biol. Coloniale Rome 3:47–54.

Marquardt, W. C. 1966. Attempted transmission of the rat coccidium *Eimeria nieschulzi* to mice. J. Parasitol. 52:691–94.

Mathis, C., and M. Leger. 1911. Plasmodium des macaques du Tonkin. Ann. Inst. Pasteur 25:593–600.

Matubayasi, H. 1938. Studies on parasitic protozoa in Japan: IV. Coccidia parasitic in wild rats *(Epimys rattus alexandrinus* and *E. norvegicus)*. Annot. Zool. Japon. 17:144–63.

Mayer, M. 1933. Über einen neuen Blutparasiten des Affen *(Entopolypoides macaci* n. g. n. sp.). Arch. Schiffs-Tropen-Hyg. 37:504–5.

———. 1934. Ein neuer, eigenartiger Blutparasit des Affen *(Entopolypoides macaci* n. g. et n. sp.). Zentr. Bakteriol. Parasitenk. Abt. I. Orig. 131:132–36.

McKissick, G. E., H. L. Ratcliffe, and A. Koestner. 1968. Enzootic toxoplasmosis in caged squirrel monkeys *Saimiri sciureus.* Pathol. Vet. 5:538–60.

McPherson, C. W., R. T. Habermann, R. R. Every, and R. Pierson. 1962. Eradication of intestinal coccidiosis from a large breeding colony of rabbits. Proc. Animal Care Panel 12:133–40.

Meier, H., Jean Holzworth, and R. C. Griffiths. 1957. Toxoplasmosis in the cat—fourteen cases. J. Am. Vet. Med. Assoc. 131:395–414.

Miklovich, N., and L. Pellérdy. 1960. Comparative investigations into the coccidiostatic effect of various sulphonamides. Acta Vet. Acad. Sci. Hung. 10:383–87.

Miller, J. H. 1959. *Hepatocystis (=Plasmodium) kochi* in the dog face baboon, *Papio doguera.* J. Parasitol. 45(Supp.):53.

Miller, Louise T., and H. A. Feldman. 1953. Incidence of antibodies for *Toxoplasma* among various animal species. J. Infect. Diseases 92:118–20.

Miller, W. W. 1908. *Hepatozoon perniciosum* (n. g., n. sp.)—a haemogregarine pathogenic for white rats; with a description of the sexual cycle in the intermediate host, a mite *(Laelaps echidninus).* U.S. Treasury Dept. Hygienic Lab. Bull. 46. 51 pp.

Møller, T. 1968. A survey on toxoplasmosis and encephalitozoonosis in laboratory animals. Z. Versuchstierk. 10:27–38.

Mooser, H. 1950. *Toxoplasma* in Zuchten weisser Mause. Schweiz. Med. Wochschr. 80:1399–1400.

Morgan, B. B., and E. F. Waller. 1940. A survey of the parasites of the Iowa cottontail *(Sylvilagus floridanus mearnsi).* J. Wildlife Management 4:21–26.

Nelson, B., G. E. Cosgrove, and N. Gengozian. 1966. Diseases of an imported primate *Tamarinus nigricollis.* Lab. Animal Care 16:255–75.

Nelson, J. B. 1962. An intracellular parasite resembling a microsporidian associated with ascites in Swiss mice. Proc. Soc. Exp. Biol. Med. 109:714–17.

Neméséri, L. 1959. Adatok a kutya coccidiosisahoz: I. *Isospora canis.* Magy. Allatorv. Lapja 14:91–92.

Niak, A. 1967. *Eimeria* in laboratory rabbits in Teheran. Vet. Record 81:549.

Nicolau, S., and G. Balmus. 1934. Toxoplasmose spontanée des souris et des cobayes. Compt. Rend. Soc. Biol. 115:959–62.

Nieschulz, O., and A. Bos. 1931. Ueber den Infektionsverlauf der Mausekokzidiosis. Z. Hyg. Infektionskrankh. Haust. 39:160–68.

Nuttall, G. H. F., and G. S. Graham-Smith. 1908. The mode of multiplication of *Piroplasma bovis, P. pitheci* in the circulating blood compared with that of *P. canis,* with notes on other species of *Piroplasma.* Parasitology 1:134–42.

Offutt, E. P., Jr., and I. R. Telford. 1945. *Sarcocystis* in the monkey. A report of two cases. J. Parasitol. 31(Supp.):15.

Orio, J., R. Depoux, P. Ravisso, and H. Cassard. 1959. Contribution à l'étude de la toxoplamose en Afrique Équatoriale: Enquête dans la population animale. Bull. Soc. Pathol. Exotique 51:607–15.

Ostler, D. C. 1961. The diseases of broiler rabbits. Vet. Record 73:1237–52.

Ott, Karen J., and L. A. Stauber. 1967. *Eperythrozoon coccoides:* Influence on course of infection of *Plasmodium chabaudi* in mouse. Science 155:1546–48.

Otto, H. 1957. Befunde an Mäusenieren bei Coccidiose *(Klossiella muris).* Frankfurter. Z. Pathol. 68:41–48.

Overdulve, J. P. 1970. The identity of *Toxoplasma* Nicolle and Manceaux, 1909 with *Isospora* Schneider, 1881. Proc. Koninkl. Ned. Akad. Wetenschap. Ser. C. 73:129–51.

Owen, Dawn. 1968. Investigations: B. Parasitological studies. Lab. Animals Centre News Letter 35:7–9.

Paget, G. E., Shirley J. Alcock, and J. F. Ryley. 1962. The pathology of *Babesia rodhaini* infections in mice. J. Pathol. Bacteriol. 84:218–20.

Pellérdy, L. 1953. Beiträge zur Kenntnis der Darmkokzidiose des Kaninchens. Die endogene Entwickelung von *Eimeria piriformis.* Acta Vet. Acad. Sci. Hung. 3:365–77.

———. 1954. Beiträge zur Spezifität der Coccidien des Hasen und Kaninchens. Acta Vet. Acad. Sci. Hung. 4:481–87.

———. 1956. On the status of the *Eimeria*

species of *Lepus europaeus* and related species. Acta Vet. Acad. Sci. Hung. 6: 451–67.

Pellérdy, L., and A. Babos. 1953. Untersuchungen über die endogene Entwicklung sowie pathologische Bedeutung von *Eimeria media*. Acta Vet. Acad. Sci. Hung. 3:173–88.

Pérard, C. 1924. Recherches sur la destruction des oocystes de coccidiés. Compt. Rend. 179:1436–38.

———. 1926. Sur la coccidiose du rat. Acad. Vet. France Bull. 102:120–24.

Perrin, T. L. 1943a. Spontaneous and experimental Encephalitozoon infection in laboratory animals. Arch. Pathol. 36:559–67.

———. 1943b. Toxoplasma and Encephalitozoon in spontaneous and in experimental infections of animals: A comparative study. Arch. Pathol. 36:568–78.

Pietrzyk, J., and J. Umiński. 1967. Malaria u malp *Cercopithecus* wywolana przez *Hepatocystis kochi*. Zwierzeta Lab. 2:72–79.

Plowright, W. 1952. An encephalitis-nephritis syndrome in the dog probably due to congenital Encephalitozoon infection. J. Comp. Pathol. Therap. 62:83–92.

Plowright, W., and G. Yeoman. 1952. Probable *Encephalitozoon* infection of the dog. Vet. Record 64:381–83.

Poelma, F. G. 1966. *Eimeria lemuris* n. sp., *E. galago* n. sp. and *E. otolicni* n. sp. from a galago *Galago senegalensis*. J. Protozool. 13:547–49.

Poisson, R. 1953. Sous-ordre des hémosporidies (Haemosporidiidea Danilewsky, 1889 emend.; Doflein, 1901), pp. 798–906. *In* P.-P. Grassé, ed. Traité de zoologie anatomie-systématique biologie. Vol. I. Fasc. II. Masson, Paris.

Poole, C. M., W. G. Keenan, D. V. Tolle, T. E. Fritz, Patricia C. Brennan, R. C. Simkins, and R. J. Flynn. 1967. Disease status of commercially produced rabbits, pp. 219–20. *In* Biological and Medical Research Division annual report, 1967. ANL-7409. Argonne National Laboratory, Argonne, Ill.

Porter, Annie. 1908. *Leucocytozoön musculi*, sp. n., a parasitic protozoön from the blood of white mice. Proc. Zool. Soc. London Part III:703–16.

Porter, J. A., Jr., C. M. Johnson, and L. De Sousa. 1966. Prevalence of malaria in Panamanian primates. J. Parasitol. 52: 669–70.

Prakash, S. 1954. Note on natural parasitic infections found in *Rattus rattus* of Delhi municipal area. Indian J. Malariol. 8:115–16.

Reichenow, E. 1949–1953. Lehrbuch der Protozoenkunde. 6th ed. 3 vol. Fischer, Jena.

Resseler, R. 1956. Un nouveau plasmodium de rat en Belgique: *Plasmodium inopinatum* n. sp. Ann. Soc. Belge Med. Trop. 36:259–63.

Riek, R. F. 1968. Babesiosis, pp. 219–68. *In* D. Weinman and M. Ristic, eds. Infectious blood diseases of man and animals: Vol. 2. The pathogens, the infections, and the consequences. Academic Press, New York.

Roberts, R. M. 1966. Encephalitis, pp. 468–69. *In* R. W. Kirk, ed. Current veterinary therapy 1966–1967: Small animal practice W. B. Saunders, Philadelphia.

Rodaniche, E. C., and T. Pinzon. 1949. Spontaneous toxoplasmosis in the guinea pig in Panama. J. Parasitol. 35:152–55.

Rodhain, J. 1933. Sur une coccidie de l'intestin de l'ouistiti: *Hapale jacchus penicillalus* (Geoffroy). Compt. Rend. Soc. Biol. 114: 1357–58.

———. 1941. Sur un Plasmodium du gibbon *Hylobates leusciscus* Geoff. Acta Biol. Belg. 1:118–23.

———. 1948. Contribution à l'étude des Plasmodiums des anthropoides africains. Transmission du *Plasmodium malariae* de l'homme au chimpanzé. Ann. Soc. Belge Med. Trop. 28:39–49.

———. 1950. Sur la pluralité des espèces de *Babesia* des rongeurs: À propos de la spécificité de *Babesia rodhaini* van den Berghe et al. Ann. Inst. Pasteur 79:777–85.

———. 1952. *Plasmodium vinckei* n. sp., un deuxième plasmodium parasite de rongeurs sauvages au Katanga. Ann. Soc. Belge Med. Trop. 32:275–79.

Rodhain, J., and L. van den Berghe. 1936. Contribution à l'étude des plasmodiums des singes africains. Ann. Soc. Belge Med. Trop. 16:521–31.

Rodhain, J., and R. Dellaert. 1943. L'infection à *Plasmodium malariae* du chimpanzé chez l'homme. Étude d'une première souche isolée de l'anthropoide *Pan satyrus verus*. Ann. Soc. Belge Med. Trop. 23:19–46.

———. 1955. Contribution à l'etude de *Plasmodium schwetzi* E. Brumpt: II. Transmission du *Plasmodium schwetzi* à l'homme. Ann. Soc. Belge Med. Trop. 35:73–76.

Rokey, N. W. 1968. Canine babesiasis, pp. 616–18. *In* R. W. Kirk, ed. Current veterinary therapy: III. Small animal practice. W. B. Saunders, Philadelphia.

Rokey, N. W., and R. Russell. 1961. Canine babesiasis (piroplasmosis)—a case report. J. Am. Vet. Med. Assoc. 138:635–38.

Ross, P. H. 1905. A note on the natural occurrence of piroplasmosis in the monkey (*Cercopithecus*). J. Hyg. 5:18–23.

Roudabush, R. L. 1937. The endogenous phases of the life cycles of *Eimeria nieschulzi, Eimeria separata*, and *Eimeria miyairii* coccidian parasites of the rat. Iowa State J. Sci. 11:135–63.

Ruch, T. C. 1959. Diseases of laboratory primates. W. B. Saunders, Philadelphia. 600 pp.

Rudzinska, Maria A., and A. Trager. 1962. Intracellular phagotrophy in *Babesia rodhaini* as revealed by electron microscopy. J. Protozool. 9:279–88.

Ruebner, B. H., J. R. Lindsey, and E. C. Melby, Jr. 1965. Hepatitis and other spontaneous liver lesions of small experimental animals, pp. 160–82. *In* W. E. Ribelin and J. R. McCoy, eds. Pathology of laboratory animals. Charles C Thomas, Springfield, Ill.

Rutherford, R. L. 1943. The life cycle of four intestinal coccidia of the domestic rabbit. J. Parasitol. 29:10–32.

Ryšavý, B. 1954. Příspěvek k poznání kokcidií našich i dovezených obratlovců. Cesk. Parasitol. 21:131–74.

Sahasrabudhe, V. K., and H. L. Shah. 1966. The occurrence of *Sarcocystis* sp. in the dog. J. Protozool. 13:531.

Sangiorgi, G. 1914. *Leucocytogregarina cuniculi,* n. sp. Giorn. Accad. Med. Torino 20:25–29.

Schmidt, L. H., R. Greenland, and Clara S. Genther. 1961a. The transmission of *Plasmodium cynomolgi* to man. Am. J. Trop. Med. Hyg. 10:679–88.

Schmidt, L. H., R. Greenland, R. Rossan, and Clara Genther. 1961b. Natural occurrence of malaria in rhesus monkeys. Science 133:753.

Scott, J. W. 1943. Life history of Sarcosporidia, with particular reference to *Sarcocystis tenella.* Wyoming Agr. Exp. Sta. Bull. 259. 63 pp.

Scott, Patricia P. 1967. The cat *(Felis catus* L.), pp. 505–67. *In* UFAW Staff, ed. The UFAW handbook on the care and management of laboratory animals. 3d ed. Livingstone and the Universities Federation for Animal Welfare, London.

Seamer, J., and F. C. Chesterman. 1967. A survey of disease in laboratory animals. Lab. Animals 1:117–39.

Seibold, H. R., and W. S. Bailey. 1957. Babesiasis (piroplasmosis) in dogs. J. Am. Vet. Med. Assoc. 130:46–48.

Sevim, I. 1967. Coccodiosis in rabbits and therapeutic trials (in Turkish). Turk Ask. vet. Hekim. Dergisi 45:40–46.

Shah, H. L. 1969. The coccidia (Protozoa: Eimeriidae) of the cat. Thesis. Univ. of Illinois. 138 pp.

Sheffield, H. G., and Marjorie L. Melton. 1969. *Toxoplasma gondii:* Transmission through feces in absence of *Toxocara cati* eggs. Science 164:431–32.

———. 1970. *Toxoplasma gondii:* The oocyst, sporozoite, and infection of cultured cells. Science 167:892–93.

Sheffy, B. E., J. A. Baker, and J. H. Gillespie. 1961. A disease-free colony of dogs. Proc. Animal Care Panel 11:208–14.

Shortt, H. E. 1948. The life cycle of *Plasmodium cynomolgi* in its insect and mammalian hosts. Trans. Roy. Soc. Trop. Med. Hyg. 42:227–30.

Shortt, H. E., and P. C. C. Garnham. 1948. The pre-erythrocytic development of *Plasmodium cynomolgi* and *Plasmodium vivax.* Trans. Roy. Soc. Trop. Med. Hyg. 41:785–95.

Shortt, H. E., G. Rao, S. S. Qadri, and R. Abraham. 1961. *Plasmodium osmaniae,* a malaria parasite of an Indian monkey *Macaca radiata.* J. Trop. Med. Hyg. 64:140–43.

Siim, J. C. 1960. Human toxoplasmosis. Williams and Wilkins, Baltimore. 220 pp.

Siim, J. C., W. M. Hutchison, and K. Work. 1969. Transmission of *Toxoplasma gondii:* Further studies on the morphology of the cystic form in cat faeces. Acta Pathol. Microbiol. Scand. 77:756–57.

Simpson, C. F., W. W. Kirkham, and J. M. Kling. 1967. Comparative morphologic features of *Babesia caballi* and *Babesia equi.* Am. J. Vet. Res. 28:1693–97.

Sinton, J. A. 1934. A quartan malaria parasite of the lower oriental monkey, *Silenus irus (Macacus cynomolgus).* Records Malaria Surv. India 4:379–410.

Smetana, H. 1933a. Coccidiosis of the liver in rabbits: I. Experimental study on the excystation of oocysts of *Eimeria stiedae.* Arch. Pathol. 15:175–92.

———. 1933b. Coccidiosis of the liver in rabbits: II. Experimental study on the mode of infection of the liver by sporozoites of *Eimeria stiedae.* Arch. Pathol. 15:330–39.

———. 1933c. Coccidiosis of the liver in rabbits: III. Experimental study of the histogenesis of coccidiosis of the liver. Arch. Pathol. 15:516–36.

Smith, H. A., and T. C. Jones. 1966. Veterinary pathology. 3d ed. Lea and Febiger, Philadelphia. 1192 pp.

Smith, T., and H. P. Johnson. 1902. On a coccidium *(Klossiella muris,* gen. et spec. nov.) parasitic in the renal epithelium of the mouse. J. Exp. Med. 6:303–16.

Stabler, R. M., and K. Welch. 1961. Research note: *Besnoitia* from an opossum. J. Parasitol. 47:576.

Stolz, G. 1962. Spontane, letal verlaufende Toxoplasmose bei einem Affen. Schweiz. Arch. Tierheilk. 104:162–66.

Strong, J. P., J. H. Miller, and H. C. McGill, Jr. 1965. Naturally occurring parasitic lesions in baboons, pp. 503–12. *In* H. Vagtborg, ed. The baboon in medical research. Univ. of Texas Press, Austin.

Sureau, P., and M. Capponi. 1955. Note sur un piroplasmide de *Rattus norvegicus* observé dans la région du centre Viet-Nam. Bull. Soc. Pathol. Exotique 48:823–28.

Szemerédi, G. 1968. Occurrence of toxoplasmosis in a Hungarian rabbit farm (in Hungarian). Magy. Allatorv. Lapja 23:176–78.

Taliaferro, W. H., and P. R. Cannon. 1936. Cellular reactions during primary infections and superinfections of *Plasmodium brasilianum* in Panamanian monkeys. J. Infect. Diseases 59:72–125.

Taliaferro, W. H., and Cessa Klüver. 1940a. The hematology of malaria *(Plasmodium brasilianum)* in Panamanian monkeys: I. Numerical changes in leucocytes. J. Infect. Diseases 67:121–61.

———. 1940b. The hematology of malaria *(Plasmodium brasilianum)* in Panamanian monkeys. II. Morphology of leucocytes and origin of monocytes and macrophages. J. Infect. Diseases 67:162–76.

Taliaferro, W. H., and Lucy G. Taliaferro. 1934. Morphology, periodicity and course of infection of *Plasmodium brasilianum* in Panamanian monkeys. Am. J. Hyg. 20:1–49.

Tanguy, Y. 1937. La piroplasmose du singe. Ann. Inst. Pasteur 59:610–23.

Thiel, P. H. van. 1964. Toxoplasmosis, pp. 495–504. *In* J. van der Hoeden, ed. Zoonoses. Elsevier, New York.

Tsuchiya, H., and L. E. Rector. 1936. Studies on intestinal parasites among wild rats caught in Saint Louis. Am. J. Trop. Med. 16:705–14.

Tsunoda, K. 1952. *Eimeria matsubayashii* sp. nov., a new species of rabbit coccidium (in Japanese). Exp. Rept. Govt. Exp. Sta. Animal Hyg. (Japan) 24:109–19.

Tuffery, A. A., and J. R. M. Innes. 1963. Diseases of laboratory mice and rats, pp. 47–108. *In* W. Lane-Petter, ed. Animals for research: Principles of breeding and management. Academic Press, New York.

Tyzzer, E. E. 1910. An extracellular coccidium, *Cryptosporidium muris* (gen. et sp. nov.), of the gastric glands of the common mouse. J. Med. Res. 23:487–509.

———. 1912. *Cryptosporidium parvum* (sp. nov.), a coccidium found in the small intestine of the common mouse. Arch. Protistenk. 26:394–412.

Varela, G., A. E. Martínez Rodríguez, and A. Trevino. 1953. Toxoplasmosis en la Republica Mexicana. Rev. Inst. Salubridad Enfermedades Trop. (Mex.) 13:217–24.

Vickers, J. H. 1966. *Hepatocystis kochi* in *Ceropithecus* monkeys. J. Am. Vet. Med. Assoc. 149:906–8.

Vincke, I. H., and M. Lips. 1948. Un nouveau *Plasmodium* d'un rongeur sauvage du Congo, *Plasmodium berghei* n. sp. Ann. Soc. Belge Med. Trop. 28:97–104.

Warner, D. E. 1933. Survival of coccidia of the chicken in soil and on the surface of eggs. Poultry Sci. 12:343–48.

Warren, McW., G. F. Bennett, A. A. Sandosham, and G. R. Coatney. 1965. *Plasmodium eylesi* sp. nov., a tertian malaria parasite from the white-handed gibbon, *Hylobates lar*. Ann. Trop. Med. Parasitol. 59:500–508.

Warren, McW., G. R. Coatney, and J. C. Skinner. 1966. *Plasmodium jefferyi* sp. n. from *Hylobates lar* in Malaya. J. Parasitol. 52: 9–13.

Warren, McW., D. E. Eyles, and R. H. Wharton. 1962. Primate malaria infections in *Mansonia uniformis*. Mosquito News 22: 303–4.

Warren, McW., and R. H. Wharton. 1963. The vectors of simian malaria: Identity, biology, and geographical distribution. J. Parasitol. 49:892–904.

Weiser, J. 1965. *Nosema muris* n. sp., a new microsporidian parasite of the white mouse *(Mus musculus* L.). J. Protozool. 12:78–83.

Wenrich, D. H. 1949. Protozoan parasites of the rat, pp. 486–501. *In* E. J. Farris and J. Q. Griffith, eds. The rat in laboratory investigation. J. B. Lippincott, Philadelphia.

Wenyon, C. M. 1926. Protozoology: A manual for medical men, veterinarians and zoologists. 2 vol. Ballière, Tindall, and Cox, London.

Wills, J. E. 1968. The establishment of an SPF guinea pig colony. J. Inst. Animal Tech. 19:99–107.

Winter, H. 1969. Fluorescent microscopy for diagnosis of babesiosis. J. Am. Vet. Med. Assoc. 154:49.

Work, K. 1969. The incidence of *Toxoplasma* antibodies among dogs and cats in Denmark. Acta Pathol. Microbiol. Scand. 75: 447–56.

Work, K., and W. M. Hutchison. 1969. A new cystic form of *Toxoplasma gondii*. Acta Pathol. Microbiol. Scand. 75:191–92.

Yakimoff, W. L., and W. F. Gousseff. 1938. The coccidia of mice *(Mus musculus)*. Parasitology 30:1–3.

Yang, Y. H., and H. C. Grice. 1964. *Klossiella muris* parasitism in laboratory mice. Can. J. Comp. Med. Vet. Sci. 28:63–66.

Yost, D. H. 1958. *Encephalitozoon* infection in laboratory animals. J. Natl. Cancer Inst. 20:957–63.

Chapter 4

CILIATES

ONLY a few ciliates affect endothermal laboratory animals. *Balantidium* is the most important genus and contains the only known pathogenic species. *Cyathodinium* is common in the guinea pig but is nonpathogenic. A third genus of possible significance is *Troglodytella,* which occurs in anthropoids from central Africa.

The ciliates which occur in endothermal laboratory animals are listed in Table 4.1. The most important species are discussed below.

Balantidium coli
(SYN. *Balantidium aragaoi, B. cunhamunizi, B. philippinensis, B. rhesum, B. simile, B. suis, B. wenrichi*)

Balantidium coli, a usually nonpathogenic ciliate, is common in the cecum and colon of several nonhuman primates, including the rhesus monkey, cynomolgus monkey, spider monkeys, howler monkeys, capuchins, baboons, orangutan, chimpanzee, and gorilla throughout the world (Benson, Fremming, and Young 1955; Gisler, Benson, and Young 1960; Habermann and Williams 1957; Hegner 1934a, b; Hegner and Chu 1930; Kuntz and Myers 1967; Poindexter 1942; Prine 1968; Van Riper et al. 1966; Young et al. 1957); it also occurs in the rat, hamster, dog, pig, and man (Bogdanovich 1955; Ewing and Bull 1966; Sheffield and Beveridge 1962). It is common in laboratory primates: incidences as

high as 87% have been reported in the rhesus monkey and 84% in the chimpanzee. It is uncommon or rare in the laboratory rat, hamster, and dog.

MORPHOLOGY

The trophozoites are ovoid, with a subterminal tubular cytostome at the smaller end (Fig. 4.1). They measure 30 to 150 μ by 25 to 120 μ, depending on the strain, and have a cytopyge near the posterior end (Auerbach 1953; Hegner 1934a; Krascheninnikow and Wenrich 1958; Lom 1955; Sen Gupta and Ray 1955). The macronucleus is kidney shaped and has a single micronucleus near the center of one of its sides. There are two contractile vacuoles and many food vacuoles containing starch grains, cell fragments, bacteria, and erythrocytes. The surface is covered by slightly oblique, longitudinal rows (kineties) of cilia. The cysts are spherical to ovoid and measure 40 to 60 μ in diameter.

LIFE CYCLE

Reproduction is by conjugation or by transverse binary fission (Nelson 1934). Infection occurs when cysts or trophozoites are ingested (Levine 1961).

PATHOLOGIC EFFECTS

Balantidium coli is usually nonpathogenic (Prine 1968; Van Riper et al. 1966). It is sometimes a secondary invader of le-

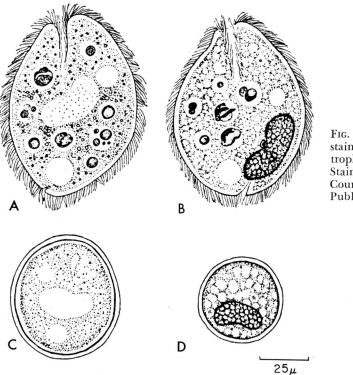

FIG. 4.1. *Balantidium coli. (A)* Unstained trophozoite. *(B)* Stained trophozoite. *(C)* Unstained cyst. *(D)* Stained cyst. (From Kudo 1966. Courtesy of Charles C Thomas, Publisher.)

25μ

sions initiated by pathogenic bacteria or viruses; occasionally it is a primary pathogen and causes diarrhea and an ulcerative enteritis in the monkey, chimpanzee, gorilla, other nonhuman primates, the dog, and rat. The ulcers sometimes extend down to the muscularis mucosae and are accompanied by lymphocytic infiltration and occasionally coagulation necrosis and hemorrhage. Organisms often occur in groups in the tissues or in the capillaries, lymphatics, and regional lymph nodes.

DIAGNOSIS

Diagnosis is made by identifying the organism in characteristic lesions. The presence of concomitant pathogenic microorganisms must be considered.

CONTROL

Sanitation will prevent infection, and the elimination of starches from the diet will control the infection by removing an important source of food for the organism. Good nutrition and the routine treatment of newly procured, asymptomatic carriers

are recommended (Bisseru 1967; Ruch 1959; Schmitt 1964). Effective treatments include carbarsone, given orally, 250 mg per day for the monkey and 500 mg per day for the chimpanzee for 10 days; and diiodohydroxyquin, given orally, 650 mg per day for the monkey and 2 g per day for the chimpanzee for 10 to 20 days (Benson, Fremming, and Young 1955; Gisler, Benson, and Young 1960; Nissen 1952; Van Riper et al. 1966; Young et al. 1957). Paromomycin (Humatin, Parke-Davis) is also reported as very effective for simians at a level of 30 mg per kg of body weight three times daily for 10 days (Schmitt 1964).

PUBLIC HEALTH CONSIDERATIONS

Because *B. coli* sometimes causes diarrhea in man, care should be taken to avoid infection.

Balantidium caviae

This apparently nonpathogenic species is common in the cecum and colon of the conventional guinea pig throughout the world (Krascheninnikow and Wenrich

1958; Nie 1950). It has not been found in cesarean-derived colonies (Calhoon and Matthews 1964). It is 55 to 115 μ by 45 to 73 μ with a mean of 92 by 65 μ, and differs from *Balantidium coli* in having a narrow, bean-shaped cytostome rather than a nearly tubular one and in having one contractile vacuole instead of two. It reproduces by transverse binary fission or sometimes conjugation, and produces spherical or slightly ovoid, thick-walled cysts 40 to 50 μ in diameter, with a mean of 45 μ.

Cyathodinium piriforme

This nonpathogenic ciliate is common in the cecum and colon of the conventional guinea pig throughout the world (Nie 1950). It has not been found in cesarean-derived colonies (Calhoon and Matthews 1964).

Trophozoites are 10 to 36 μ by 9 to 24 μ (Fig. 4.2). They are funnel shaped and have a broadly rounded anterior end bearing 11 rows of cilia, a prominent anterior concave pseudoperistomal field, and a tapered posterior end. There are 9 to 15 (usually 10 to 13) endosprits. The macronucleus is round and generally lies near the middle of the body; the micronucleus is near it. Cysts are rare; they measure 17 to 24 μ by 12 to 17 μ.

Cyathodinium cunhai

Cyathodinium cunhai is common in the cecum and colon of the conventional guinea pig throughout the world and is

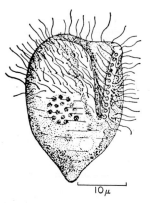

Fig. 4.2. *Cyathodinium piriforme* trophozoite. (From Kudo 1966. Courtesy of Charles C Thomas, Publisher.)

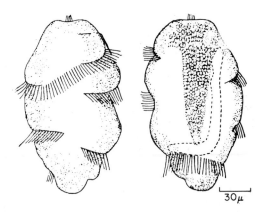

Fig. 4.3. *Troglodytella abrassarti* trophozoite. *(Left)* Ventral view. *(Right)* Dorsal view. (From Kudo 1966. Courtesy of Charles C Thomas, Publisher.)

nonpathogenic (Nie 1950). It has not been observed in cesarean-derived colonies (Calhoon and Matthews 1964).

It resembles *C. piriforme*. Its trophozoites are somewhat ovoid; the tapered end is directed anteriorly, the greatest diameter is posterior to the middle of the body, and the caudal tip is small and abrupt. Its pseudoperistomal field is very small and crescentic. No cysts have been reported.

Troglodytella abrassarti

This apparently nonpathogenic ciliate occurs in the cecum and colon of the chimpanzee in central Africa and has been reported in laboratory specimens newly imported into the United States (Brumpt and Joyeux 1912; Curasson 1929; Hegner 1934b; Kirby 1928; Nelson 1932; Van Riper et al. 1966). It is apparently commoner in recently captured chimpanzees than in those maintained in captivity.

MORPHOLOGY

Troglodytella abrassarti is ellipsoidal, flattened, and 145 to 174 μ long by 87 to 126 μ wide (Fig. 4.3) (Brumpt and Joyeux 1912). It has three zones of membranelles, or cirri, and an adoral zone. The zones of cirri are arranged in incomplete circlets which give the impression that they would form a spiral if they were continuous. There is a continuous or noncontinuous anterior zone on the ventral surface, a continuous posterior zone on the dorsal surface, and a small zone between them on each side. There are skeletal plates beneath the surface in the anterior region. The macronucleus is L-shaped, and there are about eight contractile vacuoles arranged in two circles or parallel to the bands of cirri.

LIFE CYCLE

The life cycle has not been described.

PATHOLOGIC EFFECTS

This ciliate is usually considered nonpathogenic, but it has been cited as a possible cause of colitis in the chimpanzee (Curasson 1929).

DIAGNOSIS

Tentative diagnosis is made by identifying the organism in the feces or colon in association with colitis. Since *T. abrassarti* is probably nonpathogenic, it is important that other possible causes be considered before ascribing the colitis to this organism.

CONTROL

No control or treatment has been reported.

PUBLIC HEALTH CONSIDERATIONS

Troglodytella abrassarti is of no known public health importance.

TABLE 4.1. Ciliates affecting endothermal laboratory animals

Parasite	Geographic Distribution	Endothermal Host	Location in Host	Method of Infection	Incidence — In nature	Incidence — In laboratory	Pathologic Effects	Public Health Importance	Reference
Balantidium coli*	Worldwide	Rat, hamster, dog, rhesus monkey, cynomolgus monkey, capuchins, spider monkeys, howler monkeys, baboons, orangutan, chimpanzee, gorilla, pig, man	Cecum, colon	Ingestion of cysts or trophozoites passed in feces	Common in primates; uncommon or rare in rat, hamster, dog	Common in primates; uncommon or rare in rat, hamster, dog	Usually none; sometimes enteritis, diarrhea	Sometimes causes enteritis, diarrhea	Benson et al. 1955; Bogdanovich 1955; Ewing and Bull 1966; Gisler et al. 1960; Habermann and Williams 1957; Hegner 1934a; Prine 1968; Sheffield and Beveridge 1962; Van Riper et al. 1966; Young et al. 1957
Balantidium caviae*	Worldwide	Guinea pig	Cecum, colon	Ingestion of cysts or trophozoites passed in feces	Unknown	Common	None	None	Krascheninnikow and Wenrich 1958; Nie 1950
Cyathodinium piriforme*	Worldwide	Guinea pig	Cecum, colon	Ingestion of cysts or trophozoites passed in feces	Unknown	Common	None	None	Nie 1950
Cyathodinium cunhai*	Worldwide	Guinea pig	Cecum, colon	Ingestion of trophozoites and presumably cysts passed in feces	Unknown	Common	None	None	Nie 1950
Troglodytella abrassarti*	Worldwide	Chimpanzee	Cecum, colon	Ingestion of organism passed in feces	Common	Common	Probably none; possibly colitis	None known	Brumpt and Joyeux 1912; Curasson 1929; Hegner 1934b; Kirby 1928; Nelson 1932; Van Riper et al. 1966
Troglodytella gorillae	West central Africa	Gorilla	Cecum, colon	Presumably by ingestion of organisms passed in feces	Unknown	Unknown	Unknown	None known	Reichenow 1920

* Discussed in text.

REFERENCES

Auerbach, E. 1953. A study of *Balantidium coli* Stein, 1863 in relation to cytology and behavior in culture. J. Morphol. 93:405–45.

Benson, R. E., B. D. Fremming, and R. J. Young. 1955. Care and management of chimpanzees at the Radiobiological Laboratory of the University of Texas and the United States Air Force. School Aviation Med., U.S. Air Force Rept. 55–48. 7 pp.

Bisseru, B. 1967. Diseases of man acquired from his pets. William Heinemann Medical Books, London. 482 pp.

Bogdanovich, V. V. 1955. Spontaneous balantidiasis (in Russian). Med. Parazitol. i Parazitarn. Bolezni 4:326–29.

Brumpt, E., and C. Joyeux. 1912. Sur un infusoire nouveau parasite du chimpanzé *Troglodytella abrassarti*, n.g., n. sp. Bull. Soc. Pathol. Exotique 5:499–503.

Calhoun, J. R., and P. J. Matthews. 1964. A method for initiating a colony of specific pathogen-free guinea pigs. Lab. Animal Care 14:388–94.

Curasson, G. C. M. 1929. *Troglodytella abrassarti,* infusoire pathogène du chimpanzé. Ann. Parasitol. Humaine Comparee 7:465–68.

Ewing, S. A., and R. W. Bull. 1966. Severe chronic canine diarrhea associated with *Balantidium-Trichuris* infection. J. Am. Vet. Med. Assoc. 149:519–20.

Gisler, D. B., R. E. Benson, and R. J. Young. 1960. Colony husbandry of research monkeys. Ann. N.Y. Acad. Sci. 85:758–68.

Habermann, R. T., and F. P. Williams, Jr. 1957. Diseases seen at necropsy of 708 *Macaca mulatta* (rhesus monkey) and *Macaca philippinensis* (cynomolgus monkey). Am. J. Vet. Res. 18:419–26.

Hegner, R. W. 1934a. Specificity in the genus *Balantidium* based on size and shape of body and macronucleus, with descriptions of six new species. Am. J. Hyg. 19:38–67.

———. 1934b. Intestinal protozoa of chimpanzees. Am. J. Hyg. 19:480–501.

Hegner, R. W., and H. J. Chu. 1930. A survey of protozoa parasitic in plants and animals of the Philippine Islands. Philippine J. Sci. 43:451–82.

Kirby, H., Jr. 1928. Notes on some parasites from chimpanzees. Proc. Soc. Exp. Biol. Med. 25:698–700.

Krascheninnikow, S., and D. H. Wenrich. 1958. Some observations on the morphology and division of *Balantidium coli* and *Balantidium caviae* (?). J. Protozool. 5:196–202.

Kudo, R. R. 1966. Protozoology. 5th ed. Charles C Thomas, Springfield, Ill. 1174 pp.

Kuntz, R. E., and Betty J. Myers. 1967. Microbiological parameters of the baboon *(Papio* sp.): Parasitology, pp. 741–55. *In* H. Vagtborg, ed. The baboon in medical research. Vol. 2. Univ. of Texas Press, Austin.

Levine, N. D. 1961. Protozoan parasites of domestic animals and of man. Burgess, Minneapolis. 412 pp.

Lom, J. 1955. Polysacharidové reservy nálevníku rodu *Balantidium* a *Nyctotherus.* Cesk. Biol. 4:397–409.

Nelson, E. C. 1932. The cultivation of a species of *Troglodytella*, a large ciliate, from the chimpanzee. Science 75:317–18.

———. 1934. Observations and experiments on conjugation of *Balantidium* from chimpanzee. Am. J. Hyg. 20:106–34.

Nie, D. 1950. Morphology and taxonomy of the intestinal protozoa of the guinea-pig, *Cavia porcella.* J. Morphol. 86:381–493.

Nissen, H. W. 1952. Care and handling of laboratory chimpanzees. Carworth Farms Quart. Letter 27:2–3.

Poindexter, H. A. 1942. A study of the intestinal parasites of the monkeys of the Santiago Island primate colony. Puerto Rico J. Public Health Trop. Med. 18:175–91.

Prine, J. R. 1968. Pancreatic flukes and amoebic colitis in a gorilla. Abstr. 50. 19th Ann. Meeting Am. Assoc. Lab. Animal Sci., Las Vegas.

Reichenow, E. 1920. Den Wiederkäuer-Infusorien verwandt Formen aus Gorilla und Schimpanse. Arch. Protistenk. 41:1–33.

Ruch, T. C. 1959. Diseases of laboratory primates. W. B. Saunders, Philadelphia. 600 pp.

Schmitt, J. 1964. Die Balantidiose, unter besonderer Berücksichtigung eines enzootischen Auftretens bei Menschenaffen des Zoologischen Gartens Frankfurt am Main. Deut. Tieraerztl. Wochschr. 71:68–70.

Sen Gupta, P. C., and H. N. Ray. 1955. A cytochemical study of *Balantidium coli* Malmsten, 1857. Proc. Zool. Soc. (India) 8:103–10.

Sheffield, F. W., and Elizabeth Beveridge. 1962. Prophylaxis of "wet-tail" in hamsters. Nature 196:294–95.

Van Riper, D. C., P. W. Day, J. Fineg, and J. R. Prine. 1966. Intestinal parasites of recently imported chimpanzees. Lab. Animal Care 16:360–63.

Young, R. J., B. D. Fremming, R. E. Benson, and M. D. Harris. 1957. Care and management of a *Macaca mulatta* monkey colony. Proc. Animal Care Panel 7:67–82.

Chapter 5

TREMATODES

THE trematodes, or flukes, are divided into two groups, the monogenetic and the digenetic trematodes (Dawes 1946; Morgan and Hawkins 1949; Price 1965; Skrjabin 1964; Yamaguti 1958). The monogenetic trematodes have a simple life cycle involving a single host and only affect ectothermal species. The digenetic trematodes have a complex life cycle that involves at least two hosts: a mollusk, usually a snail, in which larval reproduction occurs, and a vertebrate, in which the adult worm develops. Many are important pathogens of endothermal species, but because of the complex life cycle, infection in laboratory or commercially reared animals is rare or absent. However, some trematodes are occasionally found in endothermal laboratory animals fed food contaminated with metacercarial cysts and in animals brought into the laboratory from their natural environment.

FASCIOLIDS

Fasciolids occur in the liver, intestine, and sometimes stomach of mammals. They are found only in animals fed vegetation contaminated with metacercarial cysts and in animals obtained from their natural habitat. Species that affect endothermal laboratory animals are listed in Table 5.1; the most important, *Fasciola hepatica* and *F. gigantica*, are discussed below.

Fasciola hepatica

This trematode, which causes extensive and sometimes fatal liver damage, occurs in ruminants and the pig throughout the world (Lapage 1968). It is also found in the guinea pig (Cook 1963; Trofimov and Alyabyeva 1959), nutria (Holmes 1962; Polishchuk 1961), cottontail rabbit (Morgan and Hawkins 1949), hare (Tropilo 1965), dog, cat, rhesus monkey (Graham 1960), cynomolgus monkey (Hashimoto and Honjo 1966), man, and other mammals. It is usually rare in the guinea pig (Cook 1963), but severe outbreaks with high mortality have been reported in this species in Poland and the USSR (Golebiowski 1959; Trofimov and Alyabyeva 1959). The incidence in wild rodents and lagomorphs varies from absent or uncommon to common, depending on geographic location (Holmes 1962; Morgan and Hawkins 1949; Tropilo 1965); it is rare in the dog and cat (Burrows 1965; Scott 1967). Although usually uncommon in monkeys, with only a 0.2% incidence reported in one group of over 1,200 cynomolgus monkeys (Hashimoto and Honjo 1966), an incidence of 5% has been reported in a group of rhesus monkeys (Graham 1960).

Fasciola hepatica occurs only in laboratory-reared rodents and lagomorphs fed contaminated fresh green feeds or in specimens obtained from their natural habitat; it does not occur in laboratory animals reared and maintained on uncontaminated commercial diets.

MORPHOLOGY

The adult measures up to 30 mm long by 13 mm wide (Fig. 5.1) (Lapage 1968).

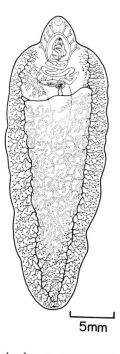

FIG. 5.1. *Fasciola hepatica* adult. (From Morgan and Hawkins 1949. Courtesy of Burgess Publishing Co.)

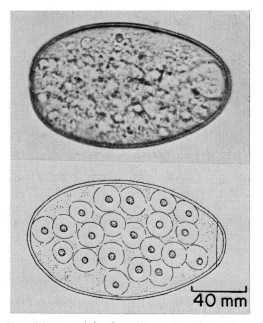

FIG. 5.2. *Fasciola hepatica* egg. Photomicrograph *(top)* and drawing *(bottom)*. *(Top* from Burrows 1965; courtesy of Yale University Press. *Bottom* courtesy of Marietta Voge, University of California.)

The surface of the body bears numerous small spines, and the intestine and gonads are extensively branched. The egg is oval and indistinctly operculated at one end and measures 130 to 150 μ by 63 to 90 μ (Fig. 5.2).

LIFE CYCLE

Eggs passed in the feces require water to hatch (Cheng 1964; Pantelouris 1965). The larvae are free-swimming and enter one of several species of snails and develop into cercariae. The cercariae leave the snail, become metacercariae, and encyst on vegetation. When ingested by the mammalian host, the metacercariae migrate through the intestinal wall and body cavity to the liver. The worms mature in the bile ducts in approximately 3 months.

PATHOLOGIC EFFECTS

Signs of infection are anorexia, debilitation, and sometimes pyrexia, jaundice, and death (Dawes and Hughes 1964; Polishchuk 1961; Renaux 1964; Trofimov and Alyabyeva 1959). Small hemorrhages are produced in the intestinal wall and peritoneum during the initial metacercarial invasion. Subsequent lesions include enlargement of the liver, with parenchymal destruction and fibrosis, and sometimes obstruction of the bile ducts.

The mortality in severely infected colonies of laboratory guinea pigs and nutria is about 50% (Polishchuk 1961; Trofimov and Alyabyeva 1959).

DIAGNOSIS

Diagnosis is based on the identification of the eggs in the feces or the adult worms in the liver at necropsy.

CONTROL

Because of the need for an intermediate mollusk host, the life cycle cannot be completed in the laboratory; however, as herbivorous laboratory animals can acquire the infection if fed contaminated greens, such feeds should be eliminated. Reportedly effective treatments include hexacloroethane, given orally in a single dose of 0.3 g per kg of body weight, for the guinea pig (Trofimov and Alyabyeva 1959), and carbon tetrachloride, given orally in a single dose of 0.3 ml per kg of body weight, for the rabbit (Ganasevich and Skovronski 1965).

Fasciola hepatica infection is rare in man (Faust, Beaver, and Jung 1968). Because of the need for an intermediate mollusk host, infected laboratory vertebrates cannot infect man.

Fasciola gigantica

This species occurs in ruminants, other mammals, and rarely man in Hawaii, the USSR, Asia, the Philippine Islands, and Africa (Soulsby 1965). Although usually rare or absent in laboratory animals, fatal ectopic fascioliasis in the laboratory guinea pig caused by this species has been reported in the Malay Peninsula (Strauss and Heyneman 1966). The outbreak was characterized by posterior paralysis and death. Fully developed flukes were found in various areas of the pelvic region, with extensive damage observed in the liver, kidneys, lungs, body wall, and hind limb musculature. Lesions included hemorrhage and fibrotic cysts filled with brown fluid.

Fasciola gigantica is morphologically similar to, but larger than, *F. hepatica* (Soulsby 1965). The adult measures 25 to 75 mm by 5 to 12 mm, and the egg, 156 to 197 μ by 90 to 104 μ. The life cycle, control, and public health aspects are the same as those of *F. hepatica*.

OPISTHORCHIDS

Opisthorchids occur in the gallbladder, bile duct, and sometimes the pancreatic duct and small intestine of mammals, birds, and reptiles. They are found only in animals that have ingested infected raw fish. Species that affect endothermal laboratory animals are listed in Table 5.2. The most important, *Opisthorchis tenuicollis* and *O. sinensis,* are discussed below.

Opisthorchis tenuicollis, Opisthorchis sinensis

These flukes are found in the bile duct and sometimes in the pancreatic duct and duodenum of the dog, cat, other mammals, and man (Lapage 1968). *Opisthorchis* has also been reported from the cynomolgus monkey (Habermann and Williams 1957). *Opisthorchis tenuicollis* occurs in North America, Europe, and Asia; *O. sinensis* occurs in Japan and southeast Asia. Neither is a serious pathogen except in heavy infections. They are rare in laboratory dogs and cats and occur only in animals that have previously eaten infected raw fish (Scott 1967). The incidence in one group of 93 cynomolgus monkeys obtained from their natural habitat was 3.2% (Habermann and Williams 1957).

The adults are lanceolate and have a smooth cuticle (Faust, Beaver, and Jung 1968; Lapage 1962; Soulsby 1965). *Opisthorchis tenuicollis* is 7 to 18 mm long by 1.5 to 3.0 mm wide, and *O. sinensis* is 10 to 25 mm long by 3 to 5 mm wide (Fig. 5.3). The eggs have a thick shell with a distinct, convex operculum and contain an asymmetrical miracidium when passed in the feces (Fig. 5.4). The egg of *O. tenuicollis* measures 26 to 30 μ by 11 to 15 μ; that of *O. sinensis* measures 27 to 35 μ by 12 to 20 μ.

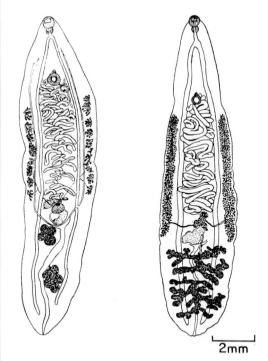

FIG. 5.3. *(Left) Opisthorchis tenuicollis. (Right) Opisthorchis sinensis.* (From Lapage 1962. Courtesy of Baillière, Tindall and Cassell.)

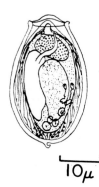

FIG. 5.4. *Opisthorchis sinensis* egg. (From Faust, Beaver, and Jung 1968. Courtesy of Lea and Febiger.)

LIFE CYCLE

Eggs passed in the feces hatch when ingested by a suitable snail (Soulsby 1965). They develop in the snail to the cercarial stage, escape, and invade the flesh of a suitable freshwater fish. The endothermal host becomes infected by eating the fish. Metacercariae are released in the duodenum and migrate up the bile duct. Egg production occurs 3 to 4 weeks after infection; the complete life cycle requires about 4 months.

PATHOLOGIC EFFECTS

Clinical signs are absent in mild infections (Soulsby 1965). The flukes cause a catarrhal inflammation and epithelial desquamation of the bile duct, sometimes cirrhosis and passive congestion of the liver, and rarely pancreatitis.

DIAGNOSIS

Diagnosis is based on identification of the eggs in the feces or the adult worms in the bile duct at necropsy.

CONTROL

Because of the complex life cycle, natural transmission cannot occur in the laboratory, and no special control procedures are required. Stibophen, 0.4 ml per kg of body weight given subcutaneously in a single dose, is reportedly an effective treatment for the cat (Renaux 1964) and is also suggested for the dog (Lapage 1962).

PUBLIC HEALTH CONSIDERATIONS

Although these flukes affect man (Faust, Beaver, and Jung 1968), infected endothermal laboratory animals are not a hazard for man because of the need for two specific intermediate hosts.

HETEROPHYIDS

The heterophyids occur in the small intestine of fish-eating mammals and birds. They are found only in animals that have ingested infected raw fish. Species that affect endothermal laboratory animals are listed in Table 5.3; none is common or important.

TROGLOTREMATIDS

The troglotrematids include the lung flukes and the fluke that transmits the agent of salmon-poisoning disease of the dog. These trematodes occur in carnivorous mammals and birds and are found only in animals that have ingested infected raw crustaceans or fishes. The species that affect endothermal laboratory animals are listed in Table 5.4; the most important are discussed below.

Paragonimus kellicotti, Paragonimus westermanii

(Lung Fluke, Oriental Lung Fluke)

These flukes usually inhabit the lungs, often causing respiratory distress in many mammals. *Paragonimus kellicotti* occurs in the dog, cat, wild carnivores, domestic animals, and rarely man in North America, particularly in the Great Lakes and Mississippi valley regions (Faust, Beaver, and Jung 1968; Soulsby 1965). *Paragonimus westermanii* occurs in the dog, cat, cynomolgus monkey, wild carnivores, domestic animals, and often man in Asia (Ruch 1959; Soulsby 1965).

Infection with *P. kellicotti* is uncommon, even in endemic areas. In a survey of 123 laboratory dogs obtained from a pound in Michigan, only one was infected (Worley 1964). *Paragonimus westermanii* infection is common in the dog but uncommon in the cynomolgus monkey. In a survey of over 1,200 cynomolgus monkeys, the infection rate was 0.1% (Hashimoto and Honjo 1966). These parasites occur only in animals permitted to eat infected raw crabs or crayfish; they cannot occur in animals reared on diets free of raw crustaceans.

MORPHOLOGY

The adults have a brown, plump, ovoid body with scale like spines (Fig. 5.5)

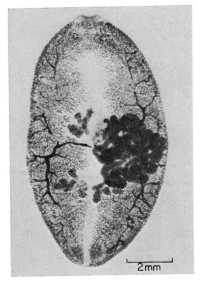

FIG. 5.5. *Paragonimus westermanii* adult. (Courtesy of Marietta Voge, University of California.)

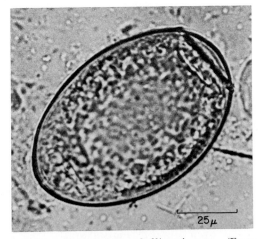

FIG. 5.6. *Paragonimus kellicotti* egg. (From Herman and Helland 1966. Courtesy of American Veterinary Medical Association.)

(Faust, Beaver, and Jung 1968). They are 7.5 to 12.0 mm long, 4 to 6 mm wide, and 3.5 to 5.0 mm thick. The oval eggs are golden brown, have a partly flattened operculum at one end, and measure 80 to 118 μ by 48 to 60 μ (Fig. 5.6).

LIFE CYCLE

Eggs in the respiratory passages are coughed up, swallowed, and passed in the feces (Fig. 5.7) (Faust, Beaver, and Jung 1968; Soulsby 1965). They hatch in water, burrow into the tissues of the first intermediate host, a snail, leave the snail, and become metacercariae in a crab or crayfish. The mammalian host is infected by ingesting the infected crustacean. The young flukes are released in the duodenum, penetrate the intestinal wall, and migrate through the peritoneal cavity and diaphragm to the lungs, where they develop to maturity in 5 to 6 weeks.

PATHOLOGIC EFFECTS

Adults occur primarily in the lungs but sometimes in the brain, liver, and other organs. Parasites in ectopic locations cause signs related to their location; those in the lungs cause coughing, wheezing, moist rales, and progressive emaciation (Bisgard and

Lewis 1964; Herman and Helland 1966). Gross lesions consist of focal areas of emphysema and soft, dark red-to-brown cysts, 2 to 3 cm in diameter, distributed throughout the parenchyma (Fig. 5.8). Incision of the cysts discloses the flukes, usually one to three in each cyst. Pleural adhesions sometimes occur. Histologic lesions include hyperplasia of the bronchial epithelium and submucosal bronchial glands and focal areas of inflammation in the lung parenchyma with clusters of fluke eggs (Fig. 5.9).

DIAGNOSIS

Diagnosis is based on demonstration of the eggs in the feces or the adult worms in the lungs at necropsy.

CONTROL

Because of the complex life cycle, natural transmission cannot occur in the laboratory, and no special control procedures are required. Bithionol, given orally at a rate of 100 to 150 mg per kg of body weight daily or every other day for 20 to 30 days, is an effective treatment for the dog (Yokogawa et al. 1961).

PUBLIC HEALTH CONSIDERATIONS

These flukes affect man; however, because of the need for specific intermediate hosts, infected endothermal animals are not a hazard for man.

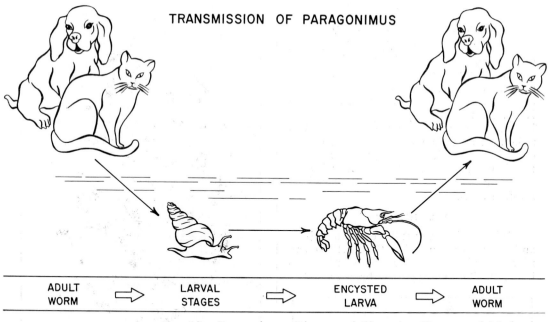

TRANSMISSION OF PARAGONIMUS

| ADULT WORM | ⇨ | LARVAL STAGES | ⇨ | ENCYSTED LARVA | ⇨ | ADULT WORM |

FIG. 5.7. *Paragonimus.* Diagram of life cycle. (Courtesy of Marietta Voge, University of California.)

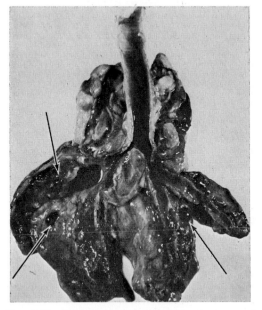

FIG. 5.8. *Paragonimus kellicotti* cysts *(arrows)* in lungs of cat. (From Herman and Helland 1966. Courtesy of American Veterinary Medical Association.)

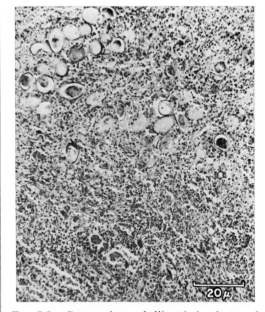

FIG. 5.9. *Paragonimus kellicotti* in lung of cat. Note inflammatory cells and fluke eggs. (From Herman and Helland 1966. Courtesy of American Veterinary Medical Association.)

Nanophyetus salmincola

(Syn. *Troglotrema salmincola*)

This fluke occurs in the small intestine of the dog, cat, and many wild rodents, carnivores, and fish-eating birds on the west coast of North America and in eastern Siberia (Schlegel, Knapp, and Millemann 1968). It is apparently not pathogenic and is important only because it transmits two rickettsial or rickettsiallike diseases of the dog. This parasite occurs only in animals that have ingested infected raw fish; it does not occur in laboratory animals reared on fish-free diets.

MORPHOLOGY

The adult is about 0.8 to 1.1 mm long and 0.3 to 0.5 mm wide (Fig. 5.10) (Bennington and Pratt 1960; Morgan and Hawkins 1949). The egg is golden brown and has

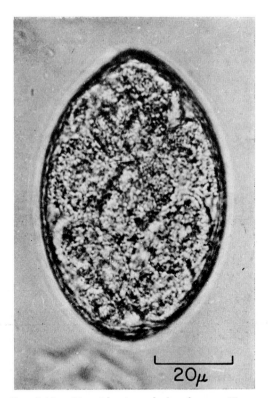

Fig. 5.11. *Nanophyetus salmincola* egg. (From Farrell 1968. Courtesy of American Veterinary Publications.)

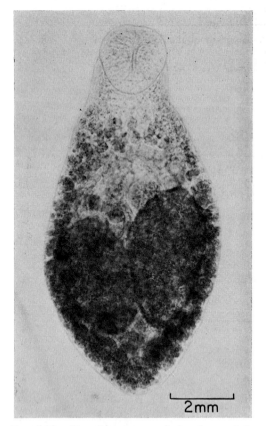

Fig. 5.10. *Nanophyetus salmincola* adult. (Courtesy of Marietta Voge, University of California.)

a small operculum at one end and a short, blunt point at the other (Fig. 5.11). It measures 64 to 80 μ by 34 to 55 μ.

LIFE CYCLE

Eggs passed in the feces hatch after about 3 months (Bennington and Pratt 1960). The first intermediate host is a snail, and the second a salmonid fish. The mammalian host is infected by eating the cercarial stages encysted in the fish. Mature worms develop in the intestine of the definitive host in 6 to 7 days.

PATHOLOGIC EFFECTS

Nanophyetus salmincola itself is apparently not pathogenic for the dog and cat (Renaux 1964; Soulsby 1965). It is important only because it transmits the rickettsia *Neorickettsia helminthoeca*, the cause of salmon-poisoning disease of the dog (Farrell, Dee, and Ott 1968; Nyberg, Knapp, and Millemann 1967), and a second rickettsiallike agent that causes Elokomin fluke fever of the dog (Farrell 1966).

DIAGNOSIS

Diagnosis is based on identification of the eggs in the feces or the adult worms in the intestine.

CONTROL

Infection is prevented by not feeding raw fish. Because of the complex life cycle, the infection cannot be disseminated in the laboratory, and no special control procedures are required.

PUBLIC HEALTH CONSIDERATIONS

Natural infection in man has been reported (Schlegel, Knapp, and Millemann 1968); however, because of the complex life cycle, infected endothermal laboratory animals are not a hazard for man.

ECHINOSTOMATIDS

These flukes usually occur in the intestine of mammals and birds. They are found only in animals that have ingested infected raw mollusks, amphibians, or fishes. Species that affect endothermal laboratory animals are listed in Table 5.5; most are uncommon and unimportant.

PLAGIORCHIDS

The plagiorchids include the oviduct flukes of the chicken and other birds. They occur only in animals that have ingested infected insects. The species that affect endothermal laboratory animals are listed in Table 5.6; the most important are discussed below.

Prosthogonimus

(Oviduct Fluke of Chicken)

Prosthogonimus is found in the bursa of Fabricius and oviduct of the chicken and other birds in most parts of the world (Price 1965; Soulsby 1965). *Prosthogonimus macrorchis* occurs in North America and is commonest in the Great Lakes region. *Prosthogonimus pellucidus* occurs in Europe; *P. ovatus* in Europe, Asia, and Africa; and *P. longus-morbificans* in Germany. None is found in laboratory-reared chickens; they occur only in chickens permitted to ingest infected dragonflies.

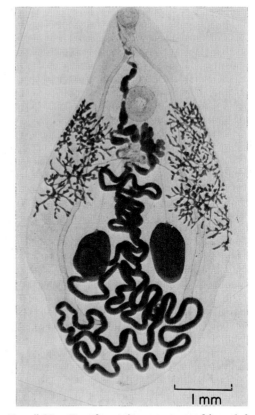

FIG. 5.12. *Prosthogonimus macrorchis* adult. (Courtesy of Marietta Voge, University of California.)

MORPHOLOGY

The adults are 6 to 8 mm long and 5 to 6 mm wide and have a spiny cuticle (Fig. 5.12) (Morgan and Hawkins 1949). The eggs have an operculum at one end and a small spine at the other. They measure 26 to 32 μ by 10 to 15 μ.

LIFE CYCLE

Eggs are passed through the cloaca (Macy 1934). Two intermediate hosts are required, a snail and a dragonfly. The bird becomes infected by ingesting the infected insect. The metacercariae are liberated in the small intestine, pass down the intestine to the cloaca, and then migrate to the bursa of Fabricius or to the oviduct, where they develop to maturity.

PATHOLOGIC EFFECTS

Signs of infection are anorexia, weight loss, reduced egg production, and malformed eggs (Soulsby 1965). Lesions include suppurative inflammation of the oviduct and often peritonitis.

DIAGNOSIS

Diagnosis is based on the clinical signs and lesions and is confirmed by identifying the eggs or adult flukes in the oviduct or in the feces (Morgan and Hawkins 1949; Soulsby 1965).

CONTROL

Because of the complex life cycle, natural transmission cannot occur in the laboratory, and no special control procedures are required. There is no effective treatment.

PUBLIC HEALTH CONSIDERATIONS

These flukes do not occur in man.

SCHISTOSOMATIDS

In the schistosomatids the sexes are separate and differ in appearance. They occur in the blood vessels of their hosts and enter through the skin or are ingested in water. They are found only in animals that have been permitted access to contaminated water. Species that affect endothermal laboratory animals are listed in Table 5.7; the most important are discussed below.

Schistosoma japonicum,
Schistosoma mansoni,
Schistosoma haematobium

(Blood Flukes)

Schistosoma japonicum occurs in the mesenteric and portal veins of the dog, cat, domestic animals, and man in eastern Asia (Lapage 1968). An incidence of 18.2% has been reported in the dog in the Philippine Islands (Soulsby 1965). Laboratory dogs and cats obtained from pounds in endemic areas are likely to be infected, but animals reared in kennels without access to snail-infested water are not.

Schistosoma mansoni occurs in the mesenteric veins of squirrel monkeys, guenons, baboons, and man in the West Indies, South America, and Africa (Fiennes 1967; Lapage 1968; Purvis, Ellison, and Husting 1965; Swellengrebel and Rijpstra 1965). It

is common in baboons obtained from their natural habitat but rare in squirrel monkeys and guenons.

Schistosoma haematobium occurs in the pelvic and mesenteric veins of guenons, baboons, the chimpanzee, and man in southern Europe, Africa, and western Asia (DePaoli 1965; Faust, Beaver, and Jung 1968; Purvis, Ellison, and Husting 1965). It is common in baboons obtained from their natural habitat but rare in guenons and the chimpanzee.

Although all three of these species of *Schistosoma* are serious pathogens for man (Faust, Beaver, and Jung 1968), they are of little importance in laboratory animals and are usually observed only at necropsy (Kuntz and Myers 1967).

MORPHOLOGY

Schistosomes occur typically in pairs with the long, slender female in the sex

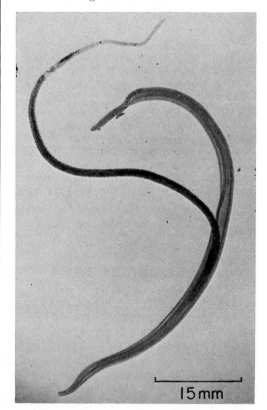

FIG. 5.13. *Schistosoma mansoni* male and female. (Courtesy of Marietta Voge, University of California.)

canal of the short, muscular male (Fig. 5.13) (Faust, Beaver, and Jung 1968).

The male of *S. japonicum* measures 12 to 20 mm by 0.5 mm; the female measures 15 to 30 mm by 0.1 to 0.3 mm. The egg is spineless, rotund, 70 to 100 μ by 50 to 65 μ, and fully embryonated when passed in the feces (Fig. 5.14*A*).

The male of *S. mansoni* is 6.4 to 9.9 mm long, and the female 7.2 to 14.0 mm. The egg is elongated-ovoid, measures 114 to 175 μ by 45 to 68 μ, is rounded at both ends, and bears a lateral spine (Fig. 5.14*B*). It is fully embryonated when passed in the feces.

The male of *S. haematobium* is 10 to 15 mm long and about 1 mm in diameter; the female is about 20 mm long and about 0.25 mm in diameter. The egg is elongated-ovoid, measures 112 to 117 μ by 40 to 70 μ, is rounded at the anterior end, and bears a posterior terminal spine (Fig. 5.14*C*). It is usually fully embryonated when excreted by the host.

LIFE CYCLE

The life cycle for all three species is similar. Eggs are excreted by the host in the feces (*S. japonicum, S. mansoni*) or in the urine (*S. haematobium*) (Faust, Beaver,

and Jung 1968). The eggs hatch in water, penetrate a snail in which they develop into cercariae, and then emerge from the snail into the surrounding water. Infection of the endothermal host occurs by skin penetration of the cercariae and possibly by ingestion of contaminated water. The cercariae develop while migrating through the tissues and eventually reach the mesenteric or pelvic vessels as young worms. The complete life cycle requires 8 to 12 weeks; adult worms sometimes live for 20 to 30 years.

PATHOLOGIC EFFECTS

The principal effects are caused by the eggs (Faust, Beaver, and Jung 1968; Smith and Jones 1966). Adult flukes in the mesenteric vessels deposit their eggs in the venules of the intestine; those in the pelvic vessels deposit their eggs in the venules of the urinary bladder. Some eggs escape from the venules, filter through the intestinal and bladder wall, and eventually break through into the lumen. Other eggs enter the circulation as emboli. These become lodged in various tissues where they often cause a severe foreign-body reaction.

Clinical signs include pyrexia, hemorrhagic diarrhea or hematuria, and ascites

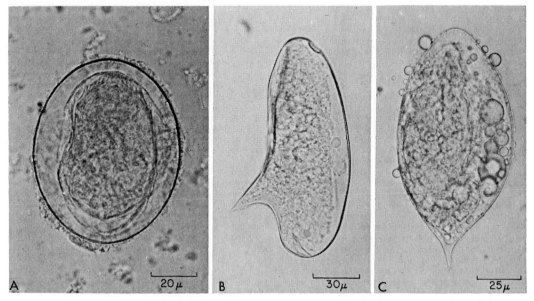

FIG. 5.14. *Schistosoma* eggs. *(A) S. japonicum. (B) S. mansoni. (C) S. haematobium.* (Courtesy of Marietta Voge, University of California.)

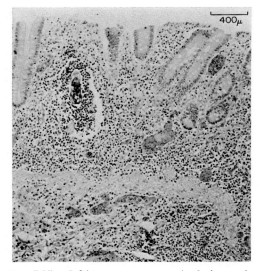

FIG. 5.15. *Schistosoma mansoni* lesions in colon of experimentally infected chimpanzee. Note dense cellularity of lamina propria, dilated and hyperemic submucosal vessels, and mature egg surrounded by leucocytes in remnants of a mucosal crypt (crypt abscess). (From Sadun et al. 1966. Courtesy of America Journal of Tropical Medicine and Hygiene.)

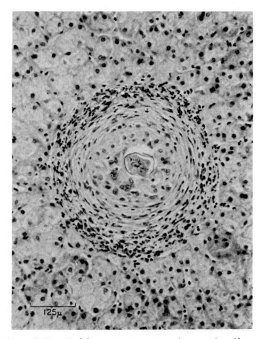

FIG. 5.16. *Schistosoma mansoni* egg in liver tissue of experimentally infected chimpanzee. (From Sadun et al. 1966. Courtesy of American Journal of Tropical Medicine and Hygiene.)

(Faust, Beaver, and Jung 1968; Sadun et al. 1966).

Thickening of the intestinal or urinary bladder wall is the commonest lesion (Fig. 5.15) (DePaoli 1965; Smith and Jones 1966). Microscopic granulomas containing eggs are also common in the liver, brain, spleen, and other organs (Fig. 5.16) (DePaoli 1965; Purvis, Ellison, and Husting 1965; Sadun et al. 1966).

DIAGNOSIS

Diagnosis is based on demonstration of the eggs in the feces or urine, or the adult worms in the blood vessels at necropsy.

CONTROL

Natural transmission cannot occur in the laboratory; therefore no special control procedures are required. There is no satisfactory treatment (Faust, Beaver, and Jung 1968).

PUBLIC HEALTH CONSIDERATIONS

Although schistosomiasis is one of the most important diseases of man (Faust, Beaver, and Jung 1968), infected laboratory animals are not a direct hazard for man because of the requirement for an intermediate mollusk host. However, because of the importance of this disease in man, excreta from infected animals should be decontaminated before being discarded.

DIPLOSTOMATIDS

These flukes usually occur in the intestine of carnivorous mammals. They are found only in animals that have ingested infected amphibians or reptiles. The species that affect endothermal laboratory animals are listed in Table 5.8. Most are uncommon and unimportant.

PARAMPHISTOMIDS

These flukes are common in the intestine of herbivorous mammals. Infection is usually by ingestion of contaminated vegetation. The species that affect endothermal laboratory animals are listed in Table 5.9. The most important are discussed below.

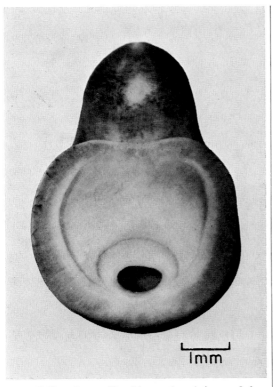

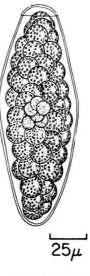

FIG. 5.18. *Gastrodiscoides hominis* egg. (From Faust 1949. Courtesy of Lea and Febiger.)

FIG. 5.17. *Gastrodiscoides hominis* adult. (From Graham 1960. Courtesy of New York Academy of Sciences.)

Gastrodiscoides hominis

This slightly pathogenic fluke occurs in the cecum and colon of the monkey, cynomolgus monkey, pig, and man in India, southeast Asia, Indonesia, and the Philippine Islands (Faust, Beaver, and Jung 1968; Graham 1960). It is common in laboratory monkeys (Graham 1960; Herman 1967; Reardon and Rininger 1968; Sasa et al. 1962; Whitney, Johnson, and Cole 1967), and in one survey it was found in 21.4% of over 1,200 cynomolgus monkeys (Hashimoto and Honjo 1966).

MORPHOLOGY

The adult is a small orange-red fluke (Fig. 5.17) (Graham 1960; Herman 1967). It measures about 6 by 3 mm and has a cuplike discoidal hind body, a cone-shaped anterior end, and a small anterior sucker. The egg is operculated and spindle shaped, has bluntly rounded ends, and measures 150 to 152 μ by 60 to 72 μ (Fig. 5.18) (Faust, Beaver, and Jung 1968). It is unembryonated when passed in the feces.

LIFE CYCLE

The life cycle involves a snail intermediate host and is similar to that of *Fasciola hepatica* (Faust, Beaver, and Jung 1968). The definitive host becomes infected by ingesting metacercariae which encyst on vegetation.

PATHOLOGIC EFFECTS

The parasite usually occurs in large numbers in infected animals (Fig. 5.19). It produces a mucous diarrhea and a mild chronic enteritis (Faust, Beaver, and Jung 1968; Herman 1967).

DIAGNOSIS

Diagnosis is based on demonstration of the eggs in the feces or adult flukes in the cecum and colon.

CONTROL

Natural transmission cannot occur in the laboratory; therefore, no special control procedures are required. No treatment is reported.

PUBLIC HEALTH CONSIDERATIONS

Although this fluke causes a mild diarrhea in man (Faust, Beaver, and Jung 1968), infected laboratory animals are not

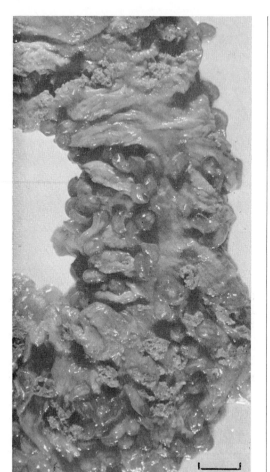

FIG. 5.19. *Gastrodiscoides hominis* adults in colon of monkey. (From Whitney, Johnson, and Cole 1967. Courtesy of R. A. Whitney, Edgewood Arsenal.)

a health hazard for man because of the need for an intermediate mollusk host.

Watsonius watsoni, Watsonius deschieni *Watsonius macaci*

Watsonius watsoni occurs in the intestine of guenons, baboons, and man in West Africa (Faust, Beaver, and Jung 1968; Fiennes 1967; Myers and Kuntz 1965; Ruch 1959). It is uncommon in guenons and baboons and rare in man. *Watsonius deschieni* occurs in the intestine of baboons in West Africa (Myers and Kuntz 1965; Ruch 1959). It is uncommon. *Watsonius macaci*

is the species reported to occur in the cynomolgus monkey (Cosgrove 1966; Fiennes 1967); however, in a survey of over 1,200 such monkeys, 0.5% were found to be infected with what was identified as *W. watsoni* (Hashimoto and Honjo 1966).

MORPHOLOGY

The adults are translucent, orange, pear shaped and about 2 to 10 mm long (Ruch 1959). The egg is light yellow, ovoid, and operculated, and measures 122 to 130 μ by 75 to 80 μ (Estes and Brown 1966).

LIFE CYCLE

The life cycle is not completely known, but it is thought to involve a snail host and to be similar to that of *Fasciola hepatica* (Faust, Beaver, and Jung 1968; Ruch 1959). The definitive host probably becomes infected by ingesting metacercariae encysted on vegetation.

PATHOLOGIC EFFECTS

Watsonius watsoni and *W. deschieni* have been associated with diarrhea and severe enteritis in baboons (Ruch 1959); otherwise, little is known of the pathologic effects of these species.

DIAGNOSIS

Diagnosis is based on identification of the eggs in the feces or the adults in the intestine at necropsy.

CONTROL

Because natural transmission cannot occur in the laboratory, no special control procedures are needed.

PUBLIC HEALTH CONSIDERATIONS

There is one report of diarrhea and death associated with *W. watsoni* infection in man (Faust, Beaver, and Jung 1968); however, because of the need for an intermediate mollusk host, infected laboratory animals are not a human health hazard.

DICROCOELIIDS

The dicrocoeliids occur in the bile and pancreatic ducts and sometimes the intestine of mammals, birds, amphibians, and reptiles. The life cycle for most of these flukes is unknown. For one species, infection of the endothermal host requires the

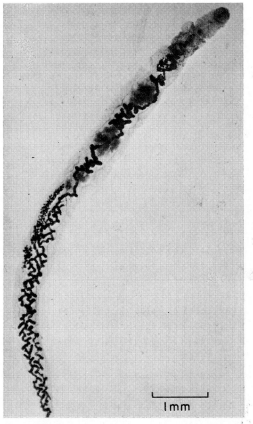

1mm

Fig. 5.20. *Athesmia foxi* adult. (Courtesy of G. E. Cosgrove, Oak Ridge National Laboratory.)

ingestion of an infected ant; for another it requires ingestion of an infected lizard. Those that affect endothermal laboratory animals are listed in Table 5.10. The most important, *Athesmia foxi* and *Platynosomum concinnum,* are discussed below.

Athesmia foxi

This moderately pathogenic fluke occurs in the bile duct of capuchins, squirrel monkeys, tamarins, and titi monkeys of northern South America, and in a wild rat (*Rattus argentiventer*) in the Malay Peninsula (Faust 1967). It is common in laboratory primates obtained from South America. Incidences of 43% in 16 capuchins (Garner, Hemrick, and Rudiger 1967) and 8% in 455 tamarins have been reported (Cosgrove, Nelsen, and Gengozian 1968).

MORPHOLOGY

The adult is long and slender, measuring about 8.5 by 0.7 mm (Fig. 5.20) (Faust 1967). The egg is ovoid and golden brown, has a thick shell and operculum, and measures 27 to 34 μ by 17 to 21 μ.

LIFE CYCLE

The life cycle is not completely known. It includes a mollusk intermediate host, but the method of infection of the vertebrate host is unknown.

PATHOLOGIC EFFECTS

The fluke frequently occurs in the bile duct, often in large numbers (Bostrom and Slaughter 1968; Ruch 1959). It causes enlargement and partial obstruction of the duct (Fig. 5.21) and inflammation and sometimes destruction of the epithelial lining (Bostrom and Slaughter 1968; Ewing et al. 1968; Garner, Hemrick, and Rudiger 1967).

DIAGNOSIS

Diagnosis is based on demonstration of the adult fluke in the bile duct either at necropsy or on examination of liver sections, or by demonstration of the eggs in the feces.

CONTROL

Because of the need for an intermediate host, transmission in the laboratory cannot occur and no special control procedures are required. No treatment is reported.

PUBLIC HEALTH CONSIDERATIONS

This parasite has not been reported from man (Fiennes 1967). Because of the need for an intermediate mollusk host, infected laboratory animals are not a direct hazard to man.

Platynosomum concinnum
(Syn. *Platynosomum fastosum*)

This fluke, the cause of so-called "lizard poisoning," occurs in the gallbladder and bile duct of the cat in Florida, Puerto Rico, the Bahama Islands, Brazil, and the Malay Peninsula (Soulsby 1965). It is common in the Caribbean area, with an incidence of about 50% in cats in the Bahama Islands (Leam and Walker 1963), but is

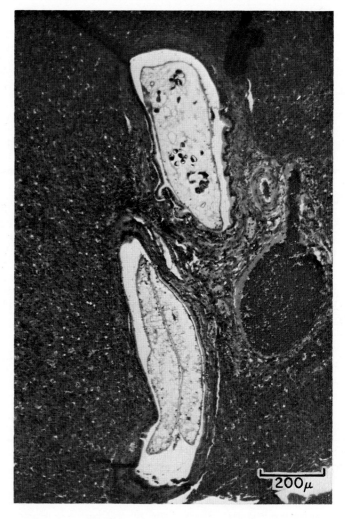

FIG. 5.21. *Athesmia foxi* in bile duct of squirrel monkey. (Courtesy of H. D. Anthony, Kansas State University.)

rare in the United States (Renaux 1964). Laboratory cats obtained from pounds in Puerto Rico, the Bahama Islands, and to a lesser extent Florida, are likely to be affected.

MORPHOLOGY

The adult is lanceolate and measures 4 to 8 mm by 1.2 to 2.5 mm (Fig. 5.22) (Soulsby 1965). The egg is brown, oval, thick shelled, and operculated, and measures 34 to 50 μ by 20 to 35 μ (Greve and Leonard 1966).

LIFE CYCLE

Eggs passed in the feces develop into cercariae in a snail; the cercariae encyst in

a lizard. The cat becomes infected by eating the lizard.

PATHOLOGIC EFFECTS

In heavy infections, the clinical signs include vomiting, diarrhea, emaciation, jaundice, and death (Greve and Leonard 1966; Soulsby 1965). The gallbladder and bile duct are distended, the wall of the bile duct is thickened, and the liver is enlarged. Histologic lesions include hyperplasia of the biliary epithelium, cellular infiltration of the lamina propria, and fibrosis of the duct wall (Fig. 5.23).

DIAGNOSIS

Diagnosis is made by demonstrating the eggs in the feces, or fluke in the gall-

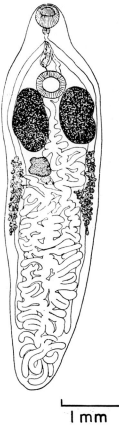

FIG. 5.22. *Platynosomum concinnum* adult. (From Lapage 1962. Courtesy of Ballière, Tindall and Cassell.)

|__1 mm__|

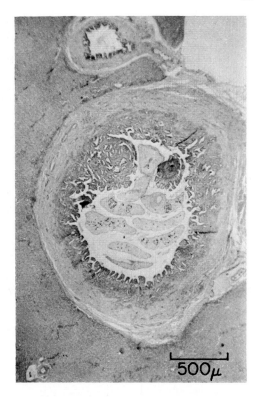

FIG. 5.23. *Platynosomum concinnum* in bile duct of cat. (From Greve and Leonard 1966. Courtesy of American Veterinary Medical Association.)

bladder or bile duct at necropsy or in histologic sections.

CONTROL

Because of the need for both a mollusk and a reptile intermediate host, natural transmission cannot occur in the laboratory. There is no treatment.

PUBLIC HEALTH CONSIDERATIONS

Infection in man has not been reported. Because of the need for intermediate hosts, infected cats are not a health hazard for man.

BRACHYLAEMIDS, LECITHODENDRIIDS, NOTOCOTYLIDS, PSILOSTOMATIDS, PHILOPHTHALMIDS

These flukes occur in various vertebrates. Those that affect endothermal laboratory animals are listed in Table 5.11. Most are uncommon or unimportant.

TABLE 5.1. Fasciolids affecting endothermal laboratory animals

Parasite	Geographic Distribution	Endothermal Host	Location in Host	Method of Infection	Incidence		Pathologic Effects	Public Health Importance	Reference
					In nature	In laboratory			
Fasciola hepatica*	Worldwide	Guinea pig, nutria, cottontail rabbits, hares, dog, cat, rhesus monkey, cynomolgus monkey, ruminants, pig, other mammals, man	Liver	Ingestion of metacercaria encysted on vegetation	Uncommon to common	Rare; occurs only in animals fed contaminated greens	Anorexia, debilitation, hepatomegaly, hepatic fibrosis; sometimes biliary obstruction, fever, icterus, death	Occurs in man; infected laboratory animals cannot infect man	Golebiowski 1959, Graham 1960, Hashimoto and Honjo 1966, Holmes 1962, Morgan and Hawkins 1949, Polishchuk 1961, Trofimov and Alyabyeva 1959, Tropilo 1965
Fasciola gigantica*	Hawaii, USSR, Asia, Philippine Islands, Africa	Guinea pig, ruminants, other mammals, man	Liver, abdominal cavity	Ingestion of metacercaria encysted on vegetation	Uncommon to common	Rare	Posterior paralysis; hemorrhage; fibrotic cysts in liver, kidneys, lungs; death	Occurs in man; infected laboratory animals cannot infect man	Soulsby 1965, Strauss and Heyneman 1966
Fasciolopsis buski	Asia	Rhesus monkey, pig, man	Duodenum, stomach	Ingestion of metacercaria encysted on vegetation	Uncommon to common	Rare	Unknown in monkey	Occurs in man; infected laboratory animals cannot infect man	Faust et al. 1968, Hartman 1961

*Discussed in text.

136

TABLE 5.2. Opisthorchids affecting endothermal laboratory animals

Parasite	Geographic Distribution	Endothermal Host	Location in Host	Method of Infection	Incidence		Pathologic Effects	Public Health Importance	Reference
					In nature	In laboratory			
Opisthorchis tenuicollis*	North America, Europe, Asia	Dog, cat, other mammals, man	Bile duct; sometimes pancreatic duct, duodenum	Ingestion of metacercaria encysted in fish	Uncommon to common	Rare	Inflammation of bile duct; sometimes hepatic cirrhosis; rarely pancreatitis	Occurs in man; infected laboratory animals cannot infect man	Faust et al. 1968 Lapage 1962 Soulsby 1965
Opisthorchis sinensis*	Japan, southeastern Asia	Dog, cat, cynomolgus monkey, other mammals, man	Bile duct; sometimes pancreatic duct, duodenum	Ingestion of metacercaria encysted in fish	Uncommon to common	Rare in dog, cat; uncommon in cynomolgus monkey	Inflammation of bile duct; sometimes hepatic cirrhosis; rarely pancreatitis	Occurs in man; infected laboratory animals cannot infect man	Faust et al. 1968 Habermann and Williams 1957 Lapage 1962 Soulsby 1965
Metorchis conjunctus	North America	Dog, cat, other carnivores, man	Bile duct, gallbladder	Ingestion of metacercaria encysted in fish	Uncommon to common	Rare in dog, cat	Inflammation of bile duct; sometimes hepatic cirrhosis; rarely pancreatitis	Occurs in man; infected laboratory animals cannot infect man	Mills and Hirth 1968 Morgan and Hawkins 1949 Soulsby 1965
Metorchis albidus	North America, Europe	Dog, cat, other carnivores	Bile duct, gallbladder	Ingestion of metacercaria encysted in fish	Uncommon to common	Rare in dog, cat	Inflammation of bile duct; sometimes hepatic cirrhosis; rarely pancreatitis	Unknown	Morgan and Hawkins 1949 Soulsby 1965
Parametorchis complexus	North America	Dog, cat, other carnivores	Bile duct	Unknown; probably by ingestion of metacercaria in fish	Unknown	Unknown; probably rare	Unknown	Unknown	Burrows 1965 Morgan and Hawkins 1949
Amphimerus pseudofelineus	United States, Panama, Ecuador, Brazil	Dog, cat, man	Bile duct	Unknown; probably by ingestion of metacercaria in fish	Unknown	Unknown; probably rare	Hepatic cirrhosis; pancreatitis	Occurs in man; infected laboratory animals cannot infect man	Faust et al. 1968 Morgan and Hawkins 1949
Pseudamphistomum truncatum	Europe, India	Dog, cat, other carnivores, man	Bile duct	Ingestion of metacercaria encysted in fish	Unknown	Unknown; probably rare	Unknown	Occurs in man; infected laboratory animals cannot infect man	Lapage 1962, 1968

*Discussed in text.

137

TABLE 5.3. Heterophyids affecting endothermal laboratory animals

Parasite	Geographic Distribution	Endothermal Host	Location in Host	Method of Infection	Incidence In nature	Incidence In laboratory	Pathologic Effects	Public Health Importance	Reference
Ascocotyle diminuta	United States	Rat	Small intestine	Ingestion of metacercaria encysted in fish	Unknown	Absent	Unknown	Unknown	Morgan and Hawkins 1949
Heterophyes heterophyes	Asia, northern Africa	Dog, cat, other carnivores, fish-eating birds, man	Small intestine	Ingestion of metacercaria encysted in fish	Unknown	Unknown; probably rare	Slight intestinal desquamation	Occurs in man; infected laboratory animals cannot infect man	Faust et al. 1968 Lapage 1962, 1968
Metagonimus yokogawai	Eastern Europe, Asia	Dog, cat, guenons, pig, fish-eating birds, man	Small intestine	Ingestion of metacercaria encysted in fish	Unknown	Unknown; probably rare	Slight intestinal desquamation	Occurs in man; infected laboratory animals cannot infect man	Cosgrove 1966 Faust et al. 1968 Lapage 1962, 1968
Stellantchasmus falcatus	Hawaii, Philippine Islands	Rat, dog, cat, man	Small intestine	Ingestion of metacercaria encysted in fish	Unknown	Unknown; probably rare	Unknown	Occurs in man; infected laboratory animals cannot infect man	Alicata 1964 Burrows 1965 Faust et al. 1968
Cryptocotyle lingua	North America, northern Europe	Dog, other carnivores, fish-eating birds	Small intestine	Ingestion of metacercaria encysted in fish	Unknown	Unknown; probably rare	Enteritis	Unknown	Lapage 1962, 1968 Morgan and Hawkins 1949 Soulsby 1965
Cryptocotyle concava	Europe	Dog, other carnivores, fish-eating birds	Small intestine	Ingestion of metacercaria encysted in fish	Uncommon	Unknown; probably rare	Enteritis	Unknown	Soulsby 1965
Phagicola longa	North America, Hawaii, southern Europe, Israel	Dog, other canids, cat	Small intestine	Ingestion of metacercaria encysted in fish	Unknown in North America; common in southern Europe	Unknown; probably rare in North America, common in southern Europe	Unknown	Unknown	Alicata 1964 Himonas 1968 Morgan and Hawkins 1949 Soulsby 1965
Phagicola italica	Italy	Dog	Small intestine	Ingestion of metacercaria encysted in fish	Unknown;	Unknown; probably rare	Unknown	Unknown	Soulsby 1965

TABLE 5.3 (continued)

Parasite	Geographic Distribution	Endothermal Host	Location in Host	Method of Infection	Incidence		Pathologic Effects	Public Health Importance	Reference
					In nature	In laboratory			
Apophallus venustus	North America, Europe	Dog, other canids, cat	Small intestine	Ingestion of metacercaria encysted in fish	Unknown	Unknown; probably rare	Unknown	Unknown	Morgan and Hawkins 1949 Soulsby 1965
Haplorchis pumilio	Israel, northern Africa, China	Dog, cat, man	Small intestine	Ingestion of metacercaria encysted in fish	Unknown	Unknown; probably rare	Unknown	Occurs in man; infected laboratory animals cannot infect man	Bisseru 1967 Soulsby 1965
Haplorchis taichui	Israel, northern Africa, China	Dog, cat, man	Small intestine	Ingestion of metacercaria encysted in fish	Unknown	Unknown; probably rare	Unknown	Occurs in man; infected laboratory animals cannot infect man	Bisseru 1967 Soulsby 1965
Haplorchis yokogawai	Asia	Macaques	Small intestine	Ingestion of metacercaria encysted in fish	Unknown	Unknown; probably rare	Unknown	Unknown	Cosgrove 1966
Pygidiopis genata	Israel, northern Africa, China	Dog, cat	Small intestine	Ingestion of metacercaria encysted in fish	Unknown	Unknown; probably rare	Unknown	Unknown	Soulsby 1965
Strictodora sawakiensis	Philippine Islands, northern Africa	Dog	Small intestine	Ingestion of metacercaria encysted in fish	Unknown	Unknown; probably rare	Unknown	Unknown	Soulsby 1965
Adleriella minutissima	Israel	Dog, cat	Small intestine	Ingestion of metacercaria encysted in fish	Unknown	Unknown; probably rare	Unknown	Unknown	Soulsby 1965

TABLE 5.4. Troglotrematids affecting endothermal laboratory animals

Parasite	Geographic Distribution	Endothermal Host	Location in Host	Method of Infection	Incidence — In nature	Incidence — In laboratory	Pathologic Effects	Public Health Importance	Reference
*Paragonimus kellicotti**	North America	Dog, cat, wild carnivores, domestic animals, man	Lungs; sometimes brain, liver, other organs	Ingestion of infected crustacean (crab, crayfish)	Uncommon	Uncommon	Cough, wheeze, rales, emphysema, emaciation, lung cysts	Rare in man; infected laboratory animals cannot infect man	Faust et al. 1968 Herman and Helland 1966 Soulsby 1965 Worley 1964
*Paragonimus westermanii**	Asia	Dog, cat, wild carnivores, domestic animals, cynomolgus monkey, man	Lungs; sometimes brain, liver, other organs	Ingestion of infected crustacean (crab, crayfish)	Common in dog; uncommon in cynomolgus monkey	Common in dog; uncommon in cynomolgus monkey	Cough, wheeze, rales, emphysema, emaciation, lung cysts	Occurs in man; infected laboratory animals cannot infect man	Faust et al. 1968 Hashimoto and Honjo 1966 Ruch 1959 Soulsby 1965
*Nanophyetus salmincola**	West coast of North America, eastern Siberia	Dog, cat, wild rodents, carnivores, fish-eating birds, man	Small intestine	Ingestion of infected salmonid fishes	Uncommon	Unknown; probably absent	Apparently none; vector of *Neorickettsia helminthoeca*; vector of agent of Elokomin fluke fever	Rare in man; infected laboratory animals cannot infect man	Bennington and Pratt 1960 Farrell 1966 Morgan and Hawkins 1949 Nyberg et al. 1967 Schlegel et al. 1968 Soulsby 1965
Collyriclum faba	United States, central Europe	Chicken, other birds	Skin, subcutaneous tissues	Unknown	Rare	Unknown; probably absent	Usually inapparent; sometimes anemia, emaciation, death	Unknown	Lapage 1962, 1968 Morgan and Hawkins 1949 Soulsby 1965

*Discussed in text.

TABLE 5.5. Echinostomatids affecting endothermal laboratory animals

Parasite	Geographic Distribution	Endothermal Host	Location in Host	Method of Infection	Incidence In nature	Incidence In laboratory	Pathologic Effects	Public Health Importance	Reference
Heterechinostomum magnovatum	United States	Rat	Small intestine	Unknown	Rare	Absent	Unknown	Unknown	Morgan and Hawkins 1949
Echinostoma guerreroi	United States	Rat	Small intestine	Unknown	Rare	Absent	Unknown	Unknown	Morgan and Hawkins 1949
Echinostoma lindoense	Indonesia	Rat, man	Small intestine	Unknown; probably by ingestion of infected mollusk	Rare	Absent	Unknown	Occurs in man	Bisseru 1967 Faust et al. 1968
Echinostoma ilocanum	Philippine Islands, China, Indonesia	Rat, dog, cat, pig, macaques, man	Small intestine	Unknown; probably by ingestion of infected mollusk	Common in dog; uncommon in other species	Unknown	Unknown	Occurs in man	Bisseru 1967 Cosgrove 1966 Faust et al. 1968
Echinostoma revolutum	North America, Europe, Asia, Indonesia	Rat, other wild rodents, chicken, other birds, man	Intestine, ceca, rectum	Ingestion of infected mollusk or amphibian	Rare in rat, chicken	Unknown; probably absent	Usually inapparent; sometimes enteritis	Occurs in man	Faust et al. 1968 Morgan and Hawkins 1949 Price 1965 Sasa et al. 1962
Echinostoma melis	Europe, Asia	Cat, other carnivores, man	Small intestine	Ingestion of infected fish	Rare	Unknown; probably absent	Enteritis	Occurs in man	Faust et al. 1968 Soulsby 1965
Echinochasmus perfoliatus	Europe, Asia	Dog, cat, fox, pig, man	Small intestine	Ingestion of infected fish	Rare	Unknown; probably absent	Enteritis	Occurs in man	Bisseru 1967 Faust et al. 1968 Soulsby 1965
Echinochasmus schwartzi	United States	Dog, muskrat	Small intestine	Unknown; probably by ingestion of infected fish	Rare	Unknown; probably rare or absent	Unknown	Unknown	Burrows 1965 Morgan and Hawkins 1949

TABLE 5.5 (continued)

Parasite	Geographic Distribution	Endothermal Host	Location in Host	Method of Infection	Incidence In nature	Incidence In laboratory	Pathologic Effects	Public Health Importance	Reference
Mesorchis denticulatus	Europe	Dog, cat	Small intestine	Unknown; probably by ingestion of infected fish	Rare	Unknown; probably rare or absent	Unknown	Unknown	Soulsby 1965
Artyfechinostomum sp.	Asia	Macaques	Intestine	Unknown	Unknown	Unknown	Unknown	Unknown	Cosgrove 1966
Reptilotrema primata	Asia	Macaques	Intestine	Unknown	Unknown	Unknown	Unknown	Unknown	Cosgrove 1966
Echinoparyphium recurvatum	North America, Europe, Asia, Africa	Chicken, other birds	Small intestine	Ingestion of infected mollusk (snail) or amphibian (tadpole)	Rare in chicken	Unknown; probably absent	Severe enteritis, anemia, emaciation	Unknown	Morgan and Hawkins 1949 Price 1965
Hypoderaeum conoideum	United States, Europe, Asia	Chicken, other birds, man	Small intestine	Ingestion of infected mollusk (snail)	Rare	Unknown; probably absent	Unknown	Occurs in man	Faust et al. 1968 Morgan and Hawkins 1949 Price 1965
Clinostomum attenuatum	United States	Chicken, pigeon	Trachea	Unknown; probably by ingestion of infected amphibian (frog)	Rare	Unknown; probably absent	Unknown	Unknown	Morgan and Hawkins 1949

TABLE 5.6. Plagiorchids affecting endothermal laboratory animals

Parasite	Geographic Distribution	Endothermal Host	Location in Host	Method of Infection	Incidence		Pathologic Effects	Public Health Importance	Reference
					In nature	In laboratory			
Plagiorchis muris	North America, Hawaii, Asia	Mouse, rat, man	Intestine	Ingestion of infected snail	Common in some areas	Absent	Unknown	Occurs in man	Ash 1962 Bisseru 1967 Olsen 1967 Sasa et al. 1962
Plagiorchis philippinensis	Philippine Islands	Mouse, rat, man	Intestine	Unknown	Common in some areas	Absent	Unknown	Occurs in man	Bisseru 1967
Plagiorchis javensis	Indonesia	Mouse, rat, man	Intestine	Unknown	Common in some areas	Absent	Unknown	Occurs in man	Bisseru 1967
Plagiorchis arcuatus	Europe	Chicken	Oviduct	Unknown; presumably by ingestion of infected insect	Unknown	Unknown; probably absent	Unknown	Unknown	Soulsby 1965
*Prosthogonimus macrorchis**	North America	Chicken, other birds	Oviduct, bursa Fabricius	Ingestion of infected insect (dragonfly)	Common in some areas	Rare or absent	Anorexia, weight loss, inflammation of oviduct, peritonitis	None	Macy 1934 Morgan and Hawkins 1949 Price 1965 Soulsby 1965
*Prosthogonimus pellucidus**	Europe	Chicken, other birds	Oviduct, bursa Fabricius	Ingestion of infected insect (dragonfly)	Common in some areas	Rare or absent	Anorexia, weight loss, inflammation of oviduct, peritonitis	None	Lapage 1968 Soulsby 1965
*Prosthogonimus ovatus**	Europe, Asia, Africa	Chicken, other birds	Oviduct, bursa Fabricius	Ingestion of infected insect (dragonfly)	Common in some areas	Rare or absent	Anorexia, weight loss, inflammation of oviduct, peritonitis	None	Lapage 1968 Soulsby 1965
*Prosthogonimus longus-morbificans**	Germany	Chicken, other birds	Oviduct, bursa Fabricius	Ingestion of infected insect (dragonfly)	Common in some areas	Rare or absent	Anorexia, weight loss, inflammation of oviduct, peritonitis	None	Soulsby 1965

*Discussed in text.

143

TABLE 5.7. Schistosomatids affecting endothermal laboratory animals

Parasite	Geographic Distribution	Endothermal Host	Method of Infection	Location in Host	Incidence In nature	Incidence In laboratory	Pathologic Effects	Public Health Importance	Reference
*Schistosoma japonicum**	Eastern Asia	Dog, cat, domestic animals, man	Skin penetration by cercaria; possibly ingestion of cercaria	Mesenteric veins, portal vein	Common in endemic areas	Rare to common, depending on source	Hemorrhagic diarrhea; thickened intestinal wall; microscopic granulomas in various organs	Causes oriental schistosomiasis; infected laboratory animals cannot infect man	Faust et al. 1968 Lapage 1968 Smith and Jones 1966
*Schistosoma mansoni**	West Indies, South America, Africa	Squirrel monkeys, guenons, baboons, man	Skin penetration by cercaria; possibly ingestion of cercaria	Mesenteric veins	Common in endemic areas	Common in baboons; rare in squirrel monkeys, guenons	Hemorrhagic diarrhea; thickened intestinal wall; microscopic granulomas in various organs	Causes intestinal schistosomiasis; infected laboratory animals cannot infect man	Faust et al. 1968 Fiennes 1967 Kuntz and Myers 1967 Lapage 1968 Purvis et al. 1965 Sadun et al. 1966 Swellengrebel and Rijpstra 1965
*Schistosoma haematobium**	Europe, Africa, western Asia	Guenons, baboons, chimpanzee, man	Skin penetration by cercaria; possibly ingestion of cercaria	Pelvic vein, mesenteric veins	Common in endemic areas	Common in baboons; rare in guenons, chimpanzee	Hematuria; thickened urinary bladder wall; microscopic granulomas in various organs	Causes urinary schistosomiasis; infected laboratory animals cannot infect man	DePaoli 1965 Faust et al. 1968 Purvis et al. 1965
Schistosoma spindale	India, Indonesia, Africa	Dog, domestic animals, man	Skin penetration by cercaria; possibly ingestion of cercaria	Mesenteric veins, portal vein	Unknown	Unknown	Intestinal nodules; hepatic cirrhosis	Occurs in man; infected laboratory animals cannot infect man	Faust et al. 1968 Lapage 1962, 1968 Soulsby 1965
Schistosoma mattheei	Africa	Baboons, other simian primates, man	Skin penetration by cercaria; possibly ingestion of cercaria	Mesenteric veins	Unknown	Unknown	Intestinal nodules; hepatic cirrhosis	Occurs in man; infected laboratory animals cannot infect man	Faust et al. 1968 Myers and Kuntz 1965

*Discussed in text.

144

TABLE 5.7 (continued)

Parasite	Geographic Distribution	Endothermal Host	Location in Host	Method of Infection	Incidence		Pathologic Effects	Public Health Importance	Reference
					In nature	In laboratory			
Schistosoma suis	India	Dog, pig, man	Mesenteric veins	Skin penetration by cercaria; possibly ingestion of cercaria	Unknown	Unknown	Intestinal nodules; hepatic cirrhosis	Occurs in in man; infected laboratory animals cannot infect man	Faust et al. 1968 Lapage 1962, 1968 Soulsby 1965
Ornithobilharzia turkestanicum	France, Asia	Cat, domestic animals	Mesenteric veins	Skin penetration by cercaria; possibly ingestion of cercaria	Unknown	Unknown	Intestinal nodules; hepatic cirrhosis	Unknown	Lapage 1962, 1968 Soulsby 1965
Heterobilharzia americana	Southern United States	Dog, raccoon, nutria	Portal vein, mesenteric veins	Skin penetration by cercaria; possibly ingestion of cercaria	Rare	Rare or absent	Diarrhea, debilitation, intestinal edema, hepatomegaly, ascites	Possibly causes dermatitis	Pierce 1963 Soulsby 1965 Thrasher 1964
Schistosomatium douthitti	Northern North America	Rat, voles, muskrat, hares	Mesenteric veins	Skin penetration by cercaria; possibly ingestion of cercaria	Uncommon in rat	Absent	Hepatic lesions	Causes dermatitis	Morgan and Hawkins 1949 Swartz 1966

TABLE 5.8. Diplostomatids affecting endothermal laboratory animals

Parasite	Geographic Distribution	Endothermal Host	Location in Host	Method of Infection	Incidence		Pathologic Effects	Public Health Importance	Reference
					In nature	In laboratory			
Alaria alata	Eastern Europe	Dog, other canids	Small intestine	Ingestion of infected frog, snake	Uncommon	Rare or absent	Usually none; sometimes catarrhal enteritis	None known	Soulsby 1965
Alaria americana	United States	Dog, other canids	Small intestine	Unknown; probably ingestion of infected frog, snake	Unknown	Unknown; probably rare	Unknown	None known	Burrows 1965 Morgan and Hawkins 1949
Alaria arisaemoides	United States	Dog, fox	Small intestine	Unknown; probably ingestion of infected frog, snake	Unknown	Unknown; probaby rare	Unknown	None known	Burrows 1965 Morgan and Hawkins 1949
Alaria canis	Southern Canada	Dog, fox	Small intestine	Unknown; probably ingestion of infected frog, snake	Unknown	Unknown; probably rare	Unknown	None known	Burrows 1965 Morgan and Hawkins 1949
Alaria marcianae	United States	Dog, cat	Small intestine	Unknown; probably ingestion of infected frog, snake	Unknown	Unknown; probably rare	Unknown	None known	Burrows 1965
Alaria michiganensis	Northern United States	Dog	Small intestine	Unknown; probably ingestion of infected frog, snake	Unknown	Unknown; probably rare	Unknown	None known	Burrows 1965 Morgan and Hawkins 1949
Alaria minnesotae	Northern United States	Cat, skunk	Small intestine	Unknown; probably ingestion of infected frog, snake	Unknown	Unknown; probably rare	Unknown	None known	Burrows 1965
Neodiplostomum tamarini	South America	Tamarins	Small intestine	Unknown	Uncommon	Unknown; probably uncommon	Unknown	None known	Cosgrove et al. 1968 Dubois 1966

TABLE 5.9. Paramphistomids affecting endothermal laboratory animals

Parasite	Geographic Distribution	Endothermal Host	Location in Host	Method of Infection	Incidence		Pathologic Effects	Public Health Importance	Reference
					In nature	In laboratory			
*Gastrodiscoides hominis**	India, southeastern Asia, Indonesia, Philippine Islands	Rhesus monkey, cynomolgus monkey, pig, man	Cecum, colon	Ingestion of metacercaria encysted on vegetation	Common	Common	Mucous diarrhea, mild enteritis	Causes mild diarrhea; infected laboratory animals cannot infect man	Faust et al. 1968 Graham 1960 Hashimoto and Honjo 1966 Herman 1967 Reardon and Rininger 1968 Sasa et al. 1962
*Watsonius watsoni**	Western Africa	Guenons, baboons, man	Intestine	Unknown; probably by ingestion of metacercaria encysted on vegetation	Uncommon	Uncommon	Diarrhea, severe enteritis	Causes diarrhea; infected laboratory animals cannot infect man	Faust et al. 1968 Fiennes 1967 Hashimoto and Honjo 1966 Myers and Kuntz 1965 Ruch 1959
*Watsonius deschieni**	Western Africa	Baboons	Intestine	Unknown; probably by ingestion of metacercaria encysted on vegetation	Uncommon	Uncommon	Diarrhea, severe enteritis	Unknown	Fiennes 1967 Myers and Kuntz 1965 Ruch 1959
*Watsonius macaci**	Asia	Cynomolgus monkey	Intestine	Unknown; probably by ingestion of metacercaria encysted on vegetation	Uncommon	Uncommon	Unknown	Unknown	Cosgrove 1966 Fiennes 1967 Hashimoto and Honjo 1966
Chiorchis noci	Asia	Macaques	Intestine	Unknown	Unknown	Unknown	Unknown	Unknown	Cosgrove 1966
Zygocotyle lunata	North America	Chicken, other birds	Ceca, small intestine	Ingestion of metacercaria encysted on vegetation	Rare	Unknown; probably absent	None	Unknown	Morgan and Hawkins 1949 Price 1965 Soulsby 1965

*Discussed in text.

147

TABLE 5.10. Dicrocoelids affecting endothermal laboratory animals

Parasite	Geographic Distribution	Endothermal Host	Location in Host	Method of Infection	Incidence In nature	Incidence In laboratory	Pathologic Effects	Public Health Importance	Reference
Athesmia foxi*	South America, Malay Peninsula	Capuchins, squirrel monkeys, tamarins, titi monkeys, wild rat (Rattus argentiventer)	Bile duct	Unknown	Common	Common	Enlargement, partial obstruction, inflammation of bile duct	None	Bostrom and Slaughter 1968 Cosgrove et al. 1966 Ewing et al. 1968 Faust 1967 Fiennes 1967 Garner et al. 1967 Ruch 1959
Brodenia laciniata	Africa	Baboons	Pancreas	Unknown	Common	Unknown	Unknown	Unknown	Cosgrove 1966 Kuntz and Myers 1966
Brodenia serrata	Africa	Mangabeys	Pancreas	Unknown	Unknown	Unknown	Unknown	Unknown	Cosgrove 1966
Controrchis biliophilus	United States	Spider monkeys	Gallbladder, intestine	Unknown	Unknown	Unknown	Unknown	Unknown	Cosgrove 1966 Fiennes 1967
Dicrocoelium dendriticum	North America, Europe, South America, Asia	Rabbit, hares, dog, cat, domestic animals, man	Bile duct	Ingestion of infected ant	Rare in rabbit, dog, cat	Unknown; probably rare	Debilitation, bile duct lesions, hepatic cirrhosis	Causes biliary lesions, hepatitis; infected laboratory animals cannot infect man	Faust et al. 1968 Soulsby 1965
Dicrocoelium colobusicola	Central Africa	Colobus monkeys	Bile duct	Unknown	Unknown	Unknown	Unknown	Unknown	Cosgrove 1966

*Discussed in text.

TABLE 5.10 (continued)

Parasite	Geographic Distribution	Endothermal Host	Location in Host	Method of Infection	Incidence		Pathologic Effects	Public Health Importance	Reference
					In nature	In laboratory			
Dicrocoelium macaci	Africa, Asia	Macaques, guenons, mangabeys, baboons, chimpanzee	Bile duct	Unknown	Unknown	Unknown	Unknown	Unknown	Cosgrove 1966 Fiennes 1967
Eurytrema procyonis	North America	Cat, fox, raccoon	Bile duct, pancreatic duct	Unknown	Unknown	Unknown	Unknown	Unknown	Burrows 1965
Eurytrema brumpti	Central Africa	Chimpanzee, gorilla	Bile duct, pancreas	Unknown	Unknown	Unknown	Enlargement, erosion of bile duct	Unknown	Cosgrove 1966 Fiennes 1967 Prine 1968
Eurytrema satoi	Japan, Africa	Cynomolgus monkey, gorilla	Bile duct, pancreas	Unknown	Unknown	Unknown	Unknown	Unknown	Cosgrove 1966 Fiennes 1967
Leipertrema rewelli	Africa	Orangutan	Pancreas	Unknown	Unknown	Unknown	Unknown	Unknown	Cosgrove 1966
Platynosomum concinnum*	Florida, Puerto Rico, Bahama Islands, Hawaii, Brazil, Malay Peninsula	Cat	Gallbladder, bile duct	Ingestion of infected lizard	Common in Caribbean area; rare in United States	Common in cats obtained from pounds in endemic areas	Vomiting, diarrhea, emaciation, icterus, biliary lesions, hepato-megaly	Unknown	Alicata 1964 Greve and Leonard 1966 Leam and Walker 1963 Soulsby 1965
Platynosomum amazonensis	South America	Tamarins	Gallbladder, bile duct	Unknown	Common	Common in tamarins obtained from natural habitat	Unknown	Unknown	Cosgrove et al. 1968 Kingston and Cosgrove 1967
Platynosomum marmoseti	South America	Tamarins	Gallbladder, bile duct	Unknown	Uncommon	Uncommon in tamarins obtained from natural habitat	Unknown	Unknown	Cosgrove et al. 1968 Kingston and Cosgrove 1967

*Discussed in text.

149

TABLE 5.11. Brachylaemids, lecithodendriids, notocotylids, psilostomatids, and philophthalmids affecting endothermal laboratory animals

Parasite	Geographic Distribution	Endothermal Host	Location in Host	Method of Infection	Incidence In nature	Incidence In laboratory	Pathologic Effects	Public Health Importance	Reference
Postharmostomum helicis	United States	Deer mice, other rodents	Cecum	Ingestion of infected snail	Common	Unknown; probably common in specimens obtained from natural habitat	Typhlitis	None	Ulmer 1951
Postharmostomum gallinum	Hawaii, Puerto Rico, Europe, northern Africa, eastern Asia	Chicken, pigeon, other birds	Small intestine, ceca	Ingestion of infected snail	Common	Unknown; probably absent	Hemorrhagic typhlitis	None	Lapage 1968 Price 1965 Soulsby 1965
Hasstilesia tricolor	United States	Cottontail rabbits	Small intestine	Unknown	Common	Unknown; probably common in specimens obtained from natural habitat	Catarrhal enteritis	None	Morgan and Hawkins 1949 Stringer et al. 1969
Phaneropsolus oviformis	South America, Asia	Macaques, slow loris	Intestine	Unknown	Common	Unknown	Unknown	Unknown	Cosgrove 1966
Phaneropsolus orbicularis	South America	Capuchins, squirrel monkeys, tamarins, night monkey	Intestine	Unknown	Common	Unknown	Unknown	Unknown	Cosgrove 1966 Cosgrove et al. 1968 G. E. Cosgrove, personal communication
Primatotrema macacae	Asia	Macaques	Intestine	Unknown	Common	Unknown	Unknown	Unknown	Cosgrove 1966
Ogmocotyle indica	Asia	Macaques	Intestine	Unknown	Uncommon	Uncommon	Unknown	Unknown	Cosgrove 1966 Graham 1960 Yoshimura et al. 1969
Catatropis verrucosa	United States, Europe	Chicken, other birds	Ceca, rectum	Ingestion of cercaria encysted on snail shell or vegetation	Unknown	Unknown	Unknown; probably slight cecal erosion	None	Lapage 1962, 1968 Price 1965 Soulsby 1965

TABLE 5.11 (continued)

Parasite	Geographic Distribution	Endothermal Host	Location in Host	Method of Infection	Incidence		Pathologic Effects	Public Health Importance	Reference
					In nature	In laboratory			
Notocotylus attenuatus	Europe, Asia	Chicken, other birds	Ceca, rectum	Ingestion of cercaria encysted on snail shell or vegetation	Common	Unknown	Slight cecal erosion	None	Lapage 1962, 1968 Price 1965 Soulsby 1965
Notocotylus thienemanni	Europe	Chicken, other birds	Ceca	Ingestion of cercaria encysted on snail shell or vegetation	Unknown	Unknown	Unknown; probably slight cecal erosion	None	Lapage 1962, 1968 Soulsby 1965
Ribeiroia ondatrae	North America	Chicken, other birds	Proventric-ulus	Ingestion of metacercaria in fish	Uncommon	Unknown; probably absent	Proventric-ulitis	None	Morgan and Hawkins 1949 Price 1965 Soulsby 1965
Phil-ophthalmus gralli	Eastern Asia, Hawaii	Chicken, other birds	Conjunctival sac	Ingestion of cercaria encysted on snail shell or vegetation	Unknown	Unknown	Congestion, erosion of conjunctiva	Occurs in man; infected laboratory animals cannot infect man	Alicata 1964 Price 1965
Phil-ophthalmus proble-maticus	Philippine Islands	Chicken	Conjunctival sac	Ingestion of cercaria encysted on snail shell or vegetation	Unknown	Unknown	Congestion, erosion of conjunctiva	None	Price 1965

151

REFERENCES

Alicata, J. E. 1964. Parasitic infections of man and animals in Hawaii. Hawaii Agr. Exp. Sta. Bull. 61. 138 pp.

Ash, L. R. 1962. The helminth parasites of rats in Hawaii and the description of *Capillaria traverae* sp. n. J. Parasitol. 48:66–68.

Bennington, E., and I. Pratt. 1960. The life history of the salmon-poisoning fluke, *Nanophyetus salmincola* (Chapin). J. Parasitol. 46:91–100.

Bisgard, G. E., and R. E. Lewis. 1964. Paragonimiasis in a dog and a cat. J. Am. Vet. Med. Assoc. 144:501–7.

Bisseru, B. 1967. Diseases of man acquired from his pets. William Heinemann Medical Books, London. 482 pp.

Bostrom, R. C., and L. J. Slaughter. 1968. Trematode *(Athesmia foxi)* infection in two squirrel monkeys *(Saimiri sciureus)*. Lab. Animal Care 18:493–95.

Burrows, R. B. 1965. Microscopic diagnosis of the parasites of man. Yale Univ. Press, New Haven, Conn. 328 pp.

Cheng, T. C. 1964. The biology of animal parasites. W. B. Saunders, Philadelphia. 727 pp.

Cook, R. 1963. Common diseases of laboratory animals, pp. 117–56. *In* D. J. Short and Dorothy P. Woodnott, eds. A.T.A. manual of laboratory animal practice and techniques. Crosby Lockwood and Son, London.

Cosgrove, G. E. 1966. The trematodes of laboratory primates. Lab. Animal Care 16:23–39.

Cosgrove, G. E., B. Nelsen, and N. Gengozian. 1968. Helminth parasites of the tamarin, *Sanguinus fuscicollis*. Lab. Animal Care 18:654–56.

Dawes, B. 1946. The Trematoda, with special reference to British and other European forms. Cambridge Univ. Press, Cambridge, England. 644 pp.

Dawes, B., and D. L. Hughes. 1964. Fascioliasis: The invasive stages of *Fasciola hepatica* in mammalian hosts. Advan. Parasitol. 2:97–168.

DePaoli, A. 1965. *Schistosoma haematobium* in the chimpanzee—a natural infection. Am. J. Trop. Med. Hyg. 14:561–65.

Dubois, G. 1966. Un Néodiplostome (Trematoda: Diplostomatidae) chez le Tamarin *Leontocebus nigricollis* (Spix). Rev. Suisse Zool. 73:37–42.

Estes, R. R., and J. C. Brown. 1966. Endoparasites of laboratory animals. U.S. Air Force School Aerospace Med. (AFSC) Brooks Air Force Base, Tex. Review 1–66. 59 pp.

Ewing, S. A., D. R. Helland, H. D. Anthony, and H. W. Leipold. 1968. Occurrence of *Athesmia* sp. in the cinnamon ringtail monkey, *Cebus albifrons*. Lab. Animal Care 18:488–92.

Farrell, R. K. 1966. Transmission of two rickettsia-like disease agents of dogs by endoparasites in northwestern U.S.A., pp. 438–39. *In* A. Corradetti, ed. Proc. First Intern. Congr. Parasitol. Pergamon Press, New York.

———. 1968. Rickettsial diseases, pp. 164–69. *In* E. J. Catcott, ed. Canine medicine. American Veterinary Publications, Santa Barbara, Calif.

Farrell, R. K., J. F. Dee, and R. L. Ott. 1968. Salmon poisoning in a dog fed kippered salmon. J. Am. Vet. Med. Assoc. 152:370–71.

Faust, E. C. 1949. Human helminthology. 3d ed. Lea and Febiger, Philadelphia. 744 pp.

———. 1967. *Athesmia* (Trematoda: Dicrocoeliidae) Odhner, 1911 liver fluke of monkeys from Colombia, South America, and other mammalian hosts. Trans. Am. Microscop. Soc. 86:113–19.

Faust, E. C., P. C. Beaver, and R. C. Jung. 1968. Animal agents and vectors of human disease. 3d ed. Lea and Febiger, Philadelphia. 461 pp.

Fiennes, R. 1967. Zoonoses of primates. Weidenfeld and Nicolson, London. 190 pp.

Ganasevich, V. I., and R. V. Skovronski. 1965. Treatment of rabbits against fascioliasis (in Russian). Probl. Parazitol. Akad. Nauk Ukr. SSR, Inst. Zool. Tr. 2-i Nauchn. Konf. Parazitologov Ukr. SSR.

Garner, E., F. Hemrick, and H. Rudiger. 1967. Multiple helminth infections in cinnamon-ringtail monkeys *(Cebus albifrons)*. Lab. Animal Care 17:310–15.

Golebiowski, S. 1959. Inwazja motylicy watrobowej u zwierzat laboratoryjnych. Med. Weterynar (Poland) 15:210–12.

Graham, G. L. 1960. Parasitism in monkeys. Ann. N.Y. Acad. Sci. 85:735–992.

Greve, J. H., and P. O. Leonard. 1966. Hepatic flukes *(Platynosomum concinnum)* in a cat from Illinois. J. Am. Vet. Med. Assoc. 149:418–20.

Habermann, R. T., and F. P. Williams, Jr. 1957. Diseases seen at necropsy of 708 *Macaca mulatta* (rhesus monkey) and *Macaca philippinensis* (cynomolgus monkey). Am. J. Vet. Res. 18:419–26.

Hartman, H. A. 1961. The intestinal fluke *(Fasciolopsis buski)* in a monkey. Am. J. Vet. Res. 11:1123–26.

Hashimoto, I., and S. Honjo. 1966. Survey of helminth parasites in cynomolgus monkeys *(Macaca irus)*. Japan. J. Med. Sci. Biol. 19:218.

Herman, L. H. 1967. *Gastrodiscoides hominis* infestation in two monkeys. Vet. Med. 62:355–56.

Herman, L. H., and D. R. Helland. 1966. Paragonimiasis in a cat. J. Am. Vet. Med. Assoc. 149:753–57.

Himonas, C. A. 1968. Parasitic helminths of dogs in Greece and their public health importance (in Greek). Epistem. Epet. kteniatrik. Skhol. Thessaloniki 9:153–390.

Holmes, R. G. 1962. Fascioliasis in Coypus *(Myocaster coypus)*. Vet. Record 74:1552.

Kingston, N., and G. E. Cosgrove. 1967. Two new species of *Platynosomum* (Trematode: Dicrocoeliidae) from South American monkeys. Proc. Helminthol. Soc. Wash. D.C. 34:147–51.

Kuntz, R. E., and Betty J. Myers. 1966. Parasites of baboons *Papio doguera* (Pucheran, 1856) captured in Kenya and Tanzania, East Africa. Primates 7:27–32.

———. 1967. Microbiological parameters of the baboon *(Papio* sp.): Parasitology, pp. 741–55. *In* H. Vagtborg, ed. The baboon in medical research. Vol. 2. Univ. Texas Press, Austin.

Lapage, G. 1962. Mönnig's veterinary helminthology and entomology. 5th ed. Williams and Wilkins, Baltimore. 600 pp.

———. 1968. Veterinary parasitology. Oliver and Boyd, Edinburgh and London. 1182 pp.

Leam, G., and I. E. Walker. 1963. Liver flukes in the Bahamas. Vet. Record 75:46–47.

Macy, R. W. 1934. *Prosthogonimus macrorchis* n. sp., the common oviduct fluke of domestic fowls in the Northern United States. Trans. Am. Microscop. Soc. 53:30–34.

Mills, J. H. L., and R. S. Hirth. 1968. Lesions caused by the hepatic trematode, *Metorchis conjunctus*, Cobbold, 1860: A comparative study in carnivora. J. Small Animal Pract. 9:1–6.

Morgan, B. B., and P. A. Hawkins. 1949. Veterinary helminthology. Burgess, Minneapolis. 400 pp.

Myers, Betty J., and R. E. Kuntz. 1965. A checklist of parasites reported for the baboon. Primates 6:137–94.

Nyberg, P. A., S. E. Knapp, and R. E. Millemann. 1967. "Salmon-poisoning" disease: IV. Transmission of the disease to dogs by *Nanophyetus salmincola* eggs. J. Parasitol. 53:694–99.

Olsen, O. W. 1967. Animal parasites: Their biology and life cycles. 2d ed. Burgess, Minneapolis. 431 pp.

Pantelouris, E. M. 1965. The common liver fluke. Pergamon Press, Oxford. 259 pp.

Pierce, K. R. 1963. *Heterobilharzia americana* infection in a dog. J. Am. Vet. Med. Assoc. 143:496–99.

Polishchuk, F. G. 1961. Acute fascioliasis in nutria (in Russian). Krolikovodstvo i Zverovodstvo 2:22–23.

Price, E. W. 1965. Trematodes of poultry, pp. 1035–55. *In* H. E. Biester and L. H. Schwarte, eds. Diseases of poultry. 5th ed. Iowa State Univ. Press, Ames.

Prine, J. R. 1968. Pancreatic flukes and amoebic colitis in a gorilla. Abstr. 50. 19th Ann. Meeting Am. Assoc. Lab. Animal Sci., Las Vegas.

Purvis, A. J., I. R. Ellison, and E. L. Husting. 1965. A short note on the findings of Schistosomes in baboons *(Papio rhodesiae)*. Central African J. Med. 11:368.

Reardon, Lucy V., and Bonny F. Rininger. 1968. A survey of parasites in laboratory primates. Lab. Animal Care 18:577–80.

Renaux, E. A. 1964. Flukes, pp. 128–30. *In* E. J. Catcott, ed. Feline medicine and surgery. American Veterinary Publications, Santa Barbara, Calif.

Ruch, T. C. 1959. Diseases of laboratory primates. W. B. Saunders, Philadelphia. 600 pp.

Sadun, E. H., F. von Lichtenberg, R. L. Hickman, J. I. Bruce, J. H. Smith, and M. J. Schoenbechler. 1966. *Schistosomiasis mansoni* in the chimpanzee: Parasitologic, clinical, serologic, pathologic and radiologic observations. Am. J. Trop. Med. Hyg. 15:496–506.

Sasa, M., H. Tanaka, M. Fukui, and A. Takata. 1962. Internal parasites of laboratory animals, pp. 195–214. *In* R. J. C. Harris, ed. The problems of laboratory animal disease. Academic Press, New York.

Schlegel, M. W., S. E. Knapp, and R. E. Millemann. 1968. "Salmon poisoning" disease: V. Definitive hosts of the trematode vector, *Nanophyetus salmincola*. J. Parasitol. 54:770–74.

Scott, Patricia P. 1967. The cat *(Felis catus* L.), pp. 505–67. *In* UFAW Staff, eds. The UFAW handbook on the care and management of laboratory animals. 3d ed. Livingstone and the Universities Federation for Animal Welfare, London.

Skrjabin, K. I. 1964. Keys to the trematodes of animals and man (English translation). H. P. Arai, ed. Univ. Illinois Press, Urbana. 351 pp.

Smith, H. A., and T. C. Jones. 1966. Veterinary pathology. 3d ed. Lea and Febiger, Philadelphia. 1192 pp.

Soulsby, E. J. L. 1965. Textbook of veterinary clinical parasitology. Vol. I. Helminths. F. A. Davis, Philadelphia. 1120 pp.

Strauss, J. M., and D. Heyneman. 1966. Fatal ectopic fascioliasis in a guinea pig breeding colony from Malacca. J. Parasitol. 52:413.

Stringer, R. P., R. Harkema, and G. C. Miller. 1969. Parasites of rabbits in North Carolina. J. Parasitol. 55:328.

Swartz, L. G. 1966. An occurrence of *Schistosomatium douthitti* (Cort, 1914) Price, 1931, in Alaska in a new natural definitive host, *Clethrionomys rutilus* (Pallas). Can. J. Zool. 44:729–30.

Swellengrebel, N. H., and A. C. Rijpstra. 1965. Lateral-spined schistosome ova in the intestine of a squirrel monkey from Surinam. Trop. Geograph. Med. 17:80–84.

Thrasher, J. P. 1964. Canine schistosomiasis. J. Am. Vet. Med. Assoc. 144:1119–26.

Trofimov, V. P., and L. L. Alyabyeva. 1959. Spontaneous fascioliasis in guinea-pigs (In Russian). Veterinariya (Moscow) 36:43–44.

Tropilo, J. 1965. Intensywność i ekstensywność inwazji *Cysticercus pisiformis* oraz *Fasciola hepatica* u zajaca *(Lepus europaeus)*. Med. Weterynar. (Poland) 20:592–4.

Ulmer, M. J. 1951. *Postharmostomum helicis* (Leidy, 1847) Robinson 1949 (Trematoda), its life history and a revision of the subfamily Brachylaeminae. Part I. Trans. Am. Microscop. Soc. 70:189–238.

Whitney, R. A., D. J. Johnson, and W. C. Cole. 1967. The subhuman primate: A guide for the veterinarian. Edgewood Arsenal, Maryland. EASP 100-26.

Worley, D. E. 1964. Helminth parasites of dogs in southeastern Michigan. J. Am. Vet. Med. Assoc. 144:42–46.

Yamaguti, S. 1958. The digenetic trematodes of vertebrates. Vol. I. 2 parts. *In* S. Yamaguti. *Systema helminthum*. Interscience, New York.

Yokogawa, M., H. Yoshimura, M. Sano, Toshihiko Okura, M. Tsuji, A. Takizawa, Y. Harada, and M. Kihata. 1961. Chemotherapy of paragonimiasis with bithionol: I. Experimental chemotherapy on the animals infected with *Paragonimus westermani* or *P. ohirai*. Japan. J. Parasitol. 10:302–16.

Yoshimura, K., Y. Hishinuma, and Mitsuko Sato. 1969. *Ogmocotyle ailuri* (Price, 1954) in the Taiwanese monkey, *Macaca cyclopis* (Swinhoe, 1862). J. Parasitol. 55:460.

Chapter 6

CESTODES

CESTODES have complex life cycles which, with few exceptions, involve at least two obligatory hosts, an invertebrate or vertebrate host in which the larval stage develops, and a vertebrate in which the adult cestode develops (Cheng 1964; Wardle and McLeod 1952). Endothermal species can be hosts for either the larval or the adult stage. Intermediate hosts are infected by the ingestion of embryonated eggs. In vertebrate intermediate hosts, the eggs hatch in the intestine, and the embryo, or oncosphere, burrows into the intestinal mucosa and is carried by the blood to the liver, lungs, brain, or other site, where further development occurs. Fully developed larvae can live in the tissues for a year or more. The definitive host is infected by ingesting infective larvae. These grow to adults in the small intestine of the host.

Most of the families of tapeworms that affect endothermal laboratory animals (Hymenolepididae, Davaineidae, Dilepididae, Mesocestoididae, Anoplocephalidae, Taeniidae) are members of the order Cyclophyllidea. The scolex of these cestodes has four cup-shaped suckers and sometimes a rostellum. The uterus is tubular with branches, or sacular, when gravid. Eggs are nonoperculated; the embryos are nonciliated and, as in all cestodes, possess three pairs of small hooks.

One family that affects endothermal laboratory animals (Diphyllobothriidae) belongs to the order Pseudophyllidea. The scolex of these cestodes usually has two grooves, or bothria. The uterus is tubular and rosettelike in appearance. Eggs are operculated; the embryos possess three pairs of small hooks and are usually ciliated.

Although hundreds of species of cestodes have been reported from endothermal animals which are sometimes acquired from their natural habitat for use in the laboratory, most have been reported only once. Some cestodes, once common in the usual laboratory animals, have become less common with the advent of cesarean-derived colonies. Others remain common and are important.

HYMENOLEPIDIDS

These small- to medium-sized tapeworms occur as the adult in the intestine of mammals and birds. Most require an arthropod as an intermediate host. Those that affect endothermal laboratory animals are listed in Table 6.1. The most important species, *Hymenolepis nana*, *H. diminuta*, and *H. carioca*, are discussed below.

Hymenolepis nana
(Syn. *Hymenolepis fraterna*)
(Dwarf Tapeworm)

This usually benign but sometimes pathogenic cestode occurs in the intestine of rodents, simian primates, and man throughout the world (Wardle and McLeod

155

1952). It is common in the wild house mouse (Sasa et al. 1962), Norway rat, and black rat (Ash 1962b), and in the conventional laboratory mouse (Heston 1941; Owen 1968; Sasa et al. 1962), rat (Ratcliffe 1949; Sasa et al. 1962), and hamster (Sheffield and Beveridge 1962; Soave 1963). Incidences of 64% (Heyneman 1961a), 87% (King and Cosgrove 1963), and 100% (Simmons, Williams, and Wright 1964) have been reported in conventional laboratory mouse colonies, with individual mice infected with as many as 2,000 worms (Heyneman 1961a). Incidences in commercially supplied rodents are also high. In one survey of mice from 12 suppliers, incidences as high as 93% were observed, with an overall average of 21% (Stone and Manwell 1966). In the same survey, incidences as high as 42% were observed in commercially supplied hamsters. This cestode does not occur in cesarean-derived, barrier-maintained colonies (Flynn, Brennan, and Fritz 1965; Foster 1963; Owen 1968), nor does it occur naturally in the guinea pig (Newton, Weinstein, and Jones 1959).

Hymenolepis nana has been reported

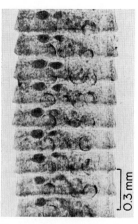

FIG. 6.2. *Hymenolepis nana*, mature proglottids. (Courtesy of Marietta Voge, University of California.)

from the rhesus monkey, squirrel monkey, and chimpanzee, but it is apparently uncommon in these species (Benson, Fremming, and Young 1954; Middleton, Clarkson, and Garner 1964; Ruch 1959). It is common in man, especially in the tropics and subtropics (Belding 1965).

MORPHOLOGY

Hymenolepis nana is a slender, white

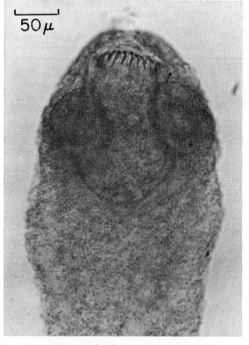

FIG. 6.1. *Hymenolepis nana* scolex with rostellum retracted. (Courtesy of Marietta Voge, University of California.)

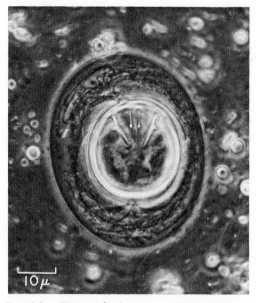

FIG. 6.3. *Hymenolepis nana*, embryonated egg. (Courtesy of Marietta Voge, University of California.)

TRANSMISSION OF HYMENOLEPIS NANA

Fig. 6.4. *Hymenolepis nana,* diagram of life cycle. Note that both
direct and indirect transmission
occur. (Courtesy of Marietta Voge,
University of California.)

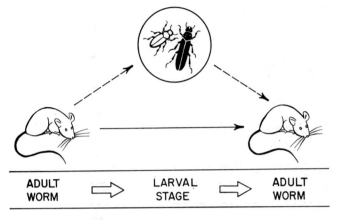

| ADULT WORM | ⇨ | LARVAL STAGE | ⇨ | ADULT WORM |

worm, usually about 25 to 40 mm long and less than 1 mm wide (Burrows 1965; Wardle and McLeod 1952). The scolex bears four suckers and a muscular structure called the rostellum, which is armed with a crown of hooks (Fig. 6.1). Mature proglottids are wider than long and trapezoidal (Fig. 6.2). The egg is oval and measures 44 to 62 μ by 30 to 55 μ. The embryo measures 24 to 30 μ by 16 to 25 μ and possesses three pairs of small hooks (Fig. 6.3).

LIFE CYCLE

The dwarf tapeworm is the only known cestode which can be transmitted directly (Cheng 1964; Wardle and McLeod 1952) (Fig. 6.4). Eggs voided in the feces of a definitive host are directly infective if ingested by another definitive host. The eggs hatch in the small intestine, and the embryos penetrate the intestinal villi and become cysticercoid larvae in 4 to 5 days. The larvae then reenter the intestinal lumen, attach to the mucosa, and develop into mature worms in 10 to 11 days. Thus the life cycle, in direct transmission, is completed in 14 to 16 days.

Indirect transmission also occurs. Infective larvae develop in flour beetles or fleas, and the definitive host becomes infected by ingestion of the infected insect (Voge and Heyneman 1957). Because the time required for larval development in the insect varies with the environmental temperature, the length of the indirect life cycle is variable.

A further variation in the life cycle is

autoinfection, or the immediate hatching of eggs within the intestine of the same host in which they were produced (Heyneman 1961b, 1962). The embryos develop into mature adults without leaving the original host.

Hymenolepis nana is also unusual in that the life-span of the adult in the intestine is usually limited to a few weeks. Successful establishment of reinfection depends on the nature of the previous infection. In direct transmission, the host tissue is invaded and a certain degree of immunity develops, whereas in indirect transmission, the initial infection is acquired by ingesting fully developed larvae in insects, the tissue phase is omitted, and immunity is not produced (Heyneman 1961b, 1962). This is especially important in relation to autoinfection, which does not usually occur in hosts initially infected by direct transmission because of the immunity produced during the tissue phase of the original infection.

PATHOLOGIC EFFECTS

The effects of this parasite depend on the number present. Heavy infection causes retarded growth and weight loss in the mouse (Tuffery and Innes 1963) and intestinal occlusion and impaction and death in the hamster (Soave 1963). In less severe cases, catarrhal enteritis occurs (Habermann and Williams 1958), and chronic inflammation and abscesses of the mesenteric lymph nodes have been reported (Simmons et al. 1967).

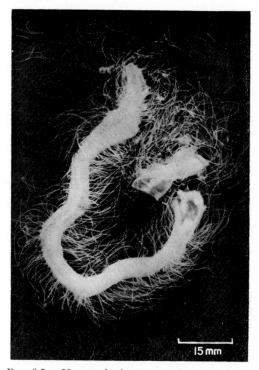

FIG. 6.5. *Hymenolepis nana,* adults in intestine of mouse. (From Heyneman 1961b. Courtesy of Journal of Infectious Diseases.)

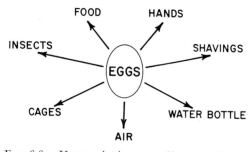

FIG. 6.6. *Hymenolepis nana,* diagram of ways in which eggs can be disseminated. (Courtesy of Marietta Voge, University of California.)

DIAGNOSIS

Diagnosis is based on the identification of the eggs in the feces or the adult worm in the intestine at necropsy (Fig. 6.5).

CONTROL

Because infection with this tapeworm can be spread in many ways (Fig. 6.6), control is extremely difficult. Complete eradication can be achieved by the cesarean-derivation, barrier-maintenance technique (Foster 1963), but measures short of this are probably of limited value. Sanitation and insect control are essential (Habermann and Williams 1958). Because of the high incidence of infection in wild rodents, effective rodent control is also important (Dove 1950). All newly acquired animals should be examined on arrival and, if infected, either treated or eliminated. Cages should be cleaned and sterilized frequently and contamination of food and water prevented.

Drugs reported to be effective for the mouse and rat and presumably for the hamster include lead arsenate, given in the diet at a level of 0.5% (Habermann and Williams 1958), and quinacrine hydrochloride, given in a single oral dose of 75 μg per g of body weight (Balazs et al. 1962). Bithionol (thiobis dichlorophenol), given in a single oral dose of 50 μg per g of body weight, is also suggested (Sasa et al. 1962), but its effectiveness is uncertain (Balazs et al. 1962). Dithiazanine, diethyltoluamide, and piperazine compounds are ineffective (Balazs et al. 1962; Habermann and Williams 1957). Effective treatments for primates include hexylresorcinol, given in a single oral dose of 0.2 g for the monkey or 0.6 to 1.0 g for the chimpanzee; gentian violet, given orally at a rate of 60 mg for the monkey or 120 to 180 mg for the chimpanzee daily for 7 to 14 days; and dichlorophen in combination with toluene (Vermiplex, Pitman-Moore), given in a single oral dose of 500 to 550 mg per kg of body weight (Benson, Fremming, and Young 1954; Ruch 1959). Niclosamide (Yomesan, Bayer), given in a single oral dose of 100 mg per kg of body weight, is effective for the removal of *H. diminuta* from the rat (Gönnert and Schraufstätter 1960) and is presumably equally effective for *H. nana* in rodents and primates (Anonymous 1968).

PUBLIC HEALTH CONSIDERATIONS

Hymenolepis nana is pathogenic for man (Faust, Beaver, and Jung 1968). Light infections are inapparent, but heavy infections cause anorexia, vomiting, diarrhea, loss of weight, abdominal pain, insomnia, apathy, irritability, nasal and anal pruritus, and sometimes neurologic signs. Although transmission from animals to man is probably uncommon, laboratory personnel working with animals should be made aware of this possibility and instructed in proper personal hygiene. Bedding and feces from infected animals should be incinerated or otherwise treated to prevent the spread of *H. nana* eggs.

Hymenolepis diminuta

(Rat Tapeworm)

Hymenolepis diminuta, a relatively benign but occasionally pathogenic cestode, occurs in the intestine of the mouse, rat, black rat, other wild rodents, the monkey, and man (Wardle and McLeod 1952). It is common in the wild Norway and black rats throughout the world, with incidences reported of 6.6% in Ceylon (Kulasiri 1954), 16.6% in eastern United States (Dove 1950), 18.4% in the black rat and 26.2% in the Norway rat in Japan (Sasa et al. 1962), 28.0% in Puerto Rico and Brazil (Heston 1941; de Léon 1964), and 50.0% in Hawaii (Ash 1962b). It is uncommon in the monkey (Ruch 1959) and rare in man (Faust,

Beaver, and Jung 1968; Stone and Manwell 1966).

Infection with the rat tapeworm has been reported in some laboratory mouse, rat, and hamster colonies, but it is uncommon (Handler 1965; Read 1951; Sasa et al. 1962; Stone and Manwell 1966). It does not occur in colonies kept free of ectoparasites and maintained on diets devoid of insects (Flynn, Brennan, and Fritz 1965; Owen 1968).

MORPHOLOGY

The adult worm measures 20 to 60 mm in length and 3 to 4 mm in width (Burrows 1965; Voge 1952). Its scolex is similar to that of *H. nana* except that it bears no hooks. Mature proglottids are much wider than long (Fig. 6.7). The egg is almost spherical, measures 62 to 88 μ by 52 to 81 μ, and contains an embryo which measures 24 to 30 μ by 16 to 25 μ and which possesses three pairs of small hooks (Fig. 6.8).

LIFE CYCLE

The life cycle of *H. diminuta* requires an insect, usually a flour beetle, moth, or flea, as an intermediate host (Fig. 6.9) (Voge and Heyneman 1957). The time necessary for development of infective larvae in insects varies with the temperature and the species of insect. At 30 C, infective

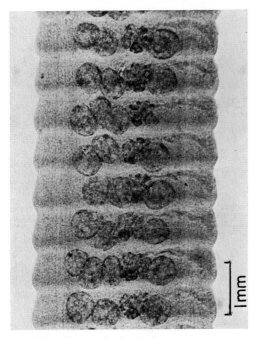

FIG. 6.7. *Hymenolepis diminuta*, mature proglottids. (Courtesy of Marietta Voge, University of California.)

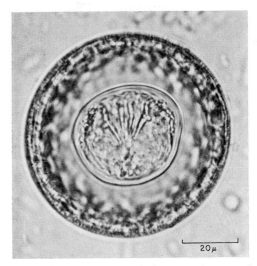

FIG. 6.8. *Hymenolepis diminuta*, embryonated egg. (Courtesy of Marietta Voge, University of California.)

FIG. 6.9. *Hymenolepis diminuta,* diagram of life cycle. Note that only indirect transmission occurs. (Courtesy of Marietta Voge, University of California.)

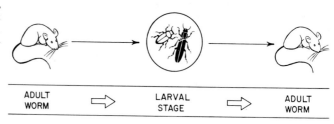

FIG. 6.10. *Hymenolepis diminuta* infection in a hamster. *(Left)* Note distention of intestine and hyperemia of serosal surface. *(Right)* Catarrhal enteritis in sections of intestine. (From Handler 1965. Courtesy of Charles C Thomas, Publisher.)

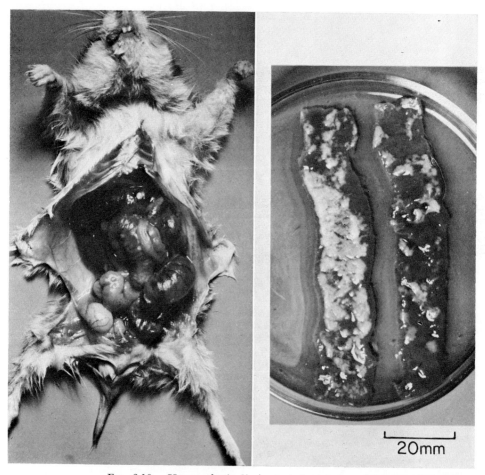

larval stages develop in the confused flour beetle *(Tribolium confusum)* in 8 days. Temperatures higher than 37 C are not suitable for development. Infective insects are ingested by a definitive host, and adult worms develop in the intestine in 16 to 19 days. Eggs are voided in the feces. Adult worms usually grow and produce eggs throughout the life of the host.

PATHOLOGIC EFFECTS

Heavy infections in rodents are rare (Belding 1965); however, when they do occur they cause either an acute catarrhal enteritis or a chronic enterocolitis (Fig. 6.10) with lymphoid hyperplasia (Fig. 6.11) (Habermann and Williams 1958; Handler 1965). The pathologic effects in simian primates have not been described; they are probably mild or inapparent, as in man.

DIAGNOSIS

Diagnosis is based on demonstration of the eggs or proglottids in the feces or the adult worm in the intestine at necropsy.

CONTROL

Elimination of the intermediate insect vector will eliminate this tapeworm from laboratory colonies. The treatments recommended for *H. nana* are also effective against this tapeworm (Habermann and Williams 1958; Ruch 1959).

PUBLIC HEALTH CONSIDERATIONS

Hymenolepis diminuta infection in man is rare and can only occur by ingestion of an infected insect (Faust, Beaver, and Jung 1968). The presence of a single worm is characteristic, and the effects are usually mild or inapparent. Laboratory animal personnel should be made aware of the method of transmission to prevent accidental infection.

Hymenolepis carioca

This apparently nonpathogenic tapeworm occurs in the intestine of the chicken and other birds throughout the United States, including Hawaii (Alicata 1964; Reid 1962; Wehr 1965). Although it is extremely common in domestic chickens, with incidences of 34.0 to 42.9% being reported (Morgan and Hawkins 1949), there are no reports of this cestode in the laboratory

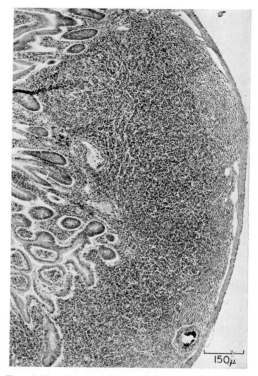

FIG. 6.11. *Hymenolepis diminuta* infection in a hamster. Lymphoid hyperplasia in a section of intestine. (From Handler 1965. Courtesy of Charles C Thomas, Publisher.)

chicken. It is unlikely to occur in facilities that practice effective insect control and would be expected only in birds brought into the laboratory from farm flocks.

MORPHOLOGY

Hymenolepis carioca is recognized by its slender, threadlike form (Wehr 1965). It measures 3 to 8 cm in length and 0.5 mm in width. The scolex does not bear hooks.

LIFE CYCLE

The life cycle involves an insect, usually a dung beetle but sometimes a stable fly or flour beetle (Fig. 6.12) (Horsfall 1938). The larval stage develops in the insect; the adult develops in the vertebrate host 2 to 4 weeks after ingestion of an infected insect.

PATHOLOGIC EFFECTS

Although several thousand of these tapeworms are sometimes found in a single

TRANSMISSION OF HYMENOLEPIS CARIOCA

FIG. 6.12. *Hymenolepis carioca*, diagram of life cycle. (Courtesy of Marietta Voge, University of California.)

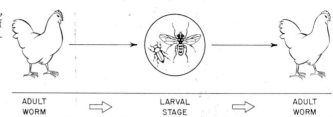

| ADULT WORM | ⇨ | LARVAL STAGE | ⇨ | ADULT WORM |

chicken, no pathologic effects have been attributed to it (Wehr 1965).

DIAGNOSIS

Diagnosis is based on demonstration of gravid proglottids in the feces or the adult worm in the intestine at necropsy.

CONTROL

Effective insect control will prevent or eliminate infection with this tapeworm. Although dibutyltin dilaurate, given orally in the feed at a level of 500 mg per kg of food for 2 to 6 days or by capsule at a dose of 125 mg per individual chicken, is an effective treatment (Edgar 1956), the elimination of insects rather than the treatment of infected animals is the recommended control (Reid 1962).

PUBLIC HEALTH CONSIDERATIONS

Hymenolepis carioca has not been reported in man.

DAVAINEIDS

These are relatively small cestodes that occur in the intestine of mammals and birds. Several are important parasites of the chicken. Those that affect endothermal laboratory animals are listed in Table 6.2. The most important species, *Davainea proglottina*, *Raillietina cesticillus*, and *R. echinobothrida*, are discussed below.

Davainea proglottina

(SYN. *Taenia proglottina*)

This very small but extremely pathogenic cestode is found in the duodenum of the chicken, pigeon, and other birds throughout the world (Reid 1962; Soulsby 1965). It is common in the domestic chicken (Soulsby 1965) but has not been reported in the laboratory chicken. Because *D. proglottina* requires a mollusk intermediate host, it is not likely to occur in laboratory-reared chickens and would only be expected to be encountered in birds brought into the laboratory from farm flocks.

MORPHOLOGY

The adult is very small, 0.5 to 3.0 mm in length, and possesses only four to nine segments (Fig. 6.13) (Lapage 1968). The scolex has a rostellum, with 80 to 90 hooks, and four suckers, which also have many small hooks. Gravid segments are barrel shaped and filled with eggs which measure 28 to 40 μ in diameter. Each egg is contained in a separate capsule.

LIFE CYCLE

Eggs passed in the feces in gravid segments hatch when ingested by a snail or slug (Olsen 1967). Development to the infective larval stage in the invertebrate host requires about 3 to 4 weeks. The chicken is infected by ingestion of the infected mollusk, and mature worms develop in about 2 weeks.

PATHOLOGIC EFFECTS

This is the most pathogenic tapeworm that affects the chicken (Soulsby 1965). Heavy infections are common, with as many as 3,000 to 4,000 worms being recovered from a single chicken (Reid 1962). Signs of infection are nonspecific and include diarrhea, weight loss, lethargy, and ruffled plumage (Morgan and Hawkins 1949; Wehr 1965). The lesions are those of a hemorrhagic enteritis. Adult worms attach to the duodenal wall and cause inflammation, with hemorrhage and thickening of the mucosa.

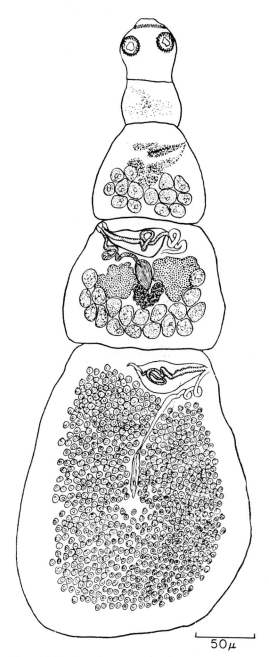

FIG. 6.13. *Davainea proglottina,* entire worm. (From Lapage 1962. Courtesy of Baillière, Tindall and Cassell.)

50μ

DIAGNOSIS

Diagnosis is based on the signs and lesions and on the identification of gravid proglottids in the feces or adult worms in scrapings or washings of the intestinal mucosa (Morgan and Hawkins 1949; Soulsby 1965). Since gravid proglottids are passed in the feces only at certain times of the day (usually in the afternoon or at night), more than one fecal examination may be required (Morgan and Hawkins 1949). Care must also be taken when examining for adult worms as they are often overlooked because of their small size (Lapage 1968).

CONTROL

Because of the need for a mollusk intermediate host, completion of the life cycle in the laboratory is unlikely, and no special control procedures are required. Treatment of infected chickens with dibutyltin dilaurate, as described for *H. carioca*, is effective (Edgar 1956).

PUBLIC HEALTH CONSIDERATIONS

This cestode has not been reported in man.

Raillietina cesticillus

This relatively nonpathogenic but sometimes debilitating tapeworm occurs in the small intestine of the chicken and other birds throughout the world (Lapage 1962, 1968). Although it is the commonest species of this genus in the domestic chicken (Soulsby 1965; Wehr 1965), its occurrence has not been reported in the laboratory chicken. Because a beetle intermediate host is required, *Raillietina cesticillus* is not likely to occur in chickens reared in the laboratory on insect-free diets, and it would be expected to be encountered only in birds brought into the laboratory from farm flocks.

MORPHOLOGY

The adult worm is usually about 4 cm in length, but sometimes measures up to 13 cm (Morgan and Hawkins 1949; Olsen 1967). The scolex has a distinctively shaped, broad rostellum which is armed with several hundred small hooks (Fig. 6.14). The suckers are unarmed and small. Gravid proglottids are filled with egg cap-

FIG. 6.14. *Raillietina cesticillus.* *(A, B)* Scolex with distinctively shaped rostellum. *(C)* Mature proglottid. *(D)* Egg. *(A, C* from Wehr 1965; courtesy of Iowa State University Press. *B, D* courtesy of W. M. Reid, University of Georgia.)

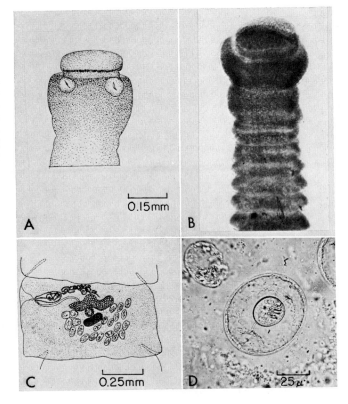

sules, each containing one egg that is 75 to 88 μ in diameter (Lapage 1968).

LIFE CYCLE

Gravid proglottids, up to 10 a day from a single worm, are passed by the chicken in the feces (Reid 1962). Several species of ground, dung, and flour beetles are intermediate hosts (Fig. 6.15). The housefly *(Musca domestica)* was once thought to be an intermediate host, but this is now recognized as incorrect (Reid 1962). Development to the infective larval stage in the beetle is dependent on the temperature and the host; at 30 C, it takes 2 weeks in the confused flour beetle *(Tribolium confusum)* (Voge 1961). The chicken is infected by ingestion of the infected beetle. Development to the adult stage in the chicken takes 2 to 4 weeks.

PATHOLOGIC EFFECTS

The severity of signs and lesions varies with the number of worms present and the

TRANSMISSION OF RAILLIETINA CESTICILLUS

FIG. 6.15. *Raillietina cesticillus,* diagram of life cycle. (Courtesy of Marietta Voge, University of California.)

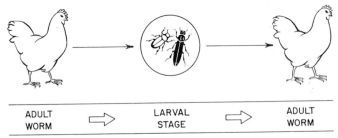

ADULT WORM ⟹ LARVAL STAGE ⟹ ADULT WORM

age of the host; young chickens are most susceptible (Wehr 1965). Light infections are usually inapparent (Morgan and Hawkins 1949). Heavy infections are uncommon, but when they occur, they cause decreased growth rate and sometimes emaciation (Reid 1962; Wehr 1965). Reduced hemoglobin and blood sugar levels and inflammation of the intestine at the point of attachment of the worm have also been reported.

DIAGNOSIS

Diagnosis is based on identification of gravid proglottids in the feces or the adult worm in the intestine at necropsy (Reid 1962).

CONTROL

This tapeworm can occur only in chickens permitted to ingest infected beetles. Because flour beetles are known intermediate hosts, care should be taken to prevent their occurrence in the laboratory. Treatment of infected chickens with dibutyltin dilaurate, as described for *H. carioca*, is effective (Edgar 1956).

PUBLIC HEALTH CONSIDERATIONS

This tapeworm has not been reported from man.

Raillietina echinobothrida

This nodule-forming tapeworm occurs in the small intestine of the chicken and other birds throughout the world (Lapage 1962; Wehr 1965). It is common in the domestic chicken (Reid 1962), but there are no reports of its occurrence in the laboratory chicken. Because of its requirement for an ant intermediate host, infection in laboratory-reared chickens is unlikely, and this tapeworm would be expected to be encountered only in birds brought into the laboratory from farm flocks.

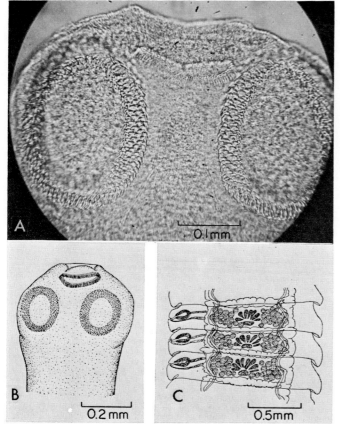

FIG. 6.16. *Raillietina echinobothrida. (A, B)* Scolex. *(C)* Gravid proglottid. *(A* courtesy of W. M. Reid, University of Georgia. *B* from Lapage 1962; courtesy of Baillière, Tindall and Cassell. *C* from Wardle and McLeod 1952; courtesy of University of Minnesota Press.)

MORPHOLOGY

The adult worm attains a length of 25 cm (Lapage 1968; Wehr 1965). The scolex bears numerous hooks; the suckers are armed with 8 to 15 rows of small hooks, and the rostellum has 2 rows of large hooks (Fig. 6.16). Gravid proglottids are either rectangular in shape or constricted longitudinally along the median line. The proglottids are filled with egg capsules containing 8 to 12 eggs each.

LIFE CYCLE

Gravid proglottids, passed in the feces, are ingested by the intermediate host, an ant (Reid 1962). The eggs hatch in the ant and develop into infective larvae in the body cavity (Olsen 1967). The chicken becomes infected by ingesting an infected ant. Development to the adult stage in the the chicken takes approximately 3 weeks (Wehr 1965).

PATHOLOGIC EFFECTS

Infection with this tapeworm causes a condition called nodular tapeworm disease (Fig. 6.17) (Lapage 1968). The young worms penetrate deeply into the intestinal mucosa, causing inflammation and nodule formation. Signs are weakness, diarrhea, emaciation, and sometimes death (Wehr 1965). The nodules are visible from the peritoneal surface and resemble tuberculosis lesions (Lapage 1968). In section, they are seen to contain caseous, necrotic material and many leucocytes (Soulsby 1965).

DIAGNOSIS

Diagnosis is based on the presence of gravid proglottids in the feces and nodules in the intestine; however, care must be taken to differentiate the lesions produced by this tapeworm from those of tuberculosis (Lapage 1968).

CONTROL

Because an ant is required as an intermediate host, completion of the life cycle in the laboratory is unlikely, and no special procedures other than routine insect control are needed. Treatment with dibutyltin dilaurate, as described for *H. carioca*, is probably effective for this tapeworm.

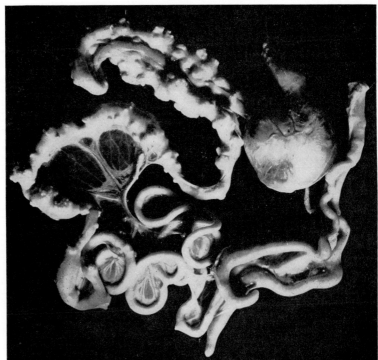

FIG.. 6.17. Nodular tapeworm disease. Lesions produced by *Raillietina echinobothrida* in chicken. (From Wehr 1965. Courtesy of Iowa State University Press.)

This cestode has not been reported from man.

Raillietina tetragona

This tapeworm, of uncertain pathogenicity, occurs in the small intestine of the chicken, pigeon, and other birds throughout the world (Olsen 1967). It is common in the domestic chicken (Wehr 1965), but it has not been reported in the laboratory chicken. Because an ant intermediate host is required, infection with this tapeworm is unlikely in laboratory-reared chickens, and it would be expected to be encountered only in birds brought into the laboratory from farm flocks.

MORPHOLOGY

The adult worm measures up to 25 cm in length and is similar to that of *R. echinobothrida* (Wehr 1965). It is distinguished by its more oval suckers and by a single row of rostellar hooks rather than a double row (Reid 1962).

LIFE CYCLE

The life cycle is also similar to that of *R. echinobothrida* (Wehr 1965).

PATHOLOGIC EFFECTS

Although this species is considered to be one of the more pathogenic tapeworms affecting the chicken, controlled experimental studies are lacking (Reid 1962). Except for a single report of intestinal nodules, little is known of the pathogenicity of this parasite in the chicken (Reid 1962; Wehr 1965).

DIAGNOSIS

Diagnosis is based on identification of the gravid proglottids in the feces or the adult worm in the intestine (Reid 1962).

CONTROL

Control is the same as that described for *R. echinobothrida* (Reid 1962). Treatment with dibutyltin dilaurate is effective (Edgar 1956).

PUBLIC HEALTH CONSIDERATIONS

Raillietina tetragona has not been reported from man.

DILEPIDIDS

These are medium-sized cestodes with unarmed suckers (Belding 1965). Those that affect endothermal laboratory animals are listed in Table 6.3. *Dipylidium caninum* is the most important species.

Dipylidium caninum

(SYN. *Taenia caninum, T. cucumerina*)
(Dog Tapeworm,
Double-pored Dog Tapeworm)

Dipylidium caninum occurs in the small intestine of the dog, cat, some wild carnivores, and rarely man throughout the world (Belding 1965; Soulsby 1965). As with most tapeworms, it is relatively harmless except in heavy infections (Lapage 1962). This is probably the commonest parasite of the dog and cat in most parts of the world (Lapage 1962). Animals obtained from pounds are usually infected. Typical incidences for the dog are 85.4% in Hawaii (Ash 1962a), 39.0% in Illinois (Cross and Allen 1948), 9.7% in Michigan (Worley 1964), 30.0% in Kenya (Murray 1968), and 20.0% in Colombia (Marinkelle 1966). In dogs used for research in New York that were obtained from various locations in eastern and southeastern United States, the incidence was 11.0% (Mann and Bjotvedt 1965). Typical incidences in the cat are 81.3% in Hawaii (Ash 1962a), 39.2% in central United States (Cross and Allen 1948), and 44.5% in Great Britain (Dubey 1966). Although common in pound animals, this parasite is uncommon in animals raised for research in kennels that practice good sanitation and parasite control (Bantin and Maber 1967; Johnson, Andersen, and Gee 1963; Morris 1963; Sheffy, Baker, and Gillespie 1961).

MORPHOLOGY

The adult worm is often 20 cm or more in length but is much shorter when large numbers are present in a host (Lapage 1968; Morgan and Hawkins 1949; Soulsby 1965). The scolex bears a rostellum with many small hooks; the suckers are unarmed. Each proglottid has two sets of male and female reproductive organs and two genital pores. Gravid proglottids are elongated, barrel shaped, and filled with egg capsules (Fig. 6.18); each capsule contains 3 to 20, usually

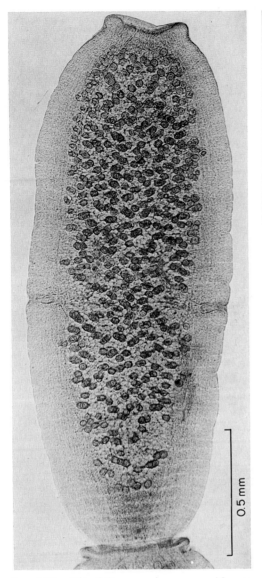

0.5 mm

FIG. 6.18. *Dipylidium caninum,* gravid proglottid. (Courtesy of Marietta Voge, University of California.)

8 to 15, eggs (Fig. 6.19). Individual eggs are spherical to oval and measure 31 to 50 μ long by 27 to 48 μ wide, the size varying inversely with the number present in a capsule (Burrows 1965). When passed in the feces, gravid proglottids are white to pink and 8 to 12 mm long by 2 to 3 mm wide. They move about vigorously, expelling egg capsules and eggs.

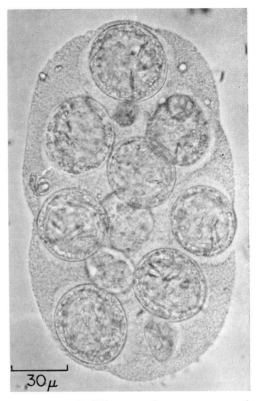

30 μ

FIG. 6.19. *Dipylidium caninum,* egg capsule with eggs. (Courtesy of TSgt R. R. Estes, USAF School of Aerospace Medicine.)

LIFE CYCLE

The life cycle requires a flea or louse as an intermediate host (Fig. 6.20) (Belding 1965; Lapage 1968). Gravid proglottids containing egg capsules and eggs either crawl out the anus of the definitive host or are passed in the feces (Olsen 1967). Flea larvae *(Ctenocephalides canis, C. felis)* in the bedding or resting places of the dog and cat ingest the egg capsules. The tapeworm embryo remains in the flea larva through the pupal stage and completes its development to the cysticercoid stage when the flea becomes an adult. The dog louse *(Trichodectes canis)* and the human flea *(Pulex irritans)* are also intermediate hosts. A definitive host is infected by ingestion of an infected flea or louse. Development to the adult cestode requires 2 to 4 weeks.

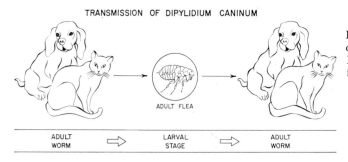

TRANSMISSION OF DIPYLIDIUM CANINUM

ADULT FLEA

| ADULT WORM | ⇨ | LARVAL STAGE | ⇨ | ADULT WORM |

Fig. 6.20. *Dipylidium caninum,* diagram of life cycle. (Courtesy of Marietta Voge, University of California.)

PATHOLOGIC EFFECTS

Infection in the dog and cat is characterized by the presence of gravid proglottids in the feces or perianal region, and sometimes by anal pruritus (Lapage 1962; Soulsby 1965) and a subtle nutritional deficiency (Silverman 1961). Occasionally heavy infections occur which cause weakness, emaciation, vomiting, diarrhea, a voracious appetite, convulsions, and a chronic, sometimes hemorrhagic, enteritis (Belding 1965; Lapage 1962; Morgan and Hawkins 1949; Mullenax and Mullenax 1962; Soulsby 1965).

DIAGNOSIS

Diagnosis is made by identification of the gravid proglottids or egg capsules in the feces or perianal region (Soulsby 1965). Gravid segments of *D. caninum* resemble those of *Mesocestoides* and are differentiated by microscopic observation of the characteristic double set of genital pores.

CONTROL

Elimination of fleas and lice from research animals will prevent the completion of the life cycle and control the infection in laboratory colonies (Johnson, Andersen, and Gee 1963).

Effective treatments include drocarbil (Nemural, Winthrop), given orally at a level of 5.0 mg per kg of body weight for the dog and 3.3 mg per kg for the cat (Habermann and Williams 1958; Siegmund 1961); niclosamide (Yomesan, Bayer), given orally at a level of 100 to 200 mg per kg of body weight for the dog and cat (Cox, Mullee, and Allen 1966; Gregor 1963; Kurelec and Rijavec 1961); dichlorophen with toluene (Vermiplex, Pitman-Moore), given orally at a level of 200 mg per kg of body

weight for the dog and cat (Soulsby 1965); and bunamidine hydrochloride (Scolaban, Burroughs Wellcome), given orally at a level of 15 to 70 mg per kg for the dog or 20 to 50 mg per kg for the cat (Burrows and Lillis 1966).

PUBLIC HEALTH CONSIDERATIONS

Dipylidium caninum infection is uncommon in man and occurs only by accidental ingestion of an infected flea or louse (Gleason 1962; Moore 1962; Turner 1962). The effects are often inapparent except for a rare, mild abdominal discomfort (Belding 1965). The elimination of fleas and lice from laboratory dogs and cats will eliminate the hazard to laboratory personnel.

MESOCESTOIDIDS

The mesocestoidids are characterized by an unarmed scolex, the absence of a rostellum, and a sparganumlike larval stage (Voge 1955a). Both the larval stages (formerly given separate generic names, such as *Tetrathyridium* and *Dithyridium*) and the adult forms occur in endothermal animals. The species that affect endothermal laboratory animals are listed in Table 6.4 and are discussed below.

Mesocestoides

Mesocestoides corti (syn. *M. variabilis*) occurs in North and Central America (Voge 1955a). The adult is found in the small intestine of the dog, cat, wild carnivores, and man (Belding 1965); it is uncommon in dogs and cats obtained from pounds and rare or absent in those raised in kennels (Johnson, Andersen, and Gee 1963; Reece, Hofstad, and Swenson 1968). The preadult, or tetrathyridial larva, occurs in the peritoneal cavity, liver, and other organs of wild rodents, the dog, cat, other mammals, amphibians, and reptiles; it is uncommon in the dog and cat (Belding 1965; Voge 1953, 1955b, 1967; Voge and Berntzen 1963).

Mesocestoides lineatus occurs in Europe, Africa, and Asia (Soulsby 1965). The adult is found in the small intestine of the dog, cat, other carnivores, and man; it is common in the dog but rare in the cat in East Africa (Fitzsimmons 1961) and uncommon or rare in both species elsewhere (Soulsby 1965). The tetrathyridial larva occurs in the peritoneal and pleural cavity of wild rodents, the dog, cat, other mammals, and ectothermal animals; it is uncommon in the dog and cat (Soulsby 1965).

A tetrathyridial *Mesocestoides* larva of unknown species has been reported in captive African and Asian primates in the United States, Europe, and Africa (Graham 1960; Myers and Kuntz 1965; Reardon and Rininger 1968). The larva occurs in the peritoneal cavity and has been observed in the rhesus monkey, cynomolgus monkey, and baboons. It is uncommon or rare.

MORPHOLOGY

The adult worm measures 30 to 150 cm in length (Lapage 1968; Soulsby 1965). The proglottids (Fig. 6.21) are similar in size and shape to those of *Dipylidium caninum,* but differ by having only one set of male and female reproductive organs and by having a single, relatively small uterine capsule which, in gravid proglottids, contains the eggs. Eggs measure 40 to 60 μ by 35 to 43 μ. The tetrathyridial larva is flat and contractile. It varies in length from 2 to 70 mm, depending on the species of parasite and species of host. In the monkey, it is proglottid shaped (Graham 1960).

LIFE CYCLE

The life cycle is not fully known. The tetrathyridial larva has been found in a variety of endothermal and ectothermal animals, but the first intermediate host is unknown (Voge 1953, 1955b, 1967). When an infected intermediate host is ingested by a suitable definitive host, the tetrathyridium develops in the intestine to an adult tapeworm in about 21 to 30 days; if ingested by an unsuitable host, the tetrathyridium persists in an encapsulated form until

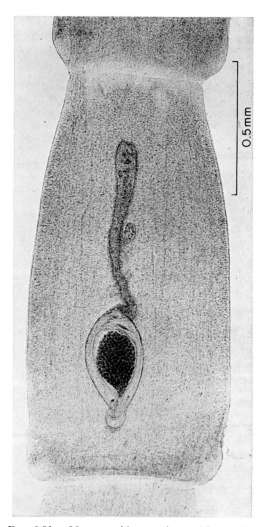

0.5 mm

FIG. 6.21. *Mesocestoides corti,* gravid proglottid. Note uterine capsule. (Courtesy of Marietta Voge, University of California.)

ingested again by another host (Soulsby 1965). Asexual multiplication of the tetrathyridial larva has also been reported (Specht and Voge 1965). Such multiplication of the larval stage sometimes occurs in the small intestine before the adult form develops (Eckert, von Brand, and Voge 1969).

PATHOLOGIC EFFECTS

The larva usually occurs free in the peritoneal or pleural cavity of the dog, cat, and monkey (Graham 1960; Soulsby 1965).

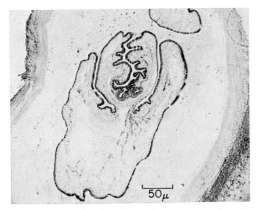

FIG. 6.22. *Mesocestoides,* larval cyst in the omentum of a monkey. (From Graham 1960. Courtesy of New York Academy of Sciences.)

When entrapped by host tissue, a small, fibrous cyst forms (Fig. 6.22). Heavy infections are uncommon (Soulsby 1965). They occasionally cause debilitation and sometimes ascites and death in the dog and cat (Soulsby 1965). No pathologic effects have been attributed to infection with the adult worm.

DIAGNOSIS

Diagnosis is based on identification of the larva in the peritoneal or pleural cavity or the typical gravid proglottids in the feces.

CONTROL

Because completion of the life cycle in the laboratory is highly unlikely, no special control procedures are required. Treatment of larval infections has not been reported. Drugs effective against *Dipylidium caninum* are probably effective against the adult.

PUBLIC HEALTH CONSIDERATIONS

This parasite rarely affects man (Belding 1965; Bisseru 1967). Because infection can occur only by ingestion of animal tissues containing larvae, infected laboratory animals are not a likely hazard for man.

ANOPLOCEPHALIDS

These cestodes have a large, unarmed, globular scolex and a relatively large strobila with wider than long proglottids (Belding 1965). The larvae of most species develop in a free-living mite; adults are parasites of mammals and birds. Those that affect endothermal laboratory animals are listed in Table 6.5. *Bertiella studeri* is the most important species.

Bertiella studeri

(SYN. *Bertiella satyri, B. conferta, B. cercopitheci, Bertia polyorchis*)

This apparently harmless tapeworm occurs in the small intestine of various primates including the rhesus monkey, cynomolgus monkey, Japanese macaque, guenons, mandrills, baboons, gibbons, chimpanzee, orangutan, and man in Africa, Asia, Indonesia, and the Philippine Islands (Fiennes 1967; Witenberg 1964). Laboratory primates obtained from their natural habitat are frequently infected. Typical incidences are 3.6 to 14.0% in the rhesus monkey (Reardon and Rininger 1968; Valerio et al. 1969), 1.4 to 5.3% in the cynomolgus monkey (Hashimoto and Honjo 1966; Tanaka et al. 1962), 7.1% in the Japanese macaque (Tanaka et al. 1962), and 7.7% in baboons (Kuntz and Myers 1966, 1967).

MORPHOLOGY

The adult worm is 10 to 30 cm in length and 1 cm in width (Wardle and McLeod 1952). The scolex is subglobose and devoid of hooks; the segments are about eight times wider than long (Fig. 6.23) and contain only one set of male and female reproductive organs. Gravid proglottids are filled with eggs enclosed in a saclike uterus. Eggs are thin shelled, measure 38 to 45 μ in diameter (Tanaka et al. 1962) and contain an embryo which is surrounded by a pyriform inner shell with a bicornate protrusion (Fig. 6.24).

LIFE CYCLE

Eggs passed in the feces are ingested by various free-living oribatid mites (Stunkard 1940). The larva develops in the mite, and the vertebrate host apparently becomes infected by accidentally ingesting an infected mite with vegetation.

PATHOLOGIC EFFECTS

Bertiella studeri causes no apparent signs or lesions.

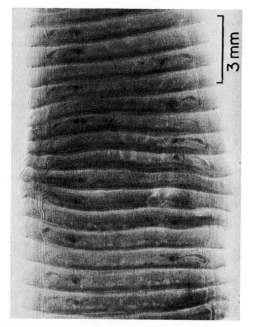

FIG. 6.23. *Bertiella studeri,* mature proglottids. (Courtesy of Marietta Voge, University of California.)

DIAGNOSIS

Diagnosis is made by finding the characteristic eggs or gravid proglottids in the feces.

CONTROL

Because completion of the life cycle in the laboratory is highly unlikely, no special control procedures are required (Kuntz and Myers 1967). No treatment of laboratory animals has been reported. Presumably drugs used against *Dipylidium caninum* would be effective against this cestode. Drocarbil (Nemural, Winthrop), when given to primates, is administered orally at a level of 4 to 5 mg per kg of body weight; dichlorophen with toluene (Vermiplex, Pitman-Moore) is given orally at a level of 200 mg per kg of body weight (Gisler, Benson, and Young 1960).

PUBLIC HEALTH CONSIDERATIONS

This parasite rarely affects man (Belding 1965; Faust, Beaver, and Jung 1968). Because infection can occur only by ingestion of an infected free-living mite, infected laboratory animals are not a direct hazard for man.

TAENIIDS

These are relatively large cestodes (Belding 1965; Lapage 1968). The scolex has a well-developed, usually armed rostellum and four unarmed suckers. The proglottids contain a single set of male and female reproductive organs and are usually longer than wide when gravid. The larval stage is either a cysticercus, coenurus, or hydatid (Fig. 6.25) (Soulsby 1965). Both larvae and adults are parasites of endothermal animals. Those that affect endothermal laboratory animals are listed in Table 6.6. The most important species are discussed below.

Taenia taeniaeformis

(SYN. *Hydatigera taeniaeformis, Taenia serrata, T. crassicollis, Cysticercus fasciolaris*)

This tapeworm occurs throughout the world (Lapage 1962). The adult worm is frequently encountered in the small intestine of the cat and wild felids and occasionally in the dog and other carnivores (Renaux 1964). The larva is common in the liver of the mouse, rat, black rat, cotton rat, voles, and other wild rodents (Alicata 1964; Cosgrove et al. 1964; Lewis 1968; Oldham 1967).

Cats obtained from pounds are frequently infected, but dogs are not. The incidence often varies widely within a small geographic area and is closely related to the local incidence in wild rodents (Ash 1962a, b; Fitzsimmons 1961). Typical reported incidences are 3.9% in central United States (Cross and Allen 1948), 4.5% in Great Britain (Dubey 1966), and 20.6% in Hawaii (Ash 1962a). In a survey of 96 stray dogs in a high incidence area (Hawaii), none was found infected (Ash 1962a). Cats raised in facilities where good sanitation and rodent control are practiced are usually free of this parasite (Morris 1963).

Wild rodents are commonly infected. Typical incidences in the rat are 19.2% in eastern United States (Dove 1950), 15.8% in Puerto Rico (de León 1964), 40.0% in Hawaii (Ash 1962b), 44.7% in Canada (Morgan and Hawkins 1949), and 58.5% in

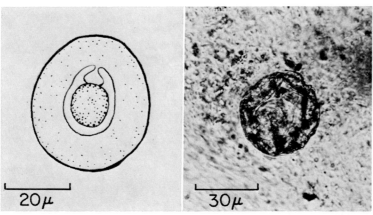

20μ   30μ

FIG. 6.24. *Bertiella studeri* egg. Diagram *(left)* shows pyriform inner shell with bicornate protrusion. *(Left* courtesy of Marietta Voge, University of California. *Right* from Tanaka et al. 1962. Courtesy of Japan Experimental Animal Research Association.)

the black rat and 74.7% in the Norway rat in Japan (Sasa et al. 1962).

The incidence in laboratory mice and rats varies from absent to common, depending on sanitation practices and diet. An incidence of over 12% has been reported in a colony of mice maintained on the same floor with laboratory cats; mice maintained on another floor with no cats had a zero incidence (Innes 1967). In another colony, a 16.6% incidence was observed in mice fed an apparently contaminated diet; other animals in the colony fed the same diet minus one ingredient (flaked maize) had a zero incidence (Duffill and Lyon 1960). In a survey of 13 commercial mouse colonies in Great Britain, approximately 50% of the mice from 4 colonies were found infected (Owen 1968); in other colonies where sanitation practices are good and uncontaminated diets are fed, the parasite is absent (Bell 1968; Flynn, Brennan, and Fritz 1965; Foster 1963; Owen 1968).

MORPHOLOGY

The adult worm is 15 to 60 cm long and 5 to 6 mm wide (Wardle and McLeod 1952). The scolex bears a rostellum with two crowns of hooks; the gravid segments contain an egg-filled uterus composed of a central, longitudinal stem with 16 to 18 lateral branches on each side (Fig. 6.26). The posterior segments are characteristically bell shaped. Eggs are typically taeniid;

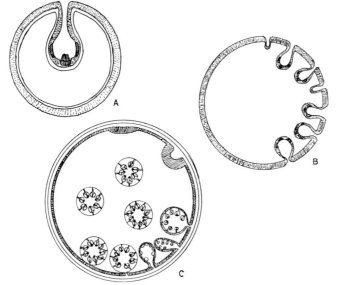

FIG. 6.25. Larval stages of taeniid cestodes: *(A)* Cysticercus. Note single invagination and scolex. *(B)* Coenurus. Note multiple invaginations, each with a developing scolex. *(C)* Hydatid. Note the several buds or brood capsules, each with a number of developing scolices. (From Soulsby 1965. Courtesy of Blackwell Scientific Publications.)

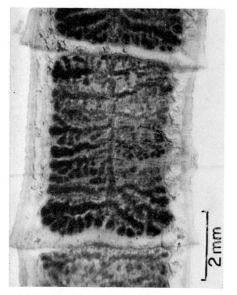

FIG. 6.26. *Taenia,* gravid proglottid. (From Soulsby 1965. Courtesy of Blackwell Scientific Publications.)

they are spherical, measure 24 to 31 μ by 22 to 27 μ (Burrows 1965), and have a striated capsule, or embryophore (Fig. 6.27). The larva is of the cysticercus type but is unique in that the scolex is not invaginated

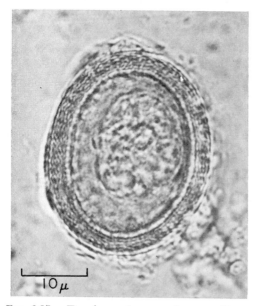

FIG. 6.27. *Taenia,* embryonated egg. (Courtesy of Marietta Voge, University of California.)

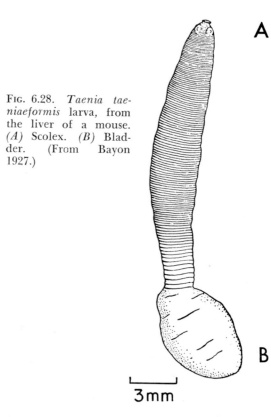

FIG. 6.28. *Taenia taeniaeformis* larva, from the liver of a mouse. *(A)* Scolex. *(B)* Bladder. (From Bayon 1927.)

into the bladder but is attached to it by a long, segmented neck (Fig. 6.28). It is sometimes several centimeters in length.

LIFE CYCLE

Embryonated eggs, when ingested by a suitable rodent, hatch in the small intestine, and the embryos pass to the liver where they develop into infective larvae in about 30 days (Wardle and McLeod 1952). Transmission to the definitive host is by ingestion of an infected rodent liver. The worms mature in a few weeks, and gravid proglottids and eggs are passed in the feces. The entire life cycle can be completed in the laboratory (Fig. 6.29).

PATHOLOGIC EFFECTS

In the cat, light infections are commonest (Burrows and Lillis 1966) and are usually inapparent (Soulsby 1965). Heavy infections, when they occur, cause chronic enteritis, diarrhea, and weight loss (Soulsby 1965). Because this tapeworm buries its scolex deep into the intestinal mucosa, it

TRANSMISSION OF TAENIA TAENIAEFORMIS

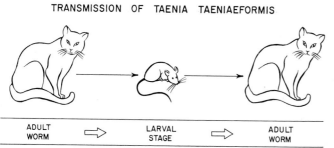

| ADULT WORM | ⇒ | LARVAL STAGE | ⇒ | ADULT WORM |

FIG. 6.29. *Taenia taeniaeformis,* diagram of life cycle. Note that entire cycle can be completed in laboratory. (Courtesy of Marietta Voge, University of California.)

produces more tissue reaction than other tapeworms (Renaux 1964). Occasionally the parasite perforates the intestinal wall and enters the peritoneal cavity (Lapage 1968). Neurologic disturbances have been associated with infection (Soulsby 1965). Their cause is uncertain although they have been attributed to toxins released by the worms.

The larval stage in rodents is characterized by the formation in the liver of white to clear cysts, 4 mm in diameter (Fig. 6.30) (Olivier 1962). In microscopic section, segmented larvae are seen in the cysts (Fig.

6.31). One or two is the usual number per animal (Morgan and Hawkins 1949). Occasionally the cysts are associated with the occurrence of hepatic sarcomas in the tissue capsule which surrounds them, especially in older animals (Jones 1967); otherwise, their presence has little effect on the health of the host (Oldham 1967).

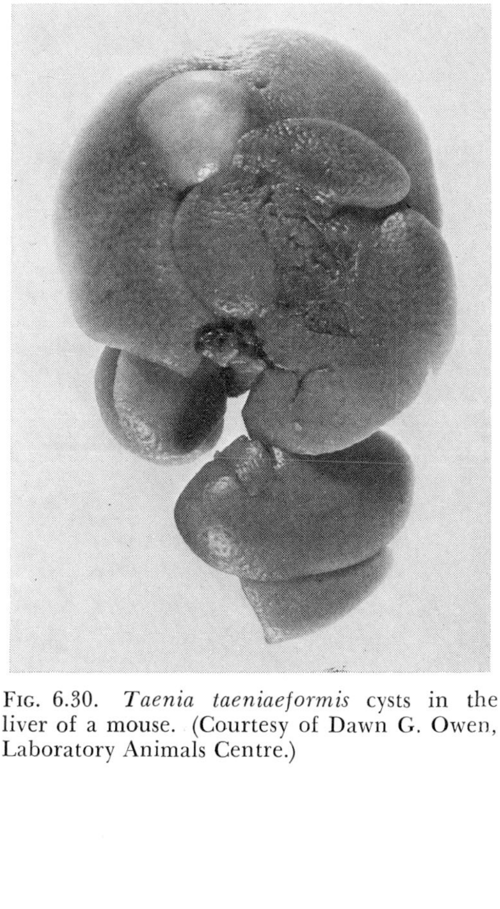

DIAGNOSIS

Diagnosis in the definitive host is based on finding the adult worm in the intestine or the eggs or gravid proglottids in the feces (Soulsby 1965). Since the eggs of the various species of *Taenia* cannot be differenti-

FIG. 6.30. *Taenia taeniaeformis* cysts in the liver of a mouse. (Courtesy of Dawn G. Owen, Laboratory Animals Centre.)

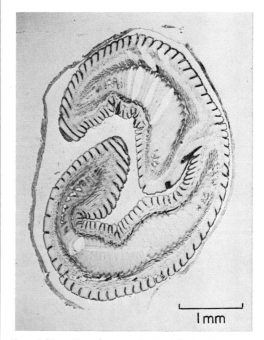

1 mm

FIG. 6.31. *Taenia taeniaeformis,* microscopic section of larva from the liver of a rat. (Courtesy of Marietta Voge, University of California.)

ated morphologically, positive identification of *T. taeniaeformis* is based on the morphology of the gravid segments. Diagnosis of infection in rodents is based on finding the characteristic hepatic cysts.

CONTROL

Proper management and sanitation are essential to prevent transmission of infection between rodents and cats and dogs maintained in the same animal facility. Food and bedding for rodents should be obtained from sources free of contamination by cat or dog feces and should be transported and stored in such a way that subsequent contamination is precluded (Oldham 1967); wild rodent control is essential in preventing the infection in cats (Lapage 1968).

Cats and dogs, especially newly acquired specimens, should be examined and treated, if infected. The drugs effective against *Dipylidium caninum* are effective against this tapeworm. Bithionol (thiobis dichlorophenol), given orally at a level of 220 mg per kg of body weight, is also effective (Enzie and Colglazier 1960). There is no treatment for the larval stage in rodents.

PUBLIC HEALTH CONSIDERATIONS

This tapeworm rarely affects man (Belding 1965). Infection can occur only by ingestion of an infected rodent.

Taenia pisiformis

(SYN. *Cysticercus pisiformis*)

Adults of this species occur in the small intestine of the dog, cat, and wild carnivores throughout the world; the larval stages occur in the liver and peritoneal cavity of the rabbit, cottontail rabbit, hares, and various wild rodents (Lapage 1968; Morgan and Hawkins 1949).

Infection is common in the dog but uncommon in the cat (Lapage 1962, 1968). It is unlikely to occur in urban animals and would not be expected to occur in those raised in kennels where the ingestion of viscera of wild rabbits is not permitted (Johnson, Andersen, and Gee 1963; Renaux 1964). Typical incidences in laboratory dogs obtained from pounds in the United States are 6.4% in Michigan (Worley 1964) and

10.0% in Illinois (Cross and Allen 1948). In dogs used for research in New York that were obtained from various locations in eastern and southeastern United States, an incidence of 37.0% was reported (Mann and Bjotvedt 1965).

Wild rabbits are usually infected, and reported incidences range from 25% in eastern United States (Holloway 1966) to almost 100% in other areas (Renaux 1964).

The incidence in laboratory rabbits varies from common to absent, depending on whether or not the diet is contaminated by dog feces (Shanks 1962). In the United States the parasite is frequently encountered; in one survey, sample rabbits from 5 of 10 commercial suppliers were found infected (Poole et al. 1967). It is also reported to be common in Great Britain (Adams, Aitken, and Worden 1967; Cushnie 1954; Napier 1963), but in a survey of sample rabbits from 16 commercial breeders, none was found infected (Owen 1968).

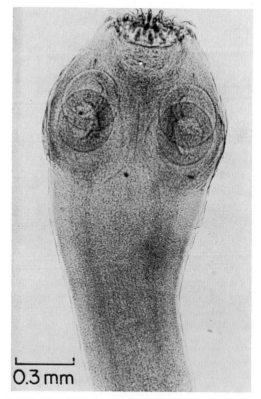

FIG. 6.32. *Taenia pisiformis* scolex. (Courtesy of Marietta Voge, University of California.)

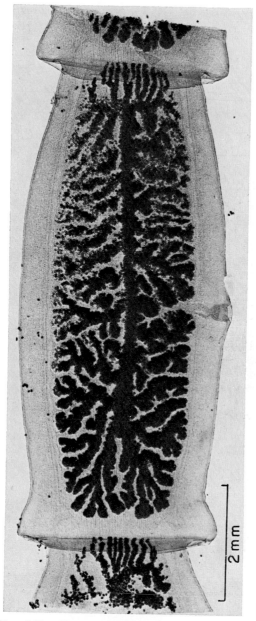

FIG. 6.33. *Taenia pisiformis*, gravid proglottid. (Courtesy of Marietta Voge, University of California.)

MORPHOLOGY

The adult worm attains a length of 20 cm and a width of several millimeters (Wardle and McLeod 1952). The scolex bears a rostellum with two crowns of hooks (Fig.

6.32). First segments are wider than long, mature segments almost square, and gravid segments longer than wide (Morgan and Hawkins 1949). Gravid proglottids are cream colored, measure 8 to 11 mm long by 4 to 5 mm wide, and contain a uterus that has 8 to 14 branches on each side of the median stem (Fig. 6.33) (Burrows 1965). Eggs are typically taeniid, dark brown, spherical to subspherical, and 34 to 41 μ by 29 to 35 μ (Burrows 1965). The larva, which is of the cysticercus type, appears as a transparent sphere about 10 mm in diameter and contains the characteristic scolex.

LIFE CYCLE

Embryonated eggs, when ingested by a suitable lagomorph or rodent, hatch in the small intestine, and the embryos pass to the liver where further development occurs (Lapage 1968). After about 15 to 30 days, the larva reaches the surface of the liver and passes into the peritoneal cavity. Transmission to the definitive host is by ingestion of the viscera of an intermediate host. The worms grow to maturity in a few weeks, and gravid proglottids and eggs are passed in the feces. Although the entire life cycle can be completed in the laboratory (Fig. 6.34), it is unlikely.

PATHOLOGIC EFFECTS

Light infections in the dog are usually inapparent (Lapage 1968); heavy infections cause abdominal discomfort and enteritis (Habermann and Williams 1958).

Infection in the rabbit is usually inapparent, and only in massive infections are abdominal distention, lethargy, and weight loss observed (Lapage 1968). The presence of the larva is usually recognized only at necropsy, when the cysts are seen either floating free in the peritoneal cavity or attached to the viscera (Fig. 6.35). Clusters of 5 to 15 cysts are usual, but as many as 250 have been observed in one rabbit (Morgan and Hawkins 1949). The migration of the larva through the liver apparently causes little damage and results in fibrous tracks through the parenchyma, or small, 1 to 3 mm, white foci on the surface (Adams, Aitken, and Worden 1967: Morgan and Hawkins 1949). Only in massive infections is extensive liver damage produced (Lapage 1968).

TRANSMISSION OF TAENIA PISIFORMIS

Fig. 6.34. *Taenia pisiformis,* diagram of life cycle. (Courtesy of Marietta Voge, University of California.)

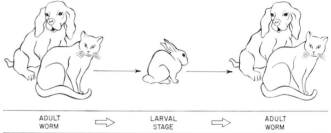

| ADULT WORM | ⇨ | LARVAL STAGE | ⇨ | ADULT WORM |

DIAGNOSIS

Diagnosis in the definitive host is based on finding the eggs and characteristic gravid proglottids in the feces (Soulsby 1965). Diagnosis in the intermediate host is made by identifying the cysts in the peritoneal cavity (Adams, Aitken, and Worden 1967).

CONTROL

Food and bedding for rabbits should be obtained from sources free of contamination by feces of dogs or other carnivores, and should be transported and stored in such a way that subsequent contamination is precluded (Adams, Aitken, and Worden 1967). Dogs should not be housed close to rabbits (Morgan and Hawkins 1949).

Newly acquired dogs and cats should be examined and treated, if infected (Habermann and Williams 1958). The drugs effective against *Dipylidium caninum* are also effective against this tapeworm. There is no treatment for the larval stage in the rabbit.

PUBLIC HEALTH CONSIDERATIONS

This tapeworm is not known to infect man.

Multiceps serialis

(Syn. *Taenia serialis, T. coenuri, Coenurus serialis, C. cuniculi*)

The adult of this species occurs in the small intestine of the dog and other canids throughout the world (Lapage 1968). The larval stage occurs in the subcutaneous tissues of wild rodents, the rabbit, hares, dog, monkey, gelada, and man (Belding 1965; Lapage 1968; Ruch 1959; Voge and Berntzen 1963).

Little is known of the incidence of this parasite in laboratory dogs. It is apparently uncommon in urban dogs and would not be expected to occur in those raised in kennels where the ingestion of tissues from wild rodents and rabbits is prevented (Galvin and Turk 1966; Johnson, Andersen, and Gee 1963). Similarly, there is little information on the incidence of infection in laboratory rabbits and simian primates. It is reported to be common in wild lagomorphs but uncommon in domestic rabbits reared on food uncontaminated with dog feces (Shanks 1962). In one survey of sample rabbits from 16 commercial breeders in Great Britain, none was found infected (Owen 1968).

MORPHOLOGY

The adult worm is up to 70 cm in length and 3 to 5 mm in width (Morgan and Hawkins 1949; Wardle and McLeod 1952). The scolex bears a rostellum with a double row of hooks. Mature segments are wider than long and contain a uterus that

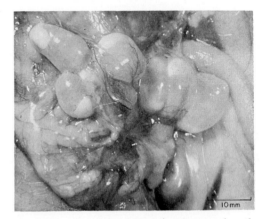

Fig. 6.35. *Taenia pisiformis,* larvae in the peritoneal cavity of a rabbit. (Courtesy of Jane K. Glaser, Argonne National Laboratory.)

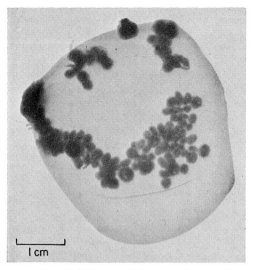

FIG. 6.36. *Multiceps serialis,* larval stage from the intermuscular connective tissue of a rabbit. Note numerous buds. (Courtesy of Marietta Voge, University of California.)

has 20 to 25 branches on each side of the median stem. Eggs are similar to those of *Taenia* and measure 31 to 34 μ by 27 to 30 μ (Burrows 1965). The larva, which is of the coenurus type, is glistening white and 4 to 5 cm in diameter. It is filled with fluid and has secondary buds protruding to the inside or outside of the original, larger cyst (Fig. 6.36). These buds usually contain a scolex.

LIFE CYCLE

The life cycle is similar to that of *Taenia pisiformis* except that the larval stage usually occurs in the subcutaneous tissues rather than in the liver and peritoneal cavity (Lapage 1962).

PATHOLOGIC EFFECTS

Infection in the dog is usually inapparent (Lapage 1968). Similarly, the larva in the rabbit usually causes no signs unless infection is massive (Morgan and Hawkins 1949). The cysts usually develop in the subcutaneous tissue and appear as swellings under the skin (Cook 1969). The flank is a common site. Rarely the cysts occur in the brain, peritoneal cavity, liver, and other organs (Ruch 1959; Voge and Berntzen 1963).

DIAGNOSIS

Diagnosis in the dog is based on identification of the gravid proglottids in the feces (Soulsby 1965). A tentative diagnosis in the rabbit is made by palpation of the characteristic, movable, subcutaneous cyst; a definitive diagnosis is based on identification of the cyst at necropsy (Adams, Aitken, and Worden 1967).

CONTROL

Control is similar to that described for *Taenia pisiformis* (Lapage 1968).

PUBLIC HEALTH CONSIDERATIONS

Since the larval stage occurs occasionally in man as a subcutaneous or cerebral cyst (Belding 1965), feces from infected dogs should be handled with caution, and laboratory personnel should be instructed in proper personal hygiene.

Echinococcus granulosus

The adult of this species occurs in the small intestine of the dog and wild canids (Matoff 1968; Smyth and Smyth 1964); the larval stage is common in the liver, lungs, and peritoneal cavity of various wild and domestic herbivores and sometimes occurs in wild rodents and lagomorphs, the dog, cat, rhesus monkey, other macaques, colobus monkeys, baboons, lemurs, Celebes ape *(Cynopithecus niger),* and man (Belding 1965; Crosby et al. 1968; Ilievski and Esber 1969; Lapage 1968).

Echinococcus granulosus is found throughout the world, particularly in areas where sheep are raised (Faust, Beaver, and Jung 1968). It is commonest in eastern and southern Europe, the Near East, southern South America, South Africa, southern Australia, New Zealand, and central Asia.

Little is known of the incidence of infection with the adult of this species in laboratory dogs. It is apparently uncommon or rare in most parts of the world and only common in dogs obtained from pounds in endemic areas. Incidences of 26% have been reported in stray dogs in southern France, 42% in Sardinia, 25% in Yugoslavia, 40% in Bulgaria, 33% in Lebanon, 25% in Jordan, 34% in Iran, 29% in India, 50% in New Zealand and southern Aus-

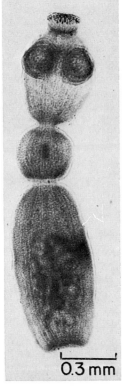

FIG. 6.37. *Echinococcus granulosus* adult. (Courtesy of Marietta Voge, University of California.)

0.3 mm

LIFE CYCLE

Eggs passed in the feces of the dog are ingested by an intermediate host and hatch in the duodenum. The embryos penetrate the intestinal wall, enter the mesenteric venules, and are carried in the bloodstream to various organs where they develop into hydatid cysts (Lapage 1968). The dog becomes infected by ingestion of the cysts in the viscera of the intermediate host. Each scolex in the ingested cyst develops into an adult worm.

PATHOLOGIC EFFECTS

It is not uncommon for one dog to harbor hundreds or thousands of adults of this species. Yet even in such heavy infections, the worms cause no clinical signs (Medda 1966; Morgan and Hawkins 1949). The effects of the larva depend on its location and size (Lapage 1968). In the monkey it sometimes causes abdominal distention or localized subcutaneous swellings (Crosby et al. 1968; Summers 1960), but usually it causes no effects and is recognized only at necropsy (Healy and Hayes 1963). It appears as a spherical mass of varying size, usually in the liver, but is sometimes embedded in the lungs or is free in the peritoneal cavity.

DIAGNOSIS

Diagnosis in the dog depends on recognition of the small worm or gravid segments in the feces; the eggs cannot be differentiated from those of *Taenia* (Morgan and Hawkins 1949). Administration of arecoline hydrobromide will cause segments to be passed for morphologic identification (Matoff 1968). Diagnosis in simian primates cannot be made from clinical signs alone and depends on demonstration of scolices, brood capsules, or daughter cysts in the hydatid fluid either on laparotomy or at necropsy (Crosby et al. 1968).

CONTROL

Although completion of the life cycle in the laboratory is unlikely, the feeding of uncooked meat containing hydatid cysts to dogs, or food contaminated with dog feces to other laboratory mammals, should be prevented (Noble and Noble 1961).

tralia, and 27% in Chile (Belding 1965; Hoghoughi and Jalayer 1967; Medda 1966).

The incidence of infection with the larva is uncommon or rare in wild rodents and lagomorphs (Belding 1965), the dog (Whitten and Shortridge 1961), cat (McDonald and Campbell 1963), and simian primates (Crosby et al. 1968; Ilievski and Esber 1969). Sporadic or occasional occurrences are reported in captive primates.

MORPHOLOGY

The adult worm is only 2 to 9 mm long and usually has only 3 to 4 proglottids (Fig. 6.37) (Soulsby 1965). The scolex bears a rostellum with hooks. The eggs are ovoid, 32 to 36 μ by 25 to 30 μ, and are indistinguishable from those of *Taenia* (Soulsby 1965). The larva is of the hydatid type and varies in size and shape, depending on the host species and the organ in which it resides. It is usually spherical or ovoid and about 5 to 10 cm in diameter (Lapage 1968). It is filled with a clear fluid and contains a multitude of tiny, infective scolices and often secondary cysts (Fig. 6.38).

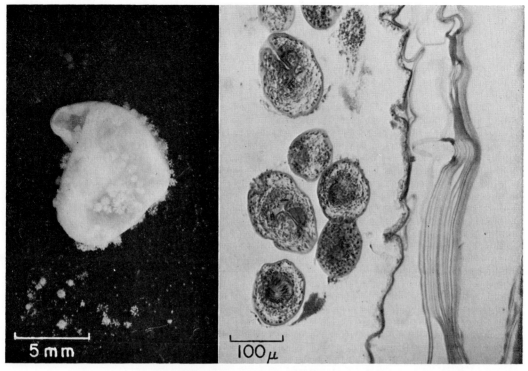

FIG. 6.38. *Echinococcus granulosus.* *(Left)* Hydatid cyst from the liver of a monkey. *(Right)* Microscopic section of hydatid cyst showing outer laminated membrane, thin germinative membrane, and several scolices. *(Left* from Healy and Hayes 1963; courtesy of American Society of Parasitologists. *Right* courtesy of Marietta Voge, University of California.)

Newly acquired dogs should be examined on arrival. Because infected animals are a serious health hazard to man, they should be destroyed unless of extreme value.

Arecoline hydrobromide, given orally at a rate of 1 to 2 mg per kg of body weight, or bunamidine hydrochloride (Scolaban, Burroughs Wellcome), given orally at a rate of 25 to 100 mg per kg of body weight, is reportedly effective against the adult worm (Forbes 1966; Shearer and Gemmell 1969; Soulsby 1965). The effectiveness of niclosamide (Yomesan, Bayer), given orally at a dosage of 100 mg per kg of body weight, is reportedly variable (Soulsby 1965).

There is no treatment for the larval infection other than surgery, which is usually impractical and, if not properly carried out, may compound the infection (Crosby et al. 1968; Lapage 1962).

PUBLIC HEALTH CONSIDERATIONS

The accidental ingestion of *E. granulosus* eggs from dog feces causes echinococcus, or hydatid disease, in man (Belding 1965). The effects of the hydatids in man, as in other animals, depend on their location and size. Often they are inapparent; sometimes they cause serious pulmonary, digestive, or neural effects and death. In endemic areas, all dogs should be assumed to be infected and their feces and cages handled with caution. Laboratory personnel should be informed of the possible hazard and instructed in proper personal hygiene.

DIPHYLLOBOTHRIIDS

These cestodes belong to the order Pseudophyllidea and are, therefore, quite different from all the other tapeworms that affect endothermal laboratory animals (Belding 1965; Lapage 1968). They have longitudinal grooves instead of rounded suckers and require two successive intermediate hosts, usually a crustacean and a fish. The adult worms vary in size; the scolex is unarmed. Both larvae and adults are parasites of endothermal animals. Those that affect endothermal laboratory animals are listed in Table 6.7. The most important species is *Diphyllobothrium latum*.

Diphyllobothrium latum

(Syn. *Bothriocephalus latus,*
Dibothriocephalus latus)
(Fish Tapeworm, Broad Fish Tapeworm)

This cestode is common in the small intestine of the dog, cat, wild carnivores, and man in areas where certain freshwater fishes, such as pike, perch, and salmonid fishes, occur (Lapage 1968; Soulsby 1965). It is most prevalent in the Great Lakes region of North America, the Baltic region of northern Europe, the lake regions of central Europe and southern Chile, and in Japan (Faust, Beaver, and Jung 1968).

Infection in laboratory dogs and cats obtained from pounds is apparently common in endemic areas and absent in others. It does not occur in laboratory dogs and cats reared on diets free of raw fish (Bantin and Maber 1967; Johnson, Andersen, and Gee 1963; Morris 1963; Sheffy, Baker, and Gillespie 1961).

MORPHOLOGY

The adult worm sometimes measures

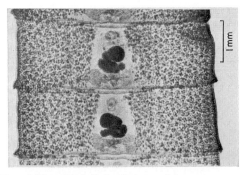

FIG. 6.39. *Diphyllobothrium latum,* mature proglottids. Note centrally located, coiled uterus. (Courtesy of Marietta Voge, University of California.)

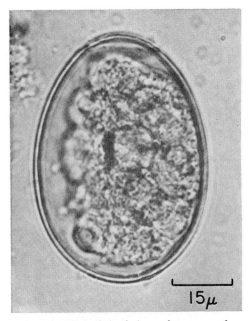

FIG. 6.40. *Diphyllobothrium latum,* embryonated egg. Note faint, inconspicuous operculum *(top).* (Courtesy of Marietta Voge, University of California.)

several meters in length (Faust, Beaver, and Jung 1968; Lapage 1968). The scolex is elongated and flat, bears a groove on each side, and has no hooks. Proglottids are wider than long. In gravid proglottids, the uterus appears as a convoluted tube in the middle of the segment (Fig. 6.39). Eggs are discharged continuously from the uterine pore, which is near the middle of the segment. The light brown, thin-shelled eggs resemble those of trematodes in that they possess a small, inconspicuous operculum (Fig. 6.40). They measure 59 to 71 μ by 42 to 49 μ.

LIFE CYCLE

The life cycle involves two obligate, intermediate hosts (Fig. 6.41) (Belding 1965; Cheng 1964; Soulsby 1965). Eggs passed in the feces of the definitive host must reach fresh water before they will hatch. In water they develop into the first larval stage, a ciliated coracidium, in about 2 weeks. The coracidium swims about in the water and must be ingested by a crustacean (copepod) within 12 to 24 hours or it will die. If ingested by a copepod, it

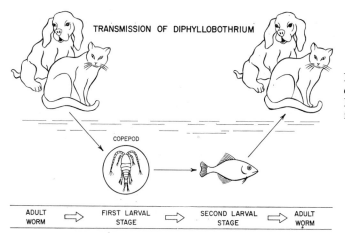

FIG. 6.41. *Diphyllobothrium latum,* diagram of life cycle. (Courtesy of Marietta Voge, University of California.)

continues its development in the hemocele and, after 14 to 18 days, it becomes a mature procercoid larva. When the crustacean is ingested by a fish, the procercoid larva migrates into the connective tissues or muscles and transforms into an infective (plerocercoid) larva. The definitive host is infected by ingesting raw or improperly cooked fish containing the infective larva. Eggs appear in the feces 5 to 6 weeks after infection.

PATHOLOGIC EFFECTS

Natural infection in the dog and cat is usually inapparent (Renaux 1964; Soulsby 1965). Massive, experimental infections produce an eosinophilia and anemia, the latter due to competition of the worms for vitamin B_{12}.

DIAGNOSIS

Diagnosis is made by finding the char- acteristic eggs in the feces (Soulsby 1965). Care must be taken to differentiate the eggs from those of the lung fluke *(Paragonimus)* and other trematodes.

CONTROL

The infection can be prevented by not feeding dogs and cats raw or improperly cooked fish (Soulsby 1965). Treatments effective against adult *Echinococcus granulosus* are also effective against this cestode.

PUBLIC HEALTH CONSIDERATIONS

This cestode causes anemia and gastrointestinal disturbances in man and is an important human parasite in many parts of the world (Belding 1965; Faust, Beaver, and Jung 1968). However, because transmission occurs only by ingestion of raw or improperly cooked fish, infected laboratory animals are not a direct hazard to man.

TABLE 6.1. Hymenolepidids affecting endothermal laboratory animals

Parasite	Geographic Distribution	Endothermal Host	Location in Host	Method of Infection	Incidence In nature	Incidence In laboratory	Pathologic Effects	Public Health Importance	Reference
*Hymenolepis nana**	Worldwide	Mouse, rat, black rat, hamster, other rodents, monkey, squirrel monkeys, chimpanzee, man	Intestine	Ingestion of intermediate host (flour beetles, fleas) or ingestion of eggs passed by definitive host	Common in rodents; uncommon in simian primates	Common in mouse, rat, hamster; uncommon in monkey, squirrel monkeys, chimpanzee	Usually inapparent; sometimes enteritis, retarded growth, weight loss, intestinal obstruction, purulent inflammation of mesenteric lymph nodes, death	Usually inapparent; heavy infections cause gastritis, anorexia, vomiting, enteritis, diarrhea, abdominal pain, weight loss, insomnia, apathy, nasal pruritus, anal pruritus, irritability, neurologic signs	Benson et al. 1954; Faust et al. 1968; Flynn et al. 1965; Habermann and Williams 1958; Heston 1941; Heyneman 1961a; King and Cosgrove 1963; Middleton et al. 1964; Owen 1968; Ratcliffe 1949; Ruch 1959; Sasa et al. 1962; Sheffield and Beveridge 1962; Simmons et al. 1964, 1967; Soave 1963; Stone and Manwell 1966; Wardle and McLeod 1952
*Hymenolepis diminuta**	Worldwide	Mouse, rat, black rat, hamster, other rodents, monkey, man	Intestine	Ingestion of intermediate host (flour beetles, moths, fleas)	Common in rodents; uncommon in monkey	Uncommon	Usually inapparent; sometimes enteritis	Rarely affects man; usually mild or inapparent	Ash 1962b; Dove 1950; Faust et al. 1968; Habermann and Williams 1958; Handler 1965; Heston 1941; Kulasiri 1954; de Léon 1964; Morgan and Hawkins 1949; Read 1951; Ruch 1959; Sasa et al. 1962; Stone and Manwell 1966; Voge 1952; Wardle and McLeod 1952

*Discussed in text.

TABLE 6.1 *(continued)*

Parasite	Geographic Distribution	Endothermal Host	Location in Host	Method of Infection	Incidence — In nature	Incidence — In laboratory	Pathologic Effects	Public Health Importance	Reference
Hymenolepis microstoma	Worldwide	Mouse, rat, cotton rat, hamster	Duodenum, bile duct, gallbladder, liver	Ingestion of intermediate host (flour beetles, fleas)	Unknown; probably uncommon	Unknown; probably uncommon	Distention, inflammation of bile duct; destruction, necrosis of liver parenchyma	None known	Heston 1941 Jones 1966
Hymenolepis citelli	Western United States	Ground squirrels, kangaroo rats	Intestine	Ingestion of intermediate host (beetles)	Common	Unknown; probably common in ground squirrels and kangaroo rats obtained from natural habitat in endemic areas	Unknown	None known	Cheng 1964 Simpson and Harmon 1968
Hymenolepis cebidarum	Central America, South America	Marmosets, titi monkeys	Intestine	Unknown	Common	Unknown; probably common in simian primates obtained from natural habitat in endemic areas	Unknown	None known	Dunn 1963 Nelson et al. 1966
*Hymenolepis carioca**	United States, Hawaii	Chicken, other birds	Small intestine	Ingestion of intermediate host (dung beetles, stable flies, flour beetles)	Common	Unknown; probably rare or absent	None	None	Alicata 1964 Horsfall 1938 Morgan and Hawkins 1949 Reid 1962 Wehr 1965
Hymenolepis cantaniana	United States, Puerto Rico, Europe, Asia	Chicken, other birds	Small intestine	Ingestion of intermediate host (dung beetles)	Uncommon to common	Unknown; probably rare or absent	None	None	Morgan and Hawkins 1949 Reid 1962 Wehr 1965
Fimbriaria fasciolaris	Worldwide	Chicken, anseriform birds	Small intestine	Ingestion of intermediate host (copepods)	Uncommon	Unknown; probably rare or absent	None known	None known	Reid 1962 Soulsby 1965 Wehr 1965

*Discussed in text.

TABLE 6.2. Davaineids affecting endothermal laboratory animals

Parasite	Geographic Distribution	Endothermal Host	Location in Host	Method of Infection	Incidence		Pathologic Effects	Public Health Importance	Reference
					In nature	In laboratory			
Davainea proglottina*	Worldwide	Chicken, pigeon, other birds	Duodenum	Ingestion of intermediate host (snails, slugs)	Common	Unknown; probably rare	Diarrhea, weight loss, ruffled plumage, enteritis	None	Edgar 1956, Lapage 1962, 1968, Morgan and Hawkins 1949, Olsen 1967, Reid 1962, Soulsby 1965, Wehr 1965
Raillietina cesticillus*	Worldwide	Chicken, other birds	Small intestine	Ingestion of intermediate host (beetles)	Common	Unknown; probably rare	Usually inapparent; sometimes decreased growth rate, emaciation	None	Edgar 1956, Lapage 1962, 1968, Morgan and Hawkins 1949, Olsen 1967, Reid 1962, Soulsby 1965, Wehr 1965
Raillietina echinobothrida*	Worldwide	Chicken, other birds	Small intestine	Ingestion of intermediate host (ants)	Common	Unknown; probably rare	Nodular enteritis, weakness, diarrhea, emaciation, sometimes death	None	Lapage 1962, 1968, Olsen 1967, Reid 1962, Soulsby 1965, Wehr 1965
Raillietina tetragona*	Worldwide	Chicken, pigeon, other birds	Small intestine	Ingestion of intermediate host (ants)	Common in chicken	Unknown; probably rare	Unknown; possibly nodular enteritis	None	Olsen 1967, Reid 1962, Wehr 1965
Raillietina celebensis	Worldwide in tropics and subtropics	Black rat, other wild rats, man	Intestine	Unknown	Common	Unknown; probably common in rats obtained from natural habitat in endemic areas	Unknown	Affects man	Belding 1965, Faust et al. 1968, Kulasiri 1954

*Discussed in text.

TABLE 6.2 (continued)

Parasite	Geographic Distribution	Endothermal Host	Location in Host	Method of Infection	Incidence In nature	Incidence In laboratory	Pathologic Effects	Public Health Importance	Reference
Raillietina alouattae	Central America, South America	Howler monkeys	Intestine	Unknown	Common	Unknown; probably common in howler monkeys obtained from natural habitat in endemic areas	Unknown	None known	Dunn 1963 Ruch 1959
Raillietina demerariensis	Central America, West Indies, South America	Howler monkeys, man	Intestine	Unknown	Common	Unknown; probably common in howler monkeys obtained from natural habitat in endemic areas	Unknown	Affects man	Belding 1965 Dunn 1963
Raillietina sp.	South America	Marmosets	Intestine	Unknown	Common	Unknown; probably common in marmosets obtained from natural habitat in endemic areas	Unknown	None known	Deinhardt et al. 1967 Nelson et al. 1966
Cotugnia digonopora	Europe, Asia, Africa	Chicken, other birds	Intestine	Unknown	Unknown	Unknown; probably rare or absent	Retarded growth, diarrhea	None known	Soulsby 1965

187

TABLE 6.3. Dilepidids affecting endothermal laboratory animals

Parasite	Geographic Distribution	Endothermal Host	Location in Host	Method of Infection	Incidence		Pathologic Effects	Public Health Importance	Reference
					In nature	In laboratory			
Dipylidium caninum*	Worldwide	Dog, cat, other carnivores, man	Small intestine	Ingestion of intermediate host (fleas, lice)	Common	Common	Usually inapparent; sometimes anal pruritus; rarely weakness, emaciation, vomiting, diarrhea, voracious appetite, convulsions, enteritis	Affects man; usually mild or inapparent infection, rarely abdominal discomfort	Ash 1962a Belding 1965 Braun and Thayer 1962 Dubey 1966 Gleason 1962 Habermann and Williams 1958 Johnson et al. 1963 Lapage 1962 Mann and Bjotvedt 1965 Marinkelle 1966 Morgan and Hawkins 1949 Silverman 1961 Soulsby 1965 Worley 1964
Joyeuxiella pasqualei	Southern Europe, Africa	Dog, cat, other carnivores	Intestine	Ingestion of transport or intermediate host (reptiles)	Common	Unknown; probably common in animals obtained from pounds in endemic areas	Unknown; probably inapparent	Unknown	Fitzsimmons 1961 Soulsby 1965
Diplopylidium noelleri	Southern Europe, southwestern Asia	Dog, cat, fox	Intestine	Ingestion of transport or intermediate host (reptiles)	Unknown	Unknown; probably rare or absent	Unknown; probably inapparent	Unknown	Soulsby 1965
Diplopylidium acanthtreta	Southern Europe, Asia, Africa	Cat, other felids	Intestine	Ingestion of transport or intermediate host (reptiles)	Unknown	Unknown; probably rare or absent	Unknown; probably inapparent	Unknown	Soulsby 1965

*Discussed in text.

188

TABLE 6.3 *(continued)*

Parasite	Geographic Distribution	Endothermal Host	Location in Host	Method of Infection	Incidence		Pathologic Effects	Public Health Importance	Reference
					In nature	In laboratory			
Diplopylidium skrjabini	USSR	Cat	Intestine	Ingestion of transport or intermediate host (reptiles)	Unknown	Unknown; probably rare or absent	Unknown; probably inapparent	Unknown	Soulsby 1965
Choanotaenia infundibulum	Worldwide	Chicken, other birds	Small intestine	Ingestion of intermediate host (flies, beetles, other insects)	Common in chicken	Unknown; probably uncommon	Unknown; probably mild or inapparent except in heavy infections	None known	Lapage 1962 Morgan and Hawkins 1949 Reid 1962 Soulsby 1965 Wehr 1965
Amoebotaenia cuneata	Worldwide	Chicken, other birds	Small intestine	Ingestion of intermediate host (earthworms)	Uncommon in chicken	Unknown; probably rare or absent	Unknown; probably mild or inapparent	None known	Lapage 1962 Morgan and Hawkins 1949 Reid 1962 Soulsby 1965 Wehr 1965
Metroliasthes lucida	North America, Africa, India	Chicken, other birds	Small intestine	Ingestion of intermediate host (grasshoppers, beetles)	Rare in chicken	Unknown; probably absent	Unknown	None known	Lapage 1962 Morgan and Hawkins 1949 Reid 1962 Soulsby 1965 Wehr 1965

TABLE 6.4. Mesocestoidids affecting endothermal laboratory animals

Parasite	Geographic Distribution	Endothermal Host	Location in Host	Method of Infection	Incidence — In nature	Incidence — In laboratory	Pathologic Effects	Public Health Importance	Reference
*Mesocestoides corti**	North America, Central America	Definitive: dog, cat, wild carnivores, man Intermediate: wild rodents, dog, cat, other mammals	Adult: small intestine Larva: peritoneal cavity, liver, other organs	Definitive host: ingestion of second intermediate host (mammals, amphibians, reptiles) Intermediate host: ingestion of first intermediate host (unknown)	Uncommon in dog, cat	Rare or absent	Adult: none known Larva: cysts in liver, other abdominal organs; occasionally debilitation; sometimes ascites, death	Rarely affects man	Belding 1965 Johnson et al. 1963 Reece et al. 1968 Voge 1953, 1955a, b, 1967 Voge and Berntzen 1963
*Mesocestoides lineatus**	Europe, Africa, Asia	Definitive: dog, cat, other carnivores, man Intermediate: wild rodents, dog, cat, other mammals	Adult: small intestine Larva: peritoneal cavity, pleural cavity	Definitive host: ingestion of second intermediate host (mammals, amphibians, reptiles) Intermediate host: ingestion of first intermediate host (unknown)	Uncommon or rare except common in dog in East Africa	Unknown; probably rare or absent except common in dogs obtained from pounds in East Africa	Adult: none known Larva: cysts in abdominal organs; occasionally debilitation; sometimes ascites, death	Rarely affects man	Bisseru 1967 Fitzsimmons 1961 Soulsby 1965
*Mesocestoides sp.**	United States Europe, Africa, Asia	Intermediate: monkey, cynomolgus monkey, baboons	Larva: peritoneal cavity	Unknown; presumably by ingestion of unknown first intermediate host	Uncommon or rare	Uncommon or rare	Larva: cysts in abdominal organs	Unknown	Graham 1960 Myers and Kuntz 1965 Reardon and Rininger 1968

*Discussed in text.

TABLE 6.5. Anoplocephalids affecting endothermal laboratory animals

Parasite	Geographic Distribution	Endothermal Host	Location in Host	Method of Infection	Incidence		Pathologic Effects	Public Health Importance	Reference
					In nature	In laboratory			
Bertiella studeri*	Africa, Asia, Indonesia, Philippine Islands	Monkey, cynomolgus monkey, Japanese macaque, guenons, mandrills, baboons, gibbons, orangutan, chimpanzee, man	Small intestine	Ingestion of intermediate host (free-living mites)	Common	Common in primates obtained from natural habitat	None known	Rarely affects man	Belding 1965 Faust et al. 1968 Fiennes 1967 Hashimoto and Honjo 1966 Kuntz and Myers 1966, 1967 Reardon and Rininger 1968 Stunkard 1940 Tanaka et al. 1962 Valerio et al. 1969 Witenberg 1964
Bertiella mucronata	South America	Capuchins, howler monkeys, titi monkeys, man	Small intestine	Unknown; probably by ingestion of infected free-living mites	Uncommon	Uncommon in primates obtained from natural habitat	None known	Rarely affects man	Belding 1965 Dunn 1963 Fiennes 1967 Pope 1966
Bertiella fallax	Africa	Capuchins (in captivity)	Small intestine	Unknown; probably by ingestion of infected free-living mites	Rare	Unknown; probably rare or absent	None known	None	Dunn 1963 Fiennes 1967
Moniezia rugosa	South America	Capuchins, howler monkeys, spider monkeys	Small intestine	Unknown; probably by ingestion of infected mites	Uncommon	Unknown; probably rare or absent	None known	None	Dunn 1963 Fiennes 1967
Atriotaenia (Oochoristica) megastoma	Central America, South America	Capuchins, howler monkeys, titi monkeys, spider monkeys, tamarins, marmosets	Small intestine	Unknown; probably by ingestion of infected insect	Common	Common in primates obtained from natural habitat	None known	None	Cosgrove et al. 1968 Deinhardt et al. 1967 Dunn 1963 Garner et al. 1967 Nelson et al. 1966
Paratriotaenia oedipomidatus	South America	Marmosets	Small intestine	Unknown; probably by ingestion of infected insect	Uncommon	Unknown; probably uncommon	None known	None known	Dunn 1968 Stunkard 1965
Oochoristica ratti	United States, Japan	Mouse, rat, black rat	Small intestine	Ingestion of intermediate host (beetles)	Rare	Unknown; probably absent	None known	None	Oldham 1967 Rendtorff 1948 Wardle and McLeod 1952

*Discussed in text.

TABLE 6.5 *(continued)*

Parasite	Geographic Distribution	Endothermal Host	Location in Host	Method of Infection	Incidence In nature	Incidence In laboratory	Pathologic Effects	Public Health Importance	Reference
Cittotaenia variabilis	North America	Rabbit, cottontail rabbits	Small intestine	Ingestion of intermediate host (free-living mites)	Uncommon in rabbit	Unknown; probably rare or absent	None known	None	Holloway 1966 Lund 1950 Morgan and Hawkins 1949 Stunkard 1941
Cittotaenia pectinata	North America, Europe, Asia	Rabbit, cottontail rabbits, hares	Small intestine	Ingestion of intermediate host (free-living mites)	Common in rabbit in Europe	Unknown; probably rare or absent	Unknown; probably digestive disturbances, emaciation	None	Cushnie 1954 Lapage 1962 Morgan and Hawkins 1949 Owen 1968
Cittotaenia ctenoides	Europe	Rabbit	Small intestine	Ingestion of intermediate host (free-living mites)	Common	Unknown; probably rare or absent	Digestive disturbances, emaciation, sometimes death	None	Cushnie 1954 Lapage 1962 Owen 1968

TABLE 6.6. Taeniids affecting endothermal laboratory animals

Parasite	Geographic Distribution	Endothermal Host	Location in Host	Method of Infection	Incidence		Pathologic Effects	Public Health Importance	Reference
					In nature	In laboratory			
*Taenia taeniaeformis**	Worldwide	Definitive: dog, cat, wild carnivores, man Intermediate: mouse, rat, cotton rat, black rat, voles, other wild rodents	Adult: small intestine Larva: liver	Definitive host: ingestion of intermediate host (rodent) Intermediate host: ingestion of embryonated egg passed by definitive host (usually cat)	Common in wild rodents, cat; uncommon in dog	Common in some rodent colonies, absent in others; common in cats obtained from pounds	Adult: enteritis, diarrhea, loss of weight; occasionally perforation of intestinal wall, neurologic disturbances Larva: cysts in liver; sometimes hepatic sarcoma	Rarely affects man	Alicata 1964 Ash 1962a, b Belding 1965 Bell 1968 Cosgrove et al. 1964 Cross and Allen 1948 Dove 1950 Dubey 1966 Dufill and Lyon 1960 Fitzsimmons 1961 Habermann and Williams 1958 Innes 1967 Jones 1967 Lapage 1962, 1968 de Léon 1964 Lewis 1968 Morgan and Hawkins 1949 Oldham 1967 Olivier 1962 Owen 1968 Renaux 1964 Sasa et al. 1962 Soulsby 1965
*Taenia pisiformis**	Worldwide	Definitive: dog, cat, wild carnivores Intermediate: rabbit, cottontail rabbits, hares, wild rodents	Adult: small intestine Larva: liver, peritoneal cavity	Definitive host: ingestion of viscera of intermediate host (lagomorphs, rodents) Intermediate host: ingestion of embryonated egg passed by definitive host (usually dog)	Common in wild lagomorphs, dog; uncommon in cat	Common in some rabbit colonies, absent in others; common in dogs obtained from rural areas	Adult: abdominal discomfort, enteritis Larva: cysts in peritoneal cavity, abdominal distention, lethargy, weight loss, liver damage	None known	Adams et al. 1967 Cross and Allen 1948 Cushnie 1954 Habermann and Williams 1958 Holloway 1966 Lapage 1962, 1968 Mann and Bjotvedt 1965 Morgan and Hawkins 1949 Napier 1963 Owen 1968 Poole et al. 1967 Renaux 1964 Soulsby 1965 Worley 1964

*Discussed in text.

193

TABLE 6.6 *(continued)*

Parasite	Geographic Distribution	Endothermal Host	Location in Host	Method of Infection	Incidence — In nature	Incidence — In laboratory	Pathologic Effects	Public Health Importance	Reference
Taenia hydatigena	Worldwide	Definitive: dog, wild carnivores; Intermediate: monkey, baboons, ruminants, pig, man	Adult: small intestine; Larva: liver, peritoneal cavity	Definitive host: ingestion of viscera of intermediate host (ruminants, pig); Intermediate host: ingestion of embryonated egg passed by definitive host (dog)	Uncommon in dog except in rural areas; rare in monkey	Unknown in dog; probably uncommon; rare in monkey	Adult: abdominal irritation, enteritis; Larva: liver damage, peritonitis	None known	Belding 1965; Fiennes 1967; Graham 1960; Lapage 1962, 1968; Myers and Kuntz 1965; Soulsby 1965
Taenia ovis	Worldwide	Dog, other canids	Small intestine	Ingestion of viscera of intermediate host (sheep, goat)	Uncommon except in rural areas	Unknown; probably uncommon	Inapparent	None known	Lapage 1962, 1968; Soulsby 1965
Taenia solium	Worldwide	Definitive: man; Intermediate: dog, monkey, baboons, pig, man	Adult: small intestine; Larva: brain, heart, muscle, subcutis	Ingestion of embryonated eggs passed by definitive host (man)	Rare in dog, monkey	Rare in dog, monkey	Usually none; sometimes brain damage	Common in many areas; adult causes mild enteritis; larva sometimes causes severe brain damage	Belding 1965; Fiennes 1967; Lapage 1968; Myers and Kuntz 1965; Ruch 1959; Vickers and Penner 1968
Taenia krabbei	Northern Europe	Dog	Small intestine	Ingestion of muscle of intermediate host (reindeer)	Uncommon	Unknown; probably rare	Inapparent	None known	Lapage 1962; Soulsby 1965
*Multiceps serialis**	Worldwide	Definitive: dog, other canids; Intermediate: wild rodents, rabbit, hares, dog, monkey, gelada, man	Adult: small intestine; Larva: subcutis	Definitive host: ingestion of tissues of intermediate host (usually lagomorphs); Intermediate host: ingestion of eggs passed by definitive host (dog)	Unknown; apparently uncommon in dog; common in wild lagomorphs	Unknown; apparently uncommon in dog and rabbit	Adult: usually inapparent; Larva: subcutaneous cysts	Rare; sometimes causes subcutaneous cysts, cerebral cysts	Adams et al. 1967; Belding 1965; Cook 1969; Lapage 1962, 1968; Morgan and Hawkins 1949; Ruch 1959; Soulsby 1965; Voge and Berntzen 1963
Multiceps multiceps	Worldwide	Dog, other canids	Small intestine	Ingestion of neural tissue of intermediate host (sheep, goat)	Unknown; apparently uncommon except in dogs in some rural areas	Unknown; probably uncommon	Usually inapparent	Rare; sometimes causes cerebral cysts, ocular cysts	Belding 1965; Galvin and Turk 1966; Lapage 1968; Soulsby 1965

*Discussed in text.

TABLE 6.6 (continued)

Parasite	Geographic Distribution	Endothermal Host	Location in Host	Method of Infection	Incidence In nature	Incidence In laboratory	Pathologic Effects	Public Health Importance	Reference
Multiceps brauni	Central and southern Africa	Definitive: dog Intermediate: wild rodents, guenons, man	Adult: small intestine Larva: subcutis, pleural cavity, abdominal cavity, brain	Definitive host: ingestion of intermediate host (rodents) Intermediate host: ingestion of eggs passed by definitive host (dog)	Uncommon in dog; common in wild rodents	Unknown; probably rare in dog	Adult: usually inapparent Larva: sub-cutaneous, pleural, abdominal, cerebral cysts	Uncommon; sometimes causes subcutaneous cysts, cerebral cysts	Belding 1965 Fain 1956
Multiceps gaigeri	India, Ceylon	Dog	Small intestine	Ingestion of neural and muscular tissues of intermediate host (goat)	Uncommon	Unknown; probably rare	Inapparent	None known	Lapage 1962, 1968 Soulsby 1965
*Echinococcus granulosus**	Worldwide; endemic in eastern and southern Europe, Near East, southern South America, southern Africa, southern Australia, New Zealand, central Asia	Definitive: dog, wild canids Intermediate: wild rodents, lagomorphs, dog, cat, domestic animals, rhesus monkey, other macaques, colobus monkey, baboons, lemurs, Celebes ape (*Cyno-pithecus niger*), man	Adult: small intestine Larva: liver, lungs, peritoneal cavity	Definitive host: ingestion of tissues of intermediate host Intermediate host: ingestion of eggs passed by definitive host (dog)	Common in dog in endemic areas; uncommon in simian primates	Rare or absent except in dogs obtained from pounds in endemic areas; rare in simian primates	Adult: inapparent Larva: usually inapparent; sometimes abdominal distention, subcutaneous swellings; cysts in liver, lungs, peritoneal cavity	Cause of hydatid disease; cysts in brain, liver, lungs	Belding 1965 Crosby et al. 1968 Faust et al. 1968 Healy and Hayes 1963 Hoghoughi and Jalayer 1967 Ilievski and Esber 1969 Lapage 1962, 1968 Matoff 1968 McDonald and Campbell 1963 Medda 1966 Morgan and Hawkins 1949 Noble and Noble 1961 Smyth and Smyth 1964 Soulsby 1965 Summers 1960 Whitten and Shortridge 1961
Echinococcus multilocularis	North central United States, northern Canada, Alaska, central Europe, Siberia	Definitive: dog, wild canids, cat Intermediate: deer mice, voles, lemmings (*Lemmus*), shrews (*Sorex*), muskrat, nutria, man	Adult: small intestine Larva: liver	Definitive host: ingestion of tissues of intermediate host Intermediate host: ingestion of eggs passed by definitive host (dog)	Common in dog and wild rodents in endemic areas	Rare or absent except in dogs obtained from pounds in endemic areas	Adult: inapparent Larva: liver cysts, death	Cause of hydatid disease; cysts in liver	Belding 1965 Carney and Leiby 1968 Cheng 1964 Faust et al. 1968 Matoff 1968 Rausch 1960 Smyth and Smyth 1964

*Discussed in text.

195

TABLE 6.7. Diphyllobothriids affecting endothermal laboratory animals

Parasite	Geographic Distribution	Endothermal Host	Location in Host	Method of Infection	Incidence In nature	Incidence In laboratory	Pathologic Effects	Public Health Importance	Reference
*Diphyllobothrium latum**	North America, Europe, southern South America, Japan	Dog, cat, wild carnivores, man	Small intestine	Ingestion of intermediate host (fresh-water fishes)	Unknown; apparently common in endemic areas	Unknown; probably rare or absent except in dogs obtained from pounds in endemic areas	Inapparent	Causes anemia, gastro-intestinal disturbances	Belding 1965 Cheng 1964 Faust et al. 1968 Lapage 1968 Renaux 1964 Soulsby 1965
Diphyllobothrium cordatum	Northwestern United States, Canada, Greenland, Iceland, Japan	Dog, wild carnivores, man	Small intestine	Unknown; probably ingestion of unknown intermediate host	Rare in dog	Unknown	Unknown	Unknown	Belding 1965 Morgan and Hawkins 1949
Diphyllobothrium dendriticum	Northern United States, Canada, Europe	Cat, wild birds, man	Small intestine	Ingestion of intermediate host (fresh-water fishes)	Rare in cat	Unknown; probably rare	Unknown	Rarely affects man	Markowski 1949 Threlfall 1969
Diphyllobothrium erinacei	Europe, Asia, Australia, South America	Definitive: dog, cat, wild felids Intermediate: wild rodents, cat, wild carnivores, monkey, other macaques, baboons, squirrel monkeys, tamarins, chicken, man	Adult: small intestine Larva: subcutis, muscle	Definitive host: ingestion of tissues of intermediate host (amphibians, reptiles, mammals) Intermediate host: ingestion of primary intermediate host (crustaceans) or secondary intermediate host (amphibians, reptiles)	Unknown	Unknown; probably uncommon in dogs obtained from pounds in endemic areas; rare in cat, monkey, chicken	Adult: inapparent Larva: cysts in subcutis, muscle; sometimes edema, anorexia, lethargy	Causes sparganosis; cysts in subcutis, muscle	Belding 1965 Cosgrove et al. 1968 Dunn 1963 Fiennes 1967 Lapin and Yakovleva 1960 Myers and Kuntz 1965 Ruch 1959 Schmidt et al. 1968 Soulsby 1965

*Discussed in text.

TABLE 6.7 (continued)

Parasite	Geographic Distribution	Endothermal Host	Location in Host	Method of Infection	Incidence		Pathologic Effects	Public Health Importance	Reference
					In nature	In laboratory			
Spirometra mansonoides	Eastern United States	Definitive: dog, cat, wild carnivores Intermediate: deer mice, voles, man	Adult: small intestine Larva: connective tissue	Definitive host: ingestion of tissues of intermediate host (wild rodents, snakes) Intermediate host: ingestion of primary intermediate host (crustaceans)	Uncommon in cat; rare in dog	Unknown; probably uncommon in cats and rare in dogs obtained from pounds in endemic areas	Adult: anemia, otherwise inapparent Larva: cysts in connective tissue	Causes sparganosis; cysts in connective tissue	Belding 1965 Burrows and Lillis 1966 Corkum 1966 Morgan and Hawkins 1949 Soulsby 1965
Spirometra reptans	South America	Intermediate: marmosets, squirrel monkeys	Larva: subcutis	Unknown; probably ingestion of unknown intermediate host	Unknown	Unknown	Larva: cysts in subcutis	Unknown	Dunn 1963, 1968
Spirometra sp.	United States, Africa	Intermediate: green monkey	Larva: abdominal cavity	Unknown; probably ingestion of unknown intermediate host	Unknown	Rare	Larva: cysts in abdominal cavity	Unknown	Morton 1969

REFERENCES

Adams, C. E., F. C. Aitken, and A. N. Worden. 1967. The rabbit, pp. 432–33. *In* UFAW Staff, ed. The UFAW handbook on the care and management of laboratory animals. 3d ed. Livingstone and the Universities Federation for Animal Welfare, London.

Alicata, J. E. 1964. Parasitic infections of man and animals in Hawaii. Hawaii Agr. Exp. Sta. Tech. Bull. 61.

Anonymous. 1968. Parasitic disease drug service. Lab. Primate Newsletter 7:21.

Ash, L. R. 1962a. Helminth parasites of dogs and cats in Hawaii. J. Parasitol. 48:63–65.

———. 1962b. The helminth parasites of rats in Hawaii and the description of *Capillaria traverae* sp. n. J. Parasitol. 48:66–68.

Balazs, T., A. M. Hatch, E. R. W. Gregory, and H. C. Grice. 1962. A comparative study of Hymenolepicides in *Hymenolepis nana* infestation of rats. Can. J. Comp. Med. Vet. Sci. 26:160–62.

Bantin, G. C., and D. F. Maber. 1967. Some parasites of the beagle. J. Inst. Animal Technicians. 18:49–59.

Bayon, H. P. 1927. Carcinoma in apposition to *Cysticercus fasciolaris* in a mouse infected with cancer cells. Parasitology 19:328–32.

Belding, D. L. 1965. Textbook of parasitology. 3d ed. Appleton-Century-Crofts, New York. 1374 pp.

Bell, Deirdre P. 1968. Disease in a caesarian-derived albino rat colony and in a conventional colony. Lab. Animals 2:1–17.

Benson, R. E., B. D. Fremming, and R. J. Young. 1954. Care and management of chimpanzees at the radiobiological laboratory of the University of Texas and the United States Air Force. Proc. Animal Care Panel 5:27–36.

Bisseru, B. 1967. Diseases of man acquired from his pets. William Heinemann Medical Books, London. 482 pp.

Braun, J. L., and C. B. Thayer. 1962. A survey for intestinal parasites in Iowa dogs. J. Am. Vet. Med. Assoc. 141:1049–50.

Burrows, R. B. 1965. Microscopic diagnosis of the parasites of man. Yale Univ. Press, New Haven, Conn. 328 pp.

Burrows, R. B., and W. G. Lillis. 1966. Treatment of canine and feline tapeworm infections with bunamidine hydrochloride. Am. J. Vet. Res. 27:1381–84.

Carney, W. P., and P. D. Leiby. 1968. *Echinococcus multilocularis* in *Peromyscus maniculatus* and *Vulpes vulpes* from Minnesota. J. Parasitol. 54:714.

Cheng, T. C. 1964. The biology of animal parasites. W. B. Saunders, Philadelphia. 727 pp.

Cook, R. 1969. Common diseases of laboratory animals, pp. 160–215. *In* D. J. Short and Dorothy P. Woodnott, eds. The I.A.T. manual of laboratory animal practice and techniques. 2d ed. Charles C Thomas, Springfield, Ill.

Corkum, K. C. 1966. Sparganosis in some vertebrates of Louisiana and observations on a human infection. J. Parasitol. 52:444–48.

Cosgrove, G. E., B. Nelson, and N. Gengozian. 1968. Helminth parasites of the tamarin, *Saguinus fuscicollis*. Lab. Animal Care 18:654–56.

Cosgrove, G. E., T. P. O'Farrell, S. V. Kaye, and P. B. Dunaway. 1964. Infection of laboratory-reared and wild cotton rats with cat tapeworm larvae. J. Tenn. Acad. Sci. 39:140–41.

Cox, D. D., M. T. Mullee, and A. D. Allen. 1966. The anthelmintic activity of Yomesan against *Taenia* spp. of dogs and cats. Vet. Med. Rev. 1:49–55.

Crosby, W. M., M. H. Ivey, W. L. Shaffer, and D. D. Holmes. 1968. *Echinococcus* cysts in the Savannah baboon. Lab. Animal Care 18:395–97.

Cross, S. X., and R. W. Allen. 1948. Incidence of intestinal helminths and trichinae in dogs and cats in Chicago. North Am. Vet. 29:27–30.

Cushnie, G. H. 1954. The life cycle of some helminth parasites of the rat, mouse and rabbit. J. Animal Technicians Assoc. 5:22–25.

Deinhardt, F., A. W. Holmes, J. Devine, and Jean Deinhardt. 1967. Marmosets as laboratory animals: IV. The microbiology of laboratory kept marmosets. Lab. Animal Care 17:48–70.

Dove, W. E. 1950. The control of laboratory pests and parasites of laboratory animals, pp. 478–87. *In* E. J. Farris, ed. The care and breeding of laboratory animals. John Wiley, New York.

Dubey, J. P. 1966. *Toxocara cati* and other intestinal parasites of cats. Vet. Record 79:506–8.

Duffill, M. L., and Mary F. Lyon. 1960. Flaked maize as a source of tapeworm infestation in mice. J. Animal Technicians Assoc. 10:148–49.

Dunn, F. L. 1963. Acanthocephalans and cestodes of South American monkeys and marmosets. J. Parasitol. 49:717–22.

———. 1968. The parasites of *Saimiri*: In the context of platyrrhine parasitism, pp. 31–

68. *In* L. A. Rosenblum and R. W. Cooper, eds. The squirrel monkey. Academic Press, New York.

Eckert, J., T. von Brand, and Marietta Voge. 1969. Asexual multiplication of *Mesocestoides corti* (Cestoda) in the intestine of dogs and skunks. J. Parasitol. 55:241–49.

Edgar, S. A. 1956. The removal of chicken tapeworms by di-n-butyltin dilaurate. Poultry Sci. 35:64–73.

Enzie, F. D., and M. L. Colglazier. 1960. Preliminary trials with bithionol against tapeworm infections in cats, dogs, sheep and chickens. Am. J. Vet. Res. 21:628–30.

Fain, A. 1956. *Coenurus* of *Taenia brauni* Setti parasitic in man and animals from the Belgian Congo and Ruanda-Urundi. Nature 178:1353.

Faust, E. C., P. C. Beaver, and R. C. Jung. 1968. Animal agents and vectors of human disease. 3d ed. Lea and Febiger, Philadelphia, 461 pp.

Fiennes, R. 1967. Zoonoses of primates. The epidemiology and ecology of simian diseases in relation to man. Weidenfeld and Nicolson, London. 190 pp.

Fitzsimmons, W. M. 1961. Observations on the parasites of the domestic cat. Vet. Med. 56:68–69.

Flynn, R. J., Patricia C. Brennan, and T. E. Fritz. 1965. Pathogen status of commercially produced laboratory mice. Lab. Animal Care 15:440–47.

Forbes, L. S. 1966. The efficiency of bunamidine hydrochloride against young *Echinococcus granulosus* infection in dogs. Vet. Record 79:306–7.

Foster, H. L. 1963. Specific pathogen-free animals, pp. 110–37. *In* W. Lane-Petter, ed. Animals for research: Principles of breeding and management. Academic Press, New York.

Galvin, T. J., and R. D. Turk. 1966. Intestinal parasitism, pp. 190–94. *In* R. W. Kirk, ed. Current veterinary therapy 1966–1967: Small animal practice. W. B. Saunders, Philadelphia.

Garner, E., F. Hemrick, and H. Rudiger. 1967. Multiple helminth infections in cinnamon-ringtail monkeys *(Cebus albifrons)*. Lab. Animal Care 17:310–15.

Gisler, D. B., R. E. Benson, and R. J. Young. 1960. Colony husbandry of research monkeys. Ann. N.Y. Acad. Sci. 85:735–992.

Gleason, Neva H. 1962. Records of human infections with *Dipylidium caninum,* the double-pored tapeworm. J. Parasitol. 48: 812.

Gönnert, R., and E. Schraufstätter. 1960. Experimentelle Untersuchungen mit N-(2'chlor-4'-nitrophenyl)-5-chlorsalicylamid, einem neuen Bandwurmmittel: I. Mitteilung: chemotherapeutische Versuche. Arzneimittel-Forsch. 10:881–84.

Graham, G. L. 1960. Parasitism in monkeys. Ann. N.Y. Acad. Sci. 85:735–992.

Gregor, W. W. 1963. Assessment of a taeniacide salicylamide. Vet. Record 75:1421–22.

Habermann, R. T., and F. P. Williams, Jr. 1957. The efficacy of some piperazine compounds and stylomycin in drinking water for the removal of oxyurids from mice and rats and a method of critical testing of anthelmintics. Proc. Animal Care Panel 7:89–97.

———. 1958. The identification and control of helminths in laboratory animals. J. Natl. Cancer Inst. 29:979–1009.

Handler, A. H. 1965. Spontaneous lesions of the hamster, pp. 210–40. *In* W. E. Ribelin and J. R. McCoy, eds. The pathology of laboratory animals. Charles C Thomas, Springfield, Ill.

Hashimoto, I., and S. Honjo. 1966. Survey of helminth parasites in cynomologus monkeys *(Macaca irus)*. Japan. J. Med. Sci. Biol. 19:218.

Healy, G. R., and N. R. Hayes. 1963. Hydatid disease in rhesus monkeys. J. Parasitol. 49:837.

Heston, W. E. 1941. Parasites, pp. 349–79. *In* G. D. Snell, ed. Biology of the laboratory mouse. Blakiston, Philadelphia.

Heyneman, D. 1961a. A natural population of anomalous branched tapeworms, *Hymenolepis nana* (Cestoda: Hymenolepididae), in a colony of DBA/1 mice. Nature 191:297–98.

———. 1961b. Studies on helminth immunity: III. Experimental verification of autoinfection from cysticercoids of *Hymenolepis nana* in the white mouse. J. Infect. Diseases 109:10–18.

———. 1962. Studies on helminth immunity: I. Comparison between lumenal and tissue phases of infection in the white mouse by *Hymenolepis nana* (Cestoda: Hymenolepididae). Am. J. Trop. Med. Hyg. 2:46–63.

Hoghoughi, N., and T. Jalayer. 1967. The prevalence of *Echinococcus granulosus* in dogs in Shiraz, Iran. Ann. Trop. Med. Parasitol. 61:437–38.

Holloway, H. L., Jr. 1966. Helminths of rabbits and opossums at Mountain Lake, Virginia. Bull. Wildlife Dis. Assoc. 2:38–39.

Horsfall, Margery W. 1938. Meal beetles as intermediate hosts of poultry tapeworms. Poultry Sci. 17:8–11.

Ilievski, V., and H. Esber. 1969. Hydatid disease in a rhesus monkey. Lab. Animal Care 19:199–204.

Innes, J. R. M. 1967. Discussion, p. 21. *In* E. Cotchin and F. J. C. Roe, eds. Pathology of laboratory rats and mice. Blackwell Scientific Publ., Oxford.

Johnson, R. M., A. C. Andersen, and W. Gee. 1963. Parasitism in an established dog kennel. Lab. Animal Care 13:731–36.

Jones, A. W. 1966. *Hymenolepis microstoma* (Dujardin, 1845) a cosmopolitan cestode of the bile duct of rodents, pp. 478–79. *In* A. Corradetti, ed. Proc. First Intern. Congr. Parasitol. Pergamon Press, New York.

Jones, T. C. 1967. Pathology of the liver of rats and mice, pp. 1–23. *In* E. Cotchin and F. J. C. Roe, eds. Blackwell Scientific Publ., Oxford.

King, Vera M., and G. E. Cosgrove. 1963. Intestinal helminths in various strains of laboratory mice. Lab. Animal Care 13:46–48.

Kulasiri, C. 1954. Some cestodes of the rat, *Rattus rattus* Linnaeus, of Ceylon and their epidemiological significance for man. Parasitology 44:349–52.

Kuntz, R. E., and Betty J. Myers. 1966. Parasites of baboons *(Papio doguera* Pucheran, 1856) captured in Kenya and Tanzania, East Africa. Primates 7:27–32.

———. 1967. Microbiological parameters of the baboon *(Papio* sp.): Parasitology, pp. 741–55. *In* H. Vagtborg, ed. The baboon in medical research. 2 vols. Univ. Texas Press, Austin.

Kurelec, B., and M. Rijavec. 1961. An anthelmintic against tapeworms. Vet. Glasnik 15:602–6.

Lapage, G. 1962. Mönnig's veterinary helminthology and entomology. 5th ed. Williams and Wilkins, Baltimore. 600 pp.

———. 1968. Veterinary parasitology. Oliver and Boyd, London. 1182 pp.

Lapin, B. A., and L. A. Yakovleva. 1960. Comparative pathology in monkeys. Charles C Thomas, Springfield, Ill. 272 pp.

Léon, D. D. de. 1964. Helminth parasites of rats in San Juan, Puerto Rico. J. Parasitol. 50:478–79.

Lewis, J. W. 1968. Studies on the helminth parasites of voles and shrews from Wales. J. Zool. 154:313–31.

Lund, E. E. 1950. A survey of intestinal parasites in domestic rabbits in six counties in in southern California. J. Parasitol. 36:13–19.

Mann, P. H., and G. Bjotvedt. 1965. The incidence of heartworms and intestinal helminths in stray dogs. Lab. Animal Care 15:102.

Marinkelle, C. J. 1966. A survey of the intestinal helminths of street dogs in Cali (Colombia, S.R.), pp. 858–59. *In* A. Corradetti, ed. Proc. First Intern. Congr. Parasitol. Vol. II. Pergamon Press, New York.

Markowski, S. 1949. On the species of *Diphyllobothrium* occurring in birds, and their relation to man and other hosts. J. Helminthol. 23:107–26.

Matoff, K. 1968. New data on the biology of *Echinococcus granulosus* and of echinococcal infestation. Angew. Parasitol. 9:65–73.

McDonald, Fay E., and A. R. Campbell. 1963. A case of cystic hydatids in the cat. New Zealand Vet. J. 11:131–32.

Medda, A. 1966. A statistical research on the presence of *Echinococcus granulosus* in dogs sacrificed in the municipal kennel of Cagliari, pp. 770–71. *In* A. Corradetti, ed. Proc. First Intern. Congr. Parasitol. Vol. II. Pergamon Press, New York.

Middleton, C. C., T. B. Clarkson, and F. M. Garner. 1964. Parasites of squirrel monkeys *(Saimiri sciureus).* Lab. Animal Care 14:335.

Moore, D. V. 1962. Human infections with *Dipylidium caninum.* Southwestern Vet. 15:283–88.

Morgan, B. B., and P. A. Hawkins. 1949. Veterinary helminthology. Burgess Publishing, Minneapolis. 400 pp.

Morris, M. L. 1963. Breeding, housing and management of cats. Cornell Vet. 53:107–30.

Morton, H. L. 1969. Sparganosis in African green monkeys *(Cercopithecus aethiops).* Lab. Animal Care 19:253–55.

Mullenax, C. H., and P. B. Mullenax. 1962. Intestinal parasitism with symptoms of chronic pancreatitis in the dog. Mod. Vet. Pract. 43:72.

Murray, M. 1968. A survey of diseases found in dogs in Kenya. Bull. Epizoot. Dis. Afr. 16:121–27.

Myers, Betty J., and R. E. Kuntz. 1965. A checklist of parasites reported for the baboon. Primates 6:137–94.

Napier, R. A. N. 1963. Rabbits, pp. 323–64. *In* W. Lane-Petter, ed. Animals for research: Principles of breeding and management. Academic Press, New York.

Nelson, B., G. E. Cosgrove, and N. Gengozian. 1966. Diseases of an imported primate *Tamarinus nigricollis.* Lab. Animal Care 16:255–75.

Newton, W. L., P. P. Weinstein, and M. F. Jones. 1959. A comparison of the development of some rat and mouse helminths in germfree and conventional guinea pigs. Ann. N.Y. Acad. Sci. 78:290–306.

Noble, E. R., and G. A. Noble. 1961. Parasitology: The biology of animal parasites. Lea and Febiger, Philadelphia. 767 pp.

Oldham, J. N. 1967. Helminths, ectoparasites and protozoa in rats and mice, pp. 641–79. *In* E. Cotchin and F. J. C. Roe, eds. Pathology of laboratory rats and mice. Blackwell Scientific Publ., Oxford.

Olivier, L. 1962. Natural resistance to *Taenia taeniaeformis:* I. Strain differences in susceptibility of rodents. J. Parasitol. 48:373–78.

Olsen, O. W. 1967. Animal parasites: Their biology and life cycles. 2d ed. Burgess, Minneapolis. 431 pp.

Owen, Dawn. 1968. Investigations: B. Parasitological studies. Lab. Animals Centre News Letter 35:7–9.

Poole, C. M., W. G. Keenan, D. V. Tolle, T. E. Fritz, Patricia C. Brennan, R. C. Simkins, and R. J. Flynn. 1967. Disease status of commercially produced rabbits, pp. 219–20. *In* Biological and Medical Research Division annual report 1967. ANL-7409. Argonne National Laboratory, Argonne, Ill.

Pope, Betty L. 1966. Some parasites of the howler monkey of northern Argentina. J. Parasitol. 52:166–68.

Ratcliffe, H. L. 1949. Metazoan parasites of the rat, pp. 502–14. *In* E. J. Farris and J. Q. Griffith, eds. The rat in laboratory investigation. J. B. Lippincott, Philadelphia.

Rausch, R. L. 1960. Recent studies on hydatid disease in Alaska. Parasitologia 2:391–98.

Read, C. P. 1951. *Hymenolepis diminuta* in the Syrian hamster. J. Parasitol. 37:324.

Reardon, Lucy V., and Bonny F. Rininger. 1968. A survey of parasites in laboratory primates. Lab. Animal Care 18:577–80.

Reece, W. O., M. S. Hofstad, and M. J. Swenson. 1968. Establishment and maintenance of an SPF beagle dog colony. Lab. Animal Care 18:509–12.

Reid, W. M. 1962. Chicken and turkey tapeworms. Georgia Agr. Exp. Sta. 71 pp.

Renaux, E. A. 1964. Metazoal and protozoal diseases, pp. 120–44. *In* E. J. Catcott, ed. Feline medicine and surgery. American Veterinary Publications, Santa Barbara, Calif.

Rendtorff, R. C. 1948. Investigations on the life cycle of *Oochoristica ratti*, a cestode from rats and mice. J. Parasitol. 34:243–52.

Ruch, T. C. 1959. Diseases of laboratory primates. W. B. Saunders, Philadelphia. 600 pp.

Sasa, M., H. Tanaka, M. Fukui, and A. Takata. 1962. Internal parasites of laboratory animals, pp. 195–214. *In* R. J. C. Harris, ed. The problems of laboratory animal disease. Academic Press, New York.

Schmidt, R. E., J. S. Reid, and F. M. Garner. 1968. Sparganosis in a cat. J. Small Animal Pract. 9:551–53.

Shanks, P. L. 1962. Common diseases in rabbits, pp. 49–53. *In* G. Porter and W. Lane-Petter, eds. Notes for breeders of common laboratory animals. Academic Press, New York.

Shearer, G. C., and M. A. Gemmell. 1969. The efficiency of bunamidine hydroxynaphthoate against *Echinococcus granulosus* in dogs. Res. Vet. Sci. 10:296–99.

Sheffield, F. W., and Elizabeth Beveridge. 1962. Prophylaxis of "wet-tail" in hamsters. Nature 196:294–95.

Sheffy, B. E., J. A. Baker, and J. H. Gillespie. 1961. A disease-free colony of dogs. Proc. Animal Care Panel 11:208–14.

Siegmund, O. H., ed. 1961. Merck veterinary manual: A handbook of diagnosis and therapy for the veterinarian. 2d ed. Merck and Co., Rahway, N.J. 1624 pp.

Silverman, P. H. 1961. The life cycles and host-parasite relations of some tapeworms of dogs. Advan. Small Animal Pract. 2:26–31.

Simmons, M. L., C. B. Richter, J. A. Franklin, and R. W. Tennant. 1967. Prevention of infectious diseases in experimental mice. Proc. Soc. Exp. Biol. Med. 126:830–37.

Simmons, M. L., H. E. Williams, and E. B. Wright. 1964. Parasite screening and therapeutic value of organic phosphates in inbred mice. Lab. Animal Care 14:326.

Simpson, R. L., and W. Harmon. 1968. Occurrence of *Hymenolepis citelli* McLeod, 1933, in the rodent genus *Dipodomys* Gray, 1841. J. Parasitol. 54:769.

Smyth, J. D., and Mildred M. Smyth. 1964. Natural and experimental hosts of *Echinococcus granulosus* and *E. multilocularis,* with comments on the genetics of speciation in the genus *Echinococcus.* Parasitology 54:493–514.

Soave, O. A. 1963. Diagnosis and control of common diseases of hamsters, rabbits, and monkeys. J. Am. Vet. Med. Assoc. 142:285–90.

Soulsby, E. J. L. 1965. Textbook of veterinary clinical parasitology: Vol. I. Helminths. F. A. Davis, Philadelphia. 1120 pp.

Specht, D., and Marietta Voge. 1965. Asexual multiplication of *Mesocestoides* tetrathyridia in laboratory animals. J. Parasitol. 51:268–72.

Stone, W. B., and R. D. Manwell. 1966. Potential helminth infections in humans from pet or laboratory mice and hamsters. Public Health Rept. 81:647–53.

Stunkard, H. W. 1940. The morphology and life history of the cestode, *Bertiella studeri*. Am. J. Trop. Med. 20:305–33.

———. 1941. Studies on the life histories of the anoplocephaline cestodes of hares and rabbits. J. Parasitol. 27:299–325.

———. 1965. *Paratriotaenia oedipomidatis* gen. et sp. n. (Cestoda), from a marmoset. J. Parasitol. 51:545–51.

Summers, W. A. 1960. A case of hydatid disease in the rhesus monkey *(Macaca mulatta)*. Allied Vet. 31:141–43.

Tanaka, H., M. Fukui, H. Yamamoto, S. Hayama and S. Kodera. 1962. Studies on the identification of common intestinal parasites of primates. Bull. Exp. Animals 11:111–16.

Threlfall, W. 1969. Further records of helminths from Newfoundland mammals. Can. J. Zool. 47:197–201.

Tuffery, A. A., and J. R. M. Innes. 1963. Diseases of laboratory mice and rats, pp. 47–108. *In* W. Lane-Petter, ed. Animals for research: Principles of breeding and management. Academic Press, New York.

Turner, J. A. 1962. Human dipylidiasis in the United States. J. Pediat. 61:763–68.

Valerio, D. A., R. L. Miller, J. R. M. Innes, K. Diane Courtney, A. J. Pallotta, and R. M. Guttmacher. 1969. *Macaca mulatta:* Management of a laboratory breeding colony. Academic Press, New York. 104 pp.

Vickers, J. H., and L. R. Penner. 1968. Cysticercosis in four rhesus brains. J. Am. Vet. Med. Assoc. 153:868–71.

Voge, Marietta. 1952. Variation in some unarmed Hymenolepididae (Cestoda) from rodents. Univ. Calif. (Berkeley) Publ. Zool. 27:1–52.

———. 1953. New host records for *Mesocestoides* (Cestoda: Cyclophyllidea) in Cali-

fornia. Am. Midland Naturalist 49:249–51.

———. 1955a. North American cestodes of the genus *Mesocestoides*. Univ. Calif. (Berkeley) Publ. Zool. 59:125–55.

———. 1955b. A list of cestode parasites of California mammals. Am. Midland Naturalist 54:413–17.

———. 1961. Observations on development and high temperature sensitivity of cysticercoids of *Raillietina cesticillus* and *Hymenolepis citelli* (Cestoda: Cyclophyllidea). J. Parasitol. 47:839–41.

———. 1967. Development in vitro of *Mesocestoides* (Cestoda) from oncosphere to young tetrathyridium. J. Parasitol. 53:78–82.

Voge, Marietta, and A. K. Berntzen. 1963. Asexual multiplication of larval tapeworms as the cause of fatal parasitic ascites in dogs. J. Parasitol. 49:983–88.

Voge, Marietta, and D. Heyneman. 1957. Development of *Hymenolepis nana* and *Hymenolepis diminuta* (Cestoda: Hymenolepididae) in the intermediate host *Tribolium confusum*. Univ. Calif. (Berkeley) Publ. Zool. 59:549–80.

Wardle, R. A., and J. A. McLeod. 1952. The zoology of tapeworms. Univ. Minnesota Press, Minneapolis. 780 pp.

Wehr, E. E. 1965. Cestodes of poultry, pp. 1006–34. *In* H. E. Biester and L. H. Schwarte, eds. Diseases of poultry. 5th ed. Iowa State Univ. Press, Ames.

Whitten, L. K., and E. H. Shortridge. 1961. Three unusual cases of secondary hydatid cysts of the peritoneal cavity of the pig, dog, and cat. New Zealand Vet. J. 9:7–8.

Witenberg, G. G. 1964. Cestodiases, pp. 649–707. *In* J. van der Hoeden, ed. Zoonoses. American Elsevier, New York.

Worley, D. C. 1964. Helminth parasites of dogs in southeastern Michigan. J. Am. Vet. Med. Assoc. 144:42–46.

Chapter 7

NEMATODES

NEMATODES comprise the largest group of helminth parasites of endothermal laboratory animals. Their importance as pathogens varies with the parasite species, migratory pathway, metabolic activity in the host, mode of feeding, and number. Equally important is the host response, often a reflection of its diet, general condition, age, and immunologic capacity. The host-parasite relationship is usually fairly well equilibrated, and most nematodes cause no apparent signs or lesions except in young animals, in those maintained in crowded conditions or otherwise stressed, or in animals with an unusually high infection level.

There are several methods of classifying nematodes. The system used in this chapter is shown in Table 7.1 (Levine 1968). In general, the nematodes are divided into 2 classes and 11 orders. Not all the orders contain species that affect endothermal laboratory animals, and only those that do are included in this table.

Most nematodes known to affect endothermal laboratory animals have been included, and only obscure or dubious species or those which are rare or of unknown incidence in unusual endothermal laboratory hosts have been omitted. No attempt has been made to include nematodes chiefly affecting nonlaboratory domestic animals as reviews of these parasites are readily available elsewhere (Lapage 1968; Levine 1968;

Mozgovoi 1953; Popova 1955, 1958; Skrjabin, Shikhobalova, and Shults 1954; Soulsby 1965, 1968).

All nematodes likely to be encountered in laboratory animals are listed in Tables 7.2 through 7.15; the most important are discussed below.

RHABDITIDS, STRONGYLOIDIDS

The rhabditids and strongyloidids belong to the order Rhabditorida (Levine 1968). Most members of this order are free-living but a few are parasitic. Those that occur in endothermal laboratory animals are listed in Table 7.2. The most important species, *Strongyloides fülleborni* and *S. cebus*, which affect laboratory primates; *S. stercoralis*, which affects man and sometimes the dog and cat; and *S. ratti*, which is often used in the laboratory for experimental infection, are discussed below.

Strongyloides fülleborni, Strongyloides cebus, Strongyloides stercoralis

Strongyloides fülleborni occurs in macaques, guenons, baboons, the chimpanzee, and rarely in man in Africa and Asia. It is common in the rhesus monkey (Guilloud, King, and Lock 1965; Habermann and Williams 1957a; Reardon and Rininger 1968; Rowland and Vandenbergh 1965; Young et al. 1957), cynomolgus monkey (Habermann and Williams 1957a; Reardon and

Rininger 1968; Sasa et al. 1962), chimpanzee (Van Riper et al. 1966), and other laboratory primates (Ruch 1959). About 50% of newly received Old World monkeys and 75% of those born in captivity at the National Primate Center, Davis, California, are infected (Ming M. Wong, personal communication). Infections in man (Ruch 1959; Wallace, Mooney, and Sanders 1948) are rare, transitory, and probably derived from primates.

Strongyloides cebus occurs in monkeys in Central and South America. It is common in squirrel monkeys, woolly monkeys, capuchins, and spider monkeys (Little 1966a).

Strongyloides stercoralis, an important parasite of man, is common in the dog in southeastern United States (Galvin and Turk 1966) but is less prevalent elsewhere (Johnson, Andersen, and Gee 1963; Thomas and Ferrebee 1961; Worley 1964). It also occurs in the chimpanzee (Desportes 1945), other apes, and the cat (Chandler 1925; Renaux 1964; Scott 1967) but is usually uncommon in these species. Infections in hosts other than man are probably transitory and die out spontaneously.

Adult worms (females only) occur in the duodenum and jejunum; larvae occur in the lungs and sometimes the pericardium. Infection is usually mild or inapparent but sometimes it is severe, especially in young dogs or in debilitated, caged primates.

MORPHOLOGY

These nematodes have two adult forms that reflect their dual life-cycle pattern: a parasitic, parthenogenetic female and a smaller, free-living, soil-dwelling male and female (Chandler and Read 1961; Little 1966a). Parasitic males are unknown.

The parasitic female (Fig. 7.1*A*) is filiform, measures 2.0 to 5.0 mm long by 30 to 80 μ wide and has a short pointed tail, a small buccal capsule, and a narrow cylindrical esophagus that extends a quarter of the length of the worm. The vulva, which is in the posterior third of the body, opens into opposed uteri with reflexed ovaries. The egg is 40 to 70 μ by 20 to 35 μ, thin-shelled, transparent, and embryonated (Fig. 7.2). The first-stage rhabditiform larvae (Fig. 7.1*B*) measure 150 to 390 μ in length when passed in the feces but grow rapidly up to 800 μ. They have a short, muscular esophagus ending in a valvulated bulb preceded by a constriction.

The free-living male (Fig. 7.1*C*) is about 0.8 to 1.1 mm long, has a gubernaculum, two short, equal spicules, and a short, conical tail; caudal alae are absent. The free-living female (Fig. 7.1*D*) is 0.9 to 1.7 mm long and has a long pointed tail, a central vulva, diverging uteri, and reflexed ovaries. The third-stage filariform, infective larva (Fig. 7.1*E*), measures 400 to 800 μ by 12 to 20 μ. It has a small genital primordium and a long, cylindrical, nonbulbar

FIG. 7.1. *Strongyloides stercoralis* life cycle. The indirect cycle includes four rhabditiform stages *(B),* an adult male *(C)* or female *(D),* whose eggs hatch and pass through two rhabditiform stages and a filariform stage *(E)* to form the parthenogenetic parasitic female adult *(A);* the direct cycle does not pass through a free-living adult stage but passes through two rhabditiform stages *(B)* and a filariform stage *(E)* to form the parthenogenetic parasitic female adult *(A).* (From Chandler and Read 1961. Courtesy of John Wiley & Sons.)

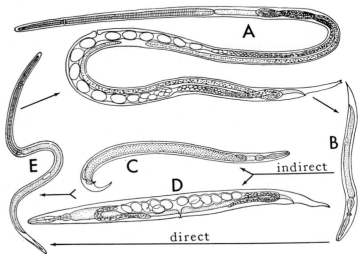

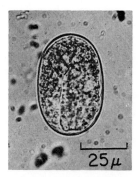

Fig. 7.2. *Strongyloides fülleborni* egg. (From Tanaka et al. 1962. Courtesy of Japan Experimental Animal Research Association.)

esophagus that extends through the anterior half of the body. Three small points located at the tip of the tail give a notched appearance when the tail is viewed ventrally.

LIFE CYCLE

Strongyloides has a dual life pattern that involves both an indirect and a direct cycle (Fig. 7.1) (Chandler and Read 1961). Soil-dwelling adults may continue through one cycle (Chang and Graham 1957) or a succession of free-living generations (Beach 1936) before initiating an indirect or heterogonic cycle by producing the distinctive filariform infective larvae. The direct or homogonic cycle results when rhabditiform larvae in the feces of parasitized hosts develop into filariform, third-stage, infective larvae without passing through a free-living adult generation in the soil.

Infective larvae resulting from either the direct or indirect route penetrate the skin or oral mucosa of the host, migrate through the bloodstream to the heart and lungs (where a later molt occurs), penetrate the alveoli into the bronchioles, pass up the trachea to the mouth, and are swallowed (Faust 1933). Completion of the last or fourth molt occurs in the duodenum and produces the adult parthenogenetic female worm.

A third pathway to parasitism is the hyperinfective route in which first-stage larvae develop within the host intestine by rapid molts into third-stage infective larvae and penetrate the bowel directly. A modification of this pattern of infection, termed autoinfection, occurs when such third-stage infective larvae pass through the anus and penetrate the perianal or perineal skin. Either route involves blood-borne migra-

tion via the portal system to the liver, heart, and lung, and then air duct passage to the mouth, followed by the intestinal phase. These self-generating processes are responsible for long, sustained infections in man (Brown and Perna 1958; Cahill 1967) and cause the most serious pathologic effects in monkeys (Ming M. Wong, personal communication).

Another route is suggested by the finding that 75% of the nursing infants at the National Primate Center, Davis, California, excrete *S. fülleborni* ova while only 16% of their mothers are positive for ova in their feces. This, together with the observation that the youngest monkeys found positive were only 12 days old, indicates that either intrauterine (Enigk 1952; Frickers 1953; Stone 1964; Supperer 1965) or transcolostral transmission (Moncol and Batte 1966; Olsen and Lyons 1965) may occur.

Immunity to reinfection has been reported with *S. stercoralis* in the dog (Sandground 1928). However, the susceptibility of young or debilitated animals and the occurrence of long-standing *S. fülleborni* infections in monkeys presumably produced by autoinfection indicate that the resistance is of a low order and serves only to contain and repress the infection.

The stimulus to produce nonfeeding infective larvae in place of free-living, bacteria-feeding rhabditiform larvae in the soil appears to be environmentally directed by such factors as previous host nutrition (Galliard 1947), temperature, and moisture or food in the soil (Beach 1936; Little 1962). Poor conditions seem to favor rapid production, conversion, or differential survival of the parasitic stage (Chandler and Read 1961; Soulsby 1965). Genetic factors are also involved (Bolla and Roberts 1968; Chang and Graham 1957; Graham 1936, 1938a, b, 1939a, b, 1940a, b, c).

Development is rapid. In the soil cycle, under optimum conditions, the four molts to adulthood are completed in 36 to 48 hours. In the parasitic cycle, newly hatched rhabditiform larvae of the next generation appear in the feces 5 to 7 days after ingestion of infective filariform larvae. Even more important than the speed with which the larvae transform is the magnification of infection made possible by the soil phase. For example, in as few as 5 days, 1,000 first-stage larvae passed in the feces can develop by the sexual soil cycle into as many as 20,000 infective larvae.

PATHOLOGIC EFFECTS

The pathologic effects are usually divided into three distinct phases, each with characteristic signs and lesions: the invasion phase, migratory phase, and intestinal phase (Soulsby 1965).

The invasion phase, when the infective larvae penetrate the skin or buccal mucosa, is sometimes accompanied by local irritation, pruritus, and erythema. This is frequently observed in man but has not been reported in the dog and is rare in simian primates (Liebegott 1962; Ruch 1959).

The migratory phase occurs when the infective larvae are carried by the venous circulation to the heart and lungs, break into the alveoli, enter the bronchi, and are coughed up and swallowed. In mild infections this phase usually produces only a sporadic cough (Morgan 1967; Renaux 1964). In massive infections, especially in young or debilitated animals, the larval migration produces an acute local inflammatory reaction around the affected alveoli and sometimes bronchopneumonia, pericarditis, massive hemorrhages in the lungs, and death (Liebegott 1962; Ruch 1959; Soulsby 1965).

During the intestinal phase, the parasite penetrates the intestinal crypts and burrows into the glandular epithelium (Fig. 7.3). Often the intestinal mucosa is riddled with worms (Soulsby 1965). This phase is characterized by a diarrhea which is sometimes hemorrhagic and occasionally chronic (Galvin and Turk 1966; Ruch 1959). The thin, watery feces are typically filled with larvae (J. D. Douglas, personal communication). Listlessness, debilitation, anorexia, emaciation, reduced growth rate, and sometimes prostration and death also occur (Faust 1936; Ruch 1959; Soulsby 1965). Lesions seen at necropsy are those of an acute enteritis, sometimes hemorrhagic and necrotic (Soulsby 1965), and are occasionally accompanied by a secondary peritonitis (Smith and Jones 1966). Eosinophilia and increased lymphoid tissue in the jejunum have also been attributed to this parasite (Vickers 1969).

The morbidity and mortality from *S.*

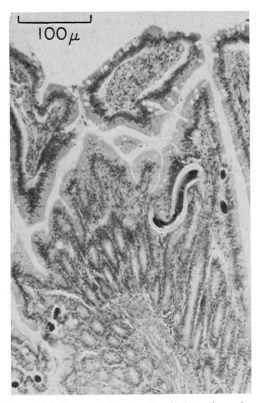

FIG. 7.3. Strongyloidosis. Small intestine of a monkey with a worm in the mucosa. (From Vickers 1969. Courtesy of New York Academy of Sciences.)

stercoralis in the dog are usually low but are sometimes high in kennels with young dogs (Soulsby 1965). Similarly, in young, debilitated or malnourished caged primates subject to massive infection and reinfection with *S. fülleborni,* mortality is sometimes high (Graham 1960; Smith and Jones 1966).

DIAGNOSIS

Diagnosis is usually based on clinical signs and identification of the larvae in the feces, using either a direct smear or the Baermann apparatus. If the fecal specimen is contaminated with soil, one must be careful to differentiate *Strongyloides* larvae from free-living rhabditiform hookworm larvae (Graham 1960). The parasitic adult females can also be demonstrated at necropsy. They are usually confined to the anterior small intestinal epithelium and are thin, transparent, and difficult to see.

Adult females, plus eggs and larvae, are best demonstrated in a scraping of the mucosa (Smith and Jones 1966; Soulsby 1965).

CONTROL

Sanitation and management are the primary methods of control. Because first-stage larvae passed in the feces can develop into third-stage infective larvae within 48 hours, it is important that feces be removed daily and that food and water be kept free of contamination (Habermann and Williams 1958; Van Riper et al. 1966). Particular care must be taken to prevent the free-living stages from breeding in kennels, runs, or cages. Because moisture is essential to the survival of larvae, keeping surfaces dry will greatly aid in controlling this parasite (Johnson, Andersen, and Gee 1963).

Newly acquired primates, dogs, and cats should be examined on arrival and either treated or eliminated, if infected. Gentian violet, phenathiazine, piperazine, and diethylcarbamazine, given orally, have been used for treatment with various results (Gisler, Benson, and Young 1960; Ruch 1959; Soulsby 1965). Dithiazanine iodide, given orally in the food at the rate of about 20 mg per kg of body weight per day for 10 to 14 days, is effective for the monkey (Gisler, Benson, and Young 1960), chimpanzee (Lang 1962; Van Riper et al. 1966), and dog (Galvin and Turk 1966) and has been recommended for the cat (Renaux 1964). Even more effective is thiabendazole, which is given orally with a stomach tube or in the food in a single dose of about 100 mg per kg of body weight for the monkey and chimpanzee (Bingham and Rabstein 1964; Guilloud, King, and Lock 1965; Van Riper et al. 1966) and about 50 mg per kg of body weight daily for 3 days for the dog and cat (Galvin and Turk 1966). Treatment should be repeated in 2 weeks (Van Riper et al. 1966).

PUBLIC HEALTH CONSIDERATIONS

Strongyloides stercoralis is pathogenic for man and, in heavy infections, causes ulcerative enteritis or pneumonia (Chandler and Read 1961; Napier, 1949a, b). Natural transmission of *S. fülleborni* from the monkey and chimpanzee to man (Ruch 1959) and experimental transmission of *S. stercoralis* from the chimpanzee to man (Desportes 1945) have been reported. It is important to alert animal care personnel of this hazard and to instruct them in proper personal hygiene and safe methods of handling infected animals and excrement.

Strongyloides ratti

Strongyloides ratti is common in the small intestine of the wild Norway rat and black rat throughout the world (Ash 1962a; Dove 1950; de León 1964) though some reports of its occurrence may be the result of infection with *S. venezuelensis*, a similar species which is also thought to be widespread in the wild Norway rat throughout the world (Little 1966a). *Strongyloides ratti* is uncommon or absent in conventional rat colonies (Sasa et al. 1962) and does not occur in cesarean-derived, barrier-sustained colonies (Foster 1963). It is important in the laboratory only as an experimental model, where it is frequently used to study in vitro cultivation of helminths, helminth development, genetics, immunity, possible transmission of viruses by helminths, and parasite metabolism (Abadie 1963; Barrett 1969; Graham 1936, 1938a, b, 1939a, b, 1940a, b, c; Ratcliffe 1949; Sheldon 1937a, b).

ANCYLOSTOMATIDS, STRONGYLIDS, SYNGAMIDS

These nematodes belong to the order Strongylorida, which is characterized by the possession of a cuticular, ray-supported bursa copulatrix in the male, and to the superfamily Strongylicae, which is characterized by a large mouth and a sturdy body (Levine 1968). Those which occur in endothermal laboratory animals are listed in Table 7.3. The most important are discussed below.

Ancylostoma caninum

(Dog Hookworm)

Ancylostoma caninum is a highly pathogenic parasite which occurs in the small intestine of the dog and other carnivores throughout the world, especially in the temperate zones. It is very common in the United States (Levine 1968), uncommon in Canada (Threlfall 1969), and uncommon or absent in the British Isles (Soulsby 1965).

Laboratory dogs obtained from pounds

are usually infected. Typical incidences reported in the United States are 58% in Hawaii (Ash 1962b), 51% in Michigan (Worley 1964), and 92% in Louisiana (Vaughn and Murphy 1962). In one survey, 60 of 100 laboratory dogs obtained from various eastern and southeastern states were infected (Mann and Bjotvedt 1965). This nematode is uncommon or absent in dogs reared in the laboratory or in kennels that practice good management and sanitation (Johnson, Andersen, and Gee 1963). It has not been observed in barrier-maintained dogs (Griesemer and Gibson 1963a).

Whether *A. caninum* occurs in the cat is uncertain. For many years it was thought that the common species of *Ancylostoma* found in the cat was *A. caninum* (Lapage 1968; Soulsby 1965). Then it was shown that the species in the cat is different from that in the dog (Burrows 1962; Fitzsimmons 1961a), that *A. caninum* is the species that commonly occurs in the dog and *A. tubaeforme* the common species in the cat, and further, that the two species are not interchangeable between the two hosts. Later, however, it was stated that both species occur in the cat (Okoshi and Murata 1966).

MORPHOLOGY

The male is 9 to 12 mm long, and the female 15 to 18 mm (Soulsby 1965). Both possess a sublobular buccal cavity with three well-developed teeth on each side. The egg is ellipsoidal and thin shelled and measures 55 to 72 μ by 34 to 45 μ (Fig. 7.4) (Burrows 1962). It is usually in the two- to eight-cell stage when passed in the feces.

LIFE CYCLE

The life cycle is direct (Morgan and Hawkins 1949; Soulsby 1965). Under optimum conditions of temperature and moisture, eggs passed in the feces hatch in 1 to 2 days and, after molting twice, develop into infective larvae in 5 to 8 days. Desiccation and temperatures below freezing or above 37 C delay hatching and are lethal to larvae. Infection occurs either by ingestion or by larval penetration of the skin. The usual method in the dog is by ingestion of contaminated food. Infective larvae that enter the body by this route develop in the gastric and intestinal mucosa and

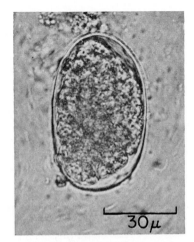

FIG. 7.4. *Ancylostoma caninum* egg. (From Ewing 1967. Courtesy of W. B. Saunders Co.)

reach maturity in the lumen of the small intestine. Infective larvae that enter the body by penetration of the skin migrate to the lungs and gain access to the intestine by the tracheal route. Should the animal be pregnant during this migratory phase, the migrating larvae sometimes enter the fetus and produce a prenatal infection. About 5 weeks are usually required to complete development from infective larva to adult.

PATHOLOGIC EFFECTS

Ancylostoma caninum is a voracious bloodsucker, often feeding from several sites in the small intestine (Soulsby 1965). The blood loss from feeding worms and hemorrhage from previous feeding locations is severe, as much as 0.2 ml per worm per day (Miller 1966a). Mature animals on an adequate diet often have no signs of infection other than a mild hypochromic anemia, but heavily infected young animals, especially those prenatally infected, develop severe signs including pallor of the mucosa, hypoproteinemia, diarrhea, weakness, progressive emaciation, cardiac failure, and death (Morgan and Hawkins 1949; Smith and Jones 1966). Other signs sometimes seen include dermatitis and itching during the period of skin penetration, especially in older, sensitized dogs, and coughing and dyspnea during the period of larval migration, especially in younger dogs.

Although small hemorrhages caused

by migrating larvae sometimes occur in the lungs in heavy infections, the most prominent lesions at necropsy are the bleeding, necrotic ulcers produced by the adult worms in the small intestine (Morgan and Hawkins 1949; Poynter 1966).

DIAGNOSIS

Diagnosis is based on the clinical signs and the demonstration of eggs in the feces or mature worms in the intestine at necropsy.

CONTROL

Complete elimination of this parasite from a research dog colony is apparently possible by raising cesarean-derived progeny in isolation (Griesemer and Gibson 1963a).

Control in a conventional colony is achieved by sanitation, by the removal of conditions favorable for the development of eggs and larvae, and by the elimination or regular treatment of infected animals (Soulsby 1965). As hot water, sunlight, and desiccation are effective larvicides, the daily cleaning of cages and pens, the elimination of roofs over runs, and the provision of well-drained concrete runs free of cracks are recommended (Lapage 1968; Morgan and Hawkins 1949). Vaccination with X-irradiated *A. caninum* larvae will produce a strong immunity (Miller 1967).

Newly acquired dogs should be examined on arrival and either treated or eliminated, if infected. Effective treatments include tetrachlorethylene, 0.2 mg per kg of body weight given orally in a single dose (Hall 1933; Miller 1966c; Morgan and Hawkins 1949); bephenium, 20 mg per kg of body weight given orally in a single dose (Burrows 1958); dithiazanine iodide, 20 mg per kg of body weight given orally daily for 5 to 7 days (Shumard and Hendrix 1962); thenium, two doses of 25 to 50 mg per kg of body weight given orally either morning and evening or on 2 consecutive days (Burrows and Lillis 1962); a mixture of equal parts toluene and dichlorophen (Vermiplex, Pitman-Moore), 440 mg per kg of body weight given orally in a single dose (Miller 1966d); DDVP (dichlorvos; Task, Shell), 35 to 40 mg per kg of body weight given orally in a single dose (Batte and Moncol 1968); and disophenol (2,6-diiodo-4-nitrophenol), 6.5 to 7.5 mg per kg of body weight given subcutaneously in a single dose (Darne and Webb 1964; Takahashi et al. 1967).

PUBLIC HEALTH CONSIDERATIONS

Infective larvae of *A. caninum* occasionally penetrate the skin of man and produce cutaneous larva migrans, a transient dermatitis and pruritus that is commonly termed creeping eruption (Faust, Beaver, and Jung 1968). A case of cutaneous larva migrans caused by *Ancylostoma* has been reported in a laboratory animal caretaker (Stone and Levy 1967). It is important, therefore, that animal care personnel be cautioned of this possibility and instructed in proper personal hygiene and safe methods of handling infected animals and excrement.

Ancylostoma tubaeforme
(Cat Hookworm)

For many years, *Ancylostoma tubaeforme*, the common hookworm of the cat, was considered to be a synonym for *A. caninum*, the common hookworm of the dog (Levine 1968; Soulsby 1965). For this reason, only recent reports in which the two species are differentiated are of value in ascertaining incidence and geographic distribution. From these reports it appears that *A. tubaeforme* is common and worldwide in distribution. It occurs in a high incidence of laboratory cats obtained as strays (Burrows 1962) but is uncommon in laboratory cats reared for research in a well-managed colony (Morris 1963).

The morphology, life cycle, pathologic effects, control, and public health aspects of this species are similar to those of *A. caninum* (Fitzsimmons 1961a; Soulsby 1965). It can be distinguished only on the basis of certain slight differences in the adults; the egg measures 55 to 76 μ by 34 to 45 μ (Fig. 7.5) and cannot be distinguished morphologically from that of *A. caninum* (Burrows 1962).

Ancylostoma braziliense

Ancylostoma braziliense occurs in the small intestine of the dog, cat, and other carnivores in southern United States, Central and South America, Asia, and southern Africa (Levine 1968; Soulsby 1965). It is frequently encountered in laboratory dogs

FIG. 7.5. *Ancylostoma tubaeforme* egg. (From Burrows 1965. Courtesy of Yale University Press.)

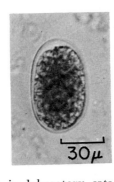

and, to a lesser extent, in laboratory cats obtained from pounds in these regions. It is uncommon or absent in dogs and cats reared in the laboratory or in those from kennels that practice good management and sanitation (Johnson, Andersen, and Gee 1963; Morris 1963), and it does not occur in cesarean-derived, barrier-maintained dogs (Griesemer and Gibson 1963a).

MORPHOLOGY

The male is 7.8 to 8.5 mm long, and the female 9.0 to 10.5 mm (Soulsby 1965). There are two teeth on each side of the buccal cavity: the outer pair is large, and the inner pair is very small. The egg measures 75 to 95 μ by 41 to 45 μ (Fig. 7.6).

LIFE CYCLE

The life cycle is similar to that of *A. caninum.*

PATHOLOGIC EFFECTS

The pathologic effects of *A. braziliense* are similar to those of *A. caninum* but are much less severe (Miller 1966b). The blood loss per worm is only about 1/100 that of *A. caninum;* heavy infections even in young dogs and cats produce no signs.

DIAGNOSIS

Diagnosis is based on demonstration of eggs in the feces or mature worms in the intestine at necropsy.

CONTROL

The control procedures for *A. caninum* are also effective for this species.

PUBLIC HEALTH CONSIDERATIONS

Ancylostoma braziliense is the commonest cause of cutaneous larva migrans in man (Faust, Beaver, and Jung 1968).

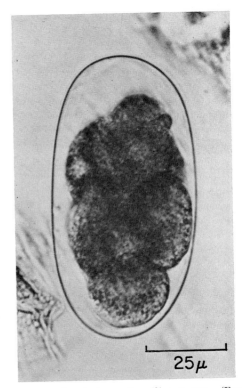

FIG. 7.6. *Ancylostoma braziliense* egg. (From Burrows 1965. Courtesy of Yale University Press.)

Ancylostoma duodenale, Necator americanus

(Human Hookworms)

These parasites are common in the small intestine of man in the tropical and subtropical parts of the world (Chandler and Read 1961; Lapage 1968). They are also occasionally reported in simian primates including the monkey, gibbons, mandrills, baboons, chimpanzee, and gorilla (Fiennes 1967; Myers and Kuntz 1965), but some of these reports may have been based on the incorrect identification of *Oesophagostomum* eggs (Ruch 1959). A few positively identified cases have been reported in the laboratory monkey and chimpanzee (Benson, Fremming, and Young 1954; Young et al. 1957). These parasites are rare or uncommon in monkeys and apes in nature and in the laboratory, and nonhuman primates are apparently only incidental hosts (Nelson 1965).

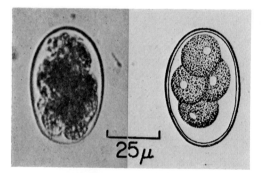

Fig. 7.7. *Ancylostoma duodenale* egg. Photomicrograph *(left)* and drawing *(right)*. *(Left* from Burrows 1965; courtesy of Yale University Press. *Right* from Yorke and Maplestone 1926.)

MORPHOLOGY

The male of *Ancylostoma duodenale* is 8 to 11 mm long, and the female 10 to 13 mm (Lapage 1968). Both have two well-developed teeth of about equal size on each side of the buccal cavity. The egg measures 60 by 40 μ (Fig. 7.7). The male of *Necator americanus* is 7 to 9 mm long, and the female 9 to 11 mm (Lapage 1968). Both have a pair of semilunar cutting plates at the margin of the buccal cavity instead of teeth. The egg is similar to that of *A. duodenale* except that it is slightly narrower and longer. It measures 64 to 76 μ by 36 to 40 μ.

LIFE CYCLE

The life cycles are similar to those of *A. caninum* except that infection with *N. americanus* is chiefly by larval penetration of skin.

PATHOLOGIC EFFECTS

Little is known of the pathologic effects of these parasites on laboratory primates, but it is assumed that they are similar to those produced by hookworms in man and other animals and include anemia and debilitation (Ruch 1959). Cutaneous larva migrans has not been reported in simian primates (Ruch 1959).

DIAGNOSIS

Diagnosis is based on demonstration of eggs in the feces or mature worms in the intestine at necropsy.

CONTROL

Control procedures are similar to those for *A. caninum*. Recommended treatments for the monkey and chimpanzee include a mixture of equal parts of toluene and dichlorophen (Vermiplex, Pitman-Moore), 550 mg per kg of body weight given orally in a single dose (Benson, Fremming, and Young 1954; Young et al. 1957), and dithiazanine iodide, 20 mg per kg of body weight given orally twice daily for 14 days (Mortelmans and Vercruysse 1962).

PUBLIC HEALTH CONSIDERATIONS

Since man is the normal host for these hookworms, infected laboratory primates should be handled with caution.

Uncinaria stenocephala

(Fox Hookworm; Northern Hookworm; European Dog Hookworm)

Uncinaria stenocephala occurs in the small intestine of the dog, cat, and fox in temperate zones throughout the world (Levine 1968; Soulsby 1965). It is commonest in northern United States, Canada, and Europe and is the only hookworm of importance in the British Isles. It is frequently seen in laboratory dogs (Bantin and Maber 1967) and, to a lesser extent, in laboratory cats (Scott 1967) in these regions. It is uncommon or absent in dogs and cats reared in the laboratory or in clean, well-managed kennels (Johnson, Andersen, and Gee 1963; Morris 1963), and it does not occur in cesarean-derived, barrier-maintained dogs (Griesemer and Gibson 1963a).

MORPHOLOGY

The male is 5 to 8 mm long, and the female 7 to 12 mm long (Soulsby 1965). It differs from *Ancylostoma* in that it has a pair of cutting plates at the ventral border of the buccal cavity instead of teeth. The egg measures 71 to 93 μ by 37 to 55 μ (Fig. 7.8) (Ehrenford 1953).

LIFE CYCLE

The life cycle is similar to that of *A. caninum* except that infection is usually acquired only by ingestion, and the larvae usually do not migrate through the lungs (Renaux 1964; Soulsby 1965).

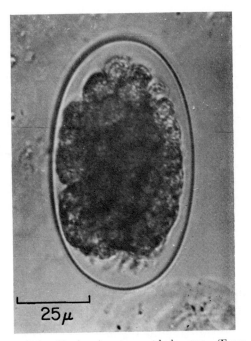

FIG. 7.8. *Uncinaria stenocephala* egg. (From Burrows 1965. Courtesy of Yale University Press.)

PATHOLOGIC EFFECTS

Uncinaria stenocephala apparently feeds on surface tissues instead of sucking blood (Renaux 1964). It sometimes inflames and erodes the intestinal mucosa (Poynter 1966), but ordinarily it produces little damage and the infection is usually inapparent (Renaux 1964).

DIAGNOSIS

Diagnosis is based on demonstration of eggs in the feces or mature worms in the intestine at necropsy.

CONTROL

Control is similar to that for *A. caninum*. Drugs effective against *A. caninum* are also effective against this hookworm except that the dosage of disophenol for *U. stenocephala* is 10 mg per kg of body weight (Soulsby 1965). Tetramisole, in a single dose of 10 mg per kg of body weight subcutaneously or 20 mg per kg orally, is also reportedly effective (Thienpont et al. 1968).

PUBLIC HEALTH CONSIDERATIONS

Uncinaria stenocephala rarely causes cutaneous larva migrans in man (Soulsby 1965).

Oesophagostomum

(Nodular Worm)

Oesophagostomum is the commonest nematode of Old World monkeys and apes (Ruch 1959). It occurs in the colon of many simian primates including the macaques, guenons, mangabeys, baboons, chimpanzee, and gorilla; it also affects man. *Oesophagostomum apiostomum* is said to be the species usually involved (Ruch 1959), but the exact incidence and geographic distribution of the various species are uncertain because identification is often limited to genus or is presumptively said to be *O. apiostomum* (Faust, Beaver, and Jung 1968). Although some authors (Faust, Beaver, and Jung 1968; Levine 1968; Sasa et al. 1962) consider *O. apiostomum*, *O. aculeatum,* and possibly *O. bifurcum* as synonyms, the proper taxonomic status of these species remains in doubt and they are treated separately here and in Table 7.3. *Oesophagostomum bifurcum* is common in Africa and Asia, and incidences of 33 to 55% have been reported in rhesus monkeys recently imported into the United States (Bingham and Rabstein 1964; Graham 1960; Guilloud, King, and Lock 1965). *Oesophagostomum aculeatum* has been reported in incidences of 28 to 62% in the Japanese macaque and cynomolgus monkey (Hashimoto and Honjo 1966; Tanaka et al. 1962). In another survey of newly imported monkeys in the United States, reported incidences of *O. apiostomum* were 70% in the rhesus monkey, 20% in the cynomolgus monkey, and none in the green monkey (Vickers 1969). A 45% incidence of an unidentified species has been reported in chimpanzees recently imported into the United States from Africa (Van Riper et al. 1966), where *O. bifurcum* and *O. stephanostomum* are common (Faust, Beaver, and Jung 1968; Levine 1968).

MORPHOLOGY

Species of *Oesophagostomum* resemble *Ancylostoma* in size and morphology, but

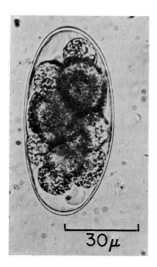

FIG. 7.9. *Oesophagostomum aculeatum* egg. (From Tanaka et al. 1962. Courtesy of Japan Experimental Animal Research Association.)

the buccal cavity is cylindrical instead of globular and has bristles or setae around the opening (Faust, Beaver, and Jung 1968). *Oesophagostomum apiostomum* males measure 8.5 to 10.5 mm by 0.2 to 0.3 mm; females are 8.0 to 10.0 mm by 0.3 mm (Habermann and Williams 1958). The eggs of *Oesophagostomum* also resemble those of hookworms in size and appearance. Those of *O. apiostomum* measure 60 to 63 μ by 27 to 40 μ, and those of *O. aculeatum* 69 to 86 μ by 35 to 55 μ (Fig. 7.9) (Habermann and Williams 1958; Tanaka et al. 1962).

LIFE CYCLE

Eggs are usually in an early division stage when passed in the feces and, under favorable conditions, hatch in 24 to 48 hours; infection is by ingestion of an infective larva (Faust, Beaver, and Jung 1968). The larva passes directly to the colon, penetrates deeply into the mucosa and induces the development of a large, firm, encapsulated nodule. No visceral migration occurs. In 5 to 8 days the nodule ruptures, and the worm escapes into the lumen and matures. In a previously infected, immune animal, the worm usually remains in the nodule, which then becomes caseous and persists for a long time (Ruch 1959).

PATHOLOGIC EFFECTS

Light infections are usually inapparent, and only in heavy infections under adverse environmental conditions are signs produced (Ruch 1959). These consist of diarrhea, loss of weight, debilitation, and increased mortality.

The typical nodules are seen at necropsy in the wall of the large intestine and occasionally in the omentum (Fig. 7.10) (Ruch 1959; Vickers 1969). They occur on the serosal surface, chiefly along the tenia, measure 2 to 4 mm in diameter and are round and glistening white or black if hemorrhage has occurred within the nodule. On incision, a motile worm is found, sometimes surrounded by hemorrhagic material. Occasionally an ulcer is seen in the intestinal mucosa with an irregular fistulous tract leading to a nodule in the muscularis (Habermann and Williams 1957a, 1958). Nodules, in which the worm is permanently encapsulated because of an immune response by the host, have caseous and often calcified centers (Habermann and Williams 1958). In severe infections, adhesions occur which sometimes cause obstruction or ascites (Ruch 1959).

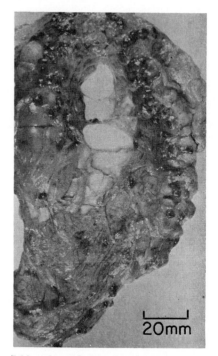

FIG. 7.10. *Oesophagostomum* nodules in the intestinal wall of a monkey. (From Whitney, Johnson, and Cole 1967. Courtesy of R. A. Whitney, Edgewood Arsenal.)

DIAGNOSIS

A tentative diagnosis is made in the living animal by identification of the eggs in the feces; however, because hookworm and *Oesophagostomum* eggs are similar, a positive identification can be made only by identifying the adult worm in the intestine.

CONTROL

Sanitation and management, the primary methods of control, will rapidly reduce the incidence of infection in a colony (Habermann and Williams 1958; Ratcliffe 1945).

Newly acquired primates should be examined on arrival and either treated or eliminated, if infected. Phenothiazine, 125 to 150 mg per kg of body weight per day given orally for 7 to 21 days, is sometimes used for both the monkey and chimpanzee (Britz et al. 1961; Gisler, Benson, and Young 1960; Young et al. 1957). A more effective treatment is thiabendazole, given orally with a stomach tube or in the food in a single dose of about 100 mg per kg of body weight, for both the monkey and chimpanzee (Bingham and Rabstein 1964; Guilloud, King, and Lock 1965; Van Riper et al. 1966). Treatment should be repeated in 2 weeks.

PUBLIC HEALTH CONSIDERATIONS

This parasite has been reported in man, and infection presumably can be contracted from simian primates (Faust, Beaver, and Jung 1968; Ruch 1959). For this reason, infected laboratory animals should be handled with caution.

Ternidens deminutus

This nematode, a close relative of *Oesophagostomum,* occurs in the cecum and colon of macaques, guenons, baboons, the chimpanzee, gorilla, and man in Asia and Africa (Amberson and Schwarz 1952; Levine 1968; Myers and Kuntz 1965; Ruch 1959). It sucks blood and sometimes causes anemia and cystic nodules in the colon wall (Levine 1968). Incidences of 60% in the green monkey and 76% in baboons have been reported in southern Africa (Nelson 1965). It is usually uncommon in laboratory monkeys (Habermann and Williams 1957a; Reardon and Rininger 1968; Ruch

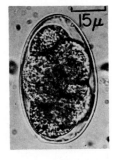

FIG. 7.11. *Ternidens deminutus* egg. (From Tanaka et al. 1962. Courtesy of Japan Experimental Animal Research Association.)

1959; Sasa et al. 1962; Tanaka et al. 1962; Valerio et al. 1969), but there is one report of an incidence of 21% (Graham 1960).

The morphology of adult worms and the egg is similar to that of *Oesophagostomum* (Ruch 1959; Tanaka et al. 1962). The egg measures 57 to 65 μ by 36 to 45 μ (Fig. 7.11). The life cycle, method of transmission, and control are also similar to those of *Oesophagostomum;* infection is by the oral route (Faust, Beaver, and Jung 1968; Valerio et al. 1969). Because this parasite is pathogenic for man, causing intestinal nodules, infected laboratory animals should be handled with caution.

Syngamus trachea

(Gapeworm)

This nematode occurs in the trachea of the chicken and many other galliform and passeriform birds throughout the world (Levine 1968; Soulsby 1965). It is likely to be found only in laboratory chickens reared in crowded, unsanitary outdoor pens; it does not occur in chickens raised in well-managed, sanitary facilities.

MORPHOLOGY

Adults have bright red bodies. The male, 2 to 6 mm long, and the female, 5 to 20 mm long, are permanently joined together in copulation (Fig. 7.12) (Soulsby 1965; Wehr 1965). The male has a characteristic orbicular mouth and hemispherical chitinous buccal capsule with eight or nine teeth at the base; six festoons form a chitinous plate around the mouth. The genital bursa is distinctly asymmetrical and obliquely truncated with short, stout rays. The spicules are slender and equal, about 57 to 64 μ long. The female has a conical tail which bears a pointed process; the vul-

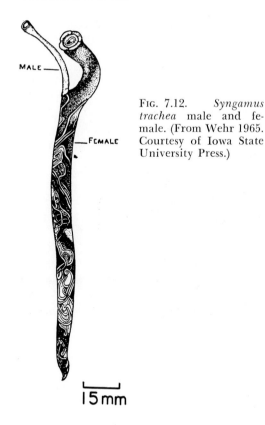

FIG. 7.12. *Syngamus trachea* male and female. (From Wehr 1965. Courtesy of Iowa State University Press.)

15 mm

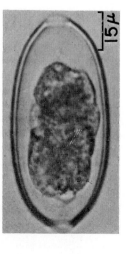

FIG. 7.13. *Syngamus trachea* egg. (From Soulsby 1965. Courtesy of Blackwell Scientific Publications.)

va is in the anterior quarter of the body. The ellipsoidal egg, usually passed in the 16- to 32-cell stage, is operculated and measures 78 to 100 μ by 43 to 46 μ (Fig. 7.13).

LIFE CYCLE

Eggs deposited by the female in the trachea are carried to the pharynx, swallowed, and passed in the feces (Wehr 1965). The eggs embryonate in 8 to 14 days, depending on the temperature and moisture. Infection is transmitted by the ingestion of an embryonated egg, an infective larva, or a transport host, usually an earthworm or snail. Larvae reach the lungs within a few hours after being ingested, probably by way of the bloodstream. They molt, migrate to the bronchi, molt again, and reach the trachea in 7 days. Eggs are found in the feces about 2 weeks after infection.

PATHOLOGIC EFFECTS

The worms in the trachea cause obstruction, tracheitis, and excess mucus pro-

duction (Lapage 1968). This results in paroxysms of dyspnea, asphyxia, a hissing sound or cough, and a characteristic extension of the head with the mouth open (gape). Anorexia and adipsia are common. In heavy infections, the bloodsucking activity of the parasites causes anemia which, in combination with the other effects, often leads to death. Young chickens are most severely affected.

Lesions produced are those of emaciation and anemia. The worms are found attached to the mucosa in the posterior part of the trachea (Fig. 7.14). The lumen of the trachea usually contains large amounts of frothy, hemorrhagic mucus.

DIAGNOSIS

Diagnosis is based on the typical signs and the demonstration of eggs in the feces of the living animal or of worms in the trachea at necropsy (Lapage 1962). Care must be taken to differentiate between the effects of this parasite and avian infectious laryngotracheitis, fowl plague, fowl pest, and aspergillosis (Soulsby 1965).

CONTROL

Sanitation and the elimination of infected chickens are the primary methods of control. Because eggs passed in the feces do not embryonate for 8 to 14 days, frequent and complete cleaning of cages and pens will prevent the dissemination of the parasite. Thiabendazole, given in the diet at a rate of 0.1%, is effective both therapeutically and prophylactically (Soulsby 1965).

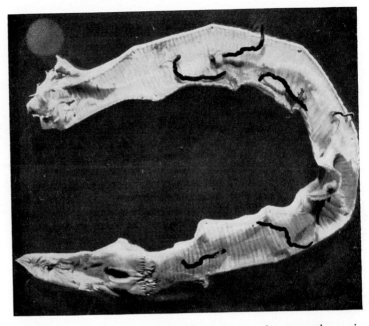

FIG. 7.14. *Syngamus trachea* adults attached to the trachea of a chicken. (From Wehr 1965. Courtesy of Iowa State University Press.)

PUBLIC HEALTH CONSIDERATIONS

This nematode does not occur in man.

TRICHOSTRONGYLIDS

Trichostrongylids are characterized by their small mouth and slender body (Levine 1968). Those which occur in endothermal laboratory animals are listed in Table 7.4. The most important are discussed below.

Molineus

Species of this trichostrongylid occur in several simian primates sometimes used in the laboratory (Dunn 1961).

Molineus torulosus occurs in the small intestine of capuchins, squirrel monkeys, and night monkeys in Brazil (Dunn 1961, 1968). It is common in capuchins obtained from their natural habitat but absent in those raised in the laboratory (Lapin and Yakovleva 1960). It inhabits the small intestine and causes a hemorrhagic, ulcerative enteritis (Lapin and Yakovleva 1960).

Molineus vexillarius occurs in the stomach and small intestine of tamarins in Peru. It is common in specimens obtained from their natural habitat, with an incidence of 95% reported (Cosgrove, Nelson, and Gengozian 1968), but it is absent in those raised in the laboratory (Deinhardt et al. 1967). It is apparently nonpathogenic (Dunn 1961, 1968).

Molineus elegans occurs in the small intestine of squirrel monkeys and capuchins in Brazil and *M. vogelianus* in pottos *(Perodicticus)* in Africa (Dunn 1961, 1968). The relative frequency and pathogenicity of these species are unknown.

MORPHOLOGY

Adults are small, slender, pale red worms (Dunn 1961; Yorke and Maplestone 1926). The male is 3.0 to 4.8 mm long, and the female 3.2 to 5.3 mm long. The egg is ellipsoidal and measures 40 to 52 μ by 20 to 29 μ (Fig. 7.15).

LIFE CYCLE

The life cycle is unknown, but transmission probably requires the ingestion of infective larvae.

PATHOLOGIC EFFECTS

Only *M. torulosus,* which causes hemorrhages and necrotic ulcers in the intestinal wall and diverticula (Lapin and Yakovleva 1960), is known to be pathogenic.

DIAGNOSIS

Diagnosis is based on demonstration of eggs in the feces or adult worms in the intestine or stomach at necropsy.

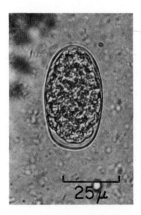

Fig. 7.15. *Molineus vexillarius* egg. (Courtesy of G. E. Cosgrove, Oak Ridge National Laboratory.)

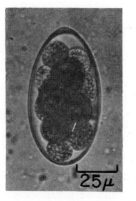

Fig. 7.16. *Trichostrongylus,* presumably *T. colubriformis,* egg. (Courtesy of Bonny F. Rininger, Bionetics Research Laboratories.)

CONTROL

Control has not been described, but sanitation and good management are apparently sufficient. Laboratories that have experienced heavy infections in newly acquired specimens report a decline in incidence with time and an absence of the parasite in laboratory-reared specimens (Cosgrove, Nelson, and Gengozian 1968; Deinhardt et al. 1967; Lapin and Yakovleva 1960).

PUBLIC HEALTH CONSIDERATIONS

Nothing is known of the public health aspects of this nematode.

Trichostrongylus colubriformis

This trichostrongylid, a common parasite of the small intestine of ruminants, occurs throughout the world (Soulsby 1965). It also affects wild rodents and lagomorphs, the dog, macaques, baboons, the chimpanzee, domestic animals, and man (Faust, Beaver, and Jung 1968; Lapage 1962, 1968; Levine 1968). It is rare in the dog but apparently common in monkeys and apes (Lapin and Yakovleva 1960). The exact incidence in laboratory primates is unknown because species identification is seldom made; however, incidences of 18 to 69% of *Trichostrongylus,* presumably *T. colubriformis,* have been reported in the rhesus monkey (Lapin and Yakovleva 1960; Reardon and Rininger 1968; Valerio et al. 1969).

MORPHOLOGY

Adults are delicate and threadlike and lack a buccal capsule and dental apparatus

(Faust, Beaver, and Jung 1968). The male is 4.5 to 5.0 mm long and the female 5.0 to 7.0 mm (Lapage 1968). The egg measures 75 to 86 μ by 34 to 45 μ and is usually in the 16- to 32-cell stage when passed in the feces (Fig. 7.16).

LIFE CYCLE

The life cycle is direct. Eggs passed in the feces embryonate and hatch in about 24 hours and reach the infective larval stage in about 3 to 4 days (Faust, Beaver, and Jung 1968). Infection is by ingestion of the infective larvae; the prepatent period is about 3 weeks.

PATHOLOGIC EFFECTS

Little is known of the effects of this parasite on laboratory animals. Light infections are inapparent in man, but heavy infections cause diarrhea and eosinophilia (Faust, Beaver, and Jung 1968). Laboratory monkeys and apes are probably similarly affected.

DIAGNOSIS

Diagnosis depends on the identification of the eggs in the feces or the adult parasites in the small intestine.

CONTROL

Sanitation and good management are probably effective in preventing the dissemination of this parasite. Because eggs passed in the feces can develop into infective larvae in as little as 3 days, the frequent removal of feces from cages and pens is important. Newly acquired animals should be examined on arrival and treated, if infected. Thiabendazole, 100 mg per kg of body weight given in a single dose and repeated in 2 weeks, is an effective treatment for the monkey (Valerio et al. 1969).

Since this parasite is sometimes pathogenic for man (Faust, Beaver, and Jung 1968), it is important that laboratory personnel be instructed in proper methods for handling infected animals and feces.

Graphidium strigosum
(Rabbit Strongyle)

This nematode occurs in the stomach of the domestic rabbit, cottontail rabbit, and hares in North America, Europe, and Australia (Enigk 1938; Hall 1916; Lapage 1968; Levine 1968). It is common in wild lagomorphs and is frequently encountered in domestic rabbits raised under conditions of poor sanitation and where wild rabbits and hares have access (Cushnie 1954). It is rare or absent in laboratory rabbits raised in facilities with good management and sanitation (Adams, Aitken, and Worden 1967).

MORPHOLOGY

Adults have a red body with many longitudinal lines and fine, transverse striations (Levine 1968). The male is 8 to 16 mm long, and the female 11 to 20 mm. The egg measures 98 to 106 μ by 50 to 58 μ (Fig. 7.17).

LIFE CYCLE

The life cycle is direct (Cushnie 1954). Eggs passed in the feces embryonate in 24 hours, hatch in another 8 to 10 hours, and then develop into infectious larvae in 4 to 6 days. Infection is by ingestion of the infective larva. When ingested, it develops rapidly in the stomach and reaches maturity in about 12 days. The average life of an adult is about 6 months.

PATHOLOGIC EFFECTS

The parasite inhabits the stomach, but whether it burrows into the mucosa and sucks blood (Neveu-Lemaire 1936) or whether it lives free in the lumen and only ingests gastric secretions (Enigk 1938) is uncertain. Light infections apparently cause few or no signs or lesions (Cushnie 1954; Lapage 1968). Heavy infections are said to cause destruction of the gastric mucosa, diarrhea, anemia, emaciation, and sometimes death (Adams, Aitken, and Worden 1967; Cushnie 1954; Lapage 1968).

DIAGNOSIS

Diagnosis is based on identification of the eggs in the feces or the adult worms in the stomach (Adams, Aitken, and Worden 1967).

CONTROL

Sanitation and the elimination of infected rabbits are the primary methods of control (Cushnie 1954). Because eggs passed in the feces do not develop into infectious larvae for 5 to 7 days, frequent and complete cleaning of cages and pens will prevent the spread of the parasite in the laboratory colony. Phenothiazine given orally (dosage not given) is suggested for treatment (Adams, Aitken, and Worden 1967).

This parasite is not known to affect man.

Nematospiroides dubius

This nematode is widely distributed among wild rodents in North America and Europe (Lepak, Thatcher, and Scott 1962; Levine 1968; Lewis 1968a, b). It does not occur naturally in laboratory rodents but is important because experimental infections are frequently used to study host-parasite relationships (Dobson 1961a, b, c, 1962a, b; Lepak, Thatcher, and Scott 1962) and to screen anthelmintics (Dobson 1961a; Thompson, Worley, and McClay 1962).

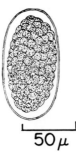

Fig. 7.17. *Graphidium strigosum* egg. (From Soulsby 1968. Courtesy of Baillière, Tindall and Cassell.)

50 μ

Nippostrongylus brasiliensis

(SYN. *Nippostrongylus muris,*
Heligmosomum muris)

This trichostrongylid is common in the small intestine of the Norway rat throughout the world (Haley 1961; Levine 1968; Sasa et al. 1962). It also occurs naturally, but much less frequently, in the black rat and rarely in the mouse. Experimental hosts in which the parasite will attain sexual maturity are the mouse, hamster, cotton rat, mongolian gerbil, rabbit, and chinchilla. The parasite does not occur naturally in laboratory rodents (Habermann and Williams 1958; Sasa et al. 1962), and its primary importance is its frequent use in studies of host-parasite relations, especially in immunology (Chandler 1939; Haley 1962; Jarrett, Jarrett, and Urquhart 1968a, b; Kassai and Aitken 1967; Ogilvie 1967; Ogilvie and Hockley 1968; Spindler 1936; Wilson and Bloch 1968), and in tests of new anthelmintics (Haley 1962; McGuire, O'Neill, and Brody 1966). It could, however, become a problem if used in an animal facility that practices poor sanitation and management.

MORPHOLOGY

Adult worms are filiform; the female is 2.5 to 6.2 mm long (Fig. 7.18*A*) and the male 2.1 to 4.5 mm (Fig. 7.18*B*) (Haley 1961). The egg is ellipsoidal and thin shelled and measures 52 to 63 μ by 28 to 35 μ (Fig. 7.18*C*).

LIFE CYCLE

The life cycle is direct. Eggs passed in the feces hatch within 24 hours and develop into infective larvae in another 3 to 4 days (Haley 1962). Infection is normally by larval penetration of the skin, but intradermal inoculation is the usual technique for experimental infection. The larvae migrate through the lungs and then, by way of the trachea, esophagus, and stomach, to the small intestine. Eggs are passed in the feces after 6 days, and adults live from a few weeks to several months.

PATHOLOGIC EFFECTS

Light infections cause an inflammation of the skin, lungs, and intestine which sub-

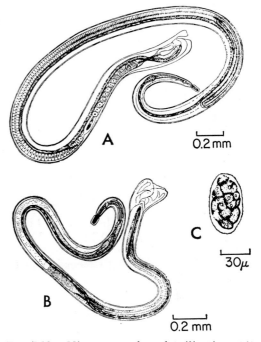

FIG. 7.18. *Nippostrongylus brasiliensis.* (*A*) Female. (*B*) Male. (*C*) Egg. (Courtesy of W. Taliaferro, Argonne National Laboratory.)

sides after a few days (Haley 1962). Severe infections cause verminous pneumonia and death.

DIAGNOSIS

Diagnosis depends on identification of the eggs in feces or adult worms in the intestine.

CONTROL

The parasite is controlled by sanitation and good management. Contaminated cages and water bottles should be effectively sanitized before being used for noninfected animals, and feces from cages of infected animals should not be permitted to contaminate cages of noninfected animals.

PUBLIC HEALTH CONSIDERATIONS

This nematode does not affect man.

Nochtia nochti

This nematode occurs in the stomach of the rhesus and cynomolgus monkeys and the stumptail macaque in India, Indonesia, and Thailand (Ruch 1959; Smetana and Orihel 1969; Yamashita 1963). Although usually rarely recognized, it was found in 4.9% of one group of over 1,200 cynomolgus monkeys (Hashimoto and Honjo 1966) and in 16 (33%) of 48 stumptail macaques (Smetana and Orihel 1969) examined for helminths at necropsy. The parasite is important because it causes a unique, neoplastic response in the host (Bonne and Sandground 1939; Graham 1960; Ruch 1959).

MORPHOLOGY

Adults are bright red and filiform (Bonne and Sandground 1939). The male is 5.7 to 6.5 mm long by 100 to 140 μ wide; the female is 7.6 to 9.9 mm by 150 to 170 μ. The egg is thin shelled and ellipsoidal and measures 60 to 80 μ by 35 to 42 μ.

LIFE CYCLE

The life cycle is direct (Bonne and Sandground 1939). Eggs laid by the female embryonate in about 12 hours, hatch soon afterward, and reach the infective larval stage in about 5 to 6 days. The method of infection is uncertain but is presumed to be by ingestion.

PATHOLOGIC EFFECTS

Nochtia nochti causes the formation of apparently benign tumors which appear as hyperemic, cauliflowerlike masses that protrude from the gastric wall at the junction of the fundus and pylorus (Fig. 7.19) (Smetana and Orihel 1969). Several worms with many eggs are found deep within each tumor, usually in the submucosa. No worms occur free in the stomach, and no tumors are produced elsewhere.

DIAGNOSIS

Diagnosis is based on recognition of gastric tumors containing *N. nochti* at necropsy.

CONTROL

Nothing is known of control, but it is probable that sanitation and good management are effective.

PUBLIC HEALTH CONSIDERATIONS

Nothing is known of the public health aspects of this nematode.

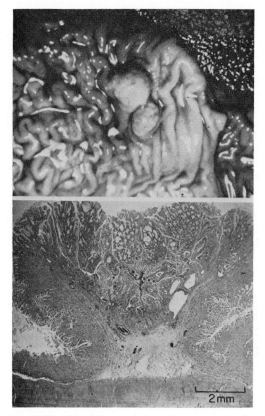

FIG. 7.19. *Nochtia nochti* in the stomach of a monkey. *(Top)* Tumor produced by parasite. *(Bottom)* Photomicrograph of tumor. *(Top* courtesy of H. F. Smetana and T. C. Orihel, Tulane University. *Bottom* from Graham 1960; courtesy of New York Academy of Sciences.)

Ollulanus tricuspis

This minute nematode occurs in the stomach of the cat, other carnivores, and the pig (Bearup 1960; Levine 1968; Soulsby 1965). It also occurs in the mouse, but this appears to be an abnormal host or transport host as development in this species is not completed (Heston 1941). It has been recognized in the cat in Canada, many parts of Europe, South Africa, Australia, and Taiwan. The incidence in the cat varies from rare or absent in some areas to 6% in Australia and 11% in southwestern Great Britain (Wales).

MORPHOLOGY

The male is 0.7 to 0.8 mm long and 35 μ wide and has stout spicules; the fe-

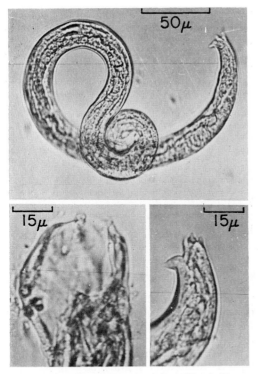

FIG. 7.20. *Ollulanus tricuspis.* *(Top)* Young female. *(Bottom)* Posterior ends of adult male *(left)* and adult female *(right).* (From Burrows 1965. Courtesy of Yale University Press.)

male is 0.8 to 1.0 mm long and 40 μ wide (Fig. 7.20) (Lapage 1968; Levine 1968).

LIFE CYCLE

The female is ovoviviparous. Larvae develop within the uterus to the infective third stage. The infective larvae are passed by emesis; infection is by ingestion of the vomitus.

PATHOLOGIC EFFECTS

The effects of infection are usually inapparent and are recognized only at necropsy (Bearup 1960; Soulsby 1965). The worms in the stomach cause increased mucus secretion and in heavy infection, hemorrhagic gastritis.

DIAGNOSIS

Diagnosis is based on recognition of the parasite, in association with gastritis, at necropsy. Infective larvae are not passed in the feces.

CONTROL

In areas where the parasite is common, dissemination of the infection can be prevented by housing cats individually. There is no treatment (Soulsby 1965).

PUBLIC HEALTH CONSIDERATIONS

This parasite is not known to affect man.

METASTRONGYLIDS

Metastrongylids have a small rudimentary mouth or none at all, generally require an intermediate host, and are usually found in the lungs of mammals (Levine 1968). Those which occur in endothermal laboratory animals are listed in Table 7.5. The most important are discussed below.

Aelurostrongylus abstrusus

(Cat Lungworm)

This pulmonary parasite is common in some parts of North America, Hawaii, South America, Europe, southwest Asia, northern Africa, and Australia (Levine 1968; Soulsby 1965). The cat appears to be the only definitive host; wild mice and other rodents are often transport hosts. Incidences of 9% in Scotland and 26% in Israel have been reported in the cat (Soulsby 1965). Although the incidence in the United States is reported to be 2%, it is suspected that the parasite is commoner but often not recognized (Renaux 1964). *Aelurostrongylus abstrusus* is likely to occur in laboratory cats obtained from pounds in endemic areas but not in cats raised in the laboratory or in catteries that practice good management and sanitation (Morris 1963). Laboratory or commercially produced rodents are not naturally infected.

MORPHOLOGY

The female is about 9 mm long, and the male 4 to 7 mm (Soulsby 1965). The female vulva lies anterior to the anus, and the tail ends bluntly; male spicules are subequal. The egg measures 80 by 70 μ. The first-stage larva passed in the feces is 360 to 400 μ long by 20 μ wide and has an undulating tail and dorsal spine (Fig. 7.21).

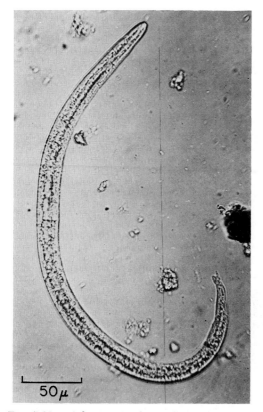

FIG. 7.21. *Aelurostrongylus abstrusus* larva. (From Burrows 1965. Courtesy of Yale University Press.)

LIFE CYCLE

Eggs passed by adult worms hatch in the lungs and the larvae pass up the trachea, down the intestinal tract, and out in the feces (Hobmaier and Hobmaier 1935). Snails and slugs are the intermediate hosts, but the cat is probably infected by ingesting transport hosts, such as wild mice, other rodents, birds, amphibians, and reptiles. The ingested larvae are liberated in the intestine, penetrate the mucosa, and migrate to the lungs. Adult worms are found in the alveolar ducts and terminal bronchioles 8 to 9 days after infection. Egg laying begins about 4 weeks after infection, and first-stage larvae are found in the feces in about 6 weeks. Adults live as long as 9 months.

PATHOLOGIC EFFECTS

Clinical signs are usually absent (Soulsby 1965). A chronic cough accompanied by progressive dyspnea, anorexia, and emaciation sometimes develops in heavy infections.

Typical gross lesions consist of gray nodules, 1 to 10 mm in diameter, either scattered over the surface of the lungs or arranged in clusters (Soulsby 1965). The nodules, when incised, exude a milky fluid which contains many eggs and larvae (Hamilton 1963; Poynter 1966). Mature worms are found at the terminal parts of the bronchioles. In microscopic sections, the embryonating eggs and larvae are seen in the alveoli, alveolar ducts, and bronchioles (Fig. 7.22) (Smith and Jones 1966). Lesions in the wild mouse and other rodents consist of larval cysts, usually in the omentum.

DIAGNOSIS

Diagnosis in the living animal is based on the respiratory signs, should they be present, and is confirmed by demonstration of the first-stage larvae in the feces (Soulsby 1965). Diagnosis at necropsy is based on the demonstration and identification of eggs and larvae in smears made from the typical pulmonary lesions.

CONTROL

Since the transmission of the disease requires the ingestion of a mollusk or a transport host, dissemination of the infection is unlikely in a clean, well-managed research animal facility. Newly acquired animals with larvae in the feces should be eliminated. Sodium iodide, 2.5 ml of a 20% solution given intravenously twice, with a 5-day interval, or methyridine, 200 mg per kg of body weight given subcutaneously, is an effective treatment (Choquette 1966). Tetramisole, given orally at a rate of 30 mg per kg of body weight every other day for about six doses, is also effective (Hamilton 1967, 1968). However, care must be taken since the margin of safety of this drug is narrow.

PUBLIC HEALTH CONSIDERATIONS

This nematode has not been reported from man.

Filaroides osleri

Filaroides osleri, a parasite that produces hemorrhagic or granular, wartlike nodules in the trachea and bronchi of the

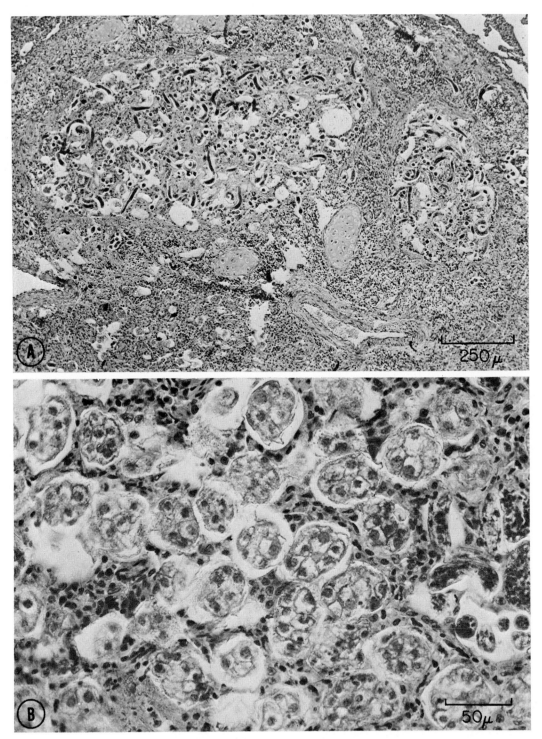

Fig. 7.22. *Aelurostrongylus abstrusus* in the lung of a cat. *(A)* Larvae in a small bronchus. *(B)* Clusters of embryonating eggs in the alveoli and larva in an alveolar duct. (From Smith and Jones 1966. Courtesy of Lea and Febiger and Armed Forces Institute of Pathology, Neg. No. 260957-2 and 260957-3.)

dog and other canids, has been reported in North and Central America, Hawaii, Europe, India, South Africa, Australia, and New Zealand (Levine 1968; Mills 1967; Soulsby 1965). It is regularly encountered in many parts of the world and is frequently reported in the United States, southern Canada, the British Isles, and South Africa. Although it has not been reported in the laboratory dog, it is likely to be encountered in specimens obtained from pounds. Because the life cycle probably involves an intermediate mollusk host, the parasite is not likely to occur in laboratory- or kennel-reared dogs.

MORPHOLOGY

The male is 5.6 to 7.0 mm long, and the female 10.0 to 13.5 mm (Mills 1967). The buccal cavity is poorly developed. The posterior end of the male is round, blunt, and almost nonbursate; the spicules are slightly unequal. The vulva and anus of the female are adjacent to one another in a cleft near the posterior end. The female is ovoviviparous; the uterus extends ante-

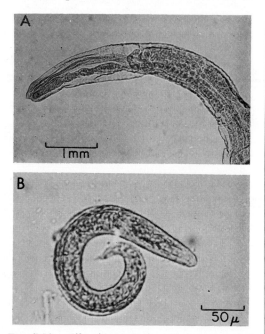

FIG. 7.23. *Filaroides osleri.* (*A*) Anterior end of adult female. Note embryonated eggs in the uterus. (*B*) First-stage larva. (From Mills and Nielsen 1966. Courtesy of American Veterinary Medical Association.)

riorly to the esophagus and is filled with embryonated eggs (Fig. 7.23*A*) which measure 80 by 50 μ. The larva passed in the feces measures up to 400 μ in length (Fig. 7.23*B*).

LIFE CYCLE

The complete life cycle is unknown. Larvae laid by the female pass up the trachea to the mouth and are swallowed and passed in the feces. Although there is some experimental evidence favoring direct infection by larvae (Urquhart, Jarrett, and O'Sullivan 1954), the findings are inconclusive (Oldham 1954). Because other species of *Filaroides* utilize slugs and land snails as intermediate hosts (Dubnitski 1955), it is reasonable to assume that this species also does (Mills 1967; Soulsby 1965), although the possibility remains of either direct infection by larvae or indirect transmission through mollusk and rodent transport hosts (Seneviratna 1959c).

PATHOLOGIC EFFECTS

The primary sign is a chronic, rasping cough (Soulsby 1965). Other signs depend on the severity of the infection. Young dogs are most acutely affected and sometimes develop respiratory distress, anorexia, and emaciation.

The gray-white, wartlike submucosal nodules range in size up to 18 mm in diameter and commonly occur at the bifurcation of the trachea (Fig. 7.24) (Poynter 1966; Urquhart, Jarrett, and O'Sullivan 1954). The nodules are usually transparent and the worms within clearly visible.

DIAGNOSIS

A diagnosis can be made in the living animal by demonstration of the typical larvae in the feces; however, even in severe infections, the number of larvae present may be small (Soulsby 1965). A more direct method is by bronchoscopic examination (Mills and Nielsen 1966). Diagnosis at necropsy is based on the demonstration of the parasite in the characteristic nodular lesions.

CONTROL

Since the life cycle probably involves the ingestion of a mollusk intermediate host, dissemination of the infection is un-

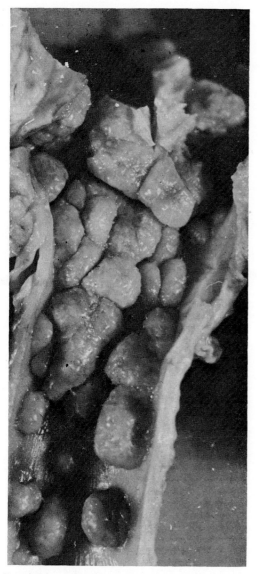

Fig. 7.24. *Filaroides osleri* lesions in the trachea of a dog. (From Mills and Nielsen 1966. Courtesy of American Veterinary Medical Association.)

likely in a research animal facility that practices good sanitation and management. Newly acquired animals with larvae in the feces should be eliminated. Arsenamide, 0.2 ml of a 1% solution per kg of body weight given intravenously daily for 21 days, appears to be the most effective treatment (Dietrich 1962).

PUBLIC HEALTH CONSIDERATIONS

This nematode has not been reported from man.

HETERAKIDS, ASCARIDIDS

These are the heterakid cecal worms, the large intestinal ascarids, and related nematodes (Levine 1968). Those that occur in endothermal laboratory animals are listed in Table 7.6. The most important are discussed below.

Heterakis spumosa

This apparently nonpathogenic nematode is common in the cecum and colon of wild Norway and black rats throughout the world (Levine 1968; Sasa et al. 1962; Smith 1953a, b, c), but it is rare in the laboratory rat (Habermann and Williams 1958; Oldham 1967). It does not occur in cesarean-derived, barrier-maintained colonies (Foster 1963).

MORPHOLOGY

Adult worms have three small lips and a cylindrical esophagus that swells posteriorly, ending in a distinct bulb (Oldham 1967). The male is 6.4 to 9.8 mm long by 200 to 260 μ in diameter; the female is 7 to 13 mm by 680 to 740 μ (Ratcliffe 1949). The egg has a thick, mammillated shell and measures 55 to 60 μ by 40 to 55 μ (Fig. 7.25A).

LIFE CYCLE

The life cycle is direct (Smith 1953c). Eggs passed in the feces embryonate in about 2 weeks. When ingested they hatch in the stomach, and the larvae migrate to the cecum and colon, where they mature in about 26 to 47 days.

PATHOLOGIC EFFECTS

No pathologic effects have been associated with this parasite.

DIAGNOSIS

Diagnosis is based on the identification of eggs in the feces or of adult worms in the large intestine.

CONTROL

Although phenothiazine, 1 g mixed with 10 ml molasses and 20 g of food, is re-

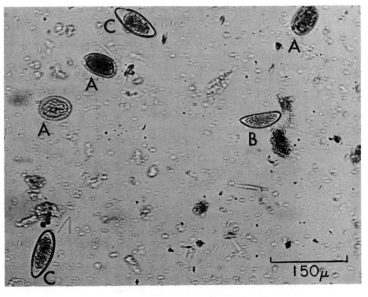

FIG. 7.25. Eggs of common nematodes of the mouse and rat. *(A)* Heterakis spumosa. *(B)* Syphacia obvelata. *(C)* Aspiculuris tetraptera. (From Habermann and Williams 1958. Courtesy of R. T. Habermann, U.S. Public Health Service.)

portedly an effective treatment (Habermann and Williams 1958), sanitation and good management should be sufficient to control this parasite as eggs passed in the feces do not embryonate for 14 days.

PUBLIC HEALTH CONSIDERATIONS

This nematode does not affect man.

Heterakis gallinarum
(Cecal Worm of Chicken)

This species is common in the ceca of the chicken and other birds throughout the world (Levine 1968; Soulsby 1965). It is relatively nonpathogenic but is important as the transport host for the pathogenic protozoan *Histomonas meleagridis,* the cause of blackhead or infectious enterohepatitis of the turkey, chicken, and other birds. *Heterakis gallinarum,* the commonest nematode of the chicken, is likely to be found in laboratory chickens reared in crowded, unsanitary outdoor pens, but not in those raised in well-managed, sanitary facilities.

MORPHOLOGY

The morphology is similar to that of *H. spumosa* (Soulsby 1965). The male is 7 to 13 mm long, and the female 10 to 17 mm (Fig. 7.26). The egg is ellipsoidal and thick shelled and measures 63 to 71 μ by 38 to 48 μ (Fig. 7.27).

LIFE CYCLE

The life cycle is direct (Levine 1968). Eggs passed in the feces embryonate in about 12 to 14 days. Birds are infected by ingestion. The eggs hatch in the crop, gizzard, or duodenum, and the larvae migrate to the ceca, where they mature in about 24 to 36 days.

PATHOLOGIC EFFECTS

No serious pathologic effects, other than its ability to transmit the agent of histomoniasis, have been ascribed to this nematode (Morgan and Hawkins 1949).

DIAGNOSIS

Diagnosis is based on identification of eggs in the feces or adult worms in the ceca.

CONTROL

Control is the same as for *H. spumosa* (Soulsby 1965). The dosage of phenothiazine for the chicken is 0.5 to 1.0 g per chicken per day. Coumaphos given in the food at a rate of 40 ppm for 10 days is also effective (Eleazer 1969).

PUBLIC HEALTH CONSIDERATIONS

This nematode does not affect man.

Paraspidodera uncinata
(Cecal Worm of Guinea Pig)

This is the only important helminth of the guinea pig (Levine 1968; Morgan and

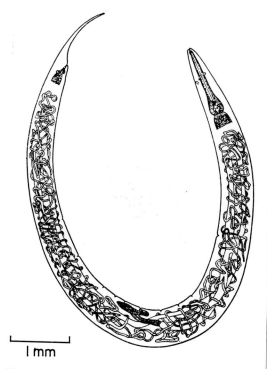

FIG. 7.26. *Heterakis gallinarum* female. (From Lapage 1968. Courtesy of Oliver and Boyd.)

Hawkins 1949). It occurs naturally in the cecum and colon of the wild guinea pig in South America and in the laboratory guinea pig throughout the world. It is uncommon in the United States, although occasional occurrences have been reported (Herlich 1959; Herlich and Dixon 1965; Porter and Otto 1934). It is common in the British Isles (Owen 1968). Guinea pigs reared in well-managed, sanitary facilities are unlikely to be infected (Habermann and Williams 1958). The parasite does not occur in cesarean-derived, barrier-maintained colonies (Calhoon and Matthews 1964; Morris 1963; Wills 1968).

MORPHOLOGY

The male is 16.3 to 17.6 mm long, and the female 18.4 to 20.9 mm (Herlich and Dixon 1965). The egg is ellipsoidal, 43 by 31 μ, and similar to that of *Heterakis gallinarum* (Fig. 7.26) (Habermann and Williams 1958).

LIFE CYCLE

The life cycle is direct (Herlich and Dixon 1965; Morgan and Hawkins 1949). Eggs passed in the feces develop into the infective stage within 3 to 5 days. When ingested, they hatch and migrate to the cecum and colon, where they mature in about 45 days.

PATHOLOGIC EFFECTS

Although this nematode is usually considered nonpathogenic (Habermann and Williams 1958), weight loss, debility, and diarrhea have been attributed to heavy infection (Cook 1969).

DIAGNOSIS

Diagnosis is based on identification of eggs in the feces or adult worms in the cecum.

CONTROL

Sanitation and good management are effective controls but, as eggs passed in the

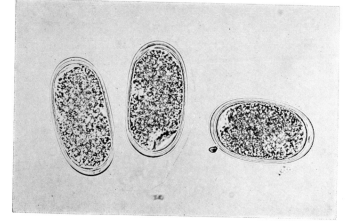

FIG. 7.27. *Heterakis gallinarum* egg. ×410. (From Benbrook and Sloss 1961. Courtesy of Iowa State University Press.)

feces can develop into the infective stage in as little as 3 days, frequent removal of feces from cages and pens is important. Treatment with phenothiazine (Habermann and Williams 1958), piperazine (Paterson 1962), or ronnel has been suggested, but none is effective (Herlich 1959). The cesarean-derivation technique is effective in eliminating this parasite (Morris 1963; Wills 1968).

PUBLIC HEALTH CONSIDERATIONS

This nematode does not affect man.

Ascaridia galli

(Large Roundworm of the Chicken)

This often debilitating parasite is common in the small intestine of the chicken and other domestic and wild birds throughout the world (Levine 1968; Wehr 1965). It is likely to be found in chickens reared in crowded, unsanitary outdoor pens, but it does not occur in laboratory chickens raised in well-managed, sanitary facilities.

MORPHOLOGY

Adults are large whitish-yellow worms (Fig. 7.28) with three prominent anterior lips, two lateral alae that run the length of the body, and no esophageal bulb (Lapage 1968; Soulsby 1965). The male is 50 to 76 mm long and has small caudal alae, 10 pairs of caudal papillae, a muscular precloacal sucker, and subequal spicules. The female is 72 to 116 mm long and has a straight,

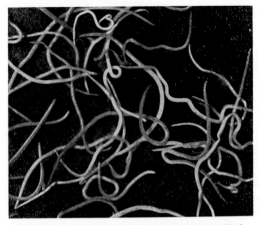

FIG. 7.28. *Ascaridia galli* from the small intestine of a chicken. (From Wehr 1965. Courtesy of Iowa State University Press.)

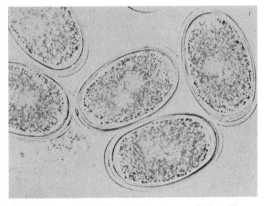

FIG. 7.29. *Ascaridia galli* eggs. ×400. (From Benbrook and Sloss 1961. Courtesy of Iowa State University Press.)

conical tail. The vulva is in the anterior part of the body. The egg is ellipsoidal, smooth, and unsegmented when passed and measures 70 to 80 μ by 45 to 50 μ (Fig. 7.29).

LIFE CYCLE

The life cycle is simple and direct (Soulsby 1965; Wehr 1965). Adults in the small intestine deposit eggs which embryonate 8 to 12 days after being passed in the feces. Infection is by the ingestion of contaminated food or water or of a mechanical transport host, such as an earthworm. Ingested eggs hatch in the proventriculus or duodenum.

The larvae remain in the intestinal lumen 6 to 9 days and then penetrate the mucosa for further development. They reenter the lumen on the 17th or 18th day and remain there until maturity. The adult stage is reached about 50 days after infection.

PATHOLOGIC EFFECTS

In severe infections in young chickens, the tissue phase of worm development causes debilitation, ruffled feathers, drooping wings, hemorrhagic diarrhea, anorexia, and reduced growth rate (Levine 1968; Soulsby 1965). Hemorrhage and inflammation of the intestinal mucosa are seen at necropsy, but adult worms are absent (Morgan and Hawkins 1949). Later, adult worms are present and, in heavy infections, sometimes cause intestinal obstruction or perforation.

Diagnosis is based on the signs and lesions and is confirmed by the identification of eggs in the feces or worms in the intestine at necropsy.

CONTROL

Piperazine adipate, given orally in the food at a dose rate of 300 to 440 mg per kg of body weight (Soulsby 1965); thiabendazole, given orally in the food at a rate of 5 g per kg of food (Wehr and Colglazier 1966); tetramisole, given orally by capsule in the food or water at a rate of 40 mg per kg of body weight (Bruynooghe, Thienpont, and Vanparijs 1968); or coumaphos, given orally in the food at a rate of 40 ppm for 10 days (Eleazer 1969), is an effective treatment but, as eggs passed in the feces do not embryonate for at least 8 days, sanitation and good management should be sufficient to control this parasite.

PUBLIC HEALTH CONSIDERATIONS

This nematode does not affect man.

Toxocara canis

This nematode occurs in the small in-

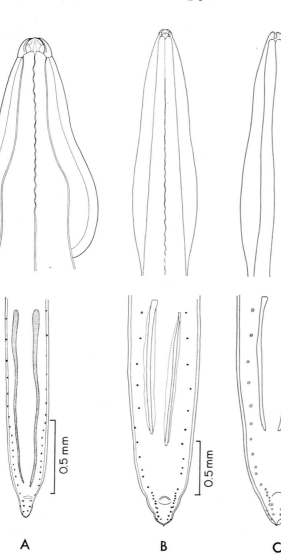

FIG. 7.30. Ascarids of the dog and cat. Ventral view. *(Top)* Anterior end. *(Bottom)* Posterior end of male. *(A) Toxocara mystax. (B) Toxocara canis. (C) Toxascaris leonina.* (From Morgan and Hawkins 1949. Courtesy of Burgess Publishing Co.)

A   B   C

testine of the dog and other canids throughout the world (Lapage 1968; Levine 1968). It is one of the two common ascarids of the dog, the other being *Toxascaris leonina*. It is an important pathogen in young dogs (Soulsby 1965) and is a common cause of visceral larva migrans in man (Faust, Beaver, and Jung 1968). Wild rodents sometimes used in the laboratory, such as ground squirrels, are often infected as paratenic hosts (Fritz, Smith, and Flynn 1968).

Laboratory dogs obtained from pounds are usually infected. Typical incidences reported in the United States are 24% in Hawaii (Ash 1962b), 36% in Michigan (Worley 1964), 22% in Louisiana (Vaughn and Murphy 1962), and 12% in dogs that were used for research in New York but were obtained from various eastern and southeastern states (Mann and Bjotvedt 1965). In the British Isles, an incidence of 21% has been reported in the London area (Woodruff, Bisseru, and Bowe 1966). *Toxocara canis* is also frequently encountered in dogs reared for the laboratory (Bantin and Maber 1967), but it is uncommon in laboratory colonies or kennels that practice good management and sanitation (Johnson, Andersen, and Gee 1963; Sheffy, Baker, and Gillespie 1961). Because infection in utero can occur, even cesarean-derived dogs are usually infected (Griesemer, Gibson, and Elsasser 1963).

The incidence in wild rodents sometimes used in the laboratory is unknown.

MORPHOLOGY

Adults are large, white worms that are curved ventrally at the anterior end and have narrow cervical alae (Fig. 7.30*B*) (Morgan and Hawkins 1949). The male is 40 to 100 mm long and has a narrow, digitiform, terminal appendage, caudal alae, and winged spicules. The female is 50 to 180 mm long and has its vulva in the anterior quarter of the body. The egg has a pitted surface, is subglobular to oval, and measures 85 by 75 μ (Fig. 7.31).

LIFE CYCLE

Transmission is usually by intrauterine infection of fetuses, but young dogs less than 3 to 5 weeks old can be infected by ingesting embryonated eggs. Mature worms develop in the intestine after larval migration by the tracheal route (Sprent 1958). Dogs over 3 to 5 weeks of age develop somatic infections only; no adults develop in the alimentary tract. Larvae in somatic tissues are activated during pregnancy, apparently by hormonal influence, and migrate to the fetus (Webster 1956). Third- and fourth-stage larvae are found in the lungs, stomach, and intestine during the first postnatal week, and adults appear in the intestine by the end of the third week (Sprent 1958). Eggs appear in the feces as early as 23 days after parturition (Douglas and Baker 1959).

Rodents infected by ingesting embry-

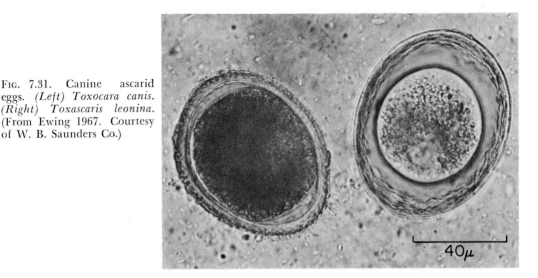

FIG. 7.31. Canine ascarid eggs. *(Left) Toxocara canis. (Right) Toxascaris leonina.* (From Ewing 1967. Courtesy of W. B. Saunders Co.)

40μ

onated eggs develop somatic infections (Sprent 1952, 1953). Whether such paratenic or transport hosts are an important source of infection for the dog is uncertain (Soulsby 1965).

Clinical signs usually occur only in young dogs (Morgan and Hawkins 1949; Soulsby 1965). The early signs are a cough and nasal discharge which usually subside after about 3 weeks. Heavy infections frequently cause vomiting. Other signs include anorexia, abdominal distention, mucoid diarrhea, debilitation, reduced growth rate, allergic pruritus, and a characteristic foul oral odor (Hoey 1968; Morgan and Hawkins 1949; Soulsby 1965). Epileptiform seizures sometimes occur and heavy infections in young dogs often cause death.

Because larvae in paratenic hosts have an affinity for the brain, the clinical signs in such hosts are usually neurologic and include hyperactivity, torticollis, opisthotonos, circling, involuntary paddling movements, debilitation, coma, and death (Fritz, Smith, and Flynn 1968).

In acute prenatal infections, migrating larvae produce lesions in the lungs (Morgan and Hawkins 1949). In light infections, these consist of petechial hemorrhages on the surface of the lung; in heavy infections, pneumonia is present. Histologically, inflammatory foci are seen throughout the lungs. Mature worms are found in the small intestine and sometimes in the stomach, bile duct, and rarely the peritoneal cavity. Mucoid enteritis is typical, and the intestine is often distended and sometimes obstructed with worms.

Often the migrating larvae are arrested in the tissues, and granulomas form around them (Fig. 7.32) (Barron and Saunders 1966). Such granulomatous lesions have been observed in the dog in a variety of tissues. Migrating larvae in rodent paratenic hosts frequently invade the brain (Fritz, Smith, and Flynn 1968). These larvae often cause no tissue reaction, but demyelination and necrosis are sometimes present (Fig. 7.33).

Diagnosis is based on demonstration of eggs in the feces, worms in the intestine

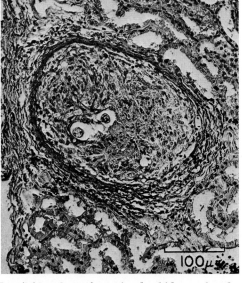

FIG. 7.32. Granuloma in the kidney of a dog with *Toxocara canis* larva in center. (From Bloom 1965. Courtesy of Charles C Thomas, Publisher.)

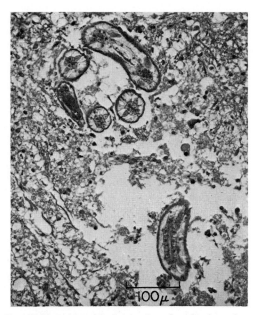

FIG. 7.33. Ascarid larva in the brain of a ground squirrel. Note demyelinization and necrosis. (From Fritz, Smith, and Flynn 1968. Courtesy of American Veterinary Medical Association.)

(Soulsby 1965), or granulomatous lesions in tissues (Barron and Saunders 1966; Fritz, Smith, and Flynn 1968).

CONTROL

Because of the intrauterine method of infection, this parasite is extremely difficult to control (Soulsby 1965). Sanitation and frequent examination and treatment will usually prevent heavy infections and will greatly reduce the incidence (Johnson, Andersen, and Gee 1963).

Newly acquired dogs should be examined on arrival and treated, if infected. Effective treatments include diethylcarbamazine given orally, 50 mg per kg of body weight in a single dose (Soulsby 1965); piperazine adipate given orally, 25 to 200 mg per kg of body weight in a single dose (Soulsby 1965); a mixture of n-butyl chloride and toluene (Nemacide, Diamond Laboratories) given orally, 0.1 ml of each drug per kg of body weight in one dose (Welter and Johnson 1963); tetramisole given orally, 7.5 to 15.0 mg per kg of body weight in a single dose (Özcan 1967); DDVP (dichlorvos; Task, Shell), 35 to 40 mg per kg of body weight given orally in a single dose (Batte and Moncol 1968); and a combination of 250 mg of thenium and 500 mg of piperazine per dog, given orally morning and evening for 1 day (Rawes and Clapham 1962).

Dogs free of *T. canis* have been obtained by raising cesarean-derived progeny in isolation and treating them orally with diethylcarbamazine, daily, for 14 to 24 months, or by maintaining bitches in isolation through several pregnancies until the larvae in their tissues are totally eliminated (Griesemer and Gibson 1963b).

There is no treatment for infected paratenic hosts.

PUBLIC HEALTH CONSIDERATIONS

Toxocara canis is a major cause of visceral larva migrans in man (Faust, Beaver, and Jung 1968; Gibson 1960; Poynter 1966; Woodruff, Bisseru, and Bowe 1966). Larvae cause granulomas in various tissues; adult worms rarely occur in the intestine (Bisseru, Woodruff, and Hutchinson 1966). Infection with this parasite, based on skin sensitivity, has also been associated with poliomyelitis and epilepsy (Woodruff, Bisseru,

and Bowe 1966). Infection is by ingestion of embryonated eggs. Persons working with laboratory dogs should be aware of these hazards and should handle infected animals and their excreta with caution. To minimize the risk, infected dogs should be treated with anthelmintics to eliminate adult worms (Faust, Beaver, and Jung 1968).

Toxocara mystax
(SYN. *Toxocara cati*)

This nematode is found in the small intestine of the cat and other felids throughout the world (Levine 1968; Sprent 1956). It is the commonest ascarid of the cat and is frequently a serious pathogen in young animals (Dubey 1966). *Toxocara mystax* is a cause of visceral larva migrans in man (Faust, Beaver, and Jung 1968). It has also been reported that eggs of this parasite can carry *Toxoplasma gondii* (Hutchison 1967). Wild rodents sometimes used in the laboratory are often infected as paratenic hosts (Fritz, Smith, and Flynn 1968).

Laboratory cats obtained from pounds or dealers are frequently infected (Scott 1967). Incidences ranging from 8 to 85% have been reported (Ash 1962b; Dubey 1966; Levine 1968; Woodruff, Bisseru, and Bowe 1966). It is uncommon in laboratory colonies that practice good management and sanitation (Morris 1963). The incidence in wild rodents sometimes used in the laboratory is unknown.

MORPHOLOGY

Adults are similar to those of *T. canis* (Morgan and Hawkins 1949). They are differentiated by their short, broad, cervical alae which end abruptly and by the long spicules of the male (Fig. 7.30A). The male is 30 to 70 mm long; the female is 40 to 120 mm long. The egg, which is smaller and more finely pitted than that of *T. canis,* measures 70 by 65 μ (Fig. 7.34).

LIFE CYCLE

The life cycle differs from that of *T. canis* in that the common method of infection is by ingestion of larvae encysted in earthworms, cockroaches, birds, rodents, and a variety of other transport hosts (Sprent 1956). Larvae derived from the tissues of the transport host develop in the alimentary tract of the cat directly, without

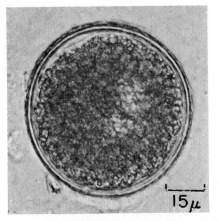

Fig. 7.34. *Toxocara mystax* egg. (From Ewing 1967. Courtesy of W. B. Saunders Co.)

undergoing a parenteral migration. Second-stage larvae enter the stomach wall and begin their final development, eventually returning to the lumen of the small intestine for the patent adult phase. Although the usual method of infection is by ingestion of larvae encysted in a transport host, infection by ingestion of embryonated eggs also sometimes occurs. Eggs passed in the feces require about 10 to 15 days to become infective. When such embryonated eggs are ingested, they hatch into larvae in the small intestine, migrate through the intestinal wall and lungs, and then return to the small intestine by way of the trachea. Larvae are sometimes found at aberrant sites in somatic tissues, but intrauterine infection does not occur.

PATHOLOGIC EFFECTS

The signs and lesions in cats are similar to those described for *T. canis* in dogs, but epileptiform seizures in young animals are commoner (Morgan and Hawkins 1949). Respiratory effects caused by larval migration through the lungs are less severe than in infections with *T. canis* (Soulsby 1965). Signs and lesions in paratenic hosts are the same as those associated with *T. canis*.

Eggs of *T. mystax* can carry the agent of toxoplasmosis (Hutchison 1967), but whether or not this is an important natural means of transmission of this agent is unknown (Frenkel, Dubey, and Miller 1969; Sheffield and Melton 1969).

DIAGNOSIS

Diagnosis is the same as described for *T. canis*.

CONTROL

Sanitation and the elimination of infected cats and transport hosts are the primary methods of control (Soulsby 1965). Because eggs passed in the feces do not become infective for 10 to 15 days, frequent and complete cleaning of cages and pens will prevent dissemination of the parasite. Newly acquired cats should be examined on arrival and treated, if infected. Treatments recommended for the cat include piperazine adipate given orally, 100 to 200 mg per kg of body weight in a single dose, and a mixture of *n*-butyl chloride and toluene (Nemacide, Diamond Laboratories) given orally, 0.1 ml of each drug per kg of body weight, in one dose (Renaux 1964). There is no treatment for infected paratenic hosts.

PUBLIC HEALTH CONSIDERATIONS

Toxocara mystax is a cause of visceral larva migrans in man (Faust, Beaver, and Jung 1968). Infection with this parasite has also been associated with poliomyelitis and epilepsy (Woodruff, Bisseru, and Bowe 1966). It has been suggested that the eggs of this nematode are an important mechanism for transmission of toxoplasmosis (Hutchison 1967), but the validity of this is uncertain. Persons working with laboratory cats should be aware of these hazards and should handle infected animals and their excreta with caution. Anthelmintic treatment of infected cats to eliminate adult worms will minimize the risk.

Toxascaris leonina

Toxascaris leonina is common in the small intestine of the dog, cat, and wild carnivores throughout the world (Levine 1968; Soulsby 1965). In heavy infections, it is a serious pathogen for young animals. Wild rodents sometimes used in the laboratory can be infected as paratenic hosts (Sprent 1959).

Dogs and cats obtained from pounds or dealers are frequently infected (Bantin and Maber 1967; Scott 1967), but the incidence, 2 to 15% (Levine 1968; Oldham 1967; Worley 1964), is lower than that for *Toxocara canis* and *T. mystax*. *Toxascaris leonina* is uncommon in laboratory dog and cat colonies that practice good management and sanitation (Johnson, Andersen, and Gee 1963; Morris 1963). It does not occur in cesarean-derived colonies (Griesemer and Gibson 1963a, b). The incidence in wild rodents sometimes used in the laboratory is unknown.

MORPHOLOGY

Adults are similar to those of *T. canis* and *T. mystax* (Morgan and Hawkins 1949). They are differentiated from *T. canis* by their straight head, from *T. mystax* by their long cervical alae, and from both species by the conical tail and heavy, wingless spicules in the male (Fig. 7.30C). The male is 20 to 70 mm long, and the female 22 to 100 mm. The egg has a smooth, nonpitted shell (Fig. 7.31) and measures 75 to 85 μ by 60 to 75 μ.

LIFE CYCLE

Eggs passed in the feces embryonate in 3 to 6 days (Soulsby 1965). Infection occurs either by ingestion of embryonated eggs or third-stage larvae encapsulated in the tissues of a paratenic host: a wild rodent, insectivore, or small carnivore (Sprent 1959). Larvae develop in the wall of the intestine and return to the lumen to mature. They do not normally migrate beyond the intestinal mucosa in the dog and cat, but in a paratenic host they sometimes enter the bloodstream and become encapsulated in various tissues. Eggs appear in the feces of the dog or cat about 74 days after infection.

PATHOLOGIC EFFECTS

The signs and lesions are similar to those of *T. canis* and *T. mystax* except that respiratory effects are not produced in the dog and cat because the larvae do not migrate through the lungs.

DIAGNOSIS

Diagnosis is the same as described for *T. canis*.

CONTROL

Sanitation and the elimination of infected dogs, cats, and transport hosts are the primary methods of control (Soulsby 1965). Because eggs passed in the feces do not become infective for 3 to 6 days, frequent and complete cleaning of cages and pens will prevent dissemination of this parasite. Newly acquired dogs and cats should be examined on arrival and treated, if infected. The agents recommended for *T. canis* and *T. mystax* are also effective for this ascarid.

PUBLIC HEALTH CONSIDERATIONS

It is assumed that *T. leonina* causes visceral larva migrans (Soulsby 1965). For this reason, infected animals should be handled with caution.

SUBULURIDS

The subulurids that occur in endothermal laboratory animals are listed in Table 7.7. Most are uncommon and none is important in laboratory animals.

OXYURIDS

These are the pinworms and related nematodes (Levine 1968). Those that occur in endothermal laboratory animals are listed in Table 7.8. The most important are discussed below.

Enterobius

Enterobius vermicularis, the common pinworm of man, has been reported in the captive chimpanzee, gibbons, and marmosets (Ruch 1959), but whether this species occurs in simian primates in their natural habitat is dubious (Hashimoto and Honjo 1966; Ruch 1959). Cross infection between simian primates and man occurs readily in captivity (Ruch 1959), but in nature, each genus of primate probably has its own species of parasite (Inglis 1961). These species, their hosts, and geographic distribution are listed in Table 7.8.

Pinworm infections in simian primates are usually not serious, but they are often irritating and are likely to induce aggressive behavior (Das 1965; Ruch 1959) just as they produce neurologic signs in children (Chandler and Read 1961). Animals obtained from their natural habitat are almost universally infected (Riopelle 1967; Ruch 1959), and it is probable that those raised in captivity are equally affected unless extensive efforts have been made to eliminate the parasite.

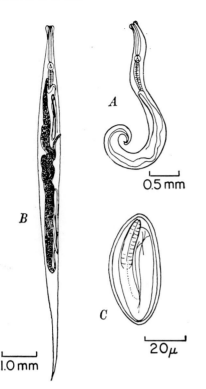

FIG. 7.35. *Enterobius vermicularis.* *(A)* Male. *(B)* Female. *(C)* Embryonated egg. (From Faust and Russell 1964. Courtesy of Lea and Febiger.)

MORPHOLOGY

The morphology of a typical species, *E. vermicularis,* is shown in Fig. 7.35 (Faust, Beaver, and Jung 1968). The male is 2.0 to 5.0 mm by 0.1 to 0.2 mm; the female is 8.0 to 13.0 mm by 0.3 to 0.5 mm. The egg is slightly flattened on one side and measures 50 to 60 μ by 20 to 30 μ.

LIFE CYCLE

The life cycle is direct (Faust, Beaver, and Jung 1968). Eggs are deposited by the adult female in the perianal or perineal region and contain fully developed larvae in 6 hours or less. Infection is by ingestion or perhaps by inhalation of infective eggs. The eggs hatch in the small intestine and reach maturity in the large intestine. The complete life cycle requires 15 to 28 days.

PATHOLOGIC EFFECTS

Perianal pruritus, restlessness, and increased aggressiveness are typical signs of infection with this parasite (Christensen 1964; Das 1965; Ruch 1959). Rarely is any enteric pathology produced even though large numbers of worms are often present in the colon at necropsy (Das 1965; Ruch 1959).

DIAGNOSIS

Diagnosis is usually made by demonstration of the adult worms emerging from the anus or by identification of eggs recovered from the perianal region with sticky cellophane tape (Faust, Beaver, and Jung 1968).

CONTROL

Control is difficult, owing to deposition of large numbers of infective eggs on the host skin and the absence of an immune response which permits repeated autoinfection or cross infection. It can be accomplished only by extreme measures of sanitation and mass treatment of all animals in a colony at the same time, or by initiating a new colony by cesarean section. Treatment of simian primates with piperazine intermittently for about a month (dosage, route, and frequency not given) (Christensen 1964); dithiazanine iodide, given twice daily for 14 days at a rate of 20 mg per kg of body weight (Mortelmans and Vercruysse 1962); DDVP (dichlorvos; Task, Shell), given orally in food at a rate of 8 to 9 mg per kg of body weight on 2 successive days (Wallach and Frueh 1968); or pyrvinium pamoate, given orally at a rate of 5 mg per kg of body weight and repeated in 14 days (Derwelis et al. 1969), is reportedly effective.

PUBLIC HEALTH CONSIDERATIONS

Not only are naturally infected primates possible sources of human infection with primate species but captive primates can acquire *E. vermicularis* from man and can thus act as reservoirs to reinfect man (Bisseru 1967).

Passalurus ambiguus

(Rabbit Pinworm)

This apparently nonpathogenic oxyurid is found, often in enormous numbers, in

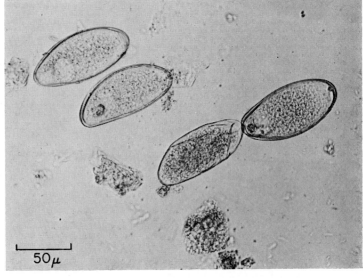

Fig. 7.36. *Passalurus ambiguus* egg. (From Habermann and Williams 1958. Courtesy of R. T. Habermann, U.S. Public Health Service.)

the cecum and colon of the rabbit, cottontail rabbit, and hares throughout the world (Lapage 1968; Levine 1968; Morgan and Hawkins 1949). It is common in the laboratory rabbit in the United States (Lund 1950; Poole et al. 1967), the British Isles (Cushnie 1954; Owen 1968), and probably throughout the world.

MORPHOLOGY

The male is 4 to 5 mm long, and the female 9 to 11 mm (Lapage 1968). Both sexes possess the typical oxyurid esophageal bulb and semitransparent body. The egg has a thin wall, is slightly flattened on one side, and measures 95 to 103 μ by 43 μ (Fig. 7.36).

LIFE CYCLE

The life cycle is direct (Boecker 1953). The egg is embryonated when laid and immediately infective. Infection is by ingestion of the embryonated egg.

PATHOLOGIC EFFECTS

No pathologic effects have been attributed to this nematode (Morgan and Hawkins 1949). Rabbits harboring as many as 3,000 adult worms develop no clinical signs. Worms are found mixed in the intestinal contents where they probably feed on bacteria. They do not ordinarily disturb the mucosa.

DIAGNOSIS

Diagnosis is made by demonstrating eggs in the feces or adult and developing worms in the cecum or colon.

CONTROL

Because eggs passed in the feces are immediately infective, control is difficult. It can be achieved only by extreme measures of sanitation and mass treatment of an entire colony or individually caged rabbits, or by initiating a new colony by cesarean section. Treatment with 1 g phenothiazine mixed with 50 g rabbit food with molasses added has been recommended (Habermann and Williams 1958), but it is not known if it is effective.

PUBLIC HEALTH CONSIDERATIONS

This nematode does not affect man.

Syphacia obvelata
(Mouse Pinworm)

This relatively nonpathogenic parasite which occurs in the cecum and, to a lesser extent, the colon, is one of the two commonest nematodes of the mouse, the other being *Aspiculuris tetraptera* (Sasa et al. 1962). Every conventional mouse colony is probably infected with this oxyurid (Hussey 1957; Owen 1968; Sasa et al. 1962; Stone and Manwell 1966) and even some cesarean-derived colonies (Flynn, Brennan, and Fritz

1965; Owen 1968). Actual incidence within a colony usually is 100% over a period of time, but the incidence observed at a specific time varies from this, depending on the diagnostic method and the age of the mice at the time of test (Sasa et al. 1962).

Although *Syphacia obvelata* has been reported from wild Norway and black rats (Ash 1962a; Sasa et al. 1962) and to be universal in laboratory rat colonies (Sasa et al. 1962), it is probable that these reports refer to *S. muris* and not to *S. obvelata* (Hussey 1957; Levine 1968).

Syphacia obvelata is also common in the laboratory hamster (Kirschenblatt 1949; Stone and Manwell 1966), the house mouse (Myers, Kuntz, and Wells 1962), and voles (Lewis 1968b; Schwentker 1957).

The monkey is susceptible to this nematode, and natural infection in the laboratory has occurred (Ruch 1959; Stone and Manwell 1966). Man is similarly susceptible and occasional natural infections are reported (Faust, Beaver, and Jung 1968; Stone and Manwell 1966).

MORPHOLOGY

Syphacia obvelata is a pointed, white, glistening worm (Fig. 7.37) (Das 1965). The male is 1.1 to 1.5 mm by 120 to 140 μ and the female 3.4 to 5.8 mm by 240 to 400 μ (Levine 1968). The mouth has three distinct lips without a buccal capsule; the esophagus has a typical oxyurid pharynx with a prebulbar swelling and a posterior, globular, valvulated bulb; small cervical alae are present (Fig. 7.38) (Oldham 1967). Three cuticular projections or mamelons are present on the ventral surface (Hussey 1957). The center mamelon of the male is near the middle of the body. The tail is long and sharply pointed. In the male, it is typically curved ventrally and about equal in length to the width of the body. It narrows abruptly behind the cloaca and has a fine terminal process. A single, slender, long spicule and a gubernaculum are present. The vulva of the female is in the anterior sixth of the body (Hussey 1957). The egg is flat on one side and measures 118 to 153 μ by 33 to 55 μ (Fig. 7.39) (Levine 1968).

LIFE CYCLE

The life cycle is direct (Chan 1952; Oldham 1967; Prince 1950; Sasa et al. 1962). The female deposits embryonated eggs within the colon and on the perianal skin. The eggs are infective in a few hours. Infection occurs in three ways: directly, by ingestion of embryonated eggs from the perianal region of an infected animal; indirectly, by ingestion of food or water contaminated with embryonated eggs; and by retroinfection, when eggs hatch in the peri-

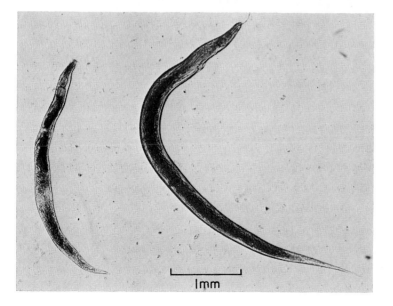

FIG. 7.37. The two commonest nematodes of the mouse. *(Left) Aspiculuris tetraptera* female. *(Right) Syphacia obvelata* female. (From Habermann and Williams 1958. Courtesy of R. T. Habermann, U.S. Public Health Service.)

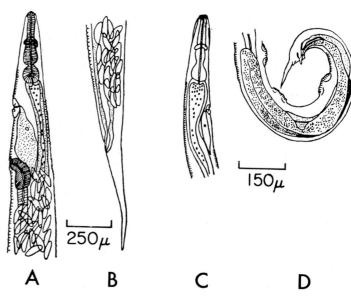

FIG. 7.38. *Syphacia obvelata.* (A) Female, head. (B) Female, tail. (C) Male, head. (D) Male, tail. (From Sasa et al. 1962. Courtesy of Academic Press.)

anal region and the larvae migrate back into the colon by way of the anus.

PATHOLOGIC EFFECTS

No specific clinical signs appear even in heavy infections (Hoag 1961). It has been suggested that infection affects weight

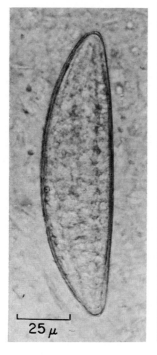

FIG. 7.39. *Syphacia obvelata* egg. (From Stone and Manwell 1966. Courtesy of W. B. Stone, State University of New York, Syracuse.)

gain, growth rate, and general health (Cook 1969; Hoag and Meier 1966), but no controlled studies to support these suggestions have been reported.

Although no specific enteric lesions have been attributed to this parasite (Habermann and Williams 1958), various disorders of the intestine have been associated with heavy infections (Harwell and Boyd 1968; Hoag 1961; Hoag and Meier 1966; Tuffery and Innes 1963). These include impaction, intussusception, and rectal prolapse. There is one report of the recovery of *S. obvelata* from the brain of a hamster (de Roever-Bonnet and Rijpstra 1961).

DIAGNOSIS

Diagnosis is based on demonstration of eggs in the feces or perianal region or of adult worms in the cecum and colon at necropsy (Sasa et al. 1962). Dependability of the different diagnostic methods varies widely. In one study, demonstration of adult worms in the intestine was the most dependable method (80.8% positive), demonstration of the eggs in the perianal region by cellophane tape the next most dependable (67.1% positive), and demonstration of eggs in fecal smears the least dependable (3.2% positive) (Sasa et al. 1962). The age of the host at the time of examination is also important. In a study using the perianal examination method, the positive rate at 3 weeks was 30% and at 4 weeks 100% (Sasa et al. 1962). Thereafter the infection rate diminished with age to 80% at 5 weeks and only 15% at 7 weeks. In another study, using a flotation technique for the examination of feces, an 80% rate of infection at 1 to 3 months of age decreased to 1% at 8 to 10 months of age (Flynn et al. 1966).

Syphacia obvelata is differentiated from *S. muris* on the basis of egg size, adult length, position of excretory pore in both sexes, position of vulva in the female, tail length, and position of the anterior and middle mamelons in the male (Hussey 1957). It is differentiated from *A. tetraptera* by size and shape of the egg, shape of the esophageal bulb, size of cervical alae, position of vulva in the female, and size and presence or absence of a spicule or gubernaculum in the male (Sasa et al. 1962).

CONTROL

Eradication of *S. obvelata* is extremely difficult. The cesarean-derivation technique is effective (Foster 1963), but reinfection is common (Flynn, Brennan, and Fritz 1965; Owen 1968). Likely sources of reinfection are egg-contaminated dust (Hoag 1961; Hoag and Meier 1966) and wild rodents (Cook 1969).

Complete control without cesarean derivation is doubtful. Frequent cage cleaning has little effect because eggs are deposited on the perianal skin and hair (Sasa et al. 1962). Many drugs are reportedly effective in removing adult worms, but often they are less efficient in eliminating immature forms (Cook 1969). Thus repeated anthelmintic treatment is necessary (Sasa et al. 1962). An entire room must be treated at one time and rigid procedures instituted to remove contamination from cages and equipment and to eliminate egg-contaminated dust (Hoag 1961; Hoag and Meier 1966). Treatment should also include concurrent washing of the perianal region of all animals with a detergent solution (Wagner 1970).

Drugs reported to be effective include piperazine adipate, given orally in the drinking water at a rate of 4 to 7 mg per ml of water for 3 to 10 days (Habermann and Williams 1957b, 1958, 1963; McPherson 1966); dithiazanine iodide, given orally

in the food at a rate of 0.1 mg per g of food for 7 days (McCowen, Callender, and Brandt 1957); stilbazium iodide, given orally in the food at a rate of 0.1 mg per g of food for 2 days (Hunt and Burrows 1963); trichlorfon combined with atropine (Freed, Ft. Dodge), given orally in the drinking water at a rate of 1.75 mg per ml of water for 14 days (Simmons, Williams, and Wright 1965); pyrvinium pamoate, given orally in the water at a rate of 0.8 mg per liter of water or in the food at a rate of 1.6 mg per kg of food for 30 days (Blair, Thompson, and Vandenbelt 1968); and DDVP (dichlorvos; Task, Shell), given orally in the food at a rate of 0.5 mg per g of food for 1 day (Wagner 1970).

PUBLIC HEALTH CONSIDERATIONS

Syphacia obvelata sometimes infects man (Faust, Beaver, and Jung 1968; Stone and Manwell 1966). Although natural infections are uncommon, persons working with laboratory rodents should be aware of this possibility and should handle infected animals and their excreta with caution.

Syphacia muris
(Rat Pinworm)

This is the common oxyurid of the rat (Hussey 1957). Because it is very similar to *Syphacia obvelata* and has been confused with this species for many years, its incidence and geographic distribution are uncertain (Levine 1968). However, it appears that it is present in most conventional rat colonies throughout the world (Hagen et al. 1968; Hussey 1957; Sasa et al. 1962; Stahl 1961) and in some cesarean-derived colonies (Bell 1968; Owen 1968). It is common in wild Norway and black rats (Ash 1962a; Sasa et al. 1962). Infection with *S. muris* in the mouse is uncommon and usually occurs only in laboratories where mice are kept in the same room with rats (Hussey 1957). It is not known if *S. muris* affects man, but the possibility has been suggested (Stone and Manwell 1966).

MORPHOLOGY

Syphacia muris is very similar to *S. obvelata* (Hussey 1957; Levine 1968). The male is 1.2 to 1.3 mm long and 100 μ wide. The tail is thin and about twice as long as the body width. The anterior mamelon is

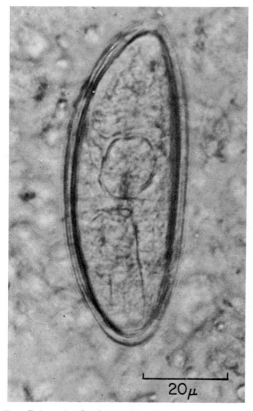

FIG. 7.40. *Syphacia muris* egg. (From Stone and Manwell 1966. Courtesy of W. B. Stone, State University of New York, Syracuse.)

near the middle of the body. The female is 2.8 to 4.0 mm long and has its vulva in the anterior quarter of the body. The egg is slightly flattened on one side and measures 72 to 82 μ by 25 to 36 μ (Fig. 7.40).

LIFE CYCLE

The life cycle appears to be identical with that of *S. obvelata* (Hussey 1957; Prince 1950; Stahl 1961).

PATHOLOGIC EFFECTS

The specific pathologic effects of this parasite are unknown, but they are probably similar to those of *S. obvelata*.

DIAGNOSIS

Diagnosis and the method of differentiating this oxyurid from other murine pinworms are the same as described for *S. obvelata* (Hussey 1957; Sasa et al. 1962).

CONTROL

The problems and methods of control are the same as for *S. obvelata*. The levels of pyrvinium pamoate recommended for the rat are 3 mg per liter in the water or 12 mg per kg in the food for 30 days (Blair and Thompson 1969).

PUBLIC HEALTH CONSIDERATIONS

Although there are no reports of *S. muris* infection in man, the possibility of such infections has been suggested (Stone and Manwell 1966). Persons working with laboratory rodents should be made aware of this potential hazard and instructed to handle infected animals with care.

Aspiculuris tetraptera

(Mouse Pinworm)

This relatively nonpathogenic oxyurid and *Syphacia obvelata* are the two commonest nematodes of the mouse (Sasa et al. 1962). *Aspiculuris tetraptera* is found in the upper colon and, to a lesser extent, in the cecum (Chan 1955; Sasa et al. 1962). It occurs in conventional mouse colonies throughout the world (Flynn, Brennan, and Fritz 1965; Sasa et al. 1962; Stone and Manwell 1966) and possibly in some cesarean-derived colonies as well (Flynn, Brennan, and Fritz 1965; Owen 1968). As with *S. obvelata*, the actual incidence within a colony over a period of time is usually 100%, but the reported incidence varies with the method of diagnosis and the age of the mice at the time of examination (Sasa et al. 1962).

Aspiculuris tetraptera occurs in the laboratory rat but is uncommon (Sasa et al. 1962). It also occurs in the house mouse, black rat, and other wild rodents throughout the world (Myers, Kuntz, and Wells 1962; Sasa et al. 1962; Yamaguti 1961).

MORPHOLOGY

Aspiculuris tetraptera (Fig. 7.36) is similar to, but readily distinguished from, *S. obvelata* (Sasa et al. 1962; Takada 1958). The esophageal bulb is oval, the esophagus club shaped, and the cuticle striated. Broad cervical alae are present; ventral mamelons are absent. The female is 3 to 4 mm long, and the vulva is in the anterior

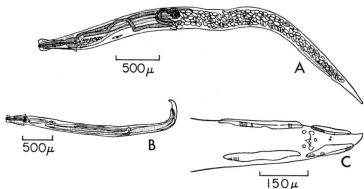

FIG. 7.41. *Aspiculuris tetraptera.* *(A)* Female. *(B)* Male. *(C)* Tail of male. (From Sasa et al. 1962. Courtesy of Academic Press.)

third of the body (Fig. 7.41*A*). The male is 2 to 4 mm long (Fig. 7.41*B*) and has a conical tail with broad caudal alae (Fig. 7.41*C*). A spicule and gubernaculum are absent. The egg is symmetrically ellipsoidal, has a thin shell, and measures 89 to 93 μ by 36 to 42 μ (Fig. 7.42).

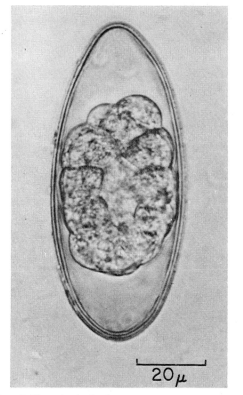

FIG. 7.42. *Aspiculuris tetraptera* egg. (From Stone and Manwell 1966. Courtesy of W. B. Stone, State University of New York, Syracuse.)

LIFE CYCLE

The life cycle is direct but distinct from that of other rodent pinworms in that the eggs are passed entirely in the feces and are not found on the perianal region of the host (Sasa et al. 1962). Furthermore, the eggs are infective only after about 6 days. Infection is by ingestion of infected eggs. Larvae develop initially in the distal portion of the colon but gradually migrate anteriorly and develop to maturity in the proximal colon (Chan 1955). Eggs appear in the feces after 23 days.

PATHOLOGIC EFFECTS

The pathologic effects associated with this pinworm are the same as those associated with *S. obvelata.*

DIAGNOSIS

Diagnosis is based on demonstration of eggs in the feces or of adult worms in the colon at necropsy (Sasa et al. 1962). The latter method is much more dependable (72.7% efficient) than the former (4.8% efficient). The cellophane-tape technique is of no value in the diagnosis of *A. tetraptera* infection as eggs of this species are not deposited in the perianal region. Age of mice at the time of the test is also important. Unlike *S. obvelata, A. tetraptera* infection is uncommon in young mice but increases in incidence with age (Sasa et al. 1962).

The method of differentiating *A. tetraptera* from other murine pinworms is the same as described for *S. obvelata* (Sasa et al. 1962).

Control of this parasite is similar to that of *S. obvelata* except that eradication is less difficult as a longer time (6 days rather than a few hours) is required before eggs passed in the feces become infective (Sasa et al. 1962). Frequent cage cleaning is effective. The cesarean-derivation technique is also effective (Foster 1963), but reinfection from egg-contaminated dust (Hoag and Meier 1966) and wild rodents (Cook 1969) is probably common (Flynn, Brennan, and Fritz 1965; Owen 1968).

Most drugs used to treat *S. obvelata* are equally effective against *A. tetraptera.*

PUBLIC HEALTH CONSIDERATIONS

This pinworm is not known to infect man (Stone and Manwell 1966).

SPIRURIDS, GNATHOSTOMATIDS, ACUARIIDS

These spirurorids are characterized by two well-developed lateral pseudolabia (Levine 1968). All require an intermediate host, usually an arthropod. Those that occur in endothermal laboratory animals are listed in Table 7.9. Most are uncommon and of little importance in laboratory specimens.

THELAZIIDS

These spirurorids are characterized by their lack of pseudolabia (Levine 1968). All require an intermediate host, usually an arthropod. Those that occur in endothermal laboratory animals are listed in Table 7.10. Only *Spirocerca lupi* and possibly *Streptopharagus armatus* and *S. pigmentatus* are important in laboratory specimens. These are discussed below.

Spirocerca lupi

(Esophageal Worm of the Dog)

This thelaziid nematode occurs in the wall of the esophagus or stomach and occasionally in other tissues of the dog and related canids in tropical and subtropical regions throughout the world (Levine 1968; Soulsby 1965). It has not been reported in the cat but occurs rarely in wild felids (Murray 1968). It is common in southern United States, with incidences usually rang-

ing from 8 to 14%, but in some local areas as high as 47% (Bailey 1963; Dodds and Garcia 1964). It is rare in northern United States (Mann and Bjotvedt 1965; Morgan and Hawkins 1949; Worley 1964) and does not occur in the British Isles (Soulsby 1965). An incidence of 18 to 32% has been reported in east central Africa (Murray 1968), 30% in India (Gupta and Pande 1962), and 43% in the Malay Peninsula (Fadzil bin Haji Yahaya 1968).

Spirocerca lupi is likely to occur in laboratory dogs obtained from pounds in areas of high incidence. It does not occur in dogs raised in the laboratory, in kennels with good management and sanitation (Johnson, Andersen, and Gee 1963), or in cesarean-derived colonies (Griesemer and Gibson 1963a).

MORPHOLOGY

Adults are bright red and usually coiled (Morgan and Hawkins 1949). The male is 30 to 54 mm long, and the female 54 to 80 mm. The egg has a thick shell and usually contains a larva when passed in the

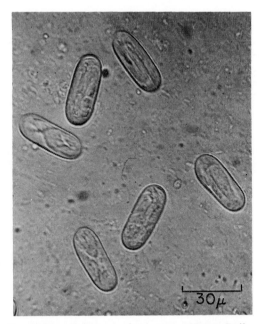

FIG. 7.43. *Spirocerca lupi* eggs. (From Bailey 1963. Courtesy of New York Academy of Sciences.)

feces (Fig. 7.43). It measures 30 to 37 μ by 11 to 15 μ.

LIFE CYCLE

The life cycle is indirect (Bailey 1963; Morgan and Hawkins 1949). Eggs are deposited into the lumen of the esophagus through a small opening and voided in the feces. Coprophagous beetles are the normal intermediate hosts, although cockroaches and many other insects have been infected experimentally. Larvae encyst in the insect and are directly infective to the final host. If the insect is ingested by an abnormal host, any of a wide variety of vertebrates, the larvae encyst in the mesentery or other tissue and remain infective. Larvae ingested by the final host penetrate the stomach, migrate in the walls of the gastric artery to the aorta, and then pass through the connective tissue to the wall of the esophagus. Eggs occur in the feces about 5 months after infection.

PATHOLOGIC EFFECTS

The adult worms usually develop in the wall of the esophagus but sometimes occur in the stomach and aorta and are occasionally found in the lungs and other tissues (Bailey 1963; Gupta and Pande 1962; Lapage 1968; Murray 1968; Soulsby 1965). They cause a granulomatous inflammatory reaction that results in a tumorlike nodular lesion. The signs produced are in proportion to the size of the nodules: small ones cause no signs whereas large pedunculated masses cause dyspnea and difficulty in swallowing. Vomiting sometimes occurs.

The characteristic nodules containing the coiled worms are seen in the esophagus and other tissues at necropsy (Fig. 7.44). The nodules, or fibrotic capsules, usually occur in the submucosa and contain, in addition to the worm, a purulent, hemorrhagic fluid. When they form in the aortic wall, they sometimes cause aneurysms which rupture and lead to fatal hemorrhage (Poynter 1966). Malignant tumors often develop at the site of the nodules either in the lumen of the esophagus or on the exterior wall. Metastasis, usually to the lungs, and hypertrophic pulmonary osteoarthropathy are frequent complications.

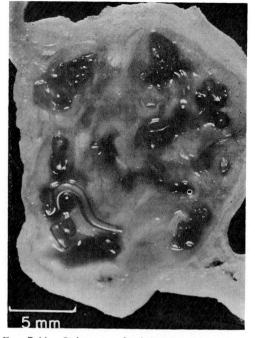

FIG. 7.44. *Spirocerca lupi* in the dog. Cross section of nodule in esophageal wall. Note adult worms. (From Bailey 1963. Courtesy of New York Academy of Sciences.)

DIAGNOSIS

Diagnosis at necropsy is based on demonstrating the parasite in the characteristic lesions (Soulsby 1965). Typical gross and histologic aortic lesions without worms or esophageal lesions are common in dogs in endemic areas and are considered presumptive evidence of spirocercosis (Murray 1968). Diagnosis in the living dog is based on clinical signs and gastroscopic or radiological examination or identification of eggs in the feces. Care must be taken to differentiate ova of *S. lupi* from those of *Physaloptera*, which are similar.

CONTROL

Since the transmission of the disease requires the ingestion of an insect or transport host, dissemination of the infection is unlikely in a research facility that practices good management and sanitation. Newly acquired animals with signs of infection or eggs in the feces should be eliminated. There is no satisfactory treatment.

PUBLIC HEALTH CONSIDERATIONS

This nematode does not affect man.

Streptopharagus armatus, Streptopharagus pigmentatus

These thelaziid nematodes occur in the stomach of monkeys and apes. *Streptopharagus armatus* occurs in the rhesus monkey, cynomolgus monkey, Japanese macaque, other macaques, guenons, patas monkey, baboons, and gibbons in the United States, Japan, and Africa. It is common in the cynomolgus monkey (10.5%) and Japanese macaque (14.3%) but uncommon in the rhesus monkey (0.5%) and other simian primates (Habermann and Williams 1957a; Tanaka et al. 1962). *Streptopharagus pigmentatus* occurs in the rhesus monkey, cynomolgus monkey, guenons, baboons, and gibbons in the United States, Europe, Africa, and Asia. It is common in the rhesus monkey (24.0%) but uncommon in the cynomolgus monkey (3.3%) and other primates (Graham 1960; Hashimoto and Honjo 1966; Reardon and Rininger 1968). Little is known of the life cycle or pathologic effects of either species. The eggs are asymmetrical, measure 28 to 38 μ by 17 to 22 μ, have a thick shell, and are embryonated when passed in the feces (Fig. 7.45) (Sasa et al. 1962).

PHYSALOPTERIDS

These spirurorids are characterized by well-developed, nonlobed pseudolabia (Levine 1968). All require an intermediate host, usually an arthropod. Those that occur in endothermal laboratory animals are listed in Table 7.11. The most important are discussed below.

Physaloptera rara, Physaloptera felidis, Physaloptera pseudopraeputialis, Physaloptera praeputialis

These nematodes occur in the stomach and duodenum of the dog, cat, and related carnivores. They are generally considered to be uncommon, but this may result from improper identification since adult worms resemble ascarids (Levine 1968; Renaux 1964).

Physaloptera rara and *P. felidis* occur in the stomach and duodenum of the dog, cat, and wild carnivores in the United States (Morgan 1946); they are common in the Midwest (Levine 1968; Morgan and Hawkins 1949; Petri 1950; Worley 1964) but uncommon or absent in other areas. *Physaloptera pseudopraeputialis* occurs in the stomach of the cat and coyote in the United States and the Philippine Islands (Levine 1968; Morgan and Hawkins 1949; Yutuc 1953). It is common in the Philippine Islands but its incidence elsewhere is unknown. *Physaloptera praeputialis* occurs in the stomach of the dog, cat, and wild felids in the United States, Hawaii, West Indies, Central America, South America, Africa, Asia, and Indonesia (Levine 1968; Soulsby 1965). It is common in Hawaii (Ash 1962b), South Africa (Fitzsimmons 1961c), Venezuela, and the Malay Peninsula (Levine 1968), but its incidence elsewhere is unknown.

These nematodes are likely to be found in laboratory dogs and cats obtained from pounds or from dealers in those areas where infection is common. They are not likely to occur in animals raised in the laboratory or obtained from kennels that practice good sanitation (Johnson, Andersen, and Gee 1963; Morris 1963), and they do not occur in cesarean-derived dogs (Griesemer and Gibson 1963a).

MORPHOLOGY

These worms are thick and muscular and resemble ascarids (Levine 1968; Morgan and Hawkins 1949; Soulsby 1965). Males measure 13 to 45 mm in length, and females 15 to 60 mm. Eggs are embryonated when passed and measure 42 to 60 μ by 29 to 42 μ (Fig. 7.46).

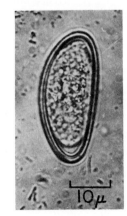

FIG. 7.45. *Streptopharagus armatus* egg. (From Tanaka et al. 1962. Courtesy of Japan Experimental Animal Research Association.)

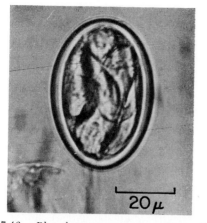

FIG. 7.46. *Physaloptera rara* egg. (From Burrows 1965. Courtesy of Yale University Press.)

LIFE CYCLE

The life cycles of these species are incompletely understood, but an arthropod intermediate host, such as a cockroach, cricket, or beetle, is always required and a second intermediate or a paratenic host may also be necessary (Soulsby 1965).

PATHOLOGIC EFFECTS

The worms firmly attach to the wall of the stomach or duodenum, feed on the mucosa, and possibly suck blood (Soulsby 1965). Early signs are vomiting and anorexia (Renaux 1964). Later signs are debilitation and dark, tarry feces. Ulcers and erosions of the gastric and intestinal mucosa are seen at necropsy.

DIAGNOSIS

Diagnosis is based on the identification of eggs in the feces or the adult worms in the stomach or duodenum.

CONTROL

Because of the need for intermediate hosts, the infection in the laboratory is self-limiting, and no control procedures other than sanitation and the elimination of possible arthropod or paratenic hosts are necessary (Soulsby 1965). Adult worms can be effectively eliminated by treatment with a mixture of *n*-butyl chloride and toluene (Nemacide, Diamond Laboratories), 0.1 ml per kg of body weight, given orally in a single dose (Renaux 1964).

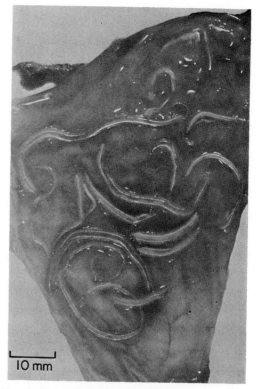

FIG. 7.47. *Abbreviata poicilometra* in the stomach of a sooty mangabey. (From Slaughter and Bostrom 1969. Courtesy of American Association for Laboratory Animal Science.)

PUBLIC HEALTH CONSIDERATIONS

The public health aspects of these parasites are unknown.

Physaloptera tumefaciens,
Physaloptera dilatata,
Abbreviata caucasica,
Abbreviata poicilometra

These physalopterids occur in the stomach of simian primates (Fig. 7.47). *Physaloptera tumefaciens* is common in macaques in Asia. In one survey of over 1,200 cynomolgus monkeys, an incidence of 27.4% was reported (Hashimoto and Honjo 1966). *Physaloptera dilatata* is found in the stomach of capuchins, woolly monkeys, and marmosets in South America (Chabaud 1954, 1955; Deinhardt et al. 1967; Yamaguti 1961). Its incidence is unknown. *Abbreviata caucasica* is found in the esophagus, stomach, and small intestine of the

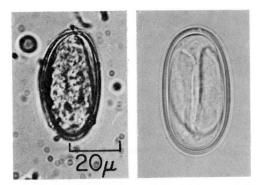

FIG. 7.48. *Physaloptera tumefaciens* egg *(left)* and *Abbreviata caucasica* egg *(right)*. *(Left* from Tanaka et al. 1962; courtesy of Japan Experimental Animal Research Association. *Right* courtesy of TSgt R. R. Estes, USAF School of Aerospace Medicine.)

rhesus monkey, baboons, orangutan, and man in southeastern Europe, southwestern Asia, and Africa (Levine 1968; Nelson 1965; Ruch 1959; Yamaguti 1961). It is common in simian primates in some areas, but rare in man. *Abbreviata poicilometra* has been found in the stomach of mangabeys and guenons in the United States and Africa; it is uncommon or rare (Slaughter and Bostrom 1969; Yamaguti 1961).

The morphology, life cycle, pathologic effects, method of diagnosis, and control of these physalopterids are similar to those of the species that affect the dog and cat. The eggs measure 39 to 50 μ by 23 to 34 μ (Fig. 7.48) (Tanaka et al. 1962).

ONCHOCERCIDS

The onchocercid or filarial nematodes are long, thin worms that live outside the intestinal tract (Levine 1968). Females produce small larvae, called microfilariae, which usually occur in the blood or lymph. All onchocercids have arthropod intermediate hosts which ingest blood or lymph. The filarial worms that occur in endothermal laboratory animals are listed in Table 7.12. The most important are discussed below.

Dirofilaria immitis

This onchocercid occurs in the right ventricle, pulmonary artery, and sometimes the vena cava of the dog, other canids, some wild carnivores, and rarely the cat (Lapage 1968; Levine 1968) and man (Abadie, Swartzwelder, and Holman 1965; Harrison

et al. 1965). It is found throughout the world, especially in the tropics and subtropics (Soulsby 1965).

Laboratory dogs obtained from pounds are often infected. Typical incidences observed in the United States are 5.7% in Michigan (Worley 1964), 7.7% in Connecticut (Hirth, Huizinga, and Nielsen 1966), 7.8% in Maryland (Wallenstein and Tibola 1960), 5.4 to 12.5% in Georgia (Thrasher et al. 1968), 15.0% in Tennessee (Parker and McCaughan 1967), 20.0% in Hawaii (Ash 1962b), 19.3% in Illinois (Marquardt and Fabian 1966), 18.1 to 55.0% in Mississippi (Garcia, Ward, and Dodds 1965; Godfrey et al. 1966), and 20.0% in dogs used for research in New York that were obtained from eastern and southeastern states (Mann and Bjotvedt 1965).

The incidence in the cat is not well documented. It is reported to be uncommon (Scott 1967) or rare (Gaafar 1964), but this may be a reflection of the rarity with which the cat is tested for microfilariae (Griffiths, Schlotthauer, and Gehrman 1962). In one survey of 107 stray cats in Hawaii, 1 cat was found positive (Ash 1962b).

Dirofilaria immitis infection is not only detrimental to the health of the laboratory dog, but it also often renders the animal useless for studies involving cardiac and pulmonary physiology or blood transfusion (Godfrey et al. 1966).

MORPHOLOGY

Adults are long, slender, threadlike worms (Fig. 7.49). The esophagus is short and has an anterior muscular part and a posterior glandular portion (Morgan and Hawkins 1949). The male is 120 to 200 mm long. It has a spirally coiled blunt tail, small caudal alae, five preanal and six postanal pairs of papillae, unequal spicules, and no bursa or gubernaculum. The female is 250 to 310 mm long. The vulva is near the posterior end of the esophagus. Microfilariae are 286 to 340 μ long and 6.1 to 7.2 μ wide (Fig. 7.50) (Lindsey 1965). The tail is straight and has no terminal hook.

LIFE CYCLE

The life cycle involves a mosquito as an intermediate host (Otto 1969a; Taylor 1960a, b). Unsheathed microfilariae released by the ovoviviparous female worm

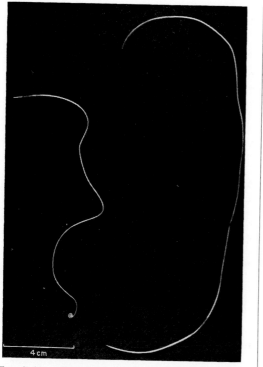

FIG. 7.49. *Dirofilaria immitis* adults. *(Left)* Male. *(Right)* Female. (Courtesy of S. H. Abadie, Louisiana State University.)

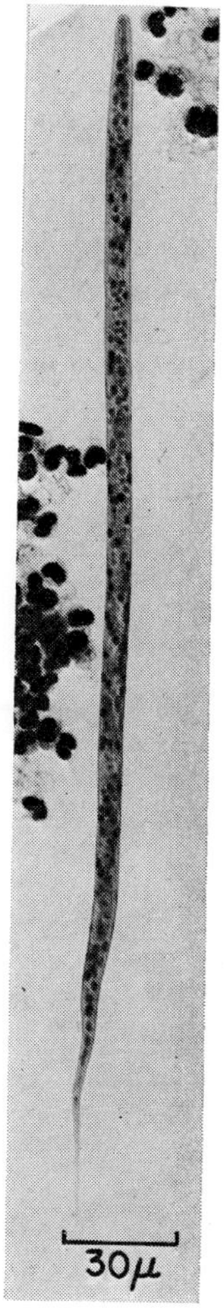

FIG. 7.50. *Dirofilaria immitis* microfilaria. (From Lindsey 1965. Courtesy of American Veterinary Medical Association.)

circulate in the blood and are ingested by the mosquito while feeding. Developmental stages are found in the Malpighian tubules of the mosquito for about 15 to 16 days (8 to 10 in the tropics). Elongate larvae then enter the body cavity of the mosquito and migrate to the thorax and head, concentrating in the cavity of the labium or cephalic spaces of the head. Infective larvae, deposited by the mosquito when it feeds, penetrate the skin either directly or more likely through the wound produced by the insect vector. Further development occurs chiefly in the deep fascia and possibly in the subcutaneous tissues, viscera, or lymphatics (Kume and Itagaki 1955). Mature worms are present in the heart in 3 to 4 months, presumably arriving by the venous route. Microfilariae are shed in 6 to 8 months.

PATHOLOGIC EFFECTS

The primary effect of the worms is a mechanical interference with blood flow and heart function, especially of the tri-cuspid valves (Jackson et al. 1966; Jackson and Wallace 1966; Otto 1962). Signs vary with the worm load and duration of infection. The usual signs are lack of endurance, cough, ascites, and heart failure. Other signs include dry hair coat, anorexia, loss of weight, increased respiration, rales, and hematuria.

Adult worms are seen at necropsy in the right auricle and ventricle, pulmonary artery, and frequently the anterior and posterior venae cavae (Fig. 7.51) (Jackson, von Lichtenberg, and Otto 1962). The mechanical interference produced by these worms causes hypertrophy and enlargement of the right ventricle, dilatation of the pulmonary arteries proximal to occlusions, and passive congestion of the lungs, liver, and spleen, accompanied by ascites (Liu, Yarns, and Tashjian 1969; Otto and Jackson 1969;

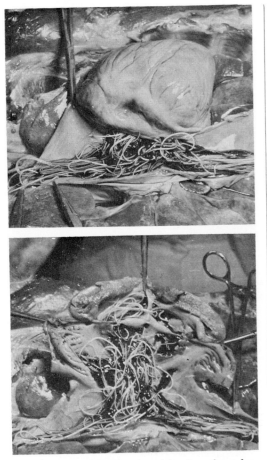

Lindsey 1965; Newton and Wright 1956, 1957).

CONTROL

Control of mosquito vectors on the premises and insectproof animal buildings are important in preventing infection. Diethylcarbamazine, given orally at a level of 2.5 to 6.5 mg per kg of body weight daily, will destroy developing larvae in dogs which cannot be otherwise protected from infection (Kume, Ohishi, and Kobayashi 1962, 1964; Otto 1969b; Warne, Tipton, and Furusho 1969). Treatment should be started 2 months prior to the mosquito season and continued until 2 months after it ends. Adult worms can be removed surgically (Jackson and Wallace 1966) or killed with arsenamide given intravenously, 2.2 mg per kg of body weight twice daily for 2 days (Jackson 1963), but such treatment is not practical for laboratory dogs.

PUBLIC HEALTH CONSIDERATIONS

Dirofilariasis, with subcutaneous, pulmonary, and cardiovascular involvement,

FIG. 7.51. *Dirofilaria immitis* in the dog. *(Top)* Worms in the right auricle and anterior and posterior venae cavae. *(Bottom)* Heart opened showing worms also in the right ventricle. (From Jackson, von Lichtenberg, and Otto 1962. Courtesy of American Veterinary Medical Association.)

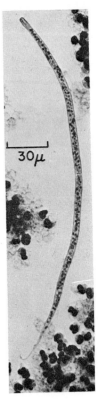

FIG. 7.52. *Dipetalonema reconditum* microfilaria. (From Lindsey 1965. Courtesy of American Veterinary Medical Association.)

30μ

Smith and Jones 1966). Histologically, changes are seen in the pulmonary arterial system and in the hepatic veins. Living microfilariae circulating in the blood and in tissues produce little damage; however, when they die, small granulomas form around them.

DIAGNOSIS

The presence of microfilariae of *D. immitis* in the bloodstream is diagnostic, but care must be taken to differentiate them from microfilariae of *Dipetalonema reconditum* (see below) (Jackson 1969;

has been reported in man in the United States but is apparently rare (Abadie, Swartzwelder, and Holman 1965; Faust, Beaver, and Jung 1968; Harrison et al. 1965). Laboratory personnel handling infected dogs should be aware of the hazard, especially if the mosquito vector is present.

Dipetalonema reconditum

This filarial nematode, which occurs in most parts of the world, is common in the dog in North America and Europe and is important because its microfilariae are frequently confused with those of *Dirofilaria immitis* (Levine 1968; Newton and Wright 1956, 1957). The adult worms are small; males are 11.5 to 15.0 mm long, and females 17.5 to 32.0 mm (Lindsey 1965). They are usually found in the subcutaneous tissues and apparently cause no serious pathology.

The microfilariae (Fig. 7.52) are very similar to those of *D. immitis* (Lindsey 1965; Morgan 1966). The presence of a curved tail is diagnostic, but this occurs only in one-third of a pure population, and it does not rule out the possibility of a concurrent dirofilariasis. Differentiation by size and shape is more reliable (Fig. 7.53). *Dipetalonema reconditum* is shorter and narrower: 258 to 292 μ by 4.7 to 5.8 μ. It also is less tapered in the anterior fifth of the body and is usually found lying in an anterior-posterior crescent shape.

Dipetalonema gracile, Dipetalonema caudispina, Dipetalonema marmosetae, Dipetalonema tamarinae

Adults of these filarial nematodes are frequently found in the peritoneal cavity of Central and South American primates, and microfilariae occur in the blood (Ruch 1959; Webber and Hawking 1955). *Dipetalonema gracile* occurs in capuchins, spider monkeys, woolly monkeys, squirrel monkeys, and marmosets; *D. caudispina* in capuchins, and squirrel monkeys; *D. marmo-*

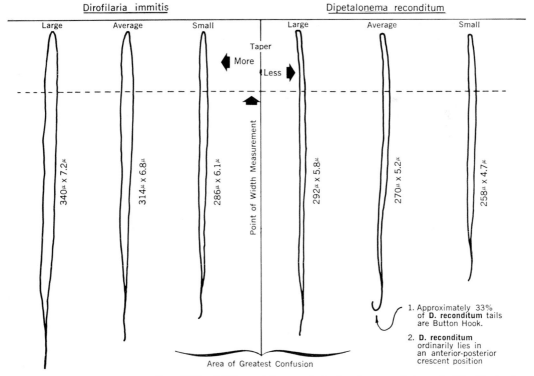

FIG. 7.53. Differential morphologic characteristics of *Dirofilaria immitis* and *Diptalonema reconditum*. (From Morgan 1966. Courtesy of Veterinary Medicine Publishing Co.)

setae in capuchins, spider monkeys, squirrel monkeys, and marmosets; and *D. tamarinae* in marmosets. All of these parasites are common in laboratory monkeys obtained from their natural habitat (Cosgrove, Nelson, and Gengozian 1968; Deinhardt et al. 1967; Dunn and Lambrecht 1963; Garner 1967; Garner, Hemrick, and Rudiger 1967; Lapin 1962).

MORPHOLOGY

Adult worms are slender and thin in the posterior region and have a smooth or finely striated cuticle (Dunn and Lambrecht 1963; Levine 1968). Males range in size from an average of 39 mm for *D. marmosetae* to 84 mm for *D. gracile,* and females range from an average of 87 to 199 mm. Microfilariae range in size from 130 μ for *D. gracile* to 406 to 430 μ for *D. tamarinae* (Fig. 7.54).

LIFE CYCLE

The life cycle is not completely known; microfilariae occur in the blood and it is presumed that they are transmitted by the bite of an arthropod, probably a mosquito.

PATHOLOGIC EFFECTS

The adult worms are usually found lying free in the peritoneal cavity (Fig. 7.55) (Garner 1967; Garner, Hemrick, and Ru-

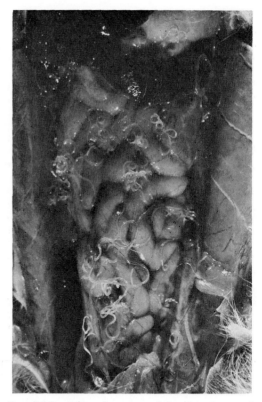

FIG. 7.55. *Dipetalonema* adults in the peritoneal cavity of a squirrel monkey. (From Whitney, Johnson, and Cole 1967. Courtesy of R. A. Whitney, Edgewood Arsenal.)

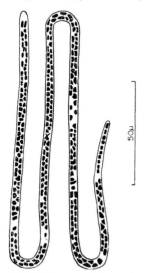

FIG. 7.54. *Dipetalonema tamarinae* microfilaria. (From Dunn and Lambrecht 1963. Courtesy of London School of Hygiene and Tropical Medicine.)

diger 1967; Whitney, Johnson, and Cole 1967). Although peritoneal adhesions have been reported in heavy infections, the worms usually cause little or no pathology.

DIAGNOSIS

Diagnosis is based on demonstration of adult worms in the peritoneal cavity or microfilariae in the blood.

CONTROL

Transmission in the laboratory is unlikely, and no special control procedures are necessary other than eliminating possible arthropod vectors.

PUBLIC HEALTH CONSIDERATIONS

Several filarial nematodes affect man (Faust, Beaver, and Jung 1968), but nothing is known of the public health aspects of these species.

Litomosoides carinii

This filarial nematode is common in the wild cotton rat in North and South America and is experimentally transmissible to the Norway rat and Mongolian gerbil (Levine 1968; Thompson, Boche, and Blair 1968). It is important only because it is frequently used in immunologic and chemotherapeutic studies of filariasis (Bertram 1966).

DRACUNCULIDS

Only two dracunculids or guinea worms occur in endothermal laboratory animals (Table 7.13). Neither is common or important.

TRICHURIDS, ANATRICHOSOMATIDS, TRICHINELLIDS

The trichurids and related nematodes differ markedly from all the previously discussed nematodes in that they have no excretory canals or phasmids, and their esophagus is not muscular (Levine 1968). Many occur in endothermal laboratory animals (Table 7.14). The most important are discussed below.

Trichuris vulpis

(Dog Whipworm)

Trichuris vulpis occurs in the cecum and colon of the dog, fox, and other canids throughout the world (Levine 1968). It is common in laboratory dogs obtained from city pounds (Mann and Bjotvedt 1965; Vaughn and Murphy 1962; Worley 1964), less common in those obtained from rural areas (Braun and Thayer 1962), uncommon in kennel-raised dogs routinely treated for worms (Johnson, Andersen, and Gee 1963), and absent in cesarean-derived, barrier-maintained colonies (Griesemer and Gibson 1963a). Light infections are usually inapparent; heavy infections cause diarrhea, anemia, loss of weight, and debility.

MORPHOLOGY

Adults are characterized by a long, slender esophageal portion that is three-fourths of the body length and a thick, blunted posterior section up to 1.3 mm wide, which contains the reproductive organs (Soulsby 1965). Both sexes are 45 to

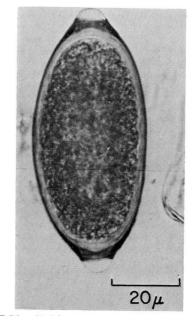

FIG. 7.56. *Trichuris vulpis* eggs. (From Burrows 1965. Courtesy of Yale University Press.)

75 mm long, but females are wider posteriorly. The male posterior end is coiled dorsally with a single spicule enclosed in a terminal sheath, which evaginates when the spicule protrudes. The vulva is near the junction of the thin and thick portions of the body. The eggs are brown and oval, measure 70 to 80 μ by 32 to 40 μ and have a thick wall with bipolar plugs (Fig. 7.56) (Habermann and Williams 1958).

LIFE CYCLE

The female parasite deposits approximately 2,000 eggs daily (Miller 1947). These are unsegmented when passed in the feces and develop into an infective stage within the eggshell if deposited on a suitable substrate. Development usually takes 3 to 4 weeks but, under ideal conditions of temperature (25 to 32 C; 77 to 89 F) and humidity, it can be accomplished in 9 to 10 days. The first-stage infective larva forms within the egg; the egg hatches only when ingested by a suitable host. After ingestion, the larva emerges from the egg and usually enters the mucosa of the anterior small intestine, aided by a 7 to 10 μ retractable lancet. It does not penetrate the mucosa and migrate parenterally but returns to

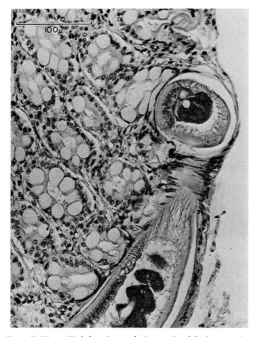

FIG. 7.57. *Trichuris vulpis* embedded in the mucosa of the colon of the dog. (From Smith and Jones 1966. Courtesy of Lea and Febiger and Armed Forces Institute of Pathology, Neg. No. 56–2349.)

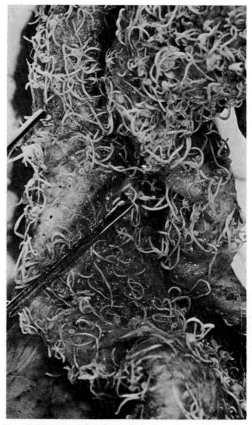

FIG. 7.58. *Trichuris vulpis* in the colon of a dog. (From Gaafar 1964. Courtesy of Veterinary Medicine Publishing Co.)

the lumen in 2 to 10 days, passes to the cecum, and matures in 70 to 90 days (Rubin 1954). Adults are usually confined to the cecum but also occur in the colon. The total life cycle requires 3 to 4 months; the longevity of adults in the host is about 16 months (Soulsby 1965).

Transmission is simple and direct: by ingestion of embryonated eggs.

PATHOLOGIC EFFECTS

The tissue migration by larvae of this parasite is limited to the mucosa of the anterior small intestine and apparently has little effect on the host (Galvin and Turk 1966). The adults in the cecum and colon embed deeply in the mucosa (Fig. 7.57). They sometimes cause thickening and inflammation (Habermann and Williams 1958) but usually produce little or no reaction (Gaafar 1964). Because of the limited inflammatory reaction, little immunity is produced, and consequently large numbers of parasites are often seen in older dogs (Fig. 7.58) (Galvin and Turk 1966).

Only in heavy infections are clinical signs seen. These consist of weight loss, abdominal pain, and mild to severe diarrhea that is sometimes hemorrhagic (Galvin and Turk 1966; Habermann and Williams 1958; Morgan 1967; Soulsby 1965).

DIAGNOSIS

Diagnosis is based on identification of the eggs in the feces or adults in the large intestine.

CONTROL

Complete elimination of this parasite from a research dog colony can be achieved by raising cesarean-derived progeny in isolation (Griesemer and Gibson 1963a).

Control in a conventional colony is achieved by sanitation, the prevention of conditions favorable to egg development, and the elimination or regular treatment of infected animals (Soulsby 1965). Eggs tolerate freezing and high temperatures but have little resistance against desiccation. Sunlight and concentrated saline solutions are lethal to unhatched larvae.

Newly acquired dogs should be examined on arrival and either treated or eliminated, if infected. Oral anthelmintics are relatively ineffective against adult worms in the cecum (Chandler and Read 1961). N-butyl chloride has been used with varying results (Soulsby 1965). It is most effective when given hourly for 5 hours at the rate of 0.1 to 10.0 ml per kg of body weight (Whitney and Whitney 1953). Phthalofyne, given intravenously, 250 to 300 mg per kg of body weight, will remove most adult worms (Burch 1954; Carlos and Directo 1962; Eshenour, Burch, and Ehrenford 1957). Temporary toxic manifestations, such as depression or ataxia, sometimes occur, but these do not alter effectiveness (Carlos and Directo 1962). Dithiazanine iodide, given orally, 20 mg per kg of body weight daily for 7 days, is also effective (McCowen, Callender, and Brandt 1957; Shumard and Hendrix 1962) but sometimes produces toxic side effects (Guilhon and Jolivet 1959). Glycobiarsol, given orally at a dose of 100 mg per kg of body weight daily for 10 days (Berberian, Poole, and Freele 1963; Edwin 1964); methyridine, given subcutaneously at a dose of 200 mg per kg of body weight (Colglazier, Enzie, and Burtner 1966); DDVP (dichlorvos; Task, Shell), given orally at a dose of 35 to 40 mg per kg of body weight (Batte and Moncol 1968); and naled (Dibrom, Chevron Chemical Co.), given orally at a dose of 15 mg per kg of body weight (Lindsey et al. 1964), are also reportedly effective.

PUBLIC HEALTH CONSIDERATIONS

Trichuris vulpis does not affect man.

Trichuris trichiura

(Human Whipworm)

This trichurid nematode occurs in the large intestine of man and in many simian primates (Faust, Beaver, and Jung 1968; Levine 1968; Ruch 1959). It is found throughout the world but is most prevalent in the tropics and subtropics. Affected laboratory primates include the rhesus monkey, cynomolgus monkey, Japanese macaque, green monkey, baboons, and chimpanzee (Britz et al. 1961; Graham 1960; Myers and Kuntz 1965; Sasa et al. 1962; Thienpont, Mortelmans, and Vercruysse 1962). An incidence of 7 to 27% has been reported in the rhesus monkey (Graham 1960; Reardon and Rininger 1968; Rowland and Vandenbergh 1965), 5 to 58% in the cynomolgus monkey (Hashimoto and Honjo 1966; Reardon and Rininger 1968; Tanaka et al. 1962), 29% in the Japanese macaque (Tanaka et al. 1962), 86% in the Formosan macaque (Kuntz et al. 1968), 6% in the green monkey (Reardon and Rininger 1968), 21 to 100% in baboons (Kuntz and Myers 1967; Reardon and Rininger 1968), and 28% in the chimpanzee (Reardon and Rininger 1968).

Although this parasite usually produces little or no pathologic effects (Graham 1960; Ruch 1959), there is one report of severe enteritis and death in the chimpanzee attributed to it (Thienpont, Mortelmans, and Vercruysse 1962).

MORPHOLOGY

Adults are similar to those of *Trichuris vulpis* (Faust, Beaver, and Jung 1968). The anterior three-fifths of the body is slender, and the posterior portion thicker and blunt. The male is 30 to 45 mm long, and the female 35 to 50 mm. The egg is oval, has bipolar plugs, measures 50 by 22 μ, and is unsegmented when passed in the feces (Fig. 7.59).

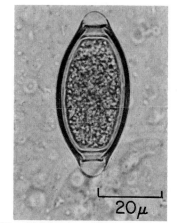

FIG. 7.59. *Trichuris trichiura* egg. (Courtesy of TSgt R. R. Estes, USAF School of Aerospace Medicine.)

LIFE CYCLE

The life cycle is direct and similar to that of *T. vulpis* (Faust, Beaver, and Jung 1968).

PATHOLOGIC EFFECTS

Light infections cause no apparent pathologic effects, but heavy infections cause anorexia, a gray, mucoid diarrhea, and sometimes death (Graham 1960; Ruch 1959; Thienpont, Mortelmans, and Vercruysse 1962).

DIAGNOSIS

Diagnosis is based on identification of the eggs in the feces or the adults in the large intestine.

CONTROL

Control is achieved by sanitation, by elimination of conditions favorable to egg development, and by regular treatment of infected animals.

Newly acquired animals should be examined on arrival and either treated or eliminated, if infected. As with *T. vulpis,* oral anthelmintics are relatively ineffective. Best results have been obtained with dithiazanine iodide, given orally in the food at the rate of about 20 mg per kg of body weight per day for 10 to 14 days (Britz et al. 1961; Lang 1962; Mortelmans and Vercruysse 1962; Shumard and Hendrix 1962). DDVP (dichlorvos; Task, Shell), given orally at a rate of 10 mg per kg of body weight in a single dose and repeated after 24 hours, is also effective (Pryor, Chang, and Raulston 1970). Thiabendazole, given in a single dose of 100 mg per kg of body weight and repeated in 14 days, is recommended as a routine treatment (Valerio et al. 1969), but it is more effective if given at a rate of 60 mg per day for 9 to 10 days (Cullum and Hamilton 1965). Other treatments are hexylresorcinol, given orally in a single dose of 200 mg and followed 2 hours later with 10 to 15 ml of a 16% solution of magnesium sulfate, for the monkey (Ruch 1959), and methyridine, given subcutaneously at a dose of 200 mg per kg of body weight, for guenons and the chimpanzee (Thienpont, Mortelmans, and Vercruysse 1962).

PUBLIC HEALTH CONSIDERATIONS

The species in monkeys and apes is similar to, if not identical with, the species in man; therefore, cross infection is possible (Ruch 1959). Because of the direct life cycle, infected animals and their excreta should be handled with caution, and laboratory personnel should be instructed in proper personal hygiene.

Capillaria hepatica
(SYN. *Hepaticola hepatica*)
(Liver Threadworm)

Capillaria hepatica occurs in the liver of a wide range of hosts throughout the world (Jones 1967; Lapage 1968; Levine 1968; Lubinsky 1956; Morgan and Hawkins 1949; Soulsby 1965). It is common in wild rodents, especially in wild rats, and occurs occasionally in other wild mammals, including simian primates, and rarely in the rabbit, dog, cat, domestic animals, and man. Because of its unusual life cycle, which requires that infected liver tissue pass through another animal or decompose to expose the eggs to air before they will embryonate, infection of laboratory rodents is unlikely. The parasite has been reported from several wild rodents sometimes used in the laboratory (Fisher 1963; Lubinsky 1956), but it has not been reported in commercially produced or laboratory-reared mice or rats (Habermann and Williams 1958; Sasa et al. 1962). It is occasionally reported in primates, including the rhesus monkey, capuchins, spider monkeys, and chimpanzee, obtained from their natural environment (Habermann and Williams 1957a; Lubinsky 1956; Ruch 1959).

The infection is usually inapparent in rodents (Lapage 1968; Lubinsky 1956; Oldham 1967), but it sometimes causes hepatitis and death in primates (Fiennes 1967; Graham 1960; Ruch 1959).

MORPHOLOGY

Males measure 17 to 32 mm by 40 to 80 μ; females reach 100 mm in length and 200 μ in width (Olsen 1967). Both sexes have a short, anterior, muscular esophagus attached to a long, glandular portion. The male has a lightly cuticularized terminal spicule up to 500 μ long, a protrusible spicule sheath that forms a funnel-shaped dilatation, and a blunt posterior end with a pair of subventral lobes. The vulva of the female lies posterior to the end of the esophagus. Eggs have bipolar plugs and

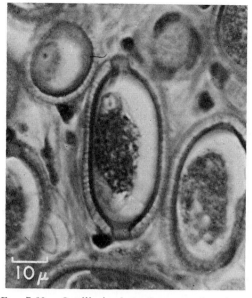

FIG. 7.60. *Capillaria hepatica* eggs in tissue section. (Courtesy of E. F. Staffeldt, Argonne National Laboratory.)

are 48 to 62 μ long and 29 to 37 μ wide (Fig. 7.60). They are similar to those of other trichurids but differ in that their shell contains many small perforations and appears striated by rodlike structures.

LIFE CYCLE

Eggs are deposited in the liver tissue but do not escape until the tissue is eaten by another host and the eggs are liberated and passed in the feces or until the first host dies and the liver decomposes (Habermann and Williams 1958; Morgan and Hawkins 1949; Olsen 1967). The eggs embryonate in 4 to 6 weeks after exposure to air. Infection occurs only when embryonated eggs are ingested. They hatch in the intestine, and the infective larvae penetrate the intestinal mucosa. In 2 to 10 days they pass via the portal system to the liver, where they develop to maturity in about 30 days.

PATHOLOGIC EFFECTS

The liver surface of infected animals contains white or yellow patches or nodules (Lubinsky 1956) which, in tissue section, are seen to contain the nematode and numerous eggs (Fig. 7.61). These large clusters of eggs cause localized liver damage and cir-

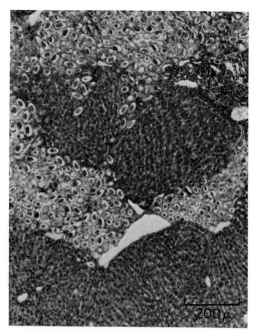

FIG. 7.61. *Capillaria hepatica* in the liver of a deer mouse. Note numerous eggs. (Courtesy of E. F. Staffeldt, Argonne National Laboratory.)

rhosis. They seldom affect the general health of rodents (Lapage 1968) but sometimes cause a fatal hepatitis in primates (Fiennes 1967; Ruch 1959).

DIAGNOSIS

Diagnosis is based on demonstration of the parasite and the typical eggs in histologic sections of liver (Jones 1967).

CONTROL

Because of the unusual life cycle, natural transmission in the laboratory is unlikely, and no special control procedures are required. There is no treatment.

PUBLIC HEALTH CONSIDERATIONS

This parasite is pathogenic for man, but cases of human infection are rare (Faust, Beaver, and Jung 1968). Transmission to man is unlikely and no special precautions are required.

Capillaria aerophila
(SYN. *Eucoleus aerophilus*)
(Fox Lungworm)

Although *Capillaria aerophila* is primarily a parasite of the respiratory tract of the fox, it has also been reported in the dog, cat, and other carnivores in North America, South America, and Europe (Lapage 1968; Levine 1968). It is rare in the cat (Renaux 1964), but little is known of its incidence in the dog. Because of the similarity of the eggs, it is suspected that *C. aerophila* is often reported as *Trichuris vulpis* (Gaafar 1964). There are no specific reports of *C. aerophila* in the laboratory; it is probably uncommon in the laboratory dog and rare in the laboratory cat.

MORPHOLOGY

Adults are long and thin. Males are 15 to 25 mm long, and females 20 to 40 mm (Habermann and Williams 1958; Lapage 1962). The male has two caudal lobes and a single spicule with a spiny sheath. The vulva of the female is near the posterior end of the esophagus. The egg is brown, oval, and 58 to 70 μ by 29 to 40 μ, and has a granular or striated shell and bipolar plugs (Fig. 7.62).

LIFE CYCLE

The life cycle is direct (Christenson 1938; Soulsby 1965). Eggs are passed in the sputum or feces and embryonate in 30 to 50

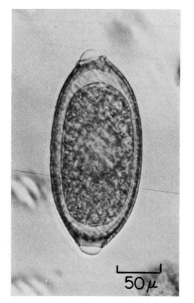

FIG. 7.62. *Capillaria aerophila* egg. (From Burrows 1965. Courtesy of Yale University Press.)

days. Infection occurs when embryonated eggs are ingested. The larvae hatch in the small intestine, penetrate the mucosa, and apparently migrate by the bloodstream to the lungs. This takes 7 to 10 days. They penetrate the alveoli, migrate up the air passages as they develop, and reach maturity about 40 days after infection. The adult worms inhabit the bronchioles, bronchi, and trachea.

PATHOLOGIC EFFECTS

Light infections are usually inapparent (Lapage 1968; Renaux 1964). Severe infections cause tracheitis, bronchitis, and sometimes pneumonia and are characterized by a cough, nasal discharge, dyspnea, anorexia, and debilitation. Young animals are the most susceptible. Tracheobronchitis, pulmonary edema, and hemorrhage, and sometimes pneumonia, are seen at necropsy (Soulsby 1965). Larvae, adult worms, and eggs are present in sections of affected tissues (Fig. 7.63) (Habermann and Williams 1958; Herman 1967).

DIAGNOSIS

Diagnosis is made by identification of the eggs in the sputum or feces. However, eggs in the feces must be differentiated from those of *T. vulpis:* those of *C. aerophila* are smaller, more ovoid, and distinctly pitted (Estes and Brown 1966).

CONTROL

Sanitation and the elimination of infected animals are the primary methods of control. Newly acquired dogs and cats should be examined on arrival and killed, if infected. Because eggs do not embryonate for 30 to 50 days, frequent and complete cleaning of cages, pens, and runs will prevent the dissemination of the parasite (Lapage 1968). There is no specific treatment.

PUBLIC HEALTH CONSIDERATIONS

This nematode does not affect man.

Capillaria plica

This relatively nonpathogenic nematode occurs in the urinary bladder and sometimes the renal pelvis of the dog and other canids (Soulsby 1965). It is also reported from the rat, cat, and wild carni-

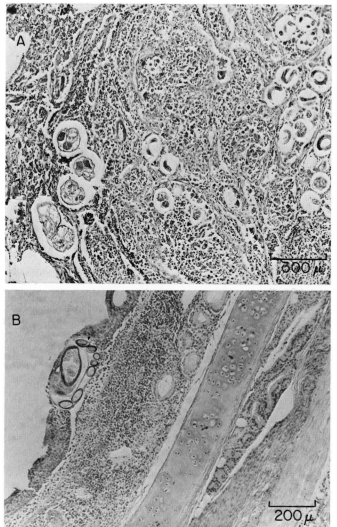

FIG. 7.63. *Capillaria aerophila* infection. *(A)* Larvae and adults in the lung of a cat. *(B)* Adult and eggs in the tracheal mucosa of a cat. *(A* from Habermann and Williams 1958; courtesy of R. T. Habermann, U.S. Public Health Service. *B* from Herman 1967; courtesy of Veterinary Medicine Publishing Co.)

vores (Chitwood and Enzie 1953; Olsen 1967; Rankin 1946). It is cosmopolitan in distribution and common in the hunting dog in Europe (Soulsby 1965) but is seldom reported in the dog elsewhere (Medway and Skelley 1961; Morgan and Hawkins 1949). This may be because of the similarity between the egg of this species and that of *Trichuris vulpis. Capillaria plica* is uncommon in the cat (Renaux 1964). There are no specific reports of this nematode in laboratory specimens; it is probably uncommon or rare in both the laboratory dog and cat and absent in laboratory-reared specimens.

MORPHOLOGY

This species is morphologically similar to *C. aerophila* (Soulsby 1965). The body is long and thin and has a finely striated cuticle. Females are 30 to 60 mm in length, and males 13 to 30 mm (Olsen 1967). The egg is typically capillarid and colorless to yellow. It measures approximately 60 by 30 μ and has characteristic bipolar plugs (Fig. 7.64).

LIFE CYCLE

Eggs passed in the urine do not develop further unless eaten by an appropriate

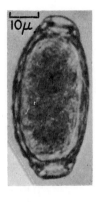

Fig. 7.64. *Capillaria plica* egg. (From Habermann and Williams 1958. Courtesy of R. T. Habermann, U.S. Public Health Service.)

earthworm (Enigk 1950; Olsen 1967). The eggs hatch in the intestine of the earthworm and the larvae burrow through the intestinal wall into the connective tissue. In about 24 hours they are infective for a vertebrate host. When an infected earthworm is ingested by the definitive host, larvae are released which molt, burrow into the intestinal wall, and molt again. The resultant third-stage larvae enter the portal circulation, pass through the liver, heart, lungs, and the general circulation to the kidneys, and migrate through the renal glomeruli, tubules, pelvis, and ureter to the bladder where they develop to adults. From infection to the adult stage takes 58 to 63 days.

PATHOLOGIC EFFECTS

Infection with *C. plica* is usually inapparent and causes little or no pathology (Renaux 1964; Soulsby 1965; Whitehead 1964).

DIAGNOSIS

Diagnosis is based on recognition of the adults in the urinary tract or the characteristic eggs in the urine. The eggs must be differentiated from those of *T. vulpis* which occasionally occur in urine contaminated with feces.

CONTROL

Control is primarily by sanitation. Phenothiazine, given orally, 0.3 to 0.5 g per kg of body weight for 3 consecutive days, is said to be effective (Soulsby 1965); however, because infection with this nematode is relatively harmless, treatment is not usually recommended (Whitehead 1964).

PUBLIC HEALTH CONSIDERATIONS

This nematode does not affect man.

Capillaria feliscati

This nematode has been found in the urinary bladder of the cat and other felids in several parts of the world (Habermann and Williams 1958; Renaux 1964; Soulsby 1965; Waddell 1968a, b). It is closely related to *Capillaria plica* and may be identical with it. Although its incidence in laboratory specimens in most parts of the world is unknown, it is common in South America (Levine 1968), and an incidence of 31% has been reported in stray cats in Australia (Waddell 1968b).

Capillaria contorta, Capillaria annulata

These two species may be synonymous (Madsen 1945, 1951, 1952). They are common inhabitants of the mucosa of the crop and esophagus of the chicken and other galliform birds throughout the world (Soulsby 1965). There are no specific reports of their occurrence in the laboratory, and they are probably rare or absent in laboratory-reared specimens.

MORPHOLOGY

These nematodes are long and threadlike. The male is 10 to 48 mm in length, and the female 25 to 70 mm (Levine 1968). The eggs are similar to those of other species of *Capillaria*. They are 46 to 70 μ by 24 to 28 μ and have typical bipolar plugs.

LIFE CYCLE

The life cycle of *C. contorta* is generally believed to be direct whereas that of *C. annulata* is thought to require an earthworm intermediary (Olsen 1967; Soulsby 1965). If, however, the two species are synonymous, then the earthworm is presumably a facultative intermediary, and the life cycle can be completed either directly or indirectly. The definitive host is infected by ingesting either eggs from soil, which become infective in 4 to 6 weeks, or third-stage larvae encysted in the body wall of earthworms, which become infective in 3 to 4 weeks. The parasites reach maturity about 3 to 4 weeks after ingestion.

PATHOLOGIC EFFECTS

Light infections are inapparent; heavy infections are characterized by anorexia, weakness, emaciation, anemia, and death (Soulsby 1965; Wehr 1965). A mild infection produces a slight inflammation and thickening of the crop wall and esophagus; marked inflammation, thickening, a mucopurulent exudate, and mucosal sloughing occur in a heavy infection. The worms with their anterior ends threaded into the mucosa are readily visible with low-power magnification. The tracks produced by the worms as they burrow into the mucosa are visible in histologic sections.

DIAGNOSIS

Diagnosis is based on demonstration of eggs in the feces or adult worms in the crop or esophagus.

CONTROL

Control is based primarily on sanitation and the elimination of infected animals. Although its use has not been reported in the chicken, methyridine, given subcutaneously at a dose of approximately 100 mg per kg of body weight, is an effective treatment in other birds (Levine 1968; Wehr et al. 1967).

PUBLIC HEALTH CONSIDERATIONS

These nematodes do not affect man.

Trichosomoides crassicauda

(Bladder Threadworm)

This relatively nonpathogenic, hairlike worm occurs in the wall of the urinary bladder and occasionally in the upper ureter and renal pelvis of wild and laboratory rats throughout the world (Ash 1962a; Dove 1950; de León 1964; Sasa et al. 1962; Snell 1967). It is frequently seen in conventional rat colonies (Bell 1968; Bone and Harr 1967; Paget and Lemon 1965; Peardon, Tufts, and Eschenroeder 1966; Sasa et al. 1962; Weisbroth and Scher 1969) but does not occur in cesarean-derived, barrier-maintained colonies (Bell 1968; Foster 1963; Paget and Lemon 1965).

MORPHOLOGY

The female is about 10 mm long and 200 μ in diameter (Morgan and Hawkins

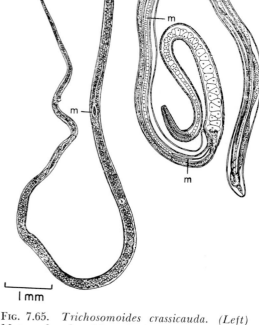

FIG. 7.65. *Trichosomoides crassicauda.* (*Left*) Mature female with male (*m*) as a permanent hyperparasite in uterus. (*Right*) Immature female with male in vagina. (From Yorke and Maplestone 1926.)

1949). The male is much smaller, 1.5 to 3.5 mm in length, and is a permanent hyperparasite harbored within the reproductive tract of the female (Fig. 7.65). Eggs are oval, 60 to 70 μ by 30 to 35 μ, and brown, with a thick shell and bipolar plugs (Fig. 7.66). They are embryonated when passed.

LIFE CYCLE

Infection is by ingestion of embryonated eggs voided in the urine (Morgan and Hawkins 1949). The primary means of transmission in the laboratory rat apparently is from parents to offspring prior to weaning (Weisbroth and Scher 1969). Eggs hatch in the stomach, and larvae penetrate the stomach wall and within a few hours are carried by the blood to the lungs and other parts of the body. Most larvae die; only those that reach the kidneys or urinary bladder survive. The complete life cycle requires 8 to 9 weeks, but eggs are not usu-

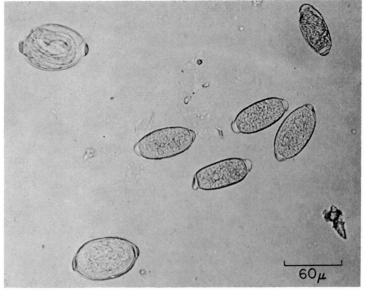

Fig. 7.66. *Trichosomoides crassicauda* eggs. (From Habermann and Williams 1958. Courtesy of R. J. Habermann, U.S. Public Health Service.)

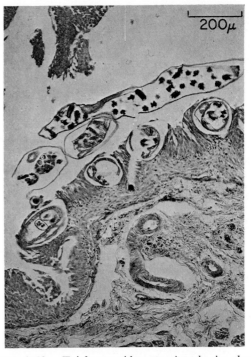

Fig. 7.68. *Trichosomoides crassicauda* in the lumen and mucosa of the urinary bladder of a rat. (From Habermann and Williams 1958. Courtesy of R. T. Habermann, U.S. Public Health Service.)

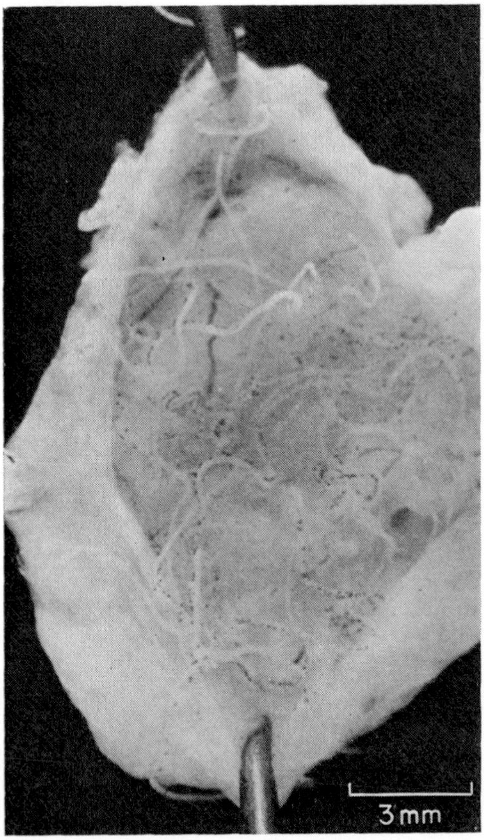

Fig. 7.67. *Trichosomoides crassicauda* females in the bladder of a rat. (Courtesy of J. M. Tufts, Ralston Purina Co.)

ally present in the urine of rats infected as neonates until 8 to 12 weeks of age.

PATHOLOGIC EFFECTS

Infection with *Trichosomoides crassicauda* is usually inapparent (Bone and Harr 1967). The females occur either free in the urinary bladder or embedded in the bladder wall (Fig. 7.67) (Peardon, Tufts, and Eschenroeder 1966). They are difficult to see without the aid of a dissecting microscope and are easily overlooked. If embedded, they produce lesions that appear grossly as white, noninflamed masses measuring about 3.0 by 0.8 mm. Microscopic examination of sections of the bladder wall show the parasite lying on or embedded in the mucosa (Fig. 7.68). Other effects of infection include granulomatous lesions in the lungs (Innes, Garner, and Stookey 1967) and eosinophilia (Ahlqvist, Rytömaa, and Borgmästars 1962). Urinary calculi and bladder tumors have been associated with infection with this parasite, but a cause and effect relationship has not been established (Chapman 1964; Smith 1946).

DIAGNOSIS

Diagnosis of the infection depends on demonstration of the parasite in the urinary bladder or in sections of the bladder wall, or on demonstration of the characteristic eggs in the urine.

CONTROL

The infection can be eliminated by the cesarean-derivation technique (Bell 1968). Control in conventional colonies depends primarily on cage sanitation and cleanliness of the drinking water (Ahlqvist and Borgmästars 1961; Bone and Harr 1967; Wahl and Chapman 1967). Newly acquired stocks should be examined and either eliminated or treated, if infected. Treatment with either nitrofurantoin, 0.2% in the food for 6 or more weeks (Chapman 1964), or methyridine, 200 mg per kg of body weight given intraperitoneally in a single dose (Peardon, Tufts, and Eschenroeder 1966), is reportedly effective.

PUBLIC HEALTH CONSIDERATIONS

This parasite does not affect man.

Anatrichosoma cutaneum

Anatrichosoma cutaneum has been encountered in the nasal mucosa and skin of the rhesus monkey (Allen 1960; Reardon and Rininger 1968; Ruch 1959). Although reported only from the United States, it undoubtedly occurs in the wild monkey in Asia. It also affects man in Asia (Faust, Beaver, and Jung 1968). Infection of the nasal passages, although usually inapparent, is common. In one study it was found in 6 of 17 monkeys examined (Allen 1960). Infection in the skin is rare and has been reported only once (Ruch 1959).

MORPHOLOGY

Little is known of the morphology of this nematode. Those observed in histologic sections are of two sizes (Allen 1960). The smaller are 60 to 72 μ in diameter, and the larger 156 to 202 μ. The larger forms with many eggs are obviously adult females. The egg is elliptical, with bipolar plugs, and measures 60 to 67 μ by 40 to 48 μ (Fig. 7.69).

LIFE CYCLE

The life cycle is unknown but is probably direct. Eggs in the nasal mucosa are embryonated when laid (Allen 1960).

PATHOLOGIC EFFECTS

The presence of this nematode in the nasal passages is usually inapparent. It produces hyperplasia and parakeratosis of the nasal mucosa but only a mild to moderate inflammation (Fig. 7.70) (Allen 1960). In

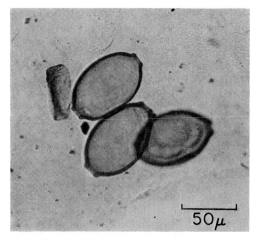

FIG. 7.69. *Anatrichosoma cutaneum* eggs. (From Allen 1960. Courtesy of American Veterinary Medical Association.)

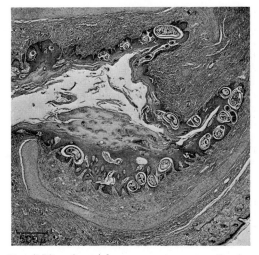

FIG. 7.70. *Anatrichosoma cutaneum*. Section from the nasal passage of a monkey. (From Allen 1960. Courtesy of American Veterinary Medical Association.)

the skin, the parasite causes a subcutaneous foreign-body reaction, but little epithelial hyperplasia and parakeratosis are seen.

DIAGNOSIS

Diagnosis is made in the living animal by identifying the eggs in scrapings of the anterior nasal mucosa or in the deceased animal by finding the parasite in histologic sections of the mucosa (Allen 1960).

CONTROL

Control is unknown; no treatment has been reported.

PUBLIC HEALTH CONSIDERATIONS

This nematode causes a form of creeping eruption in man (Faust, Beaver, and Jung 1968). Although infection in man is uncommon, laboratory personnel should handle infected animals with caution.

DIOCTOPHYMIDS, SOBOLIPHYMATIDS

Few of these nematodes occur in endothermal laboratory animals (Table 7.15), and only one species, *Dioctophyma renale*, is important.

Dioctophyma renale

(Giant Kidney Worm)

This worm, the largest nematode of terrestrial animals, occurs in the renal pel-

vis and peritoneal cavity of the dog, wild carnivores, domestic animals, and man (Woodhead 1950). It has been reported in North and South America, Europe, Asia, and Africa and is frequently found in wild mink in North America (Olsen 1967). It is uncommon in the laboratory dog (Mann and Bjotvedt 1965) as it can occur only in specimens that have eaten infected raw fish.

MORPHOLOGY

Adults are bright red. The female measures up to 1 m in length and about 12 mm in diameter; the male is 140 to 400 mm in length and 4 to 6 mm in diameter, and has a fleshy, bell-shaped terminal copulatory bursa with a single bristlelike spicule (Fig. 7.71) (Olsen 1967; Yorke and Maplestone 1926). The egg is ellipsoidal, about 74 μ long by 47 μ wide. It is yellow-brown and has a thick shell that is covered with funnel-shaped pits except at the ends (Fig. 7.72).

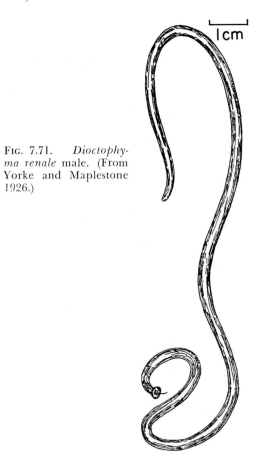

FIG. 7.71. *Dioctophyma renale* male. (From Yorke and Maplestone 1926.)

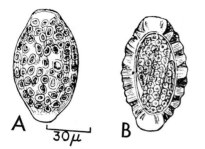

FIG. 7.72. *Dioctophyma renale* egg. *(A)* Superficial view. *(B)* Optical section. (From Yorke and Maplestone 1926.)

LIFE CYCLE

Eggs passed in the urine embryonate only in water and require 7 to 9 months to develop, depending on the temperature (Hallberg 1953; Olsen 1967; Woodhead 1950). The intermediate host is a bronchiobdellid annelid which ingests the infective eggs and later attaches to the gills of a crayfish. An ictalurid or other fish ingests the crayfish and acts as a transport host. The mammalian host becomes infected by ingesting the fish. The infective larvae are freed by digestion, penetrate the intestinal wall, enter the abdominal cavity, and usually develop into adults in the renal pelvis (chiefly in the right kidney) but sometimes in the abdominal cavity. The entire life cycle requires up to 2 years to complete.

PATHOLOGIC EFFECTS

Infection with this parasite is sometimes characterized by hematuria or other evidence of kidney disease, but usually it is inapparent and not recognized except at necropsy (Morgan and Hawkins 1949; Os-

borne et al. 1969; Soulsby 1965). Typically only one worm is present, but more than one is not uncommon. The parasite causes hydronephrosis and progressive destruction of the renal parenchyma of the infected kidney until only a fibrotic capsule containing the worm and hemorrhagic fluid remains (Hallberg 1953; Morgan and Hawkins 1949; Smith and Jones 1966). The other, noninfected kidney will often hypertrophy to twice the normal size. Worms that develop in the abdominal cavity sometimes cause peritonitis and adhesions (Soulsby 1965).

DIAGNOSIS

Diagnosis is usually made by demonstrating the parasite in the kidney or the abdominal cavity. Presence of the characteristic eggs in the urine is also diagnostic; however, if the parasite is a male or if it is in the abdominal cavity and not in the kidney, as is frequently the case in the dog, this method cannot be used (Soulsby 1965). Radiographic procedures are sometimes effective, particularly if a contrast medium is employed.

CONTROL

Because of the requirement for intermediate hosts, infection in the laboratory is self-limiting, and no control procedures are necessary. There is no treatment other than surgical removal of the worm and nephrectomy if a kidney is infected.

PUBLIC HEALTH CONSIDERATIONS

Dioctophyma renale occurs sporadically in man (Soulsby 1965). Because transmission is only by ingestion of uncooked viscera of an infected fish, infection in endothermal laboratory animals, should it occur, is not a public health problem.

TABLE 7.1. Classification of nematodes affecting endothermal laboratory animals

Class SECERNENTASIDA
  Order RHABDITORIDA
    Family RHABDITIDAE
      Subfamily RHABDITINAE
        Pelodera
    Family STRONGYLOIDIDAE
      Strongyloides
  Order STRONGYLORIDA
    Superfamily STRONGYLICAE
    Family ANCYLOSTOMATIDAE
      Subfamily ANCYLOSTOMATINAE
        Ancylostoma
      Subfamily UNCINARIINAE
        Necator
        Characostomum
        Globocephalus
        Uncinaria
    Family STRONGYLIDAE
      Subfamily OESOPHAGOSTOMINAE
        Oesophagostomum
        Ternidens
    Family SYNGAMIDAE
      Subfamily SYNGAMINAE
        Mammomonogamus
        Syngamus
    Superfamily TRICHOSTRONGYLICAE
    Family TRICHOSTRONGYLIDAE
      Subfamily TRICHOSTRONGYLINAE
        Molineus
        Obeliscoides
        Pithecostrongylus
        Trichostrongylus
      Subfamily GRAPHIDIINAE
        Graphidium
        Graphidioides
      Subfamily NEMATODIRINAE
        Nematodirus
      Subfamily HELIGMOSOMINAE
        Heligomosomum
        Nematospiroides
      Subfamily VIANNAIINAE
        Heligmonoides
        Longistriata
        Nippostrongylus
      Subfamily NOCHTIINAE
        Nochtia
      Subfamily OLLULANINAE
        Ollulanus
      Subfamily ORNITHOSTRONGYLINAE
        Ornithostrongylus
    Superfamily METASTRONGYLICAE
    Family METASTRONGYLIDAE
      Subfamily FILAROIDINAE
        Aelurostrongylus
        Anafilaroides
        Angiostrongylus
        Bronchostrongylus
        Filaroides
        Filariopsis
        Gurltia
      Subfamily VOGELOIDINAE
        Vogeloides
      Subfamily SKRJABINGYLINAE
        Crenosoma
      Subfamily PROTOSTRONGYLINAE
        Protostrongylus

  Order ASCARIDORIDA
    Superfamily ASCARIDICAE
    Family HETERAKIDAE
      Subfamily HETERAKINAE
        Heterakis
        Paraspidodera
      Subfamily ASCARIDIINAE
        Ascaridia
    Family ASCARIDIDAE
      Subfamily ASCARIDINAE
        Ascaris
        Toxocara
        Toxascaris
    Superfamily SUBULURICAE
    Family SUBULURIDAE
      Subfamily SUBULURINAE
        Subulura
    Superfamily OXYURICAE
    Family OXYURIDAE
      Subfamily HETEROXYNEMATINAE
        Dermatoxys
      Subfamily OXYURINAE
        Buckleyenterobius
        Enterobius
        Lobatorobius
        Oxyuronema
        Passalurus
      Subfamily SYPHACIINAE
        Syphacia
        Trypanoxyuris
        Wellcomia
      Subfamily ASPICULURINAE
        Aspiculuris
  Order SPIRURORIDA
    Superfamily SPIRURICAE
    Family SPIRURIDAE
      Subfamily SPIRURINAE
        Chitwoodspirura
        Mastophorus
        Spirura
        Trichospirura
      Subfamily TETRAMERINAE
        Tetrameres
    Family GNATHOSTOMATIDAE
      Subfamily GNATHOSTOMATINAE
        Gnathostoma
      Subfamily SPIROXYINAE
        Hartertia
    Superfamily ACUARIICAE
    Family ACUARIIDAE
      Subfamily ACUARIINAE
        Cheilospirura
        Dispharynx
      Subfamily SCHISTOPHORINAE
        Histiocephalus
    Superfamily THELAZIICAE
    Family THELAZIIDAE
      Subfamily THELAZIINAE
        Metathelazia
        Oxyspirura
        Thelazia
      Subfamily SPIROCERCINAE
        Spirocerca
      Subfamily ASCAROPSINAE
        Cylicospirura

TABLE 7.1 *(continued)*

Subfamily ASCAROPSINAE *(cont.)*
  Streptopharagus
Subfamily GONGYLONEMATINAE
  Gongylonema
Subfamily RICTULARIINAE
  Rictularia
Superfamily PHYSALOPTERICAE
  Family PHYSALOPTERIDAE
  Subfamily PHYSALOPTERINAE
    Physaloptera
    Abbreviata
Superfamily FILARIICAE
  Family ONCHOCERCIDAE
  Subfamily DIROFILARIINAE
    Dirofilaria
    Edesonfilaria
    Loa
    Macacanema
  Subfamily DIPETALONEMATINAE
    Brugia
    Dipetalonema
    Litomosoides
Order CAMALLANORIDA
  Family DRACUNCULIDAE

Subfamily DRACUNCULINAE
  Dracunculus
Class ADENOPHORASIDA
Order DORYLAIMORIDA
  Superfamily TRICHINELLICAE
  Family TRICHURIDAE
  Subfamily TRICHURINAE
    Trichuris
  Subfamily CAPILLARIINAE
    Capillaria
  Subfamily TRICHOSOMOIDINAE
    Trichosomoides
  Family ANATRICHOSOMATIDAE
  Subfamily ANATRICHOSOMATINAE
    Anatrichosoma
  Family TRICHINELLIDAE
    Trichinella
Order DIOCTOPHYMATORIDA
  Family DIOCTOPHYMATIDAE
  Subfamily DIOCTOPHYMATINAE
    Dioctophyma
  Family SOBOLOPHYMATIDAE
  Subfamily SOBOLOPHYMATINAE
    Soboliphyme

TABLE 7.2. Rhabditids and strongyloidids affecting endothermal laboratory animals

Parasite	Geographic Distribution	Endothermal Host	Location in Host	Method of Infection	Incidence — In nature	Incidence — In laboratory	Pathologic Effects	Public Health Importance	Reference
Pelodera strongyloides	North America, Europe	Wild rodents, dog, rhesus monkey, domestic animals	Skin lesions	Wound contamination with larva	Common in wild rodents; uncommon in dog	Uncommon or absent	Dermatitis; delayed wound healing	Unknown	Král and Schwartzman 1964; Levine 1968; Ruch 1959
Strongyloides fülleborni*	Africa, Asia (worldwide in laboratory primates)	Macaques, guenons, baboons, chimpanzee, man	Adult: duodenum, jejunum; Larva: lungs	Ingestion of infective larva or penetration of skin or buccal mucosa by larva	Common	Common	Cough, enteritis, diarrhea, debilitation; sometimes massive pulmonary hemorrhages, bronchopneumonia, death	Rare in man; effects uncertain	Guilloud et al. 1965; Habermann and Williams 1957a; Reardon and Rininger 1968; Rowland and Vandenbergh 1965; Ruch 1959; Sasa et al. 1962; Van Riper et al. 1966; Wallace et al. 1948; Young 1957
Strongyloides cebus*	Central America, South America	Squirrel monkeys, woolly monkeys, capuchins, spider monkeys	Adult: duodenum, jejunum; Larva: lungs	Ingestion of infective larva or penetration of skin or buccal mucosa by larva	Common	Common	Cough, diarrhea, pulmonary hemorrhages, bronchopneumonia	Unknown	Cosgrove et al. 1968; Little 1966a
Strongyloides stercoralis*	Worldwide, especially tropics and subtropics	Dog, cat, chimpanzee, other apes, man	Adult: duodenum, jejunum; Larva: lungs, pericardium	Ingestion of infective larva or penetration of skin or buccal mucosa by larva	Uncommon; transitory in dog, cat	Uncommon	Cough, enteritis, diarrhea, debilitation; sometimes pulmonary hemorrhages, bronchopneumonia, death	Common in man in tropics and subtropics; sometimes causes dermatitis, pruritus, ulcerative enteritis, pneumonia	Chandler 1925; Desportes 1945; Galvin and Turk 1966; Johnson et al. 1963; Levine 1968; Little 1966a, b; Renaux 1964; Scott 1967; Soulsby 1965; Worley 1964
Strongyloides ratti*	Worldwide	Rat, black rat	Adult: duodenum, jejunum; Larva: lungs	Ingestion of infective larva or penetration of skin or buccal mucosa by larva	Common	Uncommon or absent	Insignificant	Unknown	Ash 1962a; Dove 1950; de Léon 1964; Little 1966a; Sasa et al. 1962

*Discussed in text.

TABLE 7.2 *(continued)*

Parasite	Geographic Distribution	Endothermal Host	Location in Host	Method of Infection	Incidence — In nature	Incidence — In laboratory	Pathologic Effects	Public Health Importance	Reference
Strongyloides venezuelensis	Southern United States, Venezuela, Israel, probably worldwide	Rat	Adult: duodenum, jejunum, Larva: lungs	Ingestion of infective larva or penetration of skin or buccal mucosa by larva	Common	Uncommon or absent	Insignificant	Unknown	Levine 1968 Little 1966a
Strongyloides papillosus	Worldwide	Rabbit, hares, mink, rhesus monkey, gibbons, domestic animals	Adult: intestine Larva: lungs	Ingestion of infective larva or penetration of skin or buccal mucosa by larva	Common	Unknown	Unknown in laboratory animals	Unknown	Basir 1950 Levine 1968 Little 1966a Owen 1968
Strongyloides sigmodontis	Southwestern United States	Cotton rat	Adult: intestine Larva: lungs	Ingestion of infective larva or penetration of skin or buccal mucosa by larva	Common in endemic areas	Unknown	Unknown	Unknown	Melvin and Chandler 1950
Strongyloides tumefaciens	Southern United States, India	Cat	Large intestine	Ingestion of infective larva or penetration of skin or buccal mucosa by larva	Rare	Unknown; probably rare or absent	Nodular lesions in colon	Unknown	Galvin and Turk 1966 Levine 1968 Price and Dikmans 1941 Renaux 1964
Strongyloides avium	Southeastern United States, Puerto Rico, Cuba, India	Chicken, other birds	Small intestine, ceca	Ingestion of infective larva or penetration of skin by larva	Rare	Unknown; probably rare or absent	Inapparent in adults; enteritis, thickened cecal wall, hemorrhagic diarrhea in young chicken	Unknown	Cram 1929a, 1930 Levine 1968 Wehr 1965
Strongyloides oswaldoi	Puerto Rico, Brazil	Chicken	Adult: intestine Larva: lungs	Ingestion of infective larva or penetration of skin by larva	Rare	Unknown; probably rare or absent	Inapparent in adults; enteritis, thickened cecal wall, hemorrhagic diarrhea in young chicken	Unknown	Levine 1968 Travassos 1930, 1932

TABLE 7.3. Ancylostomatids, strongylids, and syngamids affecting endothermal laboratory animals

Parasite	Geographic Distribution	Endothermal Host	Location in Host	Method of Infection	Incidence — In nature	Incidence — In laboratory	Pathologic Effects	Public Health Importance	Reference
Ancylostoma caninum*	Worldwide	Dog, other carnivores, possibly cat	Small intestine	Ingestion of infective larva, skin penetration, or intrauterine	Common in dog; unknown in cat	Common in dog; unknown in cat	Anemia, hemorrhagic diarrhea, intestinal ulceration; sometimes dermatitis, cough, death	Uncommon cause of cutaneous larva migrans	Lapage 1968; Levine 1968; Mann and Bjotvedt 1965; Miller 1966a, b, c; Morgan and Hawkins 1949; Poynter 1966; Soulsby 1965
Ancylostoma tubaeforme*	Worldwide	Cat	Small intestine	Ingestion of infective larva or skin penetration	Common	Common	Anemia, fetid diarrhea, sometimes vomiting	Unknown; probable cause of cutaneous larva migrans	Burrows 1962; Levine 1968; Soulsby 1965
Ancylostoma braziliense*	Southern United States, Central America, South America, Asia, southern Africa	Dog, cat, other carnivores	Small intestine	Ingestion of infective larva or skin penetration	Common	Common	Usually inapparent; sometimes slight diarrhea	Common cause of cutaneous larva migrans	Faust et al. 1968; Levine 1968; Miller 1966b; Soulsby 1965
Ancylostoma ceylanicum	South America, Asia	Dog, cat, other carnivores	Small intestine	Ingestion of infective larva or skin penetration	Common in southeastern Asia	Unknown	Unknown	Unknown	Levine 1968
Ancylostoma duodenale*	Worldwide in tropics and subtropics	Monkey, chimpanzee, gibbons, other simian primates, man	Small intestine	Ingestion of infective larva or skin penetration	Uncommon or rare	Uncommon or rare	Unknown; presumably anemia, debilitation	Common hookworm of man; causes anemia, debilitation	Benson et al. 1954; Chandler and Read 1961; Lapage 1968; Nelson 1965; Young et al. 1957
Necator americanus*	Worldwide	Spider monkeys, patas monkey, mandrill, baboons, chimpanzee, gorilla, man	Small intestine	Chiefly larval penetration of skin	Uncommon in simian primates	Uncommon	Unknown; presumably anemia, debilitation	Common New World hookworm of man; causes anemia, debilitation	Britz et al. 1961; Fiennes 1967; Myers and Kuntz 1965; Riopelle 1967; Ruch 1959; Young et al. 1957
Characostomum asimilium	Africa, Taiwan	Macaques, guenons, slow loris	Small intestine	Unknown; probably ingestion of embryonated egg	Unknown	Unknown	Unknown	Unknown	Yamaguti 1961
Globocephalus simiae	Malay Peninsula, Indonesia	Rhesus monkey	Small intestine	Unknown; probably ingestion of embryonated egg	Unknown	Unknown	Unknown; probably anemia	Unknown	Yamaguti 1954

*Discussed in text.

TABLE 7.3 (continued)

Parasite	Geographic Distribution	Endothermal Host	Location in Host	Method of Infection	Incidence — In nature	Incidence — In laboratory	Pathologic Effects	Public Health Importance	Reference
Uncinaria stenocephala*	Worldwide, especially in temperate zones	Dog, cat, fox	Small intestine	Chiefly ingestion of infective larva	Common, especially in north temperate regions	Common	Usually inapparent; sometimes enteritis, intestinal ulceration	Rare cause of cutaneous larva migrans	Bantin and Maber 1967 Levine 1968 Poynter 1966 Renaux 1964 Scott 1967 Soulsby 1965
Uncinaria criniformis	Europe, Indonesia	Dog, other carnivores	Small intestine	Unknown; presumably by ingestion of infective larva or skin penetration	Unknown	Unknown; probably absent	Unknown	Unknown	Levine 1968 Yamaguti 1961
Oesophagostomum apiostomum*	United States, Africa, Asia, Indonesia	Macaques, man	Colon; rarely omentum	Ingestion of infective larva	Common	Common	Nodules in wall of colon; sometimes diarrhea, debilitation	Occurs in man	Faust et al. 1968 Habermann and Williams 1957a, 1958 Levine 1968 Ruch 1959
Oesophagostomum bifurcum*	United States, Africa, Asia	Macaques, guenons, mangabeys, baboons, chimpanzee, man	Colon	Ingestion of infective larva	Common	Common	Nodules in wall of colon; sometimes diarrhea, debilitation	Occurs in man	Bingham and Rabstein 1964 Faust et al. 1968 Graham 1960 Guilloud et al. 1965 Levine 1968 Myers and Kuntz 1965 Reardon and Rininger 1968 Ruch 1959 Van Riper et al. 1966
Oesophagostomum aculeatum*	United States, Asia	Macaques, man	Colon	Ingestion of infective larva	Common	Common	Nodules in wall of colon; sometimes diarrhea, debilitation	Occurs in man	Faust et al. 1968 Hashimoto and Honjo 1966 Levine 1968 Reardon and Rininger 1968 Ruch 1959 Tanaka et al. 1962
Oesophagostomum stephanostomum*	United States, Africa	Baboons, chimpanzee, gorilla, man	Colon	Ingestion of infective larva	Common	Unknown; probably common	Nodules in wall of colon; sometimes diarrhea, debilitation	Occurs in man	Faust et al. 1968 Fiennes 1967 Levine 1968 Myers and Kuntz 1965 Reardon and Rininger 1968 Ruch 1959 Van Riper et al. 1966

*Discussed in text.

269

TABLE 7.3 (continued)

Parasite	Geographic Distribution	Endothermal Host	Location in Host	Method of Infection	Incidence — In nature	Incidence — In laboratory	Pathologic Effects	Public Health Importance	Reference
Oesophagostomum blanchardi	Southeastern Asia, Indonesia	Gibbons, orangutan	Colon	Ingestion of infective larva	Unknown	Unknown	Unknown	Unknown	Yamaguti 1961
Ternidens deminutus*	United States, Africa, Asia	Macaques, guenons, baboons, chimpanzee, gorilla, man	Cecum, colon	Ingestion of infective larva	Common in some areas	Uncommon	Anemia, nodules in wall of colon	Causes nodules in wall of colon	Amberson and Schwarz 1952; Graham 1960; Habermann and Williams 1957a; Levine 1968; Myers and Kuntz 1965; Nelson 1965; Reardon and Rininger 1968; Ruch 1959; Sasa et al. 1962; Tanaka et al. 1962
Mammomonogamus ierei	West Indies	Cat	Nasal cavities	Indirect; otherwise unknown	Unknown	Unknown	Unknown	Unknown	Buckley 1934; Levine 1968; Yamaguti 1961
Mammomonogamus mcgaughei	Ceylon	Cat	Nasal cavities, pharynx	Unknown	Unknown	Unknown	Unknown	Unknown	Levine 1968; Seneviratna 1954; Yamaguti 1961
Mammomonogamus auris	China	Cat	Middle ear	Unknown	Common in some areas	Unknown	Hemorrhagic middle ear mucosa	Unknown	Faust and Tang 1934; Levine 1968; Yamaguti 1961
Syngamus trachea*	Worldwide	Chicken, other birds	Trachea	Ingestion of embryonated egg, infective larva, or transport host (earthworms, snails, slugs)	Common	Rare or absent	Tracheitis, tracheal obstruction, hissing, dyspnea, asphyxia, death	None	Lapage 1962, 1968; Levine 1968; Soulsby 1965
Syngamus skrjabinomorpha	USSR	Chicken, goose	Trachea	Ingestion of embryonated egg, infective larva, or transport host (earthworms, snails, slugs)	Unknown	Unknown	Unknown	Unknown	Shikhobalova and Ryzhikov 1956

*Discussed in text.

TABLE 7.4. Trichostrongylids affecting endothermal laboratory animals

Parasite	Geographic Distribution	Endothermal Host	Location in Host	Method of Infection	Incidence		Pathologic Effects	Public Health Importance	Reference
					In nature	In laboratory			
*Molineus torulosus**[*]	Brazil	Capuchins, squirrel monkeys, night monkey	Small intestine	Unknown; probably ingestion of larva	Common	Common	Enteritis; hemorrhages, necrotic ulcers in intestinal wall	Unknown	Dunn 1961, 1968 Lapin and Yakovleva 1960 Yorke and Maplestone 1926
*Molineus vexillarius**[*]	United States, Peru	Tamarins	Small intestine, stomach	Unknown; probably ingestion of larva	Common	Common	Apparently none	Unknown	Cosgrove et al. 1968 Dunn 1961, 1968
*Molineus elegans**[*]	Eastern Brazil	Capuchins, squirrel monkeys	Small intestine	Unknown; probably ingestion of larva	Unknown	Unknown	Unknown	Unknown	Dunn 1961, 1968
*Molineus vogelianus**[*]	Africa	Pottos (*Perodicticus*)	Small intestine	Unknown; probably ingestion of larva	Unknown	Unknown	Unknown	Unknown	Dunn 1961
Obeliscoides cuniculi	North America	Rabbit, cottontail rabbits, hares	Stomach	Ingestion of larva	Common in wild lagomorphs; rare in domestic rabbit	Rare or absent	Hemorrhagic gastritis	Unknown	Alicata 1932 Levine 1968 Lund 1950 Morgan and Hawkins 1949 Rothenbacher et al. 1964 Sollod et al. 1968
Pithecostrongylus alatus	Malay Peninsula	Guenons, orangutan	Intestine	Unknown	Unknown	Unknown	Unknown	Unknown	Skrjabin et al. 1954 Travassos 1937 Yamaguti 1961
*Trichostrongylus colubriformis**[*]	Worldwide	Wild rodents, cottontail rabbits, hares, dog, macaques, baboons, chimpanzee, domestic animals, man	Small intestine	Ingestion of larva	Common in primates; rare in dog	Common in primates; rare or absent in dog	Unknown; probably diarrhea, eosinophilia in heavy infections	Causes diarrhea, eosinophilia	Faust et al. 1968 Lapage 1962, 1968 Lapin and Yakovleva 1960 Levine 1968 Reardon and Rininger 1968 Soulsby 1965 Valerio et al. 1969
Trichostrongylus calcaratus	North America	Wild rodents, rabbit, cottontail rabbits, hares, wild carnivores, domestic animals, man	Intestine	Ingestion of larva	Common in wild lagomorphs; rare in domestic rabbit	Rare or absent	Anemia	Occurs in man	Holloway 1966 Levine 1968 Lund 1950 Sarles 1934

[*]Discussed in text.

271

TABLE 7.4 *(continued)*

Parasite	Geographic Distribution	Endothermal Host	Location in Host	Method of Infection	Incidence — In nature	Incidence — In laboratory	Pathologic Effects	Public Health Importance	Reference
Trichostrongylus retortaeformis	Europe, Asia, South America	Wild rodents, rabbit, cottontail rabbits, hares, domestic animals	Duodenum, rarely stomach	Ingestion of larva	Common in wild lagomorphs; uncommon in domestic rabbit	Uncommon	Enteritis, anemia	Unknown	Cushnie 1954 Lapage 1962 Levine 1968
Trichostrongylus sigmodontis	Southern United States	Cotton rat, rice rat	Small intestine	Ingestion of larva	Common in cotton rat	Experimental only	Unknown	Unknown	Thatcher and Scott 1962
Trichostrongylus tenuis	North America, Europe, Asia, southern Africa	Chicken, other birds	Ceca, small intestine	Ingestion of larva	Common in wild birds; rare in domestic chicken	Rare	Hemorrhagic enteritis	Unknown	Lapage 1968 Levine 1968 Soulsby 1965 Wehr 1965
*Graphidium strigosum**	North America, Europe, Australia	Rabbit, cottontail rabbits, hares	Stomach	Ingestion of larva	Common	Uncommon	Uncertain; possibly gastric trauma, diarrhea, anemia, emaciation, death	Unknown	Adams et al. 1967 Cushnie 1954 Enigk 1938 Hall 1916 Lapage 1968 Levine 1968 Neveu-Lemaire 1936
Graphidioides berlai	Brazil	Woolly monkeys, spider monkeys	Intestine	Unknown; probably ingestion of larva	Unknown	Unknown	Unknown	Unknown	Travassos 1913 Yamaguti 1961
Nematodirus leporis	North America	Rabbit, cottontail rabbit, hares	Duodenum	Ingestion of larva	Common in some areas	Uncommon	Inapparent	Unknown	Chandler 1924 Dikmans 1937 Levine 1968 Morgan and Hawkins 1949
Nematodirus weinbergi	Africa	Chimpanzee	Small intestine	Ingestion of larva	Unknown	Unknown	Unknown	Unknown	Yamaguti 1961
Heligmosomum juvenum	Western Asia	Hamster	Small intestine	Unknown; probably ingestion of larva	Unknown	Absent	Unknown	Unknown	Kirschenblatt 1949 Yamaguti 1961
*Nematospiroides dubius**	North America, Europe	Mouse, deer mice, voles, European field mouse, other rodents	Small intestine	Ingestion of larva	Common	Absent	Inapparent	Unknown	Dobson 1961a, b, c, 1962a, b Ehrenford 1954 Fahmy 1956 Lepak et al. 1962 Levine 1968 Lewis 1968a, b Thompson et al. 1962
Heligmonoides murina	West Africa	Mouse	Small intestine	Unknown; probably ingestion of larva	Unknown	Unknown	Unknown	Unknown	Baylis 1928 Yamaguti 1961

*Discussed in text.

TABLE 7.4 (continued)

Parasite	Geographic Distribution	Endothermal Host	Location in Host	Method of Infection	Incidence In nature	Incidence In laboratory	Pathologic Effects	Public Health Importance	Reference
Longistriata musculi	Southern United States	Mouse	Small intestine	Ingestion of larva or skin penetration	Unknown	Unknown	Unknown	Unknown	Dikmans 1935, Morgan and Hawkins 1949, Schwartz and Alicata 1935
Longistriata norvegica	Southern United States	Rat	Small intestine	Unknown; probably ingestion of larva or skin penetration	Unknown	Unknown	Unknown	Unknown	Dikmans 1935, Yamaguti 1961
Longistriata vexillata	North America	Rat	Small intestine	Unknown; probably ingestion of larva or skin penetration	Unknown	Unknown	Unknown	Unknown	Hall 1916, Travassos 1937, Yamaguti 1961
Longistriata dubia	United States, South America	Squirrel monkeys, tamarins, howler monkeys	Small intestine	Unknown; probably ingestion of larva or skin penetration	Unknown; probably common	Common	Unknown	Unknown	Cosgrove et al. 1968, Dunn 1968
*Nippostrongylus brasiliensis**	Worldwide	Mouse, rat, black rat	Small intestine	Larval penetration of skin	Common in rat; rare in mouse	Experimental only	Dermatitis, pneumonitis, enteritis; sometimes severe verminous pneumonia, death	None	Habermann and Williams 1958, Haley 1961, 1962, Levine 1968, Sasa et al. 1962
*Nochtia nochti**	India, Indonesia, Thailand	Rhesus monkey, cynomolgus monkey, stumptailed macaque	Stomach	Unknown; probably ingestion of larva	Uncommon to common	Uncommon in rhesus monkey; common in stumptail macaque	Gastric tumors	Unknown	Bonne and Sandground 1939, Graham 1960, Hashimoto and Honjo 1966, Ruch 1959, Smetana and Orihel 1969, Travassos and Vogelsang 1929, Yamashita 1963
*Ollulanus tricuspis**	Canada, Europe, South Africa, Australia, Taiwan	Definitive: cat, other carnivores, pig; Paratenic: mouse	Stomach	Ingestion of larva passed by emesis	Common in some areas; rare in others	Uncommon or absent	Increased gastric mucus secretion; sometimes hemorrhagic gastritis	Unknown	Bearup 1960, Cameron 1923, 1927, Heston 1941, Lapage 1968, Levine 1968, Soulsby 1965
Ornithostrongylus hastatus	Europe	Chicken, other galliforms	Intestine	Unknown; probably ingestion of larva	Unknown	Unknown	Unknown	Unknown	Yamaguti 1961
Ornithostrongylus quadriradiatus	Worldwide	Pigeon, other birds	Duodenum, crop, proventriculus	Ingestion of larva	Common	Unknown	Diarrhea, catarrhal enteritis; sometimes hemorrhage, necrosis	Unknown	Alicata 1964, Cram and Cuvillier 1931, Leibovitz 1962, Levine 1968, Soulsby 1965

*Discussed in text.

273

TABLE 7.5. Metastrongylids affecting endothermal laboratory animals

Parasite	Geographic Distribution	Endothermal Host	Location in Host	Method of Infection	Incidence		Pathologic Effects	Public Health Importance	Reference
					In nature	In laboratory			
Aelurostrongylus abstrusus *	North America, Hawaii, South America, Europe, southwestern Asia, northern Africa, Australia	Wild rodents, cat	Rodents: omentum Cat: lungs	Rodents: ingestion of intermediate host (slugs, snails) Cat: ingestion of intermediate host or transport host (rodents, birds, amphibians, reptiles)	Common in Europe; probably common in United States	Rodents: absent Cat: unknown; probably common	Rodents: cysts in omentum Cat: usually inapparent; sometimes cough, dyspnea, emaciation, nodules in lungs	Unknown	Alicata 1964 Hamilton 1963 Hobmaier and Hobmaier 1935 Levine 1968 Poynter 1966 Renaux 1964 Soulsby 1965
Anafilaroides rostratus	North America, Hawaii, Israel, Ceylon	Wild rodents, cat	Rodents: liver, thoracic muscles Cat: lungs	Rodents: ingestion of intermediate host (slugs, snails) Cat: ingestion of intermediate host or transport host (rodents)	Uncommon in cat except in Ceylon	Unknown; probably rare or absent except in Ceylon	Unknown	Unknown	Alicata 1963, 1964 Klewer 1958 Levine 1968 Seneviratna 1959a, b
Anafilaroides pararostratus	Mexico	Dog	Trachea	Unknown	Unknown	Unknown	Unknown	Unknown	Flores-Barroeta 1956 Levine 1968
Angiostrongylus cantonensis	Hawaii, other Pacific islands, Asia, Australia	Norway rat, black rat, other rats	Lungs, brain	Ingestion of intermediate host (mollusks, possibly crustaceans)	Common in endemic areas	Absent	Wheeze, cough, sneeze, emaciation, pulmonary embolisms	Causes eosinophilic meningitis	Alicata 1962, 1963, 1965 Ash 1962a Heyneman and Lim 1967 Levine 1968 Mackerras and Sandars 1955 Rosen et al. 1962 Soulsby 1965
Angiostrongylus vasorum	North America, Europe, Australia	Dog, fox, other carnivores	Heart, pulmonary artery; sometimes brain, eyes	Larvae pass in feces; method of infection unknown, probably ingestion of mollusks	Rare, except in France	Unknown; probably absent except in France	Tachypnea, dyspnea, cough, bronchitis, pulmonary embolism, tubercles in lungs	Unknown	Levine 1968 Soulsby 1965
Bronchostrongylus subcrenatus	Asia, Africa	Wild rodents, cat, other felids	Rodents: unknown Cat: lungs	Rodents: ingestion of intermediate host (mollusks) Cat: ingestion of intermediate host or transport host (rodents)	Uncommon	Rare or absent	Unknown; probably none	Unknown	Fitzsimmons 1961b Levine 1968 Soulsby 1965

*Discussed in text.

274

TABLE 7.5 (continued)

Parasite	Geographic Distribution	Endothermal Host	Location in Host	Method of Infection	Incidence — In nature	Incidence — In laboratory	Pathologic Effects	Public Health Importance	Reference
*Filaroides osleri**	North America, Hawaii, Central America, Europe, India, southern Africa, Australia, New Zealand	Dog, other canids	Trachea, bronchi	Unknown; probably ingestion of mollusks or rodents	Common in some regions; uncommon in others	Unknown; probably common in dogs obtained from pounds in some regions, uncommon in others	Cough, dyspnea, anorexia, emaciation, wartlike hemorrhagic granular nodules in trachea, bronchi	Unknown	Alicata 1964 Levine 1968 Mills 1967 Mills and Nielsen 1966 Poynter 1966 Soulsby 1965 Urquhart et al. 1954
Filaroides milksi	United States	Dog, other carnivores	Lungs	Unknown; probably ingestion of mollusks or rodents	Rare	Unknown; probably rare	Inapparent; small white foci in lungs	Unknown	Levine 1968 Mills 1967 Mills and Nielsen 1966 Poynter 1966
Filaroides barretoi	South America	Marmosets	Lungs	Unknown	Unknown; probably uncommon	Unknown; probably uncommon	Usually inapparent; sometimes atelectasis, lung hemorrhages	Unknown	Dunn 1968 Graham 1960 Ruch 1959
Filaroides gordius	South America	Squirrel monkeys	Lungs	Unknown	Unknown; probably uncommon	Unknown; probably uncommon	Usually inapparent; sometimes atelectasis, lung hemorrhages	Unknown	Dunn 1968 Graham 1960 Ruch 1959
Filaroides sp.	United States, South America	Tamarins	Lungs	Unknown	Unknown; probably common	Common	Unknown	Unknown	Cosgrove et al. 1968
Filariopsis arator	South America	Capuchins	Lungs	Unknown	Unknown	Unknown	Unknown	Unknown	Chandler 1931 Yamaguti 1961
Gurltia paralysans	South America	Cat, wild felids	Veins of lumbar lepto-meninges	Unknown	Common in southern South America	Unknown; probably absent except in southern South America	Thrombosis of veins, posterior paralysis, death	Unknown	Levine 1968 Wolffhügel 1934
Vogeloides massinoi	USSR, India	Cat	Lungs	Unknown	Common in endemic areas	Unknown; probably common in endemic areas	Unknown	Unknown	Davtjan 1933 Dougherty 1943 Levine 1968 Yamaguti 1961

*Discussed in text.

275

TABLE 7.5 (continued)

Parasite	Geographic Distribution	Endothermal Host	Location in Host	Method of Infection	Incidence — In nature	Incidence — In laboratory	Pathologic Effects	Public Health Importance	Reference
Vogeloides ramanujacharii	India	Cat	Lungs	Unknown	Common in endemic areas	Unknown; probably common in endemic areas	Unknown	Unknown	Alwar et al. 1958, Lapage 1968, Levine 1968, Yamaguti 1961
Crenosoma vulpis	North America, Europe, China	Dog, cat, fox	Lungs	Ingestion of intermediate host (slugs, snails)	Uncommon in dog, cat	Unknown; probably uncommon or absent	Cough, dyspnea, bronchitis, pulmonary edema, hemorrhage	Unknown	Lapage 1968, Levine 1968, Soulsby 1965, Wetzel 1940
Protostrongylus rufescens	North America, Europe, India, Africa, Australia	Rabbit, cottontail rabbits, domestic animals	Lungs	Ingestion of intermediate host (snails)	Rare	Unknown; probably absent	Unknown	Unknown	Davtjan 1937, Hobmaier and Hobmaier 1930, Levine 1968
Protostrongylus pulmonalis	North America, Europe, Africa	Rabbit, cottontail rabbits, hares, domestic animals	Lungs	Ingestion of intermediate host (snails)	Unknown	Unknown; probably absent except in specimens obtained from natural environment	Unknown	Unknown	Dougherty and Goble 1946, Levine 1968
Protostrongylus oryctolagi	Central Europe	Rabbit	Bronchi	Ingestion of intermediate host (probably snails, slugs)	Unknown	Unknown	Unknown	Unknown	Levine 1968
Protostrongylus boughtoni	United States	Cottontail rabbits, hares	Lungs, bronchi	Ingestion of intermediate host (probably snails, slugs)	Unknown; probably common	Unknown	Unknown	Unknown	Dougherty and Goble 1946, Levine 1968, Olsen 1954
Protostrongylus sylvilagi	Western United States	Cottontail rabbits, hares	Lungs	Ingestion of intermediate host (probably snails, slugs)	Unknown	Unknown	Unknown	Unknown	Levine 1968

TABLE 7.6. Heterakids and ascaridids affecting endothermal laboratory animals

Parasite	Geographic Distribution	Endothermal Host	Location in Host	Method of Infection	Incidence		Pathologic Effects	Public Health Importance	Reference
					In nature	In laboratory			
*Heterakis spumosa**	Worldwide	Rat, black rat	Cecum, colon	Ingestion of egg	Common	Rare	Apparently none	None	Habermann and Williams 1958 Levine 1968 Oldham 1967 Ratcliffe 1949 Smith 1953a, b, c
*Heterakis gallinarum**	Worldwide	Chicken, other birds	Ceca	Ingestion of egg	Common	Uncommon or absent	Vector of *Histomonas meleagridis*	None	Levine 1968 Morgan and Hawkins 1949 Soulsby 1965
Heterakis beramporia	Asia, Philippine Islands	Chicken	Ceca	Ingestion of egg	Unknown	Unknown	Nodules in ceca	None	Levine 1968 Soulsby 1965
*Paraspidodera uncinata**	Worldwide	Guinea pig	Cecum, colon	Ingestion of egg	Common in some regions; uncommon in others	Uncommon	Usually none; possibly weight loss, debilitation, diarrhea	None	Cook 1969 Habermann and Williams 1958 Herlich 1959 Herlich and Dixon 1965 Levine 1968 Morgan and Hawkins 1949 Paterson 1962 Porter and Otto 1934
*Ascaridia galli**	Worldwide	Chicken, other birds	Small intestine	Ingestion of embryonated egg	Common	Uncommon	Debilitation, anorexia, hemorrhagic enteritis, diarrhea	None	Lapage 1968 Levine 1968 Morgan and Hawkins 1949 Soulsby 1965 Wehr 1965
Ascaridia compar	North America, Europe, India, Philippine Islands	Chicken, other birds	Small intestine	Ingestion of embryonated egg	Unknown	Unknown; probably absent	Unknown	Unknown	Levine 1968 Wehr 1965
Ascaridia columbae	Worldwide	Pigeon	Small intestine	Ingestion of embryonated egg	Common	Uncommon	Unknown; probably none except in heavy infections	Unknown	Lapage 1968 Levine 1968 Soulsby 1965 Wehr 1965

*Discussed in text.

TABLE 7.6 (continued)

Parasite	Geographic Distribution	Endothermal Host	Location in Host	Method of Infection	Incidence		Pathologic Effects	Public Health Importance	Reference
					In nature	In laboratory			
Ascaris lumbricoides	Worldwide	Rhesus monkey, gibbons, orangutan, chimpanzee, gorilla, man	Adult: small intestine Larva: various tissues	Ingestion of embryonated egg	Uncommon	Uncommon	Usually inapparent; sometimes liver abscesses, icterus	Common large roundworm of man	Dunn and Greer 1962 Lapin and Yakovleva 1960 Levine 1968 Mortelmans and Vercruysse 1962 Pillers 1924 Reardon and Rininger 1968 Riopelle 1967 Ruch 1959
Ascaris columnaris	North America, USSR	Definitive: wild carnivores Paratenic: ground squirrels, other rodents	Adult: intestine Larva: brain, various tissues	Ingestion of embryonated egg or paratenic host	Common in ground squirrel	Common in ground squirrel	Paratenic host: abnormal motor activity, debilitation, coma, death	Unknown	Fritz et al. 1968 Levine 1968 Sprent 1968
*Toxocara canis**	Worldwide	Definitive: dog, other canids Paratenic: wild rodents	Adult: small intestine Larva: various tissues	Intrauterine; ingestion of egg (neonates only); ingestion of tissue containing larva	Common	Common	Cough, nasal discharge, vomiting, mucoid diarrhea, anorexia, debilitation, pruritus, epileptic seizures, pulmonary hemorrhages, enteritis, visceral granulomas; neurologic signs in rodents	Causes visceral larva migrans	Barron and Saunders 1966 Fritz et al. 1968 Griesemer and Gibson 1963b Griesemer et al. 1963 Hoey 1968 Levine 1968 Morgan and Hawkins 1949 Soulsby 1965 Sprent 1952, 1953, 1958 Woodruff et al. 1966
*Toxocara mystax**	Worldwide	Definitive: cat, other felids Paratenic: wild rodents	Adult: small intestine Larva: various tissues	Ingestion of egg or paratenic host (earthworms, cockroaches, birds, rodents)	Common	Common	Cough, vomiting, mucoid diarrhea, debilitation, epileptic seizures, enteritis, visceral granulomas; neurologic signs in rodents; eggs can carry *Toxoplasma gondii*	Causes visceral larva migrans; eggs can carry agent of toxoplasmosis	Dubey 1966 Frenkel et al. 1969 Fritz et al. 1968 Hutchison 1967 Levine 1968 Morgan and Hawkins 1949 Sheffield and Melton 1969 Soulsby 1965 Sprent 1956 Woodruff et al. 1966
*Toxascaris leonina**	Worldwide	Cat, dog, other carnivores	Small intestine	Ingestion of egg or paratenic host (rodents, insectivores, small carnivores)	Common	Common	Vomiting, anorexia, mucoid diarrhea, debilitation	Assumed to cause visceral larva migrans	Levine 1968 Morgan and Hawkins 1949 Soulsby 1965 Sprent 1959

*Discussed in text.

TABLE 7.7. Subulurids affecting endothermal laboratory animals

Parasite	Geographic Distribution	Endothermal Host	Location in Host	Method of Infection	Incidence In nature	Incidence In laboratory	Pathologic Effects	Public Health Importance	Reference
Subulura distans	United States, Asia, Africa	Guenons, mangabeys, mandrill, baboons	Stomach, small intestine, colon	Ingestion of intermediate host (cockroaches)	Unknown	Unknown	Unknown	Unknown	López-Neyra 1945 Myers and Kuntz 1965 Nelson 1965 Ruch 1959 Yamashita 1963
Subulura malayensis	Malay Peninsula	Cynomolgus monkey, other macaques	Colon	Unknown	Unknown	Unknown	Unknown	Unknown	López-Neyra 1945 Yamashita 1963
Subulura jacchi	United States, South America	Marmosets, tamarins	Small intestine	Ingestion of intermediate host (cockroaches)	Unknown; probably common	Common	Unknown	Unknown	Chabaud and Larivière 1955 Cosgrove et al. 1968 Deinhardt et al. 1967 Ruch 1959 Yamashita 1963
Subulura brumpti	North America, Hawaii, Central America, West Indies, Europe, Asia, Africa	Chicken, other birds	Ceca	Ingestion of intermediate host (beetles, grasshoppers, cockroaches, other arthropods)	Common	Rare or absent	Unknown	Unknown	Alicata 1964 Cuckler and Alicata 1944 Levine 1968 Wehr 1965
Subulura strongylina	United States, West Indies, Brazil	Chicken, other birds	Ceca	Ingestion of intermediate host (arthropods)	Unknown	Unknown	Unknown	Unknown	Levine 1968 Soulsby 1965 Wehr 1965
Subulura differens	Europe, southwestern Asia, Africa, South America	Chicken, other galliforms	Posterior small intestine	Ingestion of intermediate host (arthropods)	Unknown	Unknown	Unknown	Unknown	Levine 1968 Soulsby 1965
Subulura suctoria	USSR, Africa, South America	Chicken, other birds	Ceca	Ingestion of intermediate host (arthropods)	Unknown	Unknown	Unknown	Unknown	Levine 1968
Subulura minetti	India	Chicken	Ceca	Unknown	Unknown	Unknown	Unknown	Unknown	Levine 1968

TABLE 7.8. Oxyurids affecting endothermal laboratory animals

Parasite	Geographic Distribution	Endothermal Host	Location in Host	Method of Infection	Incidence In nature	Incidence In laboratory	Pathologic Effects	Public Health Importance	Reference
Dermatoxys veligera	United States, South America, Europe, Africa	Rabbit, cottontail rabbits, hares	Cecum	Ingestion of egg	Common	Rare or absent	Typhlitis	Unknown	Dikmans 1931 Holloway 1966 Levine 1968 Morgan and Hawkins 1949
Buckleyenterobius atelis	Central America, South America	Spider monkeys	Colon	Unknown; probably ingestion of egg	Unknown	Unknown	Unknown	Unknown	Buckley 1931 Cameron 1929 Sandosham 1950a Yamaguti 1961
Buckleyenterobius duplicidens	South America	Woolly monkeys	Colon	Unknown; probably ingestion of egg	Unknown	Unknown	Unknown	Unknown	Buckley 1931 Dollfus and Chabaud 1955 Yamaguti 1961
Buckleyenterobius lagothricis	South America	Woolly monkeys	Colon	Unknown; probably ingestion of egg	Unknown	Unknown	Unknown	Unknown	Buckley 1931 Yamaguti 1961
Enterobius vermicularis *	Worldwide	Marmosets, gibbons, chimpanzee, man	Large intestine	Ingestion of embryonated egg	Uncommon or absent in simian primates	Uncommon	Perianal pruritus, restlessness, aggressiveness	Common pinworm of man; causes perianal pruritus, restlessness	Cameron 1929 Christensen 1964 Hashimoto and Honjo 1966 Inglis 1961 Riopelle 1967 Sandosham 1950a
Enterobius anthropopitheci	United States, Africa	Chimpanzee	Large intestine	Ingestion of embryonated egg	Common	Common	Perianal pruritus, restlessness, aggressiveness	Unknown; probably infectious for man	Gedoelst 1916 Reardon and Rininger 1968 Riopelle 1967 Ruch 1959
Enterobius bipapillatus	Africa	Rhesus monkey, chimpanzee	Large intestine	Ingestion of embryonated egg	Common	Common	Perianal pruritus, restlessness, aggressiveness	Unknown; probably infectious for man	Gedoelst 1916 Riopelle 1967 Yamaguti 1961
Enterobius brevicauda	Africa	Baboons	Large intestine	Ingestion of embryonated egg	Unknown; probably common	Unknown; probably common	Unknown; probably causes perianal pruritus	Unknown; probably infectious for man	Sandosham 1950a Yamaguti 1961
Enterobius lerouxi	Africa	Gorilla	Large intestine	Ingestion of embryonated egg	Unknown; probably common	Unknown; probably common	Unknown; probably causes perianal pruritus	Unknown; probably infectious for man	Sandosham 1950a Yamaguti 1961

*Discussed in text.

TABLE 7.8 (continued)

Parasite	Geographic Distribution	Endothermal Host	Location in Host	Method of Infection	Incidence		Pathologic Effects	Public Health Importance	Reference
					In nature	In laboratory			
Enterobius buckleyi	Borneo	Orangutan	Large intestine	Ingestion of embryonated egg	Unknown; probably common	Unknown; probably common	Unknown; probably causes perianal pruritus	Unknown; probably infectious for man	Sandosham 1950a Yamaguti 1961
Enterobius interlabiatus	South America	Night monkey	Large intestine	Ingestion of embryonated egg	Unknown; probably common	Unknown; probably common	Unknown; probably causes perianal pruritus	Unknown; probably infectious for man	Sandosham 1950b Yamaguti 1961
Enterobius microon	South America	Night monkey	Large intestine	Ingestion of embryonated egg	Unknown; probably common	Unknown; probably common	Unknown; probably causes perianal pruritus	Unknown; probably infectious for man	Yamaguti 1961
Lobatorobius scleratus	Central America, South America	Squirrel monkeys	Cecum, colon	Unknown; probably ingestion of egg	Unknown	Unknown	Unknown	Unknown	Yamaguti 1961
Oxyuronema atelophorum	Central America	Spider monkeys	Large intestine	Unknown; probably ingestion of embryonated egg	Unknown; probably common	Unknown; probably common	Unknown; associated with hemorrhagic enteritis, abdominal discomfort	Unknown	Graham 1960 Kreis 1932 Yamaguti 1961
Passalurus ambiguus*	Worldwide	Rabbit, cottontail rabbits, hares	Cecum, colon	Ingestion of embryonated egg	Common	Common	Apparently none	None	Cushnie 1954 Habermann and Williams 1958 Lapage 1968 Levine 1968 Lund 1950 Morgan and Hawkins 1949 Owen 1968 Poole et al. 1967
Passalurus nonannulatus	North America	Cottontail rabbits, hares	Cecum, colon	Ingestion of embryonated egg	Common	Common	Unknown	Unknown	Erickson 1947 Holloway 1966 Yamaguti 1961
Syphacia obvelata*	Worldwide	Mouse, rat, black rat, hamster, voles, monkey, man	Cecum, colon	Ingestion of embryonated egg; invasion of anus by infective larva	Common in mouse, voles; rare or absent in rat, monkey	Common in mouse, hamster; uncommon in rat; rare in monkey	Usually none; sometimes associated with impaction, intussusception, rectal prolapse	Rarely occurs in man	Chan 1952 Habermann and Williams 1958 Hussey 1957 Levine 1968 Sasa et al. 1962 Stone and Manwell 1966

*Discussed in text.

TABLE 7.8 (continued)

Parasite	Geographic Distribution	Endothermal Host	Location in Host	Method of Infection	Incidence — In nature	Incidence — In laboratory	Pathologic Effects	Public Health Importance	Reference
Syphacia muris*	Worldwide	Mouse, rat, black rat	Cecum, colon	Ingestion of embryonated egg; invasion of anus by infective larva	Common in rat; rare or absent in mouse	Common in rat; uncommon in mouse	Apparently none except in heavy infections	Unknown; probably rarely occurs in man	Bell 1968 Hussey 1957 Owen 1968 Sasa et al. 1962 Stone and Manwell 1966
Trypanoxyuris minutus	South America	Capuchins, spider monkeys, howler monkeys, marmosets	Colon	Unknown; probably ingestion of egg	Unknown	Unknown	Unknown	Unknown	Menschel and Stroh 1963 Pope 1968 Yamashita 1963
Trypanoxyuris sceleratus	Central America, South America	Squirrel monkeys	Colon	Unknown; probably ingestion of egg	Unknown	Unknown	Unknown	Unknown	Dunn 1968
Trypanoxyuris tamarini	United States, South America	Tamarins	Cecum, colon	Unknown; probably ingestion of egg	Unknown; probably common	Common	None	Unknown	Cosgrove et al. 1968 Deinhardt et al. 1967
Wellcomia compar	North America	Cat	Colon	Unknown; probably ingestion of egg	Unknown	Unknown	Unknown	Unknown	Price 1930 Yamaguti 1961
Aspiculuris tetraptera*	Worldwide	Mouse, rat, black rat, other rodents	Colon	Ingestion of embryonated egg	Common in mouse; uncommon in other rodents	Common in mouse; uncommon in rat	Usually none; sometimes associated with impaction, intussusception, rectal prolapse	Unknown	Chan 1955 Flynn et al. 1965 Sasa et al. 1962 Stone and Manwell 1966 Takada 1958

*Discussed in text.

TABLE 7.9. Spirurids, gnathostomatids, and acuariids affecting endothermal laboratory animals

Parasite	Geographic Distribution	Endothermal Host	Location in Host	Method of Infection	Incidence In nature	Incidence In laboratory	Pathologic Effects	Public Health Importance	Reference
Chituoodspirura serrata	Central America	Chimpanzee, gorilla	Stomach, small intestine	Ingestion of intermediate host (insects)	Unknown	Unknown	Unknown	Unknown	Chabaud and Rousselot 1956 Yamaguti 1961
Mastophorus muricola	Europe, Africa, Asia, Central America, West Indies, Philippine Islands	Mouse, rat, black rat, hamster, other rodents, monkey	Stomach	Ingestion of intermediate host (cockroaches)	Common	Occurs only in specimens obtained from natural habitat	Unknown	Unknown	Chabaud 1954, 1955 Foster and Johnson 1939 de Léon 1964 Myers et al. 1962 Yamaguti 1961
Mastophorus muris	Worldwide	Mouse, rat, cotton rat, hamster, other rodents, cottontail rabbits	Stomach	Ingestion of intermediate host (cockroaches, fleas)	Common	Occurs only in specimens obtained from natural habitat	Unknown	Unknown	Chabaud 1954, 1955 Chitwood 1938 Cram 1926 Heston 1941 Kreis 1937 Levine 1968 Miyata 1939 Yamaguti 1961
Spirura rytipleurites	Europe, Africa	Definitive: dog, cat, fox, hedgehog Paratenic: wild rodents, birds	Adult: stomach Larva: various tissues	Ingestion of intermediate host (cockroaches, beetles) or paratenic host (rodents, birds, reptiles, amphibians)	Unknown	Unknown	Definitive host: slight local inflammation of stomach, vomiting	Unknown	Levine 1968 Soulsby 1965
Spirura guianensis	United States, South America	Tamarins	Esophagus	Unknown	Common	Common in specimens obtained from natural habitat	Slight local inflammation of esophagus	Unknown	Chitwood 1938 Cosgrove et al. 1968 Nelson et al. 1966
Trichospirura leptostoma	United States, South America	Tamarins	Pancreas	Unknown	Unknown	Unknown; probably uncommon	Unknown	Unknown	Cosgrove et al. 1968
Tetrameres americana	North America, Hawaii, South America, Africa	Chicken, other birds	Proventriculus	Ingestion of intermediate host (cockroaches, grasshoppers)	Common in some areas	Unknown; probably rare or absent	Debilitation, slight local inflammation of proventriculus	Unknown	Alicata 1964 Cram 1929b, 1931 Levine 1968 Soulsby 1965 Wehr 1965
Tetrameres fissispina	North America, West Indies, Europe, Asia	Chicken, other birds	Proventriculus	Ingestion of intermediate host (water fleas, amphipods, grasshoppers, cockroaches, earthworms)	Unknown; probably uncommon except in some areas	Unknown; probably rare or absent	Debilitation	Unknown	Chabaud 1954, 1955 Cram 1931 Levine 1968 Sugimoto and Nishiyama 1937 Wehr 1965

TABLE 7.9 *(continued)*

Parasite	Geographic Distribution	Endothermal Host	Location in Host	Method of Infection	Incidence		Pathologic Effects	Public Health Importance	Reference
					In nature	In laboratory			
Tetrameres confusa	South America, Philippine Islands	Chicken, pigeon, other birds	Proventriculus	Ingestion of unknown intermediate host	Unknown	Unknown	Debilitation, local inflammation of proventriculus	Unknown	Chabaud 1954, 1955 Cram 1931 Levine 1968
Gnathostoma spinigerum	Europe, Asia, Africa, Indonesia, Australia	Definitive: dog, cat, other carnivores Intermediate: rat, other rodents, birds	Adult: stomach wall Larva: various tissues	Definitive: ingestion of second intermediate host (fishes, amphibians, reptiles, birds, rodents) Intermediate: ingestion of first intermediate host (copepods)	Unknown	Rare or absent	Definitive: tumorlike nodules in stomach wall Intermediate: granulomatous lesions in various tissues	Larvae occur in subcutaneous tissues	Kikuchi 1956 Levine 1968 Miyazaki 1952, 1954 Soulsby 1965 Yamaguchi et al. 1955
Gnathostoma didelphis	North America, Central America	Opossum	Stomach	Ingestion of intermediate host (fishes)	Common	Common in specimens obtained from natural habitat	Gastritis, ulceration of gastric mucosa	Unknown	Babero 1960 Krupp 1962 Yamaguti 1961
Hartertia gallinarum	Africa	Chicken, other birds	Small intestine	Ingestion of intermediate host (arthropods)	Unknown	Unknown	Emaciation, diarrhea, weakness, death	Unknown	Lapage 1968 Levine 1968 Soulsby 1965
Cheilospirura hamulosa	Worldwide	Chicken, other birds	Esophagus, crop, gizzard	Ingestion of intermediate host (grasshoppers, sandhoppers, beetles, weevils)	Common	Rare or absent	Emaciation, anemia, ulceration, nodule formation	Unknown	Dotsenko 1953 Levine 1968 Morgan and Hawkins 1949 Soulsby 1965 Wehr 1965
Dispharynx nasuta	Worldwide	Chicken, pigeon, other birds	Proventriculus	Ingestion of intermediate host (sowbugs, pillbugs)	Common	Rare or absent	Tumorlike lesions, ulceration of proventriculus	Unknown	Cram 1931 Cuvillier 1937 Levine 1968 Morgan and Hawkins 1949 Wehr 1965
Histiocephalus laticaudatus	Europe	Chicken	Gizzard	Unknown	Unknown	Unknown; probably rare	Hemorrhagic inflammation, nodule formation	Unknown	Levine 1968 Soulsby 1965

TABLE 7.10. Thelaziids affecting endothermal laboratory animals

Parasite	Geographic Distribution	Endothermal Host	Location in Host	Method of Infection	Incidence In nature	Incidence In laboratory	Pathologic Effects	Public Health Importance	Reference
Metathelazia ascaroides	Unknown	Guenons	Lungs	Unknown	Unknown	Unknown	Unknown	Unknown	Dougherty 1943, 1952 Yamaguti 1961
Oxyspirura mansoni	North America, Hawaii, West Indies, South America, Asia, Africa, Australia, Pacific islands	Chicken, other birds	Conjunctival sacs	Ingestion of intermediate host (cockroaches)	Uncommon	Unknown; probably rare or absent	Irritation, lacrimation, inflammation of nictitating membranes, keratoconjunctivitis, blindness	Unknown	Alicata 1964 Levine 1968 Morgan and Hawkins 1949 Schwabe 1950a, b, 1951 Soulsby 1965
Thelazia californiensis	Western United States, Mexico	Dog, cat, other carnivores, hares, wild ruminants, man	Lacrimal ducts, conjunctival sacs, nictitating membranes	Embryonated eggs ingested by muscid fly; transferred when fly feeds on conjunctival fluids	Rare	Unknown; probably rare or absent	Scleral congestion, lacrimation, keratoconjunctivitis, photophobia	Occurs rarely in man	Burnett et al. 1957 Hosford et al. 1942 Knapp et al. 1961 Levine 1968 Morgan and Hawkins 1949 Parmelee et al. 1956 Schauffler 1966
Thelazia callipaeda	North America, Asia	Rat, rabbit, dog, monkey, man	Eyes	Embryonated eggs ingested by fly; fly probably transmits when feeding	Unknown; probably rare	Unknown; probably rare or absent	Scleral congestion, lacrimation, keratoconjunctivitis, photophobia	Occurs in man	Faust 1928 Hsü 1933 Kozlov 1963 Levine 1968 Soulsby 1965
Spirocerca lupi*	Worldwide in tropics and subtropics	Dog, other canids, wild felids	Esophagus, stomach, aorta, lungs, other organs	Ingestion of intermediate host (cockroaches, dung beetles) or paratenic hosts (reptiles, amphibians, birds, mammals)	Common in some areas; absent in others	Common in some areas; absent in others	Difficult swallowing, dyspnea, vomiting; nodules in esophagus, aorta, lungs; aortic aneurysm	None	Bailey 1963 Gupta and Pande 1962 Lapage 1968 Levine 1968 Murray 1968 Soulsby 1965
Spirocerca arctica	USSR	Dog, other canids	Esophagus, stomach	Unknown; probably ingestion of insect	Unknown	Unknown	Unknown	Unknown	Levine 1968 Soulsby 1965
Cylicospirura subaequalis	Asia, South America	Cat, wild carnivores	Stomach	Ingestion of intermediate host (arthropods)	Unknown	Unknown	Unknown	Unknown	Levine 1968 Yamaguti 1961
Cylicospirura felinea	Southern Asia, northern Africa	Cat, other felids	Stomach	Ingestion of intermediate host (arthropods)	Unknown	Unknown	Unknown	Unknown	Levine 1968 Yamaguti 1961

*Discussed in text.

285

TABLE 7.10 (continued)

Parasite	Geographic Distribution	Endothermal Host	Location in Host	Method of Infection	Incidence In nature	Incidence In laboratory	Pathologic Effects	Public Health Importance	Reference
*Streptopharagus armatus**	United States, Japan, Africa	Rhesus monkey, cynomolgus monkey, Japanese macaque, other macaques, guenons, patas monkey, baboons, gibbons	Stomach	Ingestion of intermediate host (arthropods)	Common in cynomolgus monkey, Japanese macaque	Common in cynomolgus monkey, Japanese macaque	Unknown	Unknown	Habermann and Williams 1957a; Myers and Kuntz 1965; Tanaka et al. 1962
*Streptopharagus pigmentatus**	United States, Europe, Africa, Asia	Rhesus monkey, cynomolgus monkey, guenons, baboons, gibbons	Stomach	Ingestion of intermediate host (arthropods)	Common in monkey	Common in monkey	Unknown	Unknown	Graham 1960; Hashimoto and Honjo 1966; López-Neyra 1951; Myers and Kuntz 1965; Reardon and Rininger 1968; Sasa et al. 1962
Gongylonema neoplasticum	Worldwide	Mouse, rat, black rat, hamster, voles, other rodents, rabbit, hares	Esophagus, stomach	Ingestion of intermediate host (cockroaches, mealworms, fleas)	Common	Occurs only in specimens obtained from natural habitat	Gastric ulcers	Unknown	Ash 1962a; Bacigalupo 1934; Chabaud 1954, 1955; Kirschenblatt 1949; Lapage 1968; de León 1964; Levine 1968; Oldham 1967
Gongylonema musculi	Europe	Mouse	Esophagus, stomach	Ingestion of intermediate host (insects)	Unknown	Unknown	Unknown; probably none	Unknown	Yamaguti 1961
Gongylonema macrogubernaculum	USSR	Rhesus monkey, guenons, baboons, capuchins	Lungs, esophagus, stomach	Ingestion of intermediate host (insects)	Unknown	Unknown	Unknown; probably none	Unknown	Graham 1960; Lucker 1933a; Myers and Kuntz 1965
Gongylonema pulchrum	Worldwide	Capuchins, spider monkeys, toque monkey (*Macaca sinica*), domestic animals, wild carnivores, ruminants, man	Tongue, oral cavity, esophagus, stomach	Ingestion of intermediate host (cockroaches, dung beetles)	Common	Unknown; probably rare	None	Occurs in man	Alicata 1934, 1936; Baylis 1939; Chabaud 1954, 1955; Levine 1968; Lucker 1933b

*Discussed in text.

286

TABLE 7.10 *(continued)*

Parasite	Geographic Distribution	Endothermal Host	Location in Host	Method of Infection	Incidence — In nature	Incidence — In laboratory	Pathologic Effects	Public Health Importance	Reference
Gongylonema ingluvicola	North America, Hawaii, Europe, Africa, Asia, Australia	Chicken, other birds	Crop	Ingestion of intermediate host (dung beetles, cockroaches)	Unknown	Unknown	Slight local inflammation of crop	Unknown	Alicata 1964, Chabaud 1954, 1955, Cram 1931, 1935, Levine 1968, Soulsby 1965, Wehr 1965
Rictularia muris	Europe	Mouse	Small intestine	Ingestion of intermediate host (insects)	Unknown	Unknown	Unknown	Unknown	Yamaguti 1961
Rictularia magna	Europe	Mouse	Small intestine	Ingestion of intermediate host (insects)	Unknown	Unknown	Unknown	Unknown	Yamaguti 1961
Rictularia baicalensis	USSR	Mouse, European field mouse	Small intestine	Ingestion of intermediate host (arthropods)	Unknown	Unknown	Unknown	Unknown	Chabaud 1955, Yamaguti 1961
Rictularia amurensis	USSR	Mouse	Small intestine	Ingestion of intermediate host (arthropods)	Unknown	Unknown	Unknown	Unknown	Yamaguti 1961
Rictularia ratti	India	Rat	Small intestine	Ingestion of intermediate host (arthropods)	Unknown	Unknown	Unknown	Unknown	Khera 1954, Yamaguti 1961
Rictularia citelli	North America	Ground squirrels	Small intestine	Ingestion of intermediate host (arthropods)	Common	Common	Unknown	Unknown	Fritz et al. 1968, McLeod 1933, Yamaguti 1961
Rictularia cahirensis	North America, South America, Europe, Africa, Asia	Dog, cat, other carnivores	Small intestine	Ingestion of intermediate host (arthropods)	Common in Asia	Unknown	Unknown	Unknown	Chabaud 1954, 1955, Levine 1968, Myers et al. 1962, Yamaguti 1961
Rictularia alphi	USSR	Monkey, guenons, capuchins, marmosets	Small intestine	Ingestion of intermediate host (arthropods)	Unknown	Unknown	Unknown	Unknown	Chabaud 1954, 1955, Yamaguti 1961, Yamashita 1963

TABLE 7.11. Physalopterids affecting endothermal laboratory animals

Parasite	Geographic Distribution	Endothermal Host	Location in Host	Method of Infection	Incidence In nature	Incidence In laboratory	Pathologic Effects	Public Health Importance	Reference
Physaloptera massino	North America, Europe	Mouse, ground squirrels, other rodents	Stomach	Ingestion of intermediate host (insects)	Unknown	Occurs only in specimens obtained from natural habitat	Unknown; probably gastritis	Unknown	Morgan 1943 Yamaguti 1961
Physaloptera muris-brasiliensis	North America, Hawaii, Brazil	Rat, cotton rat, other rodents	Stomach	Ingestion of intermediate host (insects)	Unknown	Occurs only in specimens obtained from natural habitat	Unknown; probably gastritis	Unknown	Ash 1962a Chabaud 1954, 1955 Morgan 1913 Yamaguti 1961
Physaloptera hispida	United States	Cotton rat	Stomach	Ingestion of intermediate host (cockroaches)	Common	Occurs only in specimens obtained from natural habitat	Unknown; probably gastritis	Unknown	Chabaud 1954, 1955 Schell 1950, 1952 Yamaguti 1961
Physaloptera bispiculata	United States, Brazil	Cotton rat, wood rats, other rodents	Stomach	Ingestion of intermediate host (insects)	Common	Occurs only in specimens obtained from natural habitat	Unknown; probably gastritis	Unknown	Chabaud 1954, 1955 Morgan 1943 Vaz and Pereira 1935 Yamaguti 1961
Physaloptera turgida	North America, South America	Opossum, wild carnivores	Stomach, duodenum	Ingestion of intermediate host (cockroaches)	Common	Common in specimens obtained from natural habitat	Hemorrhagic gastritis, hemorrhagic enteritis, ulceration	Unknown	Alicata 1937 Chabaud 1954, 1955 Hill 1940 Holloway 1966 Krupp 1962 Levine 1968
*Physaloptera rara**	United States	Dog, cat, wild carnivores	Stomach, duodenum	Ingestion of intermediate host (cockroaches, flour beetles, crickets)	Common in some areas; rare in others	Unknown; probably uncommon or absent	Vomiting, anorexia, debilitation, dark feces, gastritis, enteritis, ulceration	Unknown	Chabaud 1954, 1955 Levine 1968 Morgan 1946 Petri 1950 Petri and Ameel 1950 Worley 1964
*Physaloptera felidis**	United States	Dog, cat, wild carnivores	Stomach, duodenum	Ingestion of intermediate host (insects)	Common in some areas; rare in others	Unknown; probably rare or absent	Vomiting, debilitation, gastritis, enteritis, ulceration	Unknown	Ackert 1936 Chabaud 1954, 1955 Levine 1968 Soulsby 1965
*Physaloptera pseudopraeputialis**	United States, Philippine Islands	Cat, coyote	Stomach	Ingestion of intermediate host (insects)	Common in Philippine Islands	Unknown; probably rare	Vomiting, anorexia, debilitation, gastritis, ulceration	Unknown	Ash 1962b Levine 1968 Morgan and Hawkins 1949 Tacal and Corpuz 1962 Yutuc 1953
*Physaloptera praeputialis**	Africa, Asia, Indonesia, South America	Dog, cat, wild felids	Stomach	Ingestion of intermediate host (cockroaches, crickets)	Common in some areas	Unknown; probably uncommon or absent	Vomiting, anorexia, debilitation, gastritis, ulceration	Unknown	Ash 1962b Fitzsimmons 1961c Levine 1968 Petri and Ameel 1950 Soulsby 1965

*Discussed in text.

288

TABLE 7.11 (continued)

Parasite	Geographic Distribution	Endothermal Host	Location in Host	Method of Infection	Incidence — In nature	Incidence — In laboratory	Pathologic Effects	Public Health Importance	Reference
Physaloptera pacitae	Central America, Philippine Islands	Cat	Stomach	Ingestion of intermediate host (insects)	Unknown	Unknown, probably rare or absent	Unknown; probably gastritis	Unknown	Levine 1968
Physaloptera canis	South Africa	Dog, cat	Stomach	Ingestion of intermediate host (insects)	Unknown	Unknown; probably rare or absent	Unknown; probably gastritis	Unknown	Chabaud 1954, 1955; Levine 1968; Mönnig 1929; Soulsby 1965
Physaloptera brevispiculum	Asia	Cat, wild felids	Stomach	Ingestion of intermediate host (insects)	Unknown	Unknown; probably rare or absent	Unknown; probably gastritis	Unknown	Baylis 1939; Levine 1968
*Physaloptera tumefaciens**	Asia	Rhesus monkey, cynomolgus monkey, other macaques	Stomach	Ingestion of intermediate host (insects)	Common	Common	Hemorrhagic gastritis, ulceration	Unknown	Chabaud 1954, 1955; Hashimoto and Honjo 1966; Levine 1968; Sasa et al. 1962; Tanaka et al. 1962; Yamashita 1963
*Physaloptera dilatata**	South America	Capuchins, woolly monkeys, marmosets	Stomach	Ingestion of intermediate host (insects)	Unknown	Unknown; probably common in specimens obtained from natural habitat	Unknown; probably gastritis, ulceration	Unknown	Chabaud 1954, 1955; Deinhardt et al. 1967; Yamaguti 1961
Abbreviata gemina	Southwestern United States, Egypt	Cat, wild carnivores, chicken	Stomach	Ingestion of intermediate host (insects)	Unknown	Unknown; probably rare or absent	Unknown; probably gastritis, ulceration	Unknown	Chabaud 1954, 1955; Hannum 1941–1942; Levine 1968
*Abbreviata caucasica**	Southeastern Europe, southwestern Asia, Africa	Rhesus monkey, baboons, orangutan, man	Esophagus, stomach, duodenum	Ingestion of intermediate host (beetles)	Common in some areas	Unknown; probably uncommon	Usually inapparent; probably esophagitis, gastritis, enteritis, ulceration	Occurs in man	Chabaud 1954; Jaskoski 1960; Levine 1968; Myers and Kuntz 1965; Nelson 1965; Ruch 1959; Yamaguti 1961
*Abbreviata poicilometra**	United States, Africa	Mangabeys, guenons	Stomach	Ingestion of intermediate host (insects)	Unknown	Unknown; probably rare	Mild gastritis	Unknown	Slaughter and Bostrom 1969; Yamaguti 1961

*Discussed in text.

289

TABLE 7.12. Onchocercids affecting endothermal laboratory animals

Parasite	Geographic Distribution	Endothermal Host	Location in Host	Method of Infection	Incidence — In nature	Incidence — In laboratory	Pathologic Effects	Public Health Importance	Reference
Dirofilaria scapiceps	United States	Cottontail rabbits, hares	Adult: subcutis Microfilaria: blood	Bite of mosquito	Common	Unknown	Unknown	None	Anderson 1957 Chabaud and Anderson 1959 Crites and Phinney 1958 Highby 1943 Penner 1954
Dirofilaria uniformis	Eastern United States	Cottontail rabbits,	Adult: subcutis Microfilaria: blood	Bite of mosquito	Common	Unknown	Unknown	None	Anderson 1957 Bray and Walton 1961 Chabaud and Anderson 1959 Price 1957
*Dirofilaria immitis**	Worldwide	Dog, other canids, cat, wild carnivores, man	Adult: right ventricle, pulmonary artery, vena cava Microfilaria: blood	Bite of mosquito	Common, especially in tropics and subtropics	Common, especially in tropics and subtropics	Lack of endurance, cough, anorexia, loss of weight, increased respiration, rales, hematuria, enlargement of heart, pulmonary congestion, ascites	Occurs rarely in man	Faust et al. 1968 Jackson 1969 Jackson et al. 1962, 1966 Jackson and Wallace 1966 Levine 1968 Liu et al. 1969 Newton and Wright 1956, 1957 Otto 1962, 1969a Otto and Jackson 1969 Smith and Jones 1966 Thrasher et al. 1968
Dirofilaria repens	Europe, Asia, Africa	Dog, cat, wild carnivores, man	Adult: subcutis Microfilaria: blood	Bite of mosquito	Common in some areas	Unknown	Dermatitis, pruritus, alopecia	Occurs in man	Anderson 1957 Chabaud and Anderson 1959 Lapage 1968 Levine 1968 Nelson 1959 Soulsby 1965
Dirofilaria magnilarvatum	East Pakistan, Malay Peninsula	Rhesus monkey, cynomolgus monkey	Adult: subcutis peritoneal membranes Microfilaria: blood	Bite of mosquito	Unknown	Unknown	Unknown	Unknown	Anderson 1957 Chabaud and Anderson 1959 Hawking 1959 McCoy 1936 Price 1959 Sandosham et al. 1962 Taylor 1959 Wharton 1959

*Discussed in text.

TABLE 7.12 (continued)

Parasite	Geographic Distribution	Endothermal Host	Location in Host	Method of Infection	Incidence In nature	Incidence In laboratory	Pathologic Effects	Public Health Importance	Reference
Dirofilaria corynodes	Africa	Guenons, mangabeys, langurs	Adult: subcutis, Microfilaria: blood	Bite of mosquito	Unknown	Unknown	Unknown	None known	Anderson 1957, Chabaud and Anderson 1959, Fiennes 1967, Hawking and Webber 1955, Lapage 1968, McCoy 1936, Webber 1955a, b, c, d
Dirofilaria pongoi	Indonesia	Gibbons, orangutan	Adult: subcutis, muscle, right ventricle, Microfilaria: blood	Bite of mosquito	Unknown	Unknown	Unknown	Unknown	Anderson 1957, Chabaud and Anderson 1959, McCoy 1936, Ruch 1959
Edesonfilaria malayensis	United States, southeastern Asia	Cynomolgus monkey	Adult: peritoneal cavity, Microfilaria: blood	Unknown	Unknown	Common	Unknown	Unknown; probably none	Levine 1968, Reardon and Rininger 1968, Yamaguti and Hayama 1961, Yeh 1960
Loa loa	Africa	Guenons, mandrills, baboons, man	Adult: subcutis, mesenteries, eyes, Microfilaria: blood	Bite of tabanid fly	Unknown; probably common in some areas	Unknown	Subcutaneous swellings	Occurs in man; species in man possibly distinct	Duke 1954a, 1955, Duke and Wijers 1958, Fiennes 1967, Lavoipierre 1958, Levine 1968, Myers and Kuntz 1965, Nelson 1965, Webber 1955b
Macacanema formosana	Taiwan	Macaques	Adult: peritracheal connective tissue, Microfilaria: blood	Unknown; possibly bite of midge	Common	Unknown	Unknown	Unknown; probably nonpathogenic for man	Bergner and Jachowski 1968, Levine 1968, Schad and Anderson 1963
Brugia ceylonensis	Ceylon	Dog	Lymphatic system	Unknown; probably bite of mosquito	Uncommon	Unknown	Unknown	Unknown	Jayewardene 1962, Levine 1968
Brugia pahangi	Malay Peninsula, Africa	Dog, cat, wild felids, leaf monkeys, slow loris	Lymphatic system	Bite of mosquito	Unknown	Unknown	Unknown	Experimentally transmissible to man	Anderson 1957, Chabaud and Anderson 1959, Anderson et al. 1960, Levine 1968, Schacher 1962a, b, Soulsby 1965

TABLE 7.12 (continued)

Parasite	Geographic Distribution	Endothermal Host	Location in Host	Method of Infection	Incidence		Pathologic Effects	Public Health Importance	Reference
					In nature	In laboratory			
Brugia patei	Africa	Dog, cat	Lymphatic system	Bite of mosquito	Unknown	Unknown	Unknown	Unknown	Anderson 1957 Buckley et al. 1958 Chabaud and Anderson 1959 Laurence and Pester 1961 Levine 1968 Schacher 1962a, b Soulsby 1965
Brugia malayi	Asia, South Pacific islands	Cat, rhesus monkey, cynomolgus monkey, other macaques, slow loris, man	Adult: lymphatics, lymph nodes Microfilaria: blood	Bite of mosquito	Unknown	Unknown	Unknown	Occurs in man	Anderson 1957 Buckley 1960 Chabaud and Anderson 1959 Edeson and Wharton 1957, 1958 Fiennes 1967 Lapage 1968 Levine 1968 Sandosham et al. 1962 Soulsby 1965 Wharton 1957
Dipetalonema reconditum *	North America, Hawaii, South America, southern Europe, eastern Africa, Australia, New Zealand	Dog	Adult: subcutis Microfilaria: blood	Bite of flea or tick	Common in North America, Europe	Common	None	Unknown; possibly affects man	Lapage 1968 Levine 1968 Lindsey 1965 Newton and Wright 1956, 1957 Soulsby 1965
Dipetalonema dracunculoides	Portugal, Africa, India	Dog, other canids	Adult: peritoneal cavity Microfilaria: blood	Bite of fly	Unknown	Unknown	None	Unknown	Lapage 1968 Levine 1968 Nelson 1963 Soulsby 1965
Dipetalonema grassii	Southern Europe, eastern Africa	Dog	Adult: subcutis, peritoneal cavity Microfilaria: skin, rarely blood	Bite of tick	Unknown	Unknown	None	Unknown	Lapage 1968 Levine 1968 Soulsby 1965

*Discussed in text.

292

TABLE 7.12 (continued)

Parasite	Geographic Distribution	Endothermal Host	Location in Host	Method of Infection	Incidence In nature	Incidence In laboratory	Pathologic Effects	Public Health Importance	Reference
Dipetalonema gracile*	Central America, South America	Capuchins, spider monkeys, woolly monkeys, squirrel monkeys, marmosets, tamarins	Adult: peritoneal cavity Microfilaria: blood	Bite of arthropod, presumably mosquito	Common	Common in specimens obtained from natural habitat	Usually none; sometimes peritoneal adhesions	Unknown; possibly affects man	Cosgrove et al. 1968; Deinhardt et al. 1967; Dunn and Lambrecht 1963; Garner 1967; Lapin 1962; Levine 1968; Ruch 1959; Webber and Hawking 1955
Dipetalonema caudispina*	South America	Capuchins, squirrel monkeys	Adult: peritoneal cavity Microfilaria: blood	Bite of arthropod, presumably mosquito	Common	Common in specimens obtained from natural habitat	Slight or none	Unknown; possibly affects man	Dunn and Lambrecht 1963; Garner et al. 1967
Dipetalonema obtusa	Central America, northern South America	Capuchins, squirrel monkeys	Adult: peri-esophageal connective tissue Microfilaria: blood	Bite of arthropod, presumably mosquito	Common	Unknown	Unknown	Unknown; possibly affects man	Esslinger 1966; Levine 1968; McCoy 1936; Yeh 1957
Dipetalonema tenue	Argentina	Capuchins	Adult: subcutis, body cavity Microfilaria: blood	Bite of unknown invertebrate	Unknown	Unknown	Unknown	Unknown	Chabaud and Anderson 1959; Chabaud and Choquet 1953; Yamaguti 1961
Dipetalonema marmosetae*	Central America	Capuchins, spider monkeys, squirrel monkeys, marmosets	Adult: subcutis, body cavity Microfilaria: blood	Bite of arthropod, presumably mosquito	Common	Common in specimens obtained from natural habitat	Unknown	Unknown	Dunn and Lambrecht 1963; McCoy 1936; Ruch 1959; Webber 1955a; Yeh 1957
Dipetalonema tamarinae*	South America	Marmosets	Adult: peritoneal cavity Microfilaria: blood	Bite of arthropod, presumably mosquito	Common	Common in specimens obtained from natural habitat	Unknown	Unknown	Deinhardt et al. 1967; Dunn and Lambrecht 1963; Esslinger 1966
Dipetalonema atelense	Central America	Spider monkeys	Adult: connective tissue Microfilaria: blood	Bite of arthropod, presumably mosquito	Unknown	Unknown	Slight or none	Unknown	McCoy 1936; Ruch 1959; Yamaguti 1961; Yeh 1957
Dipetalonema parvum	South America	Capuchins, squirrel monkeys	Adult: connective tissue Microfilaria: blood	Bite of arthropod, presumably mosquito	Unknown	Unknown	Slight or none	Unknown	Dunn 1968; McCoy 1936; Ruch 1959; Yamashita 1963; Yeh 1957

*Discussed in text.

TABLE 7.12 *(continued)*

Parasite	Geographic Distribution	Endothermal Host	Location in Host	Method of Infection	Incidence — In nature	Incidence — In laboratory	Pathologic Effects	Public Health Importance	Reference
Dipetalonema perstans	Africa	Chimpanzee, gorilla, man	Adult: subcutis, body cavity Microfilaria: blood	Bite of arthropod (flies, ticks, mosquitoes)	Unknown	Unknown	Vascular occlusion	Occurs in man	Chabaud and Anderson 1959 Duke 1956 Faust et al 1968 Habermann and Menges 1968 Lapage 1968
Dipetalonema vanhoofi	Central Africa	Baboons, chimpanzee	Adult: peritoneal cavity Microfilaria: blood	Bite of arthropod	Unknown	Unknown	Peritoneal nodules	Unknown	Chabaud 1952, 1955 Levine 1968 Myers and Kuntz 1965 Peel and Chardome 1946 Ruch 1959 Yeh 1957
Dipetalonema rodhaini	Central Africa	Chimpanzee	Adult: subcutis, body cavity Microfilaria: blood	Bite of arthropod	Unknown	Unknown	Unknown	Unknown	Peel and Chardome 1947 Ruch 1959 Yamaguti 1961 Yeh 1957
Dipetalonema streptocerca	Central Africa	Chimpanzee, gorilla, man	Adult: subcutis, peritoneal cavity Microfilaria: blood	Bite of midge	Unknown	Unknown	Unknown	Occurs in man	Chardome and Peel 1949 Colbourne et al. 1950 Duke 1954b, 1956 Faust et al. 1968 Levine 1968 Ruch 1959 Yeh 1957
Dipetalonema digtatum	India	Macaques, gibbons	Adult: peritoneal cavity Microfilaria: blood	Bite of arthropod	Common	Unknown	Unknown	Unknown	Chabaud and Anderson 1959 Chabaud and Choquet 1953 Chandler 1929 Ruch 1959 Yamaguti 1961 Yeh 1957
*Litomosoides carinii**	North America, South America	Cotton rat, other wild rodents	Adult: thoracic, pericardial, peritoneal cavities Microfilaria: blood	Bite of mite	Common	Experimental only	Slight or none	Unknown	Levine 1968 Scott and MacDonald 1953 Scott et al 1951 Thompson et al. 1968

*Discussed in text.

TABLE 7.13. Dracunculids affecting endothermal laboratory animals

Parasite	Geographic Distribution	Endothermal Host	Location in Host	Method of Infection	Incidence		Pathologic Effects	Public Health Importance	Reference
					In nature	In laboratory			
Dracunculus insignis	North America	Dog, wild carnivores	Skin, subcutis, viscera	Ingestion of intermediate host (copepods)	Rare	Unknown; probably rare	Skin papules, erythema, pruritus	Unknown	Ewing and Hibbs 1966 Levine 1968 Medway and Souisby 1966
Dracunculus medinensis	USSR, Asia, New Guinea	Dog, guenons, baboons, large domestic animals, man	Skin, subcutis, viscera	Ingestion of intermediate host (copepods)	Rare	Unknown; probably rare	Skin papules, erythema, pruritus	Causes skin papules, erythema, pruritus, vomiting, diarrhea, dyspnea	Ewing and Hibbs 1966 Faust et al. 1968 Levine 1968 Myers and Kuntz 1965 Ruch 1959

TABLE 7.14. Trichurids, anatrichosomatids, and trichinellids affecting endothermal laboratory animals

Parasite	Geographic Distribution	Endothermal Host	Location in Host	Method of Infection	Incidence — In nature	Incidence — In laboratory	Pathologic Effects	Public Health Importance	Reference
Trichuris muris	Worldwide	Rat, mouse, hamster	Cecum, colon	Ingestion of embryonated egg	Common	Rare or absent	Unknown	Unknown	Fahmy 1954 Myers et al. 1962 Ratcliffe 1949
Trichuris leporis	North America, Europe	Ground squirrels, rabbit, cottontail rabbits, hares	Cecum, colon	Ingestion of embryonated egg	Common in wild and domestic rabbits	Unknown; probably uncommon	Probably none except in heavy infections	Unknown	Levine 1968 Morgan and Hawkins 1949 Tiner 1950
Trichuris sylvilagi	United States, Europe	Cottontail rabbits, hares	Cecum, colon	Ingestion of embryonated egg	Unknown	Unknown	Probably none	Unknown	Drygas and Piotrowski 1955 Tiner 1950 Yamaguti 1961
Trichuris vulpis*	Worldwide	Dog, fox, other canids	Cecum, colon	Ingestion of embryonated egg	Common	Common in pound dogs, less common in kennel dogs; absent in cesarean-derived colonies	Usually inapparent; sometimes diarrhea, anemia, loss of weight, debilitation	None	Galvin and Turk 1966 Habermann and Williams 1958 Levine 1968 Miller 1947 Morgan 1967 Soulsby 1965
Trichuris felis	North America, South America, Europe	Cat, other felids	Cecum, colon	Ingestion of embryonated egg	Uncommon	Rare or absent	Probably none except in heavy infections	Unknown	Gaafar 1964 Levine 1968 Morgan and Hawkins 1949
Trichuris trichiura*	Worldwide	Rhesus monkey, cynomolgus monkey, other macaques, baboons, chimpanzee, other primates, man	Cecum, colon	Ingestion of embryonated egg	Common in tropics and subtropics	Common in primates obtained from natural environment	Usually inapparent; sometimes anorexia, typhlitis, colitis, mucoid diarrhea, death	Whipworm of man; usually inapparent; sometimes causes colitis, typhlitis, rectal prolapse	Britz et al. 1961 Faust et al. 1968 Graham 1960 Habermann and Williams 1957a Kuntz et al. 1968 Myers and Kuntz 1965 Reardon and Rininger 1968 Ruch 1959 Tanaka et al. 1962 Yamashita 1963
Capillaria hepatica*	Worldwide	Mouse, rat, other rodents, rabbit, dog, cat, rhesus monkey, capuchins, spider monkeys, chimpanzee, domestic animals, man	Liver	Eggs in liver released after ingestion by rodent or carnivore, passed in feces, embryonated, reingested by susceptible host	Common in wild rodents; uncommon in simian primates; rare in rabbit, dog, cat	Absent except in specimens obtained from their natural habitat	Yellow nodules in liver, sometimes hepatitis, hepatic cirrhosis, death	Rarely affects man	Faust et al. 1968 Habermann and Williams 1957a, 1958 Jones 1967 Lapage 1968 Levine 1968 Lubinsky 1956 Morgan and Hawkins 1949 Olsen 1967 Ruch 1959 Soulsby 1965

*Discussed in text.

TABLE 7.14 (continued)

Parasite	Geographic Distribution	Endothermal Host	Location in Host	Method of Infection	Incidence — In nature	Incidence — In laboratory	Pathologic Effects	Public Health Importance	Reference
Capillaria bacillata	Europe	Mouse, rat, European field mouse	Esophagus	Ingestion of egg	Unknown	Absent except in specimens obtained from their natural habitat	Unknown	Unknown	Levine 1968
Capillaria muris-musculi	Europe	Mouse	Intestine	Unknown	Unknown	Absent except in specimens obtained from their natural habitat	Unknown	Unknown	Levine 1968
Capillaria traverae	Hawaii	Rat, black rat	Small intestine	Ingestion of egg or earthworm	Unknown	Absent except in specimens obtained from their natural habitat	Unknown	Unknown	Ash 1962a
Capillaria gastrica	North America, South America, Europe, Japan	Rat, black rat, European field mouse, voles	Esophagus, stomach, small intestine	Ingestion of egg	Unknown	Unknown	Unknown	Unknown	Alicata and Lucker 1932 Levine 1968
Capillaria annulosa	Europe	Rat, black rat, other rodents	Small intestine	Ingestion of egg or earthworm	Uncommon	Rare or absent	Unknown	Unknown	Hall 1916 Levine 1968 Ratcliffe 1949 Yamaguti 1961
Capillaria intestinalis	Europe	Rat, black rat	Intestine	Ingestion of egg	Uncommon	Absent except in specimens obtained from their natural habitat	Unknown	Unknown	Levine 1968
Capillaria papillosa	Europe	Rat, black rat	Urinary bladder	Ingestion of egg	Unknown	Absent except in specimens obtained from their natural habitat	Unknown	Unknown	Levine 1968
Capillaria polonica	Europe	Rat	Urinary bladder	Unknown	Unknown	Absent except in specimens obtained from their natural habitat	Unknown	Unknown	Levine 1968
Capillaria multicellularis	Japan	Rat	Small intestine	Ingestion of egg	Unknown	Unknown	Unknown	Unknown	Levine 1968

TABLE 7.14 *(continued)*

Parasite	Geographic Distribution	Endothermal Host	Location in Host	Method of Infection	Incidence — In nature	Incidence — In laboratory	Pathologic Effects	Public Health Importance	Reference
Capillaria prashadi	India	Rat	Unknown	Unknown	Unknown	Absent except in specimens obtained from their natural habitat	Unknown	Unknown	Levine 1968
Capillaria aerophila*	North America, South America, Europe	Dog, cat, fox, other carnivores	Bronchioles, bronchi, trachea	Ingestion of embryonated egg	Unknown in dog; rare in cat	Unknown; probably uncommon in dog; rare in cat	Usually inapparent; sometimes bronchitis, tracheitis, pneumonia	None	Christenson 1938 Habermann and Williams 1958 Lapage 1968 Levine 1968 Renaux 1964 Soulsby 1965
Capillaria plica*	Worldwide	Rat, dog, cat, fox	Urinary bladder, kidneys	Ingestion of earthworm	Rare to common in dog; uncommon in cat	Unknown; probably absent	Usually none	None	Chitwood and Enzie 1953 Enigk 1950 Medway and Skelley 1961 Olsen 1967 Rankin 1946 Renaux 1964 Soulsby 1965 Whitehead 1964
Capillaria feliscati*	North America, South America, Europe, China, Egypt, Australia	Cat, other felids	Urinary bladder	Unknown	Common in South America, Australia	Unknown	Unknown	Unknown	Habermann and Williams 1958 Levine 1968 Renaux 1964 Soulsby 1965 Waddell 1968a, b
Capillaria contorta*	Worldwide	Chicken, other galliforms	Esophagus, crop	Ingestion of embryonated egg or earthworm	Common	Unknown; probably rare or absent	Usually inapparent; sometimes anorexia, weakness, emaciation, anemia, esophagitis, death	None	Madsen 1945, 1951, 1952 Soulsby 1965 Wehr 1965
Capillaria annulata*	Worldwide	Chicken, other galliforms	Esophagus, crop	Ingestion of earthworm	Rare to common	Unknown; probably absent	Usually inapparent; sometimes anorexia, weakness, emaciation, anemia, esophagitis, death	None	Madsen 1945, 1951, 1952 Soulsby 1965 Wehr 1965

*Discussed in text.

TABLE 7.14 *(continued)*

Parasite	Geographic Distribution	Endothermal Host	Location in Host	Method of Infection	Incidence — In nature	Incidence — In laboratory	Pathologic Effects	Public Health Importance	Reference
Capillaria caudinflata	North America, Europe	Chicken, pigeon, other birds	Small intestine	Ingestion of earthworm	Uncommon in North America; common in Europe	Unknown; probably absent	Enteritis	Unknown	Lapage 1968 Levine 1968 Nickel 1953 Soulsby 1965 Wehr 1965
Capillaria anatis	North America, South America, Europe, Asia, Australia	Chicken, other birds	Small intestine, ceca	Unknown	Common in some areas	Unknown; probably rare or absent	Enteritis	Unknown	Lapage 1968 Levine 1968 Soulsby 1965
Capillaria obsignata	North America, South America, Europe, Asia, Australia	Chicken, pigeon, other birds	Small intestine	Ingestion of embryonated egg	Common in chicken in Great Britain; uncommon or unknown elsewhere	Unknown; probably rare or absent except in Great Britain	Hemorrhagic diarrhea, emaciation, enteritis, sometimes death	Unknown	Lapage 1968 Levine 1968 Morgan and Hawkins 1949 Soulsby 1965 Wehr 1965
Capillaria montevidensis	Uruguay	Chicken	Ceca	Unknown	Unknown	Unknown	Unknown	Unknown	Levine 1968
Capillaria uruguanensis	Uruguay	Chicken	Ceca, large intestine	Unknown	Unknown	Unknown	Unknown	Unknown	Levine 1968
*Trichosomoides crassicauda**	Worldwide	Rat, black rat	Urinary bladder, kidneys, ureters	Ingestion of embryonated egg	Common	Common	Usually inapparent; sometimes masses in bladder wall, eosinophilia, granulomatous lesions in lungs; associated with urinary calculi, tumors of bladder	None	Bell 1968 Bone and Harr 1967 Chapman 1964 Innes et al. 1967 Paget and Lemon 1965 Peardon et al. 1966 Sasa et al. 1962 Smith 1946
Trichosomoides nasalis	Europe	Rat, hamster	Nasal mucosa	Unknown	Unknown	Unknown	Unknown	Unknown	Biocca and Aurizi 1961 Chesterman and Buckley 1965 Seamer and Chesterman 1967

*Discussed in text.

TABLE 7.14 *(continued)*

Parasite	Geographic Distribution	Endothermal Host	Location in Host	Method of Infection	Incidence — In nature	Incidence — In laboratory	Pathologic Effects	Public Health Importance	Reference
*Anatrichosoma cutaneum**	United States, Asia	Rhesus monkey, man	Nasal mucosa, skin	Ingestion of egg	Common	Common	Usually inapparent; slight inflammation, hyperplasia, parakeratosis ot nasal mucosa	Causes a form of creeping eruption	Allen 1960 Faust et al. 1968 Reardon and Rininger 1968 Ruch 1959
Anatrichosoma cynomolgi	United States, Asia	Cynomolgus monkey	Nasal mucosa	Ingestion of egg	Unknown	Unknown	Unknown	Unknown	Allen 1960 Chitwood and Smith 1958
Trichinella spiralis	Worldwide	Mouse, rat, guinea pig, other rodents, dog, cat, domestic animals, man	Adult: mucosa of small intestine Larva: skeletal muscle, various organs	Ingestion of encysted larva	Common in rat; uncommon in other laboratory animals	Rare or absent	Adult: mild enteritis Larva: usually inapparent; can transmit viral infections	Important in man; causes trichinosis; infected laboratory animals not likely source of infection for man	Bisseru 1967 Cook 1969 Faust et al. 1968 Heston 1941 Levine 1968 Rausch et al. 1956 Schaeffler 1961 Smith and Jones 1966 Zimmermann and Schwarte 1958

*Discussed in text.

TABLE 7.15. Dioctophymids and soboliphymatids affecting endothermal laboratory animals

Parasite	Geographic Distribution	Endothermal Host	Location in Host	Method of Infection	Incidence In nature	Incidence In laboratory	Pathologic Effects	Public Health Importance	Reference
Dioctophyma renale[*]	North America, South America, Europe, Asia, Africa	Dog, other carnivores, domestic animals, man	Kidneys, abdominal cavity	Ingestion of uncooked viscera of fish	Unknown; probably uncommon in the dog	Uncommon	Usually inapparent; sometimes hematuria, hydronephrosis, renal hypertrophy, peritonitis	Rarely affects man	Hallberg 1953 Mann and Bjotvedt 1955 Morgan and Hawkins 1949 Olsen 1967 Smith and Jones 1966 Soulsby 1965 Woodhead 1950
Soboliphyme baturini	North America, Asia	Cat, wild carnivores	Wall of stomach	Unknown	Unknown	Unknown	Unknown	Unknown	Petrov 1930 Yamaguti 1961

*Discussed in text.

REFERENCES

Abadie, S. H. 1963. The life cycle of *Strongyloides ratti*. J. Parasitol. 49:241–48.

Abadie, S. H., J. C. Swartzwelder, and R. L. Holman. 1965. A human case of *Dirofilaria immitis* infection. Am. J. Trop. Med. Hyg. 14:117–18.

Ackert, J. E. 1936. *Physaloptera felidis* n. sp., a nematode of the cat. Trans. Am. Microscop. Soc. 55:250–54.

Adams, C. E., F. C. Aitken, and A. H. Worden. 1967. The rabbit, pp. 431–32. *In* UFAW Staff, eds. The UFAW handbook on the care and management of laboratory animals. 3d ed. Livingstone and the Universities Federation for Animal Welfare, London.

Ahlqvist, J., and H. Borgmästars. 1961. A method for getting rid of *Trichosomoides crassicauda* in laboratory rats. Ann. Med. Exp. Biol. Fenniae (Helsinki) 39:297–301.

Ahlqvist, J., T. Rytömaa, and H. Borgmästars. 1962. Blood eosinophilia caused by a common parasite in laboratory rats. Acta Haematol. 28:306–12.

Alicata, J. E. 1932. Life history of the rabbit stomach worm *Obeliscoides cuniculi*. J. Agr. Res. 44:401–19.

———. 1934. Observations on the development to egg-laying maturity of *Gongylonema pulchrum* (Nematoda: Spiruridae) in the guinea pig. Proc. Helminthol. Soc. Wash., D.C. 1:51–52.

———. 1936. Early developmental stages of nematodes occurring in swine. U.S. Dept. Agr. Tech. Bull. 489. 96 pp.

———. 1937. Larval development of the spirurid nematode, *Physaloptera turgida*, in the cockroach, *Blatella germanica*. Raboty Gel'mintol. (Skrjabin), 11–14.

———. 1962. *Angiostrongylus cantonensis* (Nematoda: Metastrongylidae) as a causative agent of eosinophilic meningoencephalitis of man in Hawaii and Tahiti. Can. J. Zool. 40:5–8.

———. 1963. Morphological and biological differences between the infective larvae of *Angiostrongylus cantonensis* and those of *Anafilaroides rostratus*. Can. J. Zool. 41:1179–83.

———. 1964. Parasitic infections of man and animals in Hawaii. Hawaii Agr. Exp. Sta. Tech. Bull. 61. 138 pp.

———. 1965. Biology and distribution of the rat lungworm, *Angiostrongylus cantonensis*, and its relationship to eosinophilic meningoencephalitis and other neurological disorders of man and animals, pp. 223–48. *In* B. Dawes, ed. Advances in parasitology. Vol. 3. Academic Press, New York.

Alicata, J. E., and J. T. Lucker. 1932. The occurrence of a species of Capillariinae in the gastric wall of rats in the United States. J. Parasitol. 18:311.

Allen, A. M. 1960. Occurrence of the nematode, *Anatrichosoma cutaneum*, in the nasal mucosae of *Macaca mulatta* monkeys. Am. J. Vet. Res. 21:389–92.

Alwar, V. S., C. M. Lalitha, and P. Seneviratna. 1958. *Vogeloides ramanujacharii* n. sp., a new lung worm from the domestic cat (*Felis catus* Linne), in India. Indian Vet. J. 35:1–5.

Amberson, J. M., and E. Schwarz. 1952. *Ternidens deminutus* Railliet and Henry, a nematode parasite of man and primates. Ann. Trop. Med. Parasitol. 46:227–37.

Anderson, R. C. 1957. The life cycles of dipetalonematid nematodes (Filaroidea: Dipetalonematidae): The problem of their evolution. J. Helminthol. 31:203–24.

Ash, L. R. 1962a. The helminth parasites of rats in Hawaii and the description of *Capillaria traverae* sp. n. J. Parasitol. 48:66–68.

———. 1962b. Helminth parasites of dogs and cats in Hawaii. J. Parasitol. 48:63–65.

Babero, B. B. 1960. On the migration of *Ascaris laevis* Leidy, 1856 in some experimentally infected hosts. Trans. Am. Microscop. Soc. 79:439–42.

Bacigalupo, J. 1934. El ciclo evolutivo del *Gongylonema neoplasticum* (Fibiger-Ditlevsen) en la Argentina. Actas Trabajos 5. Congr. Nac. Med. 3:947–49.

Bailey, W. S. 1963. Parasites and cancer: Sarcoma in dogs associated with *Spirocerca lupi*. Ann. N.Y. Acad. Sci. 108:890–923.

Bantin, G. C., and D. F. Maber. 1967. Some parasites of the beagle. J. Inst. Animal Tech. 18:49–59.

Barrett, J. 1969. The effect of ageing on the metabolism of the infective larvae of *Strongyloides ratti* Sandground, 1925. Parasitology 59:3–17.

Barron, C. N., and L. Z. Saunders. 1966. Visceral larva migrans in the dog. Pathol. Vet. 3:315–30.

Basir, M. A. 1950. The morphology and development of the sheep nematode, *Strongyloides papillosus* (Wedl, 1856). Can. J. Res. 28:173–96.

Batte, E. G., and D. J. Moncol. 1968. Intestinal nematodes of dogs, pp. 533–35. *In* R. W. Kirk, ed. Current veterinary therapy III: Small animal practice. W. B. Saunders, Philadelphia.

Baylis, H. A. 1928. On a collection of nematodes from Nigerian mammals (chiefly rodents). Parasitology 20:280–304.

————. 1939. The fauna of British India (including Ceylon and Burma): Nematoda v. 2 (Filarioidea; Dioctophymoidea; and Trichinelloidea). Secretary of State for India, London. 274 pp.

Beach, T. D. 1936. Experimental studies on human and primate species of Strongyloides. V. The free-living phase of the life cycle. Am. J. Hyg. 23:243–77.

Bearup, A. J. 1960. Parasitic infections in Australian cats. Australian Vet. J. 36:352–54.

Bell, Deirdre P. 1968. Disease in a caesarian-derived albino rat colony and in a conventional colony. Lab. Animals 2:1–17.

Benbrook, E. A., and Margaret W. Sloss. 1961. Veterinary clinical parasitology. 3d ed. Iowa State Univ. Press, Ames. 240 pp.

Benson, R. E., B. D. Fremming, and R. J. Young. 1954. Care and management of chimpanzees at the radiobiological laboratory of the University of Texas and the United States Air Force. Animal Care Panel 5:27–36.

Berberian, D. A., J. B. Poole, and H. W. Freele. 1963. Treatment of Trichuris vulpis infection of dogs with glycobiarsol. Am. J. Vet. Res. 24:819–21.

Bergner, J. F., Jr., and L. A. Jachowski, Jr. 1968. The filarial parasite, Macacanema formosana, from the Taiwan monkey and its development in various arthropods. Formosan Sci. 22:1–68.

Bertram, D. S. 1966. Dynamics of parasitic equilibrium in cotton rat filariasis, pp. 255–319. In B. Dawes, ed. Advances in parasitology. Vol. 4. Academic Press, New York.

Bingham, G. A., and M. M. Rabstein. 1964. A study of the effectiveness of thiabendazole in the rhesus monkey. Lab. Animal Care 14:357–65.

Biocca, E., and A. Aurizi. 1961. On a new parasitic nematode Trichosomoides nasalis n. sp., from the nasal cavities of Epimys norvegicus: and considerations on the family Trichosomoididae Yorke and Maplestone, 1926. J. Helminthol. R. T. Leiper Supplement, pp. 5–8.

Bisseru, B. 1967. Diseases of man acquired from his pets. William Heinemann Medical Books, London. 482 pp.

Bisseru, B., A. W. Woodruff, and R. I. Hutchinson. 1966. Infection with adult Toxocara canis. Brit. Med. J. 1:1583–84.

Blair, Lyndia S., and P. E. Thompson. 1969. Effects of pyrvinium pamoate in the ration or drinking water of rats against the pinworm Syphacia muris. Lab. Animal Care 19:639–43.

Blair, Lyndia S., P. E. Thompson, and J. M. Vandenbelt. 1968. Effects of pyrvinium pamoate in the ration or drinking water of mice against pinworms Syphacia obvelata and Aspiculuris tetraptera. Lab. Animal Care 18:314–27.

Bloom, F. 1965. Spontaneous renal lesions, pp. 93–123. In W. E. Ribelin and J. R. McCoy, eds. The pathology of laboratory animals. Charles C Thomas, Springfield, Ill.

Boecker, H. 1953. Die Entwicklung des Kaninchenoxyuren Passalurus ambiguus. Z. Parasitenk. 15:491–518.

Bolla, R. I., and L. S. Roberts. 1968. Gametogenesis and chromosomal complement in Strongyloides ratti (Nematoda: Rhabdidiasoidea). J. Parasitol. 54:849–55.

Bone, J. F., and J. R. Harr. 1967. Trichosomoides crassicauda infection in laboratory rats. Lab. Animal Care 17:321–26.

Bonne, C., and J. H. Sandground. 1939. On the production of gastric tumors, bordering on malignancy, in Javanese monkeys through the agency of Nochtia nochti, a parasitic nematode. Am. J. Cancer 37:173–85.

Braun, J. L., and C. B. Thayer. 1962. A survey for intestinal parasites in Iowa dogs. J. Am. Vet. Med. Assoc. 141:1049–50.

Bray, R. L., and B. C. Walton. 1961. The life cycle of Dirofilaria uniformis Price and transmission to wild and laboratory rabbits. J. Parasitol. 47:13–23.

Britz, W. E., Jr., J. Fineg, J. E. Cook, and E. D. Miksch. 1961. Restraint and treatment of young chimpanzees. J. Am. Vet. Med. Assoc. 138:653–58.

Brown, H. W., and V. P. Perna. 1958. An overwhelming Strongyloides infection. J. Am. Med. Assoc. 168:1648–51.

Bruynooghe, D., D. Thienpont, and O. F. J. Vanparijs. 1968. Use of tetramisole as an anthelmintic in poultry. Vet. Record 82:701–6.

Buckley, J. J. C. 1931. On two new species of Enterobius from the monkey Lagothrix humboldtii. J. Helminthol. 9:133–40.

————. 1934. On Syngamus ierei sp. nov. from domestic cats, with some observations on its life-cycle. J. Helminthol. 12:89–98.

————. 1960. On Brugia gen. nov. for Wuchereria spp. of the "malayi" group, i.e., W. malayi (Brug, 1927), W. pahangi Buckley and Edeson, 1956, and W. patei Buckley, Nelson and Heisch, 1958. Ann. Trop. Med. Parasitol. 54:75–77.

Buckley, J. J. C., G. S. Nelson, and R. B. Heisch. 1958. On Wuchereria patei n. sp. from the lymphatics of cats, dogs, and genet cats on Pate Island, Kenya. J. Helminthol. 32:73–80.

Burch, G. R. 1954. A new oral anthelmintic for canine whipworms. Vet. Med. 49:291–93.

Burnett, H. S., W. E. Parmelee, R. D. Lee, and E. D. Wagner. 1957. Observations on the life cycle of *Thelazia californiensis* Price, 1930. J. Parasitol. 43:433.

Burrows, R. B. 1958. The anthelmintic effect of bephenium on *Ancylostoma caninum*. J. Parasitol. 44:607–10.

———. 1962. Comparative morphology of *Ancylostoma tubaeforme* (Zeder, 1800) and *Ancylostoma caninum* (Ercolani, 1859). J. Parasitol. 48:715–18.

———. 1965. Microscopic diagnosis of the parasites of man. Yale Univ. Press, New Haven. 328 pp.

Burrows, R. B., and W. G. Lillis. 1962. Thenium, a new anthelmintic for dog and cat hookworms. Am. J. Vet. Res. 23:77–80.

Cahill, K. M. 1967. Thiabendazole in massive strongyloidiasis. Am. J. Trop. Med. Hyg. 16:451–53.

Calhoon, J. R., and P. J. Matthews. 1964. A method for initiating a colony of specific pathogen-free guinea pigs. Lab. Animal Care 14:388–94.

Cameron, T. W. M. 1923. On the morphology of *Ollulanus tricuspis* Leuckart 1865, a nematode parasite of the cat. J. Helminthol. 1:157–60.

———. 1927. Observations on the life history of *Ollulanus tricuspis* Leuck., the stomach worm of the cat. J. Helminthol. 5:67–80.

———. 1929. The species of *Enterobius* Leach, in primates. J. Helminthol. 7:161–82.

Carlos, E. R., and A. C. Directo. 1962. Intravenous treatment of whipworm infection in dogs. J. Am. Vet. Med. Assoc. 141:481–83.

Chabaud, A. G. 1952. Le genre *Dipetalonema* Diesing 1861: Essai de classification. Ann. Parasitol. Humaine Comparee 27:250–85.

———. 1954. Sur le cycle évolutif des spirurides et de nématodes ayant une biologie comparable. Valeur systématique des caractères biologiques. Ann. Parasitol. Humaine Comparee 29:42–88, 206–49, 358–425.

———. 1955. Essai d'interprétation phylétique des cycles évolutifs chez les nématodes parasites de vertèbres. Conclusions taxomoniques. Ann. Parasitol. Humaine Comparee 30:83–126.

Chabaud, A. G., and R. C. Anderson. 1959. Nouvel essai de classification des filaires (superfamille des Filarioidea) II. 1959. Ann. Parasitol. Humaine Comparee 34:64–87.

Chabaud, A. G., and M. T. Choquet. 1953. Nouvel essai de classification des filaires superfamille des Filarioidea. Ann. Parasitol. Humaine Comparee 28:172–92.

Chabaud, A. G., and M. Larivière. 1955. Cycle évolutif d'un ascaride: *Subulura jacchi* (Marcel, 1857) parasite de primates, chez la blatte *Blabera fusca*. Compt. Rend. Soc. Biol. 149:1416–19.

Chabaud, A. G., and René Rousselot. 1956. Un nouveau spiruride parasite du gorille, *Chitwoodspirura wehri* n. g., n. sp. Bull Soc. Pathol. Exotique 49:467–72.

Chan, K.-F. 1952. Life cycle studies on the nematode *Syphacia obvelata*. Am. J. Hyg. 56:14–21.

———. 1955. The distribution of larval stages of *Aspiculuris tetraptera* in the intestine of mice. J. Parasitol. 41:529–32.

Chandler, A. C. 1924. Some parasitic round worms of the rabbit with descriptions of two new species. Proc. U.S. Natl. Museum. 66 (Art. 16):1–6.

———. 1925. The helminthic parasites of cats in Calcutta and the relation of cats to human helminthic infections. Indian J. Med. Res. 13:213–27.

———. 1929. Some new genera and species of nematode worms, Filaroidea, from animals dying in the Calcutta Zoological Garden. Proc. U.S. Natl. Museum. 75 (Art. 6):1–10.

———. 1931. New genera and species of nematode worms. Proc. U.S. Natl. Museum. 78 (Art. 23):1–11.

———. 1939. The nature and mechanism of immunity in various intestinal nematode infections. Am. J. Trop. Med. 19:309–17.

Chandler, A. C., and C. P. Read. 1961. Introduction to parasitology, with special reference to the parasites of man. 10th ed. John Wiley, New York. 822 pp.

Chang, Patricia C. H., and G. L. Graham. 1957. Parasitism, parthenogenesis and polyploidy: The life cycle of *Strongyloides papillosus*. J. Parasitol. 43 (Supp.):13.

Chapman, W. H. 1964. The incidence of a nematode, *Trichosomoides crassicauda*, in the bladder of laboratory rats: Treatment with nitrofurantoin and preliminary report of their influence on the urinary calculi and experimental bladder tumors. Invest. Urol. 2:52–57.

Chardome, M., and E. Peel. 1949. La répartition des filaires dans la region de Coquilhatville et la transmission de *Dipetalonema streptocerca* par *Culicoides grahami*. Ann. Soc. Belge Med. Trop. 29:99–119.

Chesterman, F. C., and J. J. C. Buckley. 1965.

Trichosomoides sp. *(?nasalis* Biocca and Aurizi, 1961) from the nasal cavities of a hamster. Trans. Roy. Soc. Trop. Med. Hyg. 59:8.

Chitwood, B. G. 1938. The status of *Protospirura* vs. *Mastophorus* with a consideration of the species of these genera, pp. 115–18. *In* Livro Jub. Lauro Travassos Inst. Oswaldo Cruz.

Chitwood, M. B., and F. D. Enzie. 1953. The domestic cat, a new host for *Capillaria plica* in North America. Proc. Helminthol. Soc. Wash. D.C. 20:27–28.

Chitwood, M. B., and W. N. Smith. 1958. A redescription of *Anatrichosoma cynomolgi* Smith and Chitwood, 1954. Proc. Helminthol. Soc. Wash. D.C. 25:112–17.

Choquette, L. P. E. 1966. Parasitism of the respiratory system, pp. 369–72. *In* R. W. Kirk, ed. Current veterinary therapy 1966–1967: Small animal practice. W. B. Saunders, Philadelphia.

Christensen, L. T. 1964. Chimp and owners share worm infestation. Vet. Med. 59: 801–3.

Christenson, R. O. 1938. Life history and epidemiological studies on the fox lungworm, *Capillaria äerophila* (Creplin, 1839), pp. 119–36. *In* Livro Jub. Lauro Travassos Inst. Oswaldo Cruz.

Colbourne, M. J., G. M. Edington, M. H. Hughes, and A. Ward-Brew. 1950. A medical survey in a Gold Coast village. Roy. Soc. Trop. Med. Hyg. 44:271–90.

Colglazier, M. L., F. D. Enzie, and R. H. Burtner. 1966. The systemic action of methyridine against helminths, especially whipworms in dogs. Proc. Helminthol. Soc. Wash. D.C. 33:40–41.

Cook, R. 1969. Common diseases of laboratory animals, pp. 160–215. *In* D. J. Short and Dorothy P. Woodnott, eds. The I.A.T. manual of laboratory animal practice and techniques. 2d ed. Charles C Thomas, Springfield, Ill.

Cosgrove, G. E., B. Nelson, and N. Gengozian. 1968. Helminth parasites of the tamarin, *Saguinus fuscicollis.* Lab. Animal Care 18: 654–56.

Cram, Eloise B. 1926. A new nematode from the rat and its life history. Proc. U.S. Natl. Museum. 68 (Art. 15):1–7.

———. 1929a. New roundworm parasite, *Strongyloides avium* of chicken with observations on its life history and pathogenicity. North Am. Vet. 10:27–30.

———. 1929b. The life history of *Tetrameres americana* (Cram, 1927) Baylis, 1929, a spirurid of the proventriculus of chickens. J. Parasitol. 15:292.

———. 1930. New host records for *Strongyloides avium.* J. Parasitol. 17:55–56.

———. 1931. Developmental stages of some nematodes of the Spiruroidea parasitic in poultry and game birds. U.S. Dept. Agr. Tech. Bull. 227. 27 pp.

———. 1935. New avian and insect hosts for *Gongylonema ingluvicola* (Nematoda: Spiruridae). Proc. Helminthol. Soc. Wash. D.C. 2:59.

Cram, Eloise B., and Eugenia Cuvillier. 1931. *Ornithostrongylus quadriradiatus* of pigeons: Observations on its life history, pathogenicity and treatment. J. Parasitol. 18:116.

Crites, J. L., and G. J. Phinney. 1958. *Dirofilaria scapiceps* from the rabbit *(Sylvilagus floridanus mearnsi)* in Ohio. Ohio J. Sci. 58:128–30.

Cuckler, A. C., and J. E. Alicata. 1944. The life history of *Subulura brumpti,* a cecal nematode of poultry in Hawaii. Trans. Am. Microscop. Soc. 63:345–57.

Cullum, L. E., and B. R. Hamilton. 1965. Thiabendazole as an anthelmintic in research monkeys. Am. J. Vet. Res. 26:779–80.

Cushnie, G. H. 1954. The life cycle of some helminth parasites of the rat, mouse and rabbit. J. Animal Tech. Assoc. 5:22–25.

Cuvillier, Eugenia. 1937. Observations on the biological and morphological relationships of *Dispharynx spiralis* in bird hosts. Raboty Gel'mintol. (Skrjabin):99–104.

Darne, A., and J. L. Webb. 1964. The treatment of ancylostomiasis and of spirocercosis in dogs by the new compound, 2,6-diiiodo-4-nitrophenol. Vet. Record 76:171–72.

Das, K. M. 1965. Discussion, pp. 363–64. *In* W. E. Ribelin and J. R. McCoy, eds. Pathology of laboratory animals. Charles C Thomas, Springfield, Ill.

Davtjan, E. A. 1933. Ein neuer Nematode aus den Lungen der Hauskatze, *Osleroides massino* nov. sp. Deut. Tieraerztl. Wochschr. 41:372–74.

———. 1937. A study of the life cycle of *Synthetocaulus kochi* Schulz, Orloff and Kutass, 1933, the lungworm of sheep and goat (in Russian). Raboty Gel'mintol. (Skrjabin):105–22.

Deinhardt, F., A. W. Holmes, J. Devine, and Jean Deinhardt. 1967. Marmosets as laboratory animals: IV. The microbiology of laboratory kept marmosets. Lab. Animal Care 17:48–70.

Derwelis, S. K., J. D. Douglas, J. Fineg, and T. M. Butler. 1969. Supply, maintenance and handling of chimpanzees. Ann. N.Y. Acad. Sci. 162:311–23.

Desportes, C. 1945. Sur *Strongyloides stercoralis* (Bavay 1876) et sur les *Strongyloides* de primates. Ann. Parasitol. Humaine Comparee 20:160–90.

Dietrich, L. E., Jr. 1962. Treatment of canine lungworm infection with thiacetarsamide. J. Am. Vet. Med. Assoc. 140:572–73.

Dikmans, G. 1931. An interesting larval stage of *Dermatoxys veligera*. Trans. Am. Microscop. Soc. 50:364–65.

———. 1935. New nematodes of the genus *Longistriata* in rodents. J. Wash. Acad. Sci. 25:72–81.

———. 1937. Two new species of the nematode genus *Nematodirus* (Trichostrongylidae) from rabbits. Proc. Helminthol. Soc. Wash. D.C. 4:65–67.

Dobson, C. 1961a. Certain aspects of the host-parasite relationship of *Nematospiroides dubius* (Baylis): I. Resistance of male and female mice to experimental infections. Parasitology 51:173–79.

———. 1961b. Certain aspects of the host-parasite relationship of *Nematospiroides dubius* (Baylis): II. The effect of sex on experimental infections in the rat (an abnormal host). Parasitology 51:499–510.

———. 1961c. Certain aspects of the host-parasite relationship of *Nematospiroides dubius* (Baylis): III. The effect of a milk diet on experimental infections in the adult male mouse. Parasitology 51:511–14.

———. 1962a. Certain aspects of the host-parasite relationship of *Nematospiroides dubius* (Baylis): IV. The effect of the host's age on experimental infections in the mouse and rat. Parasitology 52:31–40.

———. 1962b. Certain aspects of the host-parasite relationship of *Nematospiroides dubius* (Baylis): V. Host specificity. Parasitology 52:41–48.

Dodds, R. P., Jr., and R. N. Garcia. 1964. Prevalence of *Spirocerca lupi* in dogs in Mississippi. J. Parasitol. 50:225.

Dollfus, R. P., and A. G. Chabaud. 1955. Cinq espèces de nématodes chez un atèle mort [*Ateles ater* (G. Cuvier 1823)] à la ménagerie du museum. Arch. Museum Nat. Hist. Nat. 7 Sér. T. 3:27–40.

Dotsenko, T. K. 1953. Determination of the biological cycle of the nematode, *Cheilospirura hamulosa*, parasite of gallinaceous birds (in Russian). Dokl. Akad. Nauk USSR 88:583–84.

Dougherty, E. C. 1943. The genus *Filaroides* van Beneden, 1858, and its relatives. Preliminary note. Proc. Helminthol. Soc. Wash. D.C. 10:69–74.

———. 1952. A note on the genus *Metathelazia* Skinker, 1931 (Nematoda: Metastrongylidae). Proc. Helminthol. Soc. Wash. D.C. 19:55–63.

Dougherty, E. C., and F. C. Goble. 1946. The genus *Protostrongylus* Kamenskii, 1905 (Nematoda: Metastrongylidae), and its relatives. Preliminary note. J. Parasitol. 32:7–16.

Douglas, J. R., and N. F. Baker. 1959. The chronology of experimental intrauterine infections with *Toxocara canis* (Werner, 1782) in the dog. J. Parasitol. 45 (Supp.): 43.

Dove, W. E. 1950. The control of laboratory pests and parasites of laboratory animals, pp. 478–87. *In* E. J. Farris, ed. The care and breeding of laboratory animals. John Wiley, New York.

Drygas, Marian, and F. Piotrowski. 1955. Morphology of *Trichuris sylvilagi* Tiner, 1950 (in Polish). Acta Parasitol. Polon. 2:343–59.

Dubey, J. P. 1966. *Toxocara cati* and other intestinal parasites of cats. Vet. Record 79:506–08.

Dubnitski, A. A. 1955. Intermediate hosts in the cycle of development of the nematode *Filaroides bronchialis* (in Russian). Karakulevod. i Zverovod. 8:51–52.

Duke, B. O. L. 1954a. The transmission of loiasis in the forest-fringe area of the British Cameroons. Ann. Trop. Med. Parasitol. 48:349–55.

———. 1954b. The uptake of the microfilariae of *Acanthocheilonema streptocerca* by *Culicoides grahamii*, and their subsequent development. Ann. Trop. Med. Parasitol. 48:416–20.

———. 1955. The development of *Loa* in flies of the genus *Chrysops* and the probable significance of the different species in the transmission of loiasis. Trans. Roy. Soc. Trop. Med. Hyg. 49:115–21.

———. 1956. The intake of the microfilariae of *Acanthocheilonema perstans* by *Culicoides grahamii* and *C. inornatipennis*, and their subsequent development. Ann. Trop. Med. Parasitol. 50:32–38.

Duke, B. O. L., and D. J. B. Wijers. 1958. Studies on loiasis in monkeys: I. The relationship between human and simian *Loa* in the rain-forest zone of the British Cameroons. Ann. Trop. Med. Parasitol. 52:158–75.

Dunn, F. L. 1961. *Molineus vexillarius* sp. n. (Nematoda: Trichostrongylidae) from a Peruvian primate, *Tamarinus nigricollis* (Spix, 1823). J. Parasitol. 47:953–56.

———. 1968. The parasites of *Saimiri* in the

context of platyrrhine parasitism, pp. 31–68. *In* L. A. Rosenblum and R. W. Cooper, eds. The squirrel monkey. Academic Press, New York.

Dunn, F. L., and W. E. Greer. 1962. Nematodes resembling *Ascaris lumbricoides* L., 1758, from a Malayan gibbon, *Hylobates agilis* F. Cuvier, 1821. J. Parasitol. 48:150.

Dunn, F. L., and F. L. Lambrecht. 1963. On some filarial parasites of South American primates, with a description of *Tetrapetalonema tamarinae* n. sp. from the Peruvian tamarin marmoset, *Tamarinus nigricollis* (Spix, 1823). J. Helminthol. 37:261–86.

Edeson, J. F. B., and R. H. Wharton. 1957. The transmission of *Wuchereria malayi* from man to the domestic cat. Trans. Roy. Soc. Trop. Med. Hyg. 51:366–70.

———. 1958. The experimental transmission of *Wuchereria malayi* from man to various animals in Malaya. Trans. Roy. Soc. Trop. Med. Hyg. 52:25–45.

Edeson, J. F. B., R. H. Wharton, and A. B. G. Laing. 1960. A preliminary account of the transmission, maintenance and laboratory vectors of *Brugia pahangi*. Trans. Roy. Soc. Trop. Med. Hyg. 54:439–49.

Edwin, J. P. 1964. The influence of glycobiarsol (Milibis) on *Trichuris vulpis*. Southwestern Vet. 17:218–20.

Ehrenford, F. A. 1953. Differentiation of the ova of *Ancylostoma caninum* and *Uncinaria stenocephala* in dogs. Am. J. Vet. Res. 14:578–80.

———. 1954. The life cycle of *Nematospiroides dubius* (Baylis) (Nematoda: Heligmosomidae). J. Parasitol. 40:480.

Eleazer, T. H. 1969. Coumaphos, a new anthelmintic for control of *Capillaria obsignata, Heterakis gallinarum,* and *Ascaridia galli* in chickens. Avian Disease 13:228–30.

Enigk, K. 1938. Ein Beitrag zur Physiologie und zum Wirt-Parasitverhältnis von *Graphidium strigosum* (Trichostrongylidae, Nematoda). Z. Parasitenk. 10:386–414.

———. 1950. Die Biologie von *Capillaria plica* (Trichuroidea, Nematodes). Z. Tropenmed. Parasitol. 1(4):560–71.

———. 1952. Zur Biologie von *Strongyloides*. Z. Tropenmed. Parasitol. 3:358–68.

Erickson, A. B. 1947. Helminth parasites of rabbits of the genus *Sylvilagus*. J. Wildlife Management 11:255–63.

Eshenour, R. W., G. R. Burch, and F. A. Ehrenford. 1957. Intravenous use of phthalofyne (Whipcide) in the treatment of canine whipworms. J. Am. Vet. Med. Assoc. 131:568–70.

Esslinger, J. H. 1966. *Dipetalonema obtusa* (McCoy, 1936) comb. n. (Filarioidea: Onchocercidae) in Colombian primates, with a description of the adult. J. Parasitol. 52:498–502.

Estes, R. R., and J. C. Brown. 1966. Endoparasites of laboratory animals. USAF School Aerospace Med. (AFSC) Brooks Air Force Base, Tex. Review 1–66. 59 pp.

Ewing, S. A. 1967. Examinations for parasites, pp. 331–91. *In* E. H. Coles, ed. Veterinary clinical pathology. W. B. Saunders, Philadelphia.

Ewing, S. A., and C. M. Hibbs. 1966. *Dracunculus insignis* (Leidy, 1858) in dogs and wild carnivores in the Great Plains. Am. Midland Naturalist 76:515–19.

Fadzil bin Haji Yahaya, M. 1968. A note on the prevalence of *Spirocerca lupi* in dogs in and around Alor Star. Kajian Vet. Singapore 1:63–65.

Fahmy, M. A. M. 1954. An investigation on the life cycle of *Trichuris muris*. Parasitology 44:50–57.

———. 1956. An investigation on the life cycle of *Nematospiroides dubius* (Nematoda: Heligmosomidae) with special reference to the free-living stages. Z. Parasitenk. 17:394–99.

Faust, E. C. 1928. Studies on *Thelazia callipaeda* Railliet and Henry, 1910. J. Parasitol. 15:75–86.

———. 1933. Experimental studies on human and primate species of *Strongyloides:* II. The development of *Strongyloides* in the experimental host. Am. J. Hyg. 18:114–32.

———. 1936. *Strongyloides* and strongyloidiasis. Rev. Parasitol. (Havana) 2:315–41.

Faust, E. C., P. C. Beaver, and R. C. Jung. 1968. Animal agents and vectors of human disease. 3d ed. Lea and Febiger, Philadelphia. 461 pp.

Faust, E. C., and P. F. Russell. 1964. Craig and Faust's clinical parasitology. 7th ed. Lea and Febiger, Philadelphia. 1099 pp.

Faust, E. C., and C. C. Tang. 1934. A new species of *Syngamus (S. auris)* from the middle ear of the cat in Foochow, China. Parasitology 26:455–59.

Fiennes, R. 1967. Zoonoses of primates: The epidemiology and ecology of simian diseases in relation to man. Weidenfeld and Nicolson, London. 190 pp.

Fisher, R. L. 1963. *Capillaria hepatica* from the rock vole in New York. J. Parasitol. 49:450.

Fitzsimmons, W. M. 1961a. The so-called cat and dog strains of *Ancylostoma caninum*. Vet. Record 73:585–86.

———. 1961b. *Bronchostrongylus subcrenatus* (Railliet and Henry, 1913) a new parasite recorded from the domestic cat. Vet. Record 73:101–2.

———. 1961c. Observations on the parasites of the domestic cat. Vet. Med. 56:68–69.

Flores-Barroeta, L. 1956. Nematodos de aves y mamiferos I. Acta Zool. Mexicana 1:1–9.

Flynn, R. J., Patricia C. Brennan, and T. E. Fritz. 1965. Pathogen status of commercially produced laboratory mice. Lab. Animal Care 15:440–47.

Flynn, R. J., R. C. Simkins, T. E. Fritz, and Patricia C. Brennan. 1966. Studies to determine the best procedure and optimum age for examining mice for *Syphacia obvelata*. Abstr. 4. 17th Ann. Meeting Animal Care Panel, Chicago.

Foster, A. O., and C. M. Johnson. 1939. A preliminary note on the identity, life cycle, and pathogenicity of an important nematode parasite of captive monkeys. Am. J. Trop. Med. 19:265–77.

Foster, H. L. 1963. Specific pathogen-free animals, pp. 110–37. *In* W. Lane-Petter, ed. Animals for research: Principles of breeding and management. Academic Press, New York.

Frenkel, J. K., J. P. Dubey, and Nancy L. Miller. 1969. *Toxoplasma gondii:* Fecal forms separated from eggs of the nematode *Toxocara cati*. Science 164:432–33.

Frickers, J. 1953. Strongyloidosis, bij het varken. Tijdschr. Diergeneesk. 78:279–99.

Fritz, T. E., D. E. Smith, and R. J. Flynn. 1968. A central nervous system disorder in ground squirrels *(Citellus tridecemlineatus)* associated with visceral larva migrans. J. Am. Vet. Med. Assoc. 153:841–44.

Gaafar, S. M. 1964. Internal parasitism of small animals. Vet. Med. 59:907–13.

Galliard, H. 1947. Les types de développement exogène de *Strongyloïdes stercoralis:* Leur transformation par passages expérimentaux. Compt. Rend. Soc. Biol., Paris. 141:102–5.

Galvin, T. J., and R. D. Turk. 1966. Intestinal parasitism, pp. 190–94. *In* R. W. Kirk, ed. Current veterinary therapy 1966–1967: Small animal practice. W. B. Saunders, Philadelphia.

Garcia, R. N., J. W. Ward, and R. Dodds. 1965. Procedures on dogs from enzootic areas of canine filariasis for bio-medical research. Abstr. 59. 16th Ann. Meeting Animal Care Panel, Philadelphia.

Garner, E. 1967. *Dipetalonema gracile* infection in squirrel monkeys *(Saimiri sciureus)*. Lab. Animal Dig. 3:16–17.

Garner, E., F. Hemrick, and H. Rudiger. 1967. Multiple helminth infections in cinnamon-

ringtail monkeys *(Cebus albifrons)*. Lab. Animal Care 17:310–15.

Gedoelst, L. 1916. Notes sur la faune parasitaire du Congo Belge. Rev. Zool. Africaine (Brussels) 5:1–90.

Gibson, T. E. 1960. *Toxocara canis* as a hazard to public health. Vet. Record 72:772–74.

Gisler, D. B., R. E. Benson, and R. J. Young. 1960. Colony husbandry of research monkeys. Ann. N.Y. Acad. Sci. 85:758–68.

Godfrey, W. D., W. A. Neely, R. L. Elliott, and J. B. Grogan. 1966. Canine heartworms in experimental cardiac and pulmonary surgery. J. Surg. Res. 6:331–36.

Graham, G. L. 1936. Studies on *Strongyloides:* I. *S. ratti* in parasitic series, each generation in the rat established with a single homogonic larva. Am. J. Hyg. 24:71–87.

———. 1938a. Studies on *Strongyloides:* II. Homogonic and heterogonic progeny of the single, homogonically derived *S. ratti* parasite. Am. J. Hyg. 27:221–34.

———. 1938b. Studies on *Strongyloides:* III. Fecundity of single *S. ratti* of homogonic origin. J. Parasitol. 24:233–43.

———. 1939a. Studies on *Strongyloides:* IV. Seasonal variation in production of heterogonic progeny by singly established *S. ratti* from homogonically derived line. Am. J. Hyg. 30:15–27.

———. 1939b. Studies on *Strongyloides:* V. Constitutional differences between a homogonic and a heterogonic line of *S. ratti*. J. Parasitol. 25:365–75.

———. 1940a. Studies on *Strongyloides:* VI. Comparison of two homogonic lines of singly established *S. ratti*. J. Parasitol. 26:207–18.

———. 1940b. Studies on *Strongyloides:* VII. Length of reproductive life in homogonic line of single established *S. ratti*. Rev. Med. Trop. Parasitol. 6:89–103.

———. 1940c. Studies on *Strongyloides:* VIII. Comparison of pure related lines of the nematode, *Strongyloides ratti*, including lines in which gigantism occurred. J. Exp. Zool. 84:241–60.

———. 1960. Parasitism in monkeys. Ann. N.Y. Acad. Sci. 85:842–60.

Griesemer, R. A., and J. P. Gibson. 1963a. The gnotobiotic dog. Lab. Animal Care 13:643–49.

———. 1963b. The establishment of an ascarid-free beagle dog colony. J. Am. Vet. Med. Assoc. 143:965–67.

Griesemer, R. A., J. P. Gibson, and D. S. Elsasser. 1963. Congenital ascariasis in gnotobiotic dogs. J. Am. Vet. Med. Assoc. 143:962–64.

Griffiths, H. J., J. C. Schlotthauer, and F. W. Gehrman. 1962. Feline dirofilariasis. J. Am. Vet. Med. Assoc. 140:61.

Guilhon, J., and G. Jolivet. 1959. Recherches sur la toxicité et les propriétés anthelminthiques de la dithiazanine. Bull. Acad. Vet. France 32:413–19.

Guilloud, N. B., A. A. King, and A. Lock. 1965. A study of the efficacy of thiabendazole and dithiazanine iodide-piperazine citrate suspension against intestinal parasites in the *Macaca mulatta*. Lab. Animal Care 15:354–58.

Gupta, V. P., and B. P. Pande. 1962. A note on pulmonary spirocercosis in a dog. J. Parasitol. 48:505–6.

Habermann, R. T., and R. W. Menges. 1968. Filariasis *(Acanthocheilonema perstans)* in a gorilla (a case history). Vet. Med. Small Anim. Clin. 63:1040–43.

Habermann, R. T., and F. P. Williams, Jr. 1957a. Diseases seen at necropsy of 708 *Macaca mulatta* (rhesus monkey) and *Macaca philippinensis* (cynomolgus monkey). Am. J. Vet. Res. 18:419–26.

———. 1957b. The efficacy of some piperazine compounds and stylomycin in drinking water for the removal of oxyurids from mice and rats and a method of critical testing of anthelmintics. Proc. Animal Care Panel 7:89–97.

———. 1958. The identification and control of helminths in laboratory animals. J. Natl. Cancer Inst. 20:979–1009.

———. 1963. Treatment of female mice and their litters with piperazine adipate in the drinking water. Lab. Animal Care 13:41–45.

Hagen, C. A., P. W. Barbera, W. H. Blair, H. M. Yamashiroya, A. M. Shefner, and S. M. Poiley. 1968. Intestinal microflora stability and the presence of murine virus antibodies in RAR defined flora rats from different sources and of different ages. Abstr. 24. 19th Ann. Meeting Am. Assoc. Lab. Animal Sci.

Haley, A. J. 1961. Biology of the rat nematode *Nippostrongylus brasiliensis* (Travassos, 1914): I. Systematics, hosts and geographic distribution. J. Parasitol. 47:727–32.

———. 1962. Biology of the rat nematode, *Nippostrongylus brasiliensis* (Travassos, 1914): II. Preparasitic stages and development in the laboratory rat. J. Parasitol. 48:13–23.

Hall, M. C. 1916. Nematode parasites of mammals of the orders Rodentia, Lagomorpha, and Hyracoidea. Proc. U.S. Natl. Museum 50:1–258.

———. 1933. Internal parasites of the dog. Vet. Med. 28:100–104.

Hallberg, C. W. 1953. *Dioctophyma renale* (Goeze, 1782): A study of the migration routes to the kidneys of mammals and resultant pathology. Trans. Am. Microscop. Soc. 72:351–63.

Hamilton, J. M. 1963. *Aelurostrongylus abstrusus* infection of the cat. Vet. Record 75:417–22.

———. 1967. The treatment of lungworm disease in the cat with tetramisole. J. Small Animal Pract. 8:325–27.

———. 1968. Treatment of experimentally induced lungworm of the cat by parenteral administration of tetramisole. Vet. Record 83:665–67.

Hannum, C. A. 1941–1942. Nematode parasites of Arizona vertebrates. Univ. Wash. Abstr. Theses 7:229–31.

Harrison, E. G., J. H. Thompson, J. C. Schlotthauer, and P. E. Zollman. 1965. Human and canine dirofilariasis in the United States. Mayo Clinical Proc. 40:906–16.

Harwell, J. F., and D. D. Boyd. 1968. Naturally occurring oxyuriasis in mice. J. Am. Vet. Med. Assoc. 153:950–53.

Hashimoto, I., and S. Honjo. 1966. Survey of helminth parasites in cynomologus *(sic)* monkeys *(Macaca irus)*. Japan. J. Med. Sci. Biol. 19:218.

Hawking, F. 1959. *Dirofilaria magnilarvatum* Price, 1959 (Nematoda: Filarioidea) from *Macaca irus* Cuvier: III. The behavior of the microfilariae in the mammalian host. J. Parasitol. 45:511–12.

Hawking, F., and W. A. F. Webber. 1955. *Dirofilaria aethiops* Webber, 1955, a filarial parasite of monkeys: II. Maintenance in the laboratory. Parasitology 45:378–87.

Herlich, H. 1959. Anthelmintic trials against *Paraspidodera uncinata* the cecal worm of the guinea pig, with observations on the length of the nematodes. J. Parasitol. 45:586.

Herlich, H., and C. F. Dixon. 1965. Growth and development of *Paraspidodera uncinata,* the cecal worm of the guinea pig. J. Parasitol. 51:300.

Herman, L. H. 1967. *Capillaria aerophila* infection in a cat. Vet. Med. 62:466–68.

Heston, W. E. 1941. Parasites, pp. 349–79. *In* The Staff, Roscoe B. Jackson Memorial Laboratory. Biology of the laboratory mouse. Blakiston, Philadelphia.

Heyneman, D., and B.-L. Lim. 1967. *Angiostrongylus cantonensis:* Proof of direct transmission with its epidemiological implications. Science 158:1057–58.

Highby, P. R. 1943. Vectors, transmission, development, and incidence of *Dirofilaria scapiceps* (Leidy, 1886) (Nematoda) from the snowshoe hare in Minnesota. J. Parasitol. 29:253–59.

Hill, W. C. 1940. The genus *Physaloptera* Rudolphi 1819 (Nematoda: Physalopteridae). Wasmann Collector 4:60–70.

Hirth, R. S., H. W. Huizinga, and S. W. Nielsen. 1966. Dirofilariasis in Connecticut dogs. J. Am. Vet. Med. Assoc. 148:1503–16.

Hoag, W. G. 1961. Oxyuriasis in laboratory mouse colonies. Am. J. Vet. Res. 22:150–53.

Hoag, W. G., and H. Meier. 1966. Infectious diseases, pp. 589–600. *In* E. L. Green, ed. Biology of the laboratory mouse. 2d ed. McGraw-Hill, New York.

Hobmaier, A., and M. Hobmaier. 1930. Life history of *Protostrongylus (Synthetocaulus) rufescens*. Proc. Soc. Exp. Biol. Med. 28:156–58.

Hobmaier, M., and A. Hobmaier. 1935. Mammalian phase of the lungworm *Aelurostrongylus abstrusus* in the cat. J. Am. Vet. Med. Assoc. 40: 191–98.

Hoey, R. 1968. Cutaneous allergy, pp. 296–301. *In* R. W. Kirk, ed. Current veterinary therapy III: Small animal practice. W. B. Saunders, Philadelphia.

Holloway, H. L., Jr. 1966. Helminths of rabbits and opossums at Mountain Lake, Virginia. Bull. Wildlife Dis. Assoc. 2:38–39.

Hosford, G. N., M. A. Stewart, and E. I. Sugarman. 1942. Eye worm *(Thelazia californiensis)* infection in man. Arch. Ophthalmol. 27:1165–70.

Hsü, H. F. 1933. On *Thelazia callipaeda* Railliet and Henry, 1910, infection in man and dog. Arch. Schiffs-Tropen-Hyg. 37:363–69.

Hunt, G. R., and R. B. Burrows. 1963. Stilbazium iodide in the mass treatment of mice infected with *Syphacia obvelata*. J. Parasitol. 49:1019–20.

Hussey, Kathleen L. 1957. *Syphacia muris* vs. *S. obvelata* in laboratory rats and mice. J. Parasitol. 43:555–59.

Hutchison, W. M. 1967. The nematode transmission of *Toxoplasma gondii*. Trans. Roy. Soc. Trop. Med. Hyg. 61:80–89.

Inglis, W. G. 1961. The oxyurid parasites (Nematoda) of primates. Proc. Zool. Soc. London 136:103–22.

Innes, J. R. M., F. M. Garner, and J. L. Stookey. 1967. Respiratory disease in rats, pp. 229–57. *In* E. Cotchin and F. J. C. Roe, eds. Pathology of laboratory rats and mice. Blackwell Scientific Publ., Oxford.

Jackson, R. F. 1963. Two-day treatment with thiacetarsamide for canine heartworm disease. J. Am. Vet. Med. Assoc. 142:23–26.

———. 1969. Diagnosis of heartworm disease by examination of the blood. J. Am. Vet. Med. Assoc. 154:374–76.

Jackson, R. F., F. von Lichtenberg, and G. F. Otto. 1962. Occurrence of adult heartworms in the venae cavae of dogs. J. Am. Vet. Med. Assoc. 141:117–21.

Jackson, R. F., G. F. Otto, P. M. Bauman, F. Peacock, W. L. Hinrichs, and J. H. Maltby. 1966. Distribution of heartworms in the right side of the heart and adjacent vessels of the dog. J. Am. Vet. Med. Assoc. 149:515–18.

Jackson, W. F., and C. R. Wallace. 1966. Canine dirofilariasis, pp. 108–11. *In* R. W. Kirk, ed. Current veterinary therapy 1966–1967: Small animal practice. W. B. Saunders, Philadelphia.

Jarrett, Ellen E. E., W. F. H. Jarrett, and G. M. Urquhart. 1968a. Immunological unresponsiveness to helminth parasites: I. The pattern of *Nippostrongylus brasiliensis* infection in young rats. Exp. Parasitol. 23:151–60.

———. 1968b. Quantitative studies on the kinetics of establishment and expulsion of intestinal nematode populations in susceptible and immune hosts. *Nippostrongylus brasiliensis* in the rat. Parasitology 58:625–39.

Jaskoski, B. J. 1960. Physalopteran infection in an orangutan. J. Am. Vet. Med. Assoc. 137:307.

Jayewardene, L. G. 1962. On two filarial parasites from dogs in Ceylon, *Brugia ceylonensis* n. sp. and *Dipetalonema* sp. inq. J. Helminthol. 36:269–80.

Johnson, R. M., A. C. Andersen, and W. Gee. 1963. Parasitism in an established dog kennel. Lab. Animal Care 13:731–36.

Jones, T. C. 1967. Pathology of the liver of rats and mice, pp. 1–23. *In* E. Cotchin and F. J. C. Roe, eds. Pathology of laboratory rats and mice. Blackwell Scientific Publ., Oxford.

Kassai, T., and I. D. Aitken. 1967. Induction of immunological tolerance in rats to *Nippostrongylus brasiliensis* infection. Parasitology 57:403–18.

Khera, S. 1954. Nematode parasites of some Indian vertebrates. Indian J. Helminthol. 6:27–133.

Kikuchi, T. 1956. An investigation into the geographical distribution of *Gnathostoma spinigerum* and an experimental study of its route of infection. Igaku Kenkyu 26:123–50.

Kirschenblatt, I. D. 1949. On the helminth fauna of *Mesocricetus auratus brandti* Nehr. (in Russian). Uch. Zap. Leningr. Gos. Univ. 101, Ser. Biol. Nauk 19:110–27.

Klewer, H. L. 1958. The incidence of helminth lung parasites of *Lynx rufus rufus* (Shreber) and the life cycle of *Anafilaroides rostratus* Gerichter, 1949. J. Parasitol. 44(Supp.):29.

Knapp, S. E., R. B. Bailey, and D. E. Bailey. 1961. Thelaziasis in cats and dogs—a case report. J. Am. Vet. Med. Assoc. 138:537–38.

Kozlov, D. P. 1963. Study on the biology of *Thelazia callipaeda* Railliet and Henry, 1910 (in Russian). Tr. Gel'mintol. Lab. Akad. Nauk SSSR 13:330–46.

Král, F., and R. M. Schwartzman. 1964. Veterinary and comparative dermatology. J. B. Lippincott, Philadelphia. 444 pp.

Kreis, H. A. 1932. A new pathogenic nematode of the family Oxyuroidea, *Oxyuronema atelophora* n. g. n. sp. in the red-spider monkey, *Ateles geoffroyi*. J. Parasitol. 18:295–302.

———. 1937. Beiträge zur Kenntnis parasitischer Nematoden: IV. Neue und wenig bekannte parasitische Nematoden. Zentr. Bakteriol. Parasitenk Abt. I. Orig. 138:487–500.

Krupp, J. H. 1962. Treatment of opossums with *Physaloptera* infections. J. Am. Vet. Med. Assoc. 141:369–70.

Kume, S., and S. Itagaki. 1955. On the life cycle of *Dirofilaria immitis* in the dog as the final host. Brit. Vet. J. 111:16–24.

Kume, S., I. Ohishi, and S. Kobayashi. 1962. Prophylactic therapy against the developing stages of *Dirofilaria immitis*. Am. J. Vet. Res. 23: 1257–59.

———. 1964. Extended studies on prophylactic therapy against the developing stages of *Dirofilaria immitis* in the dog. Am. J. Vet. Res. 25:1527–29.

Kuntz, R. E., and Betty J. Myers. 1967. Microbiological parameters of the baboon (*Papio* sp.): Parasitology, pp. 741–55. *In* H. Vagtborg, ed. The baboon in medical research. Vol. 2. Univ. Texas Press, Austin.

Kuntz, R. E., Betty J. Myers, J. F. Bergner, Jr., and D. E. Armstrong. 1968. Parasites and commensals of the Taiwan macaque (*Macaca cyclopis* Swinhoe, 1862). Formosan Sci. 22:120–36.

Lang, E. M. 1962. Erfahrungen mit neuen Anthelminthica bei Wildtieren. Schweiz. Arch. Tierheilk. 104:328–33.

Lapage, G. 1962. Mönnig's veterinary helminthology and entomology. 5th ed. Williams and Wilkins, Baltimore. 600 pp.

———. 1968. Veterinary parasitology. Oliver and Boyd, Edinburgh and London. 1182 pp.

Lapin, B. A. 1962. Disease in monkeys within the period of acclimatization, and during long-term stay in animal houses, pp. 143–49. *In* R. J. C. Harris, ed. The problems of laboratory animal disease. Academic Press, New York.

Lapin, B. A., and L. A. Yakovleva. 1960. Comparative pathology in monkeys. Charles C Thomas, Springfield, Ill. 272 pp.

Laurence, B. R., and F. R. N. Pester. 1961. The behaviour and development of *Brugia patei* (Buckley, Nelson and Heisch, 1958) in a mosquito host, *Mansonia uniformis* (Theobald). J. Helminthol. 35:285–300.

Lavoipierre, M. M. J. 1958. Studies on the host-parasite relationships of filarial-nematodes and their arthropod hosts: I. The sites of development and the migration of *Loa loa* in *Chrysops silacea*, the escape of the infective forms from the head of the fly, and the effect of the worm on its insect host. Ann. Trop. Med. Parasitol. 52:103–21.

Leibovitz, L. 1962. Thiabendazole therapy of pigeons affected with *Ornithostrongylus quadriradiatus*. Avian Diseases 6:380–84.

Léon, D. D. de. 1964. Helminth parasites of rats in San Juan, Puerto Rico. J. Parasitol. 50:478–79.

Lepak, J. W., V. E. Thatcher, and J. A. Scott. 1962. The development of *Nematospiroides dubius* in an abnormal site in the white mouse and some apparent effects on the serum proteins of the host. Texas Rept. Biol. Med. 20:374–83.

Levine, N. D. 1968. Nematode parasites of domestic animals and of man. Burgess, Minneapolis. 600 pp.

Lewis, J. W. 1968a. Studies on the helminth parasites of the long-tailed field mouse, *Apodemus sylvaticus sylvaticus* from Wales. J. Zool. 154:287–312.

———. 1968b. Studies on the helminth parasites of voles and shrews from Wales. J. Zool. 154:313–31.

Liebegott, G. 1962. Pericarditis verminosa (*Strongyloides*) beim Schimpansen. Virchows Arch. Pathol. Anat. Physiol. Klin. Med. 335:211–25.

Lindsey, A. M., A. I. Goldsby, W. F. Kuebler, Jr., and D. L. Ferguson. 1964. Whipcidal and hookcidal activity of 0,0-dimethyl-0-1, 2-dibromo-2,2-dichloroethyl phosphate in dogs. Can. J. Comp. Med. Vet. Sci. 28: 212–16.

Lindsey, J. R. 1965. Identification of canine microfilariae. J. Am. Vet. Med. Assoc. 146:1106–14.

Little, M. D. 1962. Experimental studies on the life cycle of *Strongyloides*. J. Parasitol. 48 (Supp) :41.

——. 1966a. Comparative morphology of six species of *Strongyloides* (Nematoda) and redefinition of the genus. J. Parasitol. 52:69–84.

——. 1966b. Seven new species of *Strongyloides* (Nematoda) from Louisiana. J. Parasitol. 52:85–97.

Liu, S. K., D. A. Yarns, and R. J. Tashjian. 1969. Postmortem pulmonary arteriography in canine dirofilariasis. Am. J. Vet. Res. 30:319–29.

López-Neyra, C. R. 1945. Estudios y revisión de la familia Subuluridae, con descripción de especies neuvas. Rev. Iberica Parasitol. 5:271–329.

——. 1951. Los ascaropsinae (Nematoda, Spirurata). Rev. Iberica Parasitol. 11:89–223.

Lubinsky, G. 1956. On the probable presence of parasitic liver cirrhosis in Canada. Can. J. Comp. Med. 20:457–65.

Lucker, J. T. 1933a. *Gongylonema macrogubernaculum* Lubimov, 1931: Two new hosts. J. Parasitol. 19:243.

——. 1933b. Two new hosts of *Gongylonema pulchrum* Molin, 1857. J. Parasitol. 19:248.

Lund, E. E. 1950. A survey of intestinal parasites in domestic rabbits in six counties in southern California. J. Parasitol. 36:13–19.

Mackerras, M. Josephine, and Dorothea F. Sandars. 1955. The life history of the rat lung-worm, *Angiostrongylus cantonensis* (Chen) (Nematoda: Metastrongylidae). Australian J. Zool. 3:1–21.

Madsen, H. 1945. The species of *Capillaria* (Nematodes, Trichinelloidea) parasitic in the digestive tract of Danish gallinaceous and anatine game-birds with a revised list of species of *Capillaria* in birds. Danish Rev. Game Biol. 1 (Part 1):1–112.

——. 1951. Notes on the species of *Capillaria* Zeder, 1800 known from gallinaceous birds. J. Parasitol. 37:257–65.

——. 1952. A study on the nematodes of Danish gallinaceous game-birds. Danish Rev. Game Biol. 2 (Part 1) :1–126.

Mann, P. H., and G. Bjotvedt. 1965. The incidence of heartworms and intestinal helminths in stray dogs. Lab. Animal Care 15:102.

Marquardt, W. C., and W. E. Fabian. 1966. The distribution in Illinois of filariids of dogs. J. Parasitol. 52:318–22.

McCowen, M. C., M. E. Callender, and M. C. Brandt. 1957. The anthelmintic effect of dithiazanine in experimental animals. Am. J. Trop. Med. Hyg. 6:894–97.

McCoy, O. R. 1936. Filarial parasites of monkeys of Panama. Am. J. Trop. Med. 16:383–403.

McGuire, W. C., R. C. O'Neill, and G. Brody. 1966. Anthelmintic activity of 3-methyl-5-[(P-nitrophenyl)azo]rhodanine. J. Parasitol. 52:528–37.

McLeod, J. A. 1933. A parasitological survey of the genus *Citellus* in Manitoba. Can. J. Res. 9:108–27.

McPherson, C. 1966. Diseases of mice, rats and guinea pigs, pp. 566–70. *In* R. W. Kirk, ed. Current veterinary therapy 1966–1967: Small animal practice. W. B. Saunders, Philadelphia.

Medway, W., and J. F. Skelley. 1961. *Capillaria plica* infection in a dog. J. Am. Vet. Med. Assoc. 139:907–8.

Medway, W., and E. J. L. Soulsby. 1966. A probable case of *Dracunculus medinensis* (Linnaeus, 1758) Gallandant, 1773, in a dog in Pennsylvania. J. Am. Vet. Med. Assoc. 149:176–77.

Melvin, Dorothy M., and A. C. Chandler. 1950. New helminth records from the cotton rat, *Sigmodon hispidus*, including a new species, *Strongyloides sigmodontis*. J. Parasitol. 36:505–10.

Menschel, E., and R. Stroh. 1963. Helminthologische Untersuchungen bei Pincheäffchen *(Oedipomidas oedipus)*. Z. Parasitenk. 23:376–83.

Miller, M. J. 1947. Studies on the life history of *Trichocephalus vulpis*, the whipworm of dogs. Can. J. Res. 25:1–12.

Miller, T. A. 1966a. Blood loss during hookworm infection, determined by erythrocyte labeling with radioactive [51]chromium: I. Infection of dogs with normal and with X-irradiated *Ancylostoma caninum*. J. Parasitol. 52:844–55.

——. 1966b. Blood loss during hookworm infection, determined by erythrocyte labeling with radioactive[51] chromium: II. Pathogenesis of *Ancylostoma braziliense* infection in dogs and cats. J. Parasitol. 52:856–65.

——. 1966c. Anthelmintic activity of tetrachloroethylene against various stages of *Ancylostoma caninum* in young dogs. Am. J. Vet. Res. 27:1037–40.

——. 1966d. Anthelmintic activity of toluene and dichlorophen against various stages of *Ancylostoma caninum* in young dogs. Am. J. Vet. Res. 27:1755–58.

——. 1967. Immunity of dogs to *Ancylostoma braziliense* infection following vaccination with X-irradiated *Ancylostoma caninum* larvae. J. Am. Vet. Med. Assoc. 150:508–15.

Mills, J. H. L. 1967. Filaroidiasis in the dog: A review. J. Small Animal Pract. 8:37–43.

Mills, J. H. L., and S. W. Nielsen. 1966. Canine *Filaroides osleri* and *Filaroides milksi* infection. J. Am. Vet. Med. Assoc. 149:56–63.

Miyata, I. 1939. Studies on the life history of the nematode *Protospirura muris* (Gmelin) parasitic in the stomach of the rat, especially on the relation of the intermediate hosts, cockroaches, skin moth and rat fleas (in Japanese). Jubilee Vol. Yoshida 1:101–36.

Miyazaki, I. 1952. Studies on the life history of *Gnathostoma spinigerum* Owen, 1836 in Japan (Nematoda: Gnathostomidae) (in Japanese). Igaku Kenkyu 22:1135–44.

———. 1954. Studies on *Gnathostoma* occurring in Japan (Nematoda: Gnathostomidae): II. Life history of *Gnathostoma* and morphological comparison of its larval forms. Kyushu Mem. Med. Sci. 5:123–40.

Moncol, D. J., and E. G. Batte. 1966. Transcolostral infection of newborn pigs with *Strongyloides ransomi*. Vet. Med. 61:583–86.

Mönnig, H. O. 1929. *Physaloptera canis*, n. sp. A new nematode parasite of the dog. 15th Ann. Rept. Union S. Africa Dept. Agr. 1:329–33.

Morgan, B. B. 1943. The *Physaloptera* (Nematoda) of rodents. Wasmann Collector 5:99–107.

———. 1946. Host-parasite relationships and geographical distribution of the Physalopterinae (Nematoda). Trans. Wisconsin Acad. Sci. 38:273–92.

Morgan, B. B., and P. A. Hawkins. 1949. Veterinary helminthology. Burgess, Minneapolis. 400 pp.

Morgan, H. C. 1966. Canine blood parasites: Filariasis. Vet. Med. 61:829–41.

———. 1967. The effect of helminth parasitism on the hemogram of the dog. Vet. Med. 62:218–23.

Morris, J. H. 1963. Management of a specific pathogen-free guinea pig colony. Lab. Animal Care 13:96–100.

Mortelmans, J., and J. Vercruysse. 1962. Dithiazanine iodide—anthelmintic for chimpanzee. Nord. Veterinarmed. 14 (Supp. 1): 279–83.

Mozgovoi, A. A. 1953. Ascaridata of animals and man and the diseases caused by them. Vol. 2, Part 1. *In* K. I. Skrjabin, ed. Essentials of nematodology. Acad. Sci. USSR. (English edition, Israel Program for Scientific Translations, Ltd., Jerusalem, 1968.)

Myers, Betty J., and R. E. Kuntz. 1965. A checklist of parasites reported for the baboon. Primates 6:137–94.

Myers, Betty J., R. E. Kuntz, and W. H. Wells. 1962. Helminth parasites of reptiles, birds, and mammals in Egypt: VII. Check list of nematodes collected from 1948 to 1955. Can. J. Zool. 40:531–38.

Murray, M. 1968. Incidence and pathology of *Spirocerca lupi* in Kenya. J. Comp. Pathol. 78:401–5.

Napier, L. E. 1949a. *Strongyloides stercoralis* infection: Part I. J. Trop. Med. Hyg. 52:25–30.

———. 1949b. *Strongyloides stercoralis* infection: Part II. Strongyloidiasis among ex-prisoners-of-war. J. Trop. Med. Hyg. 52:46–48.

Nelson, B., G. E. Cosgrove, and N. Gengozian. 1966. Diseases of an imported primate *Tamarinus nigricollis*. Lab. Animal Care 16:255–75.

Nelson, G. S. 1959. The identification of infective filarial larvae in mosquitoes: With a note on the species found in "wild" mosquitoes on the Kenya coast. J. Helminthol. 33:233–56.

———. 1963. *Dipetalonema dracunculoides* (Cobbold, 1870), from the dog in Kenya: With a note on its development in the louse-fly, *Hippobosca longipennis*. J. Helminthol. 37:235–40.

———. 1965. The parasitic helminths of baboons with particular reference to species transmissible to man, pp. 441–70. *In* H. Vagtborg, ed. The baboon in medical research. Univ. Texas Press, Austin.

Neveu-Lemaire, M. 1936. Traité d'helminthologie médicale et vétérinaire. Vigot, Paris. 1514 pp.

Newton, W. L., and W. H. Wright. 1956. The occurrence of a dog filariid other than *Dirofilaria immitis* in the United States. J. Parasitol. 42:246–58.

———. 1957. A reevaluation of the canine filariasis problem in the United States. Vet. Med. 52:75–78.

Nickel, E. A. 1953. Ein Beitrag zur Biologie und Pathogenität des Geflügelhaarwurms *Capillaria caudinflata* (Molin, 1858). Berlin Muench. Tieraerztl. Wochschr. 66:245–48.

Ogilvie, Bridget M. 1967. Reagin-like antibodies in rats infected with the nematode parasite *Nippostrongylus brasiliensis*. Immunology 12:113–31.

Ogilvie, Bridget M., and D. J. Hockley. 1968. Effects of immunity on *Nippostrongylus brasiliensis* adult worms: Reversible and irreversible changes in infectivity, reproduction, and morphology. J. Parasitol. 54:1073–84.

Okoshi, S., and Y. Murata. 1966. Experimental studies on *Ancylostomiasis* in cats: I. *Ancylostoma caninum* Ercolani, 1859 and *A. tubaeforme* Zeder, 1800 found in cats in Japan. Japan. J. Vet. Sci. 28:287–95.

Oldham, J. N. 1954. Infection with *Filaroides osleri*. Vet. Record 66:181.

——. 1967. Helminths, ectoparasites, and protozoa in rats and mice, pp. 641–79. *In* E. Cotchin and F. J. C. Roe, eds. Pathology of laboratory rats and mice. Blackwell Scientific Publ., Oxford.

Olsen, O. W. 1954. Occurrence of the lungworm *Protostrongylus boughtoni* Goble and Dougherty, 1943 in snowshoe hares *(Lepus americanus bairdii)* in Colorado. Proc. Helminthol. Soc. Wash. D.C. 21:52.

——. 1967. Animal parasites: Their biology and life cycles. 2d ed. Burgess, Minneapolis. 431 pp.

Olsen, O. W., and E. T. Lyons. 1965. Life cycle of *Uncinaria lucasi* Stiles, 1901 (Nematoda: Ancylostomatidae) of fur seals, *Callorhinus ursinus* Linn., on the Pribilof Islands, Alaska. J. Parasitol. 51:689–700.

Osborne, C. A., J. B. Stevens, Griselda F. Hanlon, E. Rosin, and W. J. Bemrick. 1969. *Dioctophyma renale* in the dog. J. Am. Vet. Med. Assoc. 155:605–20.

Otto, G. F. 1962. Correlation between lesions and clinical signs in heartworm infection. Proc. Ann. Florida Conf. Vet. 5th 5:33–36.

——. 1969a. Geographical distribution, vectors, and life cycle of *Dirofilaria immitis*. J. Am. Vet. Med. Assoc. 154:370–73.

——. 1969b. Chemotherapeutic agents. J. Am. Vet. Med. Assoc. 154:387–90.

Otto, G. F., and R. F. Jackson. 1969. Pathology of heartworm disease. J. Am. Vet. Med. Assoc. 154:382.

Owen, Dawn. 1968. Investigations: B. Parasitological studies. Lab. Animals Centre News Letter 35:7–9.

Özcan, C. 1967. Tetramisole treatment of ascarid infections in dogs. Ankara Univ. Vet. Fak. Derg 14:357–62.

Paget, G. E., and Phyllis G. Lemon. 1965. The interpretation of pathology data, pp. 382–405. *In* W. E. Ribelin and J. R. McCoy, eds. Pathology of laboratory animals. Charles C Thomas, Springfield, Ill.

Parker, M. V., and J. J. McCaughan, Jr. 1967. Filarias of the dog at Memphis, Tennessee. Abstr. 64. 18th Ann. Meeting Am. Assoc. Lab. Animal Sci., Wash., D.C.

Parmelee, W. E., R. D. Lee, E. D. Wagner, and

H. S. Burnett. 1956. A survey of *Thelazia californiensis*, a mammalian eye worm, with new locality records. J. Am. Vet. Med. Assoc. 129:325–27.

Paterson, J. S. 1962. Guinea-pig disease, pp. 169–84. *In* R. J. C. Harris, ed. The problems of laboratory animal disease. Academic Press, New York.

Peardon, D. L., J. M. Tufts, and H. C. Eschenroeder. 1966. Experimental treatment of laboratory rats naturally infected with *Trichosomoides crassicauda*. Invest. Urol. 4:215–19.

Peel, E., and M. Chardome. 1946. Sur des filaridés de chimpanzés "Pan paniscus" et "Pan satyrus" au Congo belge. Ann. Soc. Belge Med. Trop. 26:117–56.

——. 1947. Note complémentaire sur des filaridés de chimpanzés *Pan paniscus* et *Pan satyrus* au Congo belge. Ann. Soc. Belge Med. Trop. 27:241–50.

Penner, L. R. 1954. *Dirofilaria scapiceps* from snowshoe hare in Connecticut. J. Mammal. 35:458–59.

Petri, L. H. 1950. Life cycle of *Physaloptera rara* Hall and Wigdor, 1918 (Nematoda: Spiruroidea) with the cockroach, *Blatella germanica*, serving as the intermediate host. Trans. Kansas Acad. Sci. 53:331–37.

Petri, L. H., and D. J. Ameel. 1950. Studies on the life cycle of *Physaloptera rara* Hall and Wigdor, 1918 and *Physaloptera praeputialis* Linstow, 1889. J. Parasitol. 36(Supp.):40.

Petrov, A. M. 1930. Zur Charakteristik des Nematoden aus Kamtschatkaer Zobeln *Soboliphyme baturini* nov. gen. nov. sp. Zool. Anz. 86:265–71.

Pillers, A. W. N. 1924. *Ascaris lumbricoides* causing fatal lesions in a chimpanzee. Ann. Trop. Med. Parasitol. 18:101–2.

Poole, C. M., W. G. Keenan, D. V. Tolle, T. E. Fritz, Patricia C. Brennan, R. C. Simkins, and R. J. Flynn. 1967. Disease status of commercially produced rabbits, pp. 219–20. *In* Argonne National Laboratory Biological and Medical Research Division annual report 1967. ANL-7409. Argonne National Laboratory, Argonne, Ill.

Pope, Betty L. 1968. XV. Parasites, pp. 204–8. *In* M. R. Malinow, ed. Biology of the howler monkey *(Alouatta caraya)*. S. Karger, Basel and New York.

Popova, T. I. 1955. Strongyloids of animals and man: Strongylidae. Vol. 5. *In* K. I. Skrjabin, ed. Essentials of nematodology. Acad. Sci. USSR. (English edition, Israel Program for Scientific Translations, Ltd., Jerusalem, 1964).

——. 1958. Strongyloids of animals and man:

Trichonematidae. Vol. 7. *In* K. I. Skrjabin, ed. Essentials of nematodology. Acad. Sci. USSR. (English edition, Israel Program for Scientific Translations, Ltd., Jerusalem, 1965).

Porter, D. A., and G. F. Otto. 1934. The guinea-pig nematode, *Paraspidodera uncinata*. J. Parasitol. 20:323.

Poynter, D. 1966. Some tissue reactions to the nematode parasites of animals, pp. 321-83. *In* B. Dawes, ed. Advances in parasitology. Vol. 4. Academic Press, New York.

Price, D. L. 1957. *Dirofilaria uniformis*, n. sp. (Nematoda: Filarioidea) from *Sylvilagus floridanus mallurus* (Thomas) in Maryland. Proc. Helminthol. Soc. Wash. D.C. 24:15–19.

———. 1959. *Dirofilaria magnilarvatum* n. sp. (Nematoda: Filarioidea) from *Macaca irus* Cuvier: I. Description of the adult filarial worms. J. Parasitol. 45:499–504.

Price, E. W. 1930. *Wellcomia compar* (Leidy) the correct name for *Oxyuris compar* Leidy, 1856. J. Parasitol. 16:159.

Price, E. W., and G. Dikmans. 1941. Adenomatous tumors in the large intestine of cats caused by *Strongyloides tumefaciens*, n. sp. Proc. Helminthol. Soc. Wash. D.C. 8:41–44.

Prince, Marjorie J. R. 1950. Studies on the life cycle of *Syphacia obvelata*, a common nematode parasite of rats. Science 111:66–67.

Pryor, W. H., Jr., C.-P. Chang, and G. L. Raulston. 1970. Dichlorvos: An anthelmintic for primate trichuriasis. Lab. Animal Care 20:1118–22.

Rankin, J. S. 1946. Helminth parasites of birds and mammals in western Massachusetts. Am. Midland Naturalist 35:756–68.

Ratcliffe, H. L. 1945. Infectious diseases of laboratory animals. Ann. N.Y. Acad. Sci. 46:77–96.

———. 1949. Metazoan parasites of the rat, pp. 502–14. *In* E. J. Farris and J. Q. Griffith, Jr., eds. The rat in laboratory investigations. 2d ed. J. B. Lippincott, Philadelphia.

Rausch, R., B. B. Babero, R. V. Rausch, and E. L. Schiller. 1956. Studies on the helminth fauna of Alaska: XXVII. The occurrence of larvae of *Trichinella spiralis* in Alaskan mammals. J. Parasitol. 42:259–71.

Rawes, Deirdre A., and Phyllis A. Clapham. 1962. The efficiency of mixtures of thenium p-chlorobenzene sulfonate and piperazine against hookworms and roundworms of the dog. Vet. Record 74:383–85.

Reardon, Lucy V., and Bonny F. Rininger.

1968. A survey of parasites in laboratory primates. Lab. Animal Care 18:577–80.

Renaux, E. A. 1964. Metazoal and protozoal diseases, pp. 120–40. *In* E. J. Catcott, ed. Feline medicine and surgery. American Veterinary Publications, Santa Barbara, Calif.

Riopelle, A. J. 1967. The chimpanzee, pp. 696–708. *In* UFAW Staff, eds. The UFAW handbook on the care and management of laboratory animals. 3d ed. Livingstone and the Universities Federation for Animal Welfare, London.

Roever-Bonnet, H. de, and A. C. Rijpstra. 1961. *Syphacia obvelata* in the brain of a golden hamster. Trop. Geograph. Med. 13:167–70.

Rosen, L., R. Chappell, Gert L. Laqueur, G. D. Wallace, and P. P. Weinstein. 1962. Eosinophilic meningoencephalitis caused by a metastrongylid lung-worm of rats. J. Am. Med. Assoc. 179:620–24.

Rothenbacher. H., G. Mugera, and Sharon Tufts. 1964. Stomach worm disease, hypodermal myiasis and intestinal coccidiosis in a rabbit colony. Mich. State Univ. Vet. 24:134–36.

Rowland, Eloise, and J. G. Vandenbergh. 1965. A survey of intestinal parasites in a new colony of rhesus monkeys. J. Parasitol. 51:294–95.

Rubin, R. 1954. Studies on the common whipworm of the dog, *Trichuris vulpis*. Cornell Vet. 44:36–49.

Ruch, T. C. 1959. Diseases of laboratory primates. W. B. Saunders, Philadelphia. 600 pp.

Sandground, J. H. 1928. Some studies on susceptibility, resistance, and acquired immunity to infection with *Strongyloides stercoralis* (Nematoda) in dogs and cats. Am. J. Hyg. 8:507–38.

Sandosham, A. A. 1950a. On *Enterobius vermicularis* (Linnaeus, 1758) and some related species from primates and rodents. J. Helminthol. 24:171–204.

———. 1950b. A species of *Enterobius* from the feline douroucouli (*Aotus felineus*). Trans. Roy. Soc. Trop. Med. Hyg. 44:5–6.

Sandosham, A. A., R. H. Wharton, M. Warren, and D. E. Eyles. 1962. Microfilariae in the rhesus monkey (*Macaca mulatta*) from East Pakistan. J. Parasitol. 48:489.

Sarles, M. P. 1934. Production of fatal infestations in rabbits with *Trichostrongylus calcaratus* (Nematoda). Am. J. Hyg. 19:86–102.

Sasa, M., H. Tanaka, M. Fukui, and A. Takata. 1962. Internal parasites of laboratory animals, pp. 195–214. *In* R. J. C. Harris, ed.

The problems of laboratory animal disease. Academic Press, New York.

Schacher, J. F. 1962a. Morphology of the microfilaria of *Brugia pahangi* and of the larval stages in the mosquito. J. Parasitol. 48:679–92.

———. 1962b. Developmental stages of *Brugia pahangi* in the final host. J. Parasitol. 48: 693–706.

Schad, G. A., and R. C. Anderson. 1963. *Macacanema formosana* n. g., n. sp. (Onchocercidae: Dirofilariinae) from *Macaca cyclopsis* of Formosa. Can. J. Zool. 41:797–800.

Schaeffler, W. F. 1961. Visceral larva migrans and related diseases in animals. Part II. Illinois Vet. 4:13–18.

Schauffler, A. F. 1966. Canine thelaziasis in Arizona. J. Am. Vet. Med. Assoc. 149:521–22.

Schell, S. C. 1950. A new species of *Physaloptera* (Nematoda: Spiruroidea) from the cotton rat. J. Parasitol. 36:423–25.

———. 1952. Studies on the life cycle of *Physaloptera hispida* Schell (Nematoda: Spiruroidea) a parasite of the cotton rat (*Sigmodon hispidus littoralis* Chapman). J. Parasitol. 38:462–72.

Schwabe, C. W. 1950a. Studies on *Oxyspirura mansoni*, the tropical eyeworm of poultry: III. Preliminary observations on eyeworm pathogenicity. Am. J. Vet. Res. 11:286–90.

———. 1950b. Studies on *Oxyspirura mansoni*, the tropical eyeworm of poultry: IV. Methods for control. Proc. Hawaiian Entomol. Soc. 14:175–83.

———. 1951. Studies on *Oxyspirura mansoni* the tropical eyeworm of poultry: II. Life history. Pacific Sci. 5:18–35.

Schwartz, B., and J. E. Alicata. 1935. Life history of *Longistriata musculi*, a nematode parasitic in mice. J. Wash. Acad. Sci. 25: 128–46.

Schwentker, V. 1957. The red-backed mouse, pp. 305–8. *In* A. N. Worden and W. Lane-Petter, eds. The UFAW handbook on the care and management of laboratory animals. 2d ed. The Universities Federation for Animal Welfare, London.

Scott, J. A., and Etta M. MacDonald. 1953. Experimental filarial infections in cotton rats. Exp. Parasitol. 2:129–40.

Scott, J. A., Etta M. MacDonald, and B. Terman. 1951. A description of the stages in the life cycle of the filarial worm, *Litomosoides carinii*. J. Parasitol. 37:425–32.

Scott, Patricia P. 1967. The cat, pp. 505–67. *In* UFAW Staff, eds. The UFAW handbook on the care and management of laboratory animals. 3d ed. Livingstone

and the Universities Federation for Animal Welfare, London.

Seamer, J., and F. C. Chesterman. 1967. A survey of disease in laboratory animals. Lab. Animals 1:117–39.

Seneviratna, P. 1954. *Syngamus mcgaughei* sp. nov. in domestic cats in Ceylon. Ceylon Vet. J. 2:55–60.

———. 1959a. Studies on *Anafilaroides rostratus* Gerichter, 1949 in cats: I. The adult and its first stage larva. J. Helminthol. 33:99–108.

———. 1959b. Studies on *Anafilaroides rostratus* Gerichter, 1949 in cats: II. The life cycle. J. Helminthol. 33:109–22.

———. 1959c. Studies on the family Filaroididae Schulz, 1951. J. Helminthol. 33:123–44.

Sheffield, H. G., and Marjorie L. Melton. 1969. *Toxoplasma gondii:* Transmission through feces in absence of *Toxocara cati* eggs. Science 164:431–32.

Sheffy, B. E., J. A. Baker, and J. H. Gillespie. 1961. A disease-free colony of dogs. Proc. Animal Care Panel 11:208–14.

Sheldon, A. J. 1937a. Studies on routes of infection of rats with *Strongyloides ratti*. Am. J. Hyg. 26:358–73.

———. 1937b. Studies on active acquired resistance, natural and artificial, in the rat to infection with *Strongyloides ratti*. Am. J. Hyg. 25:53–65.

Shikhobalova, N. P., and K. M. Ryzhikov. 1956. Biology of *Syngamus skrjabinomorpha* Ryjikov, 1948 (in Russian). Tr. Gel'mintol. Lab. Akad. Nauk SSSR 8: 267–77.

Shumard, R. F., and J. C. Hendrix. 1962. Dithiazanine iodide as an anthelmintic for dogs. Vet. Med. 57:153–57.

Simmons, M. L., H. E. Williams, and Everline B. Wright. 1965. Therapeutic value of the organic phosphate trichlorfon against *Syphacia obvelata* in inbred mice. Lab. Animal Care 15:382–85.

Skrjabin, K. I., N. P. Shikhobalova, and R. S. Shults. 1954. Trichostrongylids of animals and man. Vol. 3. *In* K. I. Skrjabin, ed. Essentials of nematodology. Acad. Sci. USSR. (English edition, Israel Program for Scientific Translations, Ltd., Jerusalem, 1960).

Slaughter, L. J., and R. E. Bostrom. 1969. Physalopterid (*Abbreviata poicilometra*) infection in a sooty mangabey monkey. Lab. Animal Care 19:235–36.

Smetana, H. F., and T. C. Orihel. 1969. Gastric papillomata in *Macaca speciosa* induced by *Nochtia nochti* (Nematoda: Trichostrongyloidea). J. Parasitol. 55:349–51.

Smith, H. A., and T. C. Jones. 1966. Veterinary pathology. 3d ed. Lea and Febiger, Philadelphia. 1192 pp.

Smith, P. E. 1953a. Incidence of *Heterakis spumosa* Schneider, 1866 (Nematoda: Heterakidae) in wild rats. J. Parasitol. 39: 225–26.

———. 1953b. Host specificity of *Heterakis spumosa* Schneider, 1866 (Nematoda: Heterakidae). Proc. Helminthol. Soc. Wash. D.C. 20:19–21.

———. 1953c. Life history and host-parasite relations of *Heterakis spumosa*, a nematode parasite in the colon of the rat. Am. J. Hyg. 57:194–221.

Smith, Vivian S. 1946. Are vesical calculi associated with *Trichosomoides crassicauda*, the common bladder nematode of rats? J. Parasitol. 32:142–49.

Snell, Katharine C. 1967. Renal disease of the rat, pp. 105–47. *In* E. Cotchin and F. J. C. Roe, eds. Pathology of laboratory rats and mice. Blackwell Scientific Publ., Oxford.

Sollod, A. E., T. J. Hayes, and E. J. L. Soulsby. 1968. Parasitic development of *Obeliscoides cuniculi* in rabbits. J. Parasitol. 54:129–32.

Soulsby, E. J. L. 1965. Textbook of veterinary clinical parasitology: Vol. I. Helminths. F. A. Davis, Philadelphia. 1120 pp.

———. 1968. Helminths, arthropods and protozoa of domesticated animals (6th ed. Mönnig's veterinary helminthology and entomology). Williams and Wilkins, Baltimore. 824 pp.

Spindler, L. A. 1936. Resistance of rats to infection with *Nippostrongylus muris* following administration of the worms by duodenal tube. Am. J. Hyg. 23:237–42.

Sprent, J. F. A. 1952. On the migratory behavior of the larvae of various ascaris species in white mice: I. Distribution of larvae in tissues. J. Infect. Diseases 90:165–76.

———. 1953. On the life history of *Ascaris devosi* and its development in the white mouse and the domestic ferret. Parasitology 42:244–58.

———. 1956. The life history and development of *Toxocara cati* (Schrank 1788) in the domestic cat. Parasitology 46:54–78.

———. 1958. Observations on the development of *Toxocara canis* (Werner, 1782) in the dog. Parasitology 48:184–209.

———. 1959. The life history and development of *Toxascaris leonina* (von Linstow 1902) in the dog and cat. Parasitology 49: 330–71.

———. 1968. Notes on *Ascaris* and *Toxascaris*, with a definition of *Baylisascaris* gen. nov. Parasitology 58:185–98.

Stahl, W. 1961. *Syphacia muris*, the rat pinworm. Science 133:576–77.

Stone, O. J., and A. Levy. 1967. Creeping eruption in an animal caretaker. Lab. Animal Care 17:479–82.

Stone, W. B., and R. D. Manwell. 1966. Potential helminth infections in humans from pet or laboratory mice and hamsters. Public Health Rept. 81:647–53.

Stone, W. M. 1964. *Strongyloides ransomi* prenatal infection in swine. J. Parasitol. 50:568.

Sugimoto, M., and S. Nishiyama. 1937. On the nematode, *Tropisurus fissispinus* (Diesing, 1861), and its transmission to chicken in Formosa (in Japanese). J. Japan. Soc. Vet. Sci. 16:305–13.

Supperer, R. 1965. Untersuchungen über die Gattung *Strongyloides:* VI. Die pränatale Invasion. Berlin Muench. Tieraerztl. Wochschr. 78:108–10.

Tacal, J. V., Jr., and Z. V. Corpuz. 1962. Abnormal location of the stomach worm *Physaloptera pseudopraeputialis* in a cat. J. Am. Vet. Med. Assoc. 140:799–800.

Takada, A. 1958. Recherches sur le parasite des animaux de laboratoire. Bull. Exp. Animals 7:167–75.

Takahashi, T., O. Taniguchi, M. Nakano, T. Uchino, T. Fukushima, H. Adachi, and R. Nakamura. 1967. Experimental treatment of canine ancylostomiasis with disophenol (2,6-diiodo-4-nitrophenol) (in Japanese). Bull. Nippon Vet. Zootech. Coll. 16:43–59.

Tanaka, H. M., M. Fukui, H. Yamamoto, S. Hayama, and S. Kodera. 1962. Studies on the identification of common intestinal parasites of primates. Bull. Exp. Animals 11:111–16.

Taylor, Angela E. R. 1959. *Dirofilaria magnilarvatum* Price, 1959 (Nematoda: Filarioidea) from *Macaca irus* Cuvier: II. Microscopical studies on the microfilariae. J. Parasitol. 45:505–10.

———. 1960a. The development of *Dirofilaria immitis* in the mosquito *Aedes aegypti*. J. Helminthol. 34:27–38.

———. 1960b. The spermatogenesis and embryology of *Litomosoides carinii* and *Dirofilaria immitis*. J. Helminthol. 34:3–12.

Thatcher, V. E., and J. A. Scott. 1962. The life cycle of *Trichostrongylus sigmodontis* Baylis, 1945, and the susceptibility of various laboratory animals to this nematode. J. Parasitol. 48:558–61.

Thienpont, D., J. Mortelmans, and J. Vercruysse. 1962. Contribution à l'étude de la Trichuriose du chimpanzé et de son traitement avec la methyridine. Ann. Soc. Belge Med. Trop. 2:211–18.

Thienpont, D., O. Vanparijs, J. Spruyt, and R. Marsboom. 1968. The anthelmintic activity of tetramisole in the dog. Vet. Record 83:369–72.

Thomas, E. D., and J. W. Ferrebee. 1961. Disease-free dogs for medical research. Proc. Animal Care Panel 11:230–33.

Thompson, P. E., Linda Boche, and Lyndia S. Blair. 1968. Effects of amodiaquine against *Litomosoides carinii* in gerbils and cotton rats. J. Parasitol. 54:834–37.

Thompson, P. E., D. E. Worley, and Priscilla McClay. 1962. Effects of bis(2,4,5-trichlorophenol) piperazine salt against intestinal nematodes in laboratory animals. J. Parasitol. 48:572–77.

Thrasher, J. P., K. G. Gould, M. J. Lynch, and C. C. Harris. 1968. Filarial infections of dogs in Atlanta, Georgia. J. Am. Vet. Med. Assoc. 153:1059–63.

Threlfall, W. 1969. Further records of helminths from Newfoundland mammals. Can. J. Zool. 47:197–201.

Tiner, J. D. 1950. Two new species of *Trichuris* from North America with redescriptions of *Trichuris opaca* and *Trichuris leporis* (Nematoda: Aphasmidia). J. Parasitol. 36:350–55.

Travassos, L. P. 1930. Um novo parasita de gallinhas, *Strongyloides oswaldi* n. sp. O Campo 1:36.

———. 1932. Nota sobre *Strongyloides*. Ann. Acad. Brasil. Sci. 4:39–40.

———. 1937. Revisão da familia Trichostrongylidae Leiper, 1912. Monographias Inst. Oswaldo Cruz 1. 512 pp.

———. 1943. Un novo Trichostrongylidae de *Brachyteles arachnoides: Graphidioides berlai* n. sp. (Nematoda: Strongyloidea). Rev. Brasil. Biol. 3:199–201.

Travassos, L. P., and E. G. Vogelsang. 1929. Sobre um novo Trichostrongylidae parasito de *Macacus rhesus*. Sci. Med., Rio de Janeiro 7:509–11.

Tuffery, A. A., and J. R. M. Innes. 1963. Diseases of laboratory mice and rats, pp. 48–108. *In* W. Lane-Petter, ed. Animals for research: Principles of breeding and management. Academic Press, New York.

Urquhart, G. M., W. F. H. Jarrett, and J. G. O'Sullivan. 1954. Canine tracheo-bronchitis due to infection with *Filaroides osleri*. Vet. Record 66:143–45.

Valerio, D. A., R. L. Miller, J. R. M. Innes, K. Diane Courtney, A. J. Pallotta, and R. M. Guttmacher. 1969. *Macaca mulatta:* Man-

agement of a laboratory breeding colony. Academic Press, New York. 140 pp.

Van Riper, D. C., P. W. Day, J. Fineg, and J. R. Prine. 1966. Intestinal parasites of recently imported chimpanzees. Lab. Animal Care 16:360–63.

Vaughn, J. B., Jr., and W. S. Murphy. 1962. Intestinal nematodes in pound dogs. J. Am. Vet. Med. Assoc. 141:484–85.

Vaz, Z., and C. Pereira. 1935. Some new Brazilian nematodes. Trans. Am. Microscop. Soc. 54:36–40.

Vickers, J. H. 1969. Diseases of primates affecting the choice of species for toxicologic studies. Ann. N.Y. Acad. Sci. 162:659–72.

Waddell, A. H. 1968a. Anthelmintic treatment for *Capillaria feliscati* in the cat. Vet. Record 82:598.

———. 1968b. Further observations on *Capillaria feliscati* in the cat. Australian Vet. J. 44:33–34.

Wagner, J. E. 1970. Control of mouse pinworms, *Syphacia obvelata*, utilizing dichlorvos. Lab. Animal Care 20:39–44.

Wahl, D. V., and W. H. Chapman. 1967. The application of data on the survival of eggs of *Trichosomoides crassicauda* (Bellingham) to the control of this bladder parasite in laboratory rat colonies. Lab. Animal Care 17:386–90.

Wallace, F. G., R. D. Mooney, and A. Sanders. 1948. *Strongyloides fülleborni* in man. Am. J. Trop. Med. 28:299–302.

Wallach, J. D., and R. Frueh. 1968. Pilot study of an organophosphate anthelmintic in camels and primates. J. Am. Vet. Med. Assoc. 153:798–99.

Wallenstein, W. L., and B. J. Tibola. 1960. Survey of canine filariasis. J. Am. Vet. Med. Assoc. 137:712–16.

Warne, R. J., V. J. Tipton, and Y. Furusho. 1969. Canine heartworm disease in Japan: Screening of selected drugs against *Dirofilaria immitis in vivo*. Am. J. Vet. Res. 30:27–32.

Webber, W. A. F. 1955a. The filarial parasites of primates: A review. I. *Dirofilaria* and *Dipetalonema*. Ann. Trop. Med. Parasitol. 49:123–41.

———. 1955b. The filarial parasites of primates: A review. II. *Loa, Protofilaria,* and *Parlitomosa*, with notes on incompletely identified adult and larval forms. Ann. Trop. Med. Parasitol. 49:235–49.

———. 1955c. *Dirofilaria aethiops* Webber, 1955, a filarial parasite of monkeys: I. The morphology of the adult worms and microfilariae. Parasitology 45:369–77.

———. 1955d. *Dirofilaria aethiops* Webber, 1955, a filarial parasite of monkeys: III. The larval development in mosquitoes. Parasitology 45:388–400.

Webber, W. A. F., and F. Hawking. 1955. The filarial worms *Dipetalonema digitatum* and *D. gracile* in monkeys. Parasitology 45: 401–8.

Webster, G. A. 1956. A preliminary report on the biology of *Toxocara canis* (Werner, 1782). Can. J. Zool. 34:725–26.

Wehr, E. E. 1965. Nematodes and acanthocephalids of poultry, pp. 965–1005. *In* H. E. Biester and L. H. Schwarte, eds. Diseases of poultry. 5th ed. Iowa State Univ. Press, Ames.

Wehr, E. E., and M. L. Colglazier. 1966. Thiabendazole as an anthelmintic against *Ascaridia columbae* in pigeons. Trans. Am. Microscop. Soc. 85:164.

Wehr, E. E., M. L. Colglazier, R. H. Burtner, and L. M. Wiest, Jr. 1967. Methyridine, an effective anthelmintic for intestinal threadworm, *Capillaria obsignata,* in pigeons. Avian Diseases 11:322–26.

Weisbroth, S. H., and S. Scher. 1969. *Trichosomoides crassicauda* infection of a commercial rat breeding colony. I. Observations on life cycle and propagation. Abstr. 40. 20th Ann. Meeting Am. Assoc. Lab. Animal Sci., Dallas.

Welter, C. J., and D. R. Johnson. 1963. Anthelmintic activity of n-butyl chloride and toluene combinations in dogs and cats. Vet. Med. 58:869–72.

Wetzel, R. 1940. Zur Biologie des Fuchslungenwurmes *Crenosoma vulpis.* I. Mitteilg. Arch. Wissen. Prakt. Tierkunde 75:445–60.

Wharton, R. H. 1957. Studies on filariasis in Malaya: Observations on the development of *Wuchereria malayi* in *Mansonia (Mansonioides) longipalpis.* Ann. Trop. Med. Parasitol. 51:278–96.

———. 1959. *Dirofilaria magnilarvatum* Price, 1959 (Nematoda: Filarioidea) from *Macaca irus* Cuvier: IV. Notes on larval development in Mansonioides mosquitoes. J. Parasitol. 45:513–18.

Whitehead, J. E. 1964. Diseases of the urogenital system, pp. 255–94. *In* E. J. Catcott, ed. Feline medicine and surgery. American Veterinary Publications, Santa Barbara, Calif.

Whitney, L. F., and G. D. Whitney. 1953. Contrasting tetrachlorethylene and n-butyl chloride as canine anthelmintics. Vet. Med. 48:495–99.

Whitney, R. A., D. J. Johnson, and W. C. Cole.

1967. The subhuman primate: A guide for the veterinarian. EASP 100–26. Edgewood Arsenal, Md.

Wills, J. E. 1968. The establishment of an SPF guinea pig colony. J. Inst. Animal Tech. 19:99–107.

Wilson, R. J. M., and K. J. Bloch. 1968. Homocytotropic antibody response in the rat infected with the nematode, *Nippostrongylus brasiliensis:* II. Characteristics of the immune response. J. Immunol. 100:622–28.

Wolffhügel, K. 1934. Paraplegia cruralis parasitaria felis durch *Gurltia paralysans* nov. gen. nov. sp. (Nematoda). Z. Infectionskrankh. Haust. 46:28–48.

Woodhead, A. E. 1950. Life history of the giant kidney worm, *Dioctophyma renale* (Nematoda), of man and many other mammals. Trans. Am. Microscop. Soc. 69:21–46.

Woodruff, A. W., B. Bisseru, and J. C. Bowe. 1966. Infection with animal helminths as a factor in causing poliomyelitis and epilepsy. Brit. Med. J. 1:1576–79.

Worley, D. E. 1964. Helminth parasites of dogs in southeastern Michigan. J. Am. Vet. Med. Assoc. 144:42–46.

Yamaguchi, T., H. Toyoda, and E. Matsuo. 1955. Experimental infestation on dog with *Gnathostoma spinigerum* larvae obtained from second intermediate host, *Ophicephalus argus* Cantor (in Japanese). Shikoku Acta Med. 6:111–13.

Yamaguti, S. 1954. Studies on the helminth fauna of Japan: Part 51. Mammalian nematodes. V. Acta Med. Okayama 9:105–21.

———. 1961. The nematodes of vertebrates. Vol. III. 2 Parts. *In* S. Yamaguti. *Systema helminthum.* Interscience, New York.

Yamaguti, S., and S. Hayama. 1961. A redescription of *Edesonfilaria malayensis* Yeh, 1960, with remarks on its systematic position. Proc. Helminthol. Soc. Wash. D.C. 28:83–86.

Yamashita, J. 1963. Ecological relationships between parasites and primates: I. Helminth parasites and primates. Primates 4:1–96.

Yeh, L.-S. 1957. On a filarial parasite, *Deraïophoronema freitaslenti* n. sp., from the giant anteater, *Myrmecophaga tridactyla* from British Guiana, and a proposed reclassification of *Dipetalonema* and related genera. Parasitology 47:196–205.

———. 1960. On a new filarioid worm, *Edesonfilaria malayensis* gen. et sp. nov. from the long-tailed macaque *(Macaca irus)*. J. Helminthol. 34:125–28.

Yorke, W., and P. A. Maplestone. 1926. The nematode parasites of vertebrates. Blakiston, Philadelphia. 536 pp.

Young, R. J., B. D. Fremming, R. E. Benson, and M. D. Harris. 1957. Care and management of a *Macaca mulatta* monkey colony. Proc. Animal Care Panel 7:67–82.

Yutuc, L. M. 1953. *Physaloptera pseudopraeputialis* n. sp. a stomach worm of the cat (Nematoda: Physalopterinae). Philippine J. Sci. 82:221–26.

Zimmermann, W. J., and L. H. Schwarte. 1958. Trichiniasis in dogs and cats of Iowa. J. Parasitol. 44:520.

Chapter 8

ACANTHOCEPHALANS

ACANTHOCEPHALANS are sexually dimorphic, obligate helminth parasites of the vertebrate intestine (Hyman 1951; Meyer 1933; Van Cleave 1948; Yamaguti 1963). The adults of most species are a few millimeters in length, but some range up to 12 cm or more in size. The worms are usually sharply localized in a portion of the intestine and firmly attached to the mucosa by a deeply embedded, eversible, multiple-hooked proboscis of characteristic shape and hook arrangement. It is from the morphology of the proboscis that the name spiny- or thorny-headed worm is derived. The worms are typically white to yellow and flattened in cross section when lying against the host mucosa, but they become turgid, round in cross section, and superficially nematodelike when removed from the host to normal saline. Their resemblance to nematodes is further enhanced by the presence of a resistant cuticle with underlying syncytial hypodermis and muscle layer. Nonetheless, the group is sufficiently different to warrant the status of a distinct phylum.

The life cycle requires an arthropod intermediate host and, frequently, a second intermediate or transport host. Because cockroaches and soil-dwelling insects or crustaceans are often involved as intermediate hosts, adequate sanitation and pest control will prevent the completion of the life cycle in the laboratory. Consequently, acanthocephalan infections are important only in laboratory animals obtained from their natural habitat or in colonies with ineffective vermin control.

The acanthocephalans that affect endothermal laboratory animals are listed in Table 8.1. The most important are discussed below.

Moniliformis moniliformis

(SYN. Moniliformis dubius)

This parasite occurs in wild Norway and black rats and in other rodents throughout the world (Witenberg 1964). It is commonest in tropical and subtropical regions, especially where the cockroach is plentiful; it is less common in temperate regions (Van Cleave 1953a). Rarely, it develops accidentally in the chimpanzee (Ruch 1959), in man (Witenberg 1964), and possibly in the dog (Golvan 1962). It has not been reported in commercially or laboratory-reared rodents and is likely to be encountered only in rodents and possibly simian primates obtained from their natural habitat.

MORPHOLOGY

Moniliformis moniliformis has a thick, rounded, annulated body (Fig. 8.1) (Morgan and Hawkins 1949; Van Cleave 1953a). Males are 6 to 8 cm long, and females 10 to 32 cm. The proboscis is club shaped or cylindrical and armed with several rows of

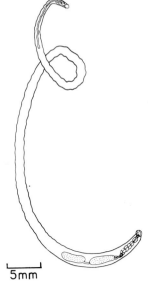

FIG. 8.1. *Moniliformis moniliformis* male. Anterior end at top. (From Olsen 1967. Courtesy of O. W. Olsen, Colorado State University.)

distinctive crescentic hooks. The egg is 90 to 125 μ by 50 to 62 μ and embryonated when passed in the feces (Fig. 8.2).

LIFE CYCLE

The life cycle is depicted in Fig. 8.3 (Moore 1946; Olsen 1967). The adult worm (*a*) produces eggs (*b*) which pass out of the

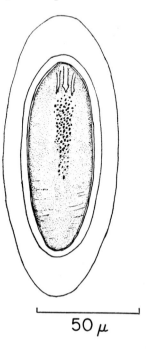

FIG. 8.2. *Moniliformis moniliformis* egg. (From Moore 1946. Courtesy of American Society of Parasitologists.)

body in the feces (*c*), are swallowed by an intermediate host (*d*), hatch in the gut (*e*) as acanthors which penetrate the gut wall (*f*), develop into immature acanthellas (*g*), and then become infective acanthellas or cystacanths (*h*). The endothermal host becomes infected by ingesting the infected invertebrate host (*i*). The invertebrate host is digested and the cystacanth released (*j*). The acanthella escapes from the cyst (*k*), attaches to the gut wall (*l*), and grows into an adult worm. Intermediate hosts are the American cockroach (*Periplaneta americana*) and various beetles. Development from egg to infective acanthella requires approximately 7 weeks; development of infective acanthella to mature worms requires approximately 5 to 6 weeks.

PATHOLOGIC EFFECTS

The worms are restricted to a small portion of the small intestine (Burlingame and Chandler 1941; Crompton and Whitfield 1968a). Light infections produce little pathology, but heavy infections cause inflammation and ulceration of the mucosa, and sometimes necrosis and penetration of the intestinal wall and secondary peritonitis (Oldham 1967).

DIAGNOSIS

Diagnosis is based on the identification of either the eggs in the feces or the adult worms in the intestine at necropsy.

CONTROL

Sanitation and insect control will prevent the completion of the life cycle and the spread of the infection in a research colony. No treatment is reported.

PUBLIC HEALTH CONSIDERATIONS

Human infections have been reported but are rare (Beck 1959; Witenberg 1964). Man can become infected only by ingestion of an infected invertebrate host, usually a cockroach.

Oncicola canis

This helminth occurs in the dog and is found only in the United States, particularly Texas, and northeastern Mexico (Lapage 1962; Morgan and Hawkins 1949; Soulsby 1965). It is locally common, with an incidence of 31.3% reported in one sur-

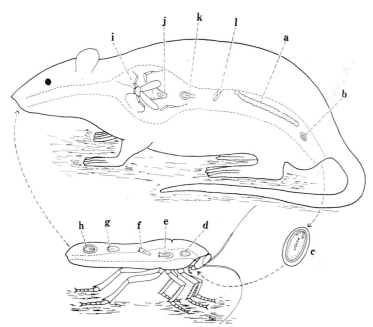

FIG. 8.3. *Moniliformis moniliformis* life cycle. See text for explanation of symbols. (From Olsen 1967. Courtesy of O. W. Olsen, Colorado State University.)

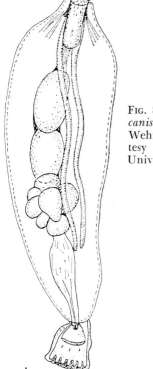

FIG. 8.4. *Oncicola canis* male. (From Wehr 1965. Courtesy of Iowa State University Press.)

1mm

vey of 134 stray dogs (Jurado-Mendoza 1966). It is rare in the laboratory dog (Braun and Thayer 1962) and is likely to occur only in those obtained from pounds in the endemic area.

MORPHOLOGY

Adults have a conical body, tapered posteriorly (Fig. 8.4), and are flat, gray, and wrinkled (Lapage 1962; Morgan and Hawkins 1949). The male is 6 to 13 mm long, and the female 7 to 14 mm. The proboscis has hooks arranged in rows. The egg is brown, oval, and 60 to 70 μ by 40 to 50 μ (Fig. 8.5). It contains an embryo that has several spines at the anterior end.

LIFE CYCLE

The life cycle is unknown but is presumed to involve an arthropod as an intermediate host and the armadillo as a second intermediate or transport host (Lapage 1962; Soulsby 1965). The dog presumably becomes infected by ingesting immature forms of the helminth encysted in muscle and connective tissue of the armadillo.

PATHOLOGIC EFFECTS

The worms attach to the wall of the small intestine of the dog (Lapage 1962).

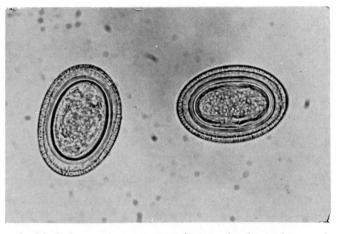

FIG. 8.5. *Oncicola canis* egg. ×410. (From Benbrook and Sloss 1961. Courtesy of Iowa State University Press.)

The proboscis is usually deeply embedded and sometimes penetrates the peritoneal surface. Clinical signs resembling rabies were observed in one heavily infected dog, but the possibility that the dog actually had rabies was not eliminated (Lapage 1962).

DIAGNOSIS

Diagnosis is based on the identification of either the eggs in the feces or the adult worms in the intestine at necropsy (Soulsby 1965).

CONTROL

Because of the probable need for a secondary intermediate or transport host, the life cycle cannot be completed in the laboratory under usual conditions. No treatment has been reported.

PUBLIC HEALTH CONSIDERATIONS

This parasite does not affect man.

Prosthenorchis

This highly pathogenic helminth is the most important intestinal parasite of Central and South American monkeys (F. Deinhardt et al. 1967; Garner, Hemrick, and Rudiger 1967; Middleton 1966; Nelson, Cosgrove, and Gengozian 1966; Richart and Benirschke 1963; Ruch 1959; Takos and Thomas 1958). *Prosthenorchis elegans* is the commonest species; *P. spirula* is less common (Dunn 1963). Both species are native to South America but are now found throughout the world, wherever New World primates are kept in captivity or where they have introduced the parasite (Chandler 1953; Dunn 1963; Ruch 1959). Although marmosets, tamarins, squirrel monkeys, spider monkeys, and capuchins are the natural hosts, transmission has occurred in captivity to macaques, the chimpanzee, gibbons, lemurs, and pottos *(Perodicticus)* (Chandler 1953; Dunn 1963). *Prosthenorchis* is important not only because it is highly pathogenic and likely to be encountered in New World monkeys obtained from their natural habitat but because the intermediate host, a cockroach, is common in primate facilities (Graham 1960).

MORPHOLOGY

The body is cylindrical, curved ventrally or spirally, and irregularly wrinkled transversely (Fig. 8.6) (Machado Filho 1950; Worms 1967). Males are 20 to 30 mm long, and the females 30 to 50 mm (Machado Filho 1950). The proboscis is globular and has five to seven rows of hooks. The eggs are large, 42 to 53 μ by 65 to 81 μ, and contain an embryo with hooks (Fig. 8.7).

LIFE CYCLE

Eggs passed in the feces of the endothermal host are ingested by the intermediate host, a cockroach (Brumpt and Urbain 1938). The development in the cockroach is similar to that of *Moniliformis moniliformis* (Dollfus 1938). The primate host is infected by ingesting an infected cockroach.

PATHOLOGIC EFFECTS

The parasite attaches to the intestinal wall by deeply embedding its spiny proboscis into the mucosa (Nelson, Cosgrove, and Gengozian 1966). The area of attachment

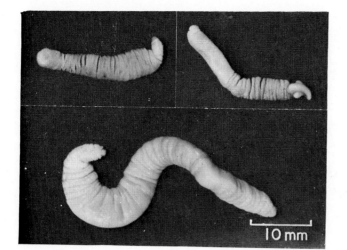

FIG. 8.6. *Prosthenorchis elegans.* *(Top)* Photograph of adult worms. *(Bottom)* Drawing of an adult male. *(Top* from Worms 1967; courtesy of Institute of Animal Technicians. *Bottom* from Machado Filho 1950; courtesy of Memórias do Instituto Oswaldo Cruz.)

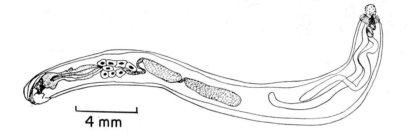

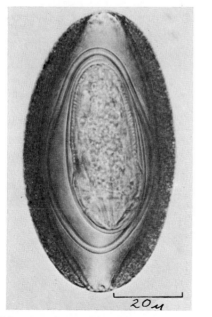

FIG. 8.7. *Prosthenorchis elegans* egg. (From Worms 1967. Courtesy of Institute of Animal Technicians.)

is usually the terminal portion of the ileum, but sometimes the cecum and colon are involved (Garner, Hemrick, and Rudiger 1967; Nelson, Cosgrove, and Gengozian 1966). Occasionally the parasite penetrates the gut wall and enters the peritoneal cavity (Dunn 1963; Nelson, Cosgrove, and Gengozian 1966).

The clinical signs vary with the degree of infection but usually include diarrhea, anorexia, debilitation, and death (Chandler 1953; F. Deinhardt et al. 1967; Nelson, Cosgrove, and Gengozian 1966; Richart and Benirschke 1963; Takos and Thomas 1958).

The most noticeable gross lesions are abscesses and granulomatous lesions that occur around the inserted proboscis of the worm (Garner, Hemrick, and Rudiger 1967; Middleton 1966; Nelson, Cosgrove, and Gengozian 1966). These appear on the serosal surface of the intestine as firm white nodules, several millimeters in diameter. Within the gut the worms are readily visible, firmly attached to the wall of the terminal ileum (Fig. 8.8). Inflammation,

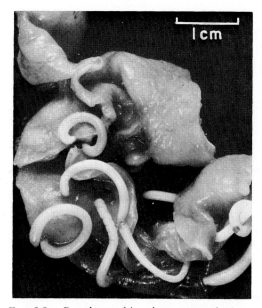

FIG. 8.8. *Prosthenorchis elegans* attached to terminal ileum of tamarin. (From Nelson, Cosgrove, and Gengozian 1966. Courtesy of American Association for Laboratory Animal Science.)

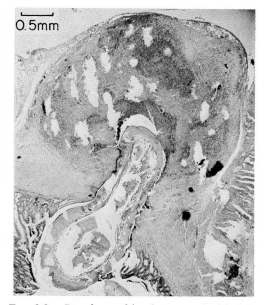

FIG. 8.9. *Prosthenorchis elegans* embedded in wall of marmoset colon. (From Ruch 1959. Courtesy of W. B. Saunders Co.)

necrosis, and ulceration of the intestinal wall are frequently seen and often perforation and peritonitis (F. Deinhardt et al. 1967; Nelson, Cosgrove, and Gengozian 1966; Richart and Benirschke 1963; Takos and Thomas 1958); intussusception or complete obstruction of the intestine in the region of the ileocecal valve sometimes occurs (Jean Deinhardt et al. 1967; Dunn 1963).

Histologically, the proboscis of the worm can be seen deeply embedded in the intestinal wall (Fig. 8.9). Inflammation, usually a granulomatous reaction, occurs at the site of attachment, accompanied by necrosis, ulceration, secondary bacterial invasion, and abscess formation.

DIAGNOSIS

Diagnosis is made by identification of either the eggs in the feces or the adult worms at necropsy (F. Deinhardt et al. 1967).

CONTROL

Sanitation and cockroach control will prevent the completion of the life cycle and the spread of the infection in a research colony. No treatment has been reported.

PUBLIC HEALTH CONSIDERATIONS

Human infections have not been reported. Although infection in man seems possible because of the broad host spectrum of this parasite, it is unlikely because it would require the ingestion of an infected cockroach.

TABLE 8.1. Acanthocephalans affecting endothermal laboratory animals

Parasite	Geographic Distribution	Endothermal Host	Location in Host	Method of Infection	Incidence In nature	Incidence In laboratory	Pathologic Effects	Public Health Importance	Reference
*Moniliformis moniliformis**	Worldwide	Rat, black rat, other rodents, dog, chimpanzee, man	Small intestine	Ingestion of intermediate host (usually a cockroach)	Common in rat, black rat; rare in dog, chimpanzee	Occurs only in animals obtained from natural habitat	Usually inapparent; sometimes enteritis, ulceration, peritonitis	Affects man; exposure in laboratory unlikely	Moore 1946 Olsen 1967 Ruch 1959 Van Cleave 1953a Witenberg 1964
Moniliformis clarki	North America	Deer mice, wood rats, ground squirrels, other rodents	Small intestine	Unknown; probably by ingestion of intermediate invertebrate host	Unknown	Occurs only in animals obtained from natural habitat	Unknown	Unknown; exposure in laboratory unlikely	Chandler 1917 Crook and Grundmann 1964 Dollfus 1938 Van Cleave 1953a
*Oncicola canis**	United States, northeastern Mexico	Dog	Small intestine	Unknown; presumably by ingestion of intermediate or transport host	Locally common; otherwise rare	Occurs in animals obtained from natural habitat in endemic areas	Trauma of intestinal wall; sometimes perforation of intestine	None	Braun and Thayer 1962 Jurado-Mendoza 1966 Lapage 1962 Price 1926 Soulsby 1965
Oncicola companulatus	South America	Cat	Small intestine	Unknown; presumably by ingestion of intermediate or transport host	Unknown	Unknown	Unknown	Unknown	Diaz-Ungria 1958 Witenberg 1938
Centrorhynchus clitorideum	North America, Europe, northern Africa, southwestern Asia	Dog, cat	Small intestine	Unknown; probably by ingestion of intermediate or transport host	Unknown	Unknown	Unknown	Unknown	Azim 1939 Witenberg 1938, 1949
Corynosoma semerme	Worldwide	Dog, other carnivores	Small intestine	Ingestion of transport host (marine fishes)	Uncommon except in Arctic	Unknown; probably absent	Unknown	Unknown	Nuorteva 1966 Yamaguti 1963
Corynosoma strumosum	Worldwide	Dog, other carnivores	Small intestine	Ingestion of transport host (marine fishes)	Uncommon except in Arctic	Unknown; probably absent	Unknown	Unknown	Nuorteva 1966 Petrochenko 1956–1958 Van Cleave 1953b Yamaguti 1963
Macracanthorhynchus catulinus	Central Asia (Turkestan)	Definitive: dog, other carnivores Transport: wild rodents	Definitive: small intestine Transport: muscle	Definitive: ingestion of transport host Transport: ingestion of intermediate host (insect)	Unknown	Unknown; probably absent	Definitive: perforation of intestinal wall; nodules in mesentery in transport host Transport: unknown	Unknown	Machulskii 1959 Meyer 1933

*Discussed in text.

TABLE 8.1 (continued)

Parasite	Geographic Distribution	Endothermal Host	Location in Host	Method of Infection	Incidence In nature	Incidence In laboratory	Pathologic Effects	Public Health Importance	Reference
*Prosthenorchis elegans**	Worldwide	Marmosets, tamarins, squirrel monkeys, spider monkeys, capuchins, macaques, gibbons	Ileum, cecum, colon	Ingestion of intermediate host (cockroach)	Common	Common	Diarrhea, enteritis, anorexia, debilitation; necrosis, ulceration, abscessation, perforation of intestinal wall; sometimes intussusception, peritonitis, death	Unknown	Chandler 1953; F. Deinhardt et al. 1967; Jean Deinhardt et al. 1967; Dunn 1963; Garner et al. 1967; Nelson et al. 1966; Richart and Benirschke 1963; Ruch 1959; Takos and Thomas 1958
*Prosthenorchis spirula**	Worldwide	Marmosets, squirrel monkeys, capuchins, macaques, chimpanzee, lemurs, pottos (*Perodicticus*)	Ileum, cecum, colon	Ingestion of intermediate host (cockroach)	Uncommon	Uncommon	Diarrhea, enteritis, anorexia, debilitation; necrosis, ulceration, abscessation, perforation of intestinal wall; sometimes intussusception, peritonitis, death	Unknown	Brumpt and Urbain 1938; Chandler 1953; Dunn 1963; Nelson et al. 1966; Ruch 1959
Mediorhynchus gallinarum	India, Philippine Islands	Chicken	Small intestine	Unknown	Rare	Unknown; probably absent	Unknown	Unknown	Van Cleave 1947, 1952
Polymorphus minutus	North America, Europe	Chicken, other birds	Small intestine	Ingestion of intermediate host (crustaceans, fishes)	Rare in chicken	Unknown; probably absent	Nodule formation in intestinal wall; sometimes death	Unknown	Crompton 1967; Crompton and Harrison 1965; Crompton and Whitfield 1968b; Lapage 1962; Soulsby 1965
Prosthorhynchus formosus	United States	Chicken, other birds	Small intestine	Ingestion of intermediate host (isopods)	Rare in chicken	Unknown; probably absent	Unknown	Unknown	Jones 1928; Sinitsin 1929; Van Cleave 1947; Ward 1950

*Discussed in text.

REFERENCES

Azim, A. 1939. Helminthes parasites des chiens et des chats en Egypte. Ann. Parasitol. Humaine Comparee 17:32–36.

Beck, J. W. 1959. Report of a possible human infection with the acanthocephalan *Moniliformis moniliformis* (syn. *M. dubius*). J. Parasitol. 45:510.

Benbrook, E. A., and Margaret W. Sloss. 1961. Veterinary clinical parasitology. 3d ed. Iowa State Univ. Press, Ames. 240 pp.

Braun, J. L., and C. B. Thayer. 1962. A survey for intestinal parasites in Iowa dogs. J. Am. Vet. Med. Assoc. 141:1049–50.

Brumpt, E., and A. Urbain. 1938. Épizootie vermineuse por Acanthocéphales *(Prosthenorchis)* ayant sévi a la singerie due Museum de Paris. Ann. Parasitol. Humaine Comparee 16:289–300.

Burlingame, P. L., and A. C. Chandler. 1941. Host-parasite relations of *Moniliformis dubius* (Acanthocephala) in albino rats, and the environmental nature of resistance to single and superimposed infections with the parasite. Am. J. Hyg. 33:1–21.

Chandler, A. C. 1947. Notes on *Moniliformis clarki* in North American squirrels. J. Parasitol. 33:278–81.

———. 1953. An outbreak of *Prosthenorchis* (Acanthocephala) infection in primates in the Houston Zoological Garden, and a report of this parasite in *Nasua narica* in Mexico. J. Parasitol. 39:226.

Crompton, D. W. T. 1967. Studies on the haemocytic reaction of *Gammarus* spp. and its relationship to *Polymorphus minutus* (Acanthocephala). Parasitology 57:389–401.

Crompton, D. W. T., and J. G. Harrison. 1965. Observations on *Polymorphus minutus* (Goeze, 1782) (Acanthocephala) from a wildfowl reserve in Kent. Parasitology 55:345–55.

Crompton, D. W. T., and P. J. Whitfield. 1968a. A hypothesis to account for the anterior migrations of adult *Hymenolepis diminuta* (Cestoda) and *Moniliformis dubius* (Acanthocephala) in the intestine of rats. Parasitology 58:227–29.

———. 1968b. The course of infection and egg production of *Polymorphus minutus* (Acanthocephala) in domestic ducks. Parasitology 58:231–46.

Crook, J. R., and A. W. Grundmann. 1964. The life history and larval development of *Moniliformis clarki* (Ward, 1917). J. Parasitol. 50:689–93.

Deinhardt, F., A. W. Holmes, J. Devine, and Jean Deinhardt. 1967. Marmosets as laboratory animals: IV. The microbiology of laboratory kept marmosets. Lab. Animal Care 17:48–70.

Deinhardt, Jean B., J. Devine, M. Passovoy, R. Pohlman, and F. Deinhardt. 1967. Marmosets as laboratory animals: I. Care of marmosets in the laboratory; pathology and outline of statistical evaluation of data. Lab. Animal Care 17:11–29.

Diaz-Ungria, C. 1958. Sobre algunos acantocefalos de mamiferos venezolanos. Rev. Med. Vet. Parasitol. (Maracay) 17:191–214.

Dollfus, R. P. 1938. Étude morphologique et systématique de deux espèces d'acanthocéphales, parasites de lemurienes et de signes revue critique du genre *Prosthenorchis* Travassos. Ann. Parasitol. Humaine Comparee 16:385–422.

Dunn, F. L. 1963. Acanthocephalans and cestodes of South American monkeys and marmosets. J. Parasitol. 49:717–22.

Garner, E., F. Hemrick, and H. Rudiger. 1967. Multiple helminth infections in cinnamon-ringtail monkeys *(Cebus albifrons)*. Lab. Animal Care 17:310–15.

Golvan, Y.-J. 1962. Le phylum des Acanthocephala (Quatrième note). La classe des Archiacanthocephala (A. Meyer 1931). Ann. Parasitol. Humaine Comparee 37:1–72.

Graham, G. L. 1960. Parasitism in monkeys. Ann. N.Y. Acad. Sci. 85:842–60.

Hyman, Libbie H. 1951. The invertebrates: Acanthocephala, Aschelminthes, and Entoprocta. The pseudocoelomate Bilateria. Vol. III. McGraw-Hill, New York. 572 pp.

Jones, Myrna. 1928. An acanthocephalid, *Plagiorhynchus formosus,* from the chicken and the robin. J. Agr. Res. 36:773–75.

Jurado-Mendoza, J. F. 1966. *Oncicola canis:* Interesante acantocephalo del perro. Proc. 5th Pan-Am. Congr. Vet. Med. Zootech., Caracas 1:289–94.

Lapage, G. 1962. Mönnig's veterinary helminthology and entomology. 5th ed. Williams and Wilkins, Baltimore. 600 pp.

Machado Filho, D. A. 1950. Revisão do gênero *Prosthenorchis* Travassos, 1915 (Acanthocephala). Mem. Inst. Oswaldo Cruz 48:495–544.

Machulskii, S. N. 1959. Helminth fauna of rodents of Buriat ASSR (in Russian). Raboty Gel'mintol. 80-Let. Skrjabin:219–24.

Meyer, A. 1933. Acanthocephala. *In* H. G. Bronn's Klassen und Ordnungen des Tierreichs. Vol. 4, Sect. 2, Bk. 2. Akademische Verlagsgesellschaft, M.B.H., Leipzig.

Middleton, C. C. 1966. Acanthocephala *(Prosthenorchis elegans)* infection in squirrel monkeys *(Saimiri sciureus)*. Lab. Animal Dig. 2:16–17.

Moore, D. V. 1946. Studies on the life history and development of *Moniliformis dubius* Meyer, 1933. J. Parasitol. 32:257–71.

Morgan, B. B., and P. A. Hawkins. 1949. Veterinary helminthology. Burgess, Minneapolis. 400 pp.

Nelson, B., G. E. Cosgrove, and N. Gengozian. 1966. Diseases of an imported primate *Tamarinus nigricollis*. Lab. Animal Care 16:255–75.

Nuorteva, P. 1966. *Corynosoma strumosum* (Rud.) and *C. semerne* (Forssell) (Acanthocephala) as pathogenic parasites of farmed minks in Finland. J. Helminthol. 40:77–80.

Oldham, J. N. 1967. Helminths, ectoparasites and protozoa in rats and mice, pp. 641–79. *In* E. Cotchin and F. J. C. Roe, eds. Pathology of laboratory rats and mice. Blackwell Scientific Publ., Oxford.

Olsen, O. W. 1967. Animal parasites: Their biology and life cycles. 2d ed. Burgess, Minneapolis. 431 pp.

Petrochenko, V. I. 1956–1958. Acanthocephala (thorn-headed worms) of domestic and wild animals (in Russian). Vol. 2. Acad. Nauk, Moskva. 458 pp.

Price, E. W. 1926. A note on *Oncicola canis* (Kaupp), an acanthocephalid parasite of the dog. J. Am. Vet. Med. Assoc. 69:704–10.

Richart, R., and K. Benirschke. 1963. Causes of death in a colony of marmoset monkeys. J. Pathol. Bacteriol. 86:221–23.

Ruch, T. C. 1959. Diseases of laboratory primates. W. B. Saunders, Philadelphia. 600 pp.

Sinitsin, D. 1929. A note on the intermediate host of *Plagiorhynchus formosus*. J. Parasitol. 15:287.

Soulsby, E. J. L. 1965. Textbook of veterinary clinical parasitology: Vol. 1. Helminths. F. A. Davis, Philadelphia. 1120 pp.

Takos, M. J., and L. J. Thomas. 1958. The pathology and pathogenesis of fatal infections due to an acanthocephalid parasite of marmoset monkeys. Am. J. Trop. Med. Hyg. 7:90–94.

Van Cleave, H. J. 1947. Thorny-headed worms (Acanthocephala) as potential parasites of poultry. Proc. Helminthol. Soc. Wash. D.C. 14:55–58.

———. 1948. Expanding horizons in the recognition of a phylum. J. Parasitol. 34:1–20.

———. 1952. Some host-parasite relationships of the Acanthocephala, with special reference to the organs of attachment. Exp. Parasitol. 1:305–30.

———. 1953a. Acanthocephala of North American mammals. Illinois Biol. Monographs 23:1–179.

———. 1953b. A preliminary analysis of the acanthocephalan genus *Corynosoma* in mammals of North America. J. Parasitol. 39:1–13.

Ward, Helen L. 1950. Acanthocephala as possible parasites of Tennessee chickens. J. Tenn. Acad. Sci. 25:242–43.

Wehr, E. E. 1965. Nematodes and acanthocephalids of poultry, pp. 965–1005. *In* H. E. Biester and L. H. Schwarte, eds. Diseases of poultry. 5th ed. Iowa State Univ. Press, Ames.

Witenberg, G. G. 1938. Studies on Acanthocephala: 3. Genus *Oncicola*, pp. 537–60. *In* Livro Jubilar Prof. Travassos, Rio de Janeiro.

———. 1949. Canine worm parasites in Palestine (in Hebrew). Refuah Vet. 5:34–40, 67–68.

———. 1964. Acanthocephala infections, pp. 708–9. *In* J. Van der Hoeden, ed. Zoonoses. Elsevier, New York.

Worms, M. J. 1967. Parasites of newly imported animals. J. Inst. Animal Technicians 18:39–47.

Yamaguti, S. 1963. Acanthocephala. Vol. V. *In* S. Yamaguti. *Systema helminthum*. Interscience, New York.

Chapter 9

LEECHES

LEECHES are aquatic or tropical rain forest annelids of the class Hirudinea (Autrum 1936; Herter 1932; Herter, Schleip, and Autrum 1939; Mann 1962; Scriban and Autrum 1934). They include scavengers that feed on nonliving material, predators that feed on tissues and fluids of soft-bodied invertebrates, and others that are blood-sucking ectoparasites of vertebrates. The soft, annulated body of a leech (2 to 16 external annuli per true internal segment) is usually flattened dorsoventrally and colorfully patterned in green, brown, or red. The leech is characterized by great powers of distension and contraction which enable it to penetrate extremely fine body openings and to ingest and store relatively large volumes of blood. A pair of suckers, one at each end of the worm, a large muscular hind sucker and a smaller anterior one surrounding the mouth, permits the looping movement and powerful adherence to prey or host during feeding.

There are two orders of leeches, Gnathobdellae and Rhynchobdellae. The order Gnathobdellae is characterized by the presence of cutting jaws. It includes the family Hirudinidae, which contains most leeches of medical and veterinary importance. The order Rhynchobdellae is characterized by a penetrating proboscis rather than by cutting jaws. It includes a number of fish parasites, chiefly in the family Piscicolidae. The presence of a strong anticoagu-

lant, capacious gut pouches which serve for long-term blood storage, and the extraordinary flexibility of the hardy body render leeches well adapted for a parasitic existence.

Leeches are occasional parasites of certain endothermal laboratory animals in their natural habitat, but they are rarely found on laboratory specimens. Those most likely to be encountered are listed in Table 9.1. The two most important species are discussed below.

Limnatus nilotica

(Horse Leech)

This leech occurs in southern and central Europe, North Africa, and southwestern Asia (Lapage 1962; Mann 1962). It occasionally attaches to the mucosa of the nasal cavities, pharynx, or larynx of the dog, domestic animals, and man. It is unlikely to occur in the laboratory except in dogs obtained from pounds in endemic areas.

MORPHOLOGY

Limnatus nilotica is 8 to 15 cm long and 1.0 to 1.5 cm wide (Fig. 9.1) (Faust, Beaver, and Jung 1968; Lapage 1962; Witenberg 1964). It is green or brown on the dorsal surface and brown to black on the ventral surface, with narrow orange stripes along the body ridges.

331

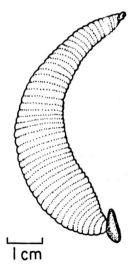

FIG. 9.1. *Limnatus nilotica.* (From Faust, Beaver, and Jung 1968. Courtesy of Lea and Febiger.)

LIFE CYCLE

This leech, like all Hirudinea, is hermaphroditic, but two specimens usually cross-fertilize to produce eggs (Witenberg 1964). The eggs are laid in cocoons and are characteristically attached to some object at the surface of a pond. The eggs hatch, and the young leeches remain at the surface of the water (Lapage 1962). Infection of an endothermal host occurs while drinking; the parasite enters either the nose or the mouth, attaches to the mucosa of the upper respiratory tract, sucks blood for days or weeks, grows, detaches, and drops out through the nostrils. Adults are not parasitic.

PATHOLOGIC EFFECTS

Signs of infection are blood or a blood-tinged froth exuding from the nose or mouth (Lapage 1962). Edema of the glottis, dyspnea, and death from asphyxiation sometimes occur.

DIAGNOSIS

Diagnosis is based on the signs and confirmed by demonstration of the leech attached to the respiratory mucosa.

CONTROL

Newly acquired dogs from endemic areas should be examined on arrival and treated, if infected. Flushing of the nasal cavities with chloroform water is reportedly effective (Lapage 1962).

PUBLIC HEALTH CONSIDERATIONS

Although this leech attacks man, exposure under laboratory conditions is unlikely.

Dinobdella ferox

This leech is widespread in southern Asia (Faust, Beaver, and Jung 1968). It frequently invades the pharynx of ruminants and occasionally the upper respiratory tract of the dog, monkeys, and man. *Dinobdella ferox* is a common inhabitant of the nasal cavities of macaques obtained from their natural habitat (Bywater and Mann 1960; Fox and Ediger 1970; Kuntz et al. 1968). Incidences as high as 6% have been observed in laboratory collections of the Formosan macaque; in one survey, 6 of 150 animals were infected (Pryor, Bergner and Raulston 1970). Because the leech is not easily detected, it is suspected that the true incidence is even higher. Laboratory monkeys obtained from endemic areas, particularly from Taiwan, are likely to be infected.

MORPHOLOGY

Dinobdella ferox is 3.5 to 6.0 cm long and 0.5 to 0.8 cm wide (Fig. 9.2). It has a

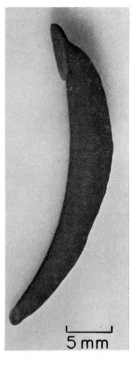

FIG. 9.2. *Dinobdella ferox.* (From Pryor, Bergner, and Raulston 1970. Courtesy of the American Veterinary Medical Association.)

dorsoventrally flattened body which is dark red when engorged (Bywater and Mann 1960; Fox and Ediger 1970).

LIFE CYCLE

The life cycle is similar to that of *L. nilotica*. Infection of the endothermal host usually occurs while drinking (Faust, Beaver, and Jung 1968). The parasite attaches to the mucosa of the upper respiratory tract or pharynx, sucks blood, and remains attached for weeks (Pryor, Bergner, and Raulston 1970) or months (Bywater and Mann 1960) until mature.

PATHOLOGIC EFFECTS

Infection with one or two parasites usually produces no signs, but severe infection causes restlessness, epistaxis, anemia, weakness, asphyxiation, and sometimes death (Pryor, Bergner, and Raulston 1970). Lesions consist of a mild, local, chronic inflammation of the nasopharyngeal mucosa with increased mucus production.

DIAGNOSIS

Diagnosis is based on recognition of the parasite. Infection in macaques is most easily detected by examining the host's nares with a flashlight (Pryor, Bergner, and Raulston 1970). When the monkey is initially handled, the parasite withdraws from view, but it will reappear if the host is held quietly (Fig. 9.3).

CONTROL

Newly acquired animals from endemic areas should be examined on arrival and treated, if infected. The leech is usually removable by gentle traction with a forceps

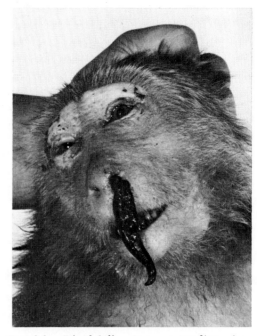

FIG. 9.3. *Dinobdella ferox* extending from nares of Formosan macaque. (From Pryor, Bergner, and Raulston 1970. Courtesy of the American Veterinary Medical Association.)

(Pryor, Bergner, and Raulston 1970). If forceps alone are insufficient, spraying the leech lightly with an insecticide is often helpful.

PUBLIC HEALTH CONSIDERATIONS

Although this leech attacks man, exposure under laboratory conditions is unlikely. However, care should be taken when removing leeches from affected animals.

TABLE 9.1. Leeches affecting endothermal laboratory animals

Parasite	Geographic Distribution	Endothermal Host	Location in Host	Method of Infection	Incidence — In nature	Incidence — In laboratory	Pathologic Effects	Public Health Importance	Reference
*Limnatus nilotica**	Southern and central Europe, North Africa, southwestern Asia	Dog, domestic animals, man	Nasal cavities, pharynx, larynx	Invasion of mouth or nares while drinking	Uncommon	Rare or absent	Loss of blood, epistaxis; sometimes edema of glottis, dyspnea, asphyxiation, death	Affects man; exposure in laboratory unlikely	Lapage 1962 Mann 1962 Witenberg 1964
Limnatus africana	West Africa	Dog, monkeys, man	Nasal cavities	Invasion of mouth or nares while drinking	Uncommon	Rare or absent	Loss of blood, epistaxis, debilitation	Affects man; exposure in laboratory unlikely	Clieng 1964 Lapage 1962
*Dinobdella ferox**	Southern Asia	Dog, rhesus monkey, Formosan macaque, ruminants, man	Nasal cavities, pharynx	Invasion of mouth or nares while drinking	Common in Formosan macaque; uncommon in dog	Common in Formosan macaque obtained from natural habitat; rare or absent in dog	Loss of blood, restlessness, epistaxis, anemia, weakness, asphyxiation, sometimes death	Affects man; exposure in laboratory unlikely	Bywater and Mann 1960 Faust et al. 1968 Fox and Ediger 1970 Kuntz et al. 1968 Pryor et al. 1970
Diestecostoma mexicanum	Central America	Dog	Upper respiratory tract	Invasion of mouth or nares while drinking	Rare	Rare or absent	Cough, dyspnea, anorexia, anemia, sometimes **death**	Unknown	Hatherill 1967

*Discussed in text.

REFERENCES

Autrum, H. 1936. Hirudineae. Part 1. *In* H. G. Bronn's Klassen und Ordnungen des Tierreichs. Vol. 4, Sect. 3, Bk. 4. Akademische Verlagsgesellschaft, M.B.H., Leipzig.

Bywater, J. E. C., and K. H. Mann. 1960. Infestation of a monkey with the leech *Dinobdella ferox*. Vet. Record 72:955.

Cheng, T. C. 1964. The biology of animal parasites. W. B. Saunders, Philadelphia. 727 pp.

Faust, E. C., P. C. Beaver, and R. C. Jung. 1968. Animal agents and vectors of human disease. 3d ed. Lea and Febiger, Philadelphia. 461 pp.

Fox, J. G., and R. D. Ediger. 1970. Nasal leech infestation in the rhesus monkey. Lab. Animal Care 20:1137–38.

Hatherill, C. W. B. 1967. *Diestecostoma mexicanum* infestation of dogs. Vet. Record 81:262.

Herter, K. 1932. Hirudinea. Egel, pp. 1–158. *In* P. Schulze, ed. Biologie der Tiere Deutschlands. Issue 35, Part 12b. Gebrüder Borntraeger, Berlin.

Herter, K., W. Schleip, and H. Autrum. 1939.

Hirudineae. Part 2. *In* H. G. Bronn's Klassen und Ordnungen des Tierreichs. Vol. 4, Sect. 3, Bk. 4. Akademische Verlagsgesellschaft, M.B.H., Leipzig.

Kuntz, R. E., Betty J. Myers, J. F. Bergner, Jr., and D. E. Armstrong. 1968. Parasites and commensals of the Taiwan macaque *(Macaca cyclopis* Swinhoe, 1862). Formosan Sci. 22:120–36.

Lapage, G. 1962. Mönnig's veterinary helminthology and entomology. 5th ed. Williams and Wilkins, Baltimore. 600 pp.

Mann, K. H. 1962. Leeches (Hirudinea), their structure, physiology, ecology, and embryology. Pergamon Press, New York. 201 pp.

Pryor, W. H. Jr., J. F. Bergner, Jr., and G. L. Raulston. 1970. Leech *(Dinobdella ferox)* infection of a Taiwan monkey *(Macaca cyclopis).* J. Am. Vet. Med. Assoc. 157: 1926–27.

Scriban, I. A., and H. Autrum. 1934. 2. Ordnung der Clitellata: Hirudinea=Egel, pp. 119–352. *In* W. Kükenthal and T. Krumbach, eds. Handbuch der Zoologie. Vol. 2, Part 2. Walter de Gruyter, Berlin and Leipzig.

Witenberg, G. G. 1964. Hirudiniases, pp. 710–19. *In* J. Van der Hoeden, ed. Zoonoses. Elsevier, New York.

Chapter 10

BUGS

THE bugs belong to the order Hemiptera, which contains approximately 77 families and about 55,000 species (James and Harwood 1969). Only 3 of these families, Polyctenidae (polyctenids), Cimicidae (cimicids), and Reduviidae (reduviids), contain species which are ectoparasites of endothermal animals.

POLYCTENIDS

Polyctenids are relatively small, morphologically peculiar, blind, pseudoplacental, viviparous ectoparasites of bats. They are quite rare and are not to be expected as pests of endothermal laboratory animals.

CIMICIDS

The family Cimicidae is comprised of some 74 species in 22 genera (Usinger 1966). These bugs are associated with man, bats, and birds throughout most of the inhabited portions of the earth. Generalized common names have been applied to the cimicids, depending upon the hosts with which they are associated (human bed bugs, bat bugs, pigeon bugs, swallow bugs, chicken bugs, etc.). Of the 22 genera, 10 are exclusively ectoparasites of bats in Asia, Africa, and North, Central, and South America (*Primicimex, Bucimex, Propicimex, Cacodmus, Aphrania, Loxaspis, Stricticimex, Crassicimex, Afrocimex,* and *Latrocimex*); 9 are exclusively ectoparasites of birds

in Europe, Asia, North and South America, Australia, and the islands of the southwest Pacific (*Oeciacus, Paracimex, Ornithocoris, Caminicimex, Psitticimex, Haematosiphon, Cimexopsis, Synxenoderus,* and *Hesperocimex*). The host for *Bertilia* from southern South America is unknown. *Leptocimex* is an ectoparasite of bats and man in Africa. The remaining and most important genus, *Cimex,* includes the common bed bug and other species that parasitize man, domestic mammals, birds, and bats.

Cimex, Haematosiphon, Hesperocimex

Cimex lectularius, the common bed bug of man, also parasitizes domestic mammals, bats, and birds (Usinger 1966). It is distributed throughout the temperate regions of the world and also occurs in tropical regions. In the tropics, *C. hemipterus* is the commoner species; man is the principal host, but it also parasitizes bats and the chicken. The common pigeon bug of Europe is *C. columbarius; C. lectularius* is also frequently associated with the pigeon. An additional 13 species of the genus *Cimex* are associated with bats.

Haematosiphon inodorus, the Mexican chicken bug, has been reported from wild birds and the chicken in southwest United States and northern Mexico (Usinger 1966). The genus *Hesperocimex* is composed of three closely related species, *H. coloradensis, H. sonorensis,* and *H. cochim-*

iensis. These species are primarily parasitic on wild birds in western United States and northern Mexico, but they can be adapted to the chicken. None has been reported as a laboratory pest, but they have the potential to become a problem.

Most of these species appear to be rather host-specific in nature, but in the laboratory they feed on a wide range of hosts. The species that has been the greatest problem in laboratory animal colonies is *C. lectularius.* This parasite has been introduced into animal colonies on infested bedding (Poiley 1950). It was once common in laboratory colonies (Heston 1941; Yunker 1964) and still is in some areas (Sasa et al. 1962; Tuffery and Innes 1963). With the advent of DDT and the improved design of animal facilities, the incidence has been greatly reduced, and infestation of laboratory colonies in the United States and northern Europe is now rare (Porter 1967; Woodnott 1963).

MORPHOLOGY

Adults are dorsoventrally flattened and have three pairs of legs, one pair of four-segmented antennae, a proboscis with three segments, wing pads but no wings, and a relatively hard, chitinous exoskeleton. The integument is usually sparsely covered with relatively short hairs or bristles. The proboscis at rest is folded back under the head. When near a prospective host, the proboscis is extended toward the host and the tip of the feeding apparatus is brought in contact with the skin. The proboscis is not inserted into the skin, as is commonly assumed, but fine stylets are extruded and forced into the tissue. Typical of these bugs is *C. lectularius* (Fig. 10.1). The eggs are white, and an operculum is located at the anterior end, which is curved upward (Fig. 10.2).

LIFE CYCLE

Most of these bugs pass through five immature instars; however, *Haematosiphon inodorus* has only four immature instars in both sexes (Lee 1955). Females of most species normally deposit three to four eggs per day in crevices (Ryckman 1958; Usinger 1966). The development time varies, depending on the temperature and the availability of food. *Cimex* develops from egg to

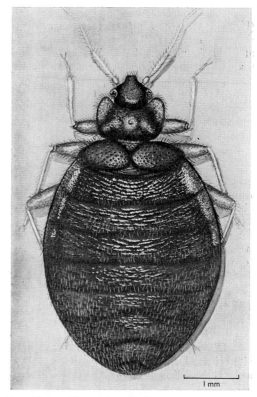

FIG. 10.1. *Cimex lectularius* female. (Courtesy of M. Dorothy Cox and Loma Linda University.)

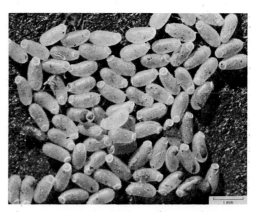

FIG. 10.2. Eggs of *Hesperocimex cochimiensis.* (Courtesy of Loma Linda University.)

adult in approximately 25 days at 30 C (Usinger 1966); *Hesperocimex sonorensis* develops from egg to adult in 39 to 42 days at 27 C (Ryckman 1958). These bugs normally live in cracks and crevices near the hosts; they feed for short periods (15 to 20 minutes) and then return to their hiding place (R. E. Ryckman, unpublished data; Usinger 1966).

PATHOLOGIC EFFECTS

Although a papular lesion, apparently an allergic response, has been reported in the guinea pig at the site of bites by these cimicids (Usinger 1966), thousands have been reared on animals in the laboratory for several years, and at no time has there been evidence of edema, erythema, or scar formation (R. E. Ryckman, unpublished data). The commonest pathologic effects of these cimicids to laboratory animals are the loss of blood and the annoyance of the bite.

DIAGNOSIS

Diagnosis is made by finding the parasite on the host or in cracks and crevices in animal buildings.

CONTROL

Because these bugs are present on the host only during feeding, control measures are directed toward their harborages and the surfaces traversed in reaching the laboratory host. The treatment of choice consists of spraying infested cracks and crevices with 5% DDT or 2% malathion (Usinger 1966). The entire animal facility should be treated. Care should be taken not to expose research animals to insecticides; therefore, they should be removed from a room before it is treated. All racks and equipment should be removed and the room carefully cleaned and then sprayed; one thorough application of an insecticide is more effective than several light applications. The racks and equipment should be cleaned and autoclaved or heat sterilized and the animals transferred to clean, sterile cages before being brought back into the room. These procedures should be repeated until all signs of the pests have disappeared. If control of these cimicids is not effected by one insecticide, it may be an indication that a resistant strain is present; in

this situation an alternate compound must be used. In institutions where laboratory animals are used as hosts to maintain colonies of arthropods, pyrethrins and a synergist should be used instead of residual insecticides.

PUBLIC HEALTH CONSIDERATIONS

The bite of these cimicids can cause a hypersensitive reaction and painful pruritus in man (Matheson 1950; R. E. Ryckman, unpublished data). The reactions may be delayed from 18 to 24 hours before clinical manifestations occur.

Although these bugs fulfill all the requirements for being effective vectors of disease (that is, they are obligate, hemophagous ectoparasites; they feed frequently and repeatedly over many months as immature and adult bugs; they may feed on many hosts during their lifetime and they have been experimentally infected with many pathogens), they have never been reported as being responsible for epidemics (James and Harwood 1969). Nevertheless, if laboratory animals are infected with pathogens, one should view with considerable concern any parasite which may feed on these animals.

REDUVIIDS

The family Reduviidae is comprised of some 20 subfamilies; all are predacious except the Triatominae, whose 14 genera and approximately 80 species are parasitic, primarily on endothermal vertebrates. The genera *Triatoma*, *Paratriatoma*, and *Rhodnius* are the most likely to affect laboratory species.

Triatoma, Paratriatoma, Rhodnius
(Kissing Bugs or Cone-nosed Bugs)

These bugs are obligate blood-feeding ectoparasites. They are usually not a problem in laboratories but have the potential to become one. The usual reservoir host for *Triatoma* and *Paratriatoma* is a pack or wood rat; however, the rock squirrel (*Citellus variegatus*) and armadillo sometimes serve as reservoir hosts (Ryckman, Christianson, and Spencer 1955; Wood and Wood 1961). The usual reservoir hosts for *Rhodnius*, in domestic situations, are domestic animals and man.

The many species of the genus *Tria-*

toma may be found throughout most of the tropical and temperate regions of the Western Hemisphere except *T. rubrofasciata*, which also occurs in tropical regions of the Eastern Hemisphere. *Paratriatoma* contains only one species, *P. hirsuta;* this species is found in southwestern United States and northwestern Mexico. Members of the genus *Rhodnius* are found in northern South America, Central America, and southern Mexico; they are common in buildings made of adobe and thatch. *Rhodnius* has been extensively reared in laboratories in Europe and North, Central, and South America.

MORPHOLOGY

Kissing bugs or cone-nosed bugs have three pairs of legs, one pair of four-segmented antennae, a three-segmented proboscis, and two compound eyes (Ryckman 1962; Usinger 1944). In addition, adults have two simple eyes or ocelli and two pairs of wings. The immature stages do not have functional wings, but the fourth and fifth instar nymphs have wing pads. Eggs are smooth or rough. *Rhodnius prolixus* (Fig. 10.3) is typical of these bugs.

LIFE CYCLE

These bugs pass through five immature instars to the adult. They usually feed for 10 to 20 minutes and then quickly return to dark, secluded areas in cracks and crevices. Immature stages require at least one blood meal and usually feed two or three times in the advanced instars before molting to the next stage. The adults live for over a year and feed at least once per week. Females require more blood than males. Eggs are laid singly and are dropped or glued to the surface at random, depending on the species.

The development period is highly variable, depending on the temperature, nutrition, and species (Ryckman 1962; Usinger 1944). At 30 C, the developmental time ranges from 4.5 months for *T. protracta* to 8 months for *P. hirsuta*. At 22 C, *P. hirsuta* requires 19 to 33 months, but at 29 C it requires 7 to 8 months. *Rhodnius* requires 3.5 months under optimum conditions.

PATHOLOGIC EFFECTS

Hundreds of these bugs have been fed on the abdomen of rabbits, weekly, for many weeks with no signs of edema, erythema, or scar formation, and with only an occasional death from an apparent anaphylactoid reaction (R. E. Ryckman, unpublished data). Severe infestations would presumably cause anemia; otherwise, these parasites have little apparent effect on their hosts.

DIAGNOSIS

Diagnosis is made by finding the parasite on the host or in cracks and crevices in animal buildings.

CONTROL

Kissing bugs are not easily killed, and they have developed resistance to a number of residual insecticides. They are relatively strong flyers and can travel long distances. They are seldom found on the host, and therefore control within animal facilities is directed toward their resting or hiding places. Source control is the most effective method when practical (James and Harwood 1969; R. E. Ryckman, unpublished data). This is accomplished by eliminating sylvatic reservoirs from the area around the laboratory and by constructing insectproof animal buildings. Residual insecticides should be applied as either sprays or dusts to those surfaces where bugs are most likely to crawl upon entering the laboratory, or to places where they hide between feedings. Lindane is effective in a concentration of 1.0% as a dust or 0.5% as a spray; malathion is effective in a concentration of 5%

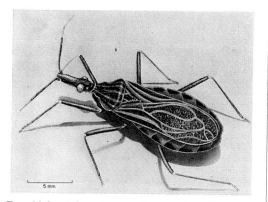

FIG. 10.3. *Rhodnius prolixus* male. (Courtesy of M. Dorothy Cox and Loma Linda University.)

as a dust or 2 to 5 % in a solution or emulsion as a spray. Dieldrin is even more effective, either at 5.0% in a dust or at 0.5% in a spray but, because of its high toxicity to mammals, it should be used only outdoors. Although a spray containing 0.2% pyrethrins with a synergist is also effective, repeated applications are necessary because it is not a residual insecticide.

PUBLIC HEALTH CONSIDERATIONS

Trypanosoma cruzi, the cause of Chagas' disease, is transmitted by kissing bugs (Gordon and Lavoipierre 1962). Repeated bites from these bugs sometimes cause hypersensitive reactions in man (Walsh and Jones 1962).

TABLE 10.1. Bugs affecting endothermal laboratory animals

Parasite	Geographic Distribution	Endothermal Host	Usual Habitat	Incidence		Pathologic Effects	Public Health Importance	Reference
				In nature	In laboratory			
Cimex lectularius*	Temperate regions, tropics	Small domestic mammals, bats, birds, man	Cracks and crevices in buildings	Formerly common; now uncommon	Formerly common; now uncommon or absent	Loss of blood, annoyance	Sometimes causes allergic reaction	Usinger 1966
Cimex hemipterus*	Tropics	Bats, chicken, man	Cracks and crevices in buildings	Common	Not reported	Loss of blood, annoyance	Sometimes causes allergic reaction	Usinger 1966
Cimex columbarius*	Western Europe	Pigeon	Cracks and crevices in buildings	Common	Not reported	Loss of blood, annoyance	Sometimes causes allergic reaction	Usinger 1966
Haematosiphon inodorus*	Southwestern United States, northern Mexico	Chicken, wild birds	Cracks and crevices in chicken houses, bird nests	Common	Not reported	Loss of blood, annoyance	Sometimes causes allergic reaction	Usinger 1966
Hesperocimex coloradensis*	Western United States, northern Mexico	Chicken, wild birds	Cavities in trees	Common in wild birds; rare in chicken	Not reported	Loss of blood, annoyance	Sometimes causes severe allergic reaction	R. E. Ryckman, unpublished data; Ryckman and Ueshima 1964; Usinger 1966
Hesperocimex sonorensis*	Western United States, northern Mexico	Chicken, wild birds	Cavities in cacti	Common in wild birds; rare in chicken	Not reported	Loss of blood, annoyance	Sometimes causes severe allergic reaction	R. E. Ryckman, unpublished data; Ryckman and Ueshima 1964; Usinger 1966
Hesperocimex cochimiensis*	Mexico (Baja California)	Chicken, wild birds	Cavities in cacti	Common in wild birds; rare in chicken	Not reported	Loss of blood, annoyance	Sometimes causes severe allergic reaction	R. E. Ryckman, unpublished data; Ryckman and Ueshima 1964; Usinger 1966
Triatoma dimidiata	Southern Mexico, Central America, northern South America	Domestic animals, man	Buildings, caves	Common	Not reported	Usually none; possibly anemia; vector of Trypanosoma cruzi, T. rangeli	Sometimes causes allergic reaction; vector of agent of trypanosomiasis	Usinger 1944
Triatoma gerstaeckeri	Southern United States, northeastern Mexico	Wood rats, armadillo	Wood rat habitats	Common	Not reported	Usually none; possibly anemia; vector of Trypanosoma cruzi	Sometimes causes allergic reaction; vector of agent of trypanosomiasis	Usinger 1944
Triatoma infestans	South America	Domestic animals, man	Buildings	Common	Not reported	Usually none; possibly anemia; vector of Trypanosoma cruzi	Sometimes causes allergic reaction; vector of agent of trypanosomiasis	James and Harwood 1969
Triatoma lecticularius	Southern United States	Wood rats	Wood rat habitats	Common	Not reported	Usually none; possibly anemia	Sometimes causes allergic reaction	Usinger 1944

*Discussed in text.

TABLE 10.1 *(continued)*

Parasite	Geographic Distribution	Endothermal Host	Usual Habitat	Incidence In nature	Incidence In laboratory	Pathologic Effects	Public Health Importance	Reference
Triatoma neotomae	Southern Texas, northeastern Mexico	Wood rats	Wood rat habitats	Common	Not reported	Usually none; possibly anemia	Sometimes causes allergic reaction	Usinger 1944
Triatoma protracta	Western North America	Wood rats	Wood rat habitats	Common	Not reported	Usually none; possibly anemia	Sometimes causes allergic reaction	Ryckman 1962
Triatoma rubida	Western North America	Wood rats	Wood rat habitats	Common	Not reported	Usually none; possibly anemia	Sometimes causes allergic reaction	Usinger 1944
Triatoma rubrofasciata	Tropics	Black rat, poultry	Buildings	Common	Not reported	Usually none; possibly anemia; vector of *Trypanosoma conorhini*	Sometimes causes allergic reaction	Usinger 1944
Triatoma sanguisuga	Southeastern United States	Wood rats, other small wild mammals, opossum	Wood rat habitats, hollow trees, stumps	Common	Not reported	Usually none; possibly anemia	Sometimes causes allergic reaction	Usinger 1944
*Paratriatoma hirsuta**	Southwestern United States, northwestern Mexico	Wood rats	Wood rat habitats	Common	Not reported	Usually none; possibly anemia	Sometimes causes allergic reaction	Usinger 1944
Rhodnius prolixus	Mexico, Central America, northern South America	Domestic animals, man	Buildings	Common	Not reported	Usually none; possibly anemia; vector of *Trypanosoma cruzi, T. rangeli*	Sometimes causes allergic reaction; vector of trypanosomiasis	James and Harwood 1969
Dipetalogaster maximus	Mexico (Baja California)	Wood rats	Exfoliative rocks	Common	Not reported	Usually none; possibly anemia	Sometimes causes allergic reaction	Ryckman and Ryckman 1967
Panstrongylus megistus	Tropical South America (south of Amazon)	Domestic animals, man	Buildings	Common	Not reported	Usually none; possibly anemia; vector of *Trypanosoma cruzi*	Sometimes causes allergic reaction; vector of agent of trypanosomiasis	James and Harwood 1969

*Discussed in text.

REFERENCES

Gordon, R. M., and M. M. J. Lavoipierre. 1962. Entomology for students of medicine. Blackwell Scientific Publ., Oxford. 353 pp.

Heston, W. E. 1941. Parasites, pp. 349–74. In G. D. Snell, ed. Biology of the laboratory mouse. Blakiston, Philadelphia.

James, M. T., and R. F. Harwood. 1969. Herms's medical entomology. 6th ed. Macmillan, New York. 484 pp.

Lee, R. D. 1955. The biology of the Mexican chicken bug, *Haematosiphon inodorus* (Duges). Pan-Pacific Entomologist 31:47–61.

Matheson, R. 1950. Medical entomology. 2d ed. Comstock, New York. 612 pp.

Poiley, S. M. 1950. Breeding and care of the Syrian hamster, pp. 118–52. In E. J. Farris, ed. The care and breeding of laboratory animals. John Wiley, New York.

Porter, G. 1967. The Norway rat, pp. 353–90. In UFAW Staff, eds. The UFAW handbook on the care and management of laboratory animals. 3d ed. Livingstone and the Universities Federation for Animal Welfare, London.

Ryckman, R. E. 1958. Description and biology of *Hesperocimex sonorensis*, new species, an ectoparasite of the purple martin. (Hemiptera: Cimicidae) Ann. Entomol. Soc. Am. 51:33–47.

———. 1962. Biosystematics and hosts of the *Triatoma protracta* complex in North America (Hemiptera: Reduviidae) (Rodentia: Cricetidae). Univ. Calif. (Berkeley) Publ. Entomol. 27:93–240.

Ryckman, R. E., C. P. Christianson, and D. Spencer. 1955. *Triatoma recurva* collected from its natural host in Sonora, Mexico. J. Econ. Entomol. 48:330–32.

Ryckman, R. E., and A. E. Ryckman. 1967. Epizootiology of *Trypanosoma cruzi* in southwestern North America. Part X: The biosystematics of *Dipetalogaster maximus*

in Mexico (Hemiptera: Reduviidae) (Kinetoplastida: Trypanosomidae). J. Med. Entomol. 4:180–88.

Ryckman, R. E., and N. Ueshima. 1964. Biosystematics of the *Hesperocimex* Complex (Hemiptera: Cimicidae) and avian hosts (Piciformes: Picidae; Passeriformes: Hirundinidae). Ann. Entomol. Soc. Am. 57: 624–38.

Sasa, M., H. Tanaka, M. Fukui, and A. Takata. 1962. Internal parasites of laboratory animals, pp. 195–214. In R. J. C. Harris, ed. The problems of laboratory animal disease. Academic Press, New York.

Tuffery, A. A., and J. R. M. Innes. 1963. Diseases of laboratory mice and rats, pp. 47–108. In W. Lane-Petter, ed. Animals for research: Principles of breeding and management. Academic Press, New York.

Usinger, R. L. 1944. The Triatominae of North and Central America and the West Indies and their public health significance. U.S. Public Health Service Bull. 288. 83 pp.

———. 1966. Monograph of Cimicidae. Entomol. Soc. Am., College Park, Md. 585 pp.

Walsh, J. D., and J. P. Jones. 1962. Public health significance of the cone-nosed bug, *Triatoma protracta* (Uhler), in the Sierra Nevada foothills of California. Calif. Vector Views 9(7):33–37.

Wood, S. F., and F. D. Wood. 1961. Observations on vectors of Chagas' disease in the United States. III. New Mexico. Am. J. Trop. Med. Hyg. 10:155–65.

Woodnott, Dorothy P. 1963. Pests of the animal house, pp. 157–68. In D. J. Short and Dorothy P. Woodnott, eds. A.T.A. manual of laboratory animal practice and techniques. Crosby Lockwood and Son, London.

Yunker, C. E. 1964. Infections of laboratory animals potentially dangerous to man: Ectoparasites and other arthropods, with emphasis on mites. Lab. Animal Care 14:455–65.

Chapter 11

FLEAS

FLEAS (Siphonaptera) are wingless insects with laterally compressed bodies and strong legs adapted for leaping. In the adult stage, all are bloodsucking ectoparasites of endothermal animals.

Fleas do not usually occur on animals raised in the laboratory since the life cycle is readily interrupted by routine sanitation. They are often found on animals obtained from their natural habitat, but even these fleas are easily controlled by isolating newly acquired animals and treating them with a suitable insecticide.

The fleas which occur on laboratory animals are listed in Table 11.1. The more important species are discussed below.

Ctenocephalides felis, Ctenocephalides canis

(Cat Flea, Dog Flea)

These are the common fleas of the dog, cat, and related carnivores (Hopkins and Rothschild 1953). They often cause a severe dermatitis and are vectors of the dog tapeworm. *Ctenocephalides felis* is usually found on the cat and dog and occasionally on other endothermal species including the mouse, rat, chicken, baboons, and man, while *C. canis* is generally restricted to the dog and feral canines (Hopkins and Rothschild 1953; Myers and Kuntz 1965). *Ctenocephalides canis* is cosmopolitan. *Ctenocephalides felis* has four distinct subspecies: *C. f. felis* occurs throughout the world; *C. f.*

strongylus is found over most of Africa, except in the Sahara region and in southwestern Africa, where *C. f. damarensis* occurs; *C. f. orientis* is found in India, Ceylon, southeastern Asia, and New Guinea.

Fleas are common on pound dogs and cats but are not usually found on those raised for research (Johnson, Andersen, and Gee 1963; Morris 1963; Sasa et al. 1962). Of the two species, *C. felis* is by far the more frequently encountered, both in nature and in the laboratory. Reasons for this are not known, but it appears that the cat flea is more vagile than the dog flea and, where the two occur together, the latter competes unfavorably with the former.

MORPHOLOGY

Fleas of these species are characteristic of most fleas (Fig. 11.1) (Hopkins and Rothschild 1953). *Ctenocephalides felis* and *C. canis* vary in size. Females sometimes exceed 2.5 mm in length while males can be less than 1.0 mm long; there is often an overlap in size between the two sexes. Both species are dark brown and possess characteristic genal and pronotal combs. *Ctenocephalides felis* usually has an elongated head, especially in the female, a single subapical bristle on the dorsal margin of the hind tibia, and three setae in the lateral metanotal area (Fig. 11.1). *Ctenocephalides canis* has a short, blunt head (Fig. 11.2), two small subapical bristles on the

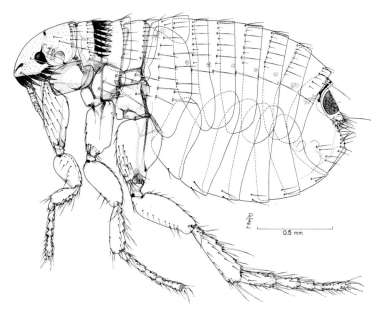

FIG. 11.1. *Ctenocephalides felis* female. (Courtesy of R. E. Lewis, Iowa State University.)

dorsal margin of the hind tibia, and usually only two setae on the lateral metanotal area. The larvae are small, white, and maggotlike, with a sclerotized head capsule and chewing mouthparts. They are legless but have a pair of caudal processes called anal struts. The eggs are small, white, and spherical.

LIFE CYCLE

Only adult fleas are found on the host, where mating and oviposition generally occur (Holland 1949). The eggs fall quickly from the pelage and often collect in the bedding. Under optimum conditions of 25 C and 80% relative humidity, the incubation period is about 2 to 4 days. There are three larval instars, but active feeding takes place only during the first and second instars. The larvae ingest organic material of both plant and animal origin, including pellets of blood excreted by adults. This material falls off the host and collects in the bedding. Shortly after molting, the third instar larva becomes quiescent and spins a cocoon. The cocoons are oval and inconspicuous. In some species they are attached to the bedding. In a few days a pupa forms. This stage lasts about 2 weeks, during which time the adult is formed. Under optimum conditions of temperature and humidity, the life cycle from egg to adult is

completed in 18 to 21 days, but in nature it probably requires a longer period. Length of life depends on the temperature, humidity, and the presence of a suitable host. Adults can live for a year or longer without food under conditions of low temperature and high humidity but expire in a few days at higher temperature and lower humidity (Bacot 1914). Apparently desiccation is as important as starvation in causing death.

A dog or cat becomes infected either by direct contact or by entering an area where adult fleas occur.

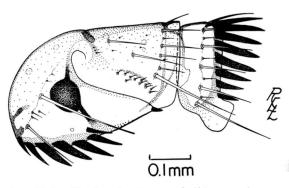

FIG. 11.2. Head of *Ctenocephalides canis*. (Courtesy of R. E. Lewis, Iowa State University.)

PATHOLOGIC EFFECTS

Flea infestation sometimes causes only minor clinical response in affected cats and dogs. More frequently, restlessness, irritability, weight loss, ruffled coat, biting, scratching, and self-induced trauma are seen (Lapage 1962; Renaux 1964). Flea bites also cause an allergic dermatitis (Goyings 1961; Kissileff 1962; Muller 1961, 1966; Walton 1968). The sensitization apparently occurs when a chemical substance is introduced by the mouthparts of the flea during feeding. Wheals and erythema occur at the site of the bite, but these are often not recognized in long-haired breeds. Sometimes small raised papules occur. Other lesions depend on the degree of self-inflicted trauma and often consist of excoriations, ulcerations, and alopecia (Král and Schwartzman 1964; Wood 1968). These lesions are usually located at the base of the tail and over the lower back. In chronic cases, the skin becomes thickened and indurated.

Histologic changes vary with the degree of trauma. Initially, the affected skin undergoes a predominantly neutrophilic inflammatory infiltration. Later, there is increased proliferation of fibroblasts and connective tissue. Acanthosis, parakeratosis, and degeneration of the pilosebaceous system often follow (Král and Schwartzman 1964; Muller 1961).

Ctenocephalides felis and *C. canis* are vectors of *Dipylidium caninum,* a tapeworm that affects the cat and dog and sometimes man (Faust and Russel 1957).

DIAGNOSIS

Infestation is diagnosed by finding either fleas or flea excrement on the host. The excrement is seen as small, dark, gritty particles in the pelage. It is important to distinguish dermatosis caused by fleas from that of other causes. Remission of signs and lesions after the parasites have been eliminated justifies a diagnosis of flea-induced dermatitis (Muller 1966).

CONTROL

Newly acquired animals should be isolated, examined, and treated, if necessary, before they are introduced into a laboratory colony. Sanitation and the use of insecti-

cides will prevent larval development and destroy adult fleas. Cages and pens should be constructed of metal, concrete, or other materials which can be readily cleaned. Pens and runs with gravel or dirt floors are not recommended; if used, they should be routinely treated with insecticides.

Most of the common insecticides are effective against *C. felis* and *C. canis* adults and larvae. Effective topical treatments for the dog include a spray containing either 0.5% methoxychlor, 0.5% malathion, 0.5 to 1.0% carbaryl, or 0.6% pyrethrins in combination with 0.5% piperonyl butoxide; a dip containing either 0.5% chlordane, 0.25% diazinon, 0.5% ronnel, or 0.025% DDVP (Vapona, Shell); or a powder containing either 5% DDT, 1% lindane, 3% chlordane, or 4% malathion in combination with 1.2% rotenone (Blakemore 1966; Muller 1966). Effective and safe treatments for the cat include powders containing either 3% rotenone, 4% malathion, 5% carbaryl, or 1% rotenone in combination with 1% pyrethrum (Blakemore 1966; Renaux 1964).

Systemic insecticides are also used to control these parasites. Ronnel, given orally at a dose of approximately 50 to 100 mg per kg of body weight every 2 to 4 days, is effective and safe for both the dog and cat (Burch 1960; Burch and Brinkman 1962; Johnston and Kerley 1962). Trichlorfon in combination with atropine, given orally twice a week at a dosage of 75 mg per kg of body weight, is recommended for treatment of the dog but not the cat (Eppley et al. 1963).

It is important that infected animal cages, pens, and runs be treated at the same time as the host; otherwise reinfestation can occur. Infected bedding should be destroyed, the cages completely sanitized, and the walls, floors, pens, and runs treated with an insecticide. A spray containing 1 to 2% malathion or 1% diazinon, lindane, or ronnel is recommended for exterior use (Wilson, Keller, and Smith 1957), and a spray containing 0.5% lindane or a dust containing 1.0% lindane is recommended for interior use (Muller 1966; Yunker 1964). Care must be taken to avoid spraying or dusting the animals, especially cats, with these more concentrated materials.

The use of a sorptive silica dust (Dri-

Die 67, FMC Corporation) has been recommended for the treatment of both animals and facilities (Tarshis 1962), but its effectiveness is questionable since several treatments are sometimes necessary.

The use of resin strips impregnated with an aerial insecticide, DDVP (Vapona, Shell), has been effective in some animal quarters, and no toxic side effects have been reported (H. Gunderson, personal communication).

Treatment of the allergic dermatitis caused by fleas consists primarily of freeing the host of the parasites (Kissileff 1962; Muller 1961). Other recommended measures include administration of corticosteroids, inoculation with flea antigen, application of topical agents for moist dermatitis, and bathing with medicated shampoos.

PUBLIC HEALTH CONSIDERATIONS

Ctenocephalides felis and *C. canis* are commonly associated with man, and in some areas of the world they replace the human flea, *Pulex irritans*. Local irritation, pruritus, and allergic responses to the bite of these parasites have been frequently reported in man (Cherney, Wheeler, and Reed 1939; Hartman 1946; Hudson, Feingold, and Kartman 1960), but not all individuals are sensitive. The usual reaction consists of a wheal, followed by induration or papule formation, which reaches maximum development in 12 to 24 hours. These fleas are not significant in the transmission of human pathogens (Pollitzer 1954). *Ctenocephalides felis* and *C. canis* can be infected with *Yersinia pestis* when fed on an infected host in the laboratory, but their vector capacity for this pathogen in nature is considered to be negligible. *Ctenocephalides canis* is an intermediate host of the tapeworm *Hymenolepis diminuta* (Simmons and Hayes 1948). Man is occasionally infected by ingestion of the flea (Yunker 1964).

Spilopsyllus cuniculi
(European Rabbit Flea)

Spilopsyllus cuniculi is commonly found on the wild hare and rabbit in Europe, particularly during the late winter and early spring (Allan and Shanks 1955), and rarely on the dog and cat (Hopkins and Rothschild 1953; Page 1952). It does not occur on lagomorphs raised in the laboratory but could be introduced on specimens obtained from their natural habitat. However, infestations in the laboratory would not be expected to persist because of the parasite's peculiar reproductive requirements.

MORPHOLOGY

Adults are dark brown. Females are about 1 mm long; males are slightly smaller. Distinguishing characteristics include a pronounced angle in the frons and the presence of genal and pronotal combs (Fig. 11.3).

LIFE CYCLE

The reproductive cycle is complicated and is intimately involved with the corticosteroid level of the host's blood (Rothschild 1960, 1965; Rothschild and Ford 1966). Eggs are deposited only after the adult female has fed on a newborn lagomorph.

PATHOLOGIC EFFECTS

Spilopsyllus cuniculi usually congregates on the ears of the host. Because of this tendency to concentrate in large numbers in a relatively restricted area, it has the potential to inflict considerable tissue damage. The irritation caused by its feeding on the ears of a rabbit has been described (Rothschild 1965). This flea is a known vector of *Trypanosoma nabiasi* (Grewal 1956) and of the virus of myxomatosis (Allan and Shanks 1955) but has not been associated with the transmission of other pathogens.

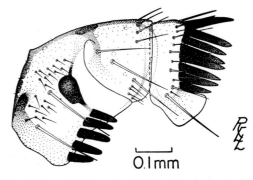

0.1 mm

FIG. 11.3. Head of *Spilopsyllus cuniculi*. (Courtesy of R. E. Lewis, Iowa State University.)

DIAGNOSIS

Diagnosis is made by identifying the parasite on the host.

CONTROL

The isolation, examination, and routine treatment of all animals brought into the laboratory from their natural habitat will prevent the introduction of this parasite into a laboratory colony. The specific topical treatments effective against *Ctenocephalides felis* and *C. canis* should be effective against *S. cuniculi*. A technique used to treat fleas in wild rats should be readily adaptable to wild rabbits and hares. Newly acquired specimens are placed for approximately 2 hours in an enclosed container with a resin strip impregnated with DDVP (Vapona, Shell) (D. R. Maddock, personal communication).

If an animal facility should become infested, the sanitation and disinfection procedures recommended for the control of the cat and dog fleas should be effective for the control of this flea.

PUBLIC HEALTH CONSIDERATIONS

Spilopsyllus cuniculi is of no known public health importance.

Xenopsylla cheopis

(Oriental or Indian Rat Flea)

Xenopsylla cheopis occurs on the Norway rat, black rat, house mouse, and other wild rodents (Hopkins and Rothschild 1953). Although its origin was probably North Africa or India, it is now found throughout the world. It occurs on a high percentage of wild rodents in urban areas in the United States, particularly in the Midwest and port cities (Heston 1941; Yunker 1964). Although it is not usually found on rodents raised in the laboratory, it can be introduced on rodents obtained from their natural habitat. It became well established in at least one laboratory mouse colony in the United States (Yunker 1964).

MORPHOLOGY

Xenopsylla cheopis adults are similar in size to those of *Ctenocephalides felis* and *C. canis* but are light amber in color and lack both genal and pronotal combs (Fig. 11.4).

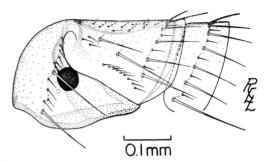

FIG. 11.4. Head of *Xenopsylla cheopis*. (Courtesy of R. E. Lewis, Iowa State University.)

LIFE CYCLE

The life cycle is similar to that of *C. canis* and *C. felis* except that the larval stages are usually limited to the nest or burrow of the host.

PATHOLOGIC EFFECTS

The pathologic effects of *X. cheopis* on its natural hosts have not been reported. It is a probable vector of *Trypanosoma lewisi* and is an intermediate host for the tapeworms *Hymenolepis diminuta* and *H. nana*.

DIAGNOSIS

Diagnosis is made by identifying the parasite on the host.

CONTROL

The inspection, isolation, and routine treatment of all newly acquired animals and the sanitation and disinfection procedures recommended for the control of *Ctenocephalides felis*, *C. canis*, and *Spilopsyllus cuniculi* should effectively control this flea.

PUBLIC HEALTH CONSIDERATIONS

Man is occasionally infected with the tapeworms *H. diminuta* and *H. nana* by ingestion of this flea (Simmons and Hayes 1948; Yunker 1964). *Xenopsylla cheopis* is also frequently associated with the transmission of *Yersinia pestis* (the cause of plague) in tropical and semitropical areas. The bite of this flea is extremely irritating to man and produces a reaction similar to that caused by the bite of the dog or cat flea.

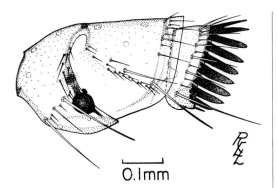

0.1mm

FIG. 11.5. Head of *Nosopsyllus fasciatus.* (Courtesy of R. E. Lewis, Iowa State University.)

Nosopsyllus fasciatus

(Northern Rat Flea)

Nosopsyllus fasciatus occurs on various species of wild rats and mice, including the Norway rat, black rat, and house mouse throughout the world (Lewis 1967). It is the flea most frequently found on wild rats in Europe, and it is common on wild rodents from urban areas in the United States (Heston 1941; Yunker 1964). Although it has not been reported from rodents raised in the laboratory, it could be introduced on rats and mice obtained from their natural environment.

MORPHOLOGY

This species is 1.5 mm to 2.5 mm long and rich amber in color. It is distinguished from other fleas by the absence of a genal comb, by the presence of a pronotal comb, and by the number of teeth in the pronotal comb (Fig. 11.5).

LIFE CYCLE

The life cycle is similar to that of *Ctenocephalides* except that the larval stages are usually limited to the nest or burrow. Adults are most plentiful during the cooler months of the year.

PATHOLOGIC EFFECTS

Nothing is known of the pathologic effects of *N. fasciatus* on its natural hosts. It is a vector of *Trypanosoma lewisi* and *T. duttoni* and an intermediate host for the tapeworms *Hymenolepis diminuta* and *H. nana.*

DIAGNOSIS

Diagnosis is made by identifying the parasite on the host.

CONTROL

The inspection, isolation, and routine treatment of all newly acquired animals and the sanitation and disinfection procedures recommended for the control of *Ctenocephalides felis, C. canis,* and *Spilopsyllus cuniculi* should be effective for the control of this flea.

PUBLIC HEALTH CONSIDERATIONS

Because this flea is an intermediate host for the tapeworms *H. diminuta* and *H. nana,* it is a potential hazard for man (Simmons and Hayes 1948; Yunker 1964). It is also an important vector of the agents of plague *(Yersinia pestis)* and typhus *(Rickettsia).* The bite of this flea is irritating to man and causes a reaction similar to that caused by the bites of the oriental rat flea and the dog and cat fleas.

Leptopsylla segnis

(Mouse Flea)

Leptopsylla segnis is a common parasite of the house mouse throughout the world (Smit 1957). It also frequently occurs on the Norway rat and the European field mouse. It has been found on a high percentage of wild rodents in Europe and in urban areas of the United States (Heston 1941; Yunker 1964). Although it has not been reported from rodents raised in the laboratory, it could be introduced on mice or rats obtained from their natural environment.

MORPHOLOGY

This species is small, 1 to 2 mm long, and is distinguished by a pair of spiniform bristles on each side of the frons and by four blunt teeth in the genal comb (Fig. 11.6).

LIFE CYCLE

The life cycle is similar to that of *Ctenocephalides* except that the larval stages are usually limited to the nest or burrow.

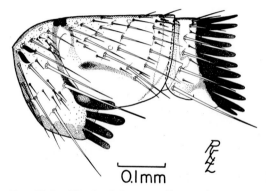

FIG. 11.6. Head of *Leptopsylla segnis*. (Courtesy of R. E. Lewis, Iowa State University.)

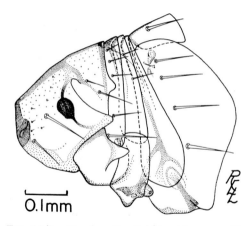

FIG. 11.7. Head of *Echidnophaga gallinacea*. (Courtesy of R. E. Lewis, Iowa State University.)

PATHOLOGIC EFFECTS

The pathologic effects of this flea on its
natural host are unknown. It is an intermediate host for the tapeworms *Hymenolepis diminuta* and *H. nana.*

DIAGNOSIS

Diagnosis is made by identifying the
parasite on the host.

CONTROL

The inspection, isolation, and routine
treatment of all newly acquired animals
and the sanitation and disinfection procedures recommended for the control of
Ctenocephalides felis, C. canis, and *Spilopsyllus cuniculi* should be effective for the
control of this flea.

PUBLIC HEALTH CONSIDERATIONS

This flea is an intermediate host for the
tapeworms *H. diminuta* and *H. nana;* consequently, it is a potential hazard for man
(Simmons and Hayes 1948; Yunker 1964).
Leptopsylla segnis is also capable of transmitting the agent of typhus (*Rickettsia*).

Echidnophaga gallinacea

(Chicken Flea, Sticktight Flea)

Echidnophaga gallinacea is a common
parasite of the chicken (Benbrook 1965). It
causes irritation, anemia, and sometimes
death, especially in young chickens. This
flea also affects other birds and occasionally
the dog, cat, rabbit, rat, mouse, numerous
other feral and domestic species, and man
(Benbrook 1965; da Costa Lima and Hatha-

way 1946). It occurs throughout the world
but is commoner in warmer climates (Hopkins and Rothschild 1953). Although it has
not been reported from laboratory colonies,
it could be introduced into a research facility on newly acquired chickens or on infected wild birds or rodents.

MORPHOLOGY

This is one of the smaller fleas, both
sexes being 1.5 mm or less in length. The
thoracic terga are small and collectively
shorter than the first abdominal tergite. The
coxae of the metathoracic legs bear
patches of spiniform bristles on the inner
surfaces, and there are spiracles on the second and third abdominal segments. The
distinguishing characteristics of the head
are shown in Figure 11.7. Neither genal
nor pronotal combs are present. The stylets
of the maxillae and epipharynx are broad,
knifelike, and equipped with several teeth
which provide firm anchorage in the tissue
of the host.

LIFE CYCLE

Females usually attach permanently to
the body; males attach less firmly (Parman
1923). Mating occurs on the host while the
female is attached and presumably feeding
(Suter 1965). One to four eggs are deposited per day, and the incubation period
is 6 to 8 days at 25 C (Parman 1923). The
larvae feed shortly after emergence, primarily on the excreta of adult fleas. After

larval development, which takes 14 to 31 days, third instar larvae spin silken cocoons. Dust and organic material adhere to the cocoons, which are frequently attached to firm objects. The pupal period ranges from 9 to 19 days. Adults are inactive for the first few days after emerging from the pupal stage and do not attach to a host for 5 to 8 days.

Infection occurs when a host enters an infested area. Direct transmission is not common because the female flea anchors itself firmly to the host and remains attached during most of its life.

PATHOLOGIC EFFECTS

Adults of *E. gallinacea* congregate in large numbers on the comb, wattles, and around the eyes of chickens, and on the lips and ears of mammals (Lapage 1962; Renaux 1964). The mouthparts of feeding females are deeply embedded in the skin and cause severe irritation, local edema, and sometimes ulcers (Lapage 1962; R. E. Lewis, unpublished data). The stylets often remain in the dermis if the fleas are forcibly removed. In the chicken, heavy infections cause anemia, decreased egg production, and sometimes death (Benbrook 1965; Lapage 1962).

This flea is not reported to transmit any pathogens, but experimental evidence indicates it is a potential vector of infectious disease agents (Benbrook 1965).

DIAGNOSIS

Diagnosis is based on clinical signs and by identifying the parasite on the host.

CONTROL

The inspection and isolation of newly acquired animals and the sanitation, individual treatments, and disinfection procedures recommended for the control of the cat and dog fleas are effective for this flea. Hanging resin strips impregnated with an aerial insecticide, DDVP (Vapona, Shell), in a chicken room will quickly eliminate any adult fleas accidentally introduced with new animals.

PUBLIC HEALTH CONSIDERATIONS

Echidnophaga gallinacea is capable of transmitting the causative agents of plague (*Yersinia pestis*) and typhus (*Rickettsia*),

and it has been found to harbor *Salmonella typhimurium* (Benbrook 1965; Yunker 1964).

Ceratophyllus gallinae

(European Chicken Flea)

Ceratophyllus gallinae is a common, extremely irritating parasite of the chicken (Lapage 1962). It also affects other birds and occasionally the rat, wild rodents, the dog, and man (Benbrook 1965; da Costa Lima and Hathaway 1946). It is found throughout the world. Although there are no reports of its occurrence in laboratory colonies, it could be introduced into a research facility on newly acquired chickens or on infected wild birds and rodents.

MORPHOLOGY

Adults are dark brown, 2 mm long, and distinguished from the other species described in this chapter by the absence of a genal comb, the presence of a pronotal comb, and the number of teeth in the pronotal comb (Fig. 11.8).

LIFE CYCLE

The life cycle is similar to that of *Ctenocephalides*. Unlike *Echidnophaga gallinacea*, this flea is not sedentary and does not firmly attach to the host. Developmental stages occur in the nest of the host, and populations of adults sometimes build up to enormous numbers. Transmission occurs by direct contact or when a host enters an infected area.

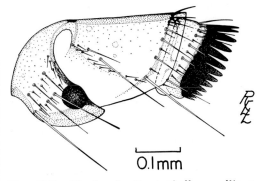

FIG. 11.8. Head of *Ceratophyllus gallinae*. (Courtesy of R. E. Lewis, Iowa State University.)

PATHOLOGIC EFFECTS

The pathologic effects of this flea are similar to those of *E. gallinacea* (Benbrook 1965).

DIAGNOSIS

Diagnosis is made by identifying the parasite on the host or in its bedding.

CONTROL

Because adults are found on the host only when feeding, eradication is greatly simplified and depends almost exclusively on sanitation. The inspection and isolation of newly acquired animals, the sanitation and disinfection procedures recommended for the control of the cat and dog fleas, and the use of DDVP recommended for the control of *E. gallinacea* are effective for the control of this flea.

PUBLIC HEALTH CONSIDERATIONS

Ceratophyllus gallinae readily bites man but little skin reaction results (R. E. Lewis, unpublished data). Otherwise, it is of no known public health importance.

Tunga penetrans

(Jigger or Chigoe)

Tunga penetrans embeds its mouthparts in the skin and causes severe irritation (Fiennes 1967). It attacks a wide variety of hosts, especially man and the pig in tropical and semitropical areas of the Western Hemisphere and Africa (Hopkins and Rothschild 1953; Matheson 1950; Tipton and Méndez 1966). Laboratory guenons and baboons obtained from their natural environment are frequently infected (Fiennes 1967).

MORPHOLOGY

The male is very small, 0.5 mm long, and brown, and never embeds in the host. The female is larger than the male, 1.0 mm long, and is also brown. The thorax is short, the three thoracic terga collectively being shorter than the first abdominal tergite. The metathoracic coxae lack patches of spiniform bristles, and females lack spiracles on the second and third abdominal segments. The head has an acute frontal angle and lacks both a genal ctenidium and large setae (Fig. 11.9).

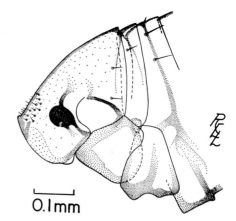

FIG. 11.9. Head of *Tunga penetrans*. (Courtesy of R. E. Lewis, Iowa State University.)

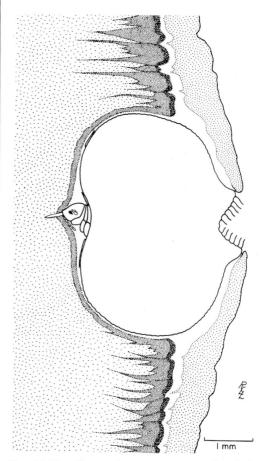

FIG. 11.10. *Tunga penetrans*, encapsulated female. (Courtesy of R. E. Lewis, Iowa State University.)

LIFE CYCLE

The life cycle is similar to that of *Echidnophaga gallinacea* (Suter 1965). Females become firmly attached to the host. The dermis of the host proliferates and encapsulates the entire body of the flea, except for the terminal abdominal segments which protrude through a small pore (Fig. 11.10). Copulation occurs after encapsulation. The female increases in size to about 5 to 7 mm. Eggs are expelled through the dermal pore, drop to the ground, and under proper conditions of temperature and humidity, hatch in a few days. Larvae apparently feed on the feces of the adults. The entire life cycle requires about 17 days (Hicks 1930).

PATHOLOGIC EFFECTS

The implanted females cause intense local irritation and pruritus. In guenons and baboons, *T. penetrans* often invades the hard skin pads on the buttocks, and secondary infection is common (Fiennes 1967).

DIAGNOSIS

Diagnosis is based on identifying the parasite in the dermal lesions.

CONTROL

Tunga penetrans is a problem only in primates obtained from their natural habitat. Once infected, the only satisfactory treatment appears to be the surgical removal of the parasite and sterilization of the wound (Fiennes 1967).

PUBLIC HEALTH CONSIDERATIONS

Man is often affected in endemic areas (Matheson 1950). Heavy infections cause debilitation and severe mutilation, usually of the feet.

TABLE 11.1.　Fleas affecting endothermal laboratory animals

Parasite	Geographic Distribution	Endothermal Host	Usual Habitat	Incidence		Pathologic Effects	Public Health Importance	Reference
				In nature	In laboratory			
Ctenocephalides felis*	Worldwide	Cat, dog, wild carnivores; occasionally mouse, rat, wild rodents, baboons, chicken, man	Pelage, plumage, bedding	Common	Common	Restlessness, irritation, allergic dermatitis, pruritus, ruffled coat, self-induced trauma, weight loss; intermediate host for Dipylidium caninum	Causes irritation, allergic dermatitis; vector of Hymenolepis diminuta	Blakemore 1966 Goyings 1961 Hopkins and Rothschild 1953 Král and Schwartzman 1964 Muller 1961, 1966 Myers and Kuntz 1965 Renaux 1964
Ctenocephalides canis*	Worldwide	Dog, wild carnivores, man	Pelage, bedding	Common	Uncommon	Restlessness, irritation, allergic dermatitis, pruritus, ruffled coat, self-induced trauma, weight loss; intermediate host for Dipylidium caninum	Causes irritation, allergic dermatitis; vector of Hymenolepis diminuta	Blakemore 1966 Goyings 1961 Hopkins and Rothschild 1953 Král and Schwartzman 1964 Muller 1961, 1966 Renaux 1964
Spilopsyllus cuniculi*	Europe	Rabbit, hares, dog, cat	Pelage, bedding	Common on rabbit, wild hare; rare on dog, cat	Rare	Dermal irritation, self-induced trauma, especially of ears; vector of myxomatosis virus; vector of Trypanosoma nabiasi	Unknown	Allan and Shanks 1955 Hopkins and Rothschild 1953 Page 1952 Rothschild 1960, 1965 Rothschild and Ford 1966
Xenopsylla cheopis*	Worldwide	Mouse, rat, black rat, wild rodents, man	Pelage, bedding	Common	Uncommon	Intermediate host for Hymenolepis diminuta, H. nana; probable vector of Trypanosoma lewisi	Causes irritation, allergic dermatitis; vector of Hymenolepis diminuta, H. nana, agent of plague	Heston 1941 Hopkins and Rothschild 1953 Simmons and Hayes 1948 Yunker 1964

*Discussed in text.

TABLE 11.1. (continued)

Parasite	Geographic Distribution	Endothermal Host	Usual Habitat	Incidence In nature	Incidence In laboratory	Pathologic Effects	Public Health Importance	Reference
Nosopsyllus fasciatus*	Worldwide	Mouse, rat, black rat, wild rodents, man	Pelage, bedding	Common	Rare	Intermediate host for Hymenolepis diminuta, H. nana; vector of Trypanosoma lewisi, T. duttoni	Causes irritation, allergic dermatitis; vector of Hymenolepis diminuta, H. nana, agent of plague, agent of typhus	Heston 1941 Lewis 1967 Simmons and Hayes 1948 Yunker 1964
Nosopsyllus londiniensis	Worldwide	Mouse, rat, black rat	Pelage, bedding	Rare	Rare	Unknown	Unknown	Lewis 1967
Leptopsylla segnis*	Worldwide	Rat, European field mouse	Pelage, bedding	Common	Rare	Intermediate host for Hymenolepis diminuta, H. nana	Vector of Hymenolepis diminuta, H. nana, agent of typhus	Heston 1941 Simmons and Hayes 1948 Smit 1957 Yunker 1964
Echidnophaga gallinacea*	Worldwide	Chicken, other birds; occasionally mouse, rat, rabbit, dog, cat, man	Skin of host; usually on head	Common	Rare	Irritation, local edema, dermal ulcer; anemia; sometimes death in chicken	Capable of transmitting agents of plague, typhus; harbors Salmonella typhimurium	Benbrook 1965 Hopkins and Rothschild 1953 Lapage 1962 Renaux 1964 Yunker 1964
Ceratophyllus gallinae*	Worldwide	Chicken, other birds; occasionally rat, wild rodents, dog, man	Bedding, plumage, pelage	Common	Rare	Irritation, local edema, dermal ulcer	Bites man, causes little reaction	Benbrook 1965 da Costa Lima and Hathaway 1946 Lapage 1962
Ceratophyllus niger	Western North America	Chicken, other birds; occasionally mouse, rat, man	Bedding	Uncommon	Unknown	Unknown	Unknown	Benbrook 1965
Tunga penetrans*	Tropical areas of Western Hemisphere and Africa	Guenons, baboons, pig, man	Imbedded in skin of host, usually in buttocks of laboratory primates	Common in endemic areas	Rare	Intense local irritation, pruritus, cysts in skin	Causes intense local irritation, pruritus, cysts in skin; mutilation of feet, debilitation	Fiennes 1967 Hopkins and Rothschild 1953 Matheson 1950 Tipton and Mendez 1966
Pulex irritans	Worldwide	Man; occasionally rat, rabbit, dog, cat, guenons, pig	Skin, pelage	Common in some areas	Rare	Intermediate host for Dipylidium caninum	Causes irritation; vector of agent of plague	Hopkins and Rothschild 1953 Yunker 1964

*Discussed in text.

REFERENCES

Allan, R. M., and P. L. Shanks. 1955. Rabbit fleas on wild rabbits and the transmission of myxomatosis. Nature 175:692.

Bacot, A. 1914. A study of the bionomics of the common rat fleas and other species associated with human habitations, with special reference to the influence of temperature and humidity at various periods of the life history of the insect. J. Hyg. (Plague Supp. III), Cambridge. 1913–1914: 447–654.

Benbrook, E. A. 1965. External parasites of poultry, pp. 925–64. In H. E. Biester and L. H. Schwarte, eds. Diseases of poultry. 5th ed. Iowa State Univ. Press, Ames.

Blakemore, J. C. 1966. Macroscopic ectoparasites, pp. 147–48. In R. W. Kirk, ed. Current veterinary therapy 1966–1967: Small animal practice. W. B. Saunders, Philadelphia.

Burch, G. R. 1960. Preliminary studies with ectoral for control of ectoparasites in small animals. Allied Vet. 31:69–72.

Burch, G. R., and D. C. Brinkman. 1962. Systemic insecticide therapy in small animals. Small Animal Clinician 2:21–27.

Cherney, L. S., C. M. Wheeler, and A. C. Reed. 1939. Flea-antigen in prevention of flea bites. Am. J. Trop. Med. 19:327–32.

Costa Lima, A. da, and C. R. Hathaway. 1946. Pulgas. Bibliografia, catálogo e animais por elas sugados. Monographias Inst. Oswaldo Cruz, (4), Dec. 522 pp.

Eppley, J. R., W. H. Hepperle, J. C. Trace, F. N. Hughes, and H. W. Larson. 1963. Controlled evaluation of systemic insecticides in the dog. Small Animal Clinician 3:394–98.

Faust, E. C., and P. F. Russel. 1957. Craig and Faust's clinical parasitology. 6th ed. Lea and Febiger, Philadelphia. 1078 pp.

Fiennes, R. 1967. Zoonoses of primates: The epidemiology and ecology of simian diseases in relation to man. Weidenfeld and Nicolson, London. 190 pp.

Goyings, L. S. 1961. Flea bite dermatitis. Mich. State Univ. Vet. 22:16–23.

Grewal, M. S. 1956. Life cycle of the rabbit trypanosome, Trypanosoma nabiasi Railliet, 1895. Trans. Roy. Soc. Trop. Med. Hyg. 50:2–3.

Hartman, M. M. 1946. Fleabite reactions: Clinical and experimental observations and effect of histamine-azoprotein therapy. Ann. Allergy 4:131–36.

Heston, W. E. 1941. Parasites, pp. 349–79. In G. D. Snell, ed. Biology of the laboratory mouse. Blakiston, Philadelphia.

Hicks, E. P. 1930. The early stages of the jigger, Tunga penetrans. Ann. Trop. Med. Parasitol. 24:575–86.

Holland, G. P. 1949. The Siphonaptera of Canada. Can. Dept. Agr. Publ. 817. Tech. Bull. 70. 306 pp.

Hopkins, G. H. E., and Miriam Rothschild. 1953. An illustrated catalogue of the Rothschild collection of fleas (Siphonaptera) in the British Museum (Nat. History): Vol. I. Tungidae and Pulicidae. British Museum (Nat. History), London. 361 pp.

Hudson, B. W., B. F. Feingold, and L. Kartman. 1960. Allergy to flea bites: II. Investigations of flea bite sensitivity in humans. Exp. Parasitol. 9:264–70.

Johnson, R. M., A. C. Andersen, and W. Gee. 1963. Parasitism in an established dog kennel. Lab. Animal Care 13:731–36.

Johnston, R. V., and T. L. Kerley. 1962. Ectoral as a systemic insecticide. Allied Vet. 33:67–72.

Kissileff, A. 1962. Relationship of dog fleas to dermatitis. Small Animal Clinician 2:132–35.

Král, F., and R. M. Schwartzman. 1964. Veterinary and comparative dermatology. J. B. Lippincott, Philadelphia. 444 pp.

Lapage, G. 1962. Mönnig's veterinary helminthology and entomology. 5th ed. Williams and Wilkins, Baltimore. 600 pp.

Lewis, R. E. 1967. Contributions to a taxonomic revision of the genus Nosopsyllus Jordan, 1933 (Siphonaptera: Ceratophyllidae): I. African species. J. Med. Entomol. 4:123–42.

Matheson, R. 1950. Medical entomology. 2d ed. Comstock, Ithaca, N.Y. 612 pp.

Morris, M. L. 1963. Breeding, housing, and management of cats. Cornell Vet. 53:107–31.

Muller, G. H. 1961. Flea allergy dermatitis. Small Animal Clinician 1:185–92.

———. 1966. Flea allergy dermatitis, pp. 125–28. In R. W. Kirk, ed. Current veterinary therapy 1966–1967: Small animal practice. W. B. Saunders, Philadelphia.

Myers, Betty J., and R. E. Kuntz. 1965. A checklist of parasites reported for the baboon. Primates 6:137–94.

Page, K. W. 1952. The ectoparasites of laboratory and domestic animals. J. Animal Tech. Assoc. 3:34–36.

Parman, D. C. 1923. Biological notes on the hen flea, Echidnophaga gallinacea. J. Agr. Res. 23:1007–9.

Pollitzer, R. 1954. Plague. World Health Organ. Monograph Ser. 22. 698 pp.

Renaux, E. A. 1964. Metazoal and protozoal diseases, pp. 121–40. In E. J. Catcott, ed.

Feline medicine and surgery. American Veterinary Publications, Santa Barbara, Calif.

Rothschild, Miriam. 1960. Observations and speculations concerning the flea vector of myxomatosis in Britain. Entomol. Month. Mag. 96:106–9.

———. 1965. The rabbit flea and hormones. Endeavour 24: 162–68.

Rothschild, Miriam, and B. Ford. 1966. Hormones of the vertebrate host controlling ovarian regression and copulation of the rabbit flea. Nature 211: 261–66.

Sasa, M., H. Tanaka, M. Fukui, and A. Takata. 1962. Internal parasites of laboratory animals, pp. 195–214. In R. J. C. Harris, ed. The problems of laboratory animal disease. Academic Press, New York.

Simmons, S. W., and W. J. Hayes, Jr. 1948. Fleas and disease. Proc. 4th Intern. Congr. Trop. Med. Malaria 2:1678–89.

Smit, F. G. A. M. 1957. Siphonaptera, pp. 1–94. In Handbooks for the identification of British insects. Vol. 1, Part 16. Roy. Entomol. Soc., London.

Suter, P. 1965. Life cycle of *Echidnophaga gallinacea*. Proc. 12th Intern. Congr. Entomol., London. 1964:830–31.

Tarshis, I. B. 1962. The use of silica aerogel compounds for the control of ectoparasites. Proc. Animal Care Panel 12:217–58.

Tipton, V. J., and E. Méndez. 1966. The fleas (Siphonaptera) of Panama, pp. 289–338. In R. L. Wenzel and V. J. Tipton, eds. The ectoparasites of Panama. Field Museum Nat. History, Chicago.

Walton, G. S. 1968. Skin diseases of domestic animals: I. Skin manifestations of allergic response in domestic animals. Vet. Record 82:204–7.

Wilson, H. G., J. C. Keller, and C. N. Smith. 1957. Control of fleas in yards. J. Econ. Entomol. 50:365–66.

Wood, J. C. 1968. III. The parasitic aspect of skin diseases. Vet. Record 82:214–23.

Yunker, C. E. 1964. Infections of laboratory animals potentially dangerous to man: Ectoparasites and other arthropods, with emphasis on mites. Lab. Animal Care 14:455–65.

Chapter 12

FLIES

Although several flies (Diptera) cause disease in endothermal animals, few are important pathogens for laboratory species. Parasitism caused by flies is highly varied and characteristically temporary. Continued parasitism of endothermal laboratory animals by such insects requires repeated contacts or invasions from outside the laboratory. Laboratory mammals or birds maintained in outdoor facilities or obtained from a wild habitat are more likely to be affected. Flies that affect endothermal laboratory animals are listed in Table 12.1. The most important are discussed below.

CUTEREBRIDS

Members of the family Cuterebridae produce primary dermal myiasis in endothermal animals. The most important genera are *Cuterebra,* which includes the rodent and rabbit botflies of the Western Hemisphere, and *Dermatobia,* which contains but one species, *D. hominis,* which affects a wide variety of endothermal hosts in tropical America.

Cuterebra
(Rodent Botflies)

This genus contains more than 40 species, all of which occur in the Western Hemisphere (Guimarães 1967; Stone et al. 1965). Most species show a high degree of host specificity (Catts 1965; Penner and Pocius 1956; Radovsky and Catts 1960). Often they are also specific as to site of larval development on their host (Catts 1965).

Cuterebra larvae produce dermal cysts in many endothermal laboratory animals (Hall 1921; Hatziolos 1967; Knipling and Bruce 1937; Maurer and Skaley 1968; Rothenbacher, Mugera, and Tufts 1964). Wild rodents, lagomorphs, and primates native to the Western Hemisphere are natural hosts; Old World rodents and hares and the dog, cat, and man are sometimes infected accidentally. Common North American species include *C. angustifrons, C. approximata, C. fontinella, C. grisea, C. latifrons,* and *C. tenebrosa,* which affect deer mice, wood rats, and related wild rodents; *C. emasculator,* which affects squirrels; and *C. cuniculi, C. horripilum, C. jellisoni, C. lepivora, C. princeps,* and *C. ruficrus,* which affect the cottontail rabbit and hares. Susceptibility of accidental hosts does not conclude their suitability as hosts in that only partial larval development sometimes occurs (Catts 1965). *Cuterebra* adults are not parasitic.

In temperate regions, the larval incidence is greatest during the summer and fall (Bennett 1955; Haas and Dicke 1958; Miller and Getz 1969). The maggots are common in rodents obtained from their natural habitats, with incidences as high as 74% reported in deer mice (Dunaway et al. 1967; Goertz 1966; Miller and Getz 1969).

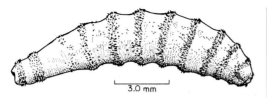

FIG. 12.1. *Cuterebra,* second-stage larva. (Courtesy of E. P. Catts, University of Delaware.)

Cuterebra larvae are uncommon in the cat and rare in the dog (Hall 1921; Hatziolos 1967). They are likely to be found only in laboratory dogs and cats previously allowed to roam free; they do not occur in dogs and cats reared in facilities with effective fly control.

MORPHOLOGY

Adults look superficially like bumblebees. They are large, 15 to 30 mm long, robust, hairy flies with uniformly dark wings (Curran 1934). Many species have conspicuous white markings or pile that contrasts with an overall black or blue-black coloration. Eggs are yellow and 1 mm long; the first-stage infective larva is minute and spindle shaped. The second stage (Fig. 12.1) is 5 to 20 mm long, and the third and final larval stage (Fig. 12.2) is dark brown and reaches 30 mm in length.

LIFE CYCLE

Gravid females often enter buildings through ground level openings and deposit their eggs either singly or in broken rows near a host, but not on the host itself (Catts 1967). The eggs hatch in 1 to 2 weeks under temperate conditions, about 25 C. Infective larvae generally enter the host through the nares and mouth (Catts 1967),

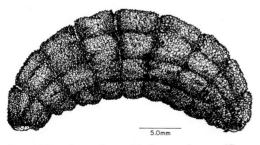

FIG. 12.2. *Cuterebra,* third-stage larva. (Courtesy of E. P. Catts, University of Delaware.)

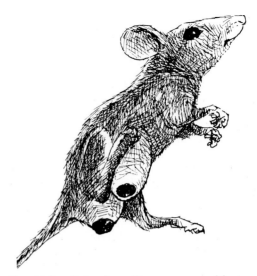

FIG. 12.3. *Cuterebra.* Deer mouse with two larval cysts or "warbles." (Courtesy of E. P. Catts, University of Delaware.)

although there is evidence that one species can penetrate intact skin (Penner 1958). The larvae apparently migrate through connective tissue and, after about 1 week, appear in the subcutaneous tissue. A small opening in the skin is produced at the posterior end of the larva for breathing and excretion. In the next 2 to 3 weeks, the larva molts and grows rapidly. This induces a large subcutaneous cyst, or "warble," to develop (Fig. 12.3). When fully grown, the third-stage larva enlarges the warble pore, backs out of the cyst, drops to the bedding, cage floor, or ground, and pupates. The total period of larval development lasts 3 to 5 weeks (Catts 1967). Pupal development takes longer, sometimes 4 to 6 months, if interrupted by winter diapause. Adult flies will not mate in a building, so continuing laboratory infestation is not likely.

PATHOLOGIC EFFECTS

There are usually one to three larvae per host (Dunaway et al. 1967). In native hosts they produce little lasting pathology. Chronic inflammation occurs around the cyst, but healing is usually rapid once the larva emerges (Catts 1965; Payne and Cosgrove 1966). Secondary infection is uncommon. Anemia, reduced hemoglobin, leucocytosis, and splenomegaly have been observed (Dunaway et al. 1967; Payne and Cosgrove 1966; Payne et al. 1965). It has been suggested that the location of larvae in inguinal and scrotal regions of male hosts results in emasculation and infertility (Dalmat 1943), but evidence of anything but physical displacement of the testes is lacking (Miller and Getz 1969; Wecker 1962). Death of the host sometimes occurs about 1 week after infection, the time the infective larvae reach the site of warble development, or when the mature larva emerges (Catts 1965). The exact cause of death is not known.

In nonnative hosts, such as the laboratory mouse, rat, rabbit, dog, and cat, the pathologic effects of *Cuterebra* are more severe (Catts 1965; Dalmat 1943). Extensive inflammation, secondary infection, and protracted healing of cysts are common (Dalmat 1943), and larval migration and development tend to be erratic (Catts 1965). Larval infection of the brain of such hosts has been reported (Hatziolos 1966, 1967).

DIAGNOSIS

Diagnosis is based on recovery of characteristic larvae from dermal cysts. Generally, there is only one maggot per cyst (Catts 1967). Accurate species identification cannot be made from larval morphology.

CONTROL

Rodent botfly infection is treated by surgically removing larvae from the dermal cysts, flushing the cyst cavity with saline or an antiseptic solution, and applying an antibiotic powder or ointment (Blakemore 1968; Conroy 1964; Hooper 1961). Control is achieved by insectproofing animal buildings. Screening of individual cages is not advised, as eggs can be deposited nearby, and larvae can infect the animals through the screen.

In temperate areas, hosts obtained from their natural habitat should be captured during midwinter, the time of lowest incidence. In warmer climates, such hosts can be isolated for 3 weeks to allow larvae to develop and to be removed.

PUBLIC HEALTH CONSIDERATIONS

Cuterebra infection has been reported in man, but it is rare (James 1947; Scott 1963). Infected laboratory animals are not a direct hazard to man.

Dermatobia hominis
(Torsalo; Human Botfly)

Dermatobia hominis is common in certain areas of Mexico and Central and South America (Guimarães and Papavero 1966). Its larvae cause dermal cysts in wild rodents, the dog, cat, monkeys, domestic animals, some birds, and man (Lapage 1968). The maggots are likely to be encountered only in laboratory rodents and monkeys obtained from their natural habitat and in dogs and cats obtained from pounds in endemic areas.

MORPHOLOGY

Adults are about 12 mm long and have a gray and metallic blue body and an orange face (James 1947). Maturing larvae are narrowed anteriorly into a characteristic bottle shape (Fig. 12.4). They are a light cream color and possess narrow belts of sparsely set spines (James 1947).

LIFE CYCLE

The life cycle is similar to that of *Cuterebra* (Guimarães and Papavero 1966), except that it probably can be completed indoors (Banegas and Mourier 1967). In nature, *D. hominis* sometimes attaches eggs to mosquitoes and other zoophilic arthropods, which then serve as vectors (Bates 1949; Matéus 1967).

PATHOLOGIC EFFECTS

The larvae produce dermal cysts, usually without marked site specificity (Guimarães and Papavero 1966); however,

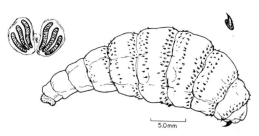

FIG. 12.4. *Dermatobia hominis,* third-stage larva. *(Insets)* Posterior spiracles *(left)* and typical spine *(right)*. (Courtesy of E. P. Catts, University of Delaware.)

in the dog and cat the cysts usually occur on the back (Král and Schwartzman 1964).

Diagnosis is based on demonstration of the parasite in a typical dermal cyst.

Treatment consists of the surgical removal of the larvae as described for *Cuterebra* or the topical application of a 1% aqueous solution of trichlorfon (Brass 1964). Effective controls include the insect-proofing of buildings and the isolation of recently captured animals.

Dermatobia hominis affects man; however, infected laboratory animals are not a direct human health hazard.

OESTRIDS

The family Oestridae includes a large group of botflies that cause either nasal or dermal myiasis in a wide variety of hosts (cattle, elephants, camels, deer, and rodents). Those of the genus *Oestromyia* attack wild rodents sometimes used as laboratory animals (Zumpt 1965). Only *Oestromyia leporina* is common.

Oestromyia leporina

(Old World Rodent Botfly)

Larvae of *Oestromyia leporina* are common dermal, cyst-producing parasites of voles and the muskrat in Europe and of pikas *(Ochotona)* in Asia. They are likely to be encountered in laboratory animals of these species obtained from their natural habitat (Zumpt 1965).

Adults have an overall blue-black appearance, with an orange and yellow head (Zumpt 1965). Larvae are 12 to 15 mm long and plump and have bands of pale, flattened spines on all segments (Fig. 12.5).

The life cycle is similar to that of *Cuterebra* except that gravid females oviposit directly on their hosts, and larvae penetrate intact skin (Zumpt 1965). In Europe, the adult flight season and egg laying occur in late summer.

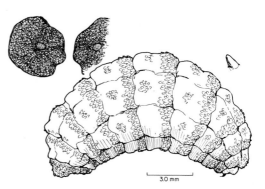

FIG. 12.5. *Oestromyia leporina* larva. *(Insets)* Posterior spiracles *(left)* and typical spine *(right)*. (Courtesy of E. P. Catts, University of Delaware.)

Larvae occur singly in cutaneous cysts, with usually only one larva per host. There is little inflammation, and the cyst heals quickly after the mature larva has emerged (Zumpt 1965).

Diagnosis is based on demonstration of the parasite in the cutaneous cysts.

Because females oviposit directly on hosts, screening is an effective method of prevention. Treatment is similar to that for *Cuterebra*.

There are no reports of infection in man (Zumpt 1965).

CALLIPHORIDS

Members of the family Calliphoridae affecting endothermal laboratory animals include the screwworm flies *(Cochliomyia* and *Chrysomya),* blowflies (other *Chrysomya* plus *Lucilia* and *Phormia),* bottle flies *(Calliphora* and *Phaenicia),* and the tumbu fly *(Cordylobia anthropophaga)* (James 1947; Stone et al. 1965; Zumpt 1965). Most of these calliphorids are cosmopolitan, with different species occurring in different parts of the world. Their larvae are distinguished from those of other flies by the characteristics of their posterior spiracles (Fig. 12.6).

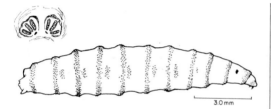

FIG. 12.6. Calliphorid larva. *(Inset)* Posterior spiracles. (Courtesy of E. P. Catts, University of Delaware.)

The vast majority of the calliphorids develop in carrion and only accidentally or facultatively cause myiasis (James 1947). Adults are attracted to decaying organic matter, such as fetid, purulent sores or soiled pelage. Their maggots feed primarily on dead or gangrenous tissue and only secondarily invade adjacent healthy tissue (Zumpt 1965).

Two species, the primary screwworm flies *Cochliomyia hominivorax* and *Chrysomya bezziana,* are obligate myiasis producers in that gravid females lay eggs on fresh wounds. These and the tumbu fly are discussed below.

Calliphorids are rare or absent in endothermal laboratory animals and are likely to affect only rodents, lagomorphs, and monkeys obtained from their natural habitat or dogs and cats obtained from pounds (Fiennes 1967; Weber 1960).

Cochliomyia hominivorax, Chrysomya bezziana

(Primary Screwworm Flies)

Cochliomyia hominivorax, the New World screwworm fly, occurs in southern United States, Mexico, and Central and South America (James 1947; Stone et al. 1965). *Chrysomya bezziana,* its Old World counterpart, occurs in Africa and southern Asia (Zumpt 1965). Both are obligate myiasis producers and will seek any fresh open wound regardless of host species. Debilitated animals are especially susceptible to attack. Screwworm fly larvae are occasional parasites of the dog and cat (Zumpt 1965). They could be encountered in animals obtained from pounds in endemic areas, but not in animals maintained in screened facilities.

MORPHOLOGY

Larvae resemble other calliphorid maggots (Fig. 12.6) (James 1947; Zumpt 1965). Adults are about 10 mm long and have a metallic blue-green body with a yellow-orange face. Eggs are elongated, about 1.25 mm long, and pearly white.

LIFE CYCLE

Eggs are deposited on fresh wounds (James 1947). Hatching occurs in 1 day or less, larval development takes about 1 week, and pupation, which occurs in the soil, requires 10 days to 8 weeks, depending on climate. Adults are active continuously in the tropics but only in warm seasons in temperate regions.

PATHOLOGIC EFFECTS

Maggots produce primary dermal myiasis without site specificity and invade deeper tissues as they develop (James 1947; Zumpt 1965). Small lacerations or puncture wounds, such as tick, fly, or mosquito feeding sites, often serve as invasion portals. Prognosis in untreated cases is grave. Usually, secondary myiasis-producing flies follow the primary screwworm invasions with fatal results.

DIAGNOSIS

Diagnosis is based on identification of the maggots in the affected tissues.

CONTROL

Larvae are killed by local application of an ointment or emulsion containing 3% lindane or a mixture of 15% chloroform and oil (Jones 1957; Stewart and Boyd 1934; Turk and Besch 1968). A 300-ppm lindane solution is used as a dip (Blakemore 1968). Dead larvae are removed, and an antibiotic ointment is applied until the wound heals. Prevention includes efficient screening of animal rooms and runs and immediate treatment of open wounds. The 3% lindane ointment is an excellent prophylactic treatment for animals with open wounds that are exposed to flies.

PUBLIC HEALTH CONSIDERATIONS

Although man is susceptible to infection (James 1947; Zumpt 1965), infected laboratory animals are not a direct hazard to human health.

Cordylobia anthropophaga
(Tumbu Fly)

This calliphorid causes dermal myiasis primarily in wild rats, but the rabbit, dog, monkeys, and man are also affected (Fiennes 1967; Lapage 1962; Zumpt 1965). It occurs in Africa south of the Sahara; the incidence varies from common in some areas to uncommon in others. This fly is likely to be found only in laboratory rats and monkeys obtained from their natural habitat, in rabbits reared in unscreened hutches, and in dogs obtained from pounds in endemic areas.

MORPHOLOGY

Adults are stout, yellow-brown flies about 6 to 12 mm long (Zumpt 1965). Mature larvae are similar to, but smaller than, *Cuterebra*. They measure 13 to 15 mm long and have fewer conspicuous body spines.

LIFE CYCLE

Females enter buildings and oviposit in shaded areas near urine and feces of potential hosts (Blacklock and Thompson 1923). Egg development takes 1 to 3 days, and infective larvae penetrate the unbroken skin of hosts making contact with oviposition sites. Larval development requires about 1 week and pupation takes 10 days. Adults feed on plant juices, fruit, and decaying matter.

PATHOLOGIC EFFECTS

The chief sites of infection are the feet, genitalia, and tail regions, but any part of the body is subject to attack (Zumpt 1965). The larvae produce swellings which are about 1 cm in diameter and have a small central opening to the exterior. Considerable irritation and distress occur when numerous larvae are involved. Secondary infection is common, and larvae often invade deeper tissues, leading to the death of the host.

DIAGNOSIS

Diagnosis is based on demonstration of the larvae in the typical swellings.

CONTROL

The screening of animal rooms, pens, and hutches and the isolation of newly acquired wild hosts are effective control measures. Larvae can also be removed surgically, as with *Cuterebra*.

PUBLIC HEALTH CONSIDERATIONS

Human infections are common in many parts of Africa (Zumpt 1965), but infected laboratory animals are not a direct hazard to man.

SARCOPHAGIDS

The family Sarcophagidae is large and includes a wide variety of biotic types (James 1947). Many are the conspicuous, large, gray tesselate flies found on carcasses of dead animals. Others breed in excrement or decaying vegetable matter, and many parasitize insects, snails, and other invertebrates.

The sarcophagids affecting endothermal laboratory animals are included in the genera *Sarcophaga* and *Wohlfahrtia*. These flies deposit tiny larvae on wounds and produce dermal myiasis.

Sarcophaga, Wohlfahrtia
(Flesh Flies)

The geographic range of flies in these genera is worldwide, but individual species have a more limited distribution and are important only locally as myiasis producers (James 1947; Stone et al. 1965; Zumpt 1965). The commonest and most widely distributed species is *S. haemorrhoidalis*, the red-tailed flesh fly. *Wohlfahrtia* species are less varied; *W. vigil* and *W. magnifica* are the New and Old World representatives, respectively. *Wohlfahrtia vigil* occurs in northern United States and Canada; *W. magnifica* occurs in southeastern Europe and southwestern Asia.

Flesh fly larvae produce dermal myiasis in a range of hosts including the wild Norway rat, hamster, rabbit, dog, cat, and man (James 1947; James and Kraft 1966; Moller 1968; Roberts 1933; Zumpt 1965). Infestation with maggots of these species is uncommon and is likely only in laboratory rodents and rabbits obtained from their natural habitat or reared in unscreened

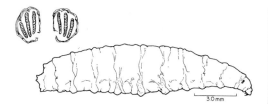

Fig. 12.7. Sarcophagid larva. *(Inset)* Posterior spiracles. (Courtesy of E. P. Catts, University of Delaware.)

facilities, or in dogs and cats obtained from pounds in endemic areas.

MORPHOLOGY

Adults are medium-to-large gray and black flies about 8 to 14 mm in length (James 1947; Zumpt 1965). Larvae are tapered, larger than those of calliphorid flies, and recognized by their characteristic posterior spiracular slits, which slant away from the midventral line (Fig. 12.7).

LIFE CYCLE

Gravid females are larviparous, depositing larvae instead of eggs on open wounds, fetid sores, and serous discharges (James 1947; Zumpt 1965). Larvae develop in 4 to 7 days, pupation requires another 4 days, and the full life cycle takes about 2 weeks to complete in temperate areas (Knipling 1936; Zumpt 1965).

PATHOLOGIC EFFECTS

The maggots of these species are usually scavengers but become facultative parasites when they occur in wounds of endothermal animals. The larvae are voracious and often actively invade healthy tissue, producing deep lesions.

DIAGNOSIS

Diagnosis is based on identification of the larvae in the dermal lesions.

CONTROL

Lindane (3%) ointment or chloroform (15%) in oil is useful in treating this type of myiasis (Jones 1957; Stewart and Boyd 1934). Prevention includes screening of animal rooms, pens, and hutches and early, thorough treatment of open wounds.

PUBLIC HEALTH CONSIDERATIONS

These flies attack man and often produce severe mutilation (Faust, Beaver, and Jung 1968; Scott 1963; Zumpt 1965), but infected laboratory animals are not a direct hazard to man.

MUSCIDS

Although most flies of the family Muscidae are nonbiting and coprophagus, a few suck blood. The commonest nonbiting genera are *Musca*, *Fannia*, and *Muscina*. The most important of those that suck blood are *Stomoxys* and *Glossina*.

Musca, Fannia, Muscina

These muscids are cosmopolitan and usually oviposit on animal wastes or decaying organic matter (James 1947; Stone et al. 1965; Zumpt 1965). They are not obligate parasites and only accidentally cause myiasis; they are, however, important vectors of disease agents (Lindsay and Scudder 1956). Common species affecting endothermal animals include the housefly *(Musca domestica)*, the lesser housefly *(Fannia canicularis)*, the latrine fly *(Fannia scalaris)*, and the false stable fly *(Muscina stabulans)*. These flies are not host-specific and will affect any endothermal laboratory animal.

MORPHOLOGY

Larvae of *Musca* and *Muscina* measure about 10 to 12 mm in length, are tapered, and have a truncated posterior (Fig. 12.8) (Zumpt 1965). *Fannia* maggots are flattened and have conspicuous lateral processes (Fig. 12.9). Adults of all three genera resemble the housefly.

LIFE CYCLE

Eggs are deposited on all kinds of decaying organic matter (Zumpt 1965). Under

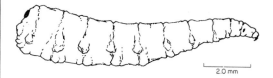

Fig. 12.8. Typical shape of muscid larva *(Musca, Muscina, Stomoxys)*. (Courtesy of E. P. Catts, University of Delaware.)

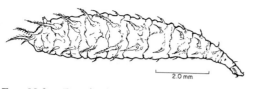

FIG. 12.9. *Fannia* larva. (Courtesy of E. P. Catts, University of Delaware.)

favorable conditions they hatch in 24 to 36 hours, pupate in 5 to 8 days, and develop into adults in another 4 to 6 days. The entire life cycle requires 10 to 14 days. Adults live about 1 month.

PATHOLOGIC EFFECTS

These flies sometimes cause a secondary or accidental myiasis in open wounds or in natural body openings (James 1947; Zumpt 1965). There is no host or site specificity; debilitated animals are the most susceptible.

Adult flies also often act as mechanical vectors for enteric pathogens, such as *Salmonella, Shigella, Escherichia,* and *Entamoeba* (Faust, Beaver, and Jung 1968; Lindsay and Scudder 1956; Yunker 1964). In some cases, they act as intermediate hosts of parasites. For example, *F. canicularis* is an intermediate host for the deer eyeworm, *Thelazia californiensis,* a nematode which sometimes occurs accidentally under the nictitating membrane of the dog in western United States (Soulsby 1965).

DIAGNOSIS

Diagnosis of myiasis caused by these flies is based on identification of the larvae in the affected tissues.

CONTROL

Screening of animal buildings and proper disposal of excrement are essential for control. Insecticidal sprays are effective in enclosed areas but, because most contain chemicals which are toxic for laboratory animals, they should be used with caution (U.S. Department of Agriculture 1967). The use of resin strips impregnated with DDVP (dichlorvos) appears to be effective and relatively nontoxic (Radeleff 1964).

Lindane (3%) ointment or chloroform (15%) in oil is used to treat the myiasis

caused by these flies (Jones 1957; Stewart and Boyd 1934).

PUBLIC HEALTH CONSIDERATIONS

The effects of these flies on man are the same as for other endothermal animals: the larvae cause myiasis and the adults transmit pathogens. Adult flies are a particular hazard in research facilities in which agents pathogenic for man are being studied. Recommended safeguards include an effective fly control program and instruction in proper personal hygiene for personnel working with laboratory animals.

Stomoxys

(Stable Flies)

Most species of this genus are found in Asia and Africa, but the commonest species, *Stomoxys calcitrans,* occurs throughout the world (Stone et al. 1965; Zumpt 1965). These flies suck blood and occasionally produce an accidental myiasis (James 1947; Zumpt 1965). They are not host-specific and will attack any endothermal laboratory animal.

MORPHOLOGY

Adults resemble the housefly but are distinguished by their darker color, more robust appearance, and modified skin-piercing mouthparts (Zumpt 1965). The larvae are similar to those of *Musca* and *Muscina* (Fig. 12.8).

LIFE CYCLE

Eggs are usually deposited deep in decaying vegetation (James and Harwood 1969). They hatch in 1 to 3 days, pupate in 7 to 21 days, and develop into adults in another 6 to 26 days.

PATHOLOGIC EFFECTS

These flies are persistent bloodsuckers (Stone et al. 1965). They usually attack the ears and legs, causing severe, painful bites and sometimes local inflammation. Occasionally they cause an accidental myiasis (Zumpt 1965).

Stomoxys adults not only act as mechanical vectors of enteric pathogens, as do other muscids, but because of their habit of feeding on one animal and then another, they can transmit blood-borne pathogens, such as *Leishmania* and *Trypanosoma* (Faust, Beaver, and Jung 1968). *Stomoxys calcitrans* is an intermediate host for *Hymenolepis carioca,* a tapeworm of the chicken (Lapage 1968).

DIAGNOSIS

Diagnosis of myiasis caused by this fly depends on identification of the larvae in affected tissue; diagnosis of the cutaneous trauma caused by adults depends on identification of the adults.

CONTROL

Control is the same as for other muscids.

PUBLIC HEALTH CONSIDERATIONS

Stomoxys readily attacks man, causing a painful bite. Otherwise, its public health aspects are similar to those described for *Musca, Fannia,* and *Muscina.*

Glossina

(Tsetse Flies)

These bloodsucking flies occur in equatorial Africa. Although they are unlikely to persist in laboratory situations, they are important because several species are intermediate hosts of trypanosomes that affect the dog, domestic animals, and man (Levine 1961). It is likely that they also transmit trypanosomiasis to African monkeys, but definitive evidence is lacking (Fiennes 1967).

HIPPOBOSCIDS

Members of the family Hippoboscidae, the louse flies, are relatively permanent ectoparasites of birds and some mammals. These flies, also called "keds," are morphologically unique; wings are absent or only temporary on several species. The most important species that affects endothermal laboratory animals is *Pseudolynchia canariensis.*

Pseudolynchia canariensis

(Pigeon Ked)

This fly occurs on the pigeon in tropical and subtropical regions throughout the world (James and Harwood 1969; Stone et al. 1965). Although it is common in southern United States and California, it is not

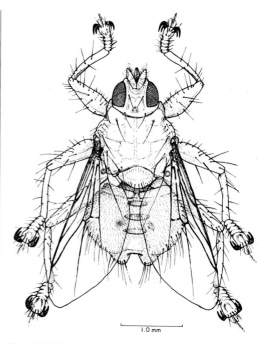

FIG. 12.10. *Pseudolynchia canariensis* adult. (Courtesy of E. P. Catts, University of Delaware.)

likely to occur on laboratory pigeons obtained from suppliers in these regions that practice good sanitation. *Pseudolynchia canariensis* sucks blood and causes painful wounds.

MORPHOLOGY

The pigeon ked is a depressed, dark brown fly, about 6.5 to 7.5 mm long, with a pair of transparent wings and strong spurred claws (Fig. 12.10) (James and Harwood 1969; Lapage 1962).

LIFE CYCLE

The female retains the larva within her body until it is ready for pupation (James and Harwood 1969; Lapage 1962). The mature larva is then deposited on the body of the host and falls off into the bedding, or it is deposited in dark crevices near the host. The larva is yellow when deposited but turns black in a few hours. The pupal stage lasts about 1 month; the adults live about 45 days (Bishopp 1929). Both sexes bite and suck blood.

PATHOLOGIC EFFECTS

This fly causes considerable annoyance as it moves through the feathers, biting and sucking blood (Bishopp 1929). In heavy infestations of young pigeons, the loss of blood retards development. In addition to its other pathologic effects, *P. canariensis* transmits *Haemoproteus columbae*, a protozoan that causes malaria of the pigeon (Baker 1967).

DIAGNOSIS

Diagnosis depends on demonstration of the parasite. The flies are often difficult to see on the host as they move rapidly through the feathers, but they are frequently found resting motionless in a head-down position on inanimate objects near the host (Bishopp 1929).

CONTROL

Newly acquired pigeons should be examined on arrival and treated, if infected. Dusting both birds and cages with a powder containing 1% pyrethrins is effective (Bishopp 1929). Because of the long pupal stage (about 1 month), weekly or semimonthly cage cleaning will eliminate the parasite.

PUBLIC HEALTH CONSIDERATIONS

Although man is not a suitable host for this parasite nor for the protozoan it transmits, persons in close contact with infected pigeons are sometimes bitten and often develop sensitivity (Bishopp 1929).

TABANIDS

The family Tabanidae comprises about 80 genera and nearly 4,000 species, including the horseflies *(Tabanus* and *Hybomitra)*, deerflies *(Chrysops)*, and clegs *(Haematopota)* (James and Harwood 1969; Stone et al. 1965). These flies are usually larger than the common housefly and often beautifully colored. Although their bite is painful, their primary importance to endothermal laboratory animals is that some are vectors of disease agents.

Tabanid flies transmit *Trypanosoma evansi*, a protozoan parasite of the dog and other endothermal animals (Levine 1961). *Chrysops discalis*, the western deerfly, can transmit *Francisella tularensis*, the causative agent of tularemia (Zumpt 1949). Several other species of *Chrysops* are vectors of *Loa loa*, an African filarial parasite that affects guenons, mandrills, baboons, and man (Zumpt 1949).

CULICIDS

Members of the family Culicidae, the mosquitoes, suck blood and are important vectors of many viral, protozoan, and helminthic diseases. The most important genera affecting endothermal laboratory animals are *Anopheles, Aedes,* and *Culex.*

Anopheles, Aedes, Culex
(Mosquitoes)

Mosquitoes occur throughout the world and attack all endothermal animals (Horsfall 1955). Their importance relates to their annoying and sometimes painful feeding habits and their ability to act as vectors of many pathogens.

MORPHOLOGY

Adults are small flies, about 2.5 to 6.0 mm long, with a slender abdomen and long proboscis (Fig. 12.11*A*) (James and Harwood 1969). The egg, larva, and pupa vary in morphology with the species. Their general appearance is shown in Figure 12.11.

LIFE CYCLE

All immature stages of mosquitoes are aquatic (James and Harwood 1969). Eggs are deposited individually or in raftlike groups on the surface of the water or on moist substrate. The hatching time and subsequent development of the larva and pupa vary widely with the species and temperature. Under ideal conditions, eggs usually hatch in 1 to 2 days; the larval stage lasts about 1 to 2 weeks, and the pupal stage 2 to 3 days. Adults live about 1 month.

PATHOLOGIC EFFECTS

Only adult female mosquitoes suck blood (James and Harwood 1969). They often enter buildings when seeking a meal. Although some species tend to prefer certain hosts, many will feed on a variety of hosts. It is generally believed that salivary secretions introduced while biting cause the local inflammation and pruritus (Bates

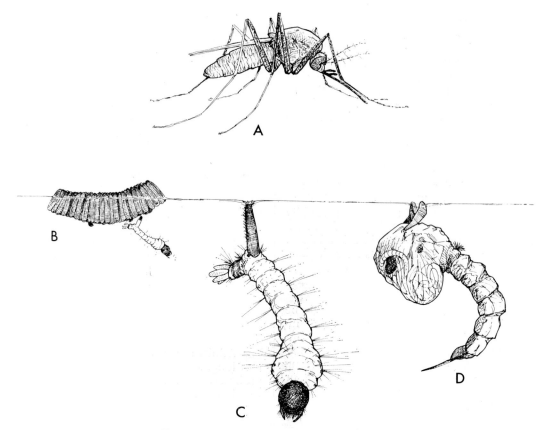

Fig. 12.11.   General morphology of mosquitoes (Culicidae). *(A)* Adult female. *(B)* Eggs. *(C)* Larva. *(D)* Pupa. (Courtesy of E. P. Catts, University of Delaware.)

1949). The amount of inflammation and irritation varies with the species of mosquito and the susceptibility of the individual animal.

Mosquitoes are vectors of many important pathogens of endothermal laboratory animals (Horsfall 1955). Some of the agents they transmit are the viruses of myxomatosis (Joubert et al. 1967), fowl pox (Benbrook 1965), western and eastern equine encephalitis, and yellow fever (Faust, Beaver, and Jung 1968). Mosquitoes are vectors of the many species of *Plasmodium* that cause malaria in laboratory primates, wild rodents, the chicken, and man (Levine 1961). They also transmit *Trypanosoma avium,* a trypanosome that affects the chicken and other birds (Bennett 1961), and filarial worms, such as *Dirofilaria, Dipetalonema, Wuchereria,* and *Brugia,* that

affect the dog, cat, many laboratory primates, and man (Fiennes 1967; Lapage 1968; Ruch 1959; Soulsby 1965).

DIAGNOSIS

Diagnosis is based on the cutaneous inflammation and identification of the parasite.

CONTROL

Insectproof construction of animal buildings with 18-mesh-per-inch screens and the use of aerial insecticides, such as resin strips containing DDVP, or surface sprays of residual insecticides, such as 5% methoxychlor, are effective controls (U.S. Department of Agriculture 1967). The flushing of floor drain traps and the emptying of water containers at least once a week will prevent indoor breeding.

Mosquitoes transmit many human pathogens (Faust, Beaver, and Jung 1968). They are particularly hazardous in research animal facilities where blood-borne pathogens are being studied. Recommended safeguards include an effective control program and instruction for animal personnel in the risks involved and the precautions to be taken.

PSYCHODIDS

The family Psychodidae consists of small mothlike flies that occur in temperate and tropical regions throughout the world (James and Harwood 1969). *Phlebotomus* (sand flies) is the most important genus because it is a vector of *Leishmania donovani* and *L. tropica,* the etiologic agents of leishmaniasis of the dog, cat, wild rodents, and man (Levine 1961).

SIMULIIDS

Members of the family Simuliidae, the blackflies, are short, stout, biting flies that occur throughout the world (James and Harwood 1969). The most important genus is *Simulium*. Species of this genus have been particularly troublesome to poultry in southern United States (Benbrook 1965) and to domestic and wild animals (including rabbits) in Europe and North America (James and Harwood 1969). They are important to endothermal laboratory animals primarily because some are vectors of pathogenic protozoans such as *Trypanosoma avium,* the cause of trypanosomiasis of the chicken and other birds (Bennett 1961). Immature stages develop in flowing streams, and adults usually abound in wooded regions. They do not normally enter buildings (James and Harwood 1969) and, consequently, are unlikely to be a problem in research animal facilities.

CERATOPOGONIDS

Flies of the family Ceratopogonidae, called midges or punkies, are minute, about 1 to 4 mm in length (James and Harwood 1969; Stone et al. 1965). *Culicoides* is the most important genus. Species of this genus occur throughout the world and, although their bite is annoying and irritating to all endothermal animals, they are important to laboratory animals primarily because they are often vectors of pathogenic agents. *Hepatocystis kochi,* a malarial parasite of guenons, mangabeys, and other primates, is known to be transmitted by midges, and *Leucocytozoon sabrazesi* and *L. caulleryi,* malarial parasites of the chicken, are thought to be transmitted by these flies (Levine 1961). *Culicoides* is also an intermediate host for filarial nematodes of simian primates and man (Faust, Beaver, and Jung 1968).

TABLE 12.1. Flies affecting endothermal laboratory animals

Parasite	Geographic Distribution	Endothermal Host	Location in Host	Incidence In nature	Incidence In laboratory	Pathologic Effects	Public Health Importance	Reference
Cuterebra*	Western Hemisphere	Deer mice, wood rats, squirrels, other New World rodents, cottontail rabbits, hares, monkeys; accidentally in Old World rodents, hares, dog, cat, man	Skin, subcutis, sometimes brain	Common	Common in animals obtained from natural habitat	Dermal cyst; sometimes anemia, leucocytosis, splenomegaly, focal encephalitis, aggressiveness, paralysis, coma, death	Affects man accidentally; infected laboratory animals cannot infect man	Bennett 1955; Catts, 1965, 1967; Dalmat 1943; Dunaway et al. 1967; Goertz 1966; Guimarães 1967; Haas and Dicke 1958; Hall 1921; Hatziolos 1966, 1967; James 1947; Knipling and Bruce 1937; Maurer and Skaley 1968; Payne and Cosgrove 1966; Payne et al. 1965; Rothenbacher et al. 1964; Wecker 1962
Dermatobia hominis*	Mexico, Central America, South America	Wild rodents, dog, cat, monkeys, domestic animals, birds, man	Skin, subcutis	Common	Common in animals obtained from natural habitat	Dermal cyst	Affects man; infected laboratory animals cannot infect man	Guimarães and Papavero 1966; James 1947; Král and Schwartzman 1964; Lapage 1968
Oestromyia leporina*	Europe, Asia	Voles, muskrat, pikas (*Ochotona*)	Skin, subcutis	Common	Common in animals obtained from natural habitat	Dermal cyst	None known	Zumpt 1965
Cochliomyia hominivorax*	Southern United States, Mexico, Central America, South America	Dog, cat, other mammals, birds	Skin, subcutis	Common; uncommon in dog, cat	Rare or absent in dog, cat	Primary myiasis	Rarely affects man; infected laboratory animals cannot directly infect man	James 1947
Other *Cochliomyia*	Western Hemisphere	Various mammals, birds	Skin, subcutis	Common	Rare or absent	Secondary myiasis	Rarely affects man; infected laboratory animals cannot directly infect man	James 1947
Chrysomyia bezziana*	Southern Asia, Africa	Dog, cat, other mammals, birds	Skin, subcutis	Common; uncommon in dog, cat	Rare or absent in dog, cat	Primary myiasis	Rarely affects man; infected laboratory animals cannot directly infect man	Zumpt 1965
Other *Chrysomyia*	Eastern Hemisphere	Various mammals, birds	Skin, subcutis	Common	Rare or absent	Secondary myiasis	Rarely affects man; infected laboratory animals cannot directly infect man	Zumpt 1965

*Discussed in text.

TABLE 12.1 (continued)

Parasite	Geographic Distribution	Endothermal Host	Location in Host	Incidence In nature	Incidence In laboratory	Pathologic Effects	Public Health Importance	Reference
Lucilia	Worldwide	Various mammals, birds	Skin, subcutis	Common	Rare or absent	Secondary myiasis	Rarely affects man; infected laboratory animals cannot directly infect man	James 1947 Zumpt 1965
Phormia	Worldwide	Various mammals, birds	Skin, subcutis	Common	Rare or absent	Secondary myiasis	Rarely affects man; infected laboratory animals cannot directly infect man	James 1947 Zumpt 1965
Calliphora	Worldwide	Various mammals, birds	Skin, subcutis	Common	Rare or absent	Secondary myiasis	Rarely affects man; infected laboratory animals cannot directly infect man	James 1947 Zumpt 1965
Phaenicia	Worldwide	Various mammals, birds	Skin, subcutis	Common	Rare or absent	Secondary myiasis	Rarely affects man; infected laboratory animals cannot directly infect man	James 1947 Zumpt 1965
Cordylobia anthropophaga*	Africa	Wild rats, rabbit, dog, monkeys, man	Skin	Uncommon to common	Rare or absent	Dermal myiasis	Causes dermal myiasis; common in endemic areas; infected laboratory animals cannot infect man	Blacklock and Thompson 1923 Fiennes 1967 Lapage 1962 Zumpt 1965
Sarcophaga*	Worldwide	Rabbit, dog, cat, other mammals, man	Skin, subcutis	Uncommon	Rare or absent	Dermal myiasis	Causes dermal myiasis; rare; infected laboratory animals cannot directly infect man	James 1947 Knipling 1936 Roberts 1933 Zumpt 1965
Wohlfahrtia vigil*	Northern United States, Canada	Rat, hamster, rabbit, dog, cat, other mammals, man	Skin, subcutis	Uncommon	Rare or absent	Dermal myiasis	Causes dermal myiasis; uncommon; laboratory animals cannot directly infect man	James 1947 James and Kraft 1966 Moller 1968
Wohlfahrtia magnifica*	Southeastern Europe, southwestern Asia, northern Africa	Rabbit, dog, cat, other mammals, man	Skin, subcutis	Uncommon	Rare or absent	Dermal myiasis	Causes dermal myiasis; uncommon; laboratory animals cannot directly infect man	Zumpt 1965
Musca domestica*	Worldwide	All endothermal animals	Skin, subcutis, natural body openings	Common	Common	Dermal, nasal, auricular, urogenital, anal myiasis; mechanical vector of pathogens	Causes myiasis; mechanical vector of pathogens	Faust et al. 1968 James 1947 Soulsby 1965 Zumpt 1965

*Discussed in text.

TABLE 12.1 *(continued)*

Parasite	Geographic Distribution	Endothermal Host	Location in Host	Incidence In nature	Incidence In laboratory	Pathologic Effects	Public Health Importance	Reference
Fannia canicularis*	Worldwide	All endothermal animals	Skin, subcutis, natural body openings	Common	Common	Dermal, nasal, auricular, urogenital, anal myiasis; mechanical vector of pathogens; intermediate host of *Thelazia californiensis*	Causes myiasis; mechanical vector of pathogens	Faust et al. 1968 James 1947 Soulsby 1965 Zumpt 1965
Fannia scalaris*	North America, Europe	All endothermal animals	Skin, subcutis, natural body openings	Common	Common	Dermal, nasal, auricular, urogenital, anal myiasis; mechanical vector of pathogens	Causes myiasis; mechanical vector of pathogens	Faust et al. 1968 James 1947 Zumpt 1965
Muscina stabulans*	North America, Europe, Asia	All endothermal animals	Skin, subcutis, natural body openings	Common	Common	Dermal, nasal, auricular, urogenital, anal myiasis; mechanical vector of pathogens	Causes myiasis; mechanical vector of pathogens	Faust et al. 1968 James 1947 Soulsby 1965 Zumpt 1965
Stomoxys calcitrans*	Worldwide	All endothermal animals	Skin, subcutis, natural body openings	Common	Common	Annoyance, trauma to skin, loss of blood; sometimes myiasis; mechanical vector of pathogens; intermediate host for *Hymenolepis carioca*	Causes annoyance, trauma to skin, loss of blood; sometimes myiasis; mechanical vector of pathogens	Faust et al. 1968 James 1947 Zumpt 1965
Glossina*	Equatorial Africa	Various mammals	Skin	Common	Absent	Vector of trypanosomes	Vector of agent of trypanosomiasis	Fiennes 1967 Levine 1961
Pseudolynchia canariensis*	Worldwide in tropics and subtropics	Pigeon	Plumage	Common	Unknown; probably rare or absent	Annoyance, trauma to skin, loss of blood, anemia, retarded growth; vector of *Haemoproteus columbae*	Causes annoyance, trauma to skin, sometimes allergic reaction	Baker 1967 Bishopp 1929 James and Harwood 1969 Lapage 1962, 1968
Tabanus	Worldwide	All endothermal mammals	Skin	Common	Unknown; probably rare or absent	Annoyance, trauma to skin; vector of trypanosomes	Causes annoyance, trauma to skin	James and Harwood 1969 Levine 1961
Hybomitra	Worldwide	All endothermal animals	Skin	Common	Unknown; probably rare or absent	Annoyance, trauma to skin; mechanical vector of blood parasites	Causes annoyance, trauma to skin	James and Harwood 1969

*Discussed in text.

TABLE 12.1 *(continued)*

Parasite	Geographic Distribution	Endothermal Host	Location in Host	Incidence — In nature	Incidence — In laboratory	Pathologic Effects	Public Health Importance	Reference
Chrysops	Worldwide	All endothermal animals	Skin	Common	Unknown; probably rare or absent	Annoyance, trauma to skin; vector of *Francisella tularensis, Loa loa*	Causes annoyance, trauma to skin; vector of agent of tularemia; vector of filarial nematode	James and Harwood 1969 Zumpt 1949
Haematopota	Worldwide	All endothermal animals	Skin	Common	Unknown; probably rare or absent	Annoyance, trauma to skin; mechanical vector of blood parasites	Causes annoyance, trauma to skin	James and Harwood 1969
*Anopheles**	Worldwide	All endothermal animals	Skin	Common	Common	Local inflammation, pruritus; vector of many viral, protozoan, helminthic agents	Causes local inflammation, pruritus; vector of many viral, protozoan, helminthic agents	Faust et al. 1968 Horsfall 1955 James and Harwood 1969
*Aedes**	Worldwide	All endothermal animals	Skin	Common	Common	Local inflammation, pruritus; vector of many viral, protozoan, helminthic agents	Causes local inflammation, pruritus; vector of many viral, protozoan, helminthic agents	Faust et al. 1968 Horsfall 1955 James and Harwood 1969
*Culex**	Worldwide	All endothermal animals	Skin	Common	Common	Local inflammation, pruritus; vector of many viral, protozoan, helminthic agents	Causes local inflammation, pruritus; vector of many viral, protozoan, helminthic agents	Faust et al. 1968 Horsfall 1955 James and Harwood 1969
Phlebotomus	Worldwide	All endothermal animals	Skin	Common	Unknown; probably rare or absent	Annoyance, trauma to skin; vector of *Leishmania donovani, L. tropica*	Causes annoyance, trauma to skin; vector of agent of leishmaniasis	James and Harwood 1969 Levine 1961
Simulium	Worldwide	All endothermal animals	Skin	Common	Unknown; probably rare or absent	Annoyance, trauma to skin; vector of *Trypanosoma avium*	Causes annoyance, trauma to skin; vector of filarial nematode	Benbrook 1965 Bennett 1961 Faust et al. 1968 James and Harwood 1969
Culicoides	Worldwide	All endothermal animals	Skin	Common	Unknown; probably rare or absent	Annoyance, trauma to skin; vector of *Hepatocystis kochi, Leucocytozoon,* filarial nematodes	Causes annoyance, trauma to skin; vector of filarial nematodes	Faust et al. 1968 James and Harwood 1969 Levine 1961

*Discussed in text.

REFERENCES

Banegas, A. D., and H. Mourier. 1967. Laboratory observations on the life history and habits of *Dermatobia hominis* (Diptera: Cuterebridae): I. Mating behavior. Ann. Entomol. Soc. Am. 60:878–81.

Baker, J. R. 1967. A review of the role played by the Hippoboscidae (Diptera) as vectors of endoparasites. J. Parasitol. 53:412–18.

Bates, M. 1949. The natural history of mosquitoes. Macmillan, New York. 379 pp.

Benbrook, E. A. 1965. External parasites of poultry, pp. 925–64. *In* H. E. Biester and L. H. Schwarte, eds. Diseases of poultry. 5th ed. Iowa State Univ. Press, Ames.

Bennett, G. F. 1955. Studies on *Cuterebra emasculator* Fitch, 1856 (Diptera: Cuterebridae) and a discussion of the status of the genus *Cephenemyia* Ltr. 1818. Can. J. Zool. 33:75–98.

———. 1961. On the specificity and transmission of some avian trypanosomes. Can. J. Zool. 39:17–33.

Bishopp, F. C. 1929. The pigeon fly—an important pest of pigeons in the United States. J. Econ. Entomol. 22:974–80.

Blacklock, B., and M. G. Thompson. 1923. A study of the tumbu fly, *Cordylobia anthropophaga* Grunberg, in Sierra Leone. Ann. Trop. Med. Parasitol. 17:443–501.

Blakemore, J. C. 1968. Macroscopic ectoparasites, pp. 268–73. *In* R. W. Kirk, ed. Current veterinary therapy III: Small animal practice. W. B. Saunders, Philadelphia.

Brass, W. 1964. Zur Behandlung des Dermatobialarvenbefalles und der Myiasis des Hundes mittels eines Phosphorsäureesters. Deut. Tieraerztl. Wochschr. 71:356–58.

Catts, E. P. 1965. Host-parasite interrelationships in rodent bot fly infections. Trans. 30th North Am. Wildlife Nat. Resources Conf. Wash., D.C. 30:184–86.

———. 1967. The biology of a California rodent bot fly *Cuterebra latifrons* Coq. (Diptera, Cuterebridae). J. Med. Entomol. 4:87–101.

Conroy, J. D. 1964. Cutaneous myiasis, pp. 143–44. *In* E. J. Catcott, ed. Feline medicine and surgery. American Veterinary Publications, Santa Barbara, Calif.

Curran, C. H. 1934. The families and genera of North American Diptera. Ballou Press, New York. 512 pp.

Dalmat, H. T. 1943. A contribution to the knowledge of the rodent warble flies (Cuterebridae). J. Parasitol. 29:311–18.

Dunaway, P. B., J. A. Payne, L. L. Lewis, and J. D. Story. 1967. Incidence and effects of *Cuterebra* in *Peromyscus*. J. Mammal. 48:38–51.

Faust, E. C., P. C. Beaver, and R. C. Jung. 1968. Animal agents and vectors of human disease. 3d ed. Lea and Febiger, Philadelphia. 461 pp.

Fiennes, R. 1967. Zoonoses of primates. Weidenfeld and Nicolson, London. 190 pp.

Goertz, J. W. 1966. Incidence of warbles in some Oklahoma rodents. Am. Midland Naturalist 75:242–45.

Guimarães, J. H. 1967. Family Cuterebridae, pp. 105.1–105.11. *In* A catalogue of the Diptera of the Americas south of the United States. Dept. Zool., Secr. Agr., Brazil.

Guimarães, J. H., and N. Papavero. 1966. A tentative annotated bibliography of *Dermatobia hominis* (Diptera, Cuterebridae). Arquiv. Zool. 14: 223–94.

Haas, G. E., and R. J. Dicke. 1958. On *Cuterebra horripilum* Clark (Diptera: Cuterebridae) parasitizing cottontail rabbits in Wisconsin. J. Parasitol. 44:527–40.

Hall, M. C. 1921. *Cuterebra* larvae from cats, with a list of those recorded from other hosts. J. Am. Vet. Med. Assoc. 12:480–84.

Hatziolos, B. C. 1966. *Cuterebra* larva in the brain of a cat. J. Am. Vet. Med. Assoc. 148:787–93.

———. 1967. *Cuterebra* larva causing paralysis in a dog. Cornell Vet. 57:129–45.

Hooper, B. E. 1961. Subcutaneous myiasis in dogs and cats. Missouri Vet. 10:19–20.

Horsfall, W. R. 1955. Mosquitoes: Their bionomics and relation to disease. Ronald, New York. 723 pp.

James, M. T. 1947. The flies that cause myiasis in man. U.S. Dept. Agr., Misc. Publ. 631. 175 pp.

James, M. T., and R. F. Harwood. 1969. Herms's medical entomology. 6th ed. Macmillan, New York. 484 pp.

James, M. T., and G. F. Kraft. 1966. The identity of the American producers of *Wohlfahrtia* myiasis, pp. 949–951. *In* A. Corradetti, ed. Proc. First Intern. Congr. Parasitol. Pergamon Press, New York.

Jones, L. M. 1957. Veterinary pharmacology and therapeutics. 2d ed. Iowa State College Press, Ames. 944 pp.

Joubert, L., J. Oudar, J. Mouchet, and C. Hannoun. 1967. Transmission de la myxomatose par les moustiques en Camargue: Rôle preëminent de *Aedes caspius* et des *Anopheles* du groupe *maculipennis*. Bull. Acad. Vet. France 40:315–22, 471.

Knipling, E. F. 1936. A comparative study of first instar larvae of the genus *Sarcophaga* (Calliphoridae, Diptera), with notes on biology. J. Parasitol. 22:417–54.

Knipling, E. F., and W. G. Bruce. 1937. Three unusual records for cuterebrine larvae (Diptera: Oestridae). Entomol. News 48: 156–58.

Král, F., and R. M. Schwartzman. 1964. Veterinary and comparative dermatology. J. B. Lippincott, Philadelphia. 444 pp.

Lapage, G. 1962. Mönnig's veterinary helminthology and entomology. 5th ed. Williams and Wilkins, Baltimore. 600 pp.

———. 1968. Veterinary parasitology. Oliver and Boyd, Edinburgh and London. 1182 pp.

Levine, N. D. 1961. Protozoan parasites of domestic animals and of man. Burgess, Minneapolis. 412 pp.

Lindsay, D. R., and H. I. Scudder. 1956. Non-biting flies and disease. Ann. Rev. Entomol. 1:323–46.

Matéus, G. 1967. El nuche y su ciclo de vida. Rev. Inst. Colomb. Agropec. 2:3–19.

Maurer, F. W., Jr., and J. E. Skaley. 1968. Cuterebrid infestation of Microtus in eastern North Dakota, Pennsylvania, and New York. J. Mammal. 49:773–74.

Miller, D. H., and L. L. Getz. 1969. Botfly infections in a population of Peromyscus leucopus. J. Mammal. 50:277–83.

Moller, A. W. 1968. Diseases and management of the golden hamster (Mesocricetus auratus), pp. 418–22. In R. W. Kirk, ed. Current veterinary therapy III: Small animal practice. W. B. Saunders, Philadelphia.

Payne, J. A., and G. E. Cosgrove. 1966. Tissue changes following Cuterebra infestation in rodents. Am. Midland Naturalist 75:205–13.

Payne, J. A., P. B. Dunaway, G. D. Martin, and J. D. Story. 1965. Effects of Cuterebra angustifrons on plasma proteins of Peromyscus leucopus. J. Parasitol. 51:1004–8.

Penner, L. R. 1958. Concerning a rabbit cuterebrid, the larvae of which may penetrate the human skin (Diptera, Cuterebridae). J. Kansas Entomol. Soc. 31:67–71.

Penner, L. R., and F. P. Pocius. 1956. Nostril entry as the mode of infection by the first stage larvae of a rodent Cuterebra. J. Parasitol. 42:(Supp.) 42.

Radeleff, R. D. 1964. Veterinary toxicology. Lea and Febiger, Philadelphia. 314 pp.

Radovsky, F. J., and E. P. Catts. 1960. Observations on the biology of Cuterebra latifrons Coquillet (Diptera: Cuterebridae). J. Kansas Entomol. Soc. 33:31–36.

Roberts, R. A. 1933. Additional notes on my-iasis in rabbits (Diptera: Calliphoridae; Sarcophagidae). Entomol. News 44:157–59.

Rothenbacher, H., G. Mugera, and S. Tufts. 1964. Stomach worm disease, hypodermal myiasis and intestinal coccidiosis in a rabbit colony. Mich. State Univ. Vet. 24:134–36.

Ruch, T. C. 1959. Diseases of laboratory primates. W. B. Saunders, Philadelphia. 600 pp.

Scott, H. G. 1963. Myiasis: Epidemiological data on human cases (North America north of Mexico: 1952–1962 inclusive). U.S. Public Health Serv., Communicable Disease Center. 14 pp.

Soulsby, E. J. L. 1965. Textbook of veterinary clinical parasitology: Vol. I. Helminths. F. A. Davis, Philadelphia. 1120 pp.

Stewart, M. A., and A. N. Boyd. 1934. A new treatment of traumatic dermal myiasis. J. Am. Med. Assoc. 103:402.

Stone, A., C. W. Sabrosky, W. W. Wirth, R. H. Foote, and J. R. Coulson. 1965. A catalog of the Diptera of America north of Mexico. U.S. Dept. Agr., Agr. Handbook 276. 1696 pp.

Turk, R. D., and E. D. Besch. 1968. Parasitic dermatoses, pp. 539–60. In E. J. Catcott, ed. Canine medicine. American Veterinary Publications, Santa Barbara, Calif.

U.S. Department of Agriculture. 1967. Suggested guide for the use of insecticides to control insects affecting crops, livestock, households, stored products, forests, and forest products. U.S. Dept. Agr., Agr. Handbook 331. 273 pp.

Weber, N. A. 1960. Visceral myiasis caused by Phaenicia sericata in the house mouse (Diptera: Calliphoridae). Proc. Entomol. Soc. Wash. D.C. 62:108.

Wecker, S. C. 1962. The effects of bot fly parasitism on a local population of the white-footed mouse. Ecology 43:561–65.

Yunker, C. E. 1964. Infections of laboratory animals potentially dangerous to man: Ectoparasites and other arthropods, with emphasis on mites. Lab. Animal Care 14:455–65.

Zumpt, F. 1949. Medical and veterinary importance of horse-flies. S. African Med. J. 23:359–62.

———. 1965. Myiasis in man and animals in the Old World: A textbook for physicians, veterinarians and zoologists. Butterworths, London. 267 pp.

Chapter 13

LICE

LICE are wingless insects that are somewhat flattened dorsoventrally. They are divided into two groups: the anoplurans, or sucking lice; and the mallophagans, or biting lice. All are obligate ectoparasites that spend their entire lives on various endothermal species (Ferris 1951; Hopkins 1949, 1957).

ANOPLURANS

The anoplurans, or sucking lice, have slender bodies, proportionately narrow, small heads, five-segmented antennae, and unique mouthparts adapted for sucking blood (Ferris 1920, 1951; James and Harwood 1969). They are frequently encountered on animals obtained from their natural habitat. They once were common on commercially produced laboratory rodents, but their incidence is now greatly reduced (Flynn 1955; Flynn, Brennan, and Fritz 1965). Laboratory animals debilitated or physically impaired either naturally or experimentally are usually more heavily infested (Bell et al. 1966; Bell, Jellison, and Owen 1962; Tuffery and Innes 1963).

The sucking lice which occur on endothermal laboratory animals are listed in Table 13.1. The most important are discussed below.

Polyplax serrata, Polyplax spinulosa

Polyplax serrata is the common louse of the laboratory mouse (Flynn 1955). It causes debilitation and anemia and is a vector of the agent of murine eperythrozoonosis. This louse is also found on the house mouse and field mice of Europe and Asia, but not on the house mouse of North America (Heston 1941; Johnson 1960). It has been reported from conventional mouse colonies throughout the world (Bateman 1961; Flynn 1955; Heine 1962; Heston 1941; Murray 1961; Sasa et al. 1962; Tuffery and Innes 1963). It is common in some colonies and rare or absent in others; it does not occur in cesarean-derived, barrier-sustained colonies (Bell 1968; Flynn, Brennan, and Fritz 1965; Foster 1963; Owen 1968).

Polyplax spinulosa, or the spined rat louse, is the common louse of the laboratory rat. It causes debilitation and anemia and is a vector of the murine haemobartonellosis agent. This louse is also found on wild Norway and black rats throughout the world (Johnson 1960; Pratt and Karp 1953) and on field mice and voles in Europe and Asia (Sasa 1950; Smetana 1962). It has been reported from conventional rat colonies in all parts of the world (Deoras and Patel 1960; Jenkins and Fletcher 1964; Olewine 1963; Sasa et al. 1962; Tarshis 1962). It is common in some colonies and rare or absent in others; it does not occur in cesarean-derived, barrier-sustained colonies (Flynn, Brennan, and Fritz 1965; Foster 1963; Owen 1968).

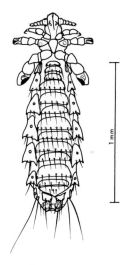

FIG. 13.1. *Polyplax serrata* female, ventral view. (Courtesy of K. C. Kim, Pennsylvania State University.)

MORPHOLOGY

Polyplax (Fig. 13.1) is a slender louse, 0.6 to 1.5 mm long, and is yellow-brown or white with a brown tinge (Farris 1950; Holmes 1959; Murray 1961; Pratt and Karp 1953). The head bears a long hair on its posterior angle. The ventral thoracic plate is well developed. It is subtriangular in *P. serrata* and pentagonal in *P. spinulosa*. The abdomen has about 7 lateral plates on each side and 7 to 13 dorsal plates. The first lateral plate is divided. The setae of the fourth lateral plate of *P. serrata* are unequal in length, the dorsal one being much longer than the ventral one; the setae of the fourth lateral plate of *P. spinulosa* are almost the same length. Eggs are elongated and fastened to the hair of the host near the skin. Nymphs resemble adults but are smaller and paler.

LIFE CYCLE

Eggs hatch in 5 to 6 days (Holmes 1959; Murray 1961). The first-stage nymphs of *P. serrata* occur over the entire body of the mouse; other stages are found predominantly on the forebody. *Polyplax spinulosa* is common on the midbody, shoulder, and neck (Holmes 1959). Self-grooming and mutual grooming control the distribution and abundance of lice on

mice and rats (Bell and Clifford 1964; Bell, Jellison, and Owen 1962). The entire life cycle is completed in about 13 days for *P. serrata* and in about 26 days for *P. spinulosa*. *Polyplax spinulosa* survives 25 to 28 days. Transmission is by direct contact (Oldham 1967).

PATHOLOGIC EFFECTS

Laboratory rodents infested with *Polyplax* are characterized by an unthrifty appearance, anemia, restlessness, and constant scratching (Heston 1941). Heavy infestations are sometimes fatal (Oldham 1967).

Polyplax serrata is known to transmit *Eperythrozoon coccoides* from mouse to mouse (Eliot 1936), and *Francisella tularensis* has been recovered from this louse (Riley and Johannsen 1938; Shaughnessy 1963; Strong 1944). *Polyplax spinulosa* transmits *Rickettsia typhi* and *Haemobartonella muris* from rat to rat (Buxton and Busvine 1957; Heston 1941) and is possibly a vector of *Brucella brucei* (Parnas, Zwolski, and Burdzy 1960a; Parnas et al. 1960b), *Borrelia duttoni* (Davis 1960, 1963; James and Harwood 1969), and *Trypanosoma lewisi* (Strong 1944).

DIAGNOSIS

Diagnosis is based on demonstration of the parasite in the pelage (Flynn 1963; Heston 1941). One should be cautious, however, about attributing any observed dermal pathology solely to lice as most infested animals are also concurrently infested with mites (Flynn 1955; Heine 1962; Owen 1968).

CONTROL

To prevent an animal facility from becoming infested, newly acquired animals should be carefully inspected on arrival and, if infested, isolated and treated with an effective insecticide. To eliminate an existing infection, all animals should be treated. Because these lice do not usually leave the host, the insecticide must be applied directly to the pelage of the animal as a dust, spray, or dip. Treatment should be repeated at weekly intervals for 2 to 3 weeks. Cages, bedding, and equipment should be cleaned and disinfected at the same time the animals are treated (Farris 1950; Pratt and Littig 1961).

Dusts containing 0.25 to 0.50% lindane, 3 to 5% malathion, 10% methoxychlor, 0.05 to 0.10% pyrethrins, or 0.5 to 1.0% rotenone, and sprays or dips containing 0.03 to 0.06% diazinon, 0.10 to 0.25% malathion, or 0.5% methoxychlor are effective treatments (Bateman 1961; Jenkins and Fletcher 1964; Roberts 1952; Symes, Muirhead-Thompson, and Busvine 1962; Tuffery and Innes 1963; U.S. Department of Agriculture 1967a). A 2% aqueous suspension of a wettable powder containing 15% butylphenoxyisopropyl chloroethyl sulfite (Aramite, Uniroyal), in combination with a wetting agent, is effective as a dip and apparently is nontoxic to mice (Flynn 1955). Also reportedly effective is the direct application to the pelage of a sorptive silica dust (Dri-Die 67, FMC Corporation) (Tarshis 1962) or a sorptive silica dust combined with pyrethrins (Drione, FMC Corporation) (Tarshis 1967). A simple method of treatment for a small number of animals, such as new additions to a colony or animals brought in from their natural environment, involves placing the animals for approximately 2 hours in a closed container with a resin strip impregnated with an aerial insecticide, DDVP (Vapona, Shell) (D. R. Maddock, personal communication).

Lice can be completely eliminated from laboratory rodents by initiating a new colony, using cesarean-derived offspring (Foster 1963).

PUBLIC HEALTH CONSIDERATIONS

These lice do not parasitize man but are an indirect hazard. *Polyplax spinulosa* can transmit *Rickettsia typhi* from rat to rat. The organisms then may be transmitted to man by a rat flea (Fox 1960). The causative agent of louse-borne typhus fever, *Rickettsia prowazeki*, can be transmitted by *P. spinulosa* (del Ponte 1958).

Hoplopleura acanthopus, Hoplopleura captiosa, Hoplopleura pacifica

Hoplopleura acanthopus is found on voles, red-backed mice, deer mice, European field mice, lemming mice *(Synaptomys)*, and pine mice *(Pitymys)* throughout the world and is occasionally found on the house mouse and laboratory mouse (Ferris 1951; Heston 1941; Johnson 1960). *Hoplo-pleura captiosa*, which has been erroneously reported as *H. hesperomydis* and *H. acanthopus,* is the only louse that may be primarily a parasite of the house mouse (Johnson 1960). It occurs in Europe, Asia, and Africa and is occasionally found on the laboratory mouse. *Hoplopleura pacifica,* or the tropical rat louse, has been incorrectly called *H. oenomydis.* It is a parasite of the black rat, Norway rat, and other wild rats throughout the world (Ferris 1951; Voss 1966). Rats brought into the laboratory from their natural habitat are frequently infested with *H. pacifica* (Sasa et al. 1962), but it has not been reported from laboratory-raised rats. None of these lice occur on cesarean-derived, barrier-sustained laboratory rodents (Flynn, Brennan, and Fritz 1965; Foster 1963; Owen 1968).

MORPHOLOGY

Hoplopleura (Fig. 13.2) is a slender louse, 1.0 to 2.0 mm long, that has seven to eight lateral plates on the abdomen (Kim 1965). Each plate is large and generally rectangular. The abdomen also has numerous ventral plates, and each abdominal segment usually bears two to three dorsal plates. The eggs are oval, about 0.5

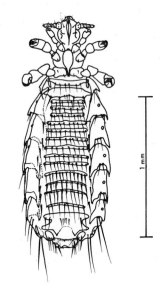

Fig. 13.2. *Hoplopleura acanthopus* female, ventral view. (Courtesy of K. C. Kim, Pennsylvania State University.)

mm long, and are attached to hairs with a drop of cement (Ferris 1951). The three nymphal stages have a characteristic heart-shaped abdomen but usually lack spiracles (Cook and Beer 1959; Kim 1966; Pratt and Karp 1953).

LIFE CYCLE

The complete life cycle is unknown. Transmission is presumably by direct contact.

PATHOLOGIC EFFECTS

The pathologic effects of *Hoplopleura* are similar to those described for *Polyplax*. *Hoplopleura acanthopus* transmits *Brucella brucei,* a common pathogen of small field rodents (Parnas et al. 1960a, b).

DIAGNOSIS

Diagnosis is based on demonstration of the parasite in the pelage.

CONTROL

The isolation, sanitation, and treatment procedures effective for *Polyplax* should be effective for *Hoplopleura* (Farris 1950; Heston 1941; Pratt and Littig 1961).

PUBLIC HEALTH CONSIDERATIONS

These lice are of no known public health importance.

Haemodipsus ventricosus

(Rabbit Louse)

Haemodipsus ventricosus has been recorded from the domestic rabbit in many parts of the world (Ferris 1951; Litvishko, Kharchenko, and Tertyshnyi 1965). It causes pruritus and alopecia and is a vector of the agent of tularemia. There are no recent reports of this louse on laboratory rabbits; it is probably rare in properly managed facilities (Meek 1943; Napier 1963).

MORPHOLOGY

Haemodipsus ventricosus (Fig. 13.3) is 1.2 to 2.5 mm long (Ferris 1932). It has a small head, a large oval abdomen, and numerous long hairs on the dorsal and ventral surfaces. The abdomen has no dorsal plates, but small lateral plates are present. The thorax has a pair of small spiracles and a ventral plate, which is about three

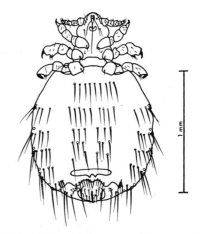

FIG. 13.3. *Haemodipsus ventricosus* female, ventral view. (Courtesy of K. C. Kim, Pennsylvania State University.)

times as wide as long. The egg is oval, measures 0.5 to 0.7 mm long, and has an apical operculum. The nymphs are yellow and translucent before feeding and red when engorged.

LIFE CYCLE

Eggs hatch in about 7 days, and the entire life cycle is completed in about 30 days (Litvishko, Kharchenko, and Tertyshnyi 1965). Transmission is apparently by direct contact.

PATHOLOGIC EFFECTS

The rabbit louse usually occurs on the dorsal and lateral surfaces of the body and pelvic area. It causes extreme pruritus, and alopecia results from rubbing and scratching (Litvishko, Kharchenko, Tertyshnyi 1965; McDougall 1929). *Haemodipsus ventricosus* usually infests young rabbits more heavily than adults, causing debility and retarded growth (Lamson 1921; Litvishko, Karchenko, and Tertyshnyi 1965). This louse is a vector of *Francisella tularensis* (Riley and Johannsen 1938; Shaughnessy 1963; Strong 1944).

DIAGNOSIS

Diagnosis is based on the clinical signs and on demonstration of the parasite or its eggs.

CONTROL

The isolation, sanitation, and treatment procedures effective for *Polypax* should be effective for *H. ventricosus*. Specific insecticides recommended for use on the rabbit include rotenone as a 1.0 to 1.5% dust, trichlorfon as a 10% dust, chlordane as a 1 to 2% dust, lindane as a 1% dust or 0.025% dip, and DDT as a 10% dust or a 5% dip (Gildow 1948; Institute of Animal Resources 1954; Litvishko, Kharchenko, and Tertyshnyi 1965; U.S. Department of Agriculture 1967a).

PUBLIC HEALTH CONSIDERATIONS

Indirectly, *H. ventricosus* is a public health hazard as it is a vector of *F. tularensis* in rabbits (Ellner 1960; Riley and Johannsen 1938). This agent causes tularemia in man.

Linognathus setosus

(Dog Sucking Louse)

Linognathus setosus is frequently found on the dog, particularly on long-hair breeds (Busvine 1966), throughout the world. It causes little irritation except in heavy infestations. This louse has also been recorded from wild canids and occasionally from the rabbit and chicken (Ferris 1951; Tarry 1967). It is sometimes found on research dogs obtained from pounds, but is usually absent from those raised in kennels.

MORPHOLOGY

Linognathus setosus (Fig. 13.4) is a large louse, 1.7 to 2.5 mm long, and is blue when fully engorged (Roberts 1952). The head is blunt, rounded anteriorly, and about as wide as long. The abdomen is oval and covered with numerous long hairs. Six spiracles are located on each side, but no plates are evident. The thoracic spiracles are large.

LIFE CYCLE

Eggs are deposited on hairs and hatch in 5 to 12 days (U.S. Departments of the Army and the Air Force 1958). Other details of the life cycle are unknown. Transmission is by direct contact. It is also possible to transfer this louse from dog to

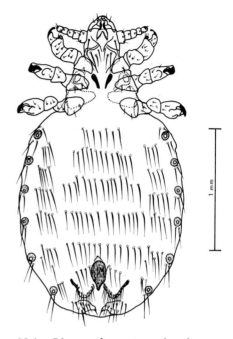

Fig. 13.4. *Linognathus setosus* female, ventral view. (Courtesy of K. C. Kim, Pennsylvania State University.)

dog on brushes, combs, or similar equipment (Blakemore 1968).

PATHOLOGIC EFFECTS

The dog louse is found primarily on the neck and shoulders, especially under a collar. A heavy infestation causes restlessness, scratching, skin inflammation, and alopecia (Roberts 1952; U.S. Departments of the Army and the Air Force 1958).

DIAGNOSIS

Diagnosis is based on the clinical signs and on demonstration of the parasite or its eggs.

CONTROL

Newly acquired dogs should be examined and, if infested, isolated and treated. Dusts containing 5% methoxychlor, chlordane, or DDT or 1% lindane applied topically to the pelage are effective treatments (Blakemore 1968; Roberts 1952; U.S. Department of Agriculture 1967a; Whitney 1950; Woodnott 1963). Lindane as a 0.01% rinse is also effective. The treated dog should be placed in a clean, disinfected cage; treatment should be repeated at weekly intervals for 2 to 3 weeks.

Systemic insecticides are also effective for the control of lice on dogs. Ronnel given orally at a dose of approximately 50 to 100 mg per kg of body weight every 2 to 4 days has given excellent results (Burch 1960; Burch and Brinkman 1962).

PUBLIC HEALTH CONSIDERATIONS

Linognathus setosus is of no known public health importance.

Pedicinus

Pedicinus eurygaster is found on macaques of tropical Asia; *P. obtusus* occurs on langurs or leaf monkeys, the green monkey, other guenons, and sometimes macaques and baboons of southeastern Asia and Africa; *P. patas* is found on guenons and colobus monkeys *(Colobus)* of India and Africa; and *P. mjobergi* occurs on howler monkeys of South America (Hopkins 1949; Kuhn and Ludwig 1967; Myers and Kuntz 1965; Pope 1966). Although Old World laboratory primates obtained from their natural environment are only occasionally infested with these relatively harmless parasites (Luck 1957; Young et al. 1957), infestation of New World specimens appears to be commoner. An incidence of 37% has been reported in the howler monkey (Pope 1966).

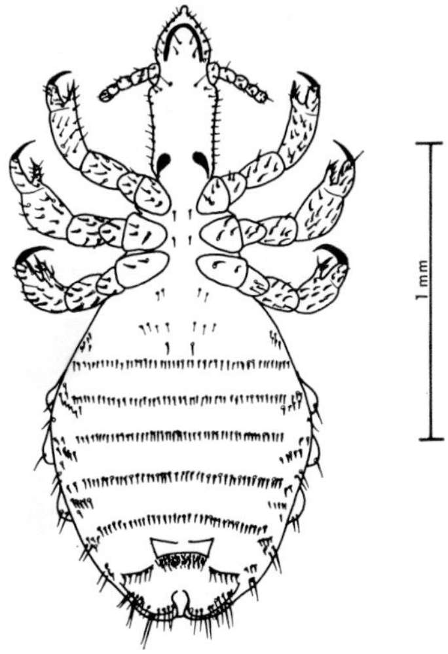

FIG. 13.5. *Pedicinus obtusus* female, ventral view. (Courtesy of K. C. Kim, Pennsylvania State University.)

MORPHOLOGY

Pedicinus (Fig. 13.5) is a slender louse, about 1.0 to 3.0 mm long, with a long head and two to three lateral plates on the abdomen (Ferris 1951; Kuhn and Ludwig 1967). The head has a pair of distinct eyes. The abdomen is membranous, except for the usual terminal and genital plates, and has several rows of minute hairs on both sides of the abdomen (Kuhn and Ludwig 1967). The egg is oval, about 0.6 to 0.9 mm long and 0.3 to 0.5 mm in diameter, and has an operculum which bears 9 to 10 cellulae. Each of the three nymphal stages has a characteristic chaetotaxy and a definite number of lateral abdominal plates.

LIFE CYCLE

The complete life cycle is unknown. Transmission is presumably by direct contact.

PATHOLOGIC EFFECTS

Pedicinus is relatively unimportant to laboratory monkeys (Luck 1957). No irritation or other clinical signs have been observed in infested monkeys.

DIAGNOSIS

Diagnosis is based on demonstration of the parasite.

CONTROL

Newly acquired monkeys should be examined and, if infested, isolated and treated. A dust containing 5.0% carbaryl, 0.1% pyrethrins, 2.0% dichlorophen, and 1.0% piperonyl butoxide (Diryl, Pitman-Moore), applied topically, has given good results (Young et al. 1957). The treated animal should be placed in a clean, disinfected cage; treatment should be repeated at weekly intervals for 2 to 3 weeks.

PUBLIC HEALTH CONSIDERATIONS

Pedicinus is of no known public health importance.

MALLOPHAGANS

The mallophagans, or biting lice, differ from the sucking lice by the presence of a pair of strong mandibles on the lower surface of the head, club-shaped or threadlike antennae with three to five segments, and a typically free first thoracic segment which is narrower than the head (Brues, Melander, and Carpenter 1954; Séguy 1944). These lice feed primarily on epidermal tissue and debris. They have been noted to ingest blood, but this is usually incidental to their other feeding.

Although a few biting lice occur on mammals, most are parasites of birds. They are not common in the laboratory but are sometimes encountered on animals obtained from their natural environment. Those which occur on endothermal laboratory animals are listed in Table 13.2. The most important are discussed below.

Gliricola porcelli, Gyropus ovalis

(Guinea Pig Lice)

Guinea pig lice are relatively benign. They are common on laboratory guinea pigs and also occur on wild species of *Cavia* in South America (Paterson 1962; Werneck 1948). Each has been reported from conventional guinea pig colonies throughout the world (Cook 1963; Deoras and Patel 1960; Meyer and Eddie 1952; Owen 1968; Sasa et al. 1962; Seamer and Chesterman 1967). These lice are common in some colonies and rare or absent in others; they do not occur in cesarean-de-

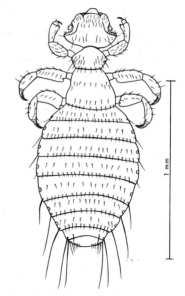

FIG. 13.7. *Gyropus ovalis* female, dorsal view. (Courtesy of R. D. Price, University of Minnesota.)

rived, barrier-sustained colonies (Calhoon and Matthews 1964; Morris 1963).

MORPHOLOGY

Gliricola porcelli, or the slender guinea pig louse (Fig. 13.6), is yellow and measures 1.0 to 1.5 mm long (Séguy 1944). Its head, which is longer than wide, has short, clubbed, and almost concealed antennae. The legs do not have distinct tarsal claws. The abdomen is long, the sides are somewhat parallel, and five pairs of spiracles are present.

Gyropus ovalis, or the oval guinea pig louse (Fig. 13.7), is light in color and 1.0 to 1.2 mm long (Séguy 1944). Its head is wider than long, and the antennae are short, club shaped, and nearly concealed. Each leg has one tarsal claw; those on the second and third pairs of legs are stout and striated. The abdomen is broad at the middle and has several rows of short, fine dorsal hairs and six pairs of spiracles.

LIFE CYCLE

Little is known of the life cycles of these lice. They live in the pelage of the guinea pig and cement their eggs to the hair (Roetti 1964). The immature stages,

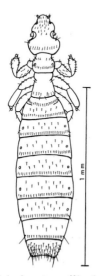

FIG. 13.6. *Gliricola porcelli* female, dorsal view. (Courtesy of R. D. Price, University of Minnesota.)

like the adults, are believed to feed principally on skin debris. Transmission is primarily by direct contact.

PATHOLOGIC EFFECTS

Mild infestations usually cause no clinical signs (Paterson 1967). Heavy infestations are characterized by general unthriftiness, a rough coat, alopecia, and scratching, especially at the back of the ears (Owen 1968).

DIAGNOSIS

Diagnosis is based on demonstration of the parasites. Infestation is often undetected until the death of the host, at which time lice occasionally are noted on the ends of hairs as the body temperature decreases.

CONTROL

The isolation, sanitation, and treatment procedures effective against *Polyplax* are recommended for the control of these lice (Cook 1963; Lane-Petter and Porter 1963; Meyer and Eddie 1952; Woodnott 1963).

Lice can be completely eliminated from laboratory guinea pigs by maintaining cesarean-derived animals and their offspring in an environment free of these parasites (Calhoon and Matthews 1964; Morris 1963).

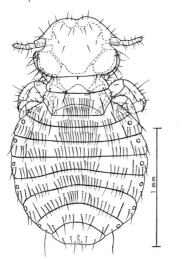

FIG. 13.8. *Trichodectes canis* female, dorsal view. (Courtesy of R. D. Price, University of Minnesota.)

PUBLIC HEALTH CONSIDERATIONS

These lice are of no known public health importance.

Trichodectes canis
(Dog Biting Louse)

Trichodectes canis is found on the dog and wild canids throughout the world (Werneck 1948). It causes little irritation except in heavy infestations; it is a vector of the dog tapeworm. Although this louse was a common parasite of pound dogs in the past and is still reported as common in some laboratory colonies (Sasa et al. 1962), it is now becoming less prevalent, especially in the United States (Dement 1965). It does not usually occur on kennel-raised dogs.

MORPHOLOGY

Trichodectes canis (Fig. 13.8) is a short, broad louse, approximately 2.0 mm long, and is yellow with dark markings (Dement 1965; Roberts 1952). The head is quadrangular and broader than long. The antennae are short, stout, three-segmented, and fully exposed; the male antennae have a much enlarged basal segment. Each leg has only one tarsal claw. The abdomen is oval and has one dorsal transverse row of medium-length hairs across each segment and six pairs of spiracles.

LIFE CYCLE

After fertilization, the female lays several eggs daily for the rest of her life, which is about 30 days (Dement 1965). The eggs are cemented near the base of the hair. They hatch in 1 to 2 weeks, molt three times, and develop into mature lice in about 2 weeks. The complete life cycle requires 3 to 4 weeks. The louse feeds on tissue debris and will survive only 3 to 7 days if separated from the host. Transmission is primarily by direct contact, but it is also possible to transfer this louse from dog to dog on brushes, combs, or similar equipment (Blakemore 1968).

PATHOLOGIC EFFECTS

This louse is usually found on the head, neck, and tail, attached by its claws or mandibles to the base of a hair (Dement

1965). Concentrations of lice seeking moisture occur near body openings or skin abrasions. The usual signs are irritation, rubbing, scratching, biting of infested areas, sleeplessness, nervousness, alopecia, and a rough, matted coat. Infestations are more prevalent on dogs which are either very young, old, debilitated, or maintained in an unsanitary environment.

Trichodectes canis is a vector for *Dipylidium caninum,* a tapeworm that affects the dog and cat and sometimes man (Dement 1965).

DIAGNOSIS

Diagnosis is based on the clinical signs and on demonstration of the parasite or its eggs.

CONTROL

Newly acquired dogs should be examined and, if infested, isolated and treated. Dusts containing up to 5% malathion, 5% methoxychlor, 1% rotenone, 1% pyrethrins, 5% DDT, 5% chlordane, or 1% lindane and sprays containing up to 0.5% malathion, 0.5% methoxychlor, 0.5% DDT, or 0.025% lindane applied topically are effective (Blakemore 1968; U.S. Department of Agriculture 1967b; Woodnott 1963). Also reportedly effective is the topical application of a sorptive silica dust (Dri-Die 67, FMC Corporation) (Tarshis 1962). The treated dog should be placed in a clean, disinfected cage; treatment should be repeated at weekly intervals for 2 to 3 weeks.

Systemic insecticides are also effective for the control of lice of dogs. Ronnel, given orally at a dose of approximately 50 to 100 mg per kg of body weight every 2 to 4 days, has given excellent results (Burch 1960; Burch and Brinkman 1962).

PUBLIC HEALTH CONSIDERATIONS

Dipylidium caninum is occasionally transmitted to man by ingestion of an infected louse.

Felicola subrostratus

(Cat Louse)

Felicola subrostratus is of little pathologic importance and is usually found in large numbers only on aged or diseased cats and some wild felids (Roberts 1952;

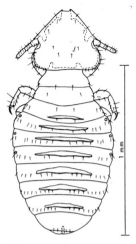

Fig. 13.9. *Felicola subrostratus* female, dorsal view. (Courtesy of R. D. Price, University of Minnesota.)

Werneck 1948). It occurs in North and South America, Europe, and Africa and is probably cosmopolitan. Although this louse is the commonest cause of lousiness of cats, infestation with it is often unnoticed; consequently, its true incidence is unknown (Renaux 1964). It probably occurs occasionally on research cats obtained from pounds.

MORPHOLOGY

Felicola subrostratus (Fig. 13.9) has a triangular head, which is pointed anteriorly, and has a median longitudinal ventral groove (Roberts 1952). The antennae are three-segmented, fully exposed, and similar in both sexes. The adults are 1.0 to 1.5 mm long and are yellow to tan. There is one tarsal claw on each leg. The abdomen is short and broad and has three pairs of spiracles and a sparse, fine, transverse row of minute dorsal hairs across each segment.

LIFE CYCLE

The eggs are laid on the fur of the cat (Renaux 1964). They hatch in 10 to 20 days and reach the adult stage in 2 to 3 weeks. The complete life cycle requires 3 to 6 weeks. The louse feeds on skin debris. Adults usually live 2 to 3 weeks but cannot survive off the host for more than a few days. Transmission is primarily by direct contact.

PATHOLOGIC EFFECTS

Heavy infestations cause restlessness, pruritus, scratching, a ruffled coat, and sometimes alopecia (Renaux 1964; Scott 1967).

DIAGNOSIS

Diagnosis is based on the clinical signs and on demonstration of the parasite or its eggs.

CONTROL

Control is similar to that for *Trichodectes canis,* except that DDT and lindane are not recommended for cats (Burch 1960; U.S. Department of Agriculture 1967b; Woodnott 1963).

PUBLIC HEALTH CONSIDERATIONS

Felicola subrostratus is of no known public health importance.

Cuclotogaster heterographa

(Chicken Head Louse)

Cuclotogaster heterographa is a common parasite of the chicken and other fowl throughout the world (Emerson 1956). It causes irritation, restlessness, and debility, especially in young chickens. There are no reports of this louse on laboratory chickens; it probably occurs infrequently in properly managed facilities.

MORPHOLOGY

Cuclotogaster heterographa (Fig. 13.10) is gray and about 2.0 mm long (Emerson 1956). Its head is longer than wide, evenly rounded in front, and widest posterior to the antennae. The antennae are five-segmented and fully exposed; those of the male have a much enlarged basal segment. The posteriodorsal margin of the thorax has four clusters of long setae. Each leg has two tarsal claws. The dorsal abdomen has a single row of hairs on each segment; the dorsal plates are divided medially on most of the segments.

LIFE CYCLE

The complete life cycle requires 2 to 3 weeks (Metcalf, Flint, and Metcalf 1962; Wilson 1934). Adults live several months on the host but only 5 to 6 days away from the host. The lice feed on tissue debris

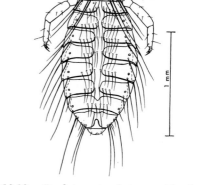

FIG. 13.10. *Cuclotogaster heterographa* female, dorsal view. (Courtesy of R. D. Price, University of Minnesota.)

and occasionally ingest blood. Transmission is primarily by direct contact.

PATHOLOGIC EFFECTS

This louse is usually found on the skin and feathers of the head and neck (Roberts and Smith 1956). It causes irritation, restlessness, damaged plumage, and weight loss or retarded growth. Young or debeaked birds and those debilitated by disease or malnutrition are more commonly affected (Benbrook 1965). Severe infestations in young chickens are sometimes fatal.

DIAGNOSIS

Diagnosis is based on the clinical signs and identification of the parasite.

CONTROL

Newly acquired chickens should be examined and, if infested, isolated and treated. Dusts containing 4 to 5% malathion, 5% carbaryl, 5% DDT, 0.25% chlordane, or 1 to 10% rotenone and sprays containing 0.5% malathion or 4.0% carbaryl applied topically to the plumage are effective (Benbrook 1965; Král and Schwartzman 1964; U.S. Department of

Agriculture 1967a). The treated chicken should be put into a clean cage; treatment should be repeated at weekly intervals for 2 to 3 weeks.

PUBLIC HEALTH CONSIDERATIONS

Cuclotogaster heterographa is of no known public health importance.

Goniocotes gallinae
(Fluff Louse)

Geniocotes gallinae is common on the chicken throughout the world (Emerson 1956). It is of little pathologic importance, causing only minor irritation except in heavy infestations. There are no reports of this louse on the laboratory chicken; it is probably rare in properly managed facilities.

MORPHOLOGY

Goniocotes gallinae (Fig. 13.11) is pale yellow and about 1.5 mm long and appears almost circular (Emerson 1956). The head is broader than long, rounded in front and angulate behind; the antennae are five-segmented, fully exposed, and the same in both sexes. There are four long hairs and several short ones on the head. Each leg

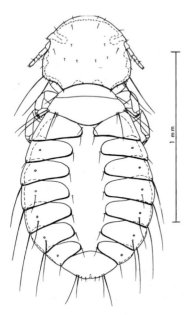

FIG. 13.11. *Goniocotes gallinae* female, dorsal view. (Courtesy of R. D. Price, University of Minnesota.)

has two tarsal claws. The dorsal abdomen has few hairs.

LIFE CYCLE

The life cycle is unknown. Transmission is presumably by direct contact.

PATHOLOGIC EFFECTS

This louse is usually found in small numbers on the down feathers anywhere on the body (Roberts and Smith 1956). It generally causes little irritation, but restlessness, damaged plumage, and weight loss sometimes accompany heavy infestations.

DIAGNOSIS

Diagnosis is based on the clinical signs and identification of the parasite.

CONTROL

The control methods described for *Cuclotogaster heterographa* are also effective for this louse (Benbrook 1965; Král and Schwartzman 1964; U.S. Department of Agriculture 1967a).

PUBLIC HEALTH CONSIDERATIONS

Goniocotes gallinae is of no known public health importance.

Goniodes dissimilis, Goniodes gigas

Goniodes dissimilis is common on the chicken and other fowl and is probably cosmopolitan in distribution (Emerson 1956). *Goniodes gigas* is also common on the chicken and other fowl. It occurs in North and Central America, Australia, Africa, Europe, and probably other parts of the world. *Goniodes dissimilis* is commoner in temperate climates, and *G. gigas* is more prevalent in the tropics. They are of little pathologic importance except in heavy infestations. These lice are seldom reported on the laboratory chicken (Deoras and Patel 1960); they are probably rare in properly managed facilities.

MORPHOLOGY

These are the largest lice occurring on the chicken; they are brown and about 3.0 mm long (Emerson 1956). The head is broadly rounded in front, angulate behind, and somewhat wider than long; the five-segmented antennae are fully exposed. Each leg has two tarsal claws. The body

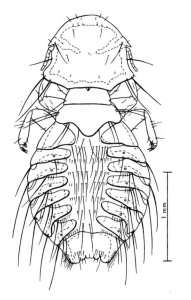

FIG. 13.12. *Goniodes dissimilis* female, dorsal view. (Courtesy of R. D. Price, University of Minnesota.)

is shaped like that of *Goniocotes* but is larger. *Goniodes dissimilis* (Fig. 13.12) has four long hairs on the posterior margin of the head. The antennae are sexually dimorphic; those of the male have a much enlarged basal segment. *Goniodes gigas* has six long hairs on the posterior margin of the head, and the antennae of the male and female are similar.

LIFE CYCLE

The life cycle of *G. gigas* requires 1 month (Conci 1956). The female lays up to 14 eggs, which hatch in about 7 days. Males live a maximum of 19 days and females a maximum of 24 after reaching maturity. The life cycle of *G. dissimilis* is unknown but is probably similar. Transmission is presumably by direct contact.

PATHOLOGIC EFFECTS

These lice occur anywhere on the body of the host. Although large in size, they generally occur in small numbers, and their effects are relatively minor.

DIAGNOSIS

Diagnosis is based on the clinical signs and identification of the parasite.

CONTROL

The control procedures suggested for *Cuclotogastra heterographa* are effective for these lice (Benbrook 1965; Král and Schwartzman 1964; U.S. Department of Agriculture 1967a).

PUBLIC HEALTH CONSIDERATIONS

Goniodes dissimilis and *G. gigas* are of no known public health importance.

Lipeurus caponis

(Wing Louse)

This louse is common on the chicken and other fowl throughout the world (Emerson 1956). It is of little pathologic importance except in heavy infestations. There are no reports of it from the laboratory chicken, but it is probably rare in properly managed animal facilities.

MORPHOLOGY

Lipeurus caponis (Fig. 13.13) is a long, slender, gray louse about 2.5 mm in length (Emerson 1956). The head is longer than wide and evenly rounded in front. The antennae are five-segmented and fully exposed; those of the male have a much enlarged basal segment. Each leg has two

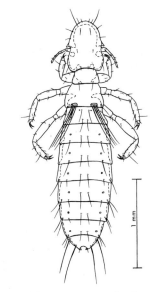

FIG. 13.13. *Lipeurus caponis* female, dorsal view. (Courtesy of R. D. Price, University of Minnesota.)

tarsal claws. The posteriodorsal margin of the thorax has two clusters of long hairs; the abdomen has relatively few dorsal hairs.

LIFE CYCLE

The life cycle requires 3 to 5 weeks in vitro (Wilson 1939); presumably the natural life cycle is of similar length. Transmission is primarily by direct contact.

PATHOLOGIC EFFECTS

This louse infests the ventral side of primary wing feathers and sometimes the tail and back feathers (Roberts and Smith 1956). It is relatively nonmotile. Heavy infestations probably cause restlessness, irritation, and unthriftiness.

DIAGNOSIS

Diagnosis is based on the clinical signs and identification of the parasite.

CONTROL

The control procedures recommended for *Cuclotogaster heterographa* are effective for this louse (Benbrook 1965; Král and Schwartzman 1964; U.S. Department of Agriculture 1967a).

PUBLIC HEALTH CONSIDERATIONS

Lipeurus caponis is of no known public health importance.

Menacanthus stramineus

(Chicken Body Louse)

This is the commonest and most destructive louse found on the chicken (Emerson 1956; Roberts and Smith 1956). It also occurs on other fowl and is worldwide in distribution. There are no reports of its occurrence on laboratory fowl; it is probably uncommon in properly managed animal facilities.

MORPHOLOGY

Menacanthus stramineus (Fig. 13.14) is yellow and 3.0 to 3.5 mm long (Emerson 1956). The head is roughly triangular. The antennae are club shaped and mostly concealed beneath the head. The ventral portion of the forehead is armed with a pair of spinelike processes, which are indicated by dashes in Figure 13.14. Each leg has

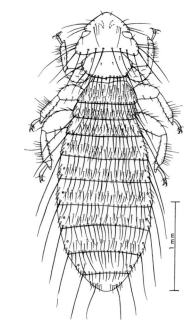

FIG. 13.14. *Menacanthus stramineus* female, dorsal view. (Courtesy of R. D. Price, University of Minnesota.)

two tarsal claws. The abdomen is elongated, broadly rounded posteriorly, and has two or more transverse rows of hairs on most dorsal plates.

LIFE CYCLE

The eggs are deposited in masses at the base of the feathers, especially around the vent. Egg incubation requires 4 to 5 days; the three nymphal stages require about 3 days each (Stockdale and Raun 1965). The female lives about 12 days and produces up to four eggs a day. The complete life cycle requires about 2 weeks. Transmission is primarily by direct contact.

PATHOLOGIC EFFECTS

This louse occurs anywhere on the body but usually on the skin of the less densely feathered parts such as the breast, thighs, and around the vent (Lapage 1962). It causes pronounced skin irritation and small blood clots near the vent (Roberts and Smith 1956). Weight gain is decreased and mortality is increased. This louse sometimes gnaws through the skin or punctures the soft quills near the base and consumes the blood that oozes out (Benbrook 1965).

The virus of equine encephalomyelitis has been isolated from this louse (Benbrook 1965).

DIAGNOSIS

Diagnosis is based on the clinical signs and identification of the parasite.

CONTROL

The control procedures recommended for *Cuclotogaster heterographa* are also effective against this louse (Benbrook 1965; Lapage 1962; U.S. Department of Agriculture 1967a).

PUBLIC HEALTH CONSIDERATIONS

Aside from its possible association with the virus of equine encephalomyelitis (Benbrook 1965), *M. stramineus* is of no known public health importance.

Menopon gallinae
(Shaft Louse)

This louse is a common parasite of the chicken and other fowl and is worldwide in distribution (Emerson 1956). It is probably of little pathologic importance. There are no reports of it from the laboratory chicken; it is probably rare in properly managed animal facilities.

MORPHOLOGY

Menopon gallinae (Fig. 13.15) is pale yellow and about 2.0 mm long (Emerson 1956). The head is roughly triangular in shape; the antennae are club shaped and almost concealed below the head. Each leg has two tarsal claws. The elongated abdomen is tapered posteriorly in the female but is rounded in the male. Only one dorsal transverse row of hairs is present on each abdominal segment.

LIFE CYCLE

Eggs are deposited one at a time at the base of a feather, sometimes several on one feather (Roberts and Smith 1956). The life cycle is unknown. Transmission is probably by direct contact.

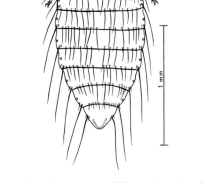

FIG. 13.15. *Menopon gallinae* female, dorsal view. (Courtesy of R. D. Price, University of Minnesota.)

PATHOLOGIC EFFECTS

This louse usually occurs on the thigh and breast feathers. Little is known of its effects, but it probably causes irritation, restlessness, and unthriftiness.

The ornithosis agent has been isolated from this louse (Benbrook 1965).

DIAGNOSIS

Diagnosis is based on the clinical signs and identification of the parasite.

CONTROL

The control procedures effective for *Cuclotogaster heterographa* are effective for this louse (Benbrook 1965; Král and Schwartzman 1964; Lapage 1962; U.S. Department of Agriculture 1967a).

PUBLIC HEALTH CONSIDERATIONS

The ornithosis agent has been isolated from this louse (Benbrook 1965); otherwise, it is of no known public health importance.

TABLE 13.1. Anoplurans affecting endothermal laboratory animals

Parasite	Geographic Distribution	Endothermal Host	Usual Habitat	Incidence — In nature	Incidence — In laboratory	Pathologic Effects	Public Health Importance	Reference
*Polyplax serrata**	Worldwide	Mouse, European field mice	Pelage, especially of shoulders	Common	Common in some colonies; rare or absent in others	Pruritus, restlessness, debilitation, anemia, sometimes death; vector of *Eperythrozoon coccoides, Francisella tularensis*	Possible vector of agent of tularemia (between rodents)	Flynn 1955 Heine 1962 Heston 1941 Murray 1961 Oldham 1967
*Polyplax spinulosa**	Worldwide	Rat, black rat, European field mice, voles	Pelage, especially of back	Common	Common in some colonies; absent in others	Pruritus, restlessness, debilitation, anemia, sometimes death; vector of *Rickettsia typhi, Haemobartonella muris;* possible vector of *Brucella brucei, Borrelia duttoni, Trypanosoma lewisi*	Vector of agent of typhus, louse-borne typhus fever (between rodents)	Holmes 1959 Jenkins and Fletcher 1964 Oldham 1967 Tarshis 1962
Polyplax alaskensis (*P. abscisa*)	Temperate regions	Voles	Pelage	Uncommon	Uncommon	Irritation	Unknown	Scanlon and Johnson 1957
Polyplax borealis	Temperate regions	Red-backed mice, tree voles (*Phenacomys*)	Pelage	Uncommon	Uncommon	Irritation	Unknown	Scanlon and Johnson 1957
*Hoplopleura acanthopus**	Worldwide	Mouse, voles, deer mice, European field mice, other rodents	Pelage	Common on voles, deer mice, European field mice; uncommon on mouse	Common on voles, deer mice, European field mice; uncommon on mouse	Pruritus, anemia; vector of *Brucella brucei*	None known	Ferris 1951 Heston 1941 Johnson 1960
*Hoplopleura captiosa**	Europe, Asia, Africa	Mouse	Pelage	Common	Uncommon	Pruritus	None known	Johnson 1960 Kim 1966
*Hoplopleura pacifica**	Worldwide	Rat, black rat, other rodents	Pelage	Common	Uncommon	Pruritus	None known	Pratt and Karp 1953
Hoplopleura hesperomydis	North America	Deer mice	Pelage	Common	Uncommon	Pruritus	Unknown	Kim 1965
Hoplopleura hirsuta	North America, Central America	Cotton rat	Pelage	Common	Uncommon	Pruritus	Unknown	Stojanovich and Pratt 1961

*Discussed in text.

TABLE 13.1 *(continued)*

Parasite	Geographic Distribution	Endothermal Host	Usual Habitat	Incidence In nature	Incidence In laboratory	Pathologic Effects	Public Health Importance	Reference
*Haemodipsus ventricosus**	Worldwide	Rabbit	Pelage, especially of back, sides	Common	Rare or absent	Pruritus, alopecia, debilitation, retarded growth; vector of *Francisella tularensis*	Vector of agent of tularemia (between rabbits)	Litvishko et al. 1965
*Linognathus setosus**	Worldwide	Rabbit, dog, wild canids, chicken	Pelage, plumage, especially of neck, shoulders	Common on dog, wild canids; uncommon on rabbit, chicken	Uncommon on dog; rare or absent on rabbit, chicken	Irritation, pruritus, restlessness, dermatitis, alopecia	None known	Busvine 1966 Roberts 1952 Tarry 1967 U.S. Dept. of Army and Air Force 1958
*Pedicinus eurygaster**	Tropical Asia	Monkey, other macaques	Pelage	Uncommon	Uncommon	None known	None known	Kuhn and Ludwig 1967
*Pedicinus obtusus**	Southeastern Asia, Africa	Langurs, green monkey, other guenons, macaques, baboons	Pelage	Uncommon	Uncommon	None known	None known	Kuhn and Ludwig 1967 Myers and Kuntz 1965
*Pedicinus patas**	India, Africa	Guenons, colobus monkeys	Pelage	Uncommon	Uncommon	None known	None known	Kuhn and Ludwig 1967
Pedicinus hamadryas	Africa	Baboons	Pelage	Uncommon	Uncommon	None known	None known	Myers and Kuntz 1965
*Pedicinus mjobergi**	South America	Howler monkeys	Pelage	Common	Common	None known	None known	Pope 1966
Pediculus schaeffi	Africa	Chimpanzee	Pelage	Rare	Rare	None known	None known	Kim and Emerson 1968

*Discussed in text.

391

TABLE 13.2. Mallophagans affecting endothermal laboratory animals

Parasite	Geographic Distribution	Endothermal Host	Usual Habitat	Incidence		Pathologic Effects	Public Health Importance	Reference
				In nature	In laboratory			
Gliricola porcelli*	Worldwide	Guinea pig, wild Cavia	Pelage	Common	Common in some colonies; rare or absent in others	Pruritus, unthriftiness, roughened coat, alopecia	None known	Meyer and Eddie 1952 Paterson 1967
Gyropus ovalis*	Worldwide	Guinea pig, wild Cavia	Pelage	Common	Common in some colonies; rare or absent in others	Pruritus, unthriftiness, roughened coat, alopecia	None known	Meyer and Eddie 1952 Paterson 1967
Trichodectes canis*	Worldwide	Dog, other canids	Pelage, especially near body openings	Common	Common in some colonies; rare or absent in others	Irritation, pruritus, restlessness, roughened coat, alopecia; vector of Dipylidium caninum	Vector of Dipylidium caninum	Dement 1965
Felicola subrostratus*	Probably worldwide	Cat, other felids	Pelage	Unknown; probably uncommon	Unknown; probably uncommon	Usually none; sometimes pruritus, restlessness, roughened coat, alopecia	None known	Renaux 1964
Cuclotogaster heterographa*	Worldwide	Chicken, other birds	Plumage, especially of head, neck	Common	Unknown; probably uncommon	Irritation, restlessness, damaged plumage, debilitation, weight loss, retarded growth	None known	Benbrook 1965 Emerson 1956 Roberts and Smith 1956
Goniocotes gallinae*	Worldwide	Chicken	Plumage, especially down feathers	Common	Unknown; probably rare	Usually slight irritation; sometimes restlessness, damaged plumage, weight loss	None known	Benbrook 1965 Emerson 1956 Roberts and Smith 1956
Goniodes dissimilis*	Worldwide, especially in temperate climates	Chicken, other birds	Plumage	Common	Unknown; probably rare	Slight irritation	None known	Benbrook 1965 Emerson 1956
Goniodes gigas*	Probably worldwide, especially in tropics	Chicken, other birds	Plumage	Common	Unknown; probably rare	Slight irritation	None known	Benbrook 1965 Deoras and Patel 1960 Emerson 1956

*Discussed in text.

TABLE 13.2 (continued)

Parasite	Geographic Distribution	Endothermal Host	Usual Habitat	Incidence		Pathologic Effects	Public Health Importance	Reference
				In nature	In laboratory			
Lipeurus caponis*	Worldwide	Chicken, other birds	Plumage, especially of wings	Common	Rare	Usually none; sometimes irritation, restlessness, unthriftiness	None known	Emerson 1956 Roberts and Smith 1956
Lipeurus laurensis	Tropics and subtropics	Chicken, other birds	Plumage	Uncommon	Uncommon	Irritation, restlessness, unthriftiness	Unknown	Arora and Chopra 1957, 1959 Emerson 1956
Menacanthus stramineus*	Worldwide	Chicken, other birds	Plumage, especially near vent	Common	Unknown; probably uncommon	Severe irritation, weight loss, sometimes death	Possible association with agent of equine encephalomyelitis	Benbrook 1965 Emerson 1956 Roberts and Smith 1956
Menacanthus cornutus	Probably worldwide	Chicken	Plumage	Uncommon	Unknown; probably rare	Irritation, unthriftiness, sometimes death	Unknown	Emerson 1956
Menacanthus pallidulus	Worldwide	Chicken	Plumage	Uncommon	Unknown; probably rare	Irritation, unthriftiness, sometimes death	Unknown	Emerson 1956
Menopon gallinae*	Worldwide	Chicken, other birds	Plumage	Common	Unknown; probably rare	Probably irritation, restlessness, unthriftiness	Associated with agent of ornithosis	Benbrook 1965 Emerson 1956 Roberts and Smith 1956
Heterodoxus spiniger	Cosmopolitan between 40 N and 40 S latitudes	Dog, other canids	Pelage	Uncommon	Unknown; probably rare	Irritation, alopecia, debilitation	Unknown	Roberts 1952
Lagopoecus sinensis	China	Chicken	Plumage	Rare	Unknown	Unknown	Unknown	Emerson 1957
Oxylipeurus dentatus	Southeastern Asia, central Pacific islands, Central America	Chicken	Plumage	Rare	Unknown	Unknown	Unknown	Emerson 1956
Trimenopon hispidum	Worldwide	Guinea pig, other Cavia	Pelage	Uncommon	Uncommon in some colonies; rare or absent in others	Irritation	None known	Cook 1963 Owen 1968 Werneck 1948

*Discussed in text.

393

REFERENCES

Arora, G. L., and N. P. Chopra. 1957. Some observations on the biology of *Lipeurus tropicalis* Peters (Mallophaga: Ischnocera). Res. Bull. Panjab Univ. 130:485–91.

———. 1959. Observations on the life-history of *Lipeurus tropicalis* Peters (Mallophaga: Ischnocera). Res. Bull. (N.S.) Panjab Univ. 10:179–87.

Bateman, N. 1961. Simultaneous eradication of three ectoparasitic species from a colony of laboratory mice. Nature 191:721–22.

Bell, Deirdre P. 1968. Disease in a caesarian-derived albino rat colony and in a conventional colony. Lab. Animals 2:1–17.

Bell, J. F., and C. Clifford. 1964. Effects of limb disability on lousiness in mice: II. Intersex grooming relationships. Exp. Parasitol. 15:340–49.

Bell, J. F., C. M. Clifford, G. J. Moore, and G. Raymond. 1966. Effects of limb disability in lousiness in mice: III. Gross aspects of acquired resistance. Exp. Parasitol. 18:49–60.

Bell, J. F., W. L. Jellison, and Cora R. Owen. 1962. Effects of limb disability on lousiness in mice: I. Preliminary studies. Exp. Parasitol. 12:176–83.

Benbrook, E. A. 1965. External parasites of poultry, pp. 925–64. In H. E. Biester and L. H. Schwarte, eds. Diseases of poultry. 5th ed. Iowa State Univ. Press, Ames.

Blakemore, J. C. 1968. Macroscopic ectoparasites, pp. 268–73. In R. W. Kirk, ed. Current veterinary therapy III: Small animal practice. W. B. Saunders, Philadelphia.

Brues, C. T., A. L. Melander, and F. M. Carpenter. 1954. Classification of insects. Vol. 108. Bull. Mus. Comp. Zool. Harvard Coll. 917 pp.

Burch, G. R. 1960. Ectoral for control of ectoparasites. Allied Vet. 31:69–72.

Burch, G. R., and D. C. Brinkman. 1962. Systemic insecticide therapy in small animals. Small Animal Clinician 2:21–27.

Busvine, J. R. 1966. Insects and Hygiene. 2d ed. Methuen, London. 467 pp.

Buxton, P. A., and J. R. Busvine. 1957. Pests of the animal house and their control, pp. 67–84. In A. N. Worden and W. Lane-Petter, eds. The UFAW handbook on the care and management of laboratory animals. 2d ed. The Universities Federation for Animal Welfare, London.

Calhoon, J. R., and P. J. Matthews. 1964. A method for initiating a colony of specific pathogen-free guinea pigs. Lab. Animal Care 14:388–94.

Conci, C. 1956. L'allevamento in condizioni sperimentali dei Mallofagi. II. *Stenocrotaphus gigas* (Taschenberg). Mem. Soc. Entomol. Ital. 35:133–50.

Cook, E. F., and J. R. Beer. 1959. The immature stages of the genus *Hoplopleura* (Anoplura: Hoplopleuridae) in North America, with descriptions of two new species. J. Parasitol. 45:405–16.

Cook, R. 1963. Common diseases of laboratory animals, pp. 117–56. In D. J. Short and Dorothy P. Woodnott, eds. A.T.A. manual of laboratory animal practice and techniques. Crosby Lockwood and Son, London.

Davis, G. E. 1960. The relapsing fever, pp. 107–18. In G. W. Hunter, III, W. W. Frye, and J. C. Swartzwelder, eds. A manual of tropical medicine. 3d ed. W. B. Saunders, Philadelphia.

———. 1963. The endemic relapsing fever, pp. 668–81. In T. G. Hull, ed. Diseases transmitted from animals to man. 5th ed. Charles C Thomas, Springfield, Ill.

Dement, W. M. 1965. Pediculosis of the canine. Southeastern Vet. 16:27–31.

Deoras, P. J., and K. K. Patel. 1960. Collection of ectoparasites of laboratory animals. Indian J. Entomol. 22:7–14.

Eliot, C. P. 1936. The insect vector for the natural transmission of *Eperythrozoon coccoides* in mice. Science 84:397.

Ellner, P. D. 1960. Tularemia, pp. 208–12. In G. W. Hunter, III, W. W. Frye, and J. C. Swartzwelder, eds. A manual of tropical medicine. 3d ed. W. B. Saunders, Philadelphia.

Emerson, K. C. 1956. Mallophaga (chewing lice) occurring on the domestic chicken. J. Kansas Entomol. Soc. 29:63–79.

———. 1957. Notes on *Lagopoecus sinensis* (Sugimoto) (Philopteridae, Mallophaga). J. Kansas Entomol. Soc. 30:9–10.

Farris, E. J. 1950. The rat as an experimental animal, pp. 43–78. In E. J. Farris, ed. The care and breeding of laboratory animals. John Wiley, New York.

Ferris, G. F. 1920. Contributions toward a monograph of the sucking lice. Part I. Stanford Univ. Publ. 52 pp.

———. 1932. Contributions toward a monograph of the sucking lice. Part V. Stanford Univ. Publ. 143 pp.

———. 1951. The sucking lice. Pacific Coast Entomol. Soc. Mem. 1:1–320.

Flynn, R. J. 1955. Ectoparasites of mice. Proc. Animal Care Panel 6:75–91.

———. 1963. The diagnosis of some forms of ectoparasitism of mice. Lab. Animal Care 13:111–25.

Flynn, R. J., Patricia C. Brennan, and T. E. Fritz. 1965. Pathogen status of commercially produced laboratory mice. Lab. Animal Care 15:440–47.

Foster, H. L. 1963. Specific pathogen-free animals, pp. 110–38. In W. Lane-Petter, ed. Animals for research: Principles of breeding and management. Academic Press, New York.

Fox, J. P. 1960. Murine typhus, pp. 79–81. In G. W. Hunter, III, W. W. Frye, and J. C. Swartzwelder, eds. A manual of tropical medicine. 3d ed. W. B. Saunders, Philadelphia.

Gildow, E. M. 1948. Success with rabbits: A practical guide to profitable rabbit raising. 2d ed. Albers Milling Co., Oconomowoc, Wis. 62 pp.

Heine, W. 1962. Zur Ektoparasitenbekämpfung bei Maus und Ratte. Z. Versuchstierk. 2:1–22.

Heston, W. E. 1941. Parasites, pp. 349–79. In G. D. Snell, ed. Biology of the laboratory mouse. Blakiston, Philadelphia.

Holmes, D. T. 1959. The life history and comparative infestations of Polyplax spinulosa (Burmeister) on normal and riboflavin-deficient rats. Diss. Abstr. 19:2693–94.

Hopkins, G. H. E. 1949. The host-associations of the lice of mammals. Proc. Zool. Soc. London 119:387–604.

———. 1957. The distribution of Phthiraptera on mammals, pp. 88–119. In Premier Symposium sur la spécificité parasitaire des parasites de Vertébrés. Intern. Union Biol. Sci., Neuchâtel.

Institute of Animal Resources Committee on Handbook. 1954. Handbook of laboratory animals. Natl. Acad. Sci.–Natl. Res. Council Publ. 317, Wash., D.C. 77 pp.

James, M. T., and R. F. Harwood. 1969. Herms's medical entomology. 6th ed. Macmillan, New York. 484 pp.

Jenkins, J. I., and F. J. Fletcher. 1964. The eradication of lice from a rat colony by means of a malathion dipping routine. J. Animal Tech. Assoc. 15:1–6.

Johnson, Phyllis T. 1960. The Anoplura of African rodents and insectivores. U.S. Dept. Agr. Tech. Bull. 1211. 116 pp.

Kim, K. C. 1965. A review of the Hoplopleura hesperomydis complex (Anoplura: Hoplopleuridae). J. Parasitol. 51:871–87.

———. 1966. A new species of Hoplopleura from Thailand, with notes and description of nymphal stages of Hoplopleura captiosa Johnson (Anoplura). Parasitology 56:603–12.

Kim, K. C., and K. C. Emerson. 1968. Descriptions of two species of Pediculidae (Anoplura) from great apes (Primates, Pongidae). J. Parasitol. 54:690–95.

Král, F., and R. M. Schwartzman. 1964. Veterinary and comparative dermatology. J. B. Lippincott, Philadelphia. 444 pp.

Kuhn, H.-J., and H. W. Ludwig. 1967. Die Affenläuse der Gattung Pedicinus. Z. Zool. Syst. Evolutionsforsch. 5:144–256.

Lamson, G. H., Jr. 1921. Lice which affect domestic animals, pp. 330–49. In W. D. Pierce, ed. Sanitary entomology. R. G. Badger, Boston.

Lane-Petter, W., and G. Porter. 1963. The guinea pig, pp. 287–321. In W. Lane-Petter, ed. Animals for research: Principles of breeding and management. Academic Press, New York.

Lapage, G. 1962. Mönnig's veterinary helminthology and entomology. 5th ed. Williams and Wilkins, Baltimore. 600 pp.

Litvishko, N. T., O. N. Kharchenko, and A. A. Tertyshnyi. 1965. Haemodipsus infestation (in Russian). Veterinariya 42:87–89.

Luck, C. R. 1957. The vervet monkey (Cercopithecus aethiops, numerous varieties), pp. 675–79. In A. N. Worden and W. Lane-Petter, eds. The UFAW handbook on the care and management of laboratory animals. 2d ed. The Universities Federation for Animal Welfare, London.

McDougall, J. B. 1929. The rabbit in health and disease. Watmoughs, London. 106 pp.

Meek, M. W. 1943. Diseases and parasites of rabbits and their control. 3d ed. Reliable Fur Industries, Montebello, Calif. 189 pp.

Metcalf, C. L., W. P. Flint, and R. L. Metcalf. 1962. Destructive and useful insects. 4th ed. McGraw-Hill, New York. 1087 pp.

Meyer, K. F., and B. Eddie. 1952. Disease problems in guinea pigs. Proc. Animal Care Panel 2:23–39.

Morris, J. H. 1963. Management of a specific pathogen-free guinea pig colony. Lab. Animal Care 13:96–100.

Murray, M. D. 1961. The ecology of the louse Polyplax serrata (Burm.) on the mouse Mus musculus L. Australian J. Zool. 9:1–13.

Myers, Betty J., and R. E. Kuntz. 1965. A checklist of parasites reported for the baboon. Primates 6:137–94.

Napier, R. A. N. 1963. Rabbits, pp. 323–64. In W. Lane-Petter, ed. Animals for research: Principles of breeding and management. Academic Press, New York.

Oldham, J. N. 1967. Helminths, ectoparasites and protozoa in rats and mice, pp. 641–79. In E. Cotchin and F. J. C. Roe, eds. Pathology of laboratory rats and mice. Blackwell Scientific Publ., Oxford.

Olewine, D. A. 1963. An effective control of Polyplax infestation without the use of insecticide. Lab. Animal Care 13:750–51.

Owen, Dawn. 1968. Investigations: B. Parasitological studies. Lab. Animals Centre News Letter 35:7–9.

Parnas, J., W. Zwolski, and K. Burdzy. 1960a. The infection of the lice *Polyplax spinulosa* and *Hoplopleura acanthopus* with the *Brucella brucei* (in Polish). Wiadomosci Parazytol. 6:441–45.

Parnas, J., W. Zwolski, K. Burdzy, and A. Koslak. 1960b. Zoological, entomological and microbiological studies on natural foci of anthropozoonozes: *Brucella brucei* and *Hoplopleura acanthopus*. Arch. Inst. Pasteur Tunis 37:195–213.

Paterson, J. S. 1962. Guinea-pig disease, pp. 169–84. *In* R. J. C. Harris, ed. The problems of laboratory animal disease. Academic Press, New York.

———. 1967. The guinea-pig or cavy (*Cavia porcellus* L.), pp. 241–87. *In* UFAW Staff, eds. The UFAW handbook on the care and management of laboratory animals. 3d ed. Livingstone and the Universities Federation for Animal Welfare, London.

Ponte, E. del. 1958. Manual de entomología médica y veterinaria argentinas. Ediciones Libreria del Colegio, Buenos Aires. 349 pp.

Pope, Betty L. 1966. Some parasites of the howler monkey of northern Argentina. J. Parasitol. 52:166–68.

Pratt, H. D., and H. Karp. 1953. Notes on the rat lice *Polyplax spinulosa* (Burmeister) and *Hoplopleura oenomydis* Ferris. J. Parasitol. 39:495–504.

Pratt, H. D., and K. S. Littig. 1961. Lice of public health importance and their control. Training Guide, Insect Control Series, Public Health Serv. Publ. 772, Part 8. 16 pp.

Renaux, E. A. 1964. Parasites of the skin, pp. 137–40. *In* E. J. Catcott, ed. Feline medicine and surgery. American Veterinary Publications, Santa Barbara, Calif.

Riley, W. A., and O. A. Johannsen. 1938. Anoplura, or lice, pp. 125–42. *In* W. A. Riley and O. A. Johannsen, eds. Medical entomology. 2d ed. McGraw-Hill, New York.

Roberts, F. H. S. 1952. Insects affecting livestock, with special reference to important species occurring in Australia. Angus and Robertson, Sydney. 267 pp.

Roberts, I. H., and C. L. Smith. 1956. Poultry lice, pp. 490–93. *In* Yearbook Agr. U.S. Dept. Agr.

Roetti, C. 1964. La mallofagosi nelle cavie. Veterinaria 13:44–46.

Sasa, M. 1950. Note on the blood-sucking lice (Anoplura) of rodents in Japan (Part 1). Japan. J. Exp. Med. 20:715–17.

Sasa, M., H. Tanaka, M. Fukui, and A. Takata. 1962. Internal parasites of laboratory animals, pp. 195–214. *In* R. J. C. Harris, ed. The problems of laboratory animal disease. Academic Press, New York.

Scanlon, J. E., and Phyllis T. Johnson. 1957. On some microtine-infesting *Polyplax* (Anoplura). Proc. Entomol. Soc. Wash. D.C. 59:279–83.

Scott, Patricia P. 1967. The cat (*Felis catus* L.), pp. 505–67. *In* UFAW Staff, eds. The UFAW handbook on the care and management of laboratory animals. 3d ed. Livingstone and the Universities Federation for Animal Welfare, London.

Seamer, J., and F. C. Chesterman. 1967. A survey of disease in laboratory animals. Lab. Animals 1:117–39.

Séguy, E. 1944. Insectes ectoparasites (Mallophages, Anoploures, Siphonaptères). Faune de France 43. Paul Lechevalier, Paris. 684 pp.

Shaughnessy, H. J. 1963. Tularemia, pp. 588–604. *In* T. G. Hull, ed. Diseases transmitted from animals to man. 5th ed. Charles C Thomas, Springfield, Ill.

Smetana, A. 1962. Beitrag zur Kenntnis der Bionomie der Mitteleuropäischen Kleinsäugerläuse (Anoplura). Cesk. Parasitol. 9: 375–411.

Stockdale, H. J., and E. S. Raun. 1965. Biology of the chicken body louse, *Menacanthus stramineus*. Ann. Entomol. Soc. Am. 58: 802–5.

Stojanovich, C. J., and H. D. Pratt. 1961. Key to the North American sucking lice in the genera *Hoplopleura* and *Neohaematopinus* with descriptions of two species. (Anoplura: Hoplopleuridae). J. Parasitol. 47:312–16.

Strong, R. P. 1944. Stitt's diagnosis, prevention and treatment of tropical diseases. 7th ed. Blakiston, Philadelphia. 1747 pp.

Symes, C. B., R. C. Muirhead-Thompson, and J. R. Busvine. 1962. Insect control in public health. Elsevier, New York. 227 pp.

Tarry, D. W. 1967. The occurrence of *Linognathus setosus* (Anoplura, Siphunculata) on poultry. Vet. Record 81:641.

Tarshis, I. B. 1962. The use of silica aerogel compounds for the control of ectoparasites. Proc. Animal Care Panel 12:217–58.

———. 1967. Silica aerogel insecticides for the prevention and control of arthropods of medical and veterinary importance. Angew. Parasitol. 8:210–37.

Tuffery, A. A., and J. R. M. Innes. 1963. Diseases of laboratory mice and rats, pp. 48–108. *In* W. Lane-Petter, ed. Animals for research: Principles of breeding and management. Academic Press, New York.

U.S. Department of Agriculture. 1967a. Suggested guide for the use of insecticides to control insects affecting crops, livestock, households, stored products, forests, and forest products. U.S. Dept. Agr., Agr. Handbook 331. 273 pp.

———. 1967b. Controlling fleas. U.S. Dept. Agr., Home Garden Bull. 121. 6 pp.

U.S. Departments of the Army and the Air Force. 1958. Care and management of laboratory animals. Tech. Bull. No. Med. 255; Air Force Pamphlet 160-12-3. 112 pp.

Voss, W. J. 1966. A lectotype designation for *Hoplopleura pacifica* Ewing (Anoplura: Hoplopleuridae). Pacific Insects 8:29–32.

Werneck, F. L. 1948. Os Malófagos de mamíferos: Parte 1: Amblycera e Ischnocera (Philopteridae e parte de Trichodectidae). Rio de Janeiro. 243 pp.

Whitney, L. F. 1950. The dog, pp. 182–201. *In* E. J. Farris, ed. The care and breeding of laboratory animals. John Wiley, New York.

Wilson, F. H. 1934. The life-cycle and bionomics of *Lipeurus heterographus* Nitzsch. J. Parasitol. 20:304–11.

———. 1939. The life-cycle and bionomics of *Lipeurus caponis* (Linn.). Ann. Entomol. Soc. Am. 32:318–20.

Woodnott, Dorothy P. 1963. Pests of the animal house: Part 1: Animal pests, pp. 157–68. *In* D. J. Short and Dorothy P. Woodnott, eds. A.T.A. manual of laboratory animal practice and techniques. Crosby Lockwood and Son, London.

Young, R. J., B. D. Fremming, R. E. Benson, and M. D. Harris. 1957. Care and management of a *Macaca mulatta* monkey colony. Proc. Animal Care Panel 7:67–82.

Chapter 14

TICKS

Ticks constitute the suborder Metastigmata of the subclass Acari. The suborder is divided into two major families: Ixodidae (ixodids) and Argasidae (argasids). All pass through four stages: egg, larva (seed tick), nymph, and adult. The larva has six legs; the nymph and adults have eight. The larva, nymph, and adults of both sexes are parasitic and feed on blood and lymph.

Not only are ticks annoying and debilitating parasites but they surpass all other arthropods in the variety of animal disease agents that they transmit. Many are also notorious for transmitting important pathogens of man.

Because of their complex ecologic requirements, ticks are uncommon in laboratory animal facilities; however, some species can become established indoors, and many species are likely to be brought into a laboratory on animals obtained from their natural habitat. Those which affect endothermal animals frequently used in the laboratory are listed in Tables 14.1 and 14.2. The most important are discussed below.

IXODIDS

All stages of ixodids, or hard ticks, have a heavy shield or scutum on the dorsum. In the adult male, the scutum extends almost to the posterior margin of the body; in the larva, nymph, and adult female, it is restricted to the anterior half of the dorsal surface. The female, nymph, and larva distend when engorged with blood.

Ixodids are known as one-, two-, or three-host ticks, depending on the number of hosts utilized. A species that attaches itself to a host as a larva and then remains for the normal sequence of feeding and molting until maturity is termed a one-host tick. A two-host tick drops off the original host as a nymph, molts to an adult on the ground, and then attaches to a second host. The larva, nymph, and adult of a three-host tick each feed on a different host; both molts occur off the host on the ground. Different host species or the same host species may be used by each of the developmental stages. Oviposition in all three types occurs on the ground or in or near the host nest.

Rhipicephalus sanguineus

(Brown Dog Tick, Kennel Tick)

This tick is important not only because its bite causes discomfort and loss of blood but because it is a vector of several important pathogens. It occurs in numerous tropical and temperate regions of the world (between 50 N and 35 S latitudes) and is common in southwestern United States, Mexico, Central and South America, southern Europe, and Africa (Bishopp and Trembley 1945; Cooley 1946; Gregson 1956; Hoogstraal 1956; Kohls and Parker 1948). In warm climates it occurs outdoors and indoors; in cool climates it is generally confined to heated buildings.

The dog and several wild carnivores are the primary hosts, the cat and man are less frequently affected, and a variety of endothermal animals, including the black rat, other wild rodents, hares, monkey, green monkey, baboons, other simian primates, and many domestic animals, are occasionally infested (Bishopp and Trembley 1945; Hoogstraal 1956, 1967; Myers and Kuntz 1965; Valerio et al. 1969). Indoors, this tick will feed on almost any endothermal animal.

Although *Rhipicephalus sanguineus* is often a serious problem in kennels and animal hospitals, there are few specific reports of its occurrence in laboratory animal facilities (Hirsh et al. 1969; Yunker 1964). It is likely to be encountered on dogs obtained from pounds in endemic areas and in laboratory buildings in which such dogs are housed. It is unlikely to be found on laboratory dogs obtained from kennels that practice good sanitation and parasite control.

MORPHOLOGY

The male is 2.2 to 3.2 mm in length, and the female 2.4 to 2.7 mm when un-
engorged, but up to 11.5 mm after feeding (Fig. 14.1) (Hoogstraal 1956). Both sexes have eyes. The male has an inornate, dark brown scutum with several parallel rows of punctations, an adanal shield, and a hexagonal basis capituli. The shield-shaped female scutum is moderately punctate.

LIFE CYCLE

Rhipicephalus sanguineus is a three-host tick (Hoogstraal 1956). Its life cycle takes a minimum of 2 months and often much longer. After feeding and mating on the final host, the female detaches, drops off, deposits 1,000 to 5,000 eggs in a protected crack or crevice, and dies. Oviposition begins 3 to 6 days after detachment. The eggs hatch after 3 weeks or more and, in a few days, the larvae seek a host. They feed 3 to 8 days, detach, drop to the ground, and in a week or more molt to nymphs. Nymphs find a new host, feed 3 to 11 days, drop off, and in 11 to 15 days molt to adults. Adult females feed for about a week; males remain attached for weeks or months.

PATHOLOGIC EFFECTS

Immature ticks are common in the pelage of the neck whereas adults attach al-

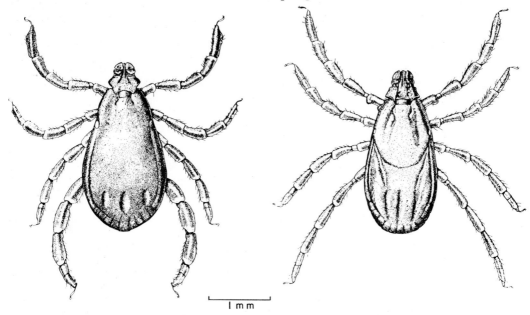

FIG. 14.1. *Rhipicephalus sanguineus.* *(Left)* Male. *(Right)* Female. (Courtesy of U.S. Department of Agriculture.)

most anywhere, frequently between the host's toes (Hoogstraal 1956).

The bite of *R. sanguineus* causes inflammation, hyperemia, edema, hemorrhage, and thickening of the skin (Belding 1965). This tick also transmits many pathogens of endothermal laboratory animals, including *Babesia canis* and *B. vogeli* (the causes of canine babesiosis or malignant jaundice), *Hepatozoon canis* (the cause of canine hepatozoonosis), *Ehrlichia canis* (the cause of canine rickettsiosis), *Salmonella enteritidis* (the cause of paratyphoid in the dog and other laboratory animals), and the filariid nematodes, *Dipetalonema reconditum* and *D. grassii* (Hoogstraal 1956; Levine 1961; Philip and Burgdorfer 1961; Soulsby 1965).

DIAGNOSIS

Diagnosis is based on the signs and on identification of the tick on the host.

CONTROL

Control is based primarily on prevention of infestation of laboratory buildings and on prompt elimination of infestation should it occur. Laboratory animal buildings should be designed in such a way that cracks and crevices are minimized, and cages and pens should be constructed of metal, concrete, or other material that can be readily cleaned and disinfected.

Newly acquired animals should be examined on arrival and treated, if infested. Effective treatments for the dog include a dip containing 0.25% diazinon, a dip or spray containing 0.15% dioxathion, or a dust containing 5.0% carbaryl (Price and McCrady 1961). An effective treatment for the monkey is a dust containing 5.0% carbaryl, 2.0% dichlorophen, 0.1% pyrethrins, and 1.0% piperonyl butoxide (Diryl, Pitman-Moore) (Valerio et al. 1969). DDT, chlordane, lindane, and malathion are relatively ineffective (Hansens 1956; Hazeltine 1959; Price 1957). Ticks can also be removed individually with a forceps (Theis 1968). If firmly clasped near the skin, the parasites' mouthparts seldom remain in the host.

Recommended treatments for infested animal buildings include diazinon as a 0.5% spray or carbaryl as a 5.0% dust (Price and McCrady 1961). DDT as a 5.0%

spray and lindane as a 0.5% spray are also recommended (McIntosh and McDuffie 1956), but their effectiveness for the brown dog tick is uncertain. Cracks and crevices likely to harbor ticks should receive particular attention. The use of a sorptive silica dust has been recommended for the treatment of both animals and buildings (Tarshis 1962, 1967), but its effectiveness is uncertain (Markov et al. 1968).

PUBLIC HEALTH CONSIDERATIONS

The brown dog tick is a vector of several important pathogens of man, including *Rickettsia rickettsi* (the cause of Rocky Mountain spotted fever), *R. siberica* (the cause of Siberian tick typhus), *R. conori* (the cause of boutonneuse fever), and *Francisella tularensis* (the cause of tularemia) (Belding 1965; Cheng 1964; Hoogstraal 1967).

Laboratory animals infested with this tick should be handled with caution, and care should be taken when removing ticks manually to prevent the contamination of open wounds or mucous membranes with blood from crushed ticks.

Dermacentor variabilis

(American Dog Tick)

The American dog tick occurs in damp, grassy, brush-covered areas of eastern, central and far western United States, southern Canada, and Mexico (Bishopp and Trembley 1945; Cooley 1938; Smith, Cole, and Gouck 1946). It is important not only because its bite is annoying and because it is a vector of the agents of Rocky Mountain spotted fever and tularemia but also because its bite sometimes causes paralysis (Robinow and Carroll 1938).

Immature stages feed on many species of wild rodents and lagomorphs, especially deer mice, voles, the cotton rat, rice rat, and cottontail rabbits (Bishopp and Trembley 1945; Hyland and Mathewson 1961; Smith, Cole, and Gouck 1946). Adults are common on the dog and wild carnivores, and they sometimes bite man.

Although this tick seldom invades research animal facilities (Yunker 1964), immature forms are likely to be found on wild rodents and lagomorphs brought into the laboratory from their natural habitat, and adults may be found on dogs obtained from

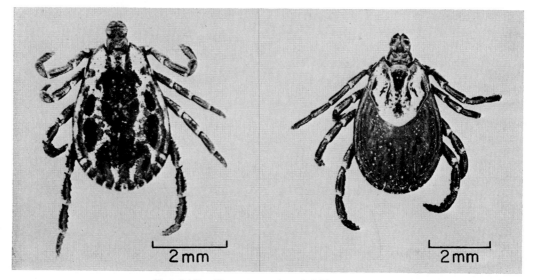

Fig. 14.2. *Dermacentor variabilis.* *(Left)* Male. *(Right)* Female. (Courtesy of G. M. Kohls, Rocky Mountain Laboratory.)

pounds in endemic areas. It is not likely to be encountered on laboratory dogs obtained from kennels that practice good sanitation and parasite control.

MORPHOLOGY

Dermacentor variabilis is a large, ornate tick (Fig. 14.2) (Cooley 1938). The male is 4 to 5 mm in length and has a gray, enameled appearance; the female is slightly larger and has a scutum which is mostly gray. This tick is differentiated from *D. andersoni* by the scutal ornamentation and the smaller, more numerous goblets in its spiracular plates.

LIFE CYCLE

Egg masses of this three-host tick are deposited in protected places on the ground and hatch in 1 or 2 months (Bishopp and Smith 1938). Unfed larvae can survive a year or more. Larvae feed on small mammals 2 to 13 days, detach, and molt 6 days to 8 months later, depending on the temperature. Nymphs feed on small mammals 3 to 11 days and molt 17 days to 10 months after feeding, again depending on the temperature. Adults attach to larger hosts. Females feed 5 to 13 days, during which time they also mate. They then detach and deposit batches of 3,000 to 6,500 eggs 3 to 58 days later. Activity is greatest in the spring and early summer in the north, but this period is more prolonged in warmer climates.

PATHOLOGIC EFFECTS

The bite of this tick causes local inflammation, edema, hemorrhage, and sometimes paralysis (Belding 1965; Robinow and Carroll 1938). Heavy infestations cause irritability and debilitation (Bishopp and Trembley 1945).

The American dog tick is a known vector of *Francisella tularensis* (Belding 1965; Robinow and Carroll 1938). The larva or nymph becomes infected while feeding on a diseased host. The infection persists to the adult stage and sometimes to the next generation. Infected larvae and nymphs transmit the agent to other small mammals; infected adults transmit it to the dog.

DIAGNOSIS

Diagnosis is based on the signs and on identification of the tick on the host.

CONTROL

Control is similar to that for *Rhipicephalus sanguineus*; the insecticides effective against that species are also effective against this tick. It is also important that underbrush, tall grass, and weeds be removed from around laboratory dog kennels and that animals on which immature stages of the tick feed be prevented access to buildings that house research dogs.

PUBLIC HEALTH CONSIDERATIONS

The American dog tick is a vector of *Rickettsia rickettsi* and *Francisella tularensis* (Hoogstraal 1967; Philip and Burgdorfer 1961; Saliba et al. 1966), and its bite sometimes causes paralysis in animals and man (Robinow and Carroll 1938). For these reasons, laboratory animals infested with this tick should be handled with caution, and care should be taken to prevent the contamination of open wounds or mucous membranes with blood from crushed ticks.

Dermacentor andersoni

(SYN. *Dermacentor venustus*)
(Rocky Mountain Wood Tick)

Dermacentor andersoni is notorious as a transmitter of disease agents that affect endothermal laboratory animals and man, and its bite sometimes causes paralysis in the dog, other animals, and man (Bishopp and Trembley 1945). This tick occurs over a wide area of western United States and Canada, especially where vegetation is low and brushy. Immature forms are found on many small wild mammals. The adults fre-quently attack large wild and domestic animals and man and, less frequently, the dog.

Although there are no specific reports of this tick on laboratory rodents or the dog, immature stages may infest wild rodents and lagomorphs brought into the laboratory from their natural habitat, and adults may be encountered on dogs obtained from pounds in the endemic area. This tick is not likely to occur on laboratory dogs obtained from kennels that practice good sanitation and rodent control.

MORPHOLOGY

Dermacentor andersoni (Fig. 14.3) closely resembles *D. variabilis*, but the goblets in its spiracular plates are larger and fewer in number, and the scutal ornamentation is different (Cooley 1938). The male is about 4 mm in length; the female is slightly larger.

LIFE CYCLE

Dermacentor andersoni is a three-host tick whose life cycle normally requires 2 years (Cooley 1932). The female lays about 6,400 eggs which hatch in about 35 days. The larvae feed on a small mammal, drop off, molt to the nymph stage, and hibernate in the soil. In the spring, the nymphs emerge from the soil, attach to a larger

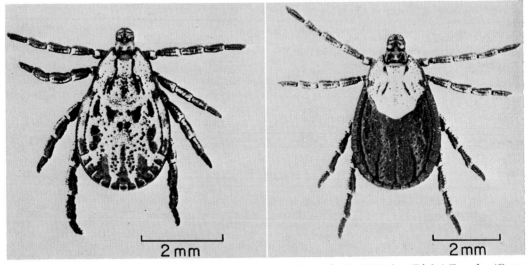

FIG. 14.3. *Dermacentor andersoni*. *(Left)* Male. *(Right)* Female. (Courtesy of G. M. Kohls, Rocky Mountain Laboratory.)

host, feed, drop off, and molt to adults. The adults attach to a third, larger host and feed.

PATHOLOGIC EFFECTS

Although there are no specific reports, heavy infestations undoubtedly cause debilitation. *Dermacentor andersoni* sometimes causes paralysis in dogs, other animals, and man, presumably by the female introducing a toxin as it feeds (Lapage 1968). The signs that develop a few days after attachment of the tick consist of progressive, ascending paralysis of the limbs, and urinary incontinence.

Dermacentor andersoni is an important vector of the agent *Francisella tularensis* (Philip and Burgdorfer 1961). It is also a possible vector of the virus of lymphocytic choriomeningitis (Hoogstraal 1966).

DIAGNOSIS

Diagnosis is based on the signs and on the presence of the attached tick, often in the dorsal cervical region.

CONTROL

Control is similar to that for *Rhipicephalus sanguineus* and *D. variabilis*.

PUBLIC HEALTH CONSIDERATIONS

This tick is an important vector of *Rickettsia rickettsi* (Hoogstraal 1967). It also transmits the virus of Colorado tick fever, *Coxiella burneti* (the cause of Q fever), *Francisella tularensis* (Hoogstraal 1966; Philip and Burgdorfer 1961), and possibly the virus of lymphocytic choriomeningitis (Hoogstraal 1966), and its bite sometimes causes tick paralysis in man (Faust, Beaver, and Jung 1968). For these reasons, laboratory animals infested with this tick should be handled with caution, and care should be taken when removing ticks individually to prevent contamination of open wounds or mucous membranes with blood from engorged ticks.

Amblyomma americanum
(Lone Star Tick)

The lone star tick is abundant in wooded areas, especially those with dense underbrush, in southeastern and south central United States and Mexico (Bishopp and Trembley 1945; Cooley and Kohls 1944b). It is also reported from Central America and Brazil. The bite of *Amblyomma americanum* is particularly annoying because of the elongated mouthparts of this tick; heavy infestations cause debilitation. *Amblyomma americanum* is a vector of several important pathogens (Bishopp and Trembley 1945; Hoogstraal 1967).

All stages occur on a variety of hosts, including wild rodents, the dog, wild carnivores, domestic animals, certain ground-inhabiting birds, and man (Bishopp and Trembley 1945).

Although there are no specific reports of the lone star tick on endothermal laboratory animals, it is likely to be encountered on wild rodents brought into the laboratory from their natural habitat and on dogs obtained from pounds in the endemic area. It is not likely to be found on laboratory dogs obtained from kennels that practice good sanitation and parasite control.

MORPHOLOGY

The male is about 3 mm long; the female is about the same length when unengorged and up to 11 mm long when engorged (Fig. 14.4) (Cooley and Kohls 1944b). The scutum of the male is a shiny reddish brown and has two posterior, U-shaped, pale markings and several narrow, pale, lateral stripes. The scutum of the female is a similar color, and it has a large pale spot posteriorly.

LIFE CYCLE

Amblyomma americanum is a three-host tick (Hooker, Bishopp, and Wood 1912; Hopla 1960). The female lays 2,000 to 10,000 eggs which hatch in 3 to 4 weeks. A few days later, the larvae climb on grass or low shrubs and form a cluster as they wait for a host. They feed 4 to 6 days, drop off, and molt to nymphs after 14 to 21 days on the ground. Two to 3 days later the nymphs are ready to feed; engorgement requires 6 to 7 days. They then fall to the ground and molt to adults after 3 to 4 weeks. A week later adults seek a new host. Females engorge in 12 to 21 days, during which time they also mate. Males remain attached for longer periods.

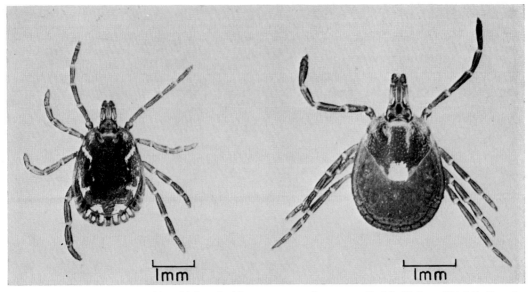

Fig. 14.4. *Amblyomma americanum. (Left)* Male. *(Right)* Female.
(Courtesy of G. M. Kohls, Rocky Mountain Laboratory.)

PATHOLOGIC EFFECTS

Heavy infestations cause exsanguination and debilitation (Bishopp and Trembley 1945). In nature, the wounds caused by the bite of this tick are often invaded by maggots of the screwworm fly. Persistent and severe irritation results if the long mouthparts remain in the host after the tick has been removed.

Amblyomma americanum is a vector of *Francisella tularensis* (Philip and Burgdorfer 1961).

DIAGNOSIS

Diagnosis is based on the signs and on identification of the tick on the host.

CONTROL

Control is similar to that of *Rhipicephalus sanguineus.* However, because of the exceptionally long mouthparts, special care must be taken when removing this tick manually (Hoogstraal 1967). By inserting a needle or scalpel under the mouthparts and applying slow, gentle traction, the tick can usually be detached intact. The topical application of camphorated phenol or 0.6% pyrethrins in methyl benzoate about 20 minutes before attempted removal reduces the amount of traction required.

PUBLIC HEALTH CONSIDERATIONS

This tick is a vector of *Rickettsia rickettsi* and *Francisella tularensis,* and it appears to be a reservoir, if not a vector, of *Coxiella burneti* (Hoogstraal 1967; Philip and Burgdorfer 1961). For these reasons, persons handling animals infested with this tick should be particularly careful not to get bitten. When removing individual ticks, care should also be taken to prevent the contamination of open wounds or mucous membranes with blood from engorged ticks.

Haemaphysalis leporispalustris

(Rabbit Tick)

The rabbit tick is common throughout the Western Hemisphere from Alaska to Argentina (Cooley 1946; Kohls 1960). All stages occur on rabbits and hares, and immature forms occur on certain wild birds and occasionally on the chicken (Bishopp and Trembley 1945). This tick rarely attacks man (Cooley 1946). Although *Haemaphysalis leporispalustris* principally affects wild lagomorphs, there are a few reports of it on the domestic rabbit and one report of it affecting the laboratory rabbit (Kohls 1960). The rabbit tick often occurs in such large numbers on its hosts (up to 4,000 to

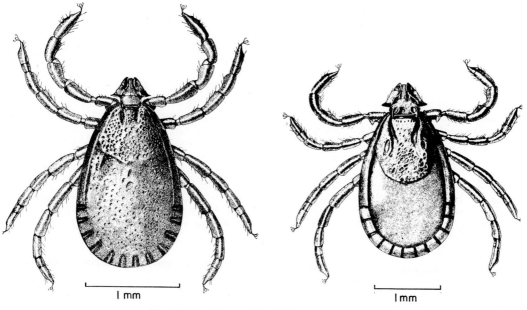

FIG. 14.5. *Haemaphysalis leporispalustris. (Left)* Male. *(Right)* Female. (Courtesy of U.S. Department of Agriculture.)

5,000) that it weakens and kills them; it is also a vector of several important pathogens (Bishopp and Trembley 1945).

MORPHOLOGY

Haemaphysalis leporispalustris is a relatively small tick (Fig. 14.5). The male is 2.2 mm long, has conical palpi and a rectangular basis capituli, and lacks eyes, ventral shields, and coxal spines (Cooley 1946). The female is about 2.6 mm long when unengorged and up to 10.0 mm in length after feeding. Its morphologic features are similar to those of the male.

LIFE CYCLE

This is a three-host tick (Bishopp and Trembley 1945; Cooley 1946). Larvae and nymphs feed about 6 to 11 days; adults feed about 19 to 26 days. Adults live about a year, and a complete life cycle varies with the temperature from 87 to 405 days (Belding 1965).

PATHOLOGIC EFFECTS

This tick usually attaches to the ears and around the eyes, but occasionally it is found between the toes or on other parts of the body (Bishopp and Trembley 1945).

It often attacks in large numbers and causes weakness, emaciation, and death.

Haemaphysalis leporispalustris is a vector of *Francisella tularensis* (Hopla 1960).

DIAGNOSIS

Diagnosis is based on the signs and on the presence of the tick on the host.

CONTROL

Control is similar to that of *Rhipicephalus sanguineus.*

PUBLIC HEALTH CONSIDERATIONS

This tick is a vector of *Rickettsia rickettsi, Francisella tularensis,* and the virus of Colorado tick fever (Hoogstraal 1966, 1967; Hopla 1960). For these reasons, persons handling infested animals should do so with caution. Care should also be taken when removing engorged ticks to prevent contamination of open wounds or mucous membranes.

Ixodes

Several species of this genus parasitize endothermal laboratory animals (Table 14.1). The commonest species in North

America are *Ixodes scapularis* (the black-legged tick) and *I. pacificus* (the California black-legged tick) (Arthur and Snow 1968; Bishopp and Trembley 1945; Cooley and Kohls 1945). *Ixodes scapularis* occurs in eastern United States and Mexico; *I. pacificus* occurs along the west coast of North America from California to British Columbia. Both principally affect the dog, domestic animals, wild ungulates, and man. Other North American species include *I. cookei, I. rugosus, I. angustus, I. kingi, I. dentatus, I. spinipalpis,* and *I. muris.* Most of these species have a broad host range; immature forms occur on wild rodents, other small mammals, and sometimes birds, and adult forms occur on the dog, domestic animals, other large mammals, and man. Exceptions are *I. dentatus* and *I. spinipalpis,* which are restricted largely to wild lagomorphs, and *I. muris,* which occurs predominantly on rodents.

Ixodes ricinus (the castor-bean tick) is the commonest species in Europe; *I. persulcatus* is commonest in eastern Europe and northern Asia (Hoogstraal 1966). *Ixodes canisuga* (the British dog tick) is common in the British Isles, *I. holocyclus* is common in Australia, and *I. pilosus, I. rubicundus, I. rasus,* and *I. schillingsi* are common in

Africa (Hoogstraal 1956, 1966, 1967; Lapage 1962, 1968).

The bite of *Ixodes* causes irritation, trauma, and sometimes paralysis (Lapage 1962). In addition, several species of this genus are vectors of important pathogens (Hoogstraal 1966, 1967).

Although there are no specific reports of the occurrence of these ticks on endothermal laboratory animals, they are likely to be encountered on wild rodents and lagomorphs brought into the laboratory from their natural habitat and on dogs obtained from pounds in endemic areas. They are not likely to be found on dogs obtained from kennels that practice good sanitation and parasite control.

MORPHOLOGY

Ticks of the genus *Ixodes* (Fig. 14.6) are characterized by anal grooves that join anterior to the anus (Cooley and Kohls 1945). Mouthparts are comparatively long, and the scutum lacks eyes, festoons, and ornamentation. The male has seven shields that almost completely cover the ventral surface. These are absent in the female. Size varies with species: males are about 2 to 3 mm long, and engorged females 7 to 16 mm.

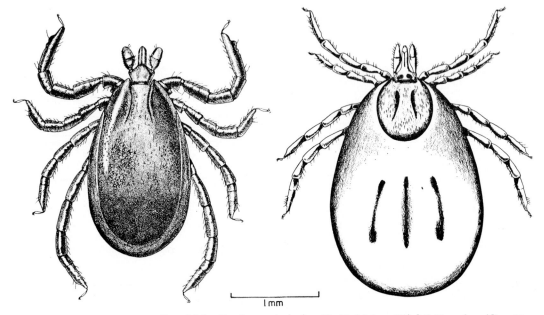

Fig. 14.6. *Ixodes scapularis. (Left)* Male. *(Right)* Female. (Courtesy of U.S. Department of Agriculture.)

LIFE CYCLE

Ixodes species are three-host ticks (Arthur and Snow 1968; Cooley and Kohls 1945). The length of time required for each stage varies with the species but is usually longer than for other ticks. *Ixodes pacificus* eggs hatch in about 54 days, and the larvae feed 4 to 9 days and molt in 37 to 38 days (Arthur and Snow 1968). Nymphs feed 7 to 11 days and molt to adults. A diapause does not appear necessary, and the entire life cycle is completed in about 7 months. On the other hand, *I. ricinus* sometimes requires as long as 3 years to complete its life cycle, each stage feeding only a few days each year (Lapage 1962, 1968). Males of several species do not feed and thus are less commonly encountered on hosts than are females.

PATHOLOGIC EFFECTS

Because of its long hypostome, the possibility of the mouthparts remaining in the host after the tick is removed is greater for *Ixodes* than for most other ticks. When this happens, persistent, severe irritation results, often with secondary bacterial invasion.

Some species frequently occur in large numbers on their hosts, causing exsanguination and debilitation. This is common in *I. dentatus* infestation of cottontail rabbits. Other species, such as *I. ricinus, I. rubicundus,* and *I. holocyclus,* cause paralysis (Lapage 1962).

Several species (*I. scapularis, I. pacificus, I. kingi, I. dentatus,* and *I. spinipalpis*) are known or suspected vectors of *Francisella tularensis* (Bishopp and Trembley 1945; Philip and Burgdorfer 1961).

DIAGNOSIS

Diagnosis is based on the signs and on identification of these ticks on a host.

CONTROL

Insecticides effective against *Rhipicephalus sanguineus* are also effective against these ticks. The method of removal of mouthparts is the same as that described for *Amblyomma americanum.*

PUBLIC HEALTH CONSIDERATIONS

Ticks of this genus are known or suspected vectors of several important pathogens of man. These include *Francisella tularensis (I. scapularis, I. pacificus, I. kingi, I. dentatus,* and *I. spinipalpis*); *Rickettsia rickettsi (I. angustus, I. dentatus,* and *I. kingi*); *R. australis,* the cause of Queensland tick typhus (*I. holocyclus*); *R. conori (I. ricinus);* and the viruses of Powassen encephalitis (*I. cookei*), Central European tick-borne encephalitis (*I. ricinus*), Russian spring-summer encephalitis (*I. persulcatus*), Omsk hemorrhagic fever (*I. persulcatus*), and Kemerovo tick-borne fever (*I. persulcatus*) (Bishopp and Trembley 1945; Philip and Burgdorfer 1961; Hoogstraal 1966, 1967). Thus, animals infested with these ticks should be handled with caution.

ARGASIDS

No scutum is present on these leathery or soft ticks. Larvae generally feed on a single animal for several days, nymphs feed on one or more different hosts for an hour or less, and adults feed on several hosts for a half hour to an hour at each meal. Adult and immature stages distend when engorged.

Argasids characteristically inhabit niches and crevices when not feeding. Usually only the larvae are transported long distances while feeding.

Argas persicus, A. sanchezi, A. radiatus, A. miniatus

(Fowl Ticks)

Ticks formerly identified as *Argas persicus* are now known to represent a complex of species: *A. persicus, A. sanchezi, A. radiatus,* and *A. miniatus* (Kohls et al. 1970). It was formerly believed that *A. persicus* occurred throughout the world, usually between latitudes 40 N and 40 S, but it now appears that this species is generally confined to the Eastern Hemisphere (Europe, Asia, and parts of Africa) and is rare in the New World. In the Western Hemisphere, *A. persicus* is known only from a few collections from eastern United States, California, and Paraguay. *Argas sanchezi* is common in southwestern United States and Mexico; *A. radiatus* is recorded from central and southern United States and Mexico; *A. miniatus* occurs in Panama and South America.

The chicken and certain wild birds are

primary hosts (Bishopp and Trembley 1945). *Argas persicus* rarely attacks man; the public health aspects of the other species are uncertain.

These ticks cause irritation, exsanguination, debilitation, and sometimes death (Bishopp and Trembley 1945; Cooley and Kohls 1944a; Hoogstraal 1956). *Argas persicus* is a vector of pathogens of the chicken and man, and its bite sometimes causes paralysis. *Argas sanchezi* also transmits a pathogen of the chicken, but pathogen transmission capabilities of the other species are uncertain.

There are no specific reports of these ticks on laboratory birds (Yunker 1964). They might be encountered on chickens obtained from farm flocks in endemic areas, but they are not likely to occur on chickens obtained from reputable commercial suppliers that practice good sanitation and parasite control.

MORPHOLOGY

Adults are ovoid and 4 to 11 mm long (Fig. 14.7) (Cooley and Kohls 1944a). A finely wrinkled integument is marked by radiating discs and laterally by quadrangular "cells." A definite suture encircles the body, dividing the dorsal and ventral surfaces.

LIFE CYCLE

The life cycle of *A. persicus* and presumably of the other species requires 4 months under favorable conditions and is extended during cool months (Hoogstraal 1956). Larvae feed 5 to 10 days, usually at the base of the host's wings, then detach, rest 4 days or more, and molt into nymphs. Nymphs have two or three instars, each of which feeds nocturnally up to 2 hours and molts about a week later. Adults are also nocturnal and feed six or seven times. When not feeding, nymphs and adults remain in crevices. After each feeding, females deposit 50 to 650 eggs which hatch in 8 days to several weeks. These species can survive 2 years without food.

PATHOLOGIC EFFECTS

Heavy infestations cause annoyance, irritation, loss of weight, weakness, anemia, and often death (Bishopp and Trembley 1945; Cooley and Kohls 1944a; Lapage 1968). *Argas persicus* and possibly the other species sometimes cause paralysis, presumably by introducing a toxin while feeding (Bishopp and Trembley 1945).

Borrelia anserina, the cause of avian spirochetosis, is transmitted by *A. persicus* and *A. sanchezi*, probably by *A. radiatus*, and possibly by *A. miniatus* (Philip and Burgdorfer 1961; G. M. Kohls, personal communication; N. W. Rokey, personal communication). *Argas persicus* also transmits the agent of aegyptianellosis (*Aegyptianella pullorum*), a disease of the chicken and other birds that occurs in southeastern Europe, Asia, and Africa (Levine 1961).

DIAGNOSIS

Diagnosis is based on signs and on identification of the tick on the host. Since the ticks occur on the host only at night, nocturnal observations are required to confirm a tentative diagnosis based on the clinical signs.

CONTROL

Control is similar to that of *Rhipicephalus sanguineus*. However, nymphs and

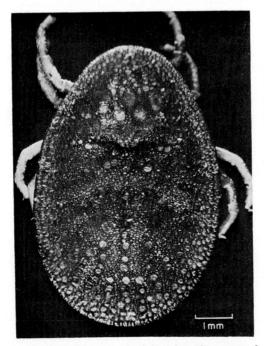

FIG. 14.7. *Argas sanchezi* female. (Courtesy of G. M. Kohls, Rocky Mountain Laboratory.)

adults spend most of their time in cracks and crevices and little time on the host (and then only at night). Thus, greater attention should be given to treatment of infested cages and buildings and less to the treatment of individual animals.

PUBLIC HEALTH CONSIDERATIONS

Although man is not a usual host for these ticks, there are a few reports of individuals being bitten (Bishopp and Trembley 1945). Since *A. persicus* and possibly the other species are reservoirs of *Coxiella burneti,* care should be taken when handling infested chickens.

Otobius megnini

(Spinose Ear Tick)

Immature forms of this tick inhabit the external ear canal and are a source of great annoyance to many animals, including the dog, cat, domestic animals, wild ungulates, and man (Bishopp and Trembley 1945; Cooley and Kohls 1944a). It also affects cottontail rabbits and hares, but the common species of this genus on lagomorphs is *Otobius lagophilus*. The original range of the spinose ear tick was probably the arid and semiarid regions of southwestern United States and Mexico (Bishopp and Trembley 1945). It is still commonest in this region, but it has often been reported in northern, central, and eastern United States, Hawaii, and western Canada; it was apparently introduced into these areas on transported livestock (Bishopp and Trembley 1945; Cooley and Kohls 1944a). The parasite now occurs also in South America, Africa, Madagascar, India, and Australia. It was probably introduced into these areas on livestock from the United States (Bishopp and Trembley 1945; Cooley and Kohls 1944a; Kohls, Sonenshine, and Clifford 1965).

The spinose ear tick is common on large domestic animals in the endemic areas but uncommon on wild lagomorphs, the dog, and cat. There are no specific reports of this tick affecting endothermal laboratory animals. It is unlikely to be encountered except possibly on lagomorphs obtained from their natural habitat or on dogs and cats obtained from pounds in endemic areas.

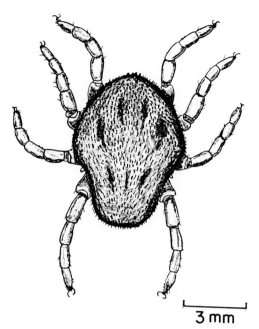

FIG. 14.8. *Otobius megnini* nymph. Note spines. (From Whitlock 1960. Courtesy of Lea and Febiger.)

MORPHOLOGY

The second nymph (Fig. 14.8), the stage ordinarily seen in the ears of endothermal animals, is about 8.5 mm long when fully fed, and has a spiny integument (Cooley and Kohls 1944a). Adults are slightly smaller and have more pronounced lateral constrictions, a vestigial hypostome, and no spines.

LIFE CYCLE

Adults inhabit cracks or crevices close to the ground, breed, and lay eggs for several months (Bishopp and Trembley 1945; Cooley and Kohls 1944a). Larvae climb the host's legs and body, enter the ears, feed 5 to 10 days, rest, and molt to first- and then second-stage nymphs. The nymphs remain in the ear and feed 1 to 7 months. The engorged second-stage nymph then leaves the host, seeks a dry protected place, and molts to an adult. Adults do not feed.

PATHOLOGIC EFFECTS

Immature stages of this tick attach deep in the external auditory canal of the host, causing extreme irritation, edema, hemorrhage, and pain (Bishopp and Trembley 1945; Lapage 1968). The ear canal is sometimes completely filled with ticks and debris. Affected animals shake their heads and scratch their ears. Secondary effects include trauma of the external ear, secondary infection of the auditory canal, deafness, and sometimes death.

DIAGNOSIS

Diagnosis is based on the clinical signs and on demonstration of *O. megnini* nymphs in the ears.

CONTROL

Newly acquired animals should be examined on arrival and treated, if infected. A mixture of 5% benzene hexachloride (containing 15% gamma isomer), 10% xylene, and 85% pine oil applied inside the ear canal is an effective treatment (McIntosh and McDuffie 1956). A sorptive silica dust (Dri-Die 67, FMC Corporation) containing 2% naled (Dibrom, Chevron Chemical Co.) deposited in the auditory canal is also reportedly effective (Tarshis and Ommert 1961). Because of the location of the parasite, deep in the ear canal, merely bathing or dipping an infected animal in an acaricide is ineffective (Bishopp and Trembley 1945).

PUBLIC HEALTH CONSIDERATIONS

Immature stages of the spinose ear tick also invade the external ear of man and cause severe pain, but such infestations are rare (Bishopp and Trembley 1945). Although this tick is not known to be a vector of any disease-producing agents, *Coxiella burneti* has been recovered from it (Philip and Burgdorfer 1961).

TABLE 14.1. Ixodids affecting endothermal laboratory animals

Parasite	Geographic Distribution	Endothermal Host	Usual Habitat	Incidence — In nature	Incidence — In laboratory	Pathologic Effects	Public Health Importance	Reference
Rhipicephalus sanguineus[*]	Worldwide in tropical and temperate regions	Black rat, other wild rodents, hares, dog, cat, wild carnivores, green monkey, monkey, baboons, other simian primates, domestic animals, man	In cracks and crevices on ground and in buildings; attached to skin of host, often between toes	Common on dog; uncommon on other animals	Common on dogs obtained from pounds in tropics and subtropics; uncommon elsewhere; uncommon on other species	Irritation; vector of *Babesia canis*, *B. vogeli*, *Hepatozoon canis*, *Ehrlichia canis*, *Salmonella enteritidis*, *Dipetalonema reconditum*, *D. grassii*	Causes irritation; vector of agents of Rocky Mountain spotted fever, Siberian tick typhus, boutonneuse fever, tularemia, other diseases	Bishopp and Trembley 1945 Cooley 1946 Gregson 1956 Hirsch et al. 1969 Hoogstraal 1956, 1967 Kohls and Parker 1948 Myers and Kuntz 1965 Yunker 1964
Rhipicephalus appendiculatus	Tropical Africa	Wild rodents, dog, baboons, domestic animals, man	Brush-covered regions; attached to skin of host	Common on dog; uncommon on other animals	Unknown; probably common on dogs obtained from pounds in endemic areas	Irritation; vector of *Hepatozoon canis*; vector of pathogens of domestic animals	Causes irritation; vector of agents of boutonneuse fever, other diseases	Hoogstraal 1956, 1967 Lapage 1962 Myers and Kuntz 1965
Rhipicephalus simus	Africa	Wild rodents, dog, cat, wild carnivores, domestic animals, man	Wide ecologic range; attached to skin of host	Common on dog; rare on cat	Unknown; probably common on dogs obtained from pounds in endemic areas	Unknown; probably irritation	Causes irritation, paralysis; vector of agent of boutonneuse fever	Hoogstraal 1956
Rhipicephalus pravus	Eastern Africa	Wild rodents, lagomorphs, dog, domestic animals, man	Bushveld; attached to skin of host	Common	Unknown; probably common on lagomorphs obtained from natural habitat and on dogs obtained from pounds in endemic areas	Unknown	Unknown	Hoogstraal 1956
Boophilus decoloratus	Tropical Africa	Dog, domestic animals, wild ungulates	Brush-covered regions; attached to skin of host	Uncommon on dog	Unknown; probably rare or absent on dog	Irritation, debilitation	Probable vector of agent of boutonneuse fever	Hoogstraal 1967 Lapage 1962
Dermacentor variabilis[*]	North America	Deer mice, voles, cotton rat, rice rat, other wild rodents, cottontail rabbits, dog, wild carnivores, man	Damp, grassy, brush-covered regions; attached to skin of host	Common	Unknown; probably common on rodents obtained from natural habitat and on dogs obtained from pounds in endemic areas	Irritation, sometimes debilitation, paralysis; vector of *Francisella tularensis*	Causes irritation, paralysis; vector of agents of Rocky Mountain spotted fever, tularemia	Bishopp and Smith 1938 Bishopp and Trembley 1945 Cooley 1938 Hyland and Mathewson 1961 Robinow and Carroll 1938 Smith et al. 1946 Yunker 1964

[*]Discussed in text.

TABLE 14.1 (continued)

Parasite	Geographic Distribution	Endothermal Host	Usual Habitat	Incidence In nature	Incidence In laboratory	Pathologic Effects	Public Health Importance	Reference
*Dermacentor andersoni**	Western North America	Wild rodents, lagomorphs, small carnivores, dog, domestic animals, man	Low brush-covered regions; attached to skin of host	Common on small mammals; uncommon on dog	Unknown; probably common on small mammals obtained from natural habitat and uncommon on dogs obtained from pounds in endemic areas	Irritation, debilitation, sometimes paralysis; vector of *Francisella tularensis*; possible vector of virus of lymphocytic choriomeningitis	Causes irritation, paralysis; vector of agents of Rocky Mountain spotted fever, Colorado tick fever, Q fever, tularemia; possible vector of virus of lymphocytic choriomeningitis	Bishopp and Trembley 1945 Cooley 1932, 1938 Faust et al. 1968 Hoogstraal 1966, 1967 Lapage 1968 Philip and Burgdorfer 1961
Dermacentor parumapertus	Southwestern United States, northern Mexico	Cottontail rabbits, hares, other small mammals, man	Arid, brush-covered regions; attached to skin of host	Common	Unknown; probably common on lagomorphs obtained from natural habitat in endemic areas	Probably irritation, debilitation; vector of *Francisella tularensis*, other pathogens	Causes irritation; vector of agents of Colorado tick fever, tularemia, an unidentified rickettsial disease	Bishopp and Trembley 1945 Cooley 1938 Hoogstraal 1966, 1967 Philip and Burgdorfer 1961
Dermacentor occidentalis	Pacific coastal region of North America	Deer mice, wood rats, other wild rodents, cottontail rabbits, hares, dog, domestic animals, man	Wooded regions; attached to skin of host	Common	Unknown; probably common on small mammals obtained from natural habitat and uncommon on dogs obtained from pounds in endemic areas	Probably irritation, debilitation; vector of *Francisella tularensis*, other pathogens	Causes irritation; vector of agents of Colorado tick fever, Rocky Mountain spotted fever, tularemia	Bishopp and Trembley 1945 Cooley 1938 Hoogstraal 1966, 1967 Philip and Burgdorfer 1961
Dermacentor pictus (*D. reticulatus*)	Central Europe, west central Asia	Wild rodents, lagomorphs, small carnivores, dog, domestic animals, man	Wooded regions, damp meadows; attached to skin of host	Common	Unknown; probably common on rodents, lagomorphs obtained from natural habitat in endemic areas	Probably irritation, debilitation; vector of *Babesia canis*	Causes irritation; vector of Omsk hemorrhagic fever; probable vector of agent of boutonneuse fever	Hoogstraal 1966, 1967 Lapage 1968
Dermacentor marginatus	Central Europe, west central Asia	Wild rodents, lagomorphs, small carnivores, dog, domestic animals, man	Brush-covered regions, low forests, marshes, alpine steppes, semidesert regions; attached to skin of host	Common	Unknown; probably common on rodents, lagomorphs obtained from natural habitat in endemic areas	Probably irritation, debilitation; probable vector of pathogens	Causes irritation; vector of agents of Russian spring-summer encephalitis, central European tick-borne encephalitis, Siberian tick typhus; probable vector of agent of boutonneuse fever	Hoogstraal 1966, 1967

*Discussed in text.

412

TABLE 14.1 (continued)

Parasite	Geographic Distribution	Endothermal Host	Usual Habitat	Incidence: In nature	Incidence: In laboratory	Pathologic Effects	Public Health Importance	Reference
Dermacentor nuttalli	North central Asia	Wild rodents, lagomorphs, small carnivores, dog, domestic animals, man	Alpine steppes, forests, desert regions; attached to skin of host	Common	Unknown; probably common on rodents, lagomorphs obtained from natural habitat in endemic areas	Probably irritation, debilitation; probable vector of pathogens	Causes irritation; vector of agent of Siberian tick typhus	Hoogstraal 1967
Dermacentor silvarum	Northern Asia	Wild rodents, lagomorphs, small carnivores, dog, domestic animals, man	Forests, steppes, brush-covered regions; attached to skin of host	Common	Unknown; probably common on rodents, lagomorphs obtained from natural habitat in endemic areas	Probably irritation, debilitation; probable vector of pathogens	Causes irritation; vector of agents of Russian spring-summer encephalitis, Siberian tick typhus	Hoogstraal 1966, 1967
*Amblyomma americanum**	Southern United States, Mexico, Central America, Brazil	Wild rodents, dog, wild carnivores, domestic animals, wild birds, man	Wooded regions; attached to skin of host	Common	Unknown; probably common on rodents obtained from natural habitat and on dogs obtained from pounds in endemic areas	Severe irritation, trauma, loss of blood, debilitation; vector of *Francisella tularensis*	Causes severe irritation, trauma; vector of agents of Rocky Mountain spotted fever, tularemia; possible vector of agent of Q fever	Bishopp and Trembley 1945 Cooley and Kohls 1944b Hoogstraal 1967 Hooker et al. 1912 Hopla 1960 Philip and Burgdorfer 1961
Amblyomma maculatum	Southern United States, Mexico, Central America, South America	Wild rodents, dog, domestic animals, wild birds	Wooded areas; attached to skin of host, often on external ear	Common	Unknown; probably uncommon on dogs obtained from pounds in endemic areas	Severe irritation, trauma; probable vector of pathogens	Unknown	Bishopp and Hixson 1936 Bishopp and Trembley 1945 Cooley and Kohls 1944b Hoogstraal 1967
Amblyomma cajennense	South central United States, Mexico, Central America, West Indies, South America	Dog, wild carnivores, domestic animals, man	Wooded areas; attached to skin of host	Common	Unknown; probably uncommon on dogs obtained from pounds in endemic areas	Severe irritation, trauma; probable vector of pathogens	Causes irritation, trauma; vector of agent of Rocky Mountain spotted fever	Bishopp and Trembley 1945 Cooley and Kohls 1944b Hoogstraal 1967
Amblyomma tuberculatum	Southeastern United States	Larva: cottontail rabbits, dog, domestic animals, chicken, wild birds	Wooded areas; attached to skin of host	Common	Unknown; probably uncommon on dogs obtained from pounds in endemic areas	Probably severe irritation, trauma; possible vector of pathogens	Unknown	Bishopp and Trembley 1945 Cooley and Kohls 1944b

*Discussed in text.

413

TABLE 14.1 *(continued)*

Parasite	Geographic Distribution	Endothermal Host	Usual Habitat	Incidence		Pathologic Effects	Public Health Importance	Reference
				In nature	In laboratory			
Amblyomma inornatum	South central United States	Cottontail rabbits, hares, dog, cattle	Wooded areas; attached to skin of host	Uncommon	Unknown; probably uncommon on dogs obtained from pounds in endemic areas	Probably severe irritation, trauma; possible vector of pathogens	Unknown	Cooley and Kohls 1944b
Amblyomma variegatum	West Indies, southwestern Asia, Africa	Wild rodents, lagomorphs, dog, domestic animals, wild birds, man	Grasslands and open forests; attached to skin of host	Common	Unknown; probably uncommon on dogs obtained from pounds in endemic areas	Probably severe irritation, trauma; vector of pathogens of domestic animals	Causes irritation, trauma; vector of agent of boutonneuse fever; possible vector of agents of lymphocytic choriomeningitis, epidemic typhus	Hoogstraal 1956, 1966, 1967
Amblyomma hebraeum	Central Africa, South Africa	Small mammals, dog, baboons, domestic animals, wild birds, man	Low wooded regions; attached to skin of host	Common	Unknown; probably uncommon on dogs obtained from pounds in endemic areas	Severe irritation, trauma; vector of pathogens of domestic animals	Causes irritation, trauma; vector of agent of boutonneuse fever	Hoogstraal 1956, 1967; Lapage 1962; Myers and Kuntz 1965
Hyalomma marginatum marginatum	Southern Europe, southwestern Asia, northern Africa	Wild rodents, hares, dog, cat, domestic animals, birds, man	Steppes and lightly forested areas; attached to skin of host	Common	Unknown; probably common on rodents obtained from natural habitat and dogs obtained from pounds in endemic areas	Severe irritation, trauma	Vector of agent of Crimean hemorrhagic fever	Hoogstraal 1956, 1966
Hyalomma marginatum rufipes	Africa, southwestern Asia	Wild rodents, hares, dog, cat, domestic animals, birds, man	Grasslands and open forests; attached to skin of host	Common	Unknown; probably common on rodents obtained from natural habitat and dogs obtained from pounds in endemic areas	Severe irritation, trauma	Vector of agent of boutonneuse fever	Hoogstraal 1956, 1966, 1967
Hyalomma excavatum	Southwestern Asia, northern Africa	Wild rodents, hares, dog, domestic animals, man	Wide ecologic range; attached to skin of host	Common on hares	Unknown; probably common on hares obtained from natural habitat in endemic areas	Unknown; probably irritation, trauma	Causes irritation, trauma; vector of agents of Uzbekistan hemorrhagic fever, Q fever	Hoogstraal 1956
Hyalomma impelatum	Southwestern Asia, northern Africa	Wild rodents, hares, dog, domestic animals, birds, man	Arid, semiarid regions; attached to skin of host	Common	Unknown; probably uncommon on dogs obtained from pounds in endemic areas	Unknown; probably irritation, trauma	Unknown	Hoogstraal 1956

TABLE 14.1 (continued)

Parasite	Geographic Distribution	Endothermal Host	Usual Habitat	Incidence		Pathologic Effects	Public Health Importance	Reference
				In nature	In laboratory			
Hyalomma truncatum	Africa	Wild rodents, lagomorphs, dog, cat, domestic animals, wild birds, man	Wooded areas; attached to skin of host	Uncommon on dog; rare on cat	Unknown; probably uncommon on dogs obtained from pounds in endemic areas	Probably severe irritation, trauma, vector of pathogens of domestic animals	Causes irritation, trauma, paralysis; vector of agent of Q fever	Hoogstraal 1956
*Haemaphysalis leporispalustris**	North America, Central America, South America	Rabbit, hares, chicken, other birds, man	Wide ecologic range; attached to skin of host	Common on rabbit, hares	Common on lagomorphs obtained from natural habitat in endemic areas; uncommon on domestic rabbit	Loss of blood, weakness, emaciation, death; vector of *Francisella tularensis*	Vector of agents of Colorado tick fever, Rocky Mountain spotted fever, tularemia	Bishopp and Trembley 1945 Cooley 1946 Hoogstraal 1966, 1967 Kohls 1960
Haemaphysalis punctata	Europe, northwestern Africa, southwestern Asia	Wild rodents, rabbit, hedgehog, other small mammals, domestic animals, birds, man	Mountainous, semidesert, and desert regions, steppes; attached to skin of host	Common	Unknown; probably common on rodents and lagomorphs obtained from natural habitat in endemic areas	Irritation, trauma, debilitation	Vector of agent of Siberian tick typhus	Hoogstraal 1967 Lapage 1968
Haemaphysalis concinna	Europe, northern Asia	Wild rodents, other small mammals, domestic animals, birds, man	Forests, swamps; attached to skin of host	Common	Unknown; probably common on rodents obtained from natural habitat in endemic areas	Unknown; probably irritation, trauma, debilitation	Vector of agents of Russian spring-summer encephalitis, Siberian tick typhus	Hoogstraal 1966, 1967
Haemaphysalis houyi	Africa	West African ground squirrel (*Euxerus*)	Grasslands; attached to skin of host	Common	Unknown; probably common on ground squirrels obtained from natural habitat in endemic areas	Unknown; probably irritation, trauma, debilitation	Unknown	Hoogstraal 1956
Haemaphysalis leachii	Africa	Wild rodents, dog, other carnivores, man	Wide ecologic range; attached to skin of host	Common	Unknown; probably common on rodents obtained from natural habitat and on dogs obtained from pounds in endemic areas	Irritation, trauma; vector of *Babesia canis*	Irritation; vector of agent of boutonneuse fever	Hoogstraal 1956, 1966, 1967 Lapage 1962 Yunker 1964
Haemaphysalis spinigera	Southern Asia	Wild rodents, other small mammals, bonnet monkey, langurs, domestic animals, man	Forests; attached to skin of host	Common	Common on rodents and monkeys obtained from natural habitat in endemic areas	Unknown; probably irritation, trauma	Vector of agent of Kyasanur forest disease	Hoogstraal 1966 Trapido et al. 1964 Valerio et al. 1969

*Discussed in text.

TABLE 14.1 *(continued)*

Parasite	Geographic Distribution	Endothermal Host	Usual Habitat	Incidence		Pathologic Effects	Public Health Importance	Reference
				In nature	In laboratory			
Haemaphysalis semermis	Southeastern Asia, Indonesia	Wild rodents, other small mammals, dog, domestic animals, man	Forests; attached to skin of host	Common	Unknown; probably common on rodents obtained from natural habitat and on dogs obtained from pounds in endemic areas	Unknown; probably irritation, trauma, debilitation	Possible vector of agent of boutonneuse fever	Hoogstraal 1967
Haemaphysalis nadchatrami	Southeastern Asia, Indonesia	Wild rodents, other small mammals, dog, domestic animals, man	Forests; attached to skin of host	Common	Unknown; probably common on rodents obtained from natural habitat and on dogs obtained from pounds in endemic areas	Unknown; probably irritation, trauma, debilitation	Possible vector of agent of boutonneuse fever	Hoogstraal 1967
*Ixodes scapularis**	Eastern United States, Mexico	Rat, voles, other wild rodents, dog, domestic animals, wild ungulates, birds, man	Attached to skin of host	Common on dog	Unknown; probably uncommon on rodents obtained from natural habitat, common on dogs obtained from pounds in endemic areas	Irritation, often severe trauma; vector of *Francisella tularensis*	Causes irritation, trauma; vector of agent of tularemia	Bishopp and Trembley 1945 Cooley and Kohls 1945 Hyland and Mathewson 1961
*Ixodes pacificus**	Pacific coastal region of North America	Wild rodents, lagomorphs; dog, cat, domestic animals, wild ungulates, birds, man	Attached to skin of host	Uncommon on rodents, lagomorphs; common on dog	Unknown; probably uncommon on rodents and lagomorphs obtained from natural habitat, common on dogs obtained from pounds in endemic areas	Irritation, trauma; possible vector of *Francisella tularensis*	Causes irritation, trauma; possible vector of agent of tularemia	Arthur and Snow 1968 Bishopp and Trembley 1945 Cooley and Kohls 1945 Philip and Burgdorfer 1961
*Ixodes cookei**	Eastern North America	Wild rodents, dog, cat, wild carnivores, domestic animals, man	Animal nests; attached to skin of host	Uncommon	Unknown; probably uncommon on rodents obtained from natural habitat and dogs obtained from pounds in endemic areas	Irritation, often severe trauma	Causes irritation, often severe trauma; possible vector of agent of Powassen encephalitis	Bishopp and Trembley 1945 Cooley and Kohls 1945 Hoogstraal 1966 Hyland and Mathewson 1961
*Ixodes rugosus**	Pacific coastal region of North America	Wild rodents, dog	Attached to skin of host	Uncommon	Unknown; probably rare on rodents obtained from natural habitat and dogs obtained from pounds in endemic areas	Irritation, trauma	Unknown	Bishopp and Trembley 1945 Cooley and Kohls 1945

*Discussed in text.

416

TABLE 14.1 (continued)

Parasite	Geographic Distribution	Endothermal Host	Usual Habitat	Incidence In nature	Incidence In laboratory	Pathologic Effects	Public Health Importance	Reference
Ixodes angustus*	Northern United States, Canada	Deer mice, voles, other wild rodents, lagomorphs, dog, cat, wild carnivores, man	Attached to skin of host	Uncommon	Unknown; probably rare on rodents obtained from natural habitat and dogs obtained from pounds in endemic areas	Irritation, trauma	Unknown; possible vector of Rocky Mountain spotted fever	Bishopp and Trembley 1945 Cooley and Kohls 1945 Hoogstraal 1967 Hyland and Mathewson 1961
Ixodes kingi*	Western North America	Wild rodents, lagomorphs, dog, wild carnivores, man	Attached to skin of host	Uncommon	Unknown; probably uncommon or rare on rodents and lagomorphs obtained from natural habitat and on dogs obtained from pounds in endemic areas	Irritation, trauma; possible vector of *Francisella tularensis*	Causes irritation, trauma; possible vector of agents of Rocky Mountain spotted fever, tularemia	Bishopp and Trembley 1945 Cooley and Kohls 1945
Ixodes dentatus*	Central and eastern United States, Mexico	Cottontail rabbits	Attached to skin of host	Common	Unknown; probably common on cottontail rabbits obtained from natural habitat in endemic areas	Severe irritation, trauma, loss of blood, debilitation; possible vector of *Francisella tularensis*	Unknown; possible vector of agents of Rocky Mountain spotted fever, tularemia	Bishopp and Trembley 1945 Cooley and Kohls 1945 Hoogstraal 1967 Hyland and Mathewson 1961
Ixodes spinipalpis*	Western North America	Wild lagomorphs, man	Attached to skin of host	Common	Unknown; probably common on lagomorphs obtained from natural habitat in endemic areas	Irritation, trauma; possible vector of *Francisella tularensis*	Unknown; possible vector of agent of tularemia	Bishopp and Trembley 1945 Cooley and Kohls 1945
Ixodes muris*	Northeastern United States; eastern Canada	Deer mice, rat, voles, other rodents, cotton-tail rabbits	Attached to skin of host	Common on deer mice, voles	Unknown; probably common on deer mice and voles obtained from natural habitat in endemic areas	Irritation, trauma; possible vector of pathogens	Unknown	Bishopp and Trembley 1945 Cooley and Kohls 1945 Hyland and Mathewson 1961 Martell et al. 1969
Ixodes ricinus*	Europe	Wild rodents, lagomorphs, dog, wild carnivores, domestic animals, birds, man	Agricultural and forest areas; attached to skin of host, often on head, neck, flanks	Common	Unknown; probably common on rodents and lagomorphs obtained from natural habitat and on dogs obtained from pounds in endemic areas	Irritation, severe trauma, paralysis; vector of pathogens of domestic animals	Causes irritation, severe trauma, paralysis; vector of agent of central European tick-borne encephalitis; possible vector of agent of boutonneuse fever	Hoogstraal 1966, 1967 Lapage 1962, 1968

*Discussed in text.

TABLE 14.1 *(continued)*

Parasite	Geographic Distribution	Endothermal Host	Usual Habitat	Incidence — In nature	Incidence — In laboratory	Pathologic Effects	Public Health Importance	Reference
*Ixodes persulcatus**	Eastern Europe, northern Asia	Wild rodents, dog, cat, wild carnivores, domestic animals, birds, man	Taiga forest; attached to skin of host	Common	Unknown; probably common on rodents obtained from natural habitat and on dogs obtained from pounds in endemic areas	Irritation, severe trauma; vector of pathogens of domestic animals	Causes irritation, trauma; vector of agents of Russian spring-summer encephalitis, Omsk hemorrhagic fever; possible vector of agent of Kemerovo tick-borne fever	Hoogstraal 1966
Ixodes hexagonus	Europe	Hedgehog, dog, wild carnivores	Agricultural and forest areas; attached to skin of host	Common on hedgehog; uncommon on dog	Unknown; probably common on hedgehogs obtained from natural habitat, uncommon on dogs obtained from pounds in endemic areas	Irritation, trauma	Unknown	Lapage 1962, 1968
*Ixodes canisuga**	British Isles	Dog, domestic animals, wild mammals	Attached to skin of host	Common on dog	Common on dog	Irritation, trauma	Unknown	Lapage 1962, 1968
*Ixodes pilosus**	South Africa	Dog, cat, domestic animals, wild mammals	"Sourveld" areas with long grass; attached to skin of host	Common	Unknown; probably common on dogs obtained from pounds in endemic areas	Irritation, trauma	Unknown	Lapage 1962
*Ixodes rubicundus**	South Africa	Wild lagomorphs, dog, wild carnivores, domestic animals	Karoo veld, hills, and mountains; attached to skin of host	Common	Unknown; probably common on lagomorphs obtained from natural habitat and on dogs obtained from pounds in rural areas	Irritation, trauma, paralysis	Unknown	Lapage 1962
*Ixodes rasus**	Africa	Wild rodents, lagomorphs, dog, wild carnivores, domestic animals, man	Wide ecologic area; attached to skin of host	Common	Unknown; probably uncommon on rodents and lagomorphs obtained from natural habitat, uncommon on dogs obtained from pounds in endemic areas	Unknown	Unknown	Hoogstraal 1956

*Discussed in text.

418

TABLE 14.1 *(continued)*

Parasite	Geographic Distribution	Endothermal Host	Usual Habitat	Incidence In nature	Incidence In laboratory	Pathologic Effects	Public Health Importance	Reference
Ixodes nairobiensis	Africa	Rat, multimammate mouse, other rodents, dog	Forest areas; attached to skin of host	Rare	Unknown; probably rare on rodents obtained from natural habitat in endemic areas	Unknown	Unknown	Hoogstraal 1956
Ixodes schillingsi*	East Africa	Colobus monkey	Wooded areas; attached to skin of host	Common	Unknown; probably common on colobus monkeys obtained from natural habitat	Unknown; probably irritation, trauma	Unknown	Hoogstraal 1956
Ixodes holocyclus*	Australia	Wild rodents, dog, cat, wild carnivores, domestic animals, birds, man	Brush- and shrub-covered regions, chiefly in coastal areas; attached to skin of host	Common	Unknown; probably common on rodents obtained from natural habitat and on dogs obtained from pounds in endemic areas	Irritation, trauma, paralysis	Causes irritation, trauma; probable vector of agent of Queensland tick typhus	Hoogstraal 1967 Lapage 1962

*Discussed in text.

419

TABLE 14.2. Argasids affecting endothermal laboratory animals

Parasite	Geographic Distribution	Endothermal Host	Usual Habitat	Incidence In nature	Incidence In laboratory	Pathologic Effects	Public Health Importance	Reference
*Argas persicus**	United States, Europe, Asia Africa, Paraguay	Chicken, other birds, man	Cracks, crevices, human dwellings; attached to skin of host	Common in Europe, Asia; rare in Western Hemisphere	Unknown; probably rare	Irritation, trauma, weight loss, weakness, anemia, sometimes paralysis, death; vector of *Borrelia anserina, Aegyptianella pullorum*	Rarely attacks man; vector of agent of Q fever	Bishopp and Trembley 1945 Cooley and Kohls 1944a Hoogstral 1956 Kohls et al. 1970 Lapage 1968 Levine 1956 Philip and Burgdorfer 1961
*Argas sanchezi**	Southwestern United States, Mexico	Chicken, other birds, possibly man	Cracks, crevices, under bark of semidesert trees; attached to skin of host, usually at base of wings	Common	Unknown; probably rare	Irritation, trauma, weight loss, weakness, anemia, sometimes death; vector of *Borrelia anserina*	Unknown; possible vector of agent of Q fever	Bishopp and Trembley 1945 Cooley and Kohls 1944a Hoogstraal 1956 Kohls et al. 1970 Lapage 1968 Levine 1956 Philip and Burgdorfer 1961
*Argas radiatus**	Central and southern United States, Mexico	Chicken, other birds, possibly man	Cracks, crevices; attached to skin of host, usually at base of wings	Common	Unknown; probably rare	Irritation, trauma, weight loss, weakness, anemia, sometimes death; probable vector of *Borrelia anserina*	Unknown; possible vector of agent of Q fever	Bishopp and Trembley 1945 Cooley and Kohls 1944a Hoogstraal 1956 Kohls et al. 1970 Lapage 1968 Levine 1956 Philip and Burgdorfer 1961
*Argas miniatus**	Panama, South America	Chicken, other birds, possibly man	Cracks, crevices; attached to skin of host, usually at base of wings	Common	Unknown; probably rare	Irritation, trauma, weight loss, weakness, anemia, sometimes death; possible vector of *Borrelia anserina*	Unknown; possible vector of agent of Q fever	Bishopp and Trembley 1945 Cooley and Kohls 1944a Hoogstraal 1956 Kohls et al. 1970 Lapage 1968 Levine 1956 Philip and Burgdorfer 1961

*Discussed in text.

TABLE 14.2 *(continued)*

Parasite	Geographic Distribution	Endothermal Host	Usual Habitat	Incidence In nature	Incidence In laboratory	Pathologic Effects	Public Health Importance	Reference
Argas reflexus	Western Europe	Pigeon, other birds, man	Cracks, crevices; attached to skin of host	Common	Unknown; probably rare	Irritation, trauma, debilitation, anemia	Causes severe irritation, trauma	Hoogstraal and Kohls 1960a Yunker 1964
Argas hermanni	Africa	Chicken, pigeon, other birds, man	Cracks, crevices; attached to skin of host	Uncommon on chicken; common on pigeon	Unknown; probably rare	Irritation, trauma, debilitation, anemia	Causes severe irritation, trauma; vector of West Nile virus	Hoogstraal 1966 Hoogstraal and Kohls 1960b Yunker 1964
Argas neghmei	Northern Chile	Chicken, pigeon, man	Cracks, crevices; attached to skin of host	Common	Unknown; probably rare	Irritation, trauma, debilitation, anemia	Causes severe irritation, trauma	Kohls and Hoogstraal 1961
Ornithodoros turicata	United States, Mexico	Wild rodents, lagomorphs, domestic animals, man	Animal burrows; attached to skin of host	Common	Unknown; probably common on rodents and lagomorphs obtained from natural habitat in endemic areas	Irritation, trauma, edema; possible vector of *Leptospira pomona*	Causes severe irritation, trauma, pruritus, local inflammation, edema, subcutaneous nodules; vector of agents of relapsing fever, possibly leptospirosis	Cooley and Kohls 1944a Philip and Burgdorfer 1961
Ornithodoros parkeri	Western United States	Wild rodents, lagomorphs, birds, man	Animal burrows; attached to skin of host	Common	Unknown; probably common on rodents and lagomorphs obtained from natural habitat in endemic areas	Unknown; probably irritation, trauma	Causes irritation, trauma; vector of agent of relapsing fever	Belding 1965 Cooley and Kohls 1944a
Ornithodoros talaje	Southern United States, Mexico, Central America, South America	Wild rodents, dog, cat, simian primates, chicken, man	Animal burrows, human dwellings; attached to skin of host	Common on wild rodents; uncommon on other animals	Unknown; probably common on rodents obtained from natural habitat in endemic areas	Unknown; probably irritation, trauma	Causes severe irritation, trauma; vector of agent of relapsing fever	Cooley and Kohls 1944a McIntosh and McDuffie 1956

TABLE 14.2 *(continued)*

Parasite	Geographic Distribution	Endothermal Host	Usual Habitat	Incidence: In nature	Incidence: In laboratory	Pathologic Effects	Public Health Importance	Reference
Ornithodoros moubata complex	Africa	Wild rodents, lagomorphs, other small mammals, dog, other carnivores, domestic animals, birds, man	Human dwellings, animal burrows; attached to skin of host	Uncommon on rodents, lagomorphs, dog, birds	Unknown; probably rare or absent	Unknown; probably irritation, trauma; possible vector of *Borrelia anserina*	Causes severe irritation, trauma, erythema, edema; vector of agents of relapsing fever, epidemic typhus	Belding 1965 Hoogstraal 1967 Lapage 1962, 1968
*Otobius megnini**	United States, Hawaii, western Canada, South America, Africa, Madagascar, India, Australia	Nymph: cottontail rabbits, hares, dog, cat, domestic animals, wild ungulates, man	Arid and semiarid regions; adult in cracks and crevices; larva and nymph in external ear canal of host	Uncommon on lagomorphs, dog, cat	Unknown; probably uncommon on lagomorphs obtained from natural habitat and on dogs, cats obtained from pounds in endemic areas	Otitis, extreme irritation, edema, hemorrhage, pain, self-inflicted trauma, secondary infection, deafness, sometimes death	Rarely affects man; causes severe pain in ear canal; possible vector of agent of Q fever	Bishopp and Trembley, 1945 Cooley and Kohls 1944a Kohls et al. 1965 Lapage 1968 McIntosh and McDuffie 1956 Philip and Burgdorfer 1961
Otobius lagophilus	Western United States, western Canada, Mexico	Nymph: cottontail rabbits, hares	Arid and semiarid regions; adult in animal burrows; larva and nymph attached to facial skin of host	Common	Unknown; probably common on lagomorphs obtained from natural habitat in endemic areas	Unknown; probably irritation, trauma	Unknown; possible vector of agents of Rocky Mountain spotted fever, Colorado tick fever	Becklund 1968 Cooley and Kohls 1944a Hoogstraal 1966, 1967

*Discussed in text.

REFERENCES

Arthur, D. R., and K. R. Snow. 1968. *Ixodes pacificus* Cooley and Kohls, 1943: Its life history and occurrence. Parasitology 58: 893–906.

Becklund, W. W. 1968. Ticks of veterinary significance found on imports in the United States. J. Parasitol. 54:622–28.

Belding, D. L. 1965. Textbook of parasitology. 3d ed. Appleton-Century-Crofts, New York. 1374 pp.

Bishopp, F. C., and H. Hixson. 1936. Biology and economic importance of the Gulf Coast tick. J. Econ. Entomol. 29:1068–76.

Bishopp, F. C., and C. N. Smith. 1938. The American dog tick, eastern carrier of Rocky Mountain spotted fever. U.S. Dept. Agr. Circ. 478. 25 pp.

Bishopp, F. C., and Helen L. Trembley. 1945. Distribution and hosts of certain North American ticks. J. Parasitol. 31:1–54.

Cheng, T. C. 1964. The biology of animal parasites. W. B. Saunders, Philadelphia. 727 pp.

Cooley, R. A. 1932. The Rocky Mountain wood tick. Montana State Coll. Agr. Exp. Sta. Bull. 268. 58 pp.

———. 1938. The genera *Dermacentor* and *Otocentor* (Ixodidae) in the United States with studies in variation. Natl. Inst. Health Bull. 171. U.S. Public Health Serv. 89 pp.

———. 1946. The genera *Boophilus, Rhipicephalus,* and *Haemaphysalis* (Ixodidae) of the New World. Natl. Inst. Health Bull. 187. U.S. Public Health Serv. 54 pp.

Cooley, R. A., and G. M. Kohls. 1944a. The Argasidae of North America, Central America and Cuba. Am. Midland Naturalist, Monograph 1. 152 pp.

———. 1944b. The genus *Amblyomma* (Ixodidae) in the United States. J. Parasitol. 30: 77–111.

———. 1945. The genus *Ixodes* in North America. Natl. Inst. Health Bull. 184. U.S. Public Health Serv. 246 pp.

Faust, E. C., P. C. Beaver, and R. C. Jung. 1968. Animal agents and vectors of human disease. 3d ed. Lea and Febiger, Philadelphia. 461 pp.

Gregson, J. D. 1956. The Ixodoidea of Canada. Can. Dept. Agr. Publ. 930. Sci. Serv. Entomol. Div. 92 pp.

Hansens, E. J. 1956. Chlordane-resistant brown dog ticks and their control. J. Econ. Entomol. 49:281–83.

Hazeltine, W. 1959. Chemical resistance of the brown dog tick. J. Econ. Entomol. 52:332–33.

Hirsch, D. C., R. L. Hickman, C. R. Burkholder, and O. A. Soave. 1969. An epizootic of babesiosis in dogs used for medical research. Lab. Animal Care 19:205–8.

Hoogstraal, H. 1956. African Ixodoidea: I. Ticks of the Sudan (With special reference to Equatoria Province and with preliminary reviews of the genera *Boophilus, Margaropus,* and *Hyalomma*). U.S. Navy Dept., Wash. D.C. Res. Rept. NM 005 050.29.07. 1101 pp.

———. 1966. Ticks in relation to human diseases caused by viruses, pp. 261–308. *In* R. F. Smith and T. E. Mittler, eds. Annual Rev. Entomol. Annual Reviews, Palo Alto, Calif.

———. 1967. Ticks in relation to human diseases caused by *Rickettsia* species, pp. 377–420. *In* R. F. Smith and T. E. Mittler, eds. Annual Rev. Entomol. Annual Reviews, Palo Alto, Calif.

Hoogstraal, H., and G. M. Kohls. 1960a. Observations on the subgenus *Argas* (Ixodoidea, Argasidae, *Argas*): 1. Study of *A. reflexus reflexus* (Fabricius, 1794), the European bird argasid. Ann. Entomol. Soc. Am. 53:611–18.

———. 1960b. Observations on the subgenus *Argas* (Ixodoidea, Argasidae, *Argas*): 3. A biological and systematic study of *Argas reflexus hermanni* Audouin, 1827 (revalidated), the African bird argasid. Ann. Entomol. Soc. Am. 53:743–55.

Hooker, W. A., F. C. Bishopp, and H. P. Wood. 1912. The life history and bionomics of some North American ticks. Bull. U.S. Bur. Entomol. 106. 239 pp.

Hopla, C. E. 1960. The transmission of tularemia organisms by ticks in the southern states. Southern Med. J. 53:92–97.

Hyland, K. E., and J. A. Mathewson. 1961. The ectoparasites of Rhode Island mammals. I. The ixodid tick fauna. Wildlife Disease 11. 14 pp. (Microcard.)

Kohls, G. M. 1960. Records and new synonymy of New World *Haemaphysalis* ticks, with descriptions of the nymph and larva of *H. juxtakochi* Cooley. J. Parasitol. 46:355–61.

Kohls, G. M., and H. Hoogstraal. 1961. Observations on the subgenus *Argas* (Ixodoidea, Argasidae, *Argas*): 4. *A. neghmei,* new species, from poultry houses and human habitations in northern Chile. Ann. Entomol. Soc. Am. 54:844–51.

Kohls, G. M., H. Hoogstraal, C. M. Clifford, and M. N. Kaiser. 1970. The subgenus *Persicargas* (Ixodoidea, Argasidae, *Argas*): 9. Redescription and New World records of *Argas (P.) persicus* (Oken), and resurrection, redescription, and records of *A.*

(P.) radiatus Railliet, *A. (P.) sanchezi* Duges, and *A. (P.) miniatus* Koch, New World ticks misidentified as *A. (P.) persicus.* Ann. Entomol. Soc. Am. 63:590–606.

Kohls, G. M., and R. R. Parker. 1948. Occurrence of the brown dog tick in the western states. J. Econ. Entomol. 41:102.

Kohls, G. M., D. E. Sonenshine, and C. M. Clifford. 1965. The systematics of the subfamily Ornithodorinae (Acarina: Argasidae): II. Identification of the larvae of the Western Hemisphere and descriptions of three new species. Ann. Entomol. Soc. Am. 58:331–64.

Lapage, G. 1962. Mönnig's veterinary helminthology and entomology. 5th ed. Williams and Wilkins, Baltimore. 600 pp.

———. 1968. Veterinary parasitology. Oliver and Boyd, Edinburgh and London. 1182 pp.

Levine, N. D. 1961. Protozoan parasites of domestic animals and of man. Burgess, Minneapolis. 412 pp.

Markov, A. A., V. A. Nabokov, B. A. Timofeev, and A. M. Mitrofanov. 1968. Effect of powdered desiccants on ticks of the family Ixodidae (in Russian). Veterinariya (Moscow) 1968:61.

Martell, A. M., R. E. Yescott, and D. G. Dodds. 1969. Some records for Ixodidae of Nova Scotia. Can. J. Zool. 47:183–84.

McIntosh, A., and W. C. McDuffie. 1956. Ticks that affect domestic animals and poultry, pp. 157–66. *In* A. Stefferud, ed. Yearbook Agr. U.S. Dept. Agr.

Myers, Betty J., and R. E. Kuntz. 1965. A checklist of parasites reported for the baboon. Primates 6:137–94.

Philip, C. B., and W. Burgdorfer. 1961. Arthropod vectors as reservoirs of microbial disease agents, pp. 391–412. *In* E. A. Steinhaus and R. F. Smith, eds. Annual Rev. Entomol. Annual Reviews, Palo Alto, Calif.

Price, M. A. 1957. Experimental control of the brown dog tick *(Rhipicephalus sanguineus).* Southwestern Vet. 11:21–23.

Price, M. A., and J. D. McCrady. 1961. Brown dog tick control. Southwestern Vet. 14:287–89.

Robinow, M., and T. B. Carroll. 1938. Tick

paralysis due to the bite of the American dog tick: Report of a case observed in Georgia. J. Am. Med. Assoc. 111:1093–94.

Saliba, G. S., F. C. Harmston, B. E. Diamond, C. L. Zymet, M. I. Goldenberg, and T. D. Y. Chin. 1966. An outbreak of human tularemia associated with the American dog tick, *Dermacentor variabilis.* Am. J. Trop. Med. Hyg. 15:531–38.

Smith, C. N., M. M. Cole, and H. K. Gouck. 1946. Biology and control of the American dog tick. U.S. Dept. Agr. Tech. Bull. 905. 74 pp.

Soulsby, E. J. L. 1965. Textbook of veterinary clinical parasitology: Vol. 1. Helminths. F. A. Davis, Philadelphia. 1120 pp.

Tarshis, I. B. 1962. The use of silica aerogel compounds for the control of ectoparasites. Proc. Animal Care Panel 12:217–58.

———. 1967. Silica aerogel insecticides for the prevention and control of arthropods of medical and veterinary importance. Angew. Parasitol. 8:210–37.

Tarshis, I. B., and W. D. Ommert. 1961. Control of the spinose ear tick, *Otobius megnini* (Duges), with an organic phosphate insecticide combined with a silica aerogel. J. Am. Vet. Med. Assoc. 138:665–69.

Theis, J. H. 1968. Mechanical removal of *Rhipicephalus sanguineus* from the dog. J. Am. Vet. Med. Assoc. 153:433–37.

Trapido, H., M. K. Goverdhan, P. K. Rajagopalan, and M. J. Rebello. 1964. Ticks ectoparasitic on monkeys in the Kyasanur Forest disease area of Shimoga District, Mysore State, India. Am. J. Trop. Med. 13: 763–72.

Valerio, D. A., R. L. Miller, J. R. M. Innes, K. Diane Courtney, A. J. Pallotta, and R. M. Guttmacher. 1969. *Macaca mulatta:* Management of a laboratory breeding colony. Academic Press, New York. 140 pp.

Whitlock, J. H. 1960. Diagnosis of veterinary parasitisms. Lea and Febiger, Philadelphia. 236 pp.

Yunker, C. E. 1964. Infections of laboratory animals potentially dangerous to man: Ectoparasites and other arthropods, with emphasis on mites. Lab. Animal Care 14:455–65.

Chapter 15

MITES

MITES are minute arachnids of the subclass Acari. Those that parasitize endothermal laboratory animals belong to the suborders Mesostigmata, Prostigmata, and Astigmata (Krantz 1970). The mites that affect endothermal laboratory animals are listed in Tables 15.1, 15.2, and 15.3. Grain mites, cheese mites, and other free-living species, which are often found in animal food and bedding, are not included.

MESOSTIGMATES (MESOSTIGMATA)

Mites of the suborder Mesostigmata are more closely related to the ticks than to other mites. They are characterized by one or more ventral sclerotized plates, a large dorsal shield or shields, and a single pair of lateral spiracles on the idiosoma (Baker and Wharton 1952). Although the great majority are nonparasitic, numerous species are animal parasites, some of which are capable of transmitting viruses, rickettsiae, bacteria, protozoans, and helminths. Twenty-eight species of Mesostigmata have been listed as parasites of the wild house mouse and 24 as parasites of the Norway rat (Strandtmann and Wharton 1958). No attempt is made here to discuss each of these. Instead, only those species likely to infest endothermal laboratory animals and those potentially capable of transmitting diseases among these animals or to man are included. These are listed in Table 15.1 and the most important are discussed below.

Ornithonyssus bacoti

(SYN. *Liponyssus bacoti, Bdellonyssus bacoti*)

(Tropical Rat Mite)

Ornithonyssus bacoti (Fig. 15.1) is a common, bloodsucking parasite that has been reported from the laboratory mouse, rat, and hamster (Harris and Stockton 1960; Keefe, Scanlon, and Wetherald 1964; Sasa et al. 1962; Scott 1958), wild rodents, the cat, wild carnivores, chicken, other birds, and man (Strandtmann and Wharton 1958). It occurs throughout the world and is common in conventional colonies in some areas (Sasa et al. 1962), but is rare in others (Flynn, Brennan, and Fritz 1965). It is not found in cesarean-derived, barrier-maintained colonies (Flynn, Brennan, and Fritz 1965; Foster 1963; Owen 1968).

Ornithonyssus bacoti often gains access to an animal building on wild rodents and lives in crevices only a short distance from laboratory rodents. If the wild rodent host deserts its nest or is captured, the mite will seek blood elsewhere. The caged laboratory rodent is an ideal host.

MORPHOLOGY

The female is white or tan and 750 μ long; when engorged with blood, it is dark red or black and over 1 mm in length (Fig. 15.2) (Baker et al. 1956). Body plates are well developed and include an elongate, narrow dorsal shield that does not cover the

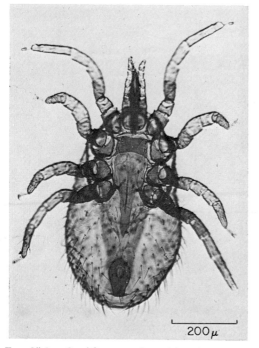

FIG. 15.1. *Ornithonyssus bacoti* female, ventral view. (Courtesy of C. Taylor, Rocky Mountain Laboratory, U.S. Public Health Service.)

entire dorsum, a rectangular sternal plate with three pairs of setae, an elongate, fingerlike epigynial plate, and an anal plate. The setae on the dorsal plate are as long as the other dorsal setae. The chelicerae are well developed, chelate, protrusible, and equal in diameter throughout. The male is smaller and possesses chelicerae modified for copulation. A fingerlike spermatodactyl, for the transfer of sperm, is on the movable chela. A single holoventral plate covers the entire intercoxal area and is usually fused with the anal shield.

LIFE CYCLE

Eggs are laid singly in the bedding or in crevices (Bertram, Unsworth, and Gordon 1946; Skaliy and Hayes 1949). The female survives about 70 days, deposits up to 100 eggs, and feeds every 2 or 3 days during this period. Larvae hatch in 1 to 4 days and molt within 1 day without feeding. The protonymph sucks blood and generally molts 5 to 14 days after feeding. It can survive for a month without food. The deutonymph is sluggish, does not feed, and molts in 1 to 2 days. Adults copulate 24 hours after emerging, and the life cycle can be completed in 13 days. Males also suck blood. *Ornithonyssus bacoti* is an obligate, intermittent bloodfeeder. All stages live in close proximity to the host, but usually

FIG. 15.2. *Ornithonyssus bacoti* female. *(Left)* Dorsal view. *(Right)* Ventral view. (From Baker et al. 1956. Courtesy of National Pest Control Association.)

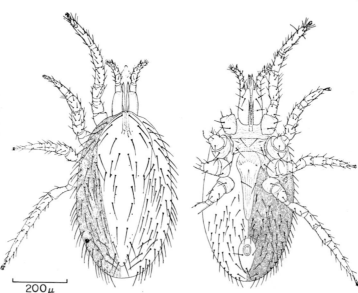

only individuals of the bloodsucking stages occur on the host.

PATHOLOGIC EFFECTS

This mite ingests blood and causes debility, anemia, decreased reproduction, and death (Harris and Stockton 1960; Keefe, Scanlon, and Wetherald 1964; Olson and Dahms 1946).

Ornithonyssus bacoti can transmit the agents of murine typhus *(Rickettsia typhi)*, rickettsialpox *(R. akari)*, Q fever *(Coxiella burneti)*, and plague *(Francisella pestis)* but is not an important natural vector of any of these pathogens (Baker et al. 1956; Strandtmann and Wharton 1958; Zemskaya and Pchelkina 1955). It is a common vector of *Litomosoides carinii*, a filarial worm of the cotton rat and other wild rodents (Bertram, Unsworth, and Gordon 1946; Williams and Brown 1945). The possibility that laboratory infestations of *O. bacoti* may circulate these or other pathogens to laboratory animals should not be discounted.

DIAGNOSIS

Infestation of an animal colony with *O. bacoti* is easily diagnosed. Engorged mites are readily seen on bedding, cages, and racks, particularly in crevices, and identification based on morphology is not difficult.

CONTROL

Effective control involves the elimination of wild rodents, the evacuation and thorough cleaning of the animal rooms and cages, and the use of chemical acaricides. Various chlorinated hydrocarbons have been found effective (Harris and Stockton 1960; Keefe, Scanlon, and Wetherald 1964; Morlan 1947; Scott 1958). These include DDT, as a 5% emulsion or 8% powder; lindane, as a 1% powder; chlordane, as a 2.0 or 2.5% emulsion; and malathion, as a 1% emulsion. A sorptive silica dust (Dri-Die 67, FMC Corporation), especially with 2% naled (Dibrom, Chevron Chemical Co.) added, is reportedly effective (Tarshis 1962). These substances are applied to surfaces that the mites traverse, such as cages, racks, floors, and walls. Treatment of bedding should be done with cau-

tion because of possible toxic effects to the animals.

Direct application of chemicals to the animals is usually not necessary because the parasite is only on the host when feeding. In severe infestations or when utilizing newly captured wild rodents, a 1% lindane dust or sorptive silica dust with 2% naled is reported to be safe for adults (Harris and Stockton 1960; Tarshis 1962). Placing infested rodents in a closed container for 24 hours with a resin strip impregnated with the aerial insecticide DDVP (dichlorvos; Vapona, Shell) (Wagner 1969) may also be effective.

PUBLIC HEALTH CONSIDERATIONS

This mite readily attacks man in the absence of its preferred hosts and is capable of inflicting an irritating to painful bite that sometimes results in an allergic dermatitis (Baker et al. 1956; Yunker 1964). *Ornithonyssus bacoti* can harbor certain pathogens for long periods following ingestion in a blood meal. These pathogens include the agents of murine typhus, rickettsialpox, Q fever, and plague (Baker et al. 1956; Strandtmann and Wharton 1958; Zemskaya and Pchelkina 1955), Coxsackie virus (Schwab, Allen, and Sulkin 1952), the tularemia bacillus *(Francisella tularensis)* (Hopla 1951), and eastern equine encephalitis virus (Clark, Lutz, and Fadness 1966). For these reasons, animals infested with this mite should be handled with caution.

Ornithonyssus sylviarum

(SYN. *Liponyssus sylviarum,* *Bdellonyssus sylviarum*)

(Northern Fowl Mite)

Ornithonyssus sylviarum is a common, bloodsucking parasite that occurs on the plumage of the chicken in temperate regions throughout the world (Baker et al. 1956). It also affects the pigeon and many wild birds (Cameron 1938; Piryanik and Akimov 1964). The mouse, rat, hamster, and man are incidental hosts. Although *O. sylviarum* is occasionally reported on the laboratory chicken (Knapp and Krause 1960), it is uncommon and is most likely to be encountered on birds obtained from farm flocks.

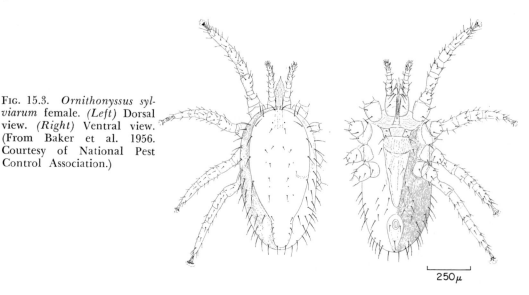

Fig. 15.3. *Ornithonyssus sylviarum* female. *(Left)* Dorsal view. *(Right)* Ventral view. (From Baker et al. 1956. Courtesy of National Pest Control Association.)

250μ

MORPHOLOGY

Adults of *O. sylviarum* are about 800 μ in length and similar to those of *O. bacoti* except that the female typically has only two pairs of setae on the sternal shield; the third pair is on the unsclerotized integument (Fig. 15.3) (Baker et al. 1956). Also,

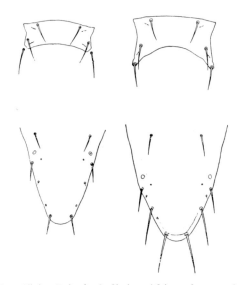

Fig. 15.4. Principal distinguishing characteristics of *Ornithonyssus sylviarum (left)* and *O. bursa (right)* females. *(Top)* Sternal plates. *(Bottom)* Posterior end of dorsal shields. (From Hirst 1922. Courtesy of British Museum—Natural History.)

in both sexes of *O. sylviarum,* most setae on the dorsal plate are smaller than those elsewhere on the dorsum, while those of *O. bacoti* are large. Confusion with *O. bursa* may also result since some specimens of *O. sylviarum* have one or both of the third pair of sternal setae on the sternal shield. An alternate distinguishing character is that *O. sylviarum* has only a single pair of well-developed setae at the posterior end of the dorsal plate, whereas *O. bursa* has two pairs in this position (Fig. 15.4).

LIFE CYCLE

The entire life cycle usually occurs on the host and can be completed in less than a week (Sikes and Chamberlain 1954). Only protonymphs and adults feed. Adults usually remain on the host, but in heavy infestations they are sometimes found on the bedding, eggs, cages, and racks, or in crevices in the floor or walls. They can survive for 2 to 3 weeks in the absence of a host.

PATHOLOGIC EFFECTS

Characteristic signs include matted and discolored feathers and thickened, scabby skin, particularly in the vent region (Baker et al. 1956). Heavy infestation has been stated to cause anemia, decreased weight gain and egg production, and sometimes death (Baker et al. 1956; Blount 1947; Siegmund 1967), but the validity of some of these statements, particularly those related to decreased egg production, has been questioned (Loomis et al. 1970).

The viruses of Newcastle disease (Hofstad 1949) and fowl pox (Brody 1936) have been recovered from *O. sylviarum* that fed on infected chickens, and those of western equine encephalitis and St. Louis encephalitis have been recovered from *O. sylviarum* taken from birds' nests (Hammon et al. 1948; Reeves et al. 1947); however, it does not appear that this mite is important in the natural transmission of these agents (Chamberlain and Sikes 1955; Chamberlain, Sikes, and Sudia 1957; Reeves et al. 1955; Sulkin et al. 1955). Nevertheless, the presence of *O. sylviarum* in laboratory facilities where experimentally infected birds are kept is an important potential hazard.

DIAGNOSIS

Infestation with *O. sylviarum* should be suspected when feathers, particularly near the vent, become matted and adjacent skin is thick and scabby. The diagnosis is confirmed by recognition of the mites on feathers that show a gray or black discoloration.

CONTROL

Effective control involves the elimination of wild birds and nests from the premises, the isolation and examination of newly acquired chickens, the sanitation of cages and shipping containers, and the use of chemical acaricides (Baker et al. 1956). Because the mite usually remains on the host's skin or plumage, it is necessary to treat the chickens as well as the cages and equipment. Several compounds are effective (Benbrook 1965; Bigley, Roth, and Eddy 1960; Foulk and Matthysse 1963; Harrison and Daykin 1965; Knapp and Krause 1960; Kraemer 1959; Kraemer and Furman 1959; Král and Schwartzman 1964; Linkfield and Reid 1958; Rodriguez and Riehl 1958; U.S. Department of Agriculture 1967; Vincent, Lindgren, and Krohne 1954). Those used to spray or paint cages and equipment include nicotine sulfate, as a 40% solution; malathion, as a 3% emulsion or 4 to 5% dust; and carbaryl, as a 4% emulsion or 5% dust. Those used directly on the chicken include malathion, as a 0.5% emulsion or 4 to 5% dust; coumaphos (Co-ral, Chemagro), as a 0.25% emulsion or 0.5% dust;

carbaryl, as a 0.25% emulsion or 5% dust; and ronnel, as a 1% dust. Care should be taken to prevent the contamination of food and water. A sorptive silica dust (Dri-Die 67, FMC Corporation), especially with 2% naled (Dibrom, Chevron Chemical Co.) added, is reportedly effective and safe when used on equipment or directly on the chicken (Tarshis 1962).

PUBLIC HEALTH CONSIDERATIONS

Ornithonyssus sylviarum will attack man in the absence of its preferred hosts. Its bite is sometimes immediately irritating and later results in erythema, induration, and pruritus (C. Yunker, unpublished data). The *Bartonella*-like agent of hemolytic-uremic syndrome, a fatal human illness, has been recovered from *O. sylviarum* collected in a patient's bedroom (Mettler 1969). This mite can also ingest and retain viable western equine encephalitis virus (Reeves et al. 1947), eastern equine encephalitis virus (Hammon et al. 1948), and the ornithosis agent (Eddie et al. 1962). Although participation of *O. sylviarum* in the maintenance or transmission of these agents in nature is questionable, infection of man through the bite of this mite or through crushing of pathogen-laden mites on his skin is a distinct possibility. For these reasons, laboratory birds infested with this mite should be handled with caution.

Ornithonyssus bursa

(SYN. *Liponyssus bursa, Bdellonyssus bursa*)

(Tropical Fowl Mite)

Ornithonyssus bursa is an important, common, bloodsucking parasite that occurs on the plumage of the chicken in tropical and subtropical parts of the world (Strandtmann and Wharton 1958). It also affects the pigeon, canary, duck, various wild birds, and occasionally man. Specific reports of this mite on the laboratory chicken are lacking. It is doubtful that it would be encountered except on birds obtained from farm flocks.

MORPHOLOGY

Ornithonyssus bursa is similar to *O. bacoti* and *O. sylviarum* (Baker et al. 1956). It is differentiated from *O. bacoti* by having dorsal plate setae that are equal to or short-

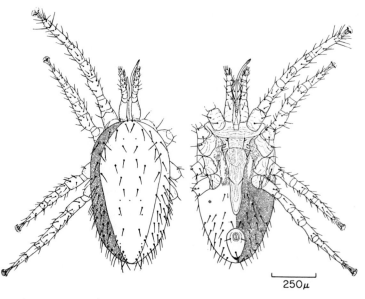

Fig. 15.5. *Ornithonyssus bursa* female. *(Left)* Dorsal view. *(Right)* Ventral view. (From Baker et al. 1956. Courtesy of National Pest Control Association.)

250μ

er than those on the adjacent integument (Fig. 15.5) and from *O. sylviarum* by having three pairs of setae on the sternal shield and two pairs of well-developed setae on the posterior end of the dorsal plate rather than one pair (Fig. 15.4).

LIFE CYCLE

Although little is known of the life cycle of this mite, it appears to be similar to that of *O. sylviarum* (Baker et al. 1956; Sikes and Chamberlain 1954; Wood 1920).

PATHOLOGIC EFFECTS

Ornithonyssus bursa causes irritation, matted feathers, anemia, and especially in young chickens, death. The mites are common on the down feathers, particularly around the vent; in young chickens they show a preference for feeding around the beak and eyes.

DIAGNOSIS

Diagnosis is based on the signs and on identification of the mite on the feathers.

CONTROL

Control is similar to that of *O. sylviarum* (Baker et al. 1956; U.S. Department of Agriculture 1967).

PUBLIC HEALTH CONSIDERATIONS

Ornithonyssus bursa readily bites man and causes skin irritation (Hirst 1916; Lodha 1969; Zimmerman 1944); otherwise, lit-

tle is known of its public health importance. However, it should be regarded as potentially capable of transmitting certain blood-borne disease agents, and birds infested with this mite should be handled with caution.

Dermanyssus gallinae

(Chicken Mite, Poultry Red Mite)

Dermanyssus gallinae is a cosmopolitan, voracious, bloodsucking parasite that occurs on the plumage of the chicken, pigeon, canary, and various other domestic and wild birds (Benbrook 1965; Strandtmann and Wharton 1958). It has also been reported from the rat, rabbit, and man, but these are probably only incidental hosts. *Dermanyssus gallinae* is the commonest mite affecting domestic birds (Benbrook 1965). It is frequently reported affecting the laboratory chicken (Bigland 1954; Harrison and Daykin 1965) and is likely to be encountered on specimens obtained from farm flocks.

MORPHOLOGY

The adult female (Fig. 15.6) is about 700 by 400 μ and, when engorged, sometimes attains a length of over 1 mm. Its elongate, whiplike chelicerae have a terminal pair of minute chelae. The ventral body plates are characteristic: the sternal shield has two pairs of setae, the genital

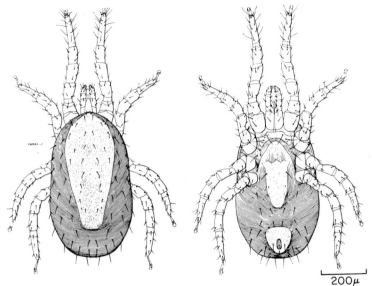

FIG. 15.6. *Dermanyssus gallinae* female. *(Left)* Dorsal view. *(Right)* Ventral view. (From Hirst 1922. Courtesy of British Museum—Natural History.)

200μ

plate is truncate, and the anal plate is a broad shield (Baker et al. 1956).

LIFE CYCLE

Eggs are laid in cracks and bedding and hatch in 2 or 3 days (Harrison and Daykin 1965; Sikes and Chamberlain 1954; Wisseman and Sulkin 1947; Wood 1917). The larvae molt within 1 to 2 days; they do not feed. Protonymphs and deutonymphs both feed, and each stage molts 1 to 2 days after ingesting blood. Adult females oviposit 12 to 24 hours after feeding. A complete cycle can occur in 9 days. Adults and nymphs hide in bedding, cage crevices, and cracks in the walls and floor during the day and feed on the host only at night. Adult mites can survive for several months without feeding (Benbrook 1965).

PATHOLOGIC EFFECTS

Clinical signs are debilitation, decreased egg production, anemia, and often death from exsanguination (Brumpt and Callot 1947; Kirkwood 1967). Skin lesions, which are uncommon (Wood 1968), consist of erythematous papular eruptions that sometimes become secondarily infected (Král and Schwartzman 1964).

The viruses of St. Louis and western and eastern equine encephalitis have been recovered from *D. gallinae* (Howitt et al. 1948; Smith, Blattner, and Heys 1944; Sul-

kin 1945), but it does not appear that this mite is important in the natural transmission of these agents (Chamberlain and Sikes 1955; Reeves et al. 1955; Sulkin et al. 1955). *Dermanyssus gallinae* is a possible vector of the agent of avian spirochaetosis *(Borrelia anserina)* (Seddon 1951) and has been shown to transmit mechanically the agent of fowl cholera *(Pasteurella multocida)* under experimental conditions (Bigland 1954). Also, *D. gallinae* transmits, experimentally, an unidentified trypanosome of canaries (Macfie and Thompson 1929; Manwell and Johnson 1931). Thus, the possibility of inadvertent transmission of blood-infecting pathogens by this mite should be kept in mind when working with experimentally infected chickens.

DIAGNOSIS

Diagnosis is based on identification of the mite in association with debilitated and anemic chickens. A "salt and pepper" appearance due to excrement, cast skins, eggs, and engorged mites is a characteristic indication of the hideaway of this parasite. Because nymphs and adults feed mainly at night, they are most easily observed and identified at this time.

CONTROL

Control is similar to that described for *Ornithonyssus sylviarum* (Baker et al. 1956;

U.S. Department of Agriculture 1967); however, because *D. gallinae* remains off the host during the day, greater emphasis should be placed on the treatment of cages, equipment, and animal rooms rather than on the treatment of individual chickens.

PUBLIC HEALTH CONSIDERATIONS

The chicken mite is an annoying pest to man. Its bite is painful and sometimes causes a papular urticaria (DeOreo 1958). It is also possible that it can transmit certain arboviruses to man. For these reasons, birds infested with this mite should be handled with caution.

Liponyssoides sanguineus

(SYN. *Allodermanyssus sanguineus*)

(House Mouse Mite)

Liponyssoides sanguineus is a bloodsucking parasite that occurs on the house mouse, wild Norway rat, other wild rodents, and man (Strandtmann and Wharton 1958). It has been found in North America, Europe, Africa, and Asia, but its distribution is localized. Although it has not yet been reported to infest laboratory rodents, such infestations may have occurred but not been recognized because the mite was confused with species of *Dermanyssus* or *Ornithonyssus*. Because of its wide distribution, its association with the house mouse and Norway rat, and its predilection for the peridomestic habitat, this mite is likely to parasitize laboratory stock. For these reasons, and because it is the vector of the agent of rickettsialpox, a disease of man, it is included here.

MORPHOLOGY

The female has elongate, whiplike chelicerae resembling those of *Dermanyssus gallinae* (Fig. 15.7) (Baker et al. 1956). It has two dorsal shields, an elongate anterior one and a reduced posterior one, and three pairs of setae on the sternal plate. Unengorged females are 650 to 750 μ long but sometimes distend to over 1 mm after feeding.

LIFE CYCLE

The female ingests blood intermittently and oviposits after each feeding (Fuller 1954; Nichols, Rindge, and Russell 1953). Eggs hatch in 4 or 5 days, and the larvae molt in 3 days without feeding. Both the protonymph and deutonymph feed only once; the former molts after 4 or 5 days and the latter after 6 to 10 days. The complete cycle requires 17 to 23 days, and the female can survive up to 51 days without feeding.

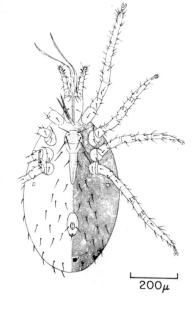

FIG. 15.7. *Liponyssoides sanguineus* female. *(Left)* Dorsal view. *(Right)* Ventral view. (From Baker et al. 1956. Courtesy of National Pest Control Association.)

200μ

Liponyssoides sanguineus is nidicolous, occurring on the host only when feeding. At other times it dwells in cracks and crevices in close proximity to the host.

PATHOLOGIC EFFECTS

The effects of *L. sanguineus* on rodent hosts are unknown. Heavy infestations probably cause debility, anemia, decreased reproduction, and death.

DIAGNOSIS

Diagnosis is based on recognition of the mite on a host or on bedding, cages, or racks, under wall moldings, or in ducts, vents, or chutes.

CONTROL

Control is not reported but is probably similar to that described for *Ornithonyssus bacoti* (Baker et al. 1956).

PUBLIC HEALTH CONSIDERATIONS

Although the bite of this mite causes a rash in man (Ewing 1942), its principal public health importance is that it is the vector of *Rickettsia akari,* the cause of rickettsialpox in man (Huebner, Jellison, and Pomerantz 1946). If a laboratory animal facility should be infested, prompt elimination is important.

Pneumonyssus simicola

(SYN. *Pneumonyssus griffithi, Pneumotuber macaci, Pneumonyssus foxi*)

(Lung Mite of Monkey)

Pneumonyssus simicola is an extremely common parasite of the lungs of the rhesus monkey (Fairbrother and Hurst 1932; Gay and Branch 1927; Habermann and Williams 1957; Ruch 1959). Incidences of 100% have been reported in this species and it is believed that no imported rhesus monkey is free of infection (Finegold, Seaquist, and Doherty 1968; Fremming et al. 1957; Innes 1965; Innes et al. 1954; Lee et al. 1954). This mite also occurs but is less common in the cynomolgus monkey (Fain 1959; Honjo et al. 1963), the pigtail macaque, and other macaques (Banks 1901; Fain 1961; Strandtmann and Wharton 1958). A single report of *P. simicola* from an African gelada baboon (Vitzthum 1930) is apparently a correct identification, but the true origin of the material has been questioned (Fain 1961).

The literature dealing with *P. simicola* is confusing, partly because some authors fail to identify monkey or mite species properly, and partly because some deal with all lung mite infections of primates as a single entity, pulmonary acariasis. It appears, however, that *P. simicola* is restricted to members of the genus *Macaca* originating in Asia and the Philippine Islands, and that the mites found in the respiratory tract of African primates, such as guenons, baboons, the chimpanzee, and gorilla, with the one exception noted above, are different species of *Pneumonyssus* (Böhm and Supperer 1955; Ewing 1929; Fain 1959).

Because of the universal occurrence of this mite in rhesus monkeys obtained from their natural habitat, its presence in laboratory monkeys should be expected and the possibility of its interfering with studies involving the pulmonary system in this species must be kept in mind (Finegold, Seaquist, and Doherty 1968; Innes 1969; Robertson et al. 1947). In contrast to its universal occurrence in rhesus monkeys obtained from their natural habitat, *P. simicola* has not been observed in laboratory-reared monkeys removed from their mothers at birth (Innes 1969; Knezevich and McNulty 1970; Valerio et al. 1969).

MORPHOLOGY

The adult is yellow-white, elongate, and ovoid (Fig. 15.8) (Fain 1961). Females are 700 to 850 μ long; males are 500 μ. Both have a single small dorsal plate which is marked by scars of muscle insertions. The female sternal plate is longer than it is wide and has three pairs of setae. An epigynial plate is absent, and the female genital opening is a transverse slit between the fourth set of coxae. Palps are composed of four free segments. Chelicerae are short with opposed chelae; the movable chela is more developed than the fixed chela. Legs are long and have small setae and terminal claws. The egg is glistening white, spherical, and about 250 to 450 μ in diameter (Grinker, Karlin, and Manalo Estrella 1962).

LIFE CYCLE

The complete life cycle is unknown (Baker et al. 1956; Hull 1956), but it has

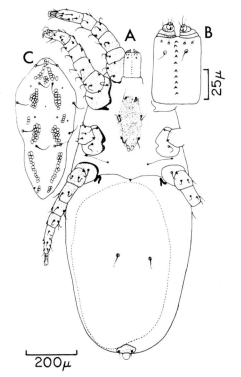

200μ

Fig. 15.8. *Pneumonyssus simicola* female. *(A)* Ventral view. *(B)* Gnathosoma (enlarged). *(C)* Dorsal shield. (From Fain 1961. Courtesy of Springer-Verlag, Berlin.)

its morphology, host distribution, and phylogenetic relationships all indicate that it is an obligate internal parasite. It has also been postulated that the mites enter the body by ingestion, reaching the lungs via the lymphatics and bloodstream (Landois and Hoepke 1914). Adult mites have been found in the pulmonary artery (Lee et al. 1954; Woodard 1968), but their presence here is uncommon and probably only a chance occurrence. Transplacental transfer of mites apparently does not occur. Mites have not been found in monkeys delivered by cesarean section or in those born naturally in the laboratory that are isolated from their mothers at birth (Fremming et al. 1957; Innes 1969; Knezevich and McNulty 1970; Valerio et al. 1969). The most plausible suggestion is that mites are transferred as larvae from the bronchi, either through direct contact, coughing, or sneezing (Baker et al. 1956).

PATHOLOGIC EFFECTS

Clinical signs are usually absent (Furman 1954; Innes et al. 1954); paroxysmal coughing and sneezing have been reported (Helwig 1925), but these signs are uncommon and may be caused by associated respiratory disease. Although earlier workers (Hamerton 1939; Helwig 1925) attributed fatalities to this mite, it is probably the direct cause of death only in massive infections (Stone and Hughes 1969).

Gross lesions range in appearance from minute, pale spots to yellowish foci a few millimeters in diameter (Fig. 15.9) (Innes et al. 1954; Stone and Hughes 1969). Their number varies from a few to hundreds. They occur in the lung parenchyma, either near the surface and elevated above it, or at depths within any lobe of the lung (Baker et al. 1956). Superficially, they resemble tubercles but are less firm. The lesions are discrete and surrounded by normal, pink crepitant lung tissue; few become approximated and confluent. Rarely is there any hemorrhage near the mites. Viewed under magnification the foci appear as pale, white jellylike masses which sometimes have a minute slit or opening in the center (Innes et al. 1954). The lesions and surrounding tissue contain a characteristic golden brown to black pigment. One to 20 mites, predominantly females but sometimes eggs,

been suggested that the entire cycle occurs in the lungs (Innes et al. 1954). Eggs presumably hatch within the female, and fully developed larvae are deposited. Larvae occur in pulmonary nodules and also in the bronchi. They are the only stage commonly found free in the bronchi and are presumed to be the infective stage (Baker et al. 1956). The protonymph and deutonymph stages are brief and have been seen only under experimental conditions (Hull 1956). Adults are found in pulmonary lesions that usually open into a bronchiole. There is evidence that the mites suck blood (Innes et al. 1954), but they also have been reported to feed on lymph and pulmonary epithelium cells (Hughes 1959).

The mode of transmission is unknown. The suggestion that *P. simicola* is normally an ectoparasite that is adventitiously inhaled (Sergeyev 1949) is refuted by the extremely high infection rates. In addition,

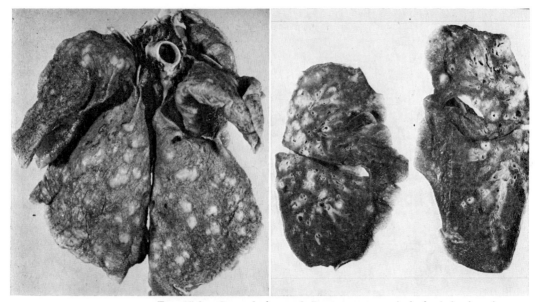

FIG. 15.9. Gross lesions of *Pneumonyssus simicola* infection in preserved lung specimens from a monkey. Note numerous pale foci beneath pleura *(left)* and on cut surface *(right)*. (Courtesy of J. R. M. Innes, Bionetics Research Laboratories.)

larvae, or males, are easily teased from the lesion (Fig. 15.10) (Baker et al. 1956; Lee et al. 1954).

Histopathology is often extensive (Innes et al. 1954). It is characterized by the

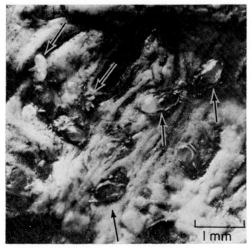

FIG. 15.10. Magnification of gross lesions of *Pneumonyssus simicola* infection in the lung of a monkey. Note mites *(arrows)* teased from typical lesions. (Courtesy of J. R. M. Innes, Bionetics Research Laboratories.)

presence of the mite in association with localized bronchiolitis and peribronchiolitis (Fig. 15.11), or focal pneumonitis in which eosinophils are prominent, and sometimes by bronchiolectasis. Pigments and double refractile needles are always present in or near the mites or their foci. This pigment, which is not seen in the lungs of normal monkeys, does not contain carbon or melanin but definitely contains iron and probably results from the mite's breakdown and excretion of the host's blood proteins (Innes et al. 1954).

DIAGNOSIS

Diagnosis of *P. simicola* infection in live monkeys is difficult. Routine roentgenographic or hematologic examinations are of no value (Innes 1965; Innes et al. 1954). Sometimes larvae can be demonstrated in tracheobronchial washings, but a negative finding does not exclude the possibility of infection (Baker et al. 1956). Gross lesions produced by the mite must be differentiated from those of tuberculosis. The finding of mites or the characteristic pigment and crystals associated with them in histologic sections is diagnostic of lung mite in-

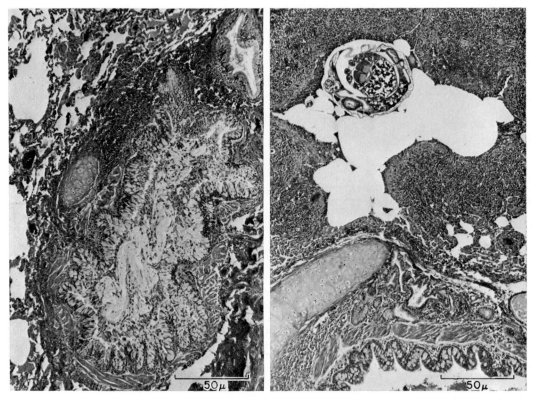

FIG. 15.11. Photomicrograph of *Pneumonyssus simicola* lesions in the lung of a monkey. *(Left)* Note thickened bronchial wall, severe peribronchial lymphocytic infiltration, hyperplasia of goblet cells, and lumen filled with cellular debris and mucus. *(Right)* Cross section of mite in parenchyma adjacent to bronchus. Note extensive chronic inflammation causing widespread consolidation and secondary emphysema. (Courtesy of T. E. Fritz, Argonne National Laboratory.)

fection, but it is not necessarily diagnostic of *P. simicola* infection. Although *P. simicola* is the usual lung mite affecting the rhesus monkey, *Rhinophaga dinolti* is sometimes found (Furman 1954). Differentiation is based primarily on morphology of the tarsal claws. The claws on the first leg of females of *R. dinolti* are much less developed than those on the third leg, whereas all tarsal claws of *P. simicola* are subequal in size. All lung mites of simian primates are similar and seldom, if ever, can be specifically identified from fragments in cross sections. Identification is a matter for the expert, who should be supplied with whole mites (as opposed to sections) whenever possible.

CONTROL

Definitive methods for control by treatment are lacking. Administration of penta-valent arsenic has yielded no significant results (Lee et al. 1954). Ronnel (Ectoral, Pitman-Moore), given intragastrically at a rate of 55 mg per kg of body weight every other day for four treatments and then weekly for 3 months, significantly reduces the number of inflamed bronchioles and active lesions in treated monkeys (as compared with untreated controls) (Finegold, Seaquist, and Doherty 1968), and DDVP (dichlorvos), used as an aerosol or vaporized in the atmosphere in conjunction with pelage dusting with lindane powder, have given encouraging results (Masse, Geneste, and Thiery 1965), but neither of these treatments is completely effective. Complete control can be achieved, however, by the development of infection-free colonies that are initiated by rearing newborn monkeys in isolation from their mothers (Innes 1969; Valerio et al. 1969).

PUBLIC HEALTH CONSIDERATIONS

Lung mite infection of monkeys has no known public health significance. Despite reports to the contrary (Fiennes 1967), mites recovered from human cases of pulmonary illness are distinctly unrelated to lung mites of monkeys, and there is no evidence that *P. simicola* is infectious to man.

Pneumonyssoides caninum

(SYN. *Pneumonyssus caninum*)

(Nasal Mite of Dog)

This relatively nonpathogenic mite inhabits the nasal cavities and sinuses of the dog and has been reported in the United States (including Hawaii), South Africa, and Australia (Baker et al. 1956; Senter 1958). Although generally uncommon and of unknown incidence in the laboratory, it is likely to be occasionally encountered in laboratory dogs throughout the world.

MORPHOLOGY

The female is similar to that of *Pneumonyssus simicola* but is slightly larger, 1.0 to 1.5 mm long (Fig. 15.12) (Baker et al. 1956; Chandler and Ruhe 1940). The male is nearly as long as the female (Furman 1954). Both sexes have palps of five segments, a small, irregular dorsal shield, an irregular sternal plate that is wider than long, and a small, ovoid anal plate. The sternal plate of the female has two pairs of setae and that of the male has three pairs. The female genital opening is a transverse slit between the fourth pair of legs; there is no epigynial plate. The first leg of both sexes has a large pair of naked, sessile, tarsal claws, dissimilar from those of other legs. Nymphs have not been found.

LIFE CYCLE

The life cycle is unknown (Baker et al. 1956). Transmission is thought to be by larval transfer on direct contact because larvae have been seen crawling from dogs' nostrils (Baker et al. 1956; Senter 1958).

PATHOLOGIC EFFECTS

Although a variety of signs, including bronchial cough, excessive nasal secretion, lacrimation, listlessness, inappetence, sudden loss of consciousness, and orbital cellulitis, have been observed (Roberts and Thompson 1969; Senter 1958), infection with this mite is usually relatively asymptomatic, with the only clinical signs being excessive mucus production and hyperemia of the nasal mucosa (Koutz, Chamberlain, and Cole 1953).

DIAGNOSIS

Although infection is usually diagnosed at necropsy, it can also be recognized by observing the mite crawling near the external nares while the dog is sleeping, or by finding the mite or its eggs in nasal washings (Carpenter 1968).

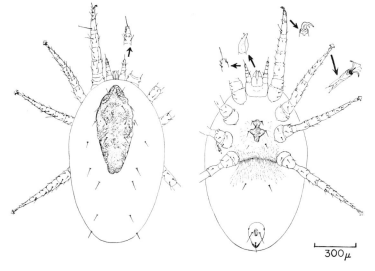

FIG. 15.12. *Pneumonyssoides caninum* female. *(Left)* Dorsal view. *(Right)* Ventral view. (From Baker et al. 1956. Courtesy of National Pest Control Association.)

300μ

Control is unknown.

This mite is of no known public health importance.

Laelaps echidninus

(SYN. *Echinolaelaps echidninus*)

(Spiny Rat Mite)

Although not an important pathogen, this mite sometimes ingests blood and is a known or potential vector of certain disease agents (Miller 1908; Parodi et al. 1959). It is a common ectoparasite of the wild Norway rat throughout the world and is occasionally found on the house mouse, cotton rat, and other wild rodents (Baker et al. 1956). *Laelaps echidninus* has been reported from the laboratory rat, but it is rare (Miller 1908; Strandtmann and Wharton 1958). It does not adapt well to the laboratory situation and is not likely to be encountered unless sanitation is extremely poor.

The female is ovoid to globular, has heavily sclerotized, reddish brown shields and is about 1 mm long (Fig. 15.13) (Strandtmann and Mitchell 1963). The ventral plates are characteristic: the sternal plate is semirectangular, slightly longer than wide, and bears three pairs of setae; the epigynial plate is elongate and flask shaped, has four pairs of setae, and is concave on its posterior margin. The anterior margin of the anal plate is convex, fitting closely within the concavity of the epigynial plate. All body setae are long and stout, and the first three pairs of coxae bear short, thick ventral spurs.

The larva is born alive, does not feed, and molts into a protonymph in 10 to 13 hours (Owen 1956). The protonymph feeds within hours after emergence and molts in 3 to 11 days; the deutonymph also feeds, and molts in 3 to 9 days. The female feeds shortly after molting and produces larvae within 5 days, sometimes by parthenogenesis. At least 16 days are required for a complete life cycle. Females live 60 to 90 days but can survive only a week without food. The mites feed at night and live in the bedding or in cage crevices during the day. Although they sometimes suck blood, they can also feed on a variety of other substances, including lacrimal secretions and serous exudate from a living host (Furman 1959), and they sometimes ingest their own larvae. Under laboratory conditions, they have never been seen to break the intact skin of their host, but they feed readily on abraded

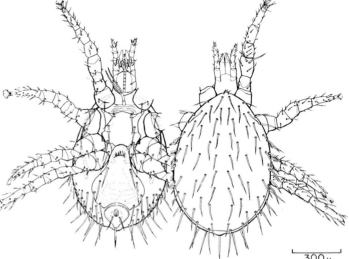

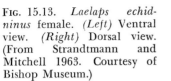

FIG. 15.13. *Laelaps echidninus* female. *(Left)* Ventral view. *(Right)* Dorsal view. (From Strandtmann and Mitchell 1963. Courtesy of Bishop Museum.)

300μ

skin (Furman 1959; Wharton and Cross 1957).

PATHOLOGIC EFFECTS

Clinical signs are unknown except that in laboratory cultures this mite has been associated with the development of footpad lesions of suckling mice (Furman 1959). *Laelaps echidninus* is the natural vector of *Hepatozoon muris* (Miller 1908), and it can also transmit the agent of tularemia *(Francisella tularensis)* among rodents under experimental conditions (Baker et al. 1956).

DIAGNOSIS

Diagnosis is based on recognition of the mite on a host or in the bedding or cage crevices.

CONTROL

Control is unknown, but measures effective against *Ornithonyssus bacoti* are probably effective against this mite.

PUBLIC HEALTH CONSIDERATIONS

Junin virus, the cause of Argentinian hemorrhagic fever, has been isolated from *L. echidninus* in South America (Parodi et al. 1959), but the significance of this in the transmission of the virus to man is uncertain as *L. echidninus* does not pierce the intact skin of man (Wharton and Cross 1957).

PROSTIGMATES (PROSTIGMATA)

Members of the suborder Prostigmata are quite different from the mesostigmates (Baker and Wharton 1952). They are structurally and biologically diverse and include some of the commonest parasites of endothermal laboratory animals. Many important plant pests also belong to this group, as well as the trombiculids (chiggers). Many trombiculids have been reported from wild rodents throughout the world (Baker et al. 1956). No attempt is made here to discuss each of these. Instead, only species likely to infest laboratory animals are included. Prostigmates that affect endothermal laboratory animals are listed in Table 15.2. The most important are discussed below.

Myobia musculi

(Fur Mite of Mouse)

Myobia musculi is a pelage-inhabiting mite that is common on the laboratory and wild house mouse throughout the world (Baker et al. 1956; Smith 1955a, b). In surveys of conventional laboratory mouse colonies in North America (Flynn 1955; Flynn, Brennan, and Fritz 1965), Europe (Blackmore and Owen 1968; Heine 1962), and Asia (Fukui et al. 1961), it has been found in incidences ranging up to 100% of the mice examined in 100% of the colonies sampled, but it is absent from cesarean-derived, barrier-maintained colonies (Flynn, Brennan, and Fritz 1965).

MORPHOLOGY

This mite is small, unsclerotized, and elongate and has transverse integumental striae (Baker et al. 1956; Grant 1942) (Fig. 15.14). The male and female differ only in size, setation, and genitalia. The gnathosoma is small, with minute, simple palpi

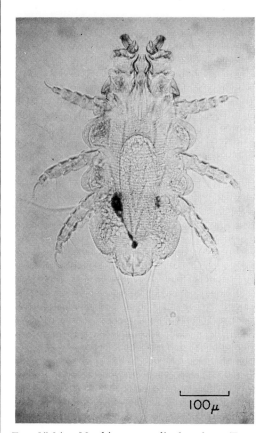

FIG. 15.14. *Myobia musculi* female. (From Flynn 1963. Courtesy of American Association for Laboratory Animal Science.)

and small, styletlike chelicerae. The first pair of legs is short, compressed, and highly adapted for hair clasping. The other three pairs are less modified; true claws are absent but each tarsus ends in a large, clawlike structure, the empodium or empodial claw. The mite is approximately twice as long as wide, and the lateral margins of the idiosoma form bulges between each pair of legs. Females are approximately 400 to 500 μ long, and males are 285 to 320 μ. The anus is dorsal. Genitalia consist of a posterior opening on the female dorsum and an elongate, dorsal, internal aedeagus in the male. The adult dorsum bears a series of large, slightly expanded, fluted setae. Eggs are oval and about 200 μ long. They resemble miniature louse nits and are attached to the bases of hairs at their lower poles. The first larva has three pairs of legs. The first pair is used for clasping hair and the second and third pairs are for walking. The mouthparts appear as a slender, whiplike proboscis. The second larva is larger and possesses a large, clawlike empodium on the third tarsi and limb buds of the developing fourth legs. Nymphs are larger than the larvae and possess three pairs of walking legs and the anterior pair of hair-clasping legs. In the protonymph, the fourth pair of legs is rudimentary while in the deutonymph this pair is well developed and possesses setae and clawlike empodia. Nymphs also have extended mouthparts.

LIFE CYCLE

Eggs hatch in 8 days (Haakh 1958). The first larva molts after 4 days; the second larva also molts in 4 days. The duration of the protonymph and deutonymph stages is not known. The entire life cycle has been reported to take 12 to 13 days (Haakh 1958), but this is no doubt an underestimate since, in that study, larvae were mistakenly called protonymphs and deutonymphs. All motile stages feed on extracellular tissue fluids (Wharton 1960). Transmission is by direct contact.

PATHOLOGIC EFFECTS

The degree of pathogenicity to mice, among strains and even in a single colony, is variable (Haakh 1958; Whiteley and Horton 1962). Light infestations cause no obvious signs and are usually inapparent (Galton 1963; Tuffery and Innes 1963). The mites ingest significant amounts of extracellular tissue fluid from the host without causing visible tissue damage (Wharton, 1960). Heavy infestations cause dermatitis, alopecia, pruritus, self-inflicted trauma, and secondary amyloidosis (Fukui et al. 1961; Galton 1963; Heston and Deringer 1948). An increase in the mitotic activity of the dermal epithelium has also been correlated with heavy infestations with this mite (Whiteley and Horton 1962).

Myobia musculi is not known to be a vector of any bacterial or viral pathogens, but its feeding habits make it well suited to such a role (Wharton 1960).

DIAGNOSIS

Diagnosis of *M. musculi* infestation is based on the demonstration of the mite (Flynn 1963). Care must be taken to distinguish *M. musculi* from *Radfordia affinis*, which is also common on the laboratory mouse (Flynn 1955). The easiest means of differentiation is by the terminal claws on the second pair of legs. *Myobia musculi* has a single empodial claw on this segment while *R. affinis* has two claws (Ewing 1938).

CONTROL

Acaricidal dips are the most widely used means of controlling *M. musculi* infestations. A 2% suspension of a wettable powder containing 15% butylphenoxyisopropyl chloroethyl sulfite (Aramite-15W, Uniroyal), combined with a wetting agent, is effective when used as a dip (Flynn 1955; Galton 1963). Treatment should be repeated in 7 to 12 days because eggs may survive. Other effective treatments include 2.0% malathion in water, applied as a dip twice, with a 12-day interval (Clark and Yunker 1964); 0.2% 4,4'dichloro-α-methylbenzhydrol (DMC, Sherwin-Williams) in 50% ethyl alcohol, applied as a dip two or three times at 5-day intervals (Stoner and Hale 1953); and a 25% proprietary solution of tetraethylthiuram monosulfide (Tetmosol, Imperial Chemicals) diluted to 1.4% in water, applied as a dip once or twice, with a 1- to 3-week interval (Cook 1953). Placing infested mice in a closed container for 24 hours with a resin strip impregnated with DDVP (dichlorvos; Vapona, Shell), or placing a small section of such a resin strip on the lid of a mouse cage for 24 hours is also effective (Wagner 1969). Because *M. musculi* feeds on interstitial fluids, control with systemic insecticides would seem feasible.

Complete eradication of *M. musculi* infestation can be achieved by initiating new colonies by cesarean section (Flynn, Brennan, and Fritz 1965).

PUBLIC HEALTH CONSIDERATIONS

Myobia musculi does not affect man.

Radfordia affinis
(SYN. *Myobia affinis*)
(Fur Mite of Mouse)

Radfordia affinis is a pelage-inhabiting mite that occurs on the laboratory and wild house mouse throughout the world (Flynn 1955; Flynn, Brennan, and Fritz 1965; Fukui et al. 1961; Heine 1962; Seamer and

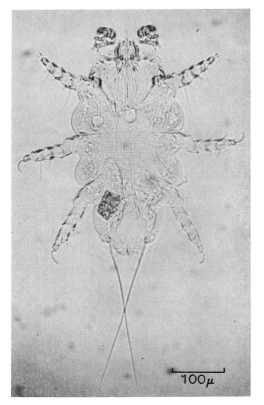

FIG. 15.15. *Radfordia affinis* female. (From Flynn 1963. Courtesy of American Association for Laboratory Animal Science.)

Chesterman 1967; Smith 1955a, b). It is common in conventional laboratory mouse colonies, but it does not occur in cesarean-derived, barrier-maintained colonies (Flynn, Brennan, and Fritz 1965). It closely resembles *Myobia musculi* with which it is undoubtedly often confused (Flynn 1963). *Radfordia affinis* is distinguished by the presence of a pair of simple terminal claws on the tarsi of the second pair of legs (Ewing 1938) (Fig. 15.15); *M. musculi* has only a single empodial claw on these segments. The life cycle, pathologic effects, diagnosis, and public health importance of *R. affinis* are unknown but are probably similar to those of *M. musculi*. Control methods used against *M. musculi* are apparently effective against this species (Flynn 1955; Heine 1962).

Radfordia ensifera
(SYN. *Myobia ensifera, Myobia ratti*)
(Fur Mite of Rat)

Radfordia ensifera is a pelage-inhabiting mite that occurs on the wild and laboratory rat throughout the world (Baker et al. 1956). It is common in some conventional laboratory rat colonies (Heine 1962; Sasa et al. 1962; Skidmore 1934), but it does not occur in cesarean-derived, barrier-maintained colonies (Blackmore and Owen 1968; Foster 1963). *Radfordia ensifera* closely resembles *Myobia musculi* and *R. affinis* (Ewing 1938) (Fig. 15.16) and is most readily distinguished by the claws on the tarsi of the second pair of legs. Those of *R. ensifera* are paired and equal, whereas those of *R. affinis* are paired and subequal; *M. musculi* has only a single empodial claw on these segments. Heavy infestations have been reported to induce self-inflicted trauma (Skidmore 1934); otherwise, little is known of its pathologic effects. Control methods effective against *M. musculi* are apparently effective against this species (Heine 1962).

Psorergates simplex
(Follicle Mite of Mouse)

Psorergates simplex is a follicle-inhabiting, sometimes scab-forming mite that has been reported from the wild mouse and frequently from the laboratory mouse in North America and Europe (Bateman 1961; Beres-

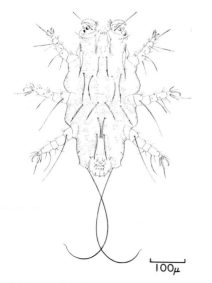

FIG. 15.16. *Radfordia ensifera* female, dorsal view. (From Baker et al. 1956. Courtesy of National Pest Control Association.)

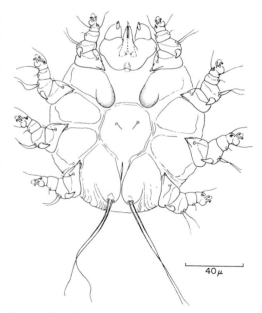

FIG. 15.17. *Psorergates simplex* female, ventral view. (Courtesy of Alma D. Smith, Rocky Mountain Laboratory, U.S. Public Health Service.)

ford-Jones 1965; Cook 1956; Flynn 1955). In one survey of commercially produced laboratory mice in the United States, incidences as high as 80% were observed (Flynn 1955). All reports of this mite in laboratory mice are from conventional colonies; it does not occur in cesarean-derived, barrier-maintained colonies (Flynn, Brennan, and Fritz 1965).

MORPHOLOGY

Psorergates simplex is a minute, rounded mite which ranges in length from 90 to 150 μ (Baker et al. 1956; Fain, Lukoschus, and Hallmann 1966) (Fig. 15.17). Adults and the nymph have four pairs of legs which are radially arranged and which have five telescoping segments; the larva has three pairs of legs (Fig. 15.18). There is a medially directed spine on the ventral surface of each femur. Each tarsus terminates in a pair of simple claws and a padlike empodium. The palpal segments are undifferentiated and coalesced. Chelicerae are minute, protrusible, styletlike and enclosed in a small conical rostrum. The anus is ventral with a tubercle on each side. The female has a pair of long, whiplike setae on each tubercle; the male has a single seta on each side and a dorsal penis.

LIFE CYCLE

The life cycle of *P. simplex* is unknown. All stages are found in a single follicle or lesion (Fig. 15.18) (Cook 1956; Flynn and Jaroslow 1956). Colonization of a follicle apparently results from the entrance of a gravid female. Transmission is by direct contact (Beresford-Jones 1967).

PATHOLOGIC EFFECTS

Follicle infection results in the formation of dermal pouches (Flynn and Jaroslow 1956). These pouches appear as small, white nodules on the visceral surface of the skin of all parts of the body, particularly the head (Fig. 15.19). Those in the dorsal neck region, where the skin is loose, are sometimes as large as 2 mm; those on the face and legs, where the skin is tight, are smaller. They are simple invaginations of the skin that open to the outside (Fig. 15.20). Occasionally these pouches become encysted and are then invaded by inflammatory cells.

An auricular mange, characterized by a thick, pale yellow crust on the inner and outer surface of the ear, has also been re-

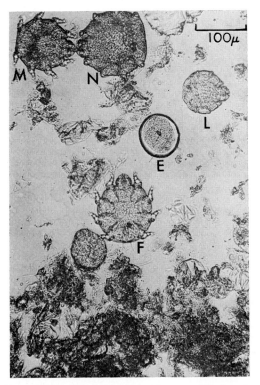

FIG. 15.18. *Psorergates simplex* egg *(E)*, female *(F)*, larva *(L)*, male *(M)*, and nymph *(N)*. (From Flynn and Jaroslow 1956. Courtesy of American Society of Parasitologists.)

ported to be caused by this mite (Cook 1956). It is apparently not common.

DIAGNOSIS

Follicular infection with *P. simplex* is easily demonstrated by examining the inner surface of the skin for macroscopic pouches (Flynn 1963). All stages of the mite can be expressed from the pouch along with caseous material (Fig. 15.18). Similarly, all stages are readily demonstrated in the scabs associated with the auricular form. Care must be taken to distinguish between psorergatic and notoedric ear mange. Definitive diagnosis is made by identification of the mite.

CONTROL

Effective treatments include weekly dipping in either a 2% suspension of a wettable powder containing 15% butylphenoxyisopropyl chloroethyl sulfite (Aramite-

15W, Uniroyal) in combination with a wetting agent (Flynn 1959a) or an aqueous emulsion containing 0.2% 4,4′dichloro-α-methylbenzhydrol (DMC, Sherwin-Williams) in combination with a 25% proprietary solution of tetraethylthiuram monosulfide (Tetmosol, Imperial Chemicals) diluted to 1.7% (Bateman 1961). Undiluted dibutyl phthalate applied topically is effective for the auricular mange caused by this mite (Cook 1956). Complete eradication can be achieved by initiating new colonies by cesarean section (Flynn, Brennan, and Fritz 1965).

PUBLIC HEALTH CONSIDERATIONS

Psorergates simplex does not affect man.

Demodex canis
(Follicle Mite of Dog)

Demodex canis is the common follicle-inhabiting mite of the dog and is the cause of demodectic mange. It occurs throughout the world in all breeds (Koutz 1954). In a

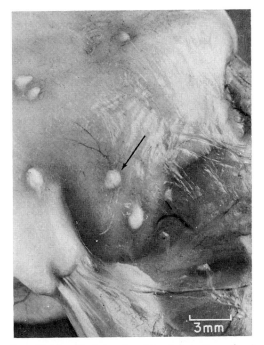

FIG. 15.19. Nodules in skin (visceral surface) of a mouse caused by *Psorergates simplex*. (From Flynn and Jaroslow 1956. Courtesy of American Society of Parasitologists.)

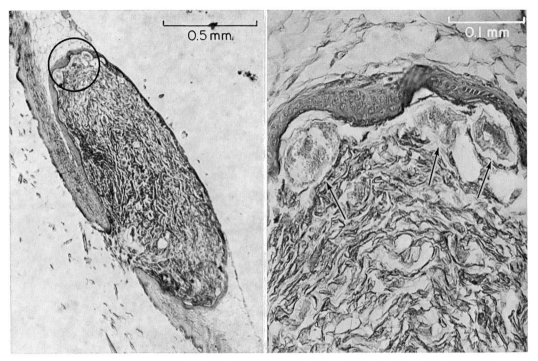

Fig. 15.20. *Psorergates simplex* lesions in the skin of a mouse. *(Left)* Section of dermal nodule. *(Right)* Magnification of circled area. Note mites in cross section *(arrows).* (From Flynn and Jaroslow 1956. Courtesy of American Society of Parasitologists.)

survey involving the examination of skin sections from 208 apparently normal dogs, 53% were found infected (Koutz, Groves, and Gee 1960). The incidence is not affected by age, sex, or length of hair, but clinical signs are commonest in dogs under 1 year of age and are most likely to be recognized in short-haired breeds (Koutz 1954). Infection is common in laboratory dogs obtained from pounds and commercial suppliers (Bantin and Maber 1967; Flynn 1959b), and only dogs obtained from colonies initiated by cesarean section (Griesemer and Gibson 1963) are free of this mite.

MORPHOLOGY

Adults are 200 to 400 μ in length and vermiform (Baker et al. 1956) (Fig. 15.21). They have four pairs of short, stumpy legs, small mouthparts, and no setae. A small, blunt rostrum contains minute styletlike chelicerae and the compressed palpal segments. The penis of the male is dorsal and anterior; the female genital opening lies between the fourth pair of legs.

LIFE CYCLE

The mite is commonly found in the sebaceous glands and hair follicles. It has also been recovered from several body tissues, but the significance of these findings is unknown (El-Gindy 1952; French 1964; Koutz 1957; Lucker and Sause 1952). Eggs require 6 days for incubation (Unsworth 1946), and the entire life cycle, which can be completed in a skin pustule, takes about 24 days (Enigk 1949).

The mode of transmission is unknown. Although attempts to transmit *D. canis* between adult dogs by direct contact have been generally unsuccessful (Cánepa and Da Graña 1945; Koutz 1957; Unsworth 1946), transmission by direct application of infected skin scraping suspensions to young dogs has been demonstrated (French, Raun, and Baker 1964). Possible neonatal trans-

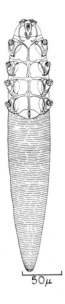

FIG. 15.21. *Demodex canis* female, ventral view. (From Baker et al. 1956. Courtesy of National Pest Control Association.)

50μ

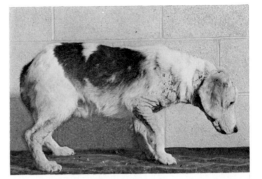

FIG. 15.22. Demodectic mange in a dog. (From Flynn 1959b. Courtesy of American Veterinary Medical Association.)

mission from nursing bitch to offspring has been reported (Greve and Gaafar 1966), and this may be the usual route (Baker 1969a). Prenatal transmission, which has been suggested as another possible route (Enigk 1949; Kirk 1950), has been recognized only once (Gowing 1964).

PATHOLOGIC EFFECTS

Since *D. canis* is often present in hair follicles in the absence of lesions, its precise role as a primary disease agent is unknown (Koutz 1966; Koutz, Groves, and Gee 1960). Intestinal parasites, malnutrition, and other debilitating diseases are possible predisposing causes of demodectic mange.

There are two types of cutaneous lesions in demodectic mange (Fig. 15.22), squamous and pustular (Koutz 1953, 1954; Král and Schwartzmann 1964). Both types are sometimes present concurrently. A localized alopecia and dry, scaly dermatitis, with mild induration, typify the squamous type. Early lesions are seen commonly on the head and sometimes on other parts of the body. The pustular type occurs as a primary condition or as a sequel to the squamous type. It is generally associated with a secondary bacterial infection and is characterized by a chronic moist dermatitis and purulent exudate. The term "red mange" is applied to a generalized hyperemia with little or no pustule formation.

Histologic lesions include capillary dilatation, epidermal acanthosis, and hyperplasia of the sebaceous glands (Baker 1969a). Inflammatory cells appear early and increase in number as the infection continues and the number of mites in a follicle increases. The follicle becomes distended and acanthosis of the follicular epidermis is seen (Fig. 15.23). Mites occlude the sebaceous ducts, inducing hyperplasia of the corresponding glands. Distended hair follicles rupture and hairs released into the dermis induce a foreign-body reaction. Rupture also permits invasion of the follicle by skin bacteria, which leads to pustule formation. Although the lesions of demodectic mange have been attributed to an allergic response on the part of the host (Hoey 1968), the histologic lesions are primarily those of a chronic inflammatory response to the mechanical presence of the mite in the follicles.

DIAGNOSIS

Diagnosis is made by microscopic identification of the mite in skin scrapings (Koutz 1953). However, demonstration of mites in association with lesions does not necessarily mean the mites cause them. *Demodex canis* is common in apparently normal dogs, and other agents (microorganisms or parasites) could be the cause of the lesions (Koutz 1966).

CONTROL

Numerous treatments are recommended for *D. canis* infection, but dogs often recover after no acaricidal therapy (Koutz

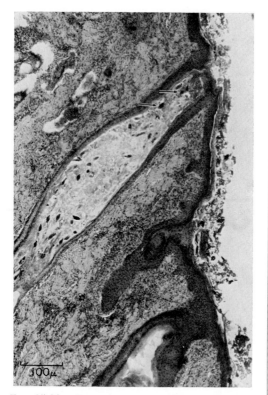

FIG. 15.23. *Demodex canis* lesions in the skin of a dog. Note infiltration of inflammatory cells, distended hair follicle, and mites *(arrows)*. (From Baker 1969a. Courtesy of Journal of Comparative Pathology.)

1955, 1966). The majority of dogs (85%) recover in a relatively short time no matter what treatment is used, an additional 10% require an extended period of time and treatment, and 5% never recover regardless of method of treatment. General measures include supportive nutrition, clipping, bathing with a nonirritating soap, and the application of medications to affected areas. An effective treatment consists of weekly bathing in a 2% aqueous suspension of a wettable powder containing 15% butylphenoxyisopropyl chloroethyl sulfite (Aramite-15W, Uniroyal) in combination with a wetting agent (Flynn 1959b). Other recommended topical treatments include the daily local application of 20 to 30% benzyl benzoate emulsion either alone or combined with lindane, rotenone, or other acaricides (Koutz 1966; Turk and Besch 1968), or weekly dipping in an aqueous solution of either 0.25% lindane or 0.25% chlordane (Camin and Rogoff 1952). Ronnel (Ectoral, Pitman-Moore), given orally at the rate of 110 mg per kg of body weight at 4-day intervals in combination with a 1% emulsion of ronnel applied topically, is reported to give fair results, but side effects, such as vomiting, coughing, or depression, are not uncommon (Koutz 1966). Supportive antibiotic and nutritional therapy is often indicated, and glucocorticoids are sometimes used to relieve inflammation (Koutz 1966). Because newborn dogs that have had no dermal contact with their mothers are generally free of infection (Greve and Gaafar 1966), complete control can probably be achieved by developing infection-free colonies initiated by cesarean section.

PUBLIC HEALTH CONSIDERATIONS

This mite does not affect man. Although infection with demodectic mites is common in man (Baker et al. 1956), *D. canis* is not the species involved.

Cheyletiella parasitivorax,
Cheyletiella yasguri

Cheyletiella parasitivorax (syn. *Ewingella americana*) is commonly reported in the pelage of the rabbit, rarely in the cat, and occasionally in the dog in North America, Europe, Asia, Australia, and New Zealand (Baker et al. 1956; Deoras and Patel 1960; Humphreys 1958; Moxham, Goldfinch, and Heath 1968). *Cheyletiella yasguri* has only recently been recognized (Smiley 1965). It has been recorded from the dog in North America (Smiley 1965) and Europe (Baker 1969b), and it is possible that previous reports of *C. parasitivorax* from the dog were in fact *C. yasguri* (Ewing, Mosier, and Foxx 1967; Foxx and Ewing 1969). The pathogenicity of these mites is uncertain (Baker et al. 1956). They appear to be obligatory parasites which live in the keratin layer of the dermis and feed on tissue fluids (Barr 1955; Foxx and Ewing 1969; Mykytowycz 1957; Olsen and Roth 1947).

Cheyletiella parasitivorax has been reported from the laboratory rabbit in Great Britain and India (Deoras and Patel 1960; Seamer and Chesterman 1967). It is uncommon in Great Britain but common in India, where 78 of 112 rabbits examined (69.6%)

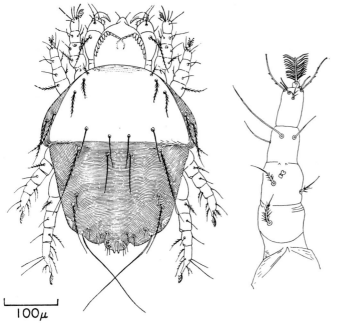

100μ

FIG. 15.24. *Cheyletiella. (Left)*
C. parasitivorax female, dorsal
view. *(Right)* First leg of *C. yas-*
guri female. Note apically
cleaved sensory organ on genu.
(Left from Baker et al. 1956;
courtesy of National Pest Control Association. *Right* from
Smiley 1965; courtesy of R. L.
Smiley, U.S. Department of
Agriculture.)

were infected. This mite has not been reported from the laboratory rabbit in North
America but heavy infestations of this species, which may be referable to *C. yasguri*,
have been reported in some dog-breeding
kennels in the United States (Reed 1961;
Weitkamp 1964). Laboratory dogs acquired
from such kennels are likely to be infected.

MORPHOLOGY

The female of either species is oval,
measures 350 to 500 μ long (Fig. 15.24), and
is larger than the male (Baker et al. 1956;
Foxx and Ewing 1969). Both sexes have a
single semicircular dorsal shield and a
large gnathosoma. The palpal tibia has a
heavy curved claw that is dentate on its in-
ferior margin. Chelicerae are styletlike and
usually enclosed within the rostrum. The
legs have six segments and terminate in an
empodium that has a double row of tenent
hairs. Tarsal claws are absent. *Cheyletiella
parasitivorax* has an ovate sensory organ or
seta on the genu of the first leg, whereas
that of *C. yasguri* is apically cleaved (Fig.
15.24) (Smiley 1965).

LIFE CYCLE

Although the complete life cycle is unknown, studies of *P. yasguri* indicate that
these mites are nonburrowing, obligatory

parasites (Foxx and Ewing 1969). All stages, including the egg, larva, first nymph,
second nymph, and adult male and female,
occur on the host. Apparently the life cycle is completed on one host and transmission is by direct contact.

PATHOLOGIC EFFECTS

Although these mites are often found
on healthy animals (Baker et al. 1956; Conroy 1964) they are sometimes associated with
dermatosis and mange (Barr 1955; Ewing,
Mosier, and Foxx 1967; Favati and Galliano 1962; Foxx and Ewing 1969; Humphreys 1958; Král and Schwartzman 1964;
Strasser 1963). Signs include mild hair loss,
scaling, hyperemia, pruritus, serous exudation, and thickening of the skin. A subacute, nonsuppurative dermatitis with cellular infiltration and mild hyperkeratosis
is seen in tissue section (Foxx and Ewing
1969).

Cheyletiella parasitivorax has been
shown capable of transmitting myxomatosis
virus among wild domestic rabbits in Australia (Mykytowycz 1958).

DIAGNOSIS

Diagnosis is made by identifying the
mites in skin scrapings or on tufts of hair
(Ewing, Mosier, and Foxx 1967; Strasser

1963.) When the host is examined with low magnification, mites, mite exuviae, and tissue debris are seen (Barr 1955; Wood 1968).

CONTROL

Cheyletiella parasitivorax is susceptible to many externally applied acaricides, whose choice depends largely on the host involved (Baker 1969b). A benzyl benzoate emulsion (concentration not given) applied topically (frequency not given) is recommended for the rabbit (Barr 1955); a solution of rotenone or other derris extracts in oil or a dust containing rotenone and pyrethrum (concentrations not given) is recommended for the topical treatment (frequency not given) of the cat (Conroy 1964; Olsen and Roth 1947). Since commercial rotenone preparations are usually irritating to the cat, dilution to one-half or less of the original concentration is suggested. The local topical application of a 20 to 30% benzyl benzoate emulsion, alone or in combination with lindane or other acaricides, or bathing with a 0.16% concentration of an organic phosphate compound, supona (Dermaton, William Cooper and Nephews) (Ewing, Mosier, and Foxx 1967; Link 1965), or with a lindane solution (concentration not given) (Weitkamp 1964; Yasgur 1968) two or three times at 4- to 7-day intervals, is recommended for the dog. Because this mite may inhabit litter and bedding, it is advisable that cages, equipment, and rooms be treated at the same time. Thorough cleaning of the building and equipment and spraying with 0.5% chlordane, 0.5% diazinon, or 4.0% malathion are effective (Yasgur 1968).

PUBLIC HEALTH CONSIDERATIONS

There are several reports of dermatitis in owners of dogs and cats infested with these mites (Humphreys 1958; Moxham, Goldfinch, and Heath 1968; Olsen and Roth 1947). For these reasons, infested animals should be handled with caution.

ASTIGMATES (ASTIGMATA)

Mites of the suborder Astigmata are closely related to the prostigmates but are quite different from the mesostigmatic mites and the ticks. The astigmates include numerous free-living species, such as the cheese mites and grain mites, and several species that parasitize animals, the most important of which are the itch mites or mange mites. Members of this suborder are soft bodied in all stages. Sexual dimorphism is common, and the males usually have prominent adanal suckers. Astigmates that affect endothermal laboratory animals are listed in Table 15.3. The most important are discussed below.

Sarcoptes scabiei

(SYN. *Acarus siro*)

(Itch Mite, Sarcoptic Mange Mite)

Sarcoptes scabiei causes sarcoptic mange, or scabies, of many domestic and wild mammals throughout the world (Baker et al. 1956; Baker and Wharton 1952). It exists as a number of populations or races which, while morphologically alike, differ in their ability to utilize various hosts. These populations are given subspecific names. Thus *S. scabiei hominis* is the common itch mite of man, *S. scabiei canis* infects dogs, and *S. scabiei cuniculi*, rabbits. Although interhost transmission sometimes occurs, such infections are usually transient and mild (Král and Schwartzman 1964). In addition to the dog and rabbit, other laboratory animals in which this mite has been reported are the hamster (Enigk and Grittner 1951), cynomolgus monkey (Leerhoy and Jensen 1967), orangutan (Weidman 1923), chimpanzee (Van Stee 1964), and gibbons (Goldman and Feldman 1949).

Sarcoptes scabiei infection is common in the laboratory dog obtained from pounds and some commercial suppliers (Flynn 1959b). It is particularly common in young dogs, and the incidence is highest in short-haired breeds (Gregor 1965). Laboratory dogs obtained from colonies initiated by cesarean section and maintained in isolation from conventional colonies (Griesemer and Gibson 1963) are probably free of this mite.

This mite is also common in some rabbit colonies (Adams, Aitken, and Worden 1967; Cook 1969; Hagan and Lund 1962) but uncommon or absent in others, and it is unlikely to be encountered in the laboratory except in stocks obtained from sup-

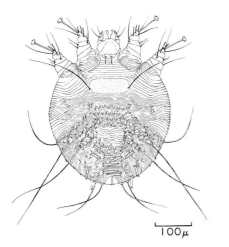

|‾100μ‾|

FIG. 15.25. *Sarcoptes scabiei* female, dorsal view. (From Baker et al. 1956. Courtesy of National Pest Control Association.)

pliers which do not have effective sanitation and parasite control programs.

The hamster and simian primates are only rarely infected.

MORPHOLOGY

The female is broadly oval, about 380 μ long by 270 μ wide, translucent, white, and covered with fine parallel striae (Fig. 15.25) (Buxton 1921; Fain 1968a). A pair of body setae, the verticals, are located anterodorsally. Middorsally, the female possesses a shieldlike plastron, a number of transverse rows of triangular scales, and three pairs of thick, cone-shaped setae. Posterodorsally, seven pairs of long, bladelike setae are present. The anus is a terminal, longitudinal slit, and the genital opening is a simple, transverse ventral slit between the third and fourth pairs of legs. The first and second pairs of legs possess five free segments and a stalked ambulacral sucker; the third and fourth pairs possess four free segments and terminate in long, stiff setae. The palpi have three segments and contain large, chelate chelicerae. The male is similar to but smaller than the female. It measures 220 by 170 μ and is further distinguished from the female and immature forms by the presence of an ambulacral sucker on the fourth pair of legs and a sclerotized, bell-shaped genital opening be-

tween this pair of legs. The second active nymphs (tritonymphs) resemble females but lack a genital opening. Those that will develop into females measure 340 by 270 μ, and those that will become males measure 295 by 220 μ. The first nymph (protonymph) is similar but measures only 270 by 195 μ. The larva is 215 by 156 μ and has only three pairs of legs.

LIFE CYCLE

A fertilized female burrows into the epidermis and deposits eggs in the tunnel behind her (Fain 1968a; Mellanby 1943). The eggs hatch in 3 to 8 days, and the larvae migrate to the skin surface and molt, successively, to protonymphs, tritonymphs, and adults. The adult stage is reached 4 to 6 days after the eggs hatch. Males and unfertilized females also burrow in the skin, but mating occurs on the skin surface. The entire life cycle takes 10 to 14 days.

Transmission is by direct contact (Gordon, Unsworth, and Seaton 1943; Mellanby 1943).

PATHOLOGIC EFFECTS

Sarcoptic mange in the dog (Fig. 15.26) is characterized by a papular dermatitis with subsequent rupture and crusting of the lesions, pruritus, and automutilation (Conroy 1968; Král and Schwartzman 1964). Initial lesions usually occur in the inguinal or axillary regions or along the margins of the ears. The skin becomes dry, rough, and thickened, and a generalized alopecia develops. Secondary pyoderma is not uncommon (Smith and Claypoole 1967), and dogs with extensive scabies sometimes become

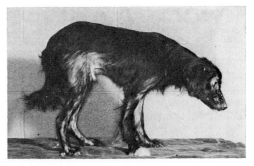

FIG. 15.26. Sarcoptic mange in a dog. (From Flynn 1959b. Courtesy of American Veterinary Medical Association.)

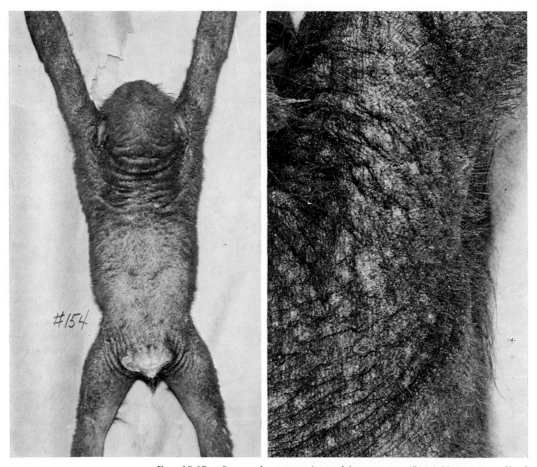

FIG. 15.27. Sarcoptic mange in a chimpanzee. *(Left)* Note generalized parakeratosis over neck and shoulders. *(Right)* Close-up view of right shoulder. (From Van Stee 1964. Courtesy of E. W. Van Stee, U.S. Air Force.)

cachectic and die (Král and Schwartzman 1964).

In the rabbit, lesions occur first on the head, ears, and legs and then become generalized (Camin and Rogoff 1952). The disease in this species is similar to notoedric mange but is frequently more serious. It is characterized by intense pruritus and scratching, accompanied by erythema, scaling of the skin, some loss of fur, and self-inflicted trauma (Adams, Aitken, and Worden 1967; Hagan and Lund 1962).

In simian primates, scabies is characterized by thickening of the skin, usually over the back, neck, and shoulders (Fig. 15.27), but sometimes over the lower trunk

and extremities (Goldman and Feldman 1949; Leerhoy and Jensen 1967; Van Stee 1964; Weidman 1923, 1935). Other signs include scaling of the skin, pruritus, alopecia, and emaciation.

In histologic sections of infected skin, hyperkeratosis, parakeratosis, and crusting, and, within the epidermis, burrows containing many parasites and eggs are seen (Fig. 15.28) (Fuerstenberg 1861; Goldman and Feldman 1949).

DIAGNOSIS

A tentative diagnosis is based on the signs and lesions and confirmed by demonstrating the parasite or eggs in deep skin

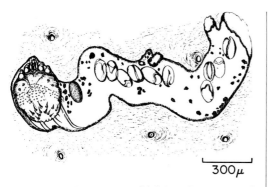

$\overline{300\mu}$

FIG. 15.28. *Sarcoptes scabiei* female, eggs, and debris in burrow in skin. (From Fuerstenberg 1861.)

scrapings. The suspected lesion is scraped vigorously with a sharp curved knife until the skin is roseate. Scrapings are transferred to a microscope slide with a drop of glycerine, immersion oil, or water, covered with a cover glass, and examined under the low power objective of a microscope. In dogs, scrapings of the tips of the ears often yield mites even though the ears may be free of lesions (Smith and Claypoole 1967). If burrows are evident in intact skin, adult female mites can often be teased out with a needle (Mellanby 1943). In the dog (Smith and Claypoole 1967) and primate (Van Stee 1964; Weidman 1923), scrapings are often negative for mites, and only a presumptive diagnosis can be made based on pruritic, papular eruptions and alopecia.

Differential diagnosis in the dog should involve consideration of seborrhea, eczema, contact dermatitis, dermatophytosis and demodectic mange (caused by *Demodex canis*), notoedric mange (caused by *Notoedres cati*), and otodectic mange (caused by *Otodectes cynotis*) (Conroy 1968; Smith and Claypoole 1967). In the rabbit, sarcoptic mange must be differentiated from notoedric mange (caused by *N. cati*) and ear canker (caused by *Psoroptes cuniculi*). *Sarcoptes scabiei* females differ from all other mange mites of laboratory animals by possessing the following combination of characteristics: vertical setae; ambulacral suckers on the tarsi of the first and second legs only; a dorsum with scales, cones, and bladelike setae; and a terminal anus.

CONTROL

General control measures include supportive nutrition, clipping, bathing with a nonirritating soap, and the weekly application of medication to affected areas (Conroy 1968; Van Stee 1964). Effective treatments for the dog include 0.25% chlordane or 0.03 to 0.06% lindane suspension in water (Link 1965), a lotion containing 0.05% lindane in combination with 0.06% rotenone (Smith and Claypoole 1967), a 1% solution of ronnel (Burch and Brinkman 1962), a 2% aqueous suspension of a wettable powder containing 15% butylphenoxyisopropyl chloroethyl sulfite (Aramite-15W, Uniroyal) in combination with a wetting agent (Flynn 1959b), and placing a resin strip impregnated with DDVP (dichlorvos; Vapona, Shell) in the cage for 2 weeks (Whitney 1969). Effective treatments for the rabbit include 0.05% solution of lindane (Cook 1969), 10% DDT in talc (Hagan and Lund 1962), benzyl benzoate (concentration not given) (Adams, Aitken, and Worden 1967; Cook 1969), and a 25% proprietary solution of tetraethylthiuram monosulfide (Tetmosol, Imperial Chemicals) (dilution not given) (Adams, Aitken, and Worden 1967). Effective treatments for simian primates include 25% emulsion of benzyl benzoate (Rewell 1948) and 0.1% solution of lindane (Van Stee 1964).

PUBLIC HEALTH CONSIDERATIONS

Subspecies of *S. scabiei* from lower vertebrates (Král and Schwartzman 1964) and primates (Goldman and Feldman 1949; Weidman 1923) are transmissible to man by direct contact. Although human infections with animal subspecies are generally believed to be mild and self-limiting (Král and Schwartzman 1964), severe pruritus and prolonged papular eruption have been reported in human infection of canine origin (Smith and Claypoole 1967; Tannenbaum 1965; Thomsett 1963, 1968). For these reasons, infected laboratory animals should be handled with caution.

Notoedres muris

(SYN. *Notoedres alepis*)

(Ear Mange Mite of Rat)

Notoedres muris, the cause of ear mange in the rat, has also been reported

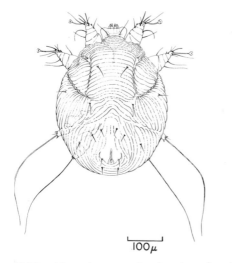

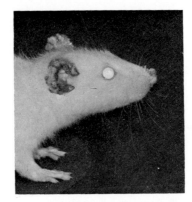

FIG. 15.30. Notoedric mange in rat. (From Flynn 1960. Courtesy of Jane K. Glaser, Argonne National Laboratory.)

FIG. 15.29. *Notoedres muris* female, dorsal view. (From Baker et al. 1956. Courtesy of National Pest Control Association.)

Transmission is by direct contact, but experimental transmission by the housefly has been demonstrated (Holz 1955).

from the black rat, multimammate mouse, and wild rodents (Fain 1965a, 1968a). It has been recognized in North America, Europe, and Africa and probably occurs throughout the world. *Notoedres muris* is common in some rat colonies but uncommon in others (Fain 1965a; Flynn 1960; Sasa et al. 1962). It has not been reported in cesarean-derived, barrier-maintained colonies (Foster 1963; Owen 1968).

MORPHOLOGY

The female measures 400 by 350 μ (Fig. 15.29) and resembles that of *Sarcoptes scabiei* but differs by the dorsal position of its anal opening and by the absence of heavy dorsal spines, cones, and triangular scales (Baker et al. 1956). The middorsal integumental striations are not scalelike, paragenital setae are absent, and the perianal setae are relatively small (Fain 1965a; Watson 1962). The male and immature forms resemble those of *S. scabiei*.

LIFE CYCLE

Eggs are laid in burrows in the stratum corneum and hatch in 4 or 5 days (Gordon, Unsworth, and Seaton 1943). Preadult stages (larva and first and second nymphs) live an average of 14.5 days and the entire life cycle takes 19 to 21 days. Fertilization is thought to occur in the burrows.

PATHOLOGIC EFFECTS

Notoedric mange of the rat affects the ear pinnae, nose, and tail and sometimes the external genitalia and limbs (Flynn 1960; Hirst 1922). Lesions of the ears appear as papillomalike horny excrescences and yellowish crusts (Fig. 15.30). Those of the nose are also wartlike and horny, but caudal and dermal lesions are erythematous and vesicular or papular.

The mites are usually restricted to the stratum corneum but occasionally they penetrate this layer, giving rise to a more severe skin reaction and serum exudation (Gordon, Unsworth, and Seaton 1943). Epidermal cells in affected areas proliferate and gradually cornify (Watson 1962). Encapsulation of the mite by fibrous tissue does not occur. Localized inflammation, characterized by an increase in polymorphonuclear leucocytes and lymphocytes, is sometimes so intense as to obscure the dermal fibrous tissues beneath the lesion. The central cartilage is apparently not affected.

DIAGNOSIS

Differential diagnosis should involve consideration of dermatitic and eczematic causes, mycotic infections, and self-inflicted trauma. Although the presence of mites and eggs in skin scrapings is diagnostic for mange, care must be taken to differentiate notoedric mange of the rat from that caused by *Trixacarus diversus* (Guilhon 1946a, b). *Notoedres muris* differs from *T. diversus* by lacking a shield and triangular scales on the dorsum.

CONTROL

Effective treatments include the topical application of a 0.10 to 0.25% lindane solution once, or twice with a 6-day interval (Camin and Rogoff 1952; Taylor 1945); or dipping weekly, for 3 weeks, in a 2% aqueous suspension of a wettable powder containing 15% butylphenoxyisopropyl chloroethyl sulfite (Aramite-15W, Uniroyal) (Flynn 1960). Complete eradication of *N. muris* infection can probably be achieved by initiating new colonies by cesarean section (Foster 1963; Owen 1968).

PUBLIC HEALTH CONSIDERATIONS

Notoedres muris does not affect man.

Notoedres sp.

(Ear Mange Mite of Hamster)

This mite, the cause of ear mange in the hamster, is known from the United States and Europe (Băies, Suteu, and Klemm 1968; Hindle 1947; C. Yunker, unpublished information). Although it is apparently uncommon (Wantland 1968), about 60% of the animals in one colony were affected (Băies, Suteu, and Klemm 1968).

MORPHOLOGY

The morphologic characteristics of this mite are similar to those of other species of *Notoedres* (Băies, Suteu, and Klemm 1968). The female measures about 265 by 198 μ and the male about 124 by 106 μ.

LIFE CYCLE

The life cycle appears to be similar to that of *S. scabiei* and *N. muris* (Băies, Suteu, and Klemm 1968; Wantland 1968). Eggs laid in burrows in the skin hatch in 3 to 4 days. The larva transforms into a nymph which burrows into the skin and molts, once or twice, to become an adult. The complete cycle requires 6 to 10 days.

Transmission is presumed to be by direct contact, but attempts to confirm this experimentally have failed.

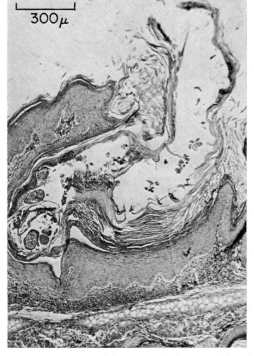

FIG. 15.31. Notoedric mange lesions in skin of a hamster. Note mite and debris in stratum corneum. (Courtesy of W. Klemm, Facultatea de Medicina Veterinara, Romania.)

PATHOLOGIC EFFECTS

Notoedric mange of the hamster is similar to that of the rat (Băies, Suteu, and Klemm 1968; Hindle 1947). In the female hamster, usually only the ears are affected, but in the male, lesions occur on the ears, nose, genitalia, tail, and feet. In histologic sections of affected skin, there are numerous mites and eggs and much debris (Fig. 15.31).

DIAGNOSIS

Mange of the hamster caused by *Notoedres* sp. must be differentiated from that caused by *Sarcoptes scabiei* (Enigk and Grittner 1951). *Notoedres* sp. differs from *S. scabiei* by having a dorsal anus and by lacking large dorsal spines, cones, and triangular scales.

CONTROL

Effective treatments include the topical application of a 25% proprietary solution of tetraethylthiuram monosulfide (Tetmo-

sol, Imperial Chemicals) diluted to 2.5%
and applied every 2 to 3 days for four treatments (Fulton 1943; Hindle 1947) or dipping in a 0.5% solution of lindane once, or
twice with a 6- to 7-day interval (Băies,
Suteu, and Klemm 1968).

PUBLIC HEALTH CONSIDERATIONS

The ear mange mite of the hamster
does not affect man (Wantland 1968).

Notoedres cati
(SYN. Notoedres caniculi)
(Notoedric Mange Mite)

Notoedres cati, the cause of head
mange in the cat (Conroy 1964; English
1960; Holzworth 1968) and rabbit (Adams,
Aitken, and Worden 1967; Camin and Rogoff 1952; Osborne 1947), is common in the
cat but uncommon in the rabbit in North
America, Europe, Africa, and probably
throughout the world (Fain 1965a, 1968a).
It is likely to be encountered in laboratory
cats obtained from pounds, but unlikely to
be found in the laboratory rabbit except in
stocks obtained from suppliers who do not
have effective sanitation and parasite control programs. Rarely, this mite also infects
the dog (Hirst 1922).

MORPHOLOGY

The female (Fig. 15.32) measures 275
by 230 μ and resembles that of *N. muris* except that it has scalelike, middorsal integumental striations, a single pair of paregeni-
tal setae, and large perianal setae (Fain
1965a). The male and immature stages resemble those of *Sarcoptes scabiei*.

LIFE CYCLE

The life cycle is similar to that of *S.
scabiei* (Baker et al. 1956) and *N. muris*
(English 1960; Gordon, Unsworth, and
Seaton 1943). Transmission is by direct
contact.

PATHOLOGIC EFFECTS

The mite burrows into the epidermis
of the ears, neck, and face, and sometimes
the legs, ventral abdomen, and genital region, especially in younger animals (Camin
and Rogoff 1952; Conroy 1964; Osborne
1947). There is a persistent pruritus and
alopecia, and self-inflicted trauma is common (Adams, Aitken, and Worden 1967;

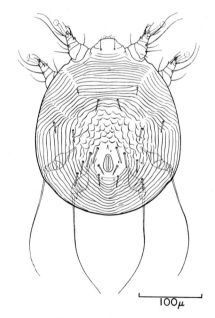

FIG. 15.32. *Notoedres cati* female, dorsal view.
(From Hirst 1922. Courtesy of British Museum—
Natural History.)

Holsworth 1968). A grayish yellow crust develops on the ears, face, and neck, and the
skin becomes thickened and wrinkled. Involvement of the entire body sometimes occurs, with subsequent dehydration and
death (English 1960; Hirst 1922).

DIAGNOSIS

Other diseases that must be distinguished from notoedric mange include
dermatomycoses, superficial pyoderma, and
chronic eczematous dermatitis (Conroy
1964). The presence of the parasite or eggs
in deep skin scrapings is diagnostic for
mange. In the cat, notoedric mange must
be distinguished from mange caused by
Otodectes cynotis, the ear mite. *Notoedres
cati* differs from *O. cynotis* by having a pair
of anterodorsal body setae, the verticals,
situated on a dorsal flap over the mouthparts; no dorsal body shields or elongate
terminal body setae; and well-developed
third and fourth pairs of legs. In the rabbit notoedric mange must be differentiated
from sarcoptic mange caused by *S. scabiei*
and psoroptic mange caused by *Psoroptes
cuniculi*. *Notoedres cati* differs from *S.
scabiei* by having a dorsal anus and by lack-

ing large dorsal spines, cones, and triangular scales. It differs from *P. cuniculi* in possessing vertical setae and lacking dorsal shields, long terminal body setae, and ambulacral suckers on the tarsi of the fourth pair of legs.

CONTROL

General control measures include supportive nutrition, clipping, bathing in warm soapy water, and the weekly application of medication to affected areas (Conroy 1964; Holzworth 1968; Král and Schwartzman 1964). Effective agents for the cat include 0.25 to 1.25% malathion in an aqueous suspension (Conroy 1964; English 1960) and 3 to 10% sulfur as an ointment or lotion (Conroy 1964; Holzworth 1968). Effective agents for the rabbit include a 0.05% lindane solution (Cook 1969), 10% DDT in talcum powder (Hagan and Lund 1962), a 25% proprietary solution of tetraethylthiuram monosulfide (Tetmosol, Imperial Chemicals) (dilution not given) (Adams, Aitken, and Worden 1967), benzyl benzoate (concentration not given) (Adams, Aitken, and Worden 1967), and dimethyl phthalate (concentration not given) (Osborne 1947).

PUBLIC HEALTH CONSIDERATIONS

Notoedres cati sometimes causes a transient dermatitis in man (Davies 1941; Sequeira and Dowdeswell 1942). For this reason, infected animals should be handled with caution.

Knemidokoptes mutans

(Scaly-leg Mite)

Knemidokoptes mutans, the cause of scaly leg of the chicken, has been reported from North America, Europe, and Africa and probably occurs throughout the world (Baker et al. 1956; Fain and Elsen 1967; Král and Schwartzman 1964). It is common in domestic poultry (Benbrook 1965), but has not been reported from the laboratory chicken and is not likely to be encountered except on birds obtained from farm flocks.

MORPHOLOGY

The female is round and measures 350 to 450 μ by 280 to 380 μ (Fain and Elsen 1967; Nevin 1935) (Fig. 15.33). It resembles that of *Sarcoptes scabiei* in the shape

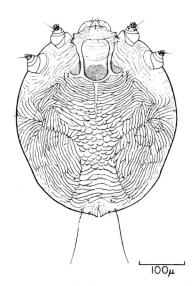

FIG. 15.33. *Knemidokoptes mutans* female, dorsal view. (From Hirst 1922. Courtesy of British Museum—Natural History.)

and position of its anal and genital openings but dorsal spines, cones, and triangular scales are absent. The pattern of dorsal striae is scalelike. Elongate body setae are not present except for a single terminal pair. A dorsal shield, the plastron, is present but vertical setae are absent. The tarsus of each leg is fused with the tibia; all tarsi are clawlike and lack ambulacral claws, pretarsal stalks, and elongate setae. The male measures 200 to 240 μ by 145 to 160 μ. Immature stages resemble those of *S. scabiei.*

LIFE CYCLE

The life cycle is similar to that of *S. scabiei* (Baker et al. 1956; Fain and Elsen 1967).

PATHOLOGIC EFFECTS

The mites burrow beneath the epidermal scales of the legs and feet, causing irritation, inflammation, vesicle formation, serous exudation, and crust formation (Griffiths and O'Rourke 1950). The crust sometimes covers the entire limb (Fig. 15.34) (Nevin 1935). The condition progresses slowly. If untreated, pronounced distortion of the legs, lameness, and sometimes loss of terminal digits result (Bishopp and Wood 1931).

DIAGNOSIS

The identification of the causative mite in typical lesions is diagnostic. Care must be taken to distinguish *K. mutans* from the depluming itch mite, *Neocnemidocoptes laevis gallinae.*

CONTROL

Effective control involves the isolation and examination of newly acquired chickens, elimination of affected and exposed individuals, and sanitation of cages and shipping containers. Treatment, when indicated, consists of removing the crusts after softening with warm soapy water, oil, or glycerine (Král and Schwartzman 1964) and then applying 0.1 to 0.5% lindane in water (Cleland 1953; Cook 1969; Griffiths and O'Rourke 1950). A single application is sufficient for mild cases but severe ones should be treated twice.

PUBLIC HEALTH CONSIDERATIONS

This mite does not affect man.

Knemidokoptes pilae

(Scaly-face Mite)

Knemidokoptes pilae, the cause of scaly face and scaly leg of the parakeet, has been reported from North America, South America, Europe, and Africa and probably occurs throughout the world (Fain and Elsen 1967; Yunker and Ishak 1957). It is common in caged parakeets (Altman 1968; Kutzer 1964; Wichmann and Vincent 1958) and is likely to be encountered in the parakeet in the laboratory.

MORPHOLOGY

Adults and immature stages resemble those of *K. mutans* and *Sarcoptes scabiei* (Fain and Elsen 1967). The female (Fig. 15.35) measures 315 to 428 μ by 252 to 378 μ. The male measures 200 to 219 μ by 143 to 152 μ.

LIFE CYCLE

The life cycle is similar to that of *S. scabiei* (Blackmore 1963; Wichmann and Vincent 1958). The mite apparently completes its entire life cycle within the lesions it produces (Yunker and Ishak 1957).

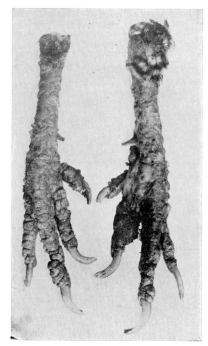

FIG. 15.34. Scaly leg of the chicken caused by *Knemidokoptes mutans.* (From Benbrook and Sloss 1961. Courtesy of Iowa State University Press.)

PATHOLOGIC EFFECTS

The mite invades the feather follicles, skin folds, and smooth epidermis of the face, foot, and cere by direct penetration, producing primary and secondary pouch-like cavities (Altman 1968; Fain and Elsen 1967; Kutzer 1964; Wichmann and Vincent 1958; Yunker and Ishak 1957). The first signs are a gray-white to yellow, powdery, crusty mass over the affected area which, on close examination, is seen to be pitted and to resemble a honeycomb (Fig. 15.36). The lesions usually appear first at the base of the cere and the corners of the mouth. Later they extend to cover the eyes, forehead, cere, and adjacent areas. The beak often becomes distorted and friable. Early leg infections resemble those of *K. mutans* in the chicken in that gross lesions are absent. Lesions on the legs usually appear first at the point of the hock and progress to cover all the nonfeathered portions. Pruritus is probably absent as scratching or rubbing of the beak is not common.

In histologic sections, the mites are

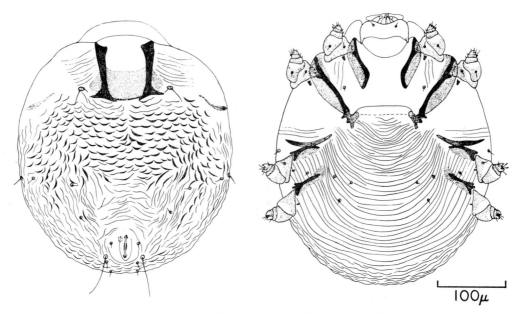

FIG. 15.35. *Knemidokoptes pilae* female. *(Left)* Dorsal view. *(Right)* Ventral view. (From Fain and Elsen 1967. Courtesy of A. Fain, Institut de Médecine Tropicale Prince Léopold.)

seen in the deeper layers of the stratum corneum (Blackmore 1963; Yunker and Ishak 1957). Hyperkeratosis and sloughing of the keratin are common.

DIAGNOSIS

Diagnosis is based on the typical lesions and confirmed by identification of the mite.

CONTROL

Effective control involves the isolation and examination of newly acquired parakeets, the elimination of any affected birds, and sanitation of cages and shipping containers. Treatment is rarely indicated; however, when appropriate, it consists of the topical application of 12.5 to 25.0% benzyl benzoate emulsion (Wichmann and Vincent 1958), a cream containing 10% crotamiton (Eurax, Geigy), or a cream containing rotenone in combination with orthophenylphenol (concentrations not given) (Goodwinol, Goodwinol) (Altman 1968) to the affected areas, one to three times a week until the lesions are healed.

PUBLIC HEALTH CONSIDERATIONS

This mite does not affect man.

Neocnemidocoptes laevis gallinae

(SYN. *Knemidokoptes laevis* var. *gallinae*)

(Depluming Itch Mite)

This mite affects the feathered skin of the chicken (Baker et al. 1956; Benbrook 1965). It has been reported from North America, Europe, and Africa (Fain and Elsen 1967) and probably occurs throughout the world. It is uncommon in the domestic chicken and is not likely to be encountered in the laboratory.

MORPHOLOGY

The female measures 340 to 435 μ by 310 to 390 μ and is similar to that of *Knemidokoptes mutans* but differs by having dorsal striae that are transverse and unbroken, discrete tibiae and tarsi, and vestigial pretarsal stalks (Fig. 15.37) (Baker et al. 1956; Fain and Elsen 1967). The male measures 204 to 210 μ by 144 to 150 μ. Immature forms resemble those of *Sarcoptes scabiei*.

LIFE CYCLE

The life cycle is similar to that of *S. scabiei* (Baker et al. 1956; Fain and Elsen 1967).

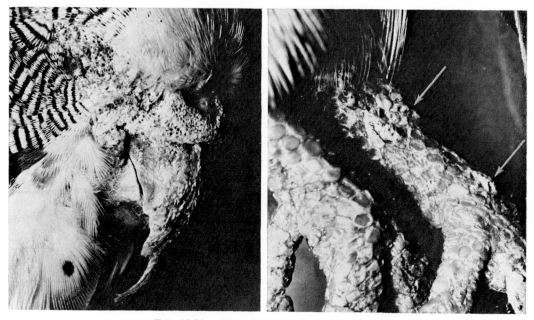

FIG. 15.36. *Knemidokoptes pilae* lesions on the face *(left)* and leg *(right)*. (From Fain and Elsen 1967. Courtesy of A. Fain, Institut de Médecine Tropicale Prince Léopold.)

PATHOLOGIC EFFECTS

The mites burrow into the skin and cause an intense pruritus (Bishopp and Wood 1931). Feathers in affected areas, especially of the back, head, neck, abdomen, and upper legs, fall out, break off, or are plucked out by the bird (Hirst 1922; Král and Schwartzman 1964). Wing and tail feathers are not affected. Scales and small papules are produced, and the skin becomes thick and wrinkled, particularly on the neck. Severe infections sometimes lead to emaciation and death.

DIAGNOSIS

Demonstration of *Neocnemidocoptes laevis gallinae* beneath the scales or at the base of quills is diagnostic. Care must be taken to distinguish this mite from the scaly-leg mite, *K. mutans.*

CONTROL

Control is based on isolation and examination of newly acquired chickens, elimination of affected and exposed individuals, and sanitation of cages and shipping containers. Treatments effective against *K. mutans* are probably effective against this mite (Baker et al. 1956).

PUBLIC HEALTH CONSIDERATIONS

Neocnemidocoptes laevis gallinae is not known to infect man.

Cytodites nudus

(SYN. *Cytoleichus nudus*)

(Air-sac Mite)

Cytodites nudus is an internal parasite of the respiratory tract of the chicken and other birds throughout the world (Baker et al. 1956; Fain and Bafort 1964). It is uncommon in farm flocks (Benbrook 1965) and is not likely to be encountered in the laboratory chicken.

MORPHOLOGY

This mite is long and oval (Fig. 15.38) (Fain 1960). The female measures 480 to 650 μ by 325 to 500 μ and has a few short setae, a smooth dorsal integument, and a gnathosoma that is modified to form a tube for the chelicerae. The legs are short and unmodified; they end in stalked ambulacral suckers and have a pair of small, unequal

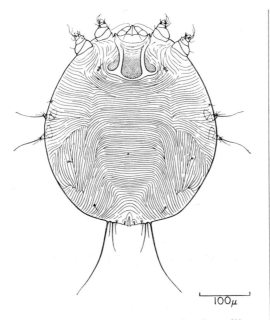

FIG. 15.37. *Neocnemidocoptes laevis gallinae* female, dorsal view. (From Hirst 1922. Courtesy of British Museum—Natural History.)

claws. The female genital opening is a simple longitudinal slit located between the third pair of legs. The male resembles the female in size and general appearance. It differs in having reduced, sessile ambulacral suckers and in the position of the genital opening, which is located between the fourth pair of legs.

LIFE CYCLE

Larvae are born alive and are succeeded by two nymphal stages; otherwise little is known of the life cycle (Baker et al. 1956; Fain and Bafort 1964).

Although this mite is readily transmitted, the mechanism is unknown (Baker et al. 1956); it is thought to be spread by coughing.

PATHOLOGIC EFFECTS

Signs of infection are coughing, weakness, incoordination, loss of weight, and occasionally death (Baker et al. 1956; Benbrook 1965). Other effects include mucus accumulation in the trachea and bronchi, pulmonary edema, emphysema, pneumonia, enteritis, and peritonitis (Lindt and Kutzer 1965).

DIAGNOSIS

Because the respiratory signs are nonspecific, a definitive diagnosis based on recognition of the mite in association with pulmonary lesions can be made only at necropsy.

CONTROL

Control based on elimination of affected and exposed birds is probably effective. Treatment of infected individuals is rarely indicated; however, when appropriate, inhalation of a dust containing lindane or DDT (concentration not given) has been suggested (Baker et al. 1956).

PUBLIC HEALTH CONSIDERATIONS

This mite is of no known public health importance. Two specimens, supposedly of *C. nudus*, were recovered from the omentum of an East African native on autopsy, but the significance of this finding is unknown (Castellani 1907).

Laminosioptes cysticola

(Fowl Cyst Mite; Flesh Mite)

Laminosioptes cysticola occurs in the subcutaneous tissues of the chicken, pigeon, and other birds in North America, South America, Europe, and Australia and probably throughout the world (Baker et al. 1956). It is uncommon in farm flocks (Benbrook 1965; Bishopp and Wood 1931) and

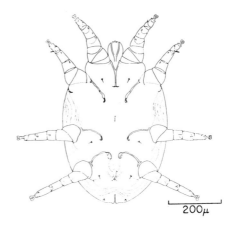

FIG. 15.38. *Cytodites nudus* male, ventral view. (From Baker et al. 1956. Courtesy of National Pest Control Association.)

is not likely to be encountered in the laboratory chicken.

MORPHOLOGY

Adults measure 200 to 260 μ, are elongate, and have a smooth dorsal integument and few setae (Baker et al. 1956) (Fig. 15.39). The gnathosoma is small and not visible from a dorsal view. The first two pairs of legs are short, and their tarsi are clawlike. The third and fourth pairs of legs are longer, and their tarsi terminate in long padlike post-tarsi.

LIFE CYCLE

The life cycle and mode of transmission are unknown (Baker et al. 1956).

PATHOLOGIC EFFECTS

The mite occurs in the subcutaneous tissues and forms a small nodule that calcifies after the mite dies (Lindquist and Belding 1949). Mild infection is believed to do no harm, but heavy infection is sometimes fatal (Baker et al. 1956).

DIAGNOSIS

The subcutaneous nodules produced by this mite are easily demonstrated in the living chicken by wetting the breast, parting the feathers, and moving the skin back and forth (Lindquist and Belding 1949). Identification of mites excised from the nodules is confirmatory.

CONTROL

Nothing is known of control.

PUBLIC HEALTH CONSIDERATIONS

This mite does not affect man.

Psoroptes cuniculi

(SYN. *Psoroptes communis* var. *cuniculi*
Psoroptes equi var. *cuniculi,*
Psoroptes equi var. *caprae*)

(Ear Canker Mite of Rabbit)

Psoroptes cuniculi, the cause of ear canker in the rabbit, is common throughout the world (Adams, Aitken, and Worden 1967; Alicata 1964; Giorgi 1968; Hirst 1922; Lund 1951). It is frequently encountered in laboratory rabbits obtained from commercial sources, occurring in most shipments from most suppliers (Poole et al. 1967).

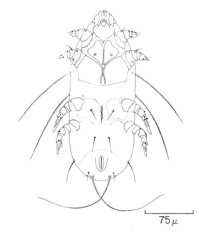

FIG. 15.39. *Laminosioptes cysticola* female, ventral view. (Courtesy of Institute of Acarology).

MORPHOLOGY

Psoroptes cuniculi is morphologically indistinguishable from *P. equi* (Fig. 15.40) (Sweatman 1958a). The female is relatively large, 400 to 750 μ long, rounded, and a translucent, brownish white. The idiosoma is striated and has a small rectangular anterodorsal shield, a pair of long lateral setae, and two pairs of long terminal setae; other body setae are relatively small. The genital opening is a slit resembling an inverted U located between the apodemes of the second pair of legs. The anus is a simple terminal slit. All legs are long and consist of five free segments. The first, second, and fourth tarsi are clawlike and each has an ambulacral sucker on a segmented stalk; the third tarsus ends in a pair of long, whiplike setae. The male is 370 to 550 μ long and the idiosoma is bilobed posteriorly. Each lobe has two long setae and three shorter ones. A small anterodorsal plate similar to that of the female is present, as well as a larger, hexagonal, posterodorsal one. The heavily sclerotized male genitalia are located ventrally between the apodemes of the fourth pair of legs. The anus is a ventroterminal slit that has a large copulatory sucker on either side.

LIFE CYCLE

Psoroptes cuniculi is a nonburrowing, obligate parasite and all forms feed on the

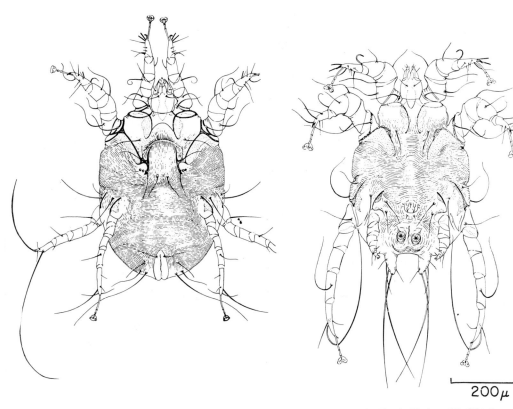

200μ

Fig. 15.40. *Psoroptes equi* (morphologically indistinguishable from *P. cuniculi*). *(Left)* Female, ventral view. *(Right)* Male, ventral view. (From Baker et al. 1956. Courtesy of National Pest Control Association.)

host by piercing the epidermis and ingesting tissue fluids. The entire life cycle occurs under the margins of the scab that forms at the site of infection (Baker et al. 1956). Eggs hatch in 4 days and three immature stages (larva, protonymph, and tritonymph) ensue (Fain 1964a; Sweatman 1958a). The adult male attaches to the female tritonymph for 2 or more days, awaiting her final molt, at which time copulation occurs (Sweatman 1958a). The complete cycle requires about 21 days.

This mite is transmitted readily among rabbits by direct contact. It has also been experimentally transmitted on the housefly (Holz 1955).

PATHOLOGIC EFFECTS

Signs of infection in rabbits are shaking of the head, scratching of the ears, hyperemia, and crust formation in the pinna and a brown, malodorous discharge in the external ear canal (Fig. 15.41) (Adams, Aitken, and Worden 1967; Lund 1951; Marine 1924). Lesions sometimes spread to the face, neck, and legs. Severely affected animals become debilitated. Pyogenic otitis media, characterized by a loss of equilibrium and torticollis, is common (Streeter 1945), and fatal meningitis is occasionally seen.

DIAGNOSIS

Isolation of *P. cuniculi* from the typical lesions is diagnostic. Mites of the genus *Psoroptes* differ from all other mange mites in that the stalks from which their ambulacral suckers arise are segmented.

CONTROL

Control is based on eradication by treatment. The most effective procedure involves the examination and treatment of

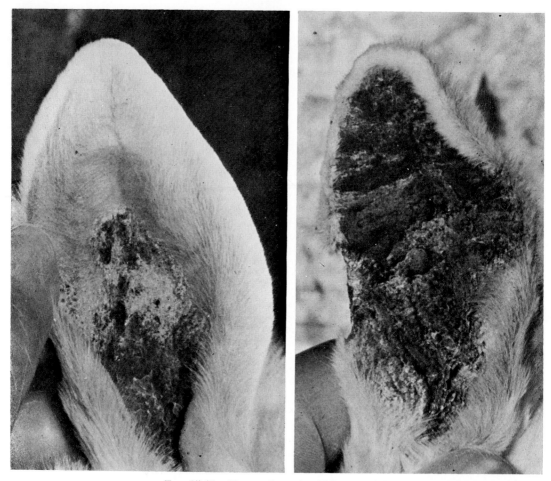

Fig. 15.41.   Ear canker of rabbit caused by *Psoroptes cuniculi*. *(Left)* Usual appearance. *(Right)* Extreme case. (Courtesy of B. Matanic, State University of New York.)

all newly acquired rabbits (Lund 1951). Those showing no signs of infection should be treated once; those showing visible lesions should be treated weekly until completely cured. In severe cases, treatment is facilitated if scabs and crusts are first removed after softening with a few drops of hydrogen peroxide (Streeter 1945) or a mixture of oil and ether (Král and Schwartzman 1964). Agents effective against this mite include 0.25% lindane solution (Lund 1951), 0.5% DDT in aqueous emulsion (Král and Schwartzman 1964), 25 to 30% benzyl benzoate emulsion (Hagan and Lund 1962), 10% aqueous solution of a proprietary solution containing 25% tetra-ethylthiuram monosulfide (Tetmosol, Imperial Chemicals) (Cook 1969), and a sorptive dust impregnated with 2% naled (Dibrom, Chevron Chemical Co.) (Tarshis 1962). Because the housefly is potentially capable of transmitting this mite, an effective program should also include fly control.

PUBLIC HEALTH CONSIDERATIONS

Psoroptes cuniculi does not affect man.

"*Chorioptes cuniculi*"

This mite is generally regarded as a cause of ear canker of the rabbit (Adams, Aitken, and Worden 1967; Cook 1969; Hagan and Lund 1962; Streeter 1945; Woodnott 1963). It reportedly also infests the body skin, where it causes mange (Hagan and Lund 1962). However, in a classical study of the bionomics and systematics of mites of the genus *Chorioptes* (Sweatman 1957), the existence of *C. cuniculi* could not be verified, indicating that the original record of chorioptic mites from a rabbit (Zuern, 1874) may have been erroneous. This name has been perpetuated without its validity being questioned. Only two species of *Chorioptes*, *C. bovis* and *C. texanus*, are presently recognized; both are parasites of ungulates. Survival of the former species on foreign host epidermal material has been demonstrated, so it is possible that *C. bovis* is capable of infesting rabbits and may be the species in question. However, it is also possible that no species of *Chorioptes* is a rabbit parasite. It is suggested that collections from rabbits of mites presumed to be chorioptic be submitted to a taxonomic acarologist for definitive identification.

Otodectes cynotis

(Ear Canker Mite of Carnivores)

Otodectes cynotis, the cause of ear canker in the dog, cat, and other carnivores, is extremely common throughout the world (Berg and Shomer 1963; Sweatman 1958b). In the United States, a 27 to 100% incidence has been reported in the dog (Tonn 1961), and it is estimated that 75% of the cats are infected (Staggs 1961). In Great Britain, incidences of 2.5 to 3.5% have been reported in the dog and 20.2 to 28.4% in the cat (Beresford-Jones 1955). An incidence of 29.1% has been reported in the dog in Australia (Grono 1969). *Otodectes cynotis* is uncommon in laboratory dogs and cats reared in colonies that have effective control programs (Johnson, Andersen, and Gee 1963; Morris 1963), and it does not occur in cesarean-derived, barrier-maintained colonies (Griesemer and Gibson 1963). However, laboratory dogs and cats obtained from pounds or from kennels that do not have effective control programs are likely to be infected.

MORPHOLOGY

The female is similar to that of *Psoroptes cuniculi* except that the fourth pair of legs is much smaller (Fig. 15.42) (Sweatman 1958b). The male possesses large, stalked, ambulacral suckers on the fourth pair of legs whereas those of *P. cuniculi* are small and vestigial. In addition, the ambulacral suckers of both sexes of *O. cynotis* arise from short, unsegmented stalks.

LIFE CYCLE

The life cycle is similar to that of *P. cuniculi*, except that male and female nymphal stages are indistinguishable (Sweatman 1958b). The complete cycle requires about 18 to 28 days.

The mite is transmitted by direct contact, especially during nursing (Baker et al. 1956). Transmission between the dog and cat also occurs (Tonn 1961).

PATHOLOGIC EFFECTS

This mite is usually found deep in the external auditory meatus (Berg and Shomer 1963), but sometimes secondary foci occur on the feet and tip of the tail (Conroy 1964). It is uncertain if the mite pierces the epidermis and feeds on lymph (Camin and Rogoff 1952) or if it feeds on desquamated epithelial cells and possibly cerumen (Evans, Sheals, and MacFarlane 1961). Nevertheless, intense irritation results, and inflammatory exudates, cerumen, and mites accumulate in the auditory canal (Fig. 15.43) (Baker et al. 1956; Camin and Rogoff 1952; Staggs 1961). The infection is usually bilateral. The host shakes its head and scratches its ears. Ulceration of the auditory canal is common and auricular hematoma, otitis media with torticollis and circling, and convulsions sometimes occur. Otodectic mange is thought to be the most frequent cause of convulsive seizures in the cat (Staggs 1961). The mite has been identified in 37 to 59% of otitis externa cases in the dog (Frost and Beresford-Jones 1960; Grono 1969).

DIAGNOSIS

Diagnosis is based on signs and lesions and is confirmed by identification of the mite. *Otodectes cynotis* is often visible with the aid of an otoscope, but microscopic examination of scrapings from the ear is indicated when otoscopy fails to demonstrate mites (Frost and Beresford-Jones 1960). In the dog, *O. cynotis* must be differentiated

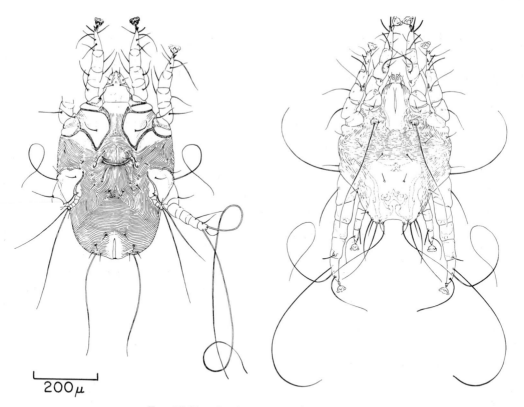

200μ

FIG. 15.42. *Otodectes cynotis.* *(Left)* Female, ventral view. *(Right)* Male, dorsal view. (From Baker et al. 1956. Courtesy of National Pest Control Association.)

from *Sarcoptes scabiei* and *Notoedres cati,* and in the cat, from *N. cati. Otodectes cynotis* is distinguishable from these other mites by its lack of vertical setae and by having a greatly reduced fourth pair of legs.

CONTROL

Control is usually based on eradication by treatment (Cook 1969). The most effective procedure involves the examination of all newly acquired dogs and cats and the periodic reexamination of all animals in the colony. Any dog or cat showing even mild otitis externa should be treated weekly until cured or until it is certain that the otitis is not caused by *O. cynotis* (Berg and Shomer 1963; Page 1952); and if the mite is identified on any animal in the colony, all should be treated at least once (Conroy 1964). Treatment is facilitated if the ears are first freed of cerumen and debris by in-

stilling a bland oil into the outer ear canal and floating the material to the outside by gentle massage (Conroy 1964). Agents effective against *O. cynotis* include 0.5% to 1.0% rotenone in oil (Camin and Rogoff 1952; Conroy 1964) and 24% dimethyl phthalate in oil (Ridamite, Parlam Corp.) (Berg and Shomer 1963; Conroy 1964). Also effective, but possibly contraindicated for the cat because of toxicity, are 0.25% lindane solution (Camin and Rogoff 1952) and 1% ronnel solution applied topically (Burch and Brinkman 1962). When treating the cat, it is recommended that the tip of the tail and all feet be included (Berg and Shomer 1963). Complete eradication can probably be achieved by the development of infection-free colonies initiated either by cesarean section (Griesemer and Gibson 1963) or by rearing natural-born offspring in isolation from their mothers.

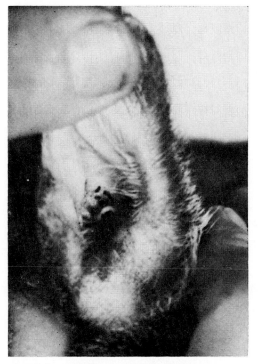

FIG. 15.43. Otodectic mange in cat. Note accumulation of exudate and cerumen in auditory canal. (Courtesy of G. R. Burch, Pitman-Moore.)

PUBLIC HEALTH CONSIDERATIONS

This mite does not affect man.

Myocoptes musculinus

(Myocoptic Mange Mite)

Myocoptes musculinus, a pelage-inhabiting mite that occurs on the laboratory and wild house mouse throughout the world (Baker et al. 1956; Smith 1955a, b), is the commonest ectoparasite of the laboratory mouse. In a survey of commercially produced, conventional laboratory mice in the United States, nearly all mice from seven different sources were found to be infested (Flynn 1955). In other surveys of conventional laboratory mice in Europe (Blackmore and Owen 1968; Heine 1962) and Asia (Fukui et al. 1961), similar high incidences have been observed. However, despite this high incidence in conventional colonies, this mite does not occur in cesarean-derived, barrier-maintained colonies (Flynn, Brennan, and Fritz 1965). *Myocop-*

tes musculinus has been reported on a single occasion from the guinea pig (Sengbusch 1960), but the significance of this is unknown.

MORPHOLOGY

The female is white, oval, and approximately 300 μ long by 130 μ wide (Watson 1960) (Fig. 15.44). The body is striated; the dorsal striae are scalelike and the ventral ones appear as minute denticles. The genital opening is triangular but, when closed, appears as a transverse slit between the fourth pair of legs. The anus is posteroventral and associated with a pair of long terminal setae. The chelicerae are large and chelate. The first and second legs have six free segments and terminate in short stalks bearing ambulacral suckers. The third and fourth pairs of legs have six segments, but ambulacral suckers are absent. The femur and genu are modified for clasping hairs; they are enlarged and strongly chitinized, and the tibia and tarsus fold over these segments. The male is smaller (about 190 by 135 μ), less striated, and more heavily sclerotized than the female. Anterior to the third pair of legs it resembles the female, but the posterior portion differs. The aedeagus is located in a deltoid genital opening, the anus is accompanied by a small pair of suckers, and the idiosoma is posteriorly bilobate. The fourth pair of legs is greatly enlarged and has five free segments, none of which are modified for hair-clasping.

LIFE CYCLE

The stages of the life cycle include egg, first larva, second larva (sometimes called deutonymph), nymph, and adult (Watson 1960, 1961). All stages occur in the pelage and a complete cycle requires about 14 days. The mite apparently feeds on epidermal tissue but not on tissue fluids.

Transmission is by direct contact (Watson 1961).

PATHOLOGIC EFFECTS

Signs are usually absent or unnoticed (Tuffery and Innes 1963). When present they include alopecia and erythema in the cervical region and occasionally on the shoulders and dorsum (Gambles 1952; Watson 1961). Pruritus and traumatic derma-

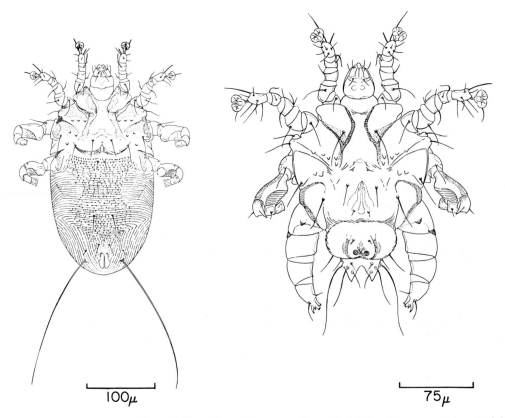

FIG. 15.44. *Myocoptes musculinus. (Left)* Female, ventral view. *(Right)* Male, ventral view. (From Baker et al. 1956. Courtesy of National Pest Control Association.)

titis, especially of the abdomen, also occur. The coat becomes gray (Watson 1961) and loses its sheen (Tuffery 1962). Skin of adult mice, in the areas of mite attachment, shows increased mitotic activity; this is not seen in younger mice (Watson 1961). In the guinea pig, *M. musculinus* is reported to cause a suppurative mange (Sengbusch 1960).

DIAGNOSIS

Diagnosis of infestation is based on recognition and identification of the mite. Mites, if present in large numbers, are easily found by killing a mouse and placing the carcass overnight on a piece of black paper bordered by cellophane tape, sticky side up (Fig. 15.45) (Flynn 1963). The next day the mites will have migrated onto the paper or tape. *Myocoptes musculinus* must be distinguished from *Trichoecius rom-boutsi, Myobia musculi,* and *Radfordia affinis,* all of which are common on the laboratory mouse. The last two species are readily separated from *M. musculinus* in that only their first pair of legs is modified for clasping hairs. *Myocoptes musculinus* is larger than *T. romboutsi,* the female has a broader body, and the male has two long and two short rather than four long terminal setae (Flynn 1955).

CONTROL

The control procedures given for *Myobia musculi* will also control this mite (Clark and Yunker 1964; Cook 1953; Davis 1957; Flynn 1955; Flynn, Brennan, and Fritz 1965; Sengbusch 1960; Wagner 1969).

PUBLIC HEALTH CONSIDERATIONS

Myocoptes musculinus does not affect man.

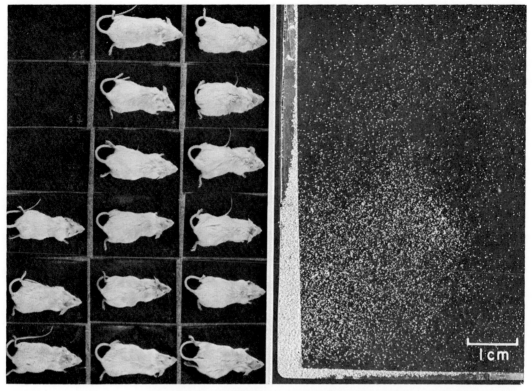

Fig. 15.45. Method of recovering *Myocoptes musculinus* from a mouse. *(Left)* Mice on black paper surrounded by cellophane tape, sticky side up. *(Right)* Typical paper with mites which migrated from one mouse carcass during 18 hours. *(Left* from Flynn 1955; courtesy of Jane K. Glaser, Argonne National Laboratory. *Right* from Flynn 1963; courtesy of the American Association for Laboratory Animal Science.)

Trichoecius romboutsi

(SYN. *Myocoptes romboutsi*)

Trichoecius romboutsi, a pelage-inhabiting mite, has been reported from the mouse in the United States and Europe (Fain, Munting, and Lukoschus 1970; Flynn 1955). Its incidence in laboratory mouse colonies in the United States was high in 1955, but a survey in 1965 failed to disclose it (Flynn, Brennan, and Fritz 1965). It is similar to *M. musculinus,* and failure to identify it may account for the lack of reports of its occurrence.

MORPHOLOGY

Trichoecius romboutsi (Fig. 15.46) is similar to *M. musculinus* but smaller; the female is about 260 μ and the male about 170 μ long (Flynn 1955). The female is more elliptical than that of *M. musculinus* and the male has four long rather than two long and two short terminal setae.

LIFE CYCLE

The life cycle is unknown, but is probably similar to that of *M. musculinus.*

PATHOLOGIC EFFECTS

This mite usually occurs simultaneously with *M. musculinus, Myobia musculi,* and *Radfordia affinis* (Flynn 1955); consequently its specific pathologic effects are unknown.

DIAGNOSIS

Diagnosis is based on recognition and identification of the mite. The black paper and cellophane tape technique used to

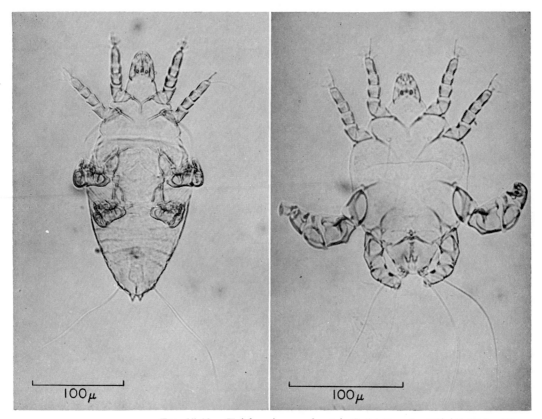

FIG. 15.46. *Trichoecius romboutsi. (Left)* Female. *(Right)* Male. (From Flynn 1963. Courtesy of the American Association for Laboratory Animal Science.)

demonstrate *M. musculinus* infestation is also effective for this mite (Flynn 1963).

CONTROL

Control measures effective against *M. musculi* are also effective against *T. romboutsi* (Flynn 1955).

PUBLIC HEALTH CONSIDERATIONS

This mite is not known to affect man.

Chirodiscoides caviae

(SYN. *Campylochirus caviae, Indochirus utkalensis*)

(Fur Mite of Guinea Pig)

Chirodiscoides caviae is a common pelage-inhabiting parasite of the guinea pig (Blackmore and Owen 1968; Deoras and Patel 1960; Harrison and Daykin 1965;

Hirst 1922; Patnaik 1965; Sasa et al. 1962). Although it has been reported only from Europe and Asia, it probably occurs throughout the world. In a survey in Great Britain, 18 of 80 guinea pigs from 20 different colonies were found infected (Blackmore and Owen 1968), and incidences of 52.8 to 100.0% have been observed in India (Deoras and Patel 1960).

MORPHOLOGY

Both sexes are elongate and about 350 to 500 μ long (Fig. 15.47) (Hirst 1917a). The mouthparts are compressed, the sternal region is modified as a striated, hair-clasping organ, and the first and second pairs of legs are modified for clasping hair but the third and fourth pairs are more elongate and less modified.

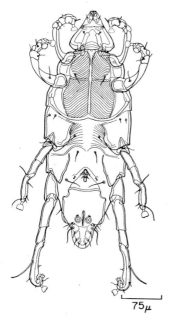

75μ

FIG. 15.47. *Chirodiscoides caviae* female, ventral view. (From Hirst 1922. Courtesy of British Museum—Natural History.)

LIFE CYCLE

The life cycle has not been studied, but an egg, larva, and two nymphal stages are known (Hirst 1917a).

PATHOLOGIC EFFECTS

The parasite attaches to the hairs of the entire body, but the posterodorsal area is most heavily infested (Deoras and Patel 1960; Hirst 1922). Infestation often goes unnoticed, but severe pruritus and alopecia sometimes occur (Harrison and Daykin 1965; Patnaik 1965).

DIAGNOSIS

Diagnosis is based on recognition and identification of the mite in the pelage.

CONTROL

Only control based on treatment with acaricides has been reported. Several thorough treatments with a pyrethrin aerosol (concentration not given) reduces the degree of infestation but does not eliminate it (Harrison and Daykin 1965). A more effective treatment consists of dipping affected guinea pigs weekly for 3 weeks either in 0.2% 4,4'-dichloro-α-methylbenzhydrol (DMC, Sherwin-Williams) in 50% ethyl alcohol, or in a 2% suspension of a wettable powder containing 15% butylphenoxyisopropyl choroethyl sulfite (Aramite-15W, Uniroyal) plus a wetting agent (Sengbusch 1960).

PUBLIC HEALTH CONSIDERATIONS

Chirodiscoides caviae is of no known public health significance.

TABLE 15.1. Mesostigmates affecting endothermal laboratory animals

Parasite	Geographic Distribution	Endothermal Host	Usual Habitat	Incidence In nature	Incidence In laboratory	Pathologic Effects	Public Health Importance	Reference
*Ornithonyssus bacoti**	Worldwide	Mouse, rat, hamster, wild rodents, wild carnivores, cat, chicken, wild birds, man	Bedding, wild rodent burrows, cracks and crevices in animal buildings; skin of host while feeding	Common on mouse, rat, other wild rodents	Common in some conventional colonies; rare or absent in others	Loss of blood, debilitation, anemia, decreased reproduction, death; vector of filarial worm of cotton rat	Affects man; causes irritation, sometimes dermatitis; potential vector of agents of murine typhus, rickettsial pox, Q fever, eastern equine encephalitis, plague, tularemia	Baker et al. 1956 Harris and Stockton 1960 Keefe et al. 1964 Olson and Dahms 1946 Sasa et al. 1962 Scott 1958 Yunker 1964
*Ornithonyssus sylviarum**	Worldwide in temperate zones	Mouse, rat, hamster, chicken, pigeon, wild birds, man	Skin, feathers; sometimes cracks and crevices in animal buildings	Common on chicken; rare on mouse, rat, hamster, man	Uncommon on chicken	Matted feathers, scab formation, thickened skin, anemia, retarded growth, death; possible vector of pathogens	Causes pruritus, dermatitis; possible vector of agents of equine encephalitides, ornithosis	Baker et al. 1956 Cameron 1938 Knapp and Krause 1960 Pirvanik and Akimov 1964 Sikes and Chamberlain 1954
*Ornithonyssus bursa**	Worldwide in tropics and subtropics	Chicken, pigeon, canary, duck, wild birds, man	Skin, feathers; sometimes cracks and crevices in animal buildings	Common on chicken	Unknown; probably rare or absent	Irritation, matted feathers, anemia, death	Causes irritation; possible vector of pathogens	Baker et al. 1956 Sikes and Chamberlain 1954 Strandtmann and Wharton 1958
*Dermanyssus gallinae**	Worldwide	Rat, rabbit, chicken, pigeon, canary, other birds, man	Cracks and crevices in animal buildings; skin of host while feeding	Common on chicken; rare on rat, rabbit, man	Common on chicken	Irritation, loss of blood, debilitation, decreased egg production, anemia, papules in skin, sometimes death; potential vector of agents of avian spirochaetosis, avian malaria	Causes irritation, sometimes papular urticaria; potential vector of viral encephalitides	Baker et al. 1956 Benbrook 1965 Bigland 1954 Brumpt and Callot 1947 Harrison and Daykin 1965 Kirkwood 1967 Sikes and Chamberlain 1954 Strandtmann and Wharton 1958
*Liponyssoides sanguineus**	North America, Europe, Africa, Asia	Mouse, rat, other rodents, man	Cracks and crevices in animal buildings, wild rodent burrows; skin of host while feeding	Uncommon	Unknown	Unknown; probably debilitation, anemia, decreased reproduction, death	Causes dermatitis; vector of *Rickettsia akari*	Baker et al. 1956 Fuller 1954 Huebner et al. 1946 Nichols et al. 1953 Strandtmann and Wharton 1958
Hirstionyssus butantanensis	South America	Mouse	Skin, pelage	Unknown	Unknown; probably rare or absent	Unknown	None known	da Fonseca 1932

*Discussed in text.

TABLE 15.1 *(continued)*

Parasite	Geographic Distribution	Endothermal Host	Usual Habitat	Incidence In nature	Incidence In laboratory	Pathologic Effects	Public Health Importance	Reference
*Pneumonyssus simicola**	Asia, Philippine Islands	Rhesus monkey, cynomolgus monkey, pigtail macaque, other macaques	Lungs	Common	Common	Foci in lungs, sometimes death	None known	Baker et al. 1956; Fain 1959, 1961; Fairbrother and Hurst 1932; Finegold et al. 1968; Fremming et al. 1957; Furman 1954; Gay and Branch 1927; Habermann and Williams 1957; Honjo et al. 1963; Innes 1969; Innes et al. 1954; Lee et al. 1954; Masse et al. 1965; Robertson et al. 1947; Strandtmann and Wharton 1958; Valerio et al. 1969; Vitzthum 1930
Pneumonyssus duttoni	Africa	Guenons	Trachea	Common	Unknown	Tracheitis	None known	Fain 1959
Pneumonyssus santos-diasi	Africa	Guenons, baboons	Lungs	Common	Unknown	Unknown	None known	Fain 1959; Myers and Kuntz 1965
Pneumonyssus longus	Africa	Guenons, chimpanzee	Lungs	Common	Unknown	Unknown	None known	Fain 1959
Pneumonyssus oudemansi	Africa	Guenons, chimpanzee, gorilla	Lungs	Uncommon	Unknown	Unknown	None known	Fain 1959
Pneumonyssus africanus	Africa	Guenons	Bronchi	Rare	Unknown	Unknown	None known	Fain 1959
Pneumonyssus mossambicencis	Africa	Baboons	Lungs	Uncommon	Unknown	Unknown	None known	Fain 1959
Pneumonyssus congoensis	Africa	Baboons	Lungs	Rare	Unknown	Unknown	None	Fain 1959; Myers and Kuntz 1965
Rhinophaga dinolti	Asia	Rhesus monkey	Lungs	Rare	Unknown	Unknown	None known	Fain 1955; Furman 1954; Oudemans 1935
Rhinophaga cercopitheci	Africa	Guenons	Lungs	Uncommon	Unknown	Chronic pneumonitis, excessive mucus production	None	Fain et al. 1958; Strandtmann and Wharton 1958

*Discussed in text.

TABLE 15.1 *(continued)*

Parasite	Geographic Distribution	Endothermal Host	Usual Habitat	Incidence In nature	Incidence In laboratory	Pathologic Effects	Public Health Importance	Reference
Rhinophaga papionis	Africa	Baboons	Lungs	Uncommon	Unknown	Chronic pneumonitis, excessive mucus production	None	Fain et al. 1958 Myers and Kuntz 1965 Strandtmann and Wharton 1958
*Pneumonyssoides caninum**	United States, South Africa, Australia	Dog	Nasal cavities, sinuses	Uncommon	Unknown	Hyperemia of nasal mucosa, excessive mucus production	None known	Baker et al. 1956 Chandler and Ruhe 1940 Furman 1954 Koutz et al. 1953 Roberts and Thompson 1969 Senter 1958
Pneumonyssoides stammeri	South America	Woolly monkey	Nasal cavities, sinuses	Rare	Unknown	Unknown	None known	Fain 1961 Vitzthum 1930
Haemogamasus pontiger	North America, Europe, Asia, Africa, Australia	Mouse, rat, other rodents, man	Skin, pelage; wild rodent burrows, bedding, buildings	Common	Rare	Unknown	Sometimes causes dermatitis	Baker et al. 1956 Hill and Gordon 1945
Eulaelaps stabularis	North America, Europe, Asia	Mouse, rat, other rodents, other small mammals, man	Skin, pelage; wild rodent burrows, bedding	Common	Unknown	Potential vector of *Francisella tularensis*	Sometimes causes dermatitis	Baker et al. 1956
*Laelaps echidninus**	Worldwide	Mouse, rat, cotton rat, other rodents	Skin, pelage; bedding, cage crevices, wild rodent burrows	Common on rat	Rare	Unknown; vector of *Hepatozoon muris*	Potential vector of Argentinian hemorrhagic fever virus	Baker et al. 1956 Furman 1959 Miller 1908 Owen 1956 Strandtmann and Mitchell 1963 Strandtmann and Wharton 1958
Laelaps nuttalli	Worldwide in tropics and subtropics	Mouse, rat, other rodents	Skin, pelage; rodent burrows	Common on rat	Unknown	Unknown	None	Strandtmann and Wharton 1958 Tipton 1960
Haemolaelaps glasgowi	Worldwide	Mouse, rat, other rodents, wild lagomorphs, other small mammals, carnivores, birds	Skin, pelage, plumage; rodent burrows, other animal nests	Common	Uncommon	Unknown	None	Baker et al. 1956 Strandtmann 1949
Haemolaelaps casalis	Worldwide	Mouse, rat, other rodents, chicken, wild birds, man	Skin, pelage, plumage; rodent burrows, other animal nests, bedding	Common	Uncommon	Unknown	Sometimes causes dermatitis	Baker et al. 1956 Strandtmann and Wharton 1958

*Discussed in text.

TABLE 15.2. Prostigmates affecting endothermal laboratory animals

Parasite	Geographic Distribution	Endothermal Host	Usual Habitat	Incidence In nature	Incidence In laboratory	Pathologic Effects	Public Health Importance	Reference
Myobia musculi[*]	Worldwide	Mouse	Skin, pelage	Common	Common	Dermatitis, alopecia, pruritus, self-inflicted dermal trauma, secondary amyloidosis	None	Blackmore and Owen 1968 Flynn 1955, 1963 Flynn et al. 1965 Fukui et al. 1961 Galton 1963 Grant 1942 Haakh 1958 Heine 1962 Whiteley and Horton 1962
Radfordia affinis[*]	Worldwide	Mouse	Skin, pelage	Common	Common	Unknown; probably dermatitis, alopecia, pruritus	None	Flynn 1955, 1963 Flynn et al. 1965 Fukui et al. 1961 Heine 1962 Seamer and Chesterman 1967
Radfordia ensifera[*]	Worldwide	Rat	Skin, pelage	Common	Common	Self-inflicted dermal trauma	None	Baker et al. 1956 Heine 1962 Sasa et al. 1962 Skidmore 1934
Psorergates simplex[*]	North America, Europe; probably worldwide	Mouse	Hair follicles	Unknown	Common	Caseous nodules in skin, dermal cysts, sometimes scabby dermatitis of ears	None	Bateman 1961 Beresford-Jones 1965, 1967 Cook 1956 Fain et al. 1966 Flynn 1955, 1959a, 1963 Flynn and Jaroslow 1956
Psorergates oettlei	South Africa	Multimammate mouse	Skin	Unknown	Rare	Scabby dermatitis, alopecia	None	Fain et al. 1966 Till 1960
Psorergates cercopitheci	United States, Africa	Guenons, mangabeys	Skin	Rare	Rare	Dermatitis, alopecia	None	Lavoipierre and Crewe 1955 Sheldon 1966 Zumpt and Till 1954
Demodex canis[*]	Worldwide	Dog	Hair follicles	Common	Common	Sometimes dry, scaly dermatitis, alopecia, induration; sometimes moist dermatitis, pustule formation, serous exudation	None	Baker 1969a Baker et al. 1956 Bantin and Maber 1967 Enigk 1949 Koutz 1953, 1954, 1955, 1957, 1966 Koutz et al. 1960 Král and Schwartzman 1964
Demodex musculi	Unknown; probably worldwide	Mouse	Skin	Rare	Unknown; probably rare	Unknown	None	Hirst 1917b

[*]Discussed in text.

473

TABLE 15.2 (continued)

Parasite	Geographic Distribution	Endothermal Host	Usual Habitat	Incidence In nature	Incidence In laboratory	Pathologic Effects	Public Health Importance	Reference
Demodex ratti	Unknown; probably worldwide	Rat	Skin	Rare	Unknown; probably rare	Unknown	None	Hirst 1917b
Demodex criceti	United States; probably worldwide	Hamster	Skin	Rare	Uncommon	Epidermal cell destruction; dry, scaly, scabby dermatitis; alopecia	None	Flatt and Kerber 1968 Nutting 1961, 1965 Nutting and Rauch 1958
Demodex aurati	United States; probably worldwide	Hamster	Skin	Rare	Uncommon	Perifollicular hyperpigmentation; dry, scaly, scabby dermatitis; alopecia	None	Flatt and Kerber 1968 Nutting 1961, 1965 Nutting and Rauch 1963
Demodex sp.	United States	Mongolian gerbil	Skin	Rare	Uncommon	Alopecia, scabby dermatitis	Unknown	Reynolds and Gainer 1968
Demodex caviae	Unknown; probably worldwide	Guinea pig	Skin	Unknown	Unknown; probably rare	Unknown	None	Bacigalupo and Roveda 1954
Demodex cuniculi	Unknown; probably worldwide	Rabbit	Skin	Rare	Unknown; probably rare	Unknown	None	Král and Schwartzman 1964
Demodex cati	Unknown; probably worldwide	Cat	Skin	Rare	Unknown; probably rare	Scabby dermatitis, alopecia	None	Hirst 1922 Král and Schwartzman 1964 Trimmier 1966
*Cheyletiella parasitivorax**	North America, Europe, Asia, Australia, New Zealand	Rabbit, cat, man, possibly dog	Skin, pelage	Common on rabbit; rare on cat	Common on rabbit in some areas	Alopecia, scaly dermatitis, pruritus, serous, exudation, thickening of skin	Causes dermatitis	Baker et al. 1956 Barr 1955 Deoras and Patel 1960 Ewing et al. 1967 Moxham et al. 1968 Mykytowycz 1957 Olsen and Roth 1947 Seamer and Chesterman 1967 Strasser 1963
*Cheyletiella yasguri**	North America, Europe	Dog, man	Skin, pelage	Uncommon	Unknown	Alopecia, scaly dermatitis, pruritus	Causes dermatitis	Baker 1969b Ewing et al. 1967 Favati and Galliano 1962 Humphreys 1958 Reed 1961 Smiley 1965 Wetkamp 1964 Yasgur 1968

*Discussed in text.

TABLE 15.2 (continued)

Parasite	Geographic Distribution	Endothermal Host	Usual Habitat	Incidence		Pathologic Effects	Public Health Importance	Reference
				In nature	In laboratory			
Syringophilus bipectinatus	Eastern United States, Europe; probably worldwide	Chicken, other birds	Quills of wing and body feathers	Uncommon	Unknown; probably rare or absent	Partial or entire loss of feathers	None	Benbrook 1965 Hwang 1959 Jones 1956 Rebrassier and Martin 1932 Schwabe 1956
Eutrombicula alfreddugesi	North America, South America	Various mammals, chicken, other birds, man	Grass; skin of host	Common	Absent; occurs only on animals obtained from natural habitat or on chickens penned outdoors	Heavy infestations cause weakness, anorexia, death in young chickens	Human pest (chigger); causes irritation, local inflammation, pruritus	Baker et al. 1956 Wharton and Fuller 1952
Eutrombicula batatas	Southwestern United States, Central America, South America	Chicken, other birds, domestic animals, man	Grass; skin of host	Common	Absent; occurs only on chickens penned outdoors	None	Human pest (chigger); causes irritation, local inflammation, pruritus	Baker et al. 1956 Wharton and Fuller 1952
Neotrombicula autumnalis	Europe	Wild rodents, rabbit, hares, dog, cat, chicken, other birds, domestic animals, man	Grass; skin of host	Common	Absent; occurs only on animals obtained from natural habitat or on chickens penned outdoors	None	Human pest (chigger); causes irritation, local inflammation, pruritus	Baker et al. 1956 Wharton and Fuller 1952 U.S. Dept. Agr. 1967
Neoschoengastia americana	North America, Central America, West Indies	Chicken, other birds	Grass; skin of host	Common	Absent; occurs only on chickens penned outdoors	Irritation	None	Baker et al. 1956 Wharton and Fuller 1952 U.S. Dept. Agr. 1967

TABLE 15.3. Astigmates affecting endothermal laboratory animals

Parasite	Geographic Distribution	Endothermal Host	Usual Habitat	Incidence — In nature	Incidence — In laboratory	Pathologic Effects	Public Health Importance	Reference
*Sarcoptes scabiei**	Worldwide	Hamster, rabbit, dog, other canids, cynomolgus monkey, orangutan, chimpanzee, gibbons, domestic animals, man	Skin	Common in dog, rabbit; uncommon in other animals	Common in dog; uncommon in rabbit; rare in hamster, simian primates	Scabby papular dermatitis, pruritus, self-inflicted trauma, alopecia, thickening of skin, emaciation, sometimes death	Occasionally causes severe dermatitis	Adams et al. 1967 Baker et al. 1956 Camin and Rogoff 1952 Cook 1969 Enigk and Grittner 1951 Fain 1968a Goldman and Feldman 1949 Hagan and Lund 1962 Král and Schwartzman 1964 Leerhoy and Jensen 1967 Van Stee 1964 Weidman 1923
Prosarcoptes pitheci	Africa, Europe	Guenons, baboons, capuchins (in captivity)	Skin	Unknown	Unknown; probably rare or absent	Scabby papular dermatitis, pruritus, alopecia	Unknown	Fain 1963, 1968a Phillipe 1948
Pithesarcoptes talapoini	Africa, Europe	Guenons	Skin	Rare	Unknown	Scabby dermatitis, alopecia	Unknown	Fain 1965b, 1968a
Cosarcoptes scanloni	Southeastern Asia	Cynomolgus monkey	Skin	Rare	Unknown	Unknown	Unknown	Fain 1968a
Trixacarus diversus	Europe	Rat	Skin	Unknown	Rare	Scabby dermatitis, alopecia	Unknown	Fain 1968a Guilhon 1946a, b
Notoedres musculi	Europe	Mouse	Skin	Uncommon	Uncommon	Unknown	None	Fain 1965a
*Notoedres muris**	North America, Europe, Africa; probably worldwide	Rat, black rat, multimammate mouse, wild rodents	Skin, usually of ears	Common	Common in some colonies, uncommon or absent in others	Wartlike, horny excrescences on ears, nose; papular dermatitis	None	Fain 1965a, 1968a Flynn 1960 Gordon et al. 1943 Hirst 1922 Watson 1962
Notoedres sp.*	North America, Europe	Hamster	Skin, usually of ears	Unknown	Uncommon	Scaly dermatitis, particularly of ears	None	Bâies et al. 1968 Hindle 1947 Wantland 1968
Notoedres jamesoni	Southeastern Asia	Rat	Skin	Rare	Unknown; probably absent	Unknown	None	Fain 1965a, 1968a Lavoipierre 1964

*Discussed in text.

476

TABLE 15.3 (continued)

Parasite	Geographic Distribution	Endothermal Host	Usual Habitat	Incidence In nature	Incidence In laboratory	Pathologic Effects	Public Health Importance	Reference
Notoedres cati*	North America, Europe, Africa; probably worldwide	Rabbit, cat, dog, man	Skin, usually of ears, head, neck	Common in cat; uncommon in rabbit; rare in dog	Common in cat; uncommon in rabbit; rare in dog	Scaly dermatitis; pruritus; alopecia; self-inflicted trauma; crusts on ears, face, neck; thickening of skin; sometimes death	Causes transient dermatitis	Adams et al. 1967 Baker et al. 1956 Camin and Rogoff 1952 Conroy 1964
Notoedres galagoensis	Central Africa	Galagos	Skin	Rare	Unknown; probably rare	Unknown	None	Fain 1963, 1965a, 1968b
Knemidokoptes mutans*	North America, Europe, Africa; probably worldwide	Chicken	Skin, beneath epidermal scales of legs	Common	Unknown; probably uncommon	Irritation, inflammation, vesicles, crusts on legs; deformity of legs; lameness	None	Baker et al. 1956 Benbrook 1965 Bishopp and Wood 1931 Fain and Elsen 1967 Griffiths and O'Rourke 1950 Král and Schwartzman 1964 Nevin 1935
Knemidokoptes pilae*	North America, South America, Europe, Africa; probably worldwide	Parakeet	Skin, usually base of beak, legs	Common	Unknown; probably common	Crust formation on face, legs; deformity of beak	None	Altman 1968 Blackmore 1963 Fain and Elsen 1967 Kutzer 1964 Wichmann and Vincent 1958 Yunker and Ishak 1957
Neocnemidocoptes laevis gallinae*	North America, Europe, Africa; probably worldwide	Chicken	Skin of body, head, upper legs	Uncommon	Unknown; probably rare or absent	Dermatitis, pruritus, loss of feathers, dermal scales, papules	None	Baker et al. 1956 Benbrook 1965 Fain and Elsen 1967 Hirst 1922 Král and Schwartzman 1964
Neocnemidocoptes laevis laevis	Europe	Pigeon	Skin	Uncommon	Unknown	Dermatitis, pruritus, loss of feathers	None	Fain and Elsen 1967
Cytodites nudus*	Worldwide	Chicken, other birds	Trachea, bronchi, lungs	Uncommon	Unknown; probably rare or absent	Cough, weakness, incoordination, loss of weight; sometimes pneumonia, death	None	Baker et al. 1956 Benbrook 1965 Fain and Bafort 1964 Lindt and Kutzer 1965

*Discussed in text.

TABLE 15.3 *(continued)*

Parasite	Geographic Distribution	Endothermal Host	Usual Habitat	Incidence		Pathologic Effects	Public Health Importance	Reference
				In nature	In laboratory			
*Laminosioptes cysticola**	North America, South America, Europe, Australia; probably worldwide	Chicken, pigeon, other birds	Subcutis	Uncommon	Unknown; probably rare or absent	Subcutaneous nodules, sometimes death	None	Baker et al. 1956 Benbrook 1965 Bishopp and Wood 1931 Lindquist and Belding 1919
*Psoroptes cuniculi**	Worldwide	Rabbit	External ear canal; skin of face, neck, legs	Common	Common	Otitis, dermatitis, pruritus, crusts on ears, face, neck, legs; sometimes loss of equilibrium, torticollis, meningitis, death	None	Adams et al. 1967 Alicata 1964 Baker et al. 1956 Giorgi 1968 Hirst 1922 Král and Schwartzman 1964 Lund 1951 Marine 1924 Poole et al. 1967 Streeter 1945 Sweatman 1958a
*Otodectes cynotis**	Worldwide	Dog, cat, other carnivores	External ear canal; sometimes skin of feet, tail	Common	Common	Otitis, dermatitis, pruritus, self-inflicted trauma, ulceration of auditory canal; sometimes auricular hematoma, torticollis, circling, convulsions	None	Baker et al. 1956 Beresford-Jones 1955 Berg and Shomer 1963 Camin and Rogoff 1952 Conroy 1964 Evans et al. 1961 Frost and Beresford-Jones 1960 Grono 1969 Johnson et al. 1963 Král and Schwartzman 1964 Morris 1963 Staggs 1961 Sweatman 1958b Tonn 1961
Alouattalges corbeti	South America	Howler monkeys, night monkey	Skin	Uncommon	Unknown; probably uncommon	Unknown	None	Fain 1966
Fonsecalges saimirii	South America	Squirrel monkeys, tamarins	Skin	Uncommon	Uncommon	Unknown; possibly dermatitis	None	Cosgrove et al. 1968 Dunn 1968 Fain 1966 Flatt and Patton 1969

*Discussed in text.

TABLE 15.3 (continued)

Parasite	Geographic Distribution	Endothermal Host	Usual Habitat	Incidence		Pathologic Effects	Public Health Importance	Reference
				In nature	In laboratory			
Paracoroptes gordoni	Africa	Guenons	Skin of body, ears	Uncommon	Unknown; probably rare	Dermatitis, crusts, scales	Unknown	Fain 1963 Lavoipierre 1955
Pangorillages pani	Africa	Chimpanzee	Skin	Rare	Unknown; probably rare or absent	Unknown	Unknown	Fain 1962
*Myocoptes musculinus**	Worldwide	Mouse, possibly guinea pig	Skin, pelage	Common in mouse	Common in mouse	Usually none, sometimes erythema, self-inflicted trauma, dermatitis, alopecia	None	Baker et al. 1956 Blackmore and Owen 1968 Flynn 1955 Flynn et al. 1965 Fukui et al. 1961 Gambles 1952 Heine 1962 Sengbusch 1960 Smith 1955a, b Watson 1960, 1961
*Trichoecius romboutsi**	United States, Europe	Mouse	Skin, pelage	Unknown	Unknown; was common, now apparently uncommon	Unknown	None	Fain et al. 1970 Flynn 1955, 1963
Trichoecius muris	Europe	Rat	Skin, pelage	Unknown; probably rare	Unknown; probably absent	Unknown	Unknown	Fain et al. 1970
*Chirodiscoides caviae**	Europe, Asia; probably worldwide	Guinea pig	Skin, pelage	Common	Common	Usually none; sometimes pruritus, alopecia	None	Blackmore and Owen 1968 Deoras and Patel 1960 Harrison and Daykin 1965 Hirst 1917a 1922 Patnaik 1965
Listrophorus gibbus	Asia; probably worldwide	Rabbit	Skin, pelage	Common	Common in India; otherwise unknown	Unknown	None	Deoras and Patel 1960 Evans et al. 1961 Hirst 1922
Listrocarpus cosgrovei	South America	Marmosets, tamarins	Skin	Unknown; probably rare	Unknown; probably rare	Unknown	None	Cosgrove et al. 1968 Fain 1967
Listrocarpus hapalei	South America	Marmosets	Skin	Unknown; probably rare	Unknown; probably rare	Unknown	None	Fain 1967

*Discussed in text.

TABLE 15.3 (continued)

Parasite	Geographic Distribution	Endothermal Host	Usual Habitat	Incidence — In nature	Incidence — In laboratory	Pathologic Effects	Public Health Importance	Reference
Listrocarpus saimirii	South America	Squirrel monkeys	Skin	Unknown; probably rare	Unknown; probably rare	Unknown	None	Fain 1967
Listrocarpus lagothrix	South America	Woolly monkeys	Skin	Unknown; probably rare	Unknown; probably rare	Unknown	None	Fain 1967
Megninia cubitalis	North America, Hawaii, Europe, South Africa; probably worldwide	Chicken, other birds	Down feathers, contour feathers	Common	Unknown; probably rare or absent	Usually none; sometimes dermal irritation	None	Alicata et al. 1947 Baker et al. 1956 Benbrook 1965 Hirst 1922 Zumpt 1966
Megninia ginglymura	Unknown; probably worldwide	Chicken, other birds	Down feathers, contour feathers	Uncommon	Unknown; probably rare or absent	Usually none; sometimes feather pulling	None	Baker et al. 1956 Hirst 1922
Pterolichus obtusus	Unknown; probably worldwide	Chicken	Wing feathers, tail feathers	Unknown; probably common	Uncommon	Usually none; sometimes reduced vigor	None	Alicata et al. 1946 Baker et al. 1956 Deoras and Patel 1960 Hirst 1922
Dermoglyphus minor	Unknown; probably worldwide	Chicken, other birds	Quill feathers	Uncommon	Unknown; probably rare or absent	None	None	Baker et al. 1956 Evans et al. 1961 Hirst 1922
Dermoglyphus elongatus	Unknown; probably worldwide	Chicken, other birds	Quill feathers	Uncommon	Unknown; probably rare or absent	Loss of feathers	None	Baker et al. 1956 Hirst 1922
Rivoltasia bifurcata	North America, South America, Europe; probably worldwide	Chicken	Skin, downy parts of quill feathers	Uncommon	Unknown	Pruritus, feather damage	None	Baker et al.1956 Benbrook 1965 Bishopp and Wood 1931 Evans et al. 1961 Fain 1965c
Epidermoptes bilobatus	North America, South America, Europe; probably worldwide	Chicken	Skin	Uncommon	Unknown	Desquamation, scabby dermatitis, loss of feathers	None	Baker et al. 1956 Benbrook 1965 Fain 1965c
Rhyncoptes anastosi	South America	Marmosets, tamarins	Skin	Rare	Unknown; probably rare	Unknown	None	Fain 1965d

TABLE 15.3 *(continued)*

Parasite	Geographic Distribution	Endothermal Host	Usual Habitat	Incidence In nature	Incidence In laboratory	Pathologic Effects	Public Health Importance	Reference
Rhyncoptes cebi	South America	Capuchins	Skin	Rare	Unknown; probably rare	Unknown	None	Fain 1965d
Rhyncoptes cercopitheci	Africa	Guenons	Skin	Rare	Unknown; probably rare	Unknown	None	Fain 1965d
Samirioptes paradoxus	South America	Squirrel monkeys	Skin	Unknown; probably rare	Unknown; probably rare	Unknown	None	Fain 1968b
Audycoptes greeri	South America	Squirrel monkeys	Hair follicles	Unknown; probably rare	Rare	Unknown	None	Dunn 1968 Fain 1968b Lavoipierre 1964
Audycoptes lawrenci	South America	Squirrel monkeys	Hair follicles	Unknown; probably rare	Rare	Unknown	None	Dunn 1968 Fain 1968b Lavoipierre 1964
Lemurnyssus galagoensis	Africa	Galagos	Nasal cavities	Rare	Unknown; probably rare	Unknown	None	Fain 1964b
Mortelmansia brevis	South America	Squirrel monkeys	Nasal cavities	Rare	Unknown; probably rare	Unknown	None	Dunn 1968 Fain 1964b
Mortelmansia longis	South America	Squirrel monkeys	Nasal cavities	Rare	Unknown; probably rare	Unknown	None	Dunn 1968 Fain 1964b
Mortelmansia duboisi	South America	Marmosets	Nasal cavities	Rare	Unknown; probably rare	Unknown	None	Dunn 1968 Fain 1964b

REFERENCES

Adams, C. E., F. C. Aitken, and A. N. Worden. 1967. The rabbit (*Oryctolagus cuniculus* L.), pp. 396–448. *In* UFAW Staff, ed. The UFAW handbook on the care and management of laboratory animals. 3d ed. Livingstone and the Universities Federation for Animal Welfare, London.

Alicata, J. E. 1964. Parasitic infections of man and animals in Hawaii. Technical Bull. 61. Hawaii Agricultural Experiment Station, University of Hawaii, Honolulu. 138 pp.

Alicata, J. E., F. G. Holdaway, J. H. Quisenberry, and D. D. Jensen. 1946. Observations on the comparative efficacy of certain old and new insecticides in the control of lice and mites of chickens. Poultry Sci. 25:376–80.

Alicata, J. E., L. Kartman, T. Nishida, and A. L. Palafox. 1947. Efficacy of certain sprays in control of lice and mites of chickens. J. Econ. Entomol. 40:922–23.

Altman, R. B. 1968. Parasitic diseases of caged birds, pp. 360–63. *In* R. W. Kirk, ed. Current veterinary therapy III: Small animal practice. W. B. Saunders, Philadelphia.

Bacigalupo, J., and R. J. Roveda. 1954. *Demodex caviae* n. sp. Rev. Med. Vet. 36:149–53.

Băies, A., I. Suteu, and W. Klemm. 1968. *Notoëdres*-Räude des Goldhamsters. Z. Versuchstierk. 10:251–57.

Baker, E. W., T. M. Evans, D. J. Gould, W. B. Hull, and H. L. Keegan. 1956. A manual of parasitic mites of medical or economic importance. Tech. Publ. Natl. Pest Control Assoc., Inc., New York. 170 pp.

Baker, E. W., and G. H. Wharton. 1952. An introduction to acarology. Macmillan, New York. 465 pp.

Baker, K. P. 1969a. The histopathology and pathogenesis of demodecosis of the dog. J. Comp. Pathol. 79:321–27.

———. 1969b. Infestation of domestic animals with the mite *Cheyletiella parasitivorax*. Vet. Record 84:561.

Banks, N. 1901. A new genus of endoparasitic acarians. Geneesk. Tijdschr. Nederl.-Indië. 41:334–36.

Bantin, G. C., and D. F. Maber. 1967. Some parasites of the beagle. J. Inst. Animal Tech. 18:49–59.

Barr, A. R. 1955. A case of "mange" of the domestic rabbit due to *Cheyletiella parasitivorax* (Megnin). J. Parasitol. 41:323.

Bateman, N. 1961. Simultaneous eradication of three ectoparasitic species from a colony of laboratory mice. Nature 191:721–22.

Benbrook, E. A. 1965. External parasites of poultry, pp. 925–64. *In* H. E. Biester and and L. H. Schwarte, eds. Diseases of poultry. 5th ed. Iowa State Univ. Press, Ames.

Benbrook, E. A., and Margaret W. Sloss. 1961. Veterinary clinical parasitology. 3d ed. Iowa State Univ. Press, Ames. 240 pp.

Beresford-Jones, W. P. 1955. Observations on the incidence of *Otodectes cynotis* (Hering) on dogs and cats in the London area. Vet. Record 67:716–17.

———. 1965. Occurrence of the mite *Psorergates simplex* in mice. Aust. Vet. J. 41:289–90.

———. 1967. Observations on the transmission of the mite *Psorergates simplex* Tyrrell 1883 in laboratory mice, pp. 277–80. *In* E. J. L. Soulsby, ed. The reaction of the host to parasitism. Vet. Med. Rev., N. G. Elwert Universitäts und Verlagsbuchhandlung, Marburg/Lahn.

Berg, P., and R. R. Shomer. 1963. Otocariasis in the dog and cat. J. Am. Vet. Med. Assoc. 143:1224–26.

Bertram, D. S., K. Unsworth, and R. M. Gordon. 1946. The biology and maintenance of *Liponyssus bacoti* Hirst, 1913, and an investigation into its role as a vector of *Litomosoides carinii* to cotton rats and white rats, together with some observations on the infection in white rats. Ann. Trop. Med. Parasitol. 40:228–54.

Bigland, C. H. 1954. A rabbit infestation with poultry mites and experimental mite transmission of fowl cholera. Can. J. Comp. Med. 18:213–14.

Bigley, W. S., A. R. Roth, and G. W. Eddy. 1960. Laboratory and field tests against mites and lice attacking poultry. J. Econ. Entomol. 53:12–14.

Bishopp, F. C., and H. P. Wood. 1931. Mites and lice on poultry. U.S. Dept. Agr. Farmers' Bull. 801. 19 pp.

Blackmore, D. K. 1963. Some observations on *Cnemidocoptes pilae,* together with its effect on the budgerigar *(Melopsittacus undulatus).* Vet. Record 75:592–95.

Blackmore, D. K., and D. G. Owen. 1968. Ectoparasites: The significance in British wild rodents. Symp. Zool. Soc. London No. 24:197–220.

Blount, W. P. 1947. Diseases of poultry. Baillière, Tindall, and Cox, London. 562 pp.

Böhm, L. K., and R. Supperer. 1955. Zwei neue Lungenmilben aus Menschenaffen, *Pneumonyssus oudemansi* und *Pneumonyssus vitzthumi* (Acarina: Halarachnidae). Österr. Zool. Zeitschr. 6:11–29.

Brody, A. L. 1936. The transmission of fowl-pox. Cornell Univ. Agr. Exp. Sta. Mem. 195. 37 pp.

Brumpt, E., and J. Callot. 1947. Rôle pathogène de l'acarien *Dermanyssus gallinae*. Compt. Rend. Soc. Biol. 141:1253–54.

Burch, G. R., and D. C. Brinkman. 1962. Systemic insecticide therapy. Small Animal Clinician 2:21–27.

Buxton, P. A. 1921. The external anatomy of the *Sarcoptes* of the horse. Parasitology 13:114–45.

Cameron, D. 1938. The northern fowl mite (*Liponyssus sylviarum* C. and F., 1877). Can. J. Res. 16:230–54.

Camin, J. H., and W. M. Rogoff. 1952. Mites affecting domesticated mammals. S. Dakota State Coll. Agr. Exp. Sta. Bull. 10. 12 pp.

Cánepa, E., and A. Da Graña. 1945. Investigaciones sobre demodeccia del perro. Rev. Med. Cien. Afines 7:801–13.

Carpenter, J. L. 1968. Sinusitis, pp. 151–53. *In* R. W. Kirk, ed. Current veterinary therapy III: Small animal practice. W. S. Saunders, Philadelphia.

Castellani, A. 1907. Note on an acarid-like parasite found in the omentum of a negro. Zentr. Bakteriol. Parasitenk. Abt. I. Orig. 43:372.

Chamberlain, R. W., and R. K. Sikes. 1955. Laboratory investigations on the role of bird mites in the transmission of Eastern and Western equine encephalitis. Am. J. Trop. Med. Hyg. 4:106–18.

Chamberlain, R. W., R. K. Sikes, and W. D. Sudia. 1957. Attempted laboratory infection of bird mites with the virus of St. Louis encephalitis. Am. J. Trop. Med. Hyg. 6:1047–53.

Chandler, W. L., and D. S. Ruhe. 1940. *Pneumonyssus caninum* n. sp., a mite from the frontal sinus of the dog. J. Parasitol. 26: 59–70.

Clark, G. M., A. E. Lutz, and LaVerne Fadness. 1966. Observations on the ability of *Haemogamasus liponyssoides* Ewing and *Ornithonyssus bacoti* (Hirst) (Acarina, Gamasina) to retain Eastern equine encephalitis virus. Am. J. Trop. Med. Hyg. 15:107–12.

Clark, G. M., and C. E. Yunker. 1964. Control of fur mites on mice in entomological laboratories, pp. 235–36. Proc. First Intern. Congr. Acarol., Ft. Collins, Colo.

Cleland, J. W. 1953. A preliminary note on the control of *Cnemidocoptes mutans* Robin. New Zealand Entomologist 1:17–18.

Conroy, J. D. 1964. Acariasis, pp. 140–43. *In* E. J. Catcott, ed. Feline medicine and surgery. American Veterinary Publications, Santa Barbara, Calif.

———. 1968. Sarcoptic mange (sarcoptic scabies, sarcoptic acariasis), pp. 263–65. *In* R. W. Kirk, ed. Current veterinary therapy III: Small animal practice. W. B. Saunders, Philadelphia.

Cook, R. 1953. Murine mange: The control of *Myocoptes musculinus* and *Myobia musculi* infestations. Brit. Vet. J. 109:113–16.

———. 1956. Murine ear mange: The control of *Psorergates simplex* infestation. Brit. Vet. J. 112:22–25.

———. 1969. Common diseases of laboratory animals, pp. 160–215. *In* D. J. Short and D. P. Woodnott, eds. The I.A.T. manual of laboratory animal practice and techniques. 2d ed. Charles C Thomas, Springfield, Ill.

Cosgrove, G. E., B. Nelson, and N. Gengozian. 1968. Helminth parasites of the tamarin, *Saguinus fuscicollis*. Lab. Animal Care 18:654–56.

Davies, J. H. T. 1941. Cat itch: *Cheyletiella* and *Notoedres* compared. Brit. J. Dermatol. Syphilis 53:18–24.

Davis, R. 1957. Control of the myocoptic mange mite, *Myocoptes musculinus* (Koch), on laboratory mice. J. Econ. Entomol. 50: 695.

Deoras, P. J., and K. K. Patel. 1960. Collection of ectoparasites of laboratory animals. Indian J. Entomol. 22:7–14.

DeOreo, G. A. 1958. Pigeons acting as vector in acariasis caused by *Dermanyssus gallinae* (De Geer, 1778). Arch. Dermatol. 77:422–29.

Dunn, F. L. 1968. The parasites of *Saimiri*, pp. 31–68. *In* L. A. Rosenblum and R. W. Cooper, eds. The squirrel monkey. Academic Press, New York.

Eddie, B., K. F. Meyer, F. L. Lambrecht, and D. P. Furman. 1962. Isolation of *Ornithosis bedsoniae* from mites collected in turkey quarters and from chicken lice. J. Infect. Diseases 110:231–37.

El-Gindy, H. 1952. The presence of *Demodex canis* in lymphatic glands of dogs. J. Am. Vet. Med. Assoc. 121:181–82.

English, P. B. 1960. Notoedric mange in cats, with observations on treatment with malathion. Austral. Vet. J. 36:85–88.

Enigk, K. 1949. Zur Kenntnis der Demodexräude des Hundes. Zentr. Bakteriol. Parasitenk. 153:76–90.

Enigk, K., and I. Grittner. 1951. Die Sarcoptesräude des Goldhamsters. Z. Parasitenk. 15:25–33.

Evans, G. O., J. G. Sheals, and D. MacFarlane. 1961. The terrestrial Acari of the British Isles: An introduction to their morphology, biology and classification: Vol. I. Introduction and biology. British Museum (Nat. Hist.), London. 219 pp.

Ewing, H. E. 1929. Notes on the lung mites of primates (Acarina: Dermanyssidae), including the description of a new species. Proc. Entomol. Soc. Wash. D.C. 31:126–30.

———. 1938. North American mites of the subfamily Myobiinae, new subfamily (Arachnida). Proc. Entomol. Soc. Wash. D.C. 40:180–97.

———. 1942. A second introduced rat mite becomes annoying to man. Proc. Helminthol. Soc. Wash. D.C. 9:74–75.

Ewing, S. A., J. E. Mosier, and Teralene S. Foxx. 1967. Occurrence of *Cheyletiella* spp. on dogs with skin lesions. J. Am. Vet. Med. Assoc. 151:64–67.

Fain, A. 1955. Deux nouveaux acariens de la famille Halarachnidae Oudemans, parasites des fosses nasales des singes au Congo Belge et au Ruanda-Urandi. Rev. Zool. Bot. Afr. 51:307–24.

———. 1959. Les acariens du genre *Pneumonyssus* Banks, parasites endopulmonaires des singes au Congo Belge (Halarchnidae: Mesostigmata). Ann. Parasitol. Humaine Comparee 34:126–48.

———. 1960. Révision du genre Cytodites (Megnin) et description de deux espèces et un genre nouveaux dans la famille Cytoditidae Oudemans (Acarina: Sarcoptiformes). Acarologia 2:238–49.

———. 1961. Sur le statut de deux espèces d'acariens du genre *Pneumonyssus* Banks déscrites par H. Vitzthum. Désignation d'un neotype pour *Pneumonyssus simicola* Banks, 1901 (Mesostigmata: Halarachnidae). Z. Parasitenk. 21:141–50.

———. 1962. *Pangorillages pani* g. n., sp. n. Acarien psorique du Chimpanzé (Psoralgidae: Sarcoptiformes). Rev. Zool. Bot. Afr. 66:283–90.

———. 1963. Les acariens producteurs de gale chez les lemuriens et les singes avec une étude des Psoroptidae (Sarcoptiformes). Bull. Inst. Roy. Sci. Nat. Belg. 39:1–125.

———. 1964a. Le développement postembryonnaire chez les Acaridiae parasites cutanés des mammifères et des oiseaux (Acarina: Sarcoptiformes). Bull. Sci. Acad. Roy. Belg. (5) 50:19–34.

———. 1964b. Les Lemurnyssidae parasites nasicoles des Lorisidae africains et des Cebidae sud-américains. Description d'une espèce nouvelle (Acarina: Sarcoptiformes). Ann. Soc. Belg. Med. Trop. 44:453–58.

———. 1965a. Notes sur le genre *Notoedres* Railliet, 1893 (Sarcoptidae: Sarcoptiformes). Acarologia 7:321–42.

———. 1965b. Nouveaux genres et espèces d'Acariens Sarcoptiformes parasites (Note préliminaire). Rev. Zool. Bot. Afr. 72:252–56.

———. 1965c. A review of the family Epidermoptidae Trouessart parasitic on the skin of birds (Acarina: Sarcoptiformes). 2 Parts. Koninklijke Vlaamse Academie voor Wetenschappen, Letteren en Schone Kunsten van België, Brussels.

———. 1965d. A review of the family Rhyncoptidae Lawrence parasitic on porcupines and monkeys (Acarina: Sarcoptiformes), pp. 135–59. *In* J. A. Naegele, ed. Advances in acarology. Vol. II. Cornell Univ. Press, Ithaca, N.Y.

———. 1966. Les acariens producteurs de gale chez les lémuriens et les singes: II. Nouvelles observations avec description d'une espèce nouvelle. Acarologia 8:94–114.

———. 1967. Diagnoses d'Acariens Sarcoptiformes nouveaux. Rev. Zool. Bot. Afr. 65:378–82.

———. 1968a. Étude de la variabilite de *Sarcoptes scabiei* avec une revision des Sarcoptidae. Acta Zool. Pathol. Antverpiensia 47:3–196.

———. 1968b. Notes sur trois acariens remarquables (Sarcoptiformes). Acarologia 10:276–91.

Fain, A., and J. Bafort. 1964. Les acariens de la famille Cytoditidae (Sarcoptiformes) description de sept espèces nouvelles. Acarologia 6:504–28.

Fain, A., and P. Elsen. 1967. Les acariens de la famille Knemidokoptidae producteurs de gale chez les oiseaux (Sarcoptiformes). Acta Zool. Pathol. Antverpiensia 45:3–142.

Fain, A., F. Lukoschus, and P. Hallmann. 1966. Le genre *Psorergates* chez les muridés description de trois espèces nouvelles (Psorergatidae: Trombidiformes). Acarologia 8:251–74.

Fain, A., G. Mignolet, and Y. Bereznay. 1958. L'acariase des voies respiratoires chez les singes du Zoo d'Anvers. Bull. Soc. Roy. Zool. Anvers 9:15–19.

Fain, A., A. J. Munting, and F. Lukoschus. 1970. Les Myocoptidae parasites des rongeurs en Hollande et en Belgique. Acta Zool. Pathol. Antverpiensia 50:67–172.

Fairbrother, R. W., and E. W. Hurst. 1932. Spontaneous diseases observed in 600 monkeys. J. Pathol. Bacteriol. 35:867–73.

Favati, V., and I. Galliano. 1962. Infestione da *Cheyletiella parasitivorax* (Megnin, 1878) nel cane. Parassitologia 4:69–73.

Fiennes, R. 1967. Zoonoses of primates. The epidemiology and ecology of simian diseases in relation to man. Weidenfeld and Nicolson, London. 190 pp.

Finegold, M. J., M. E. Seaquist, and M. J. Doherty. 1968. Treatment of pulmonary acariasis in rhesus monkeys with an organic phosphate. Lab. Animal Care 18:127–30.

Flatt, R. E., and W. T. Kerber. 1968. Demodectic mite infestation in golden hamsters. Lab. Animal Digest 4:6–7.

Flatt, R. E., and N. M. Patton. 1969. A mite infestation in squirrel monkeys *(Saimiri sciureus)*. J. Am. Vet. Med. Assoc. 155: 1233–35.

Flynn, R. J. 1955. Ectoparasites in mice. Proc. Animal Care Panel 6:75–91.

———. 1959a. Follicular acariasis of mice caused by *Psorergates simplex* successfully treated with Aramite. Am. J. Vet. Res. 20: 198–200.

———. 1959b. Demodectic and sarcoptic mange of dogs successfully treated with Aramite. J. Am. Vet. Med. Assoc. 134:177–79.

———. 1960. *Notoedres muris* infestation of rats. Proc. Animal Care Panel 10:69–70.

———. 1963. The diagnosis of some forms of ectoparasitism of mice. Proc. Animal Care Panel 13:111–25.

Flynn, R. J., Patricia C. Brennan, and T. E. Fritz. 1965. Pathogen status of commercially produced laboratory mice. Lab. Animal Care 15: 440–47.

Flynn, R. J., and B. N. Jaroslow. 1956. Nidification of a mite *(Psorergates simplex* Tyrrell 1883: Myobiidae) in the skin of mice. J. Parasitol. 42:49–52.

Fonseca, F. O. R. da. 1933. Notas de acareologia II: *Ichoronyssus butantanensis* sp. n. (Acarina, Dermanyssidae). Mem. Inst. Butantan. 7:135–38.

Foster, H. L. 1963. Specific pathogen-free animals, pp. 109–38. *In* W. Lane-Petter, ed. Animals for research: Principles of breeding and management. Academic Press, New York.

Foulk, J. D., and J. G. Matthysse. 1963. Experiments on control of the northern fowl mite. J. Econ. Entomol. 56:321–26.

Foxx, Teralene S., and S. A. Ewing. 1969. Morphologic features, behavior, and life history of *Cheyletiella yasguri*. Am. J. Vet. Res. 30:269–85.

Fremming, B. D., M. D. Harris, Jr., R. J. Young, and R. E. Benson. 1957. Preliminary investigation into the life cycle of the monkey lung mite *(Pneumonyssus foxi)*. Am. J. Vet. Res. 18:427–28.

French, F. E. 1964. *Demodex canis* in canine tissues. Cornell Vet. 54:271–90.

French, F. E., E. S. Raun, and D. L. Baker. 1964. Transmission of *Demodex canis* Leydig to pups. Iowa State J. Sci. 38:291–98.

Frost, R. C., and W. P. Beresford-Jones. 1960. Otodectic mange in the dog. Vet. Record 72:375.

Fuerstenberg, M. H. F. 1861. Die Krätzmilben der Menschen und Tiere. Wilhelm Engelmann, Leipzig. 240 pp.

Fukui, M., S. Matsuzaki, H. Tanaka, T. Nomura, H. Tozawa, and Y. Takagaki. 1961. Studies on the acaric dermatitis of albino mice in Japan (in Japanese). Bull. Exp. Animals 10:83–90.

Fuller, H. S. 1954. Studies of rickettsialpox: III. Life cycle of the mite vector, *Allodermanyssus sanguineus*. Am. J. Hyg. 59: 236–39.

Fulton, J. D. 1943. The treatment of *Notoedres* infections in golden hamsters *(Cricetus auratus)* with dimethyl diphenylene disulphide (Mitigal) and tetraethylthiuram monosulphide. Vet. Record 55:219.

Furman, D. P. 1954. A revision of the genus *Pneumonyssus* (Acarina: Halarachnidae). J. Parasitol. 40:31–42.

———. 1959. Feeding habits of symbiotic mesostigmatid mites of mammals in relation to pathogen-vector potentials. Am. J. Trop. Med. Hyg. 8:5–12.

Galton, M. 1963. Myobic mange in the mouse leading to skin ulceration and amyloidosis. Am. J. Pathol. 43:855–65.

Gambles, M. R. 1952. *Myocoptes musculinus* (Koch) and *Myobia musculi* (Schranck), two species of mite commonly parasitising the laboratory mouse. Brit. Vet. J. 108:194–203.

Gay, D. M., and A. Branch. 1927. Pulmonary acariasis in monkeys. Am. J. Trop. Med. 7:49–55.

Giorgi, W. 1968. Doencas observadas em coelhos durante o quinquênio 1963–1967, no Estado de São Paulo. O Biológico 34:71–82.

Goldman, L., and M. D. Feldman. 1949. Human infestation with scabies of monkeys. Arch. Dermatol. Syphilol. 59:175–78.

Gordon, R. M., K. Unsworth, and D. R. Seaton. 1943. The development and transmission of scabies as studied in rodent infections. Ann. Trop. Med. Parasitol. 37: 174–94.

Gowing, G. M. 1964. Advanced demodectic dermatitis in 4-day-old dachshund puppies. Mod. Vet. Pract. 45:70.

Grant, C. D. 1942. Observations on *Myobia musculi* (Schrank) (Arachnida: Acarina: Cheyletidae). Microentomology 7:64–76.

Gregor, W. W. 1965. The incidence of skin disease in small animal practice, pp. 33–69. *In* A. J. Rook and G. S. Walton, eds. Comparative physiology and pathology of the skin. F. A. Davis, Philadelphia.

Greve, J. H., and S. M. Gaafar. 1966. Natural

transmission of *Demodex canis* in dogs. J. Am. Vet. Med. Assoc. 148:1043–45.

Griesemer, R. A., and J. P. Gibson. 1963. The gnotobiotic dog. Lab. Animal Care 13: 643–49.

Griffiths, R. B., and F. J. O'Rourke. 1950. Observations on the lesions caused by *Cnemidocoptes mutans* and their treatment, with special reference to the use of "Gammexane." Ann. Trop. Med. Parasitol. 44:93–100.

Grinker, J. A., D. A. Karlin, and P. Manalo Estrella. 1962. Lung mites: Pulmonary acariasis in the primate. Aerospace Med. 33:841–45.

Grono, L. R. 1969. Studies of the ear mite, *Otodectes cynotis*. Vet. Record 85:6–8.

Guilhon, J. 1946a. Un nouvel acarien parasite du rat blanc. Compt. Rend. Acad. Sci. 223:108–9.

———. 1946b. Une nouvelle affection cutanée du rat. Bull. Acad. Vet. France 19:285–96.

Haakh, U. 1958. Ektoparasitenfreie Laboratoriumsmäuse; die *Myobia*-Räude der weissen Mäuse und ihre Bekämpfung. Z. Tropenmed. Parasitol. 9:75–87.

Habermann, R. T., and F. P. Williams. 1957. Diseases seen at necropsy of 708 *Macaca mulatta* (rhesus monkey) and *Macaca philippinensis* (cynomolgus monkey). Am. J. Vet. Res. 18:419–26.

Hagen, K. W., Jr., and E. E. Lund. 1962. Common diseases of domestic rabbits. U.S. Dept. Agr. Publ. 45-53. 8 pp.

Hamerton, A. E. 1939. Pulmonary acariasis in monkeys. Fourth Congr. Intern. Pathol. Comp., Rome 2:271–73.

Hammon, W. McD., W. C. Reeves, R. Cunha, C. Espana, and G. Sather. 1948. Isolation from wild bird mites *(Liponyssus sylviarum)* of a virus or mixture of viruses from which St. Louis and Western equine encephalitis viruses have been obtained. Science 107:92–93.

Harris, J. M., and J. J. Stockton. 1960. Eradication of the tropical rat mite *Ornithonyssus bacoti* (Hirst, 1913) from a colony of mice. Am. J. Vet. Res. 21:316–18.

Harrison, I. R., and M. M. Daykin. 1965. The biology and control of ectoparasites of laboratory animals with special reference to poultry parasites. J. Inst. Animal Tech. 16: 69–73.

Heine, W. 1962. Zur Ektoparasitenbekämpfung bei Maus und Ratte. Z. Versuchstierk. 2:1–22.

Helwig, F. C. 1925. Arachnid infection in monkeys. Am. J. Pathol. 1:389–95.

Heston, W. E., and Margaret K. Deringer. 1948.

Hereditary renal disease and amyloidosis in mice. Arch. Pathol. 46:49–58.

Hill, M. A., and R. M. Gordon. 1945. An outbreak of dermatitis amongst troops in North Wales caused by rodent mites. Ann. Trop. Med. Parasitol. 39:46–52.

Hindle, E. 1947. The golden hamster *(Mesocricetus auratus)*, pp. 196–202. *In* A. N. Worden, ed. The care and management of laboratory animals. Williams and Wilkins, Baltimore.

Hirst, S. 1916. On the occurrence of the tropical fowl mite *(Liponyssus bursa,* Berlese) in Australia, and a new instance of its attacking man. Ann. Mag. Nat. Hist. Ser. 8, 18:243–44.

———. 1917a. On three new parasitic acari. Ann. Mag. Nat. Hist. Ser. 8, 20:431–34.

———. 1917b. Remarks on certain species of the genus *Demodex* Owen (the *Demodex* of man, the horse, dog, rat, and mouse). Ann. Mag. Nat. Hist. Ser. 8, 20:232–35.

———. 1922. Mites injurious to domestic animals. Brit. Museum (Nat. Hist.) Econ. Ser. 13. 107 pp.

Hoey, R. 1968. Cutaneous allergy, pp. 296–301. *In* R. W. Kirk, ed. Current veterinary therapy III: Small animal practice. W. B. Saunders, Philadelphia.

Hofstad, M. S. 1949. Recovery of Newcastle disease (pneumoencephalitis) virus from mites, *Liponyssus sylviarum,* after feeding upon Newcastle-infected chickens. Am. J. Vet. Res. 10:370–71.

Holz, J. 1955. Untersuchungen über die Möglichkeit der Übertragung von milben *(Psoroptes* und *Notoedres)* und Läusen *(Polyplax spinulosa)* durch *Musca domestica.* Tieraerztl. Umschau 10:248–49.

Holzworth, Jean. 1968. Notoedric mange of cats (head mange), pp. 265–66. *In* R. W. Kirk, ed. Current veterinary therapy III: Small animal practice. W. B. Saunders, Philadelphia.

Honjo, S., K. Muto, T. Fujiwara, Y. Suzuki, and K. Imaizumi. 1963. Statistical survey of internal parasites in cynomolgus monkeys *(Macaca irus)*. Japan. J. Med. Sci. Biol. 16:217–24.

Hopla, C. E. 1951. Experimental transmission of tularemia by the tropical rat mite. Am. J. Trop. Med. 31:768–82.

Howitt, B. F., H. R. Dodge, L. K. Bishop, and R. H. Gorrie. 1948. Virus of Eastern equine encephalomyelitis isolated from chicken mites *(Dermanyssus gallinae)* and chicken lice *(Eomenocanthus stramineus)*. Proc. Soc. Exp. Biol. Med. 68:622–25.

Huebner, R. J., W. L. Jellison, and C. Pomerantz. 1946. Rickettsialpox—a newly recognized rickettsial disease: IV. Isolation of a rickettsia apparently identical with the causative agent of rickettsialpox from *Allodermanyssus sanguineus,* a rodent mite. Public Health Rept. (U.S.) 61:1677–82.

Hughes, T. E. 1959. Mites, or the Acari. Athlone Press, London. 225 pp.

Hull, W. B. 1956. The nymphal stages of *Pneumonyssus simicola* Banks, 1901 (Acarina: Halarachnidae). J. Parasitol. 42:653–56.

Humphreys, M. 1958. *Cheyletiella parasitivorax* infestation of the dog. Vet. Record 70:442.

Hwang, J. C. 1959. Case reports of the quill mite, *Syringophilus bipectinatus,* in poultry. Proc. Helminthol. Soc. Wash. D.C. 26:47–50.

Innes, J. R. M. 1965. Personal communication, p. 33. *In* R. Fiennes. 1967. Zoonoses of primates: The epidemiology and ecology of simian diseases in relation to man. Weidenfeld and Nicolson, London.

——. 1969. "Discussion," p. 36. *In* W. I. B. Beveridge, ed. Using primates in medical research: Part I. Husbandry and technology. *In* E. I. Goldsmith and J. Moor-Jankowski, eds. Primates in medicine. Vol. 2. S. Karger, New York.

Innes, J. R. M., M. W. Colton, P. P. Yevich, and C. L. Smith. 1954. Pulmonary acariasis as an enzootic disease caused by *Pneumonyssus simicola* in imported monkeys. Am. J. Pathol. 30:813–35.

Johnson, R. M., A. C. Andersen, and W. Gee. 1963. Parasitism in an established dog kennel. Lab. Animal Care 13:731–36.

Jones, O. G. 1956. Common diseases of cage birds and other less usual pets. Vet. Record 68:918–32.

Keefe, T. J., J. E. Scanlon, and L. D. Wetherald. 1964. *Ornithonyssus bacoti* (Hirst) infestation in mouse and hamster colonies. Lab. Animal Care 14:366–69.

Kirk, H. 1950. Phenamidine in demodectic mange in dogs. J. Am. Vet. Med. Assoc. 116:300.

Kirkwood, A. C. 1967. Anaemia in poultry infested with the red mite *Dermanyssus gallinae.* Vet. Record 80:514.

Knapp, F. W., and G. F. Krause. 1960. Control of the northern fowl mite, *Ornithonyssus sylviarum* (C. and F.), with Ronnel, Bayer L13/59 and Bayer 21/199. J. Econ. Entomol. 53:4–5.

Knezevich, A. L., and W. P. McNulty, Jr. 1970. Pulmonary acariasis *(Pneumonyssus simicola)* in colony-bred *Macaca mulatta.* Lab. Animal Care 20:693–96.

Koutz, F. R. 1953. *Demodex folliculorum* studies: II. Comparison of various diagnostic methods. Speculum (Ohio State Univ.) 6:8–9, 23, 26, 44.

——. 1954. *Demodex folliculorum* studies: III. A survey of clinical cases in dogs. J. Am. Vet. Med. Assoc. 124:131–33.

——. 1955. *Demodex folliculorum* studies: IV. Treatment methods. North Am. Vet. 36:129–31, 136.

——. 1957. *Demodex folliculorum* studies: VI. The internal phase of canine demodectic mange. J. Am. Vet. Med. Assoc. 131:45–48.

——. 1966. Demodectic mange, pp. 156–58. *In* R. W. Kirk, ed. Current veterinary therapy 1966–1967: Small animal practice. W. B. Saunders, Philadelphia.

Koutz, F. R., D. M. Chamberlain, and C. R. Cole. 1953. *Pneumonyssus caninum* in the nasal cavity and paranasal sinuses. J. Am. Vet. Med. Assoc. 122:106–9.

Koutz, F. R., H. F. Groves, and Carolyn M. Gee. 1960. A survey of *Demodex canis* in the skin of clinically normal dogs. Vet. Med. 55:52–53.

Kraemer, P. 1959. Relative efficacy of several materials for control of poultry ectoparasites. J. Econ. Entomol. 52:1195–99.

Kraemer, P., and D. P. Furman. 1959. Systemic activity of Sevin in control of *Ornithonyssus sylviarum* (C. and F.). J. Econ. Entomol. 52:170–71.

Král, F., and R. M. Schwartzman. 1964. Veterinary and comparative dermatology. J. B. Lippincott, Philadelphia. 44 pp.

Krantz, G. W. 1970. A manual of acarology. Oregon State University Book Stores, Corvallis, Ore. 335 pp.

Kutzer, E. 1964. Knemidocoptes-Räude bei Ziervögeln. Wien. Tieraerztl. Monatsschr. 51:36–43.

Landois, F., and H. Hoepke. 1914. Eine endoparasitäre Milbe in der Lunge von *Macacus rhesus.* Zentr. Bakteriol. Parasitenk. Abt. I. Orig. 73:384–95.

Lavoipierre, M. M. J. 1955. A description of a new genus of sarcoptiform mites and of three new species of Acarina parasitic on primates in the British Cameroons. Ann. Trop. Med. Parasitol. 49:299–307.

——. 1964. A new family of Acarines belonging to the suborder Sarcoptiformes parasitic in the hair follicles of primates. Ann. Natal Museum 16:191–208.

Lavoipierre, M. M. J., and W. Crewe. 1955. Miscellanea: The occurrence of a mange-mite, *Psorergates* sp. (Acarina), in a West African monkey. Ann. Trop. Med. Parasitol. 49:351.

Lee, R. E., R. B. Williams, Jr., W. B. Hull,

and S. N. Stein. 1954. Significance of pulmonary acariasis in rhesus monkeys *(Macaca mulatta).* Federation Proc. 13:85–86.

Leerhoy, J., and H. S. Jensen. 1967. Sarcoptic mange in a shipment of cynomolgus monkeys. Nord. Veterinarmed. 19:128–30.

Lindquist, W. D., and R. C. Belding. 1949. A report on the subcutaneous or flesh mite of chickens. Mich. State Coll. Vet. 10:20–21.

Lindt, S., and E. Kutzer. 1965. Luftsackmilben *(Cytodites nudus)* als Ursache einer granulomatösen Pneumonie beim Huhn. Pathol. Vet. 2:264–76.

Link, R. P. 1965. Uses of insecticides on domestic animals, pp. 727–39. *In* L. M. Jones, ed. Veterinary pharmacology and therapeutics. Iowa State Univ. Press, Ames.

Linkfield, R. L., and W. M. Reid. 1958. Newer acaricides and insecticides in the control of ectoparasites of poultry. J. Econ. Entomol. 51:188–90.

Lodha, K. R. 1969. The occurrence of tropical fowl mite, *Ornithonyssus (Bdellonyssus, Liponyssus) bursa* on man in Rajasthan (India). Vet. Record 84:363–65.

Loomis, E. G., E. L. Bramhall, J. A. Allen, R. A. Ernest, and L. L. Dunning. 1970. Effects of the northern fowl mite on white leghorn chickens. J. Econ. Entomol. 63: 1885–89.

Lucker, J. T., and M. P. Sause. 1952. The occurrence of demodectic mites, *Demodex folliculorum,* in the internal tissues and organs of the dog. North Am. Vet. 33:787–96.

Lund, E. E. 1951. Ear mange in domestic rabbits. Small Stock Mag. 35:18–19.

Macfie, J. W. S., and J. G. Thomson. 1929. A trypanosome of the canary *(Serinus canarius* Koch). Trans. Roy. Soc. Trop. Med. Hyg. 23:5–6.

Manwell, R. D., and C. M. Johnson. 1931. A natural trypanosome of the canary. Am. J. Hyg. 14:231–34.

Marine, D. 1924. The cure and prevention of ear canker in rabbits. Science 60:158.

Masse, R., M. Geneste, and G. Thiery. 1965. Acariose pulmonaire du singe traitement, prophylaxie. Rec. Méd. Vét. Ecole Alfort 141:1227–34.

Mellanby, K. 1943. Scabies. Oxford Univ. Press, London. 81 pp.

Mettler, Norma E. 1969. Isolation of a microtatobiote from patients with hemolytic-uremic syndrome and thrombotic thrombocytopenic purpura and from mites in the United States. New Eng. J. Med. 281: 1023–27.

Miller, W. W. 1908. *Hepatozoon perniciosum*

(n. g., n. sp.); a haemogregarine pathogenic for white rats; with a description of the sexual cycle in the intermediate host, a mite *(Lelaps echidninus).* U.S. Treasury Dept. Marine Hosp. Serv. Bull. 46. 51 pp.

Morlan, H. B. 1947. Dusts containing combinations of DDT, sulfur, and hydroxy pentamethyl flavan to control rat ectoparasites. J. Econ. Entomol. 40:917–18.

Morris, M. L. 1963. Breeding, housing and management of cats. Cornell Vet. 53:107–31.

Moxham, J. W., T. T. Goldfinch, and A. C. G. Heath. 1968. *Cheyletiella parasitivorax* infestation of cats associated with skin lesions of man. New Zealand Vet. J. 16:50–52.

Myers, Betty J., and R. E. Kuntz. 1965. A checklist of parasites reported for the baboon. Primates 6:137–94.

Mykytowycz, R. 1957. Short contributions: Parasitic habit of the rabbit mite, *Cheyletiella parasitivorax* (Megnin). C.S.I.R.O. Wildlife Res. 2:164.

———. 1958. Contact transmission of infectious myxomatosis of the rabbit *Oryctolagus cuniculus* (L). C.S.I.R.O. Wildlife Res. 3:1–6.

Nevin, F. R. 1935. Anatomy of *Cnemidocoptes mutans* (R. and L.), the scaly-leg mite of poultry. Ann. Entomol. Soc. Am. 28:338–67.

Nichols, E., M. E. Rindge, and G. G. Russell. 1953. The relationship of the habits of the house mouse and the mouse mite *(Allodermanyssus sanguineus)* to the spread of rickettsialpox. Ann. Internal Med. 39:92–102.

Nutting, W. B. 1961. *Demodex aurati* sp. nov., and *D. criceti,* ectoparasites of the golden hamster *(Mesocricetus auratus).* Parasitology 51:515–22.

———. 1965. Host-parasite relations: Demodicidae. Acarologia 7:301–17.

Nutting, W. B., and H. Rauch. 1958. *Demodex criceti* n. sp. (Acarina: Demodicidae) with notes on its biology. J. Parasitol. 44:328–33.

———. 1963. Distribution of *Demodex aurati* in the host *(Mesocricetus auratus)* skin complex. J. Parasitol. 49:323–29.

Olsen, S. J., and H. Roth. 1947. On the mite *Cheyletiella parasitivorax,* occurring on cats, as a facultative parasite of man. J. Parasitol. 33:444–45.

Olson, T. A., and R. G. Dahms. 1946. Observations on the tropical rat mite, *Liponyssus bacoti,* as an ecto-parasite of laboratory animals and suggestions for its control. J. Parasitol. 32:56–60.

Osborne, H. G. 1947. Dimethyl phthalate for the treatment of mange in rabbits caused by *Notoedres cati* var. *cuniculi* (Gerlach, 1857). Can. J. Comp. Med. 11:144–45.

Oudemans, A. C. 1935. Kritische Literatur-übersicht zur Gattung *Pneumonyssus*. Beschreibung dreier Arten, darunter einer Neuen. Z. Parasitenk. 7: 466–512.

Owen, B. L. 1956. Life history of the spiny rat mite under artificial conditions. J. Econ. Entomol. 49:702–3.

Owen, Dawn. 1968. Investigation: B. Parasitological studies. Lab. Animals Centre News Letter 35:7–9.

Page, K. W. 1952. The ectoparasites of laboratory and domestic animals. J. Animal Tech. Assoc. 3:34–36.

Parodi, A. S., H. R. Rugiero, D. J. Greenway, N. Mettler, A. Martinez, M. Boxaca, and J. M. de la Barrera. 1959. Aislamiento del virus Junin (F.H.E.) de los acaros de la zona epidemica *(Echinolaelaps echidninus,* Berlese). Prensa Med. Arg. 46:2242–44.

Patnaik, M. M. 1965. On the validity of *Indochirus utkalensis* (Listrophoridae: Acarina). J. Parasitol. 51:301–2.

Phillipe, J. 1948. Note sur les gales du singe. Bull. Soc. Pathol. Exotique 41:597–600.

Piryanik, G. I., and I. A. Akimov. 1964. Gamasid mites of birds and their nests in the Ukrainian SSR (in Russian). Zool. Zh. 43: 671–79.

Poole, C. M., W. G. Keenan, D. V. Tolle, T. E. Fritz, Patricia C. Brennan, R. C. Simkins, and R. J. Flynn. 1967. Disease status of commercially produced rabbits, pp. 219–20. *In* Biological and Medical Research Division Annual Report 1967. ANL-7409. Argonne National Laboratory, Argonne, Ill.

Rebrassier, R. E., and E. D. Martin. 1932. *Syringophilus bi-pectinatus* a quill mite of poultry. Science 76:128.

Reed, C. M. 1961. *Cheyletiella parasitovorax (sic)* infestation of pups. J. Am. Vet. Med. Assoc. 138:306–7.

Reeves, W. C., W. McD. Hammon, W. H. Doetschman, H. E. McClure, and G. Sather. 1955. Studies on mites as vectors of Western equine and St. Louis encephalitis viruses in California. Am. J. Trop. Med. Hyg. 4:90–105.

Reeves, W. C., W. McD. Hammon, D. P. Furman, H. E. McClure, and B. Brookman. 1947. Recovery of Western equine encephalomyelitis virus from wild bird mites *(Liponyssus sylviarum)* in Kern County, California. Science 105:411–12.

Rewell, R. E. 1948. Diseases of tropical origin in captive wild animals. Trans. Roy. Soc. Trop. Med. Hyg. 42:17–25.

Reynolds, S. L., and J. H. Gainer. 1968. Dermatitis of Mongolian gerbils *(Meriones unguiculatus)* caused by *Demodex* sp. Abstr. 150. 19th Ann. Meeting American Association for Laboratory Animal Science, Las Vegas.

Roberts, S. R., and T. J. Thompson. 1969. *Pneumonyssus caninum* and orbital cellulitis in the dog. J. Am. Vet. Med. Assoc. 155:731–34.

Robertson, O. H., C. G. Loosli, T. T. Puck, H. Wise, H. M. Lemon, and W. Lester, Jr. 1947. Tests for the chronic toxicity of propylene glycol and triethylene glycol on monkeys and rats by vapor inhalation and oral administration. J. Pharmacol. Exp. Therap. 91:52–76.

Rodriguez, J. L., Jr., and L. A. Riehl. 1958. Malathion for control of chicken mites on hens in wire cages. J. Econ. Entomol. 51: 158–60.

Ruch, T. C. 1959. Diseases of laboratory primates. W. B. Saunders, Philadelphia. 600 pp.

Sasa, M., H. Tanaka, M. Fukui, and A. Takata. 1962. Internal parasites of laboratory animals, pp. 195–214. *In* R. J. C. Harris, ed. The problems of laboratory animal disease. Academic Press, New York.

Schwab, Marjorie, Rae Allen, and S. E. Sulkin. 1952. The tropical rat mite *(Liponyssus bacoti)* as an experimental vector of Coxsackie virus. Am. J. Trop. Med. Hyg. 1: 982–86.

Schwabe, O. 1956. A quill mite of poultry: A case report. J. Am. Vet. Med. Assoc. 129: 481–82.

Scott, H. G. 1958. Control of mites on hamsters. J. Econ. Entomol. 51: 412–13.

Seamer, J., and F. C. Chesterman. 1967. A survey of disease in laboratory animals. Lab. Animals 1:117–39.

Seddon, H. R. 1951. Diseases of domestic animals in Australia: Part 3. Tick and mite infestations. Div. Vet. Hyg. Dept. Public Health, Commonwealth Australia 7. 200 pp.

Sengbusch, H. G. 1960. Control of *Myocoptes musculinus* on guinea pigs. J. Econ. Entomol. 53:168.

Senter, H. G. 1958. *Pneumonyssus caninum:* A case report. Mod. Vet. Practice. May 15, pp. 55–56.

Sequeira, J. H., and R. M. Dowdeswell. 1942. "Cat-itch" from a pet lynx. E. African Med. J. 18:345–47.

Sergeyev, A. N. 1949. Mite invasion of lungs in *Macacus rhesus* (in Russian). Tr. Sukhumi Biol. Sta. Akad. Med. Nauk SSSR 1: 295–98.

Sheldon, W. G. 1966. Psorergatic mange in the

sooty mangabey *(Cercocebus torquates atys)* monkey. Lab. Animal Care 16:276–79.

Siegmund, O. H. 1967. The Merck veterinary manual: A handbook of diagnosis and therapy for the veterinarian. 3d ed. Merck and Co., Rahway, N.J. 1674 pp.

Sikes, R. K., and R. W. Chamberlain. 1954. Laboratory observations on three species of bird mites. J. Parasitol. 40:691–97.

Skaliy, P., and W. J. Hayes, Jr. 1949. The biology of *Liponyssus bacoti* (Hirst, 1913) (Acarina, Liponyssidae). Am. J. Trop. Med. 29:759–72.

Skidmore, L. V. 1934. Acariasis of the white rat *(Rattus norvegicus* form *albinus).* Can. Entomologist 66:110–15.

Smiley, R. L. 1965. Two new species of the genus *Cheyletiella* (Acarina: Cheyletidae). Proc. Entomol. Soc. Wash. D.C. 67:75–79.

Smith, E. B., and T. F. Claypoole. 1967. Canine scabies in dogs and humans. J. Am. Med. Assoc. 199:95–100.

Smith, Margaret G., R, J. Blattner, and Florence M. Heys. 1944. The isolation of the St. Louis encephalitis virus from chicken mites *(Dermanyssus gallinae)* in nature. Science 100:362–63.

Smith, W. W. 1955a. The abundance and distribution of the ectoparasites of the house mouse in Mississippi. J. Parasitol. 41:58–62.

———. 1955b. Relation of certain environmental factors to the abundance and distribution of house mouse ectoparasites in Mississippi. Trans. Am. Microscop. Soc. 74:170–75.

Staggs, T. W. 1961. *Otodectes cynotis* in the cat. Southeastern Vet. 12: 152–55.

Stone, W. B., and J. A. Hughes. 1969. Massive pulmonary acariasis in the pig-tailed macaque. Bull. Wildlife Dis. Assoc. 5:20–22.

Stoner, R. D., and W. M. Hale. 1953. A method for eradication of the mite, *Myocoptes musculinus,* from laboratory mice. J. Econ. Entomol. 46:692–93.

Strandtmann, R. W. 1949. The blood-sucking mites of the genus *Haemolaelaps* (Acarina: Laelaptidae) in the United States. J. Parasitol. 35:325–52.

Strandtmann, R. W., and C. J. Mitchell. 1963. The laelaptine mites of the *Echinolaelaps* complex from the Southwest Pacific area (Acarina: Mesostigmata). Pacific Insects 5:541–76.

Strandtmann, R. W., and G. W. Wharton. 1958. A manual of mesostigmatid mites parasitic on vertebrates. Contrib. No. 4 Inst. Acarology Univ. Maryland, College Park. 330 pp.

Strasser, H. 1963. Kaninchenräude durch Be-

fall mit der Raubmilbe *Cheyletiella parasitivorax.* Kleintier Praxis 8:212–14.

Streeter, W. R. 1945. Parasitic otorrhea. Vet. Med. 40:412–13.

Sulkin, S. E. 1945. Recovery of equine encephalomyelitis virus (Western type) from chicken mites. Science 101:381–83.

Sulkin, S. E., C. L. Wisseman, Jr., E. M. Izumi, and Christine Zarafonetis. 1955. Mites as possible vectors or reservoirs of equine encephalomyelitis in Texas. Am. J. Trop. Med. Hyg. 4:119–35.

Sweatman, G. K. 1957. Life history, non-specificity, and revision of the genus *Chorioptes,* a parasitic mite of herbivores. Can. J. Zool. 35:641–89.

———. 1958a. On the life history and validity of the species in *Psoroptes,* a genus of mange mites. Can. J. Zool. 36:905–29.

———. 1958b. Biology of *Otodectes cynotis,* the ear canker mite of carnivores. Can. J. Zool. 36:849–62.

Tannenbaum, M. H. 1965. Canine scabies in man: A report of human mange. J. Am. Med. Assoc. 193:321–22.

Tarshis, I. B. 1962. The use of silica aerogel compounds for the control of ectoparasites. Proc. Animal Care Panel 12:217–58.

Taylor, E. L. 1945. Benzenehexachloride: A promising new acaricide. Vet. Record 57: 210–11.

Thomsett, L. R. 1963. Diseases transmitted to man by dogs and cats. Practitioner 191:630–40.

———. 1968. Mite infestations of man contracted from dogs and cats. Brit. Med. J. (July 13):93–95.

Till, W. M. 1960. *"Psorergates oettlei"* n. sp., a new mange-causing mite from the multimammate rat. Acarologia 2:75–79.

Tipton, V. J. 1960. The genus *Laelaps,* with a review of the Laelaptinae and a new subfamily Alphalaelaptinae (Acarina: Laelaptidae). Univ. Calif. (Berkeley) Publ. Entomol. 16:233–356.

Tonn, R. J. 1961. Studies on the ear mite *Otodectes cynotis,* including life cycle. Ann. Entomol. Soc. Am. 54:416–21.

Trimmier, B. R. 1966. Demodicosis in a cat. Southwestern Vet. (Fall, 1966): 57–58.

Tuffery, A. A. 1962. Mite eradication, pp. 158–61. *In* G. Porter and W. Lane-Petter, eds. Notes for breeders of common laboratory animals. Academic Press, New York.

Tuffery, A. A., and J. R. M. Innes. 1963. Diseases of laboratory mice and rats, pp. 46–108. *In* W. Lane-Petter, ed. Animals for research: Principles of breeding and management. Academic Press, New York.

Turk, R. D., and E. D. Besch. 1968. Parasitic

dermatoses, pp. 539–60. *In* E. J. Catcott, ed. Canine medicine. American Veterinary Publications, Santa Barbara, Calif.

U.S. Department of Agriculture. 1967. Suggested guide for the use of insecticides to control insects affecting crops, livestock, households, stored products, forests, and forest products. U.S. Dept. Agr., Agr. Handbook 331. 273 pp.

Unsworth, K. 1946. Studies on the clinical and parasitological aspects of canine demodectic mange. J. Comp. Pathol. Therap. 56:114–27.

Valerio, D. A., R. L. Miller, J. R. M. Innes, K. Diane Courtney, A. J. Pallotta, and R. M. Guttmacher. 1969. *Macaca mulatta:* Management of a laboratory breeding colony. Academic Press, New York. 140 pp.

Van Stee, E. W. 1964. Some observations on the clinical management of the chimpanzee. USAF School Aerospace Med. (AFSC) Brooks Air Force Base, Tex. Tech. Doc. Rept. SAM–TDR 64-45. 44 pp.

Vincent, L. E., D. L. Lindgren, and H. E. Krohne. 1954. Toxicity of malathion to the northern fowl mite. J. Econ. Entomol. 47:943–44.

Vitzthum, H. 1930. *Pneumonyssus stammeri,* ein neuer Lungenparasit. Z. Parasitenk. 2:595–615.

Wagner, J. E. 1969. Control of mouse ectoparasites with resin vaporizer strips containing Vapona. Lab. Animal Care 19:804–7.

Wantland, W. W. 1968. Parasitology, pp. 171–83. *In* R. A. Hoffman, P. F. Robinson, and Hulda Magalhaes, eds. The golden hamster: Its biology and use in medical research. Iowa State Univ. Press, Ames.

Watson, D. P. 1960. On the adult and immature stages of *Myocoptes musculinus* (Koch) with notes on its biology and classification. Acarologia 2:335–44.

———. 1961. The effect of the mite *Myocoptes musculinus* (C. L. Koch, 1840) on the skin of the white laboratory mouse and its control. Parasitology 51:373–78.

———. 1962. On the immature and adult stages of *Notoedres alepis* (Railliet and Lucet, 1893) and its effect on the skin of the rat. Acarologia 4:64–77.

Weidman, F. D. 1923. Certain dermatoses of monkeys and an ape. Pemphigus, scabies, sebaceous cyst, local subcutaneous edema, benign superficial blastomycotic dermatosis and tinea capitis and cercinata. Arch. Dermatol. Syphilol. 7:289–302.

———. 1935. Dermatoses of monkeys and apes. Ninth Intern. Congr. Dermatol. 1:600–606.

Weitkamp, R. A. 1964. *Cheyletiella parasiti-*

vorax parasitism in dogs. J. Am. Vet. Med. Assoc. 144:597–99.

Wharton, G. W., Jr. 1960. Host-parasite relationships between *Myobia musculi* (Schrank, 1781) and *Mus musculus* Linnaeus, 1758. Libro Hom. Caballero y Caballero Jubileo 1930–1960. Sec. Educ. Publ., Mexico, D.F.

Wharton, G. W., Jr., and H. F. Cross. 1957. Studies on the feeding habits of three species of laelaptid mites. J. Parasitol. 43:45–50.

Wharton, G. W., Jr., and H. S. Fuller. 1952. A manual of the chiggers: The biology, classification, distribution, and importance to man of the larvae of the family Trombiculidae (Acarina). Mem. Entomol. Soc. Wash. D.C. 185 pp.

Whiteley, H. J., and Daphne L. Horton. 1962. The effect of *Myobia musculi* on the epidermis and hair regrowth cycle in the ageing CBA mouse. J. Pathol. Bacteriol. 83:509–14.

Whitney, L. F. 1969. Vapona bars—a possible treatment for sarcoptic mange? Vet. Med. Small Animal Clin. 64:993.

Wichmann, R. W., and D. J. Vincent. 1958. Cnemidocoptic mange in the budgerigar (*Melopsittacus undulatus*). J. Am. Vet. Med. Assoc. 133:522–24.

Williams, R. W., and H. W. Brown. 1945. The development of *Litomosoides carinii* filariid parasite of the cotton rat in the tropical rat mite. Science 102:482–83.

Wisseman, C. L., Jr., and S. E. Sulkin. 1947. Observations on the laboratory care, life cycle, and hosts of the chicken mite, *Dermanyssus gallinae*. Am. J. Trop. Med. 27:463–69.

Wood, H. P. 1917. The chicken mite (*Dermanyssus gallinae* Redi): Its life history and habits. U.S. Dept. Agr. Tech. Bull. 553. 15 pp.

———. 1920. Tropical fowl mite in the United States, with notes on life history and control. U.S. Dept. Agr. Circ. 79. 8 pp.

Wood, J. C. 1968. Skin diseases of domestic animals. III. The parasitic aspect of skin diseases. Vet. Record 82:214–23.

Woodard, J. C. 1968. Acarous (*Pneumonyssus simicola*) arteritis in rhesus monkeys. J. Am. Vet. Med. Assoc. 153:905–9.

Woodnott, Dorothy P. 1963. Pests of the animal house, pp. 157–68. *In* D. J. Short and Dorothy P. Woodnott, eds. The A.T.A. manual of laboratory animal practice and techniques. Crosby Lockwood and Son, London.

Yasgur, I. 1968. Cheyletiella dermatitis, pp. 226–67. *In* R. W. Kirk, ed. Current veterinary therapy III: Small animal practice. W. B. Saunders, Philadelphia.

Yunker, C. E. 1964. Infections of laboratory animals potentially dangerous to man: Ectoparasites and other arthropods, with emphasis on mites. Lab. Animal Care 14: 455–65.

Yunker, C. E., and K. G. Ishak. 1957. Histopathological observations on the sequence of infection in knemidokoptic mange of budgerigars *(Melopsittacus undulatus).* J. Parasitol. 43:664–72.

Zemskaya, A. A., and A. A. Pchelkina. 1955. Experimental infection of the bird mite *Dermanyssus gallinae* Redi and the rat mite *Bdellonyssus bacoti* Hirst by the causative agent of Q fever (in Russian). Dokl. Akad. Nauk SSSR 101:391–92.

Zimmerman, E. C. 1944. A case of bovine auricular myiasis and some ectoparasites new to Hawaii. Proc. Hawaiian Entomol. Soc. 12:199–200.

Zuern, F. A. 1874. Räudemilben im Ohr der Hunde und bei Kaninchen. Wochschr. Tieraerztl. Viehzucht. 18:277–83.

Zumpt, F. 1966. The feather mite, *Megninia cubitalis* (Megnin), as a cause of "depluming-itch," pp. 1027–28. *In* A. Corradetti, ed. Proc. First Intern. Congr. Parasitol. Vol. II. Pergamon Press, New York.

Zumpt, F., and W. M. Till. 1954. The lung and nasal mites of the genus *Pneumonyssus* Banks (Acarina: Laelaptidae) with description of two new species from African primates. J. Entomol. Soc. S. Africa 17:195–212.

Chapter 16

PENTASTOMIDS

PENTASTOMIDS constitute a highly aberrant group of arthropods (Fain 1961; Heymons 1935). They have a wormlike and generally annulated appearance. The body is white, legless, and either cylindrical or flat.

These arthropods are typically heteroxenous parasites. In the most evolved species, the adults live in the respiratory tract of carnivorous animals, usually snakes, and the larvae develop in the tissues of various animals, usually mammals.

The intermediate host becomes infected by drinking water or eating food contaminated by fecal material or by mucus from the respiratory tract of an animal harboring adult pentastomids; the definitive host becomes infected by eating animals or viscera containing nymphs.

The development in the intermediate host generally takes several months. The developmental stages include a primary or migrating larva; a secondary or resting larva which molts several times; and a tertiary larva or nymph which encysts in the tissues of the host, generally in the peritoneal cavity. The tertiary larva usually remains encysted until ingested by the definitive host, but sometimes, for reasons not clearly understood, it escapes from its cystic envelope and migrates through the tissues of the intermediate host, causing acute peritonitis and possibly death (Chalmers 1899).

Natural infections have been reported in some endothermal species occasionally used in the laboratory. Experimental infections have also been produced. The pentastomids that may be encountered in endothermal laboratory species are listed in Table 16.1. The most important species are described below.

Linguatula serrata
(Tongue Worm)

Linguatula serrata, a relatively benign parasite, is found throughout the world, but its exact incidence is unknown. It is commonest in Europe, especially eastern Europe (Heymons 1942), and has been reported from the United States (Stiles 1895), South America (Gelormini and Roveda 1938), South Africa (Ortlepp 1934), Asia (Faust 1927; Heymons 1935), the Philippine Islands (Tubangui and Masiluñgan 1936), Australia (Pullar 1936), and New Zealand (Gurr 1953).

Adults occur in the nasal passages of the dog and other canids, and rarely in domestic farm species and man (Heymons 1942). The nymph sometimes occurs in the wild Norway rat, black rat, guinea pig, rabbit, cat, titi monkey, gelada baboon, and man (Bochefontaine 1876; Heymons 1942; Kuntz, Myers, and Vice 1967; Strong, Shattuck, and Wheeler 1926). It is common in domestic farm species. A report of canine nymphal linguatulosis in Japan

493

is of doubtful validity (Yamashita and Ohbayashi 1954). The nymph was probably *Armillifer moniliformis.*

The incidence of *L. serrata* in laboratory specimens is unknown. It is not likely to be encountered except in dogs obtained from pounds or in rodents obtained from their natural habitat. The mouse, guinea pig, and rock squirrel *(Otospermophilus beecheyi)* have been infected experimentally (Heymons 1942; Hobmaier and Hobmaier 1940; Koch 1907).

MORPHOLOGY

The adults have a transparent, tongue-shaped body with approximately 90 annuli (Fig. 16.1) (Sambon 1922). The anterior end has two pairs of simple retractile hooks. The female is 80 to 130 mm long and 10 mm wide, and reddish orange eggs are visible along the median line of the

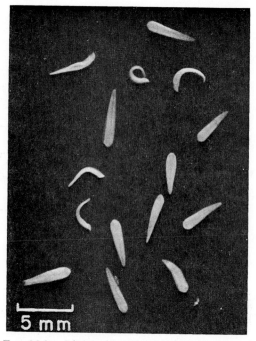

FIG. 16.2. *Linguatula serrata* nymphs. (Courtesy of A. Fain, Institut de Médecine Tropicale Prince Léopold.)

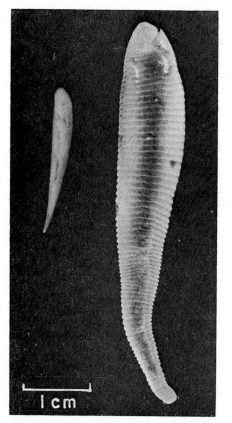

FIG. 16.1. *Linguatula serrata.* *(Left)* Male. *(Right)* Female. (Courtesy of A. Fain, Institut de Médecine Tropicale Prince Léopold.)

body; the male is 20 mm long and 3 to 4 mm wide. The nymph, sometimes called *Pentastomum denticulatum,* is 4 to 6 mm long and 1 mm wide (Fig. 16.2). It has spinous body rings and two pairs of binate hooks (Fig. 16.3). The egg is oval, about 70 to 90 μ in diameter, and is individually enclosed in a thin bladderlike envelope containing a clear fluid. It has a thick chitinous shell containing an embryo with rudimentary mouthparts and four short legs, each bearing two clawlike hooks. On the back of the embryo is the so-called dorsal organ or facette.

LIFE CYCLE

Eggs are expelled from the definitive host in the nasal mucus or are swallowed and passed in the feces (Hobmaier and Hobmaier 1940). When ingested by an intermediate host, they hatch in the intestine. The resultant larvae migrate to the internal organs, usually the mesenteric lymph nodes, and after about 6 months and nine molts, they develop into infective nymphs. These nymphs remain viable in

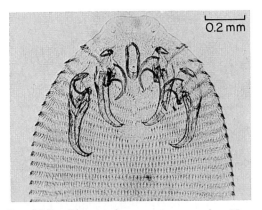

FIG. 16.3. *Linguatula serrata* nymph. Note spinous body rings and the two pairs of binate hooks. (Courtesy of A. Fain, Institut de Médecine Tropicale Prince Léopold.)

the intermediate host for over 2 years. The definitive host becomes infected by ingesting viscera containing the infective stage, but the method by which nymphs get to the nasal cavities is unknown. This may occur while contaminated food is being masticated or possibly later during emesis. Adults survive about 2 years in the definitive host. They feed on nasal mucus and secretions and occasionally on blood (Heymons 1942).

PATHOLOGIC EFFECTS

Usually there are no signs of infection, but a severe catarrhal or suppurative rhinitis and epistaxis sometimes occur (Enigk and Düwel 1957; Heymons 1942). Restlessness, sneezing, and difficult breathing are occasionally seen. The sense of smell is often reduced or abolished.

The nymph generally does not produce signs and is an incidental necropsy finding, appearing as a small fibrous or calcified tubercle in the viscera. A massive infection has caused peritonitis in an experimentally infected guinea pig (Koch 1907).

DIAGNOSIS

Diagnosis is based on clinical signs and the presence of *L. serrata* eggs in the feces or nasal mucus.

CONTROL

Newly acquired dogs showing signs of upper respiratory disease should be exam-

ined for this parasite. Infected dogs can be treated by spraying the nasal passages with an aerosol containing ascaridol (the active ingredient in chenopodium oil) (Enigk and Düwel 1957), or the parasites can be removed surgically (Olt and Ströse 1914).

There is no treatment for nymphal infections.

PUBLIC HEALTH CONSIDERATIONS

This parasite is not an important public health problem (Fain 1960). The nymph and, very rarely, the adults have been reported in man.

Porocephalus

Porocephalus crotali occurs in North and South America, *P. clavatus* occurs in South America, and *P. subulifer* is confined to tropical Africa (Fain 1961, 1966; Heymons 1935). *Porocephalus* nymphs are occasionally found in the viscera of some endothermal laboratory species. They are relatively benign parasites. Adults usually live in the lung of large snakes.

The *P. crotali* nymph has been found in deer mice and the cotton rat in the United States (Layne 1967; Self and McMurry 1948), and there is a doubtful record in a marmoset *(Saguinus)* (Heymons 1935). The nymph of *P. clavatus* has been reported from the common marmoset (Heymons 1935), from laboratory tamarins *(Saguinus nigricollis)* in the United States (Cosgrove, Nelson, and Gengozian 1968; Nelson, Cosgrove, and Gengozian 1966), and, erroneously, from African primates and man (Fiennes 1967). The nymph of *P. subulifer* has been found in a guenon (Heymons 1935) and in a galago (Fain 1961), and nymphs of an unidentified species of *Porocephalus* have been recovered from a squirrel monkey (A. Fain, unpublished data).

The rat, mouse, and hamster have been experimentally infected with eggs of *P. crotali* (Esslinger 1962a, b), and the mouse, rat, and guinea pig have been experimentally infected with eggs of *P. clavatus* (da Fonseca 1939).

Porocephalus clavatus is apparently common in laboratory tamarins obtained from their natural habitat, and an incidence of 29% has been reported (Self and

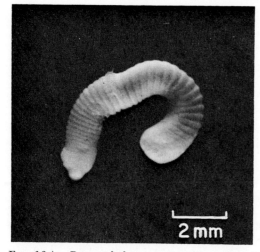

FIG. 16.4. *Porocephalus* nymph. (Courtesy of A. Fain, Institut de Médecine Tropicale Prince Léopold.)

Cosgrove 1968). The incidence of *P. crotali* and *P. subulifer* in laboratory specimens is unknown. They are not likely to be encountered except in some primates and wild rodents obtained from endemic areas.

MORPHOLOGY

The *Porocephalus* nymph has a cylindrical, smoothly annulated body which is often club shaped (Fig. 16.4) (Heymons 1935). Nymphs of *P. crotali* and *P. clavatus* are about 8 to 14 mm long; the nymph of *P. subulifer* is 7 to 15 mm long and 1.2 to 1.5 mm wide. Each nymph has approximately 30 to 45 annuli. Two unequal pairs of hooks are located at the anterior end around the mouth. The inner pair is simple; each of the outer hooks has an accessory spine. The adults are similar, only larger.

LIFE CYCLE

The life cycle resembles that of *Linguatula serrata* except that the adults occur in snakes instead of in the dog and other canids. Adults of *P. crotali* are common in rattlesnakes *(Crotalus)* and also occur in the cottonmouth water moccasin *(Ancistrodon piscivorus);* adults of *P. clavatus* occur in boas *(Boa, Epicrates* and *Eunectes);* and those of *P. subulifer* occur only in file snakes *(Mehelya)* (Fain 1961,

1966; Heymons 1935; Penn 1942; Self and McMurry 1948).

PATHOLOGIC EFFECTS

In deer mice and the cotton rat, the nymph locates in the viscera, mesentery, and abdominal and thoracic walls (Layne 1967). It produces no signs or serious pathology.

In primates, the nymph encysts in many tissues (Fig. 16.5, 16.6), including the liver, lungs, peritoneum, and meninges, but produces little or no injury (A. Fain, unpublished data; Nelson, Cosgrove, and Gengozian 1966). Inflammatory reaction is minimal (Fig. 16.7) unless the nymph dies; then a foreign body reaction and gradual resorption occur (Fig. 16.8).

DIAGNOSIS

Since this parasite usually does not produce signs or lesions, diagnosis is made by finding the nymph at necropsy.

CONTROL

No special procedures other than routine sanitation are necessary. The *Porocephalus* nymph can occur only in laboratory species permitted to ingest food contaminated with feces of infected snakes. There is no treatment.

PUBLIC HEALTH CONSIDERATIONS

Porocephalus is of no known public health importance. All reports of the nymph in man are of doubtful validity (Fain 1960).

Armillifer armillatus

This relatively benign parasite occurs naturally only in tropical Africa, where it is common. The nymphs develop in various endothermal species and are frequently found in the rhesus monkey, other macaques, galagos, guenons, mangabeys, baboons, the chimpanzee, dog, and man (Fain 1960, 1961, 1966; Fiennes 1967; Heymons 1935). There is a report of the occurrence of the nymphs in a New World monkey, a capuchin, from a European zoo (Desportes and Roth 1943), but this infection was probably acquired in the zoo. Adults of *Armillifer armillatus* live in the lung of large snakes.

The incidence of *A. armillatus* in lab-

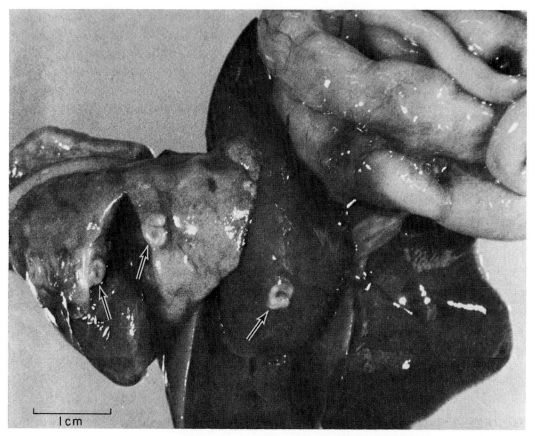

FIG. 16.5. *Porocephalus clavatus* nymphs *(arrows)* in the liver and lungs of a tamarin *(Saguinus nigricollis)*. (From Nelson, Cosgrove, and Gengozian 1966. Courtesy of American Association for Laboratory Animal Science.)

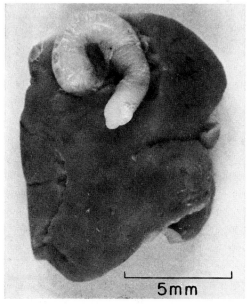

FIG. 16.6. *Porocephalus* nymph on the liver of a squirrel monkey. (Courtesy of A. Fain, Institut de Médecine Tropicale Prince Léopold.)

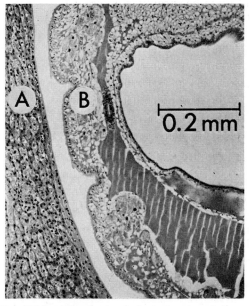

FIG. 16.7. Histologic section of encysted *Porocephalus clavatus* nymph in the liver of a tamarin. *(A)* Liver tissue. *(B)* Parasite. Note absence of inflammation. (From Nelson, Cosgrove, and Gengozian 1966. Courtesy of American Association for Laboratory Animal Science.)

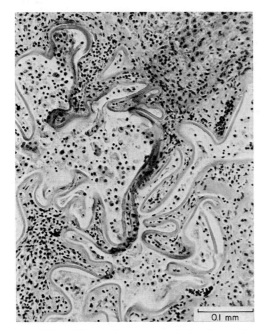

FIG. 16.8. Histologic section of the liver of a tamarin containing degenerating *Porocephalus clavatus* nymph. Note inflammatory reaction. (From Nelson, Cosgrove, and Gengozian 1966. Courtesy of American Association for Laboratory Animal Science.)

oratory specimens is unknown. It is not likely to be encountered except in primates obtained from tropical Africa.

MORPHOLOGY

The nymphs have a cylindrical, annulated body about 13 to 23 mm long (Fig. 16.9) (Fain 1961). The annuli are thick and projecting, and their number varies from 15 to 19 in the male nymph and from 18 to 22 in the female nymph. The hooks are simple. Adults closely resemble the nymphs but are larger.

LIFE CYCLE

The adults live in the lung of large African snakes *(Python, Bitis)* (Broden and Rodhain 1907, 1908–1909, 1910). The intermediate host becomes infected by swallowing food contaminated by snake feces or saliva.

PATHOLOGIC EFFECTS

Encysted nymphs are commonly found in the peritoneal cavity (Fig. 16.10) (Fain

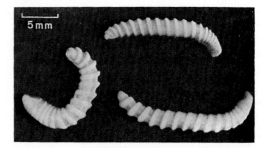

FIG. 16.9. *Armillifer armillatus* nymphs. (From Fain 1961. Courtesy of Musée royal de l'Afrique Centrale.)

1961). Often they are located beneath the capsule or are embedded in the superficial layers of the liver. They usually cause little or no reaction in the host even at high levels of infection, but there is one report of peritonitis and death caused by *Armillifer* nymphs in 7 of 24 laboratory mangabeys (Whitney and Kruckenberg 1967).

DIAGNOSIS

Diagnosis is based on finding nymphs at necropsy.

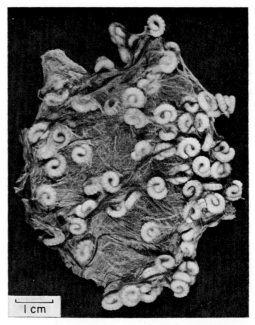

FIG. 16.10. *Armillifer armillatus* nymphs encysted in the omentum of a green monkey. (From Fain 1961. Courtesy of Musée royal de l'Afrique Centrale.)

CONTROL

Other than routine sanitation, no special control procedures are necessary. Infection can only occur if laboratory species are permitted to ingest eggs passed in the feces or saliva of infected snakes. There is no treatment.

PUBLIC HEALTH CONSIDERATIONS

In some parts of tropical Africa man is frequently infected (Bouckaert and Fain 1959; Cannon 1942), but the parasite in endothermal laboratory species is of no public health importance. Man can only be infected by ingesting eggs passed in snake feces or saliva.

TABLE 16.1. Pentastomids affecting endothermal laboratory animals

Parasite	Geographic Distribution	Endothermal Host	Location in Host	Method of Infection	Incidence In nature	Incidence In laboratory	Pathologic Effects	Public Health Importance	Reference
Linguatula serrata*	Worldwide	Definitive: dog, other canids, domestic animals, man Intermediate: rat, black rat, guinea pig, rabbit, cat, titi monkey, gelada baboon, domestic animals, man	Adult: nasal cavity Nymph: mesenteric lymph nodes, viscera	Definitive: ingestion of encysted nymphs in viscera of intermediate host Intermediate: ingestion of eggs passed by definitive host	Common in dog in eastern Europe; rare in rat, rabbit, cat, titi monkey	Unknown; probably rare	Usually none; sometimes rhinitis, epistaxis, restlessness, sneezing, dyspnea in dog; tubercles in viscera in rat, rabbit, cat	Rare in man	Bochefontaine 1876 Enigk and Duwel 1957 Heymons 1942 Hobmaier and Hobmaier 1940 Kuntz et al. 1967 Strong et al. 1926
Porocephalus crotali*	North America, South America	Intermediate: deer mice, cotton rat	Viscera, mesentery, abdominal wall, thoracic wall	Ingestion of eggs passed by definitive host (pit vipers)	Common in some areas; uncommon in others	Unknown	Benign cysts in viscera, mesentery, abdominal wall, thoracic wall	None	Layne 1967 Self and McMurry 1948
Porocephalus clavatus*	South America	Intermediate: tamarins, marmosets	Liver, lungs, peritoneum, meninges, other tissues	Ingestion of eggs passed by definitive host (boas, other large snakes)	Unknown	Common in tamarins, marmosets obtained from natural habitat	Benign cysts in liver, lungs, peritoneum, meninges, other tissues	None	Cosgrove et al. 1968 Heymons 1935 Nelson et al. 1966 Self and Cosgrove 1968
Porocephalus subulifer*	Tropical Africa	Intermediate: guenons, galagos	Viscera	Ingestion of eggs passed by definitive host (file snakes)	Unknown	Unknown	Benign cysts in viscera	None	Fain 1961 Heymons 1935
Porocephalus sp.*	South America	Intermediate: squirrel monkeys	Liver	Unknown; presumably by ingestion of eggs passed by definitive host	Unknown	Unknown	Benign cysts in viscera	Unknown	A. Fain, unpublished data

*Discussed in text.

500

TABLE 16.1 *(continued)*

Parasite	Geographic Distribution	Endothermal Host	Location in Host	Method of Infection	Incidence In nature	Incidence In laboratory	Pathologic Effects	Public Health Importance	Reference
Gigliolella brumpti	Madagascar	Intermediate: lemur ape (*Cheirogaleus medius*)	Mesentery	Unknown; presumably by ingestion of eggs passed by definitive host	Unknown	Unknown	Benign cysts in mesentery	None	Chabaud and Choquet 1954
*Armillifer armillatus**	Tropical Africa	Intermediate: dog, monkey, other macaques, galagos, guenons, mangabeys, baboons, chimpanzee, man	Peritoneal cavity	Ingestion of eggs passed by definitive host (pythons, vipers)	Common	Unknown	Usually benign cysts in peritoneal cavity; rarely peritonitis, death	Common in man in endemic areas; infected endothermal laboratory animals cannot infect man	Desportes and Roth 1943 Fain 1960, 1961 Fiennes 1967 Heymons 1935 Whitney and Kruckenberg 1967
Armillifer moniliformis	Asia, Australia	Intermediate: various mammals, possibly dog, cat, cynomolgus monkey, man	Viscera, peritoneal cavity	Ingestion of eggs passed by definitive host (pythons)	Unknown	Unknown	Unknown	Rare in man	Fain 1966 Worms 1967 Yamashita and Ohbayashi 1954

*Discussed in text.

REFERENCES

Bochefontaine, M. 1876. Pentastome denticulé provenant du poumon d'un cobaye. Compt. Rend. Mem. Soc. Biol. Paris 28:261.

Bouckaert, L., and A. Fain. 1959. Een geval van nymphale porocephalose met dodelijk verloop. Ann. Soc. Belge Med. Trop. 39: 793–98.

Broden, A., and J. Rodhain. 1907. Contribution à l'étude de Porocephalus moniliformis. Ann. Trop. Med. Parasitol. 1907: 493–504.

———. 1908–1909. Contribution à l'étude de Porocephalus moniliformis. Ann. Trop. Med. Parasitol. 1908–1909: 303–13.

———. 1910. Contribution à l'étude de Porocephalus moniliformis. Ann. Trop. Med. Parasitol. 1910:167–76.

Cannon, D. A. 1942. Linguatulid infestation of man. Ann. Trop. Med. Parasitol. 36: 160–66.

Chabaud, A. G., and Marie-Therese Choquet. 1954. Nymphes du Pentastome Gigliolella (n. gen.) brumpti (Giglioli 1922) chez un Lemurien. Riv. Parassitologia 15:331–36.

Chalmers, A. J. 1899. A case of Pentastoma constrictum. Zentr. Bakteriol. Parasitenk. 26:518.

Cosgrove, G. E., B. Nelson, and N. Gengozian. 1968. Helminth parasites of the tamarin, Saguinus fuscicollis. Lab. Animal Care 18:654–56.

Desportes, C., and P. Roth. 1943. Helminthes récoltés an cours d'autopsies pratiquées sur différents mammifères morts a la ménagerie du Museum de Paris. Bull. Museum Hist. Nat. Paris 15:108–14.

Enigk, K., and D. Düwel. 1957. Feststellung und Behandlung des Linguatula-Befalles beim Hund. Deut. Tieraerztl. Wochschr. 64:401–3.

Esslinger, J. H. 1962a. Development of Porocephalus crotali (Humboldt, 1808) (Pentastomida) in experimental hosts. J. Parasitol. 48:452–56.

———. 1962b. Hepatic lesions in rats experimentally infected with Porocephalus crotali (Pentastomida). J. Parasitol. 48:631–38.

Fain, A. 1960. La pentastomose chez l'homme. Bull. Acad. Roy. Med. Belg., Ser. VI, 25: 516–32.

———. 1961. Les pentastomidés de l'Afrique Centrale. Ann. Musee Roy. Afrique Centrale, Ser. 8, Sci. Zool. 92:1–115.

———. 1966. Pentastomida of snakes—their parasitological role in man and animals. Mem. Inst. Butantan (Sao Paulo) 33:167–74.

Faust, E. C. 1927. Linguatulids from man and other hosts in China. Am. J. Trop. Med. 7:311–25.

Fiennes, R. 1967. Zoonoses of primates: The epidemiology and ecology of simian diseases in relation to man. Weidenfeld and Nicolson, London. 190 pp.

Fonseca, F. da. 1939. Observaçoes sobre o ciclo evolutivo de Porocephalus clavatus, especialmente sobre o seu orquidotropismo em cobaias. Mem. Inst. Butantan (Sao Paulo) 12:185–90.

Gelormini, N., and R. J. Roveda. 1938. Linguatula serrata. Inst. Parasitol. Enferm. Parasit. Univ. Buenos Aires 1:3–12.

Gurr, L. 1953. A note on the occurrence of Linguatula serrata (Frohlich, 1789) in the wild rabbit, Oryctolagus cuniculus, in New Zealand. New Zealand J. Sci. Technol. 35: 49–50.

Heymons, R. 1935. Pentastomida, pp. 1–268. In H. G. Bronn's Klassen und Ordnungen des Tierreichs. Vol. 5, Sect. 4, Bk. 1. Akademische Verlagsgesellschaft M.B.H., Leipzig.

———. 1942. Der Nasenwurm des Hundes (Linguatula serrata Froelich), seine Wirte und Beziechungen zur europäischen Tierwelt, seine Herkunft und praktische bedeutung auf Grund unserer bisherigen Kenntnisse. Z. Parasitenk. 12:607–38.

Hobmaier, A., and M. Hobmaier. 1940. On the life-cycle of Linguatula rhinaria. Am. J. Trop. Med. 20:199–210.

Koch, M. 1907. Zur Kenntnis des Parasitismus der Pentastomen. Verhandl. Deut. Ges. Pathol. 17:265–79.

Kuntz, R. E., Betty J. Myers, and T. E. Vice. 1967. Intestinal protozoans and parasites of the gelada baboon (Theropithecus gelada Rüppel, 1835). Proc. Helminthol. Soc. Wash. D.C. 34:65–66.

Layne, J. N. 1967. Incidence of Porocephalus crotali (Pentastomida) in Florida mammals. Bull. Wildlife Dis. Assoc. 3:105–9.

Nelson, B., G. E. Cosgrove, and N. Gengozian. 1966. Diseases of an imported primate Tamarinus nigricollis. Lab. Animal Care 16:255–75.

Olt, A. and A. Ströse. 1914. Die Wildkrankheiten und ihre Bekämpfung. J. Neumann, Neudamm. 649 pp.

Ortlepp, R. J. 1934. Note on the occurrence of the tongue-worm, Linguatula serrata, in a dog in South Africa. J. S. African Vet. Med. Assoc. 5:113–14.

Penn, G. H., Jr. 1942. The life history of Porocephalus crotali, a parasite of the Louisiana muskrat. J. Parasitol. 28:277–83.

Pullar, E. M. 1936. A note on the occurrence of

Linguatula serrata (Frohlich, 1789) in Australia. Australian Vet. J. 12:61–64.

Sambon, L. W. 1922. A synopsis of the family Linguatulidae. J. Trop. Med. Hyg. 25: 188–206, 391–428.

Self, J. T., and G. E. Cosgrove. 1968. Pentastome larvae in laboratory primates. J. Parasitol. 54:969.

Self, J. T., and F. B. McMurry. 1948. *Porocephalus crotali* Humboldt (Pentastomida) in Oklahoma. J. Parasitol. 34:21–23.

Stiles, C. W. 1895. On the recent occurrence of *Linguatula rhinaria*, Railliet, 1886, and *Taenia echinococcus*, v. Siebold, 1853, in the United States of North America. Trans. First Pan-Am. Med. Congr. Wash., D.C. (Part 2):1163–65.

Strong, R. P., G. C. Shattuck, and R. E. Wheeler. 1926. Other parasitic infections of animals, pp. 118–47. *In* Medical Report of the Hamilton Rice Expedition to the Amazon. Harvard Univ. Press, Cambridge, Mass.

Tubangui, M. A., and Victoria A. Masiluñgan. 1936. Notes on Philippine linguatulids (Arthropoda: Pentastomida). Philippine J. Sci. 60:399–403.

Whitney, R. A., Jr., and S. M. Kruckenberg. 1967. Pentastomid infection associated with peritonitis in mangabey monkeys. J. Am. Vet. Med. Assoc. 151:907–8.

Worms, M. J. 1967. Parasites in newly imported animals. J. Inst. Animal Tech. 18: 39–47.

Yamashita, J., and M. Ohbayashi. 1954. On a tongue worm, *Linguatula serrata* Frölich, 1789, showing the same parasitism as in the intermediate host within a dog body (in Japanese). Mem. Fac. Agr. Hokkaido Univ. 2:146–48.

P A R T 2

Parasites of Laboratory Reptiles and Amphibians

Chapter 17

PROTOZOANS

NUMEROUS protozoans occur in reptiles and amphibians. Most are non-pathogenic and little is known of others. Where information is relatively complete and the organism is thought to be important, it is discussed in detail. Otherwise, it is described more briefly or listed in the tables only.

FLAGELLATES

The flagellates that affect laboratory reptiles and amphibians are listed in Table 17.1. Some occur in the blood, some on the skin or gills, and many in the intestine (Walton 1964). *Trypanosoma*, the commonest hemoflagellate, and *Oodinium*, a common ectoparasite of fishes that sometimes affects aquatic amphibians, are pathogenic in heavy infections (Barrow 1958; Geus 1960; Reichenbach-Klinke and Elkan 1965). None of the enteric flagellates is known to be pathogenic and most are probably commensals. *Trypanosoma, Oodinium*, and some of the commonest enteric flagellates are described below.

Trypanosoma

Many species of *Trypanosoma* have been described from amphibians and several from reptiles (Table 17.1) (Diamond 1965; Walton 1964; Woo 1969a). Most are either nonpathogenic or their pathogenicity is unknown, but a few are highly pathogenic. *Trypanosoma pipientis, T. rana-rum,* and *T. chattoni* are the species commonest in frogs and toads in North America, and *T. rotatorium, T. loricatum,* and *T. inopinatum* are the commonest species in anurans in Europe. Incidences as high as 38% of *T. pipientis* have been observed in the leopard frog in Minnesota (Diamond 1965) and 14% in Ontario (Woo 1969a). *Trypanosoma diemyctyli,* which occurs in the red-spotted newt and other newts in the United States, is also common (Nigrelli 1929b). Laboratory frogs and red-spotted newts obtained from their natural habitat are usually infected.

MORPHOLOGY

Trypanosoma pipientis is about 70 μ long by about 4 μ wide (Fig. 17.1*A*) (Diamond 1965). It has a round or elliptical nucleus near the center of the body, a medium-sized kinetoplast, a narrow undulating membrane, and a long flagellum. *Trypanosoma ranarum* has two adult forms, one that is about 74 μ long by 5 μ wide (Fig. 17.1*B*) and one that is about 71 μ long by 8 μ wide (Fig. 17.1*C*). In the narrow form the nucleus is located in the anterior one-third of the body, but in the wide form, it is in the middle third of the body. In both forms the kinetoplast is large, the undulating membrane is wide, and the flagellum is less than one-half the body length. *Trypanosoma chattoni* occurs in vertebrates only in a spherical form; it has

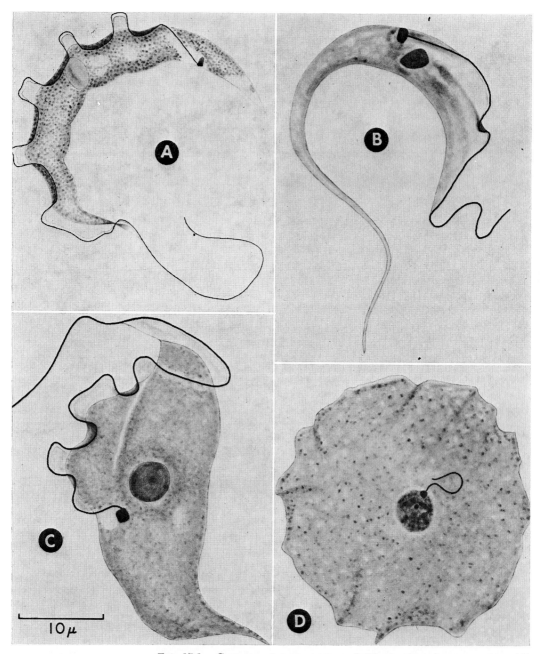

FIG. 17.1. Common trypanosomes of North American anurans. *(A) Trypanosoma pipientis* adult. *(B) T. ranarum* adult, narrow form. *(C) T. ranarum* adult, wide form. *(D) T. chattoni* adult. (From Diamond 1965. Courtesy of L. S. Diamond, U.S. Public Health Service.)

no undulating membrane and the flagellum, when present, is very short (Fig. 17.1*D*). *Trypanosoma diemyctyli* is long and slender, 45 to 116 μ long by 2 to 5 μ wide (Barrow 1958; Kudo 1966).

LIFE CYCLE

The life cycle requires an invertebrate vector (Kudo 1966; Wenyon 1926; Woo 1969b). For most trypanosomes of aquatic reptiles and amphibians it is probably a leech; for terrestrial reptiles and possibly for some adult amphibians it is probably a bloodsucking arthropod. Although anurans are usually thought to be infected during the tadpole stage by the bite of an infected leech, there is some evidence that adult frogs can be infected by the bite of an infected mosquito (Walton 1964), and adult toads have been infected by ingestion of an infected sand fly (*Phlebotomus*) (Anderson and Ayala 1968).

PATHOLOGIC EFFECTS

The pathogenicity of the species affecting frogs and toads is varied (Diamond 1965). *Trypanosoma inopinatum* is one of the most pathogenic species. It causes either an acute or chronic infection. In acute infection, an excessive and continuous production of juvenile forms of the parasite is characteristic; in chronic infection, adult forms predominate. Acute infection causes spleen destruction and the host almost always dies. *Trypanosoma pipientis* causes spleen enlargement but death is uncommon. *Trypanosoma ranarum* causes no recognizable pathologic effects. *Trypanosoma diemyctyli* causes debilitation, anorexia, erythrocyte degeneration, and death; the degree of parasitemia and resultant pathologic effects are related to the environmental temperature, with pathogenicity greatest at 15 C and least at 20 to 25 C (Barrow 1958; Nigrelli 1929b).

DIAGNOSIS

Diagnosis is based on identification of the parasite in the blood (Diamond 1965). A small amount of blood, mixed with an equal amount of citrate-saline solution (0.5% sodium citrate, 0.65% sodium chloride), is placed on a glass slide and examined microscopically. The living trypanosomes are usually readily recognized by their rapid, wavy motion. *Trypanosoma chattoni* is diagnosed by recognizing it in Giemsa-stained smears of peripheral blood.

CONTROL

Because of the need for an invertebrate intermediate host, it is unlikely that the life cycle would be completed in the laboratory, and no special control procedures are needed. There is no treatment.

PUBLIC HEALTH CONSIDERATIONS

The trypanosomes of reptiles and amphibians are not known to affect man.

Oodinium

Members of this genus are common on the skin and gills of marine fishes in their natural habitat and are occasionally encountered on freshwater fishes in aquariums (Jacobs 1946; Reichenbach-Klinke and Elkan 1965). It is not known if any reptiles or amphibians are affected with this dinoflagellate in nature, but one species, *Oodinium pillularis*, has been reported as an ectoparasite on the skin and gills of captive frog tadpoles, newts, and the axolotl in Europe (Geus 1960; Reichenbach-Klinke and Elkan 1965). The source of infection is unknown. Likely sources are contaminated water, contaminated live food, or infected, newly acquired fishes (Jacobs 1946). The incidence and likelihood of infection of laboratory amphibians are unknown.

MORPHOLOGY

The parasitic stage, the form found on amphibians, is oval to piriform, measures 12 to 150 μ in the longest dimension, and has pseudopodia but no flagella (Fig. 17.2) (Geus 1960; Jacobs 1946; Reichenbach-Klinke and Elkan 1965). The free-swimming stage, or gymnodinium, is oval to round, measures 10 to 19 μ in diameter, and has a posterior and an equatorial flagellum but no pseudopodia.

LIFE CYCLE

The mature parasitic form drops off the host and, after a series of binary divisions, develops into many free-swimming gymnodinia (Geus 1960; Jacobs 1946; Reichenbach-Klinke and Elkan 1965). A gymnodinium must reach a suitable host

FIG. 17.2. *Oodinium pillularis*, parasitic stage. (From Reichenbach-Klinke and Elkan 1965. Courtesy of Academic Press.)

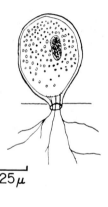

25 μ

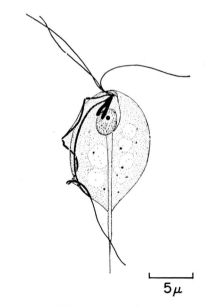

5 μ

FIG. 17.3. *Trichomitus batrachorum*. (From Honigberg 1953. Courtesy of American Society of Parasitologists.)

within 24 to 48 hours or die. If it reaches a host, it attaches and changes into the parasitic form. The parasitic stage grows for about a week before reaching maturity.

PATHOLOGIC EFFECTS

Heavy infections cause the formation of a gray coating on the skin and gills, debilitation, impaired respiration, and sometimes death (Geus 1960; Reichenbach-Klinke and Elkan 1965). Young animals are most susceptible (Jacobs 1946).

DIAGNOSIS

Diagnosis is based on the signs and on identification of the parasite on the skin or gills.

CONTROL

Because the source of infection in captive amphibians is unknown, no specific control procedures can be recommended. Copper sulfate, 2 ppm, or acriflavine, 10 ppm, in the water is an effective treatment (Geus 1960; Reichenbach-Klinke and Elkan 1965).

PUBLIC HEALTH CONSIDERATIONS

Oodinium is not known to affect man.

Tritrichomonas, Trichomitus, Tetratrichomonas

These genera are morphologically similar. *Tritrichomonas* and *Trichomitus* (Fig. 17.3) typically have three anterior flagella and *Tetratrichomonas* has four (Honigberg 1963). All have a piriform body, an undulating membrane, an axostyle that protrudes from the posterior end, and a costa. Reproduction is by simple binary fission and no cysts are formed.

The commonest species are *Tritrichomonas augusta* (syn. *Trichomonas augusta*), *Trichomitus batrachorum* (syn. *Tritrichomonas batrachorum*, *Trichomonas batrachorum*, *Trichomonas natricis*), and *Tetratrichomonas prowazeki* (syn. *Trichomonas prowazeki*). None is known to be pathogenic.

Tritrichomonas augusta is common in the large intestine of frogs, toads, salamanders, newts, and lizards in North, Central, and South America, Europe, and Asia (Reichenbach-Klinke and Elkan 1965; Walton 1964). Incidences as high as 100% have been reported in salamanders in eastern United States (Rankin 1937). It is elongate, spindle shaped, and 15 to 27 μ long by 5 to 13 μ wide, and has an axostyle that contains dark-staining granules and a rod- or sausage-shaped parabasal body (Honigberg 1950b, 1953, 1963). This flagellate has been associated with liver lesions in the leopard frog (Walton 1964); otherwise, nothing is known of its pathogenicity.

Trichomitus batrachorum occurs in the large intestine of many species of frogs, toads, salamanders, newts, the axolotl, snakes, and lizards throughout the world

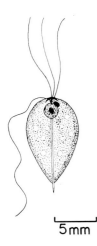

Fig. 17.4. *Monocercomonas.* (From Levine 1961. Courtesy of N. D. Levine and Burgess Publishing Co.)

5mm

(Honigberg 1950b, 1953, 1963; Moskowitz 1951; Reichenbach-Klinke and Elkan 1965; Walton 1964). It is ovoid, measures 6 to 21 μ long by 4 to 20 μ wide, and has an axostyle without granules and a V-shaped parabasal body.

Tetratrichomonas prowazeki occurs in the large intestine of frogs, toads, salamanders, newts, amphiuma, and snakes in the United States, Europe, and South America (Honigberg 1951, 1963). It is frequently elongate and measures 5.5 to 22.0 μ long by 3.5 to 18.5 μ wide.

Monocercomonas

This flagellate of unknown pathogenicity is similar to *Tritrichomonas* except that it lacks an undulating membrane and a costa (Fig. 17.4) (Honigberg 1963; Levine 1961). It is piriform and has three anterior flagella, one trailing flagellum, a parabasal body, and a projecting axostyle. Reproduction is by simple binary fission. It does not form cysts.

Monocercomonas batrachorum (syn. *Eutrichomastix batrachorum*) is the commonest species in laboratory amphibians (Reichenbach-Klinke and Elkan 1965; Walton 1964). It occurs in the large intestine of frogs, toads, salamanders, and the red-spotted newt in the United States, Europe, Asia, and Africa. Incidences as high as 77% have been reported in the red-spotted newt in eastern United States (Rankin 1937). Its length, from anterior end to tip of axostyle, is about 15 μ; its width is about 6 μ (Dobell 1909).

Monocercomonas colubrorum (syn.

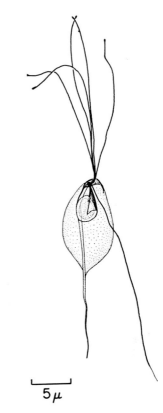

5μ

Fig. 17.5. *Hexamastix batrachorum.* (From Honigberg and Christian 1954. Courtesy of American Society of Parasitologists.)

Trichomastix lacertae, T. serpentis, Eutrichomastix serpentis) is the commonest species in laboratory snakes and lizards (Honigberg 1963; Moskowitz 1951). It occurs in the large intestine of racers, rat snakes, hognose snakes, kingsnakes, water snakes, bullsnakes, garter snakes, other snakes, chameleons, and other lizards in North America, Europe, Africa, and Asia. Its length, including the projecting axostyle, is 9 to 20 μ; its width is 5 to 10 μ.

Hexamastix

Hexamastix is similar to *Monocercomonas* except that it has five anterior flagella and one trailing flagellum (Fig. 17.5) (Honigberg 1963). Its pathogenicity is unknown. Reproduction is by binary fission. It is not known to produce cysts.

Hexamastix batrachorum (syn. *Polymastix batrachorum*) is the most frequently encountered species in laboratory reptiles

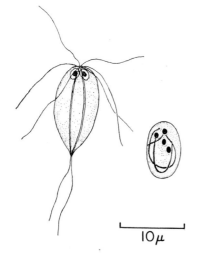

FIG. 17.6. *Hexamita intestinalis. (Left)* Trophozoite. *(Right)* Cyst. (From Cheng 1964. Courtesy of W. B. Saunders Co.)

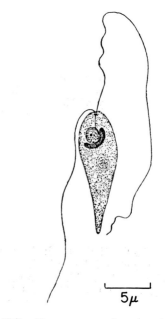

FIG. 17.7. *Proteromonas lacertae-viridis.* (From Kudo 1966. Courtesy of Charles C Thomas, Publisher.)

and amphibians. It is common in the intestine of salamanders and newts in the United States and Europe (Rankin 1937; Reichenbach-Klinke and Elkan 1965; Walton 1964, 1966); it measures 7.0 to 15.5 μ by 5.0 to 10.5 μ (Honigberg and Christian 1954).

Hexamita

The trophozoites of this genus are piriform and bilaterally symmetrical, with two nuclei, two axostyles, and six anterior and two posterior flagella (Fig. 17.6) (Kudo 1966). Some species form cysts.

Hexamita intestinalis and *H. batrachorum* are the commonest species in laboratory reptiles and amphibians (Honigberg 1950a; Walton 1964). Neither is known to be pathogenic. *Hexamita intestinalis* occurs in the large intestine of frogs, toads, salamanders, newts, and the axolotl in the United States, Europe, and Asia; incidences as high as 38% have been reported in the marbled salamander in eastern United States (Rankin 1937). Its trophozoites are 10 to 16 μ long. *Hexamita batrachorum* occurs in the large intestine of frogs, toads, salamanders, and newts in the United States. Incidences as high as 42% have been reported in the dusky salamander in eastern United States (Rankin 1937).

Proteromonas

The trophozoites of this genus are elongated piriform, with two flagella on the anterior end, one directed forward and the other trailing posteriorly (Fig. 17.7) (Honigberg 1950a; Kudo 1966; Moskowitz 1951). It forms cysts which are unusual in that they are capable of increasing in size (Wenyon 1926).

Proteromonas longifila (possible syn. *P. lacertae-viridis*) is the commonest species in laboratory amphibians (Reichenbach-Klinke and Elkan 1965; Walton 1964). It occurs in the rectum of frogs, toads, salamanders, and newts in North America, South America, and Europe, with incidences as high as 89% reported in the red-spotted newt in eastern United States (Rankin 1937). Nothing is known of it pathogenicity.

Proteromonas lacertae-viridis (possible syn. *P. longifila*) is the commonest species in laboratory lizards (Honigberg 1950a; Moskowitz 1951). It occurs in the rectum of snakes, iguanas, horned lizards, spiny lizards, European lizards, European chameleons, night lizards, and other lizards throughout the world. Trophozoites are

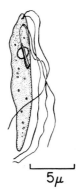

FIG. 17.8. *Karotomorpha bufonis.* (From Cheng 1964. Courtesy of W. B. Saunders Co.)

11 to 22 μ long by 2 to 5 μ wide. Nothing is known of its pathogenicity.

Karotomorpha

This flagellate is elongated, spindle shaped, and about 12 to 16 μ long by 2 to 6 μ wide (Fig. 17.8) (Kudo 1966; Wenyon 1926). It has two pairs of flagella at the anterior end.

Karotomorpha bufonis (syn. *Monocercomonas bufonis; Polymastix bufonis*) and *K. swezyi* are the commonest species in laboratory reptiles and amphibians (Rankin 1937; Walton 1964). Neither is known to be pathogenic. *Karotomorpha bufonis* occurs in the rectum of the leopard frog, European toad, other toads, tiger salamander, palmate newt, other newts, and the axolotl in North America and Europe. *Karotomorpha swezyi* occurs in the rectum of the leopard frog, other frogs, American toad, other toads, dusky salamanders, other salamanders, red-spotted newt, and California newt in the United States.

OPALINIDS

Because these organisms have some characteristics of the ciliates and some of the flagellates, they are classified separately in a position between the other two groups (Honigberg et al. 1964). Sexual reproduction is by fusion and not conjugation; asexual multiplication is by longitudinal fission. The whole body is uniformly covered with longitudinally arranged, parallel rows of cilia (Wenyon 1926). There is no cytostome.

Many opalinids occur in laboratory

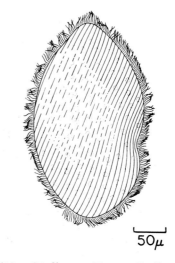

FIG. 17.9. *Opalina.* (From Corliss 1959b. Courtesy of Society of Systematic Zoology.)

amphibians (Table 17.2), but none in laboratory reptiles. All are commensals and nonpathogenic (Kudo 1966).

Opalina, Protoopalina

Opalina (Fig. 17.9) is flattened and oval and has many nuclei; *Protoopalina* (Fig. 17.10) is cylindrical or spindle shaped and has two nuclei. The species most likely to be encountered in the laboratory are *O. obtrigonoidea, O. ranarum, P. intestinalis,* and *P. mitotica.*

Opalina obtrigonoidea is common in the intestine of the leopard frog, wood frog, pickerel frog, green treefrog, spring peeper, cricket frogs, chorus frogs, other frogs, American toad, and other toads in the United States; it measures about 400 to 840 μ in length and 175 to 180 μ in width.

Opalina ranarum is common in the

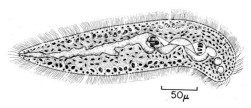

FIG. 17.10. *Protoopalina intestinalis.* (From Wenyon 1926.)

intestine of the grass frog, edible frog, European treefrog, other frogs, European toad, other toads, and the alpine newt in Europe; it is about 300 μ in length.

Protoopalina intestinalis is common in the intestine of the grass frog, edible frog, European treefrog, other frogs, toads, common newt, and palmate newt in Europe, Africa, and Australia; it is about 330 μ long by 68 μ wide. *Protoopalina mitotica* occurs in the intestine of the tiger salamander in central United States; it is about 300 μ long by 37 μ wide.

SARCODINES

Relatively few sarcodines affect laboratory reptiles and amphibians. Of these, only *Entamoeba invadens* and possibly *E. ranarum* are known pathogens. These two species are described below. The others are listed in Table 17.3.

Entamoeba invadens

(SYN. *Entamoeba serpentis*)

This sarcodine, the cause of amebiasis of reptiles, is the most important known pathogen of captive snakes and lizards (Marcus 1968; Page 1966; Ratcliffe 1961). It occurs in the intestine and sometimes the stomach and liver of racers, kingsnakes, water snakes, garter snakes, other snakes, painted turtles, Greek tortoise, softshell turtles, the green iguana, and other lizards throughout the world (Fantham and Porter 1953–1954; Meerovitch 1958; Ratcliffe 1961). It is common in reptiles in captivity and often causes a high morbidity and mortality in captive snakes and lizards (Page 1966; Ratcliffe and Geiman 1938). Turtles carry the organism with no ill effects and, consequently, are a reservoir of infection for snakes (Meerovitch 1957, 1958). Laboratory snakes, lizards, and turtles are likely to be infected.

MORPHOLOGY

Entamoeba invadens (Fig. 17.11) closely resembles *E. histolytica,* the cause of amebiasis of man (Geiman and Ratcliffe 1936). Living trophozoites are ameboid and actively motile and have a continually varying size and shape. The average diameter of fixed specimens is about 16 μ. The endoplasm is dense and contains a nucleus and food vacuoles that are filled with host-

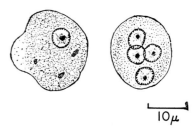

FIG. 17.11.   *Entamoeba invadens. (Left)* Trophozoite. *(Right)* Cyst. (From Fantham and Porter 1953–1954. Courtesy of Zoological Society of London.)

cell debris, leucocytes, or bacteria. Cysts are indistinguishable from those of *E. histolytica.* They are 11 to 20 μ in diameter and contain one to four nuclei, a glycogen vacuole, and chromatoid bodies.

LIFE CYCLE

Reproduction is by binary fission; cysts are formed (Geiman and Ratcliffe 1936). Before encysting, the trophozoite becomes round and small. It produces a cyst wall and the nucleus divides twice, producing four small nuclei. The quadrinucleate cyst is passed in the feces, and when it is ingested by a suitable host, an ameba with four nuclei emerges. It divides several times and produces eight small uninucleate amebas, each of which develops into a trophozoite.

PATHOLOGIC EFFECTS

Signs of infection are usually nonspecific and consist of anorexia, weight loss, and sometimes blood-stained mucus in the excreta (Ratcliffe and Geiman 1938). Death usually occurs in 2 to 10 weeks. Although the organisms sometimes cause minor damage in the lungs, spleen, pancreas, and kidneys (Ratcliffe and Geiman 1938; Zwart 1964), the severest lesions occur in the gastrointestinal tract and liver (Ratcliffe and Geiman 1934, 1938). Lesions in the colon and liver are typical and appear to be primary; those in the small intestine and stomach appear to be secondary. In the colon, discrete, irregular ulcers, from 1 to 5 mm in width, develop in the mucosa. Adjacent tissues are first congested and edematous and later necrotic. The initial lesions rapidly extend to the entire colonic mucosa, and the wall becomes thickened, intensely congested, and nonelastic. The submucosa and muscularis become involved, and the organism enters the blood and lymph vessels. Lesions in the small intestine (ileum) appear to be extensions of those in the large intestine. They are often as widespread as those in the colon, but the necrosis usually involves only the mucosa and superficial submucosa. Blood-stained mucus, containing large numbers of cysts, and trophozoites fill the lumen. Initial lesions in the stomach consist of cone-shaped ulcers, about 2 mm in diameter and 1 mm in depth. They extend into the submucosa, and are filled with a soft, friable, blood-stained mass of exudate and debris containing many trophozoites. Although the ulcers increase in size and number, they rarely coalesce. The liver is mottled, pale brown to dark red, and usually swollen and friable. Focal necrosis of the hepatic parenchyma occurs but is often obscured by the massive necrosis caused by obstruction of the branches of the portal vein by thrombi and emboli. Macroscopically, the hepatic lesions appear as necrotic foci that range in size from less than 1 mm to 3 to 4 cm in diameter.

DIAGNOSIS

Diagnosis is based on the microscopic demonstration of cysts and trophozoites in the feces of the living animal or in the lesions at necropsy (Marcus 1968). Saline enemas are helpful in detecting this protozoan in fecal excretions (Fantham and Porter 1953–1954).

CONTROL

Control is based on sanitation and prophylactic treatment with antibiotics (Cowan 1968). An effective prophylaxis for newly acquired reptiles consists of the oral administration of tetracycline at a rate of 400 to 800 mg per meter of body length (Ratcliffe 1961). The drug is mixed in the feed for animals that accept such food or it is inserted in capsules in the body cavity of food animals. Diloxanide (Entamide, Boots Pure Drug Co.), given orally at a rate of 0.5 g per kg of body weight or emetine hydrochloride at a rate of 40 mg per kg of body weight combined with a diiodohydroxyquin enema (Wallach 1969), is an effective treatment (Marcus 1968). Because turtles are reservoirs of infection for snakes, the two types of reptiles should not be housed in proximity. Water from turtle enclosures should be prevented from reaching snakes, and separate cleaning and feeding utensils should be used for the two types.

PUBLIC HEALTH CONSIDERATIONS

Although *E. invadens* and the human pathogen, *E. histolytica,* are morphologically indistinguishable, biological, biochemical, and immunologic studies have shown that they are not identical and, consequently, there is no danger of human infection with *E. invadens* (E. Meerovitch, personal communication).

Entamoeba ranarum

This sarcodine occurs in the intestine of the leopard frog, green frog, bullfrog, grass frog, edible frog, other frogs, European toad, other toads, red-spotted newt, common newt, palmate newt, and other newts in the United States, Europe, India, and the Philippine Islands (Walton 1964, 1966). Although it has been reported once (in 1922) as being associated with a hepatic abscess in a grass frog, an etiologic relationship was not established, and the organism is considered to be nonpathogenic (Geiman and Ratcliffe 1936; Kudo 1966). It is morphologically similar to *Entamoeba invadens* and *E. histolytica* (Kudo 1966; Wenyon 1926). Trophozoites are 10 to 50 μ in diameter; cysts usually contain 4 nuclei but sometimes as many as 16.

SPOROZOANS

Many sporozoans occur in laboratory reptiles and amphibians (Reichenbach-Klinke and Elkan 1965; Walton 1964). Some are found in the intestine, some in the blood, and others in the kidneys, gallbladder, muscle, skin, and other tissues. Although most are probably pathogenic, few produce overt signs of disease.

Sporozoans likely to be encountered in laboratory reptiles and amphibians are listed in Table 17.4. The most important are described below.

Eimeria

Several species of this coccidian parasite occur in laboratory reptiles and amphibians but none is common (Table 17.4)

(Fantham and Porter 1953–1954; Pellérdy 1963; Reichenbach-Klinke and Elkan 1965; Saxe 1955; Walton 1964). Most inhabit the intestine, but some that occur in snakes are found in the gallbladder and bile duct. Although most species probably cause some pathologic effects, only *Eimeria bitis,* which occurs in the garter snake and other snakes, is a known pathogen.

MORPHOLOGY

Eimeria is characterized by an oocyst that produces four sporocysts, each with two sporozoites (Fig. 17.12) (Kudo 1966).

LIFE CYCLE

The life cycle is direct (Kudo 1966; Levine 1961). Infection is by ingestion of an oocyst passed in the feces. Schizogony and gametogony occur in the same host.

PATHOLOGIC EFFECTS

The pathologic effects of most species of *Eimeria* that occur in laboratory reptiles and amphibians are unknown. Schizogony and gametogony, which occur in the epithelial cells of the intestine, gallbladder, or bile duct, probably cause tissue damage in the host, but these effects are known only in *E. bitis* infection of garter snakes (Fantham and Porter 1953–1954). Infection with this species causes denuding of the mucosa and extensive fibrosis of the submucosa of the gallbladder.

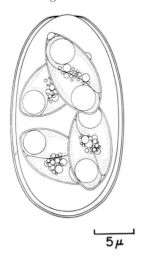

5 μ

FIG. 17.12. *Eimeria scriptae* oocyst. (From Sampson and Ernst 1969. Courtesy of Society of Protozoologists.)

DIAGNOSIS

Diagnosis is based on recognition of lesions and identification of the oocyst in feces or intestinal contents.

CONTROL

Sulfamethazine in the drinking water at a level of 7 gm per liter has been suggested as a treatment for reptiles, but its effectiveness is unknown (Wallach 1969).

PUBLIC HEALTH CONSIDERATIONS

None of the species of *Eimeria* that occur in reptiles and amphibians is transmissible to man.

Isospora

Isospora is differentiated from *Eimeria* by the fact that its oocyst produces two sporocysts, each with four sporozoites (Fig. 17.13) (Kudo 1966). Several species occur in laboratory reptiles and amphibians (Pellérdy 1963; Reichenbach-Klinke and Elkan 1965; Walton 1964). The commonest species is *I. lieberkühni,* which occurs in the kidneys of the grass frog, edible frog, and toads in Europe (Walton 1964; Wenyon 1926). Its pathogenicity has not been described, but heavy infections probably cause extensive kidney damage. The other species found in laboratory reptiles and amphibians occur in the intestine. None is known to be pathogenic.

Haemogregarina

Hemogregarines are the commonest sporozoans in the blood of laboratory snakes and turtles. They also occur in amphibians but are less common (Walton 1964). Although usually considered nonpathogenic (Marcus 1968; O'Connor 1966), heavy infections sometimes cause anemia (Fantham and Porter 1953–1954).

Haemogregarina stepanowi is the species usually found in turtles (Acholonu 1966; Edney 1949; Marquardt 1966; Marzinowsky 1927; Roudabush and Coatney 1937; Wang and Hopkins 1965). It has been reported from the snapping turtle, painted turtle, red-eared turtle, other cooters, box turtles, softshell turtles, European pond terrapin, and other turtles in the United States and Europe. Incidences of 45 to 75% have been observed in cen-

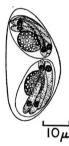

FIG. 17.13. *Isospora lieberkühni* oocyst. (From Wenyon 1926.)

tral and southern United States (Herban and Yaeger 1969; Marquardt 1966; Wang and Hopkins 1965). It is commonest in aquatic turtles and less common in terrestrial species.

Haemogregarina sp. has been reported from the racer, rat snake, kingsnakes, water snakes, bullsnakes, garter snakes, and other snakes in North America. An incidence of 40% has been observed in a survey of 50 snakes of nine species in central United States (Marquardt 1966) and 31% in 600 snakes in central and southwestern United States (Hull and Camin 1960).

MORPHOLOGY

The forms found in the blood of laboratory reptiles and amphibians (Fig. 17.14) vary with the stage of the life cycle and species of host (Hull and Camin 1960; Kudo 1966). They range in size from 10 to 17 μ long by 2 to 4 μ wide.

LIFE CYCLE

The life cycle is shown in Figure 17.14 (Kudo 1966). Schizogony and gametogony occur in the erythrocytes of the reptile or amphibian; sexual reproduction occurs in a bloodsucking invertebrate, usually a leech.

PATHOLOGIC EFFECTS

The presence of a hemogregarine in an erythrocyte causes extreme distortion of the blood cell, including nuclear displacement and cytoplasmic attenuation (Fantham and Porter 1953–1954). The number of erythrocytes affected varies up to 80% or more (Hull and Camin 1960). In snakes,

and presumably in turtles, when more than about 4% of the erythrocytes are affected, anemia usually results (Fantham and Porter 1953–1954).

DIAGNOSIS

Diagnosis is based on detection of anemia and on demonstration of the parasite in stained blood smears (Fantham and Porter 1953–1954).

CONTROL

No treatment has been reported.

PUBLIC HEALTH CONSIDERATIONS

Haemogregarina does not affect man.

Pleistophora myotrophica

This pathogenic microsporidan occurs in the skeletal muscle of the European toad (Canning, Elkan, and Trigg 1964; Reichenbach-Klinke and Elkan 1965). It is common in laboratory toads in Great Britain (Canning, Elkan, and Trigg 1964).

MORPHOLOGY

The morphology varies with the stage of the life cycle (Fig. 17.15) (Canning, Elkan, and Trigg 1964). Schizonts contain up to 8 nuclei. Small sporonts have 2 or 3 nuclei but, when mature, they contain up to 100 nuclei. Spores are oval and measure 3.5 to 6.7 μ long by 2.0 to 3.0 μ wide. On one side of the anterior pole of each spore is a small granule to which is attached a filament. When extended, this filament is 80 to 220 μ long.

LIFE CYCLE

The life cycle of *Pleistophora myotrophica* is illustrated in Figure 17.15 (Canning, Elkan, and Trigg 1964). The sporoplasm is thought to hatch in the gut (*a*) and to migrate to the muscles by way of the blood vascular system. Eighteen days later, granular bodies are found in the muscle capillaries (*b*). Between 18 and 23 days, the parasite multiplies, first by binary fission (*c, d*), then by multiple fission (*e, f, g*), and finally by plasmotomy (*h, i*) until multinuclear sporonts are formed (*j–n*). Separation into sporoblasts (*o*) precedes spore formation (*p, q*). Spores are released on the death and decomposition of the host (Canning 1966; Canning, Elkan, and Trigg

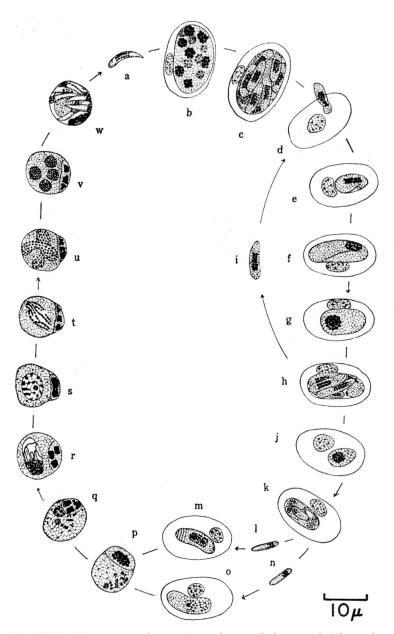

Fig. 17.14. *Haemogregarina stepanowi,* morphology and life cycle. a–o, schizogony and gametogony in turtle; p–w, sexual reproduction in bloodsucking invertebrate. (From Kudo 1966. Courtesy of Charles C Thomas, Publisher.)

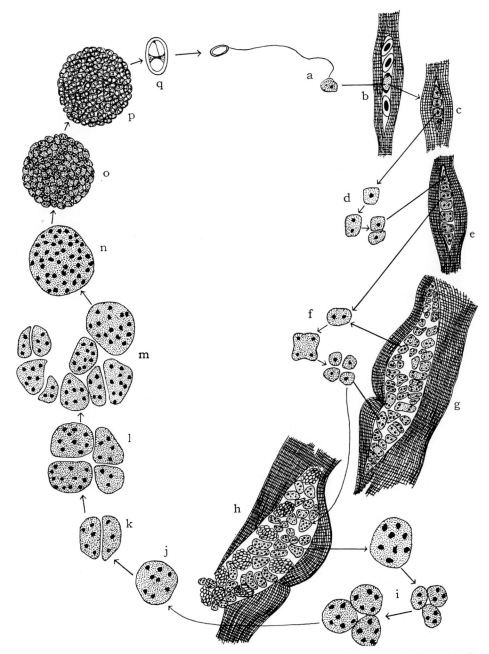

FIG. 17.15. *Pleistophora myotrophica,* morphology and life cycle in skeletal muscle of a toad. See explanation in text. (From Canning, Elkan, and Trigg 1964. Courtesy of Society of Protozoologists.)

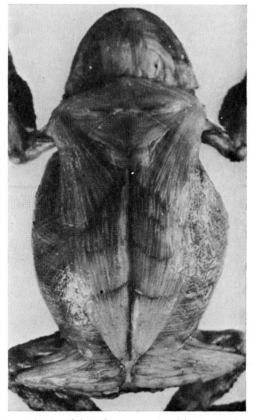

FIG. 17.16. *Pleistophora myotrophica* infection in European toad. Spores packed between muscle fibers appear as white lines. (Courtesy of E. Elkan, London.)

1964). Infection occurs by ingestion of a contaminated invertebrate that acts as a mechanical vector.

PATHOLOGIC EFFECTS

Infection with *P. myotrophica* causes anorexia, emaciation, and death (Canning, Elkan, and Trigg 1964). The skeletal muscle is atrophied and packed with spores, which appear at necropsy as white lines (Fig. 17.16). All stages of the parasite are seen in sections of muscle.

DIAGNOSIS

Diagnosis is based on the clinical signs and gross lesions and confirmed by demonstration of the parasite in histologic sections of muscle.

CONTROL

No treatment is known.

PUBLIC HEALTH CONSIDERATIONS

Pleistophora myotrophica does not affect man.

Dermocystidium, Dermosporidium

These parasites are of uncertain classification; they have some characteristics of a fungus and some of a sporozoan (Hoffman 1967; Reichenbach-Klinke and Elkan 1965). *Dermocystidium ranae* occurs in the grass frog, edible frog, and other frogs and *D. pusula* in newts in Europe. *Dermosporidium granulosum* occurs in the grass frog and *D. multigranulosum* in the edible frog in Europe. They are uncommon and are important only because they cause dermal cysts.

MORPHOLOGY

The immature stage appears as a hyaline-walled cyst filled with an amorphous mass containing chromatin granules (Hoffman 1967). Spores of *Dermocystidium* are round, measure 3 to 12 μ in diameter, and contain a nucleus and a large eccentric vacuole (Fig. 17.17). Those of *Dermosporidium* are 9 to 18 μ in diameter (Reichenbach-Klinke and Elkan 1965).

LIFE CYCLE

The life cycle is unknown (Hoffman 1967; Reichenbach-Klinke and Elkan

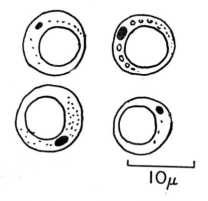

FIG. 17.17. *Dermocystidium.* (*Left*) *D. ranae* spores. (*Right*) *D. pusula* spores. (From Reichenbach-Klinke and Elkan 1965. Courtesy of Academic Press.)

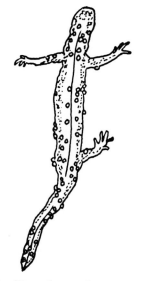

FIG. 17.18. Dermal cysts in a newt caused by *Dermocystidium pusula*. (From Reichenbach-Klinke and Elkan 1965. Courtesy of Academic Press.)

1965). Chromatin granules in the immature stage coalesce to form nuclei, and the protoplasmic mass reforms into spores. The method of transmission is unknown.

PATHOLOGIC EFFECTS

Both *D. ranae* and *D. pusula* cause the formation of dermal cysts (Fig. 17.18) (Reichenbach-Klinke and Elkan 1965). These cysts are often numerous and greatly debilitate the host. In histologic section they are seen to contain numerous spores. *Dermosporidium granulosum* and *D. multigranulosum* also cause the formation of spore-filled dermal cysts (Reichenbach-Klinke and Elkan 1965). Those of *D. granulosum* are semispherical and about 4 to 8 mm in diameter; those of *D. multigranulosum* are cylindrical and about 0.4 to 2.0 mm in diameter.

DIAGNOSIS

Diagnosis is based on the gross appearance of the cysts and identification of the causative agent in tissue sections.

CONTROL

Nothing is known of control.

PUBLIC HEALTH CONSIDERATIONS

These agents are not known to affect man.

CILIATES

The ciliates likely to be encountered in laboratory reptiles and amphibians are listed in Table 17.5. Most occur in the intestine and some on the skin and gills or in the urinary bladder or nervous tissue (Walton 1964). Most are commensals and none is known to be a pathogen (Kudo 1966; Wenyon 1926). The commonest are described below.

Balantidium

This nonpathogenic ciliate has an oval, ellipsoidal, or subcylindrical body with longitudinally, spirally arranged rows of cilia, a peristome at or near the anterior end, a poorly developed cytopharynx, an elongated or spherical macronucleus, and a micronucleus (Fig. 17.19) (Kudo 1966; Wenyon 1926). Reproduction is by conjugation and binary fission. Cysts are formed.

Balantidium entozoon, *B. elongatum*, and *B. duodeni* are the species most likely to be encountered in laboratory reptiles and amphibians (Reichenbach-Klinke and Elkan 1965; Walton 1964). *Balantidium entozoon* occurs in the intestine of the grass frog, edible frog, other frogs, European toad, common newt, and crested newt in Europe and measures about 100 to 300 μ in length. *Balantidium elongatum* occurs in the intestine of the grass frog, edible

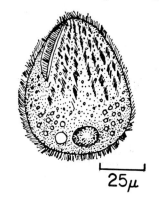

FIG. 17.19. *Balantidium duodeni*. (From Kudo 1966. Courtesy of Charles C Thomas, Publisher.)

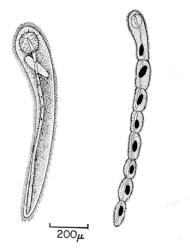

FIG. 17.20. *Haptophrya gigantea.* *(Left)* Single organism. *(Right)* Chain of organisms. (From Wenyon 1926.)

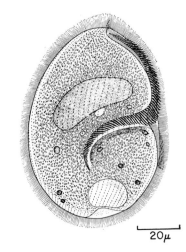

FIG. 17.21. *Nyctotherus cordiformis.* (From Wenyon 1926.)

frog, other frogs, alpine newt, common newt, and crested newt in Europe and Asia; it measures about 100 to 300 μ in length. *Balantidium duodeni,* which occurs in the intestine of the grass frog, edible frog, and other frogs in Europe and Asia, measures about 70 to 80 μ in length.

Haptophrya

This protozoan has an elongated, uniformly ciliated body with an anterior circular sucker and a long contractile canal (Fig. 17.20) (Kudo 1966; Wenyon 1926; Woodhead 1928). It multiplies by budding and often occurs as a chain of individuals. Nothing is known of its pathogenicity.

Haptophrya michiganensis and *H. gigantea* are the species most likely to be encountered in laboratory reptiles and amphibians (Reichenbach-Klinke and Elkan 1965; Walton 1964). *Haptophrya michiganensis* occurs in the intestine of the leopard frog, wood frog, and American toad and is common in the Jefferson salamander, marbled salamander, dusky salamander, axolotl, and other salamanders in the United States; it measures about 1.1 to 1.6 mm in length. *Haptophrya gigantea,* which is common in the intestine of the edible frog, other frogs, and toads in Europe and Africa and which has been reported from the slimy salamander *(Pletho-*

don glutinosus) in the United States (Rankin 1937), sometimes reaches 1.3 to 1.6 mm in length.

Nyctotherus

This nonpathogenic ciliate has an oval or reniform body, with a peristome that begins at the anterior end and extends along the side to about the middle of the body, a long esophagus, an elongated macronucleus, a small micronucleus, and a posterior contractile vacuole (Fig. 17.21) (Golikova 1963; Kudo 1966; Wenyon 1926). It varies in length from about 60 to 190 μ and from about 30 to 60 μ in width. Reproduction is by binary fission; cysts are sometimes formed.

Nyctotherus cordiformis is the commonest species. It occurs in the intestine of the leopard frog, green frog, bullfrog, grass frog, wood frog, pickerel frog, edible frog, cricket frogs, European treefrog, green treefrog, spring peeper, chorus frogs *(Pseudacris),* other frogs, American toad, European toad, other toads, red-spotted newt, California newt, and other newts throughout the world (Reichenbach-Klinke and Elkan 1965; Walton 1964).

Trichodina

This protozoan has a bell-shaped body with a highly developed basal adhesive disc, a skeletal ring with radially arranged denticles, and an adoral zone of cilia arranged in a spiral (Fig. 17.22) (Corliss 1959a; Kudo 1966; Lom 1958, 1970). Asexual reproduction is by binary fission and sexual reproduction by conjugation (Davis 1947).

Trichodina urinicola, T. pediculus, and T. fultoni are the species most likely to be encountered in laboratory amphibians (Kudo 1966; Lom 1958, 1970; Reichenbach-Klinke and Elkan 1965; Walton 1964). Trichodina urinicola occurs in the urinary bladder of the edible frog, toads, and newts in North America, Europe, and Africa. Trichodina pediculus occurs on the skin of the edible frog and other frogs in North America, Europe, and Asia. Trichodina fultoni occurs on the gills of mudpuppies in the United States; it measures 35 to 60 μ in diameter and 25 to 55 μ in height. None is common or of known pathogenicity.

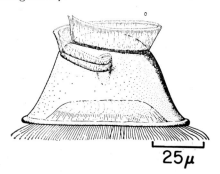

FIG. 17.22. Trichodina urinicola. (From Corliss 1959a. Courtesy of Society of Protozoologists.)

TABLE 17.1. Flagellates affecting laboratory reptiles and amphibians

Parasite	Geographic Distribution	Reptilian or Amphibian Host	Location in Host	Method of Infection	Incidence in Nature	Remarks	Reference
*Trypanosoma pipientis**	North America	Leopard frog, wood frog	Blood	Bite of leech	Common	Causes spleen enlargement	Diamond 1965 Woo 1969a
*Trypanosoma ranarum**	North America, Europe, Asia	Leopard frog, green frog, bullfrog, edible frog	Blood	Unknown; probably by bite of leech; possibly by bite of or ingestion of arthropod	Common	Apparently nonpathogenic	Diamond 1965 Woo 1969a
*Trypanosoma chattoni**	North America, Europe, Asia, Africa, South America	Leopard frog, green frog, bullfrog, treefrogs, other frogs, toads	Blood	Unknown; probably by bite of leech; possibly by bite of or ingestion of arthropod	Common	Pathologic effects unknown	Diamond 1965
Trypanosoma schmidti	Southeastern United States	Leopard frog	Blood	Unknown; probably by bite of leech; possibly by bite of or ingestion of arthropod	Unknown	Pathologic effects unknown	Diamond 1965
*Trypanosoma rotatorium**	Canada, Europe, Asia, Africa, South America	Leopard frog, green frog, bullfrog, edible frog, treefrogs, other frogs, European toad, other toads	Blood	Unknown; probably by bite of leech or bite of or ingestion of arthropod	Common in Europe; uncommon in Canada	Pathologic effects unknown	Diamond 1965 Woo 1969a
Trypanosoma canadensis	Canada	Leopard frog	Blood	Unknown; probably by bite of leech; possibly by bite of or ingestion of arthropod	Uncommon	Pathologic effects unknown	Diamond 1965 Woo 1969a
Trypanosoma gaumontis	Canada	Leopard frog, American toad	Blood	Unknown; probably by bite of leech; possibly by bite of or ingestion of arthropod	Uncommon	Pathologic effects unknown	Diamond 1965 Woo 1969a
Trypanosoma clamatae	North America	Green frog	Blood	Unknown; probably by bite of leech; possibly by bite of or ingestion of arthropod	Uncommon	Pathologic effects unknown	Diamond 1965 Woo 1969a
Trypanosoma parvum	North America	Green frog	Blood	Unknown; probably by bite of leech; possibly by bite of or ingestion of arthropod	Uncommon	Pathologic effects unknown	Diamond 1965 Woo 1969a
*Trypanosoma loricatum**	Europe, Asia	Edible frog, other frogs	Blood	Unknown; probably by bite of leech or bite of or ingestion of arthropod	Common	Pathologic effects unknown	Diamond 1965
*Trypanosoma inopinatum**	Southern Europe, northern Africa, India	Grass frog, edible frog, other frogs	Blood	Bite of leech	Common	Causes spleen destruction, death	Diamond 1965
Trypanosoma grylli	Southeastern United States	Cricket frogs	Blood	Unknown; probably by bite of leech; possibly by bite of or ingestion of arthropod	Uncommon	Pathologic effects unknown	Diamond 1965 Woo 1969a

* Discussed in text.

524

TABLE 17.1 (continued)

Parasite	Geographic Distribution	Reptilian or Amphibian Host	Location in Host	Method of Infection	Incidence in Nature	Remarks	Reference
Trypanosoma lavalia	Canada	American toad	Blood	Unknown; probably by bite of leech; possibly by bite of or ingestion of arthropod	Uncommon	Pathologic effects unknown	Diamond 1965 Woo 1969a
Trypanosoma montrealis	Canada	American toad	Blood	Unknown; probably by bite of leech; possibly by bite of or ingestion of arthropod	Uncommon	Pathologic effects unknown	Diamond 1965 Woo 1969a
*Trypanosoma diemyctyli**	United States	Red-spotted newt, other newts	Blood	Unknown; probably by bite of leech; possibly by bite of or ingestion of arthropod	Common	Heavy infections cause debilitation, anorexia, erythrocyte degeneration, death	Barrow 1958 Nigrelli 1929b Woo 1969a
Trypanosoma ambystomae	United States	Mole salamanders, California newt, other newts	Blood	Unknown; probably by bite of leech; possibly by bite of or ingestion of arthropod	Uncommon	Pathologic effects unknown	Walton 1964 Woo 1969a
Trypanosoma barbari	United States	California newt	Blood	Unknown; probably by bite of leech; possibly by bite of or ingestion of arthropod	Uncommon	Pathologic effects unknown	Walton 1964, 1966 Woo 1969a
Trypanosoma tritonis	Japan	Newts	Blood	Unknown; probably by bite of leech; possibly by bite of or ingestion of arthropod	Common	Pathologic effects unknown	Matubayasi 1937c
Trypanosoma chrysemydis	North America	Painted turtles, map turtle	Blood	Bite of leech	Uncommon	Pathologic effects unknown	Roudabush and Coatney 1937 Wenyon 1926 Woo 1969a, b
Trypanosoma thamnophis	North America	Garter snakes	Blood	Unknown; probably by bite of arthropod	Uncommon	Pathologic effects unknown	Fantham and Porter 1953–1954 Page 1966 Woo 1969a
Leishmania sp.	Western United States	Desert night lizard	Intestine	Unknown; probably by ingestion of invertebrate	Uncommon	Pathologic effects unknown	Honigberg 1950a
Leishmania henrici	West Indies	Anoles	Blood, intestine	Unknown; probably by bite of or ingestion of invertebrate	Uncommon	Pathologic effects unknown	Honigberg 1950a Wenyon 1926
Leishmania chamaeleonis	Africa	Chameleons	Intestine	Unknown; probably by ingestion of invertebrate	Uncommon	Pathologic effects unknown	Honigberg 1950a
Cryptobia sp.	United States	Marbled salamander, dusky salamanders, other salamanders, red-spotted newt	Blood	Unknown; probably by bite of invertebrate	Common	Incidence of 59% reported in red-spotted newt in eastern United States. Pathologic effects unknown	Rankin 1937 Walton 1964

*Discussed in text.

525

TABLE 17.1 (continued)

Parasite	Geographic Distribution	Reptilian or Amphibian Host	Location in Host	Method of Infection	Incidence in Nature	Remarks	Reference
Oodinium pillularis*	Europe	Frogs, newts, axolotl	Skin, gills	Direct contact with free-living stage in water	Unknown	Reported only in aquarium amphibians. Heavy infections cause gray coating on skin, gills; debilitation; impaired respiration; sometimes death	Geus 1960 Reichenbach-Klinke and Elkan 1965
Tritrichomonas augusta*	North America, Central America, South America, Europe, Asia	Leopard frog, green frog, bullfrog, grass frog, wood frog, edible frog, pickerel frog, cricket frogs, green treefrog, spring peeper, other frogs, American toad, common toad, European toad, other toads, Jefferson salamander, spotted salamander, marbled salamander, tiger salamander, dusky salamanders, other salamanders, red-spotted newt, California newt, other newts, European lizards	Large intestine	Ingestion of organism passed in feces	Common	Syn. Trichomonas augusta. Incidence of 100% reported in salamanders in eastern United States. Associated with liver lesions in leopard frog; otherwise, pathologic effects unknown	Honigberg 1950b, 1953, 1963 Rankin 1937 Reichenbach-Klinke and Elkan 1965 Walton 1964
Tritrichomonas nonconforma	Southeastern United States, West Indies	Green anole	Intestine	Ingestion of organism passed in feces	Common	Syn. Trichomonas hoplodactyli. Pathologic effects unknown	Honigberg 1963 Moskowitz 1951
Trichomitus batrachorum*	Worldwide	Leopard frog, bullfrog, edible frog, treefrogs, other frogs, American toad, common toad, European toad, South African clawed toad, other toads, Jefferson salamander, spotted salamander, tiger salamander, European salamanders, other salamanders, alpine newt, other newts, axolotl, water snakes, bullsnakes, garter snakes, other snakes, spiny lizards, horned lizards, European lizards, other lizards	Large intestine	Ingestion of organism passed in feces	Common	Syn. Tritrichomonas batrachorum, Trichomonas batrachorum, Trichomonas natricis. Pathologic effects unknown	Honigberg 1950b, 1953, 1963 Moskowitz 1951 Reichenbach-Klinke and Elkan 1965 Walton 1964, 1966

*Discussed in text.

TABLE 17.1 (continued)

Parasite	Geographic Distribution	Reptilian or Amphibian Host	Location in Host	Method of Infection	Incidence in Nature	Remarks	Reference
*Tetratrichomonas prowazeki**	United States, Europe, South America	Bullfrog, grass frog, other frogs, common toad, European toad, European salamanders, red-spotted newt, California newt, crested newt, amphiuma, water snakes, garter snakes	Large intestine	Ingestion of organism passed in feces	Common	Syn. *Trichomonas prowazeki*. Pathologic effects unknown	Honigberg 1951, 1963
Hypotrichomonas acosta	North America, Central America, South America, northern Africa, Asia	Racers, rat snakes, hognose snakes, kingsnakes, water snakes, bullsnakes, garter snakes, other snakes, beaded lizard, gila monster, other lizards	Large intestine	Ingestion of organism passed in feces	Common	Syn. *Trichomonas acosta*. Pathologic effects unknown	Honigberg 1963 Lee 1960 Moskowitz 1951
*Monocercomonas batrachorum**	United States, Europe, Asia, Africa	Grass frog, other frogs, toads, marbled salamander, dusky salamanders, other salamanders, red-spotted newt	Large intestine	Ingestion of organism passed in feces	Common	Syn. *Eutrichomastix batrachorum*. Incidence of 77% reported in red-spotted newt in eastern United States. Pathologic effects unknown	Honigberg 1963 Rankin 1937 Reichenbach-Klinke and Elkan 1965 Walton 1964
*Monocercomonas colubrorum**	North America, Europe, Asia, Africa	Racers, rat snakes, hognose snakes, kingsnakes, water snakes, bullsnakes, garter snakes, other snakes, chameleons, lizards	Large intestine	Ingestion of organism passed in feces	Common	Syn. *Trichomastix lacertae, T. serpentis, Eutrichomastix serpentis*. Pathologic effects unknown	Honigberg 1963 Moskowitz 1951
Monocercomonas moskowitz	North America, South America, Asia	Racers, other snakes, spiny lizards, other lizards	Intestine	Ingestion of organism passed in feces	Uncommon	Syn. *Monocercomonas mabuiae*. Pathologic effects unknown	Honigberg 1963 Moskowitz 1951
*Hexamastix batrachorum**	United States, Europe	Spotted salamander, marbled salamander, dusky salamanders, other salamanders, red-spotted newt, common newt	Intestine	Ingestion of organism passed in feces	Common	Syn. *Polymastix batrachorum*. Pathologic effects unknown	Honigberg 1963 Honigberg and Christian 1954 Rankin 1937 Reichenbach-Klinke and Elkan 1965 Walton 1964, 1966
Hexamastix kirbyi	Southwestern United States, Mexico	Horned lizards, spiny lizards, other lizards	Intestine	Ingestion of organism passed in feces	Uncommon	Pathologic effects unknown	Honigberg 1955
Hexamastix crassus	Southwestern United States, Mexico	Horned lizards, other lizards	Intestine	Ingestion of organism passed in feces	Uncommon	Pathologic effects unknown	Honigberg 1955

*Discussed in text.

TABLE 17.1 (continued)

Parasite	Geographic Distribution	Reptilian or Amphibian Host	Location in Host	Method of Infection	Incidence in Nature	Remarks	Reference
Trimitus parvus	United States, Europe	Leopard frog, grass frog, European toad, red-spotted newt, garter snakes	Intestine	Ingestion of organism passed in feces	Uncommon	Pathologic effects unknown	Grassé 1952 Honigberg 1963 Reichenbach-Klinke and Elkan 1965 Walton 1964, 1967
Retortamonas dobelli	United States, Europe	Leopard frog, grass frog, green frog, bullfrog, cricket frogs, other frogs, European toad, other toads, European salamanders, newts	Intestine	Ingestion of organism passed in feces	Uncommon	Apparently nonpathogenic	Bishop 1931 Reichenbach-Klinke and Elkan 1965 Walton 1964
Retortamonas saurarum	United States, Europe	Water snakes, pine snake, garter snakes, other snakes, gila monster, other lizards	Intestine	Ingestion of organism passed in feces	Uncommon	Pathologic effects unknown	Honigberg 1950a Moskowitz 1951
Retortamonas sp.	South America	Tortoises	Intestine	Ingestion of organism passed in feces	Uncommon	Pathologic effects unknown	Honigberg 1950a Wenyon 1926
Chilomastix caulleryi	United States, Europe	Leopard frog, European toad, other toads, spotted salamander, tiger salamander, European salamanders, newts, axolotl	Intestine	Ingestion of organism passed in feces	Uncommon	Syn. *Bodo ludibundus.* Apparently nonpathogenic	Reichenbach-Klinke and Elkan 1965 Walton 1964
Chilomastix sp.	United States	Tortoises, other turtles	Intestine	Ingestion of organism passed in feces	Uncommon	Pathologic effects unknown	Honigberg 1950a
Chilomastix bursa	Western United States, Mexico	Horned lizards, spiny lizards, night lizards, other lizards	Intestine	Ingestion of organism passed in feces	Uncommon	Pathologic effects unknown	Honigberg 1950a Moskowitz 1951
Chilomastix sp.	Northern Africa	European lizards, other lizards	Intestine	Ingestion of organism passed in feces	Uncommon	Pathologic effects unknown	Honigberg 1950a
Monocercomonoides rotunda	Europe	European toad, European salamanders	Intestine	Ingestion of organism passed in feces	Uncommon	Syn. *Retortamonas rotunda.* Pathologic effects unknown	Bishop 1932 Reichenbach-Klinke and Elkan 1965 Walton 1964
Monocercomonoides lacertae	North America, Asia	Gopher snake, other snakes, iguanas, horned lizards, spiny lizards, night lizards, other lizards	Intestine	Ingestion of organism passed in feces	Uncommon	Pathologic effects unknown	Honigberg 1950a Moskowitz 1951 Tanabe 1933
Trepomonas sp.	United States	Leopard frog, tiger salamander, dusky salamander, other salamanders	Intestine	Ingestion of organism passed in feces	Uncommon	Pathologic effects unknown	Honigberg 1950a Honigberg and Christian 1952 Walton 1964
Trepomonas agilis	Europe	Grass frog, edible frog, other frogs, newts	Intestine	Ingestion of organism passed in feces	Uncommon	Pathologic effects unknown	Honigberg 1950a Walton 1964

TABLE 17.1 (continued)

Parasite	Geographic Distribution	Reptilian or Amphibian Host	Location in Host	Method of Infection	Incidence in Nature	Remarks	Reference
Trepomemas sp.	United States	Box turtles, snapping turtles, other turtles	Intestine	Ingestion of organism passed in feces	Uncommon	Pathologic effects unknown	Honigberg 1950a
Hexamita intestinalis*	United States, Europe, Asia	Leopard frog, bullfrog, grass frog, edible frog, spring peeper, other frogs, European toad, other toads, spotted salamander, marbled salamanders, dusky salamanders, other salamanders, red-spotted newt, crested newt, California newt, other newts, axolotl	Large intestine	Ingestion of organism passed in feces	Common	Incidence of 88% reported in marbled salamander in eastern United States. Pathologic effects unknown	Honigberg 1950a Rankin 1937 Walton 1964
Hexamita batrachorum*	United States	Leopard frog, other frogs, common toad, other toads, spotted salamander, tiger salamander, dusky salamander, other salamanders, red-spotted newt, California newt	Large intestine	Ingestion of organism passed in feces	Common	Incidence of 42% reported in dusky salamanders in eastern United States. Pathologic effects unknown	Honigberg 1950a Rankin 1937 Walton 1964
Hexamita sp.	United States	Cricket frogs, toads, dusky salamander, other salamanders	Large intestine	Ingestion of organism passed in feces	Uncommon	Pathologic effects unknown	Honigberg 1950a
Hexamita sp.	Europe	Newts	Large intestine	Ingestion of organism passed in feces	Uncommon	Pathologic effects unknown	Honigberg 1950a
Hexamita parvus	North America, Europe, northern Africa, Asia	Pond turtles, European pond terrapin, tortoises, other turtles	Intestine, urinary bladder	Ingestion of organism passed in feces or urine	Uncommon	Pathologic effects unknown	Honigberg 1950a Walton 1964
Hexamita sp.	North America, Europe	Box turtles, snapping turtles, tortoises, other turtles	Large intestine	Ingestion of organism passed in feces	Uncommon	Pathologic effects unknown	Honigberg 1950a
Hexamita natrix	Japan	Water snakes	Stomach, small intestine	Ingestion of organism passed in feces	Uncommon	Pathologic effects unknown	Honigberg 1950a Matubayasi 1937a
Octomitus sp.	United States	Frogs	Large intestine	Ingestion of organism passed in feces	Uncommon	Pathologic effects unknown	Honigberg 1950a
Octomitus sp.	United States	Dusky salamander	Large intestine	Ingestion of organism passed in feces	Uncommon	Pathologic effects unknown	Honigberg 1950a
Octomitus sp.	Europe, Africa	European lizards, other lizards	Large intestine	Ingestion of organism passed in feces	Uncommon	Pathologic effects unknown	Honigberg 1950a

*Discussed in text.

TABLE 17.1 (continued)

Parasite	Geographic Distribution	Reptilian or Amphibian Host	Location in Host	Method of Infection	Incidence in Nature	Remarks	Reference
Giardia agilis	United States, Europe, Africa	Edible frog, other frogs, toads	Intestine	Ingestion of organism passed in feces	Uncommon	Syn. Giardia alata, G. gracilis, G. xenopi, G. xenopodis. Apparently nonpathogenic	Reichenbach-Klinke and Elkan 1965 Walton 1964
Giardia sp.	Europe	European pond terrapin	Small intestine	Ingestion of organism passed in feces	Uncommon	Pathologic effects unknown	Honigberg 1950a
Giardia sp.	North America	Kingsnakes	Small intestine	Ingestion of organism passed in feces	Unknown	Pathologic effects unknown	Fantham and Porter 1953–1954
Proteromonas longifila*	North America, South America, Europe	Leopard frog, other frogs, toads, Jefferson salamander, spotted salamander, marbled salamander, dusky salamander, European salamanders, other salamanders, red-spotted newt, other newts, axolotl	Rectum	Ingestion of organism passed in feces	Common	Possible syn. Proteromonas lacertae-viridis. Incidence of 89% reported in red-spotted newt in eastern United States. Pathologic effects unknown	Honigberg 1950a Rankin 1937 Reichenbach-Klinke and Elkan 1965 Walton 1964
Proteromonas regnardi	Europe	European pond terrapin	Rectum	Ingestion of organism passed in feces	Uncommon	Pathologic effects unknown	Honigberg 1950a
Proteromonas lacertae-viridis*	Worldwide	Snakes, iguanas, horned lizards, spiny lizards, European lizards, European chameleon, night lizards, other lizards	Rectum	Ingestion of organism passed in feces	Common in lizards	Possible syn. Proteromonas longifila. Pathologic effects unknown	Honigberg 1950a Moskowitz 1951
Karotomorpha bufonis*	North America, Europe	Leopard frog, European toad, other toads, tiger salamander, palmate newt, other newts, axolotl	Rectum	Ingestion of organism passed in feces	Common	Syn. Monocercomonas bufonis, Polymastix bufonis. Pathologic effects unknown	Rankin 1937 Walton 1964
Karotomorpha swezyi*	United States	Leopard frog, other frogs, American toad, other toads, dusky salamanders, other salamanders, red-spotted newt, California newt	Rectum	Ingestion of organism passed in feces	Common	Pathologic effects unknown	Rankin 1937 Walton 1964

*Discussed in text.

TABLE 17.2. Opalinids affecting laboratory amphibians

Parasite	Geographic Distribution	Reptilian or Amphibian Host	Location in Host	Method of Infection	Incidence in Nature	Remarks	Reference
Opalina obtrigonoidea[*]	United States	Leopard frog, wood frog, pickerel frog, green treefrog, spring peeper, cricket frogs, other frogs, American toad, other toads	Intestine	Ingestion of organism passed in feces	Common	Nonpathogenic	Kudo 1966 Walton 1964, 1966
Opalina carolinensis	United States	Leopard frog, other frogs, toads	Intestine	Ingestion of organism passed in feces	Uncommon	Nonpathogenic	Kudo 1966 Walton 1964
Opalina virguloidea	United States	Wood frog, spring peeper, other frogs	Intestine	Ingestion of organism passed in feces	Uncommon	Nonpathogenic	Walton 1964
Opalina ranarum[*]	Europe, Asia, northern Africa, South America	Grass frog, edible frog, European treefrog, other frogs, European toad, other toads, alpine newt	Intestine	Ingestion of organism passed in feces	Common	Nonpathogenic	Reichenbach-Klinke and Elkan 1965 Walton 1964, 1966 Wenyon 1926
Opalina chlorophili	United States	Spring peeper, other frogs	Intestine	Ingestion of organism passed in feces	Uncommon	Nonpathogenic	Kudo 1966 Walton 1964
Opalina hylaxena	United States	Spring peeper, other frogs	Intestine	Ingestion of organism passed in feces	Uncommon	Nonpathogenic	Kudo 1966 Walton 1964
Opalina discophrya	United States	American toad, other toads	Intestine	Ingestion of organism passed in feces	Uncommon	Nonpathogenic	Walton 1964
Opalina triangulata	United States	Common toad, other toads	Intestine	Ingestion of organism passed in feces	Uncommon	Nonpathogenic	Walton 1964
Opalina obtrigona	Europe	European treefrog	Intestine	Ingestion of organism passed in feces	Uncommon	Nonpathogenic	Reichenbach-Klinke and Elkan 1965 Walton 1964
Opalina cincta	Europe	European toad	Intestine	Ingestion of organism passed in feces	Uncommon	Nonpathogenic	Walton 1964
Protoopalina intestinalis[*]	Europe, Africa, Australia	Grass frog, edible frog, European treefrog, other frogs, toads, common newt, palmate newt	Intestine	Ingestion of organism passed in feces	Common	Nonpathogenic	Kudo 1966 Reichenbach-Klinke and Elkan 1965 Walton 1964 Weynon 1926
Protoopalina australis	Europe	European treefrog	Intestine	Ingestion of organism passed in feces	Uncommon	Nonpathogenic	Walton 1964
Protoopalina hylarum	Europe	European treefrog	Intestine	Ingestion of organism passed in feces	Uncommon	Nonpathogenic	Walton 1964
Protoopalina xenopodos	Africa	Clawed toads	Intestine	Ingestion of organism passed in feces	Uncommon	Nonpathogenic	Walton 1964
Protoopalina mitotica[*]	Central United States	Tiger salamander	Intestine	Ingestion of organism passed in feces	Uncommon	Nonpathogenic	Kudo 1966 Rankin 1937 Reichenbach-Klinke and Elkan 1965 Walton 1964

[*]Discussed in text.

531

TABLE 17.3. Sarcodines affecting laboratory reptiles and amphibians

Parasite	Geographic Distribution	Reptilian or Amphibian Host	Location in Host	Method of Infection	Incidence in Nature	Remarks	Reference
Entamoeba invadens*	Worldwide	Racers, kingsnakes, water snakes, garter snakes, other snakes, painted turtles, Greek tortoise, softshell turtles, green iguana, other lizards	Intestine, stomach, liver	Ingestion of organism passed in feces	Common	Syn. Entamoeba serpentis. Important pathogen of snakes, lizards. Causes anorexia; weight loss; ulcers in colon, ileum, stomach; necrotic foci in liver; death	Cowan 1968 Fantham and Porter 1953–1954; Geiman and Ratcliffe 1936 Marcus 1968 Meerovitch 1957, 1958 Page 1966 Ratcliffe 1961 Ratcliffe and Geiman 1934, 1938 Zwart 1964
Entamoeba ranarum*	United States, Europe, India, Philippine Islands	Leopard frog, green frog, bullfrog, grass frog, edible frog, other frogs, European toad, other toads, red-spotted newt, common newt, palmate newt, other newts	Intestine	Ingestion of organism passed in feces	Common	Considered to be nonpathogenic; associated once with liver abscess in grass frog	Geiman and Ratcliffe 1936 Kudo 1966 Walton 1964, 1966 Wenyon 1926
Entamoeba currens	Europe	Edible frog, European toad, other toads	Intestine	Ingestion of organism passed in feces	Uncommon	Pathologic effects unknown	Walton 1964
Entamoeba pyrrhogaster	United States	Red-spotted newt	Intestine	Ingestion of organism passed in feces	Uncommon	Pathologic effects unknown	Reichenbach-Klinke and Elkan 1965 Walton 1964
Entamoeba testudinis	United States, Europe	Greek tortoise, other tortoises, box turtles	Intestine	Ingestion of organism passed in feces	Uncommon	Pathologic effects unknown	Geiman and Wichterman 1937 Kudo 1966 Wenyon 1926
Entamoeba barreti	United States	Snapping turtles	Intestine	Ingestion of organism passed in feces	Uncommon	Pathologic effects unknown	Geiman and Wichterman 1937 Kudo 1966 Wenyon 1926
Entamoeba terrapinae	United States	Red-eared turtle	Intestine	Ingestion of organism passed in feces	Uncommon	Pathologic effects unknown	Geiman and Wichterman 1937 Kudo 1966
Entamoeba sp.	Canada, Great Britain	Garter snakes	Intestine	Ingestion of organism passed in feces	Uncommon	Pathologic effects unknown	Fantham and Porter 1953–1954
Endolimax ranarum	United States, Philippine Islands	Leopard frog, green frog, other frogs	Intestine	Ingestion of organism passed in feces	Uncommon	Pathologic effects unknown	Kudo 1966 Walton 1964, 1966
Endolimax clevelandi	United States	Cooter, box turtles	Intestine	Ingestion of organism passed in feces	Uncommon	Pathologic effects unknown	Gutierrez-Ballesteros and Wenrich 1950 Kudo 1966

*Discussed in text.

532

TABLE 17.3 *(continued)*

Parasite	Geographic Distribution	Reptilian or Amphibian Host	Location in Host	Method of Infection	Incidence in Nature	Remarks	Reference
Vahlkampfia ranarum	Europe	Frogs	Intestine	Ingestion of organism passed in feces	Uncommon	Pathologic effects unknown	Reichenbach-Klinke and Elkan 1965 Walton 1964 Wenyon 1926
Vahlkampfia froschi	Europe	Frogs	Intestine	Ingestion of organism passed in feces	Uncommon	Pathologic effects unknown	Walton 1964 Wenyon 1926
Vahlkampfia salamandrae	United States	Newts	Intestine	Ingestion of organism passed in feces	Uncommon	Pathologic effects unknown	Reichenbach-Klinke and Elkan 1965 Walton 1964
Vahlkampfia reynoldsi	United States	Eastern fence lizard	Intestine	Ingestion of organism passed in feces	Uncommon	Pathologic effects unknown	Reichenbach-Klinke and Elkan 1965
Vahlkampfia dobelli	Europe	Wall lizard	Intestine	Ingestion of organism passed in feces	Uncommon	Pathologic effects unknown	Reichenbach-Klinke and Elkan 1965
Copramoeba salamandrae	United States	Red-spotted newt	Intestine	Ingestion of organism passed in feces	Uncommon	Pathologic effects unknown	Reichenbach-Klinke and Elkan 1965 Walton 1964
Mastigamoeba hylae	United States, Europe, South America	Leopard frog, green frog, bullfrog, edible frog, treefrogs, toads, common newt	Intestine	Ingestion of organism passed in feces	Uncommon	Pathologic effects unknown	Kudo 1966 Reichenbach-Klinke and Elkan 1965 Walton 1964, 1967 Wenyon 1926

TABLE 17.4. Sporozoans affecting laboratory reptiles and amphibians

Parasite	Geographic Distribution	Reptilian or Amphibian Host	Location in Host	Method of Infection	Incidence in Nature	Remarks	Reference
Eimeria ranarum	United States, Europe	Grass frog, edible frog, marbled salamander	Intestine	Ingestion of oocyst passed in feces	Uncommon	Incidence of 6% reported in marbled salamander in eastern United States. Pathologic effects unknown	Pellérdy 1963 Rankin 1937 Reichenbach-Klinke and Elkan 1965 Saxe 1955 Walton 1964
Eimeria ranae	Europe	Grass frog, edible frog	Intestine	Ingestion of oocyst passed in feces	Uncommon	Pathologic effects unknown	Dobell 1909 Pellérdy 1963 Saxe 1955 Walton 1964
Eimeria neglecta	Europe	Grass frog, edible frog	Intestine	Ingestion of oocyst passed in feces	Uncommon	Pathologic effects unknown	Pellérdy 1963 Saxe 1955 Walton 1964
Eimeria prevoti	Europe	Edible frog	Intestine	Ingestion of oocyst passed in feces	Uncommon	Pathologic effects unknown	Pellérdy 1963 Saxe 1955 Walton 1964
Eimeria belawini	Europe	Treefrogs	Intestine	Ingestion of oocyst passed in feces	Uncommon	Pathologic effects unknown	Pellérdy 1963 Saxe 1955 Walton 1964
Eimeria mazai	Europe, Asia	European toad, other toads	Intestine	Ingestion of oocyst passed in feces	Uncommon	Syn. *Eimeria transcaucasia.* Pathologic effects unknown	Pellérdy 1963 Saxe 1955 Walton 1964
Eimeria grobbeni	United States, Europe	Tiger salamander, European salamanders, California newt	Intestine	Ingestion of oocyst passed in feces	Uncommon	Pathologic effects unknown	Doran 1953 Pellérdy 1963 Saxe 1955 Walton 1964
Eimeria ambystomae	United States	Tiger salamander, dusky salamanders	Intestine	Ingestion of oocyst passed in feces	Uncommon	Pathologic effects unknown	Pellérdy 1963 Saxe 1955 Walton 1964
Eimeria distorta	United States	Tiger salamander	Intestine	Ingestion of oocyst passed in feces	Uncommon	Pathologic effects unknown	Pellérdy 1963 Saxe 1955 Walton 1964
Eimeria kingi	United States	Tiger salamander	Intestine	Ingestion of oocyst passed in feces	Uncommon	Pathologic effects unknown	Pellérdy 1963 Saxe 1955 Walton 1964
Eimeria waltoni	United States	Tiger salamander	Intestine	Ingestion of oocyst passed in feces	Uncommon	Pathologic effects unknown	Pellérdy 1963 Saxe 1955 Walton 1964
Eimeria longaspora	United States	Red-spotted newt	Intestine	Ingestion of oocyst passed in feces	Uncommon	Pathologic effects unknown	Barrow and Hoy 1960 Pellérdy 1963 Walton 1964

TABLE 17.4 *(continued)*

Parasite	Geographic Distribution	Reptilian or Amphibian Host	Location in Host	Method of Infection	Incidence in Nature	Remarks	Reference
Eimeria megaresidua	United States	Red-spotted newt	Intestine	Ingestion of oocyst passed in feces	Uncommon	Pathologic effects unknown	Barrow and Hoy 1960 Pellérdy 1963 Walton 1964
Eimeria propria	Europe, Asia	European salamanders, common newt, alpine newt, crested newt, palmate newt, other newts	Intestine	Ingestion of oocyst passed in feces	Uncommon	Pathologic effects unknown	Matubayasi 1937c Pellérdy 1963 Saxe 1955 Walton 1964
Eimeria salamandrae	Europe	European salamanders	Intestine	Ingestion of oocyst passed in feces	Uncommon	Pathologic effects unknown	Pellérdy 1963 Saxe 1955 Walton 1964
Eimeria salamandra atrae	Europe	European salamanders	Intestine	Ingestion of oocyst passed in feces	Uncommon	Pathologic effects unknown	Pellérdy 1963 Saxe 1955 Walton 1964
Eimeria canaliculata	Europe	Common newt, alpine newt, crested newt, palmate newt	Intestine	Ingestion of oocyst passed in feces	Uncommon	Pathologic effects unknown	Pellérdy 1963 Saxe 1955 Walton 1964
Eimeria spherica	Europe, Asia	Common newt, alpine newt, crested newt, palmate newt, other newts	Intestine	Ingestion of oocyst passed in feces	Uncommon	Pathologic effects unknown	Matubayasi 1937c Pellérdy 1963 Saxe 1955 Walton 1964
Eimeria tertia	Europe	Alpine newt, crested newt	Intestine	Ingestion of oocyst passed in feces	Uncommon	Pathologic effects unknown	Pellérdy 1963 Saxe 1955 Walton 1964
*Eimeria bitis**	Canada	Garter snakes, other snakes	Gallbladder, bile duct	Ingestion of oocyst passed in feces	Uncommon	Causes denuding of mucosa, fibrosis of submucosa of gallbladder	Fantham and Porter 1953–1954 Pellérdy 1963
Eimeria annea	Canada	Garter snakes, green snakes	Unknown	Ingestion of oocyst passed in feces	Uncommon	Pathologic effects unknown	Vetterling and Widmer 1968
Eimeria zamenis	United States	Racers, kingsnakes, other snakes	Gallbladder	Ingestion of oocyst passed in feces	Uncommon	Pathologic effects unknown	Anderson et al. 1968 Roudabush 1937 Vetterling and Widmer 1968
Eimeria lampropeltis	Central United States	Kingsnakes	Unknown; oocyst found in feces	Ingestion of oocyst passed in feces	Uncommon	Pathologic effects unknown	Anderson et al. 1968
Eimeria tropidonoti	Europe	Water snakes	Intestine	Ingestion of oocyst passed in feces	Uncommon	Pathologic effects unknown	Pellérdy 1963 Vetterling and Widmer 1968 Wenyon 1926

*Discussed in text.

535

TABLE 17.4 (continued)

Parasite	Geographic Distribution	Reptilian or Amphibian Host	Location in Host	Method of Infection	Incidence in Nature	Remarks	Reference
Eimeria cystisfelleae	Europe	Water snakes	Bile duct	Ingestion of oocyst passed in feces	Uncommon	Pathologic effects unknown	Pellérdy 1963 Vetterling and Widmer 1968
Eimeria persica	Europe	Water snakes	Gallbladder	Ingestion of oocyst passed in feces	Uncommon	Pathologic effects unknown	Pellérdy 1963 Vetterling and Widmer 1968
Eimeria chrysemydis	United States	Painted turtle	Intestine	Ingestion of oocyst passed in feces	Uncommon	Pathologic effects unknown	Pellérdy 1963 Sampson and Ernst 1969
Eimeria delagei	United States, Europe	Painted turtle, European pond terrapin	Intestine	Ingestion of oocyst passed in feces	Uncommon	Pathologic effects unknown	Pellérdy 1963
Eimeria scriptae	Central United States	Red-eared turtle	Intestine	Ingestion of oocyst passed in feces	Uncommon	Pathologic effects unknown	Sampson and Ernst 1969
Eimeria pseudemydis	Central America	Cooters	Intestine	Ingestion of oocyst passed in feces	Uncommon	Pathologic effects unknown	Lainson 1968
Eimeria brodeni	Europe	Greek tortoise	Intestine	Ingestion of oocyst passed in feces	Uncommon	Pathologic effects unknown	Pellérdy 1963 Sampson and Ernst 1969
Eimeria chelydrae	Southeastern United States	Snapping turtle	Intestine	Ingestion of oocyst passed in feces	Uncommon	Pathologic effects unknown	Ernst et al. 1969
Eimeria amydae	United States	Softshell turtles	Intestine	Ingestion of oocyst passed in feces	Uncommon	Pathologic effects unknown	Pellérdy 1963 Roudabush 1937
Eimeria dericksoni	United States	Softshell turtles	Intestine	Ingestion of oocyst passed in feces	Uncommon	Pathologic effects unknown	Pellérdy 1963 Roudabush 1937
Eimeria crocodyli	Central America	American crocodile	Intestine	Ingestion of oocyst passed in feces	Uncommon	Pathologic effects unknown	Lainson 1968
Eimeria sceloporis	Southwestern United States, Mexico	Spiny lizards	Intestine	Ingestion of oocyst passed in feces	Uncommon	Pathologic effects unknown	Bovee and Telford 1965
Isospora lieberkühni*	Europe	Grass frog, edible frog, toads	Kidneys	Ingestion of oocyst passed in urine	Common	Pathologic effects unknown; heavy infections probably cause kidney damage	Pellérdy 1963 Reichenbach-Klinke and Elkan 1965 Walton 1964 Wenyon 1926
Isospora ranae	Europe	Edible frog	Intestine	Ingestion of oocyst passed in feces	Uncommon	Pathologic effects unknown	Pellérdy 1963 Walton 1964
Isospora hylae	Europe	Treefrogs	Intestine	Ingestion of oocyst passed in feces	Uncommon	Pathologic effects unknown	Pellérdy 1963 Walton 1964

*Discussed in text.

TABLE 17.4 (continued)

Parasite	Geographic Distribution	Reptilian or Amphibian Host	Location in Host	Method of Infection	Incidence in Nature	Remarks	Reference
Isospora wladimirovi	Europe	Treefrogs	Intestine	Ingestion of oocyst passed in feces	Uncommon	Pathologic effects unknown	Pellérdy 1963 Walton 1964
Isospora jeffersonianum	United States	Jefferson salamander	Intestine	Ingestion of oocyst passed in feces	Uncommon	Pathologic effects unknown	Doran 1953 Pellérdy 1963 Walton 1964
Isospora phisalix	Europe	Rat snakes	Intestine	Ingestion of oocyst passed in feces	Uncommon	Pathologic effects unknown	Pellérdy 1963
Isospora sp.	Asia	Rat snakes	Intestine	Ingestion of oocyst passed in feces	Common	Pathologic effects unknown	Matubayasi 1937b Pellérdy 1963
Isospora natricis	Europe	Water snakes	Intestine	Ingestion of oocyst passed in feces	Uncommon	Pathologic effects unknown	Pellérdy 1963
Isospora dirumpens	United States	Racer, rat snake, gopher snake	Intestine	Ingestion of oocyst passed in feces	Uncommon	Pathologic effects unknown	Pellérdy 1963 Roudabush 1937
Isospora wilkiei	Central America	American crocodile	Intestine	Ingestion of oocyst passed in feces	Uncommon	Pathologic effects unknown	Lainson 1968
Isospora basilisci	Central America	Basilisks	Intestine	Ingestion of oocyst passed in feces	Uncommon	Pathologic effects unknown	Lainson 1968
Isospora fragilis	Europe	Old World vipers,	Intestine	Ingestion of oocyst passed in feces	Uncommon	Pathologic effects unknown	Pellérdy 1963
Tyzzeria natrix	Asia	Water snakes	Intestine	Ingestion of oocyst passed in feces	Common	Pathologic effects unknown	Matubayasi 1937b Pellérdy 1963
Cyclospora viperae	Europe	Old World vipers, other snakes	Intestine	Ingestion of oocyst passed in feces	Uncommon	Pathologic effects unknown	Pellérdy 1963
Caryospora lampropeltis	Central United States	Kingsnakes	Unknown; oocysts found in feces	Ingestion of oocyst passed in feces	Uncommon	Pathologic effects unknown	Anderson et al 1968
Caryospora japonicum	Asia	Water snakes	Intestine	Ingestion of oocyst passed in feces	Common	Pathologic effects unknown	Matubayasi 1937b Pellérdy 1963
Caryospora simplex	Europe	Old World vipers	Intestine	Ingestion of oocyst passed in feces	Uncommon	Pathologic effects unknown	Kudo 1966 Pellérdy 1963
Cryptosporidium lampropeltis	Central United States	Kingsnakes	Unknown; oocysts found in feces	Unknown; probably ingestion of oocyst passed in feces	Uncommon	Uncertain if parasite of snakes; possibly parasite of rodent ingested by snake	Anderson et al. 1968 Duszynski 1969
Haemogregarina clamatae	United States	Leopard frog, green frog	Blood	Bite of leech or other bloodsucking invertebrate	Uncommon	Pathologic effects unknown	Walton 1964

537

TABLE 17.4 *(continued)*

Parasite	Geographic Distribution	Reptilian or Amphibian Host	Location in Host	Method of Infection	Incidence in Nature	Remarks	Reference
Haemogregarina catesbianae	United States	Bullfrog	Blood	Bite of leech or other bloodsucking invertebrate	Uncommon	Pathologic effects unknown	Walton 1964
Haemogregarina hortai	Europe	Edible frog	Blood	Bite of leech or other bloodsucking invertebrate	Uncommon	Pathologic effects unknown	Walton 1964
Haemogregarina boueti	Africa	Toads	Blood	Bite of leech or other bloodsucking invertebrate	Common	Incidence of 30% reported in northeastern Africa. Pathologic effects unknown	Mohammed and Mansour 1966
Haemogregarina aegyptia	Africa	Toads	Blood	Bite of leech or other bloodsucking invertebrate	Common	Pathologic effects unknown	Mohammed and Mansour 1966
Haemogregarina pestanae	Africa	Toads	Blood	Bite of leech or other bloodsucking invertebrate	Uncommon	Pathologic effects unknown	Mansour and Mohammed 1966a
Haemogregarina faiyumensis	Africa	Toads	Blood	Bite of leech or other bloodsucking invertebrate	Uncommon	Pathologic effects unknown	Mansour and Mohammed 1966b
*Haemogregarina stepanowi**	United States, Europe	Snapping turtle, painted turtles, Blanding's turtle, red-eared turtle, other cooters, box turtles, softshell turtles, European pond terrapin, other turtles	Blood	Bite of leech or tick	Common	Incidences of 45 to 75% reported in central and southern United States. Pathologic effects unknown; heavy infections probably cause anemia	Acholonu 1966 Edney 1949 Herban and Yaeger 1969 Krasilnikov 1965 Marquardt 1966 Marzinowsky 1927 Roudabush and Coatney 1937 Wang and Hopkins 1965
Haemogregarina ibera	Europe	Greek tortoise	Blood	Bite of leech or tick	Uncommon	Pathologic effects unknown	Krasilnikov 1965
*Haemogregarina sp.**	North America	Racer, rat snake, king-snakes, water snakes, bullsnakes, garter snakes, other snakes	Blood	Bite of leech or other bloodsucking invertebrate	Common	Incidence of 40% reported in central United States, 31% in central and southwestern United States. Heavy infections cause anemia	Fantham and Porter 1953–1954 Hull and Camin 1960 Marquardt 1966 Roudabush and Coatney 1937
Karyolysus lacertae	Europe	Wall lizard	Blood	Ingestion of mite	Uncommon	Pathologic effects unknown	Kudo 1966 Reichenbach-Klinke and Elkan 1965
Karyolysus bicapsulatus	Europe	Wall lizard	Blood	Ingestion of mite	Uncommon	Pathologic effects unknown	Reichenbach-Klinke and Elkan 1965

*Discussed in text.

TABLE 17.4 (continued)

Parasite	Geographic Distribution	Reptilian or Amphibian Host	Location in Host	Method of Infection	Incidence in Nature	Remarks	Reference
Karyolysus lacazei	Europe	Wall lizard	Blood	Ingestion of mite	Uncommon	Pathologic effects unknown	Reichenbach-Klinke and Elkan 1965
Karyolysus zuluetai	Europe	Wall lizard	Blood	Ingestion of mite	Uncommon	Pathologic effects unknown	Reichenbach-Klinke and Elkan 1965
Hepatozoon mauritanicum	Europe, Africa	Greek tortoise	Blood	Ingestion of tick	Uncommon	Pathologic effects unknown	Reichenbach-Klinke and Elkan 1965
Lankesterella minima	Europe, Africa, Asia, Central America, South America	Grass frog, edible frog, other frogs, toads	Blood	Bite of leech	Common	Syn. Dactylosoma ranarum. Incidence of 60% reported in edible frog in central Europe. Pathologic effects unknown	Kudo 1966 Pellérdy 1963 Wenyon 1926
Lankesterella canadensis	Canada	Bullfrog	Blood	Bite of leech	Uncommon	Pathologic effects unknown	Pellérdy 1963 Walton 1964
Lankesterella bufonis	Africa	Toads	Blood	Unknown; probably bite of leech	Uncommon	Pathologic effects unknown	Pellérdy 1963
Lankesterella tritonis	Europe	Crested newt	Blood	Unknown; probably bite of leech	Uncommon	Pathologic effects unknown	Pellérdy 1963
Plasmodium floridense	Southeastern United States, Central America	Green anole, spiny lizards	Blood	Bite of bloodsucking arthropod	Common	Heavy infections sometimes cause death	Garnham 1966 Jordan 1964
Plasmodium mexicanum	Southwestern United States, Mexico	Spiny lizards	Blood	Bite of bloodsucking arthropod	Common	Pathologic effects unknown	Ayala 1970 Ayala and Lee 1970 Garnham 1966 Pelaez et al. 1948
Plasmodium rhadinurum	Mexico, Central America, South America	Iguanas, other lizards	Blood	Bite of bloodsucking arthropod	Common	Causes discoloration of spleen, splenomegaly	Carini 1945 Garnham 1966
Simondia metchnikowi	North America, Europe, Asia, Africa, Australia	Painted turtle, Blanding's turtle, map turtle, red-eared turtle, softshell turtles, other turtles	Blood	Bite of bloodsucking invertebrate	Common	Pathologic effects unknown	DeGiusti 1965 Garnham 1966 Marquardt 1966 Wang and Hopkins 1965
Haemohormidium stableri	United States	Leopard frog	Blood	Bite of unknown bloodsucking arthropod	Uncommon	Pathologic effects unknown	Laird and Bullock 1969 Schmittner and McGhee 1961 Walton 1964
Haemohormidium jahni	United States	Red-spotted newt	Blood	Bite of unknown bloodsucking arthropod	Uncommon	Causes degeneration of erythrocytes	Laird and Bullock 1969 Nigrelli 1929a, b Walton, 1964

TABLE 17.4 (continued)

Parasite	Geographic Distribution	Reptilian or Amphibian Host	Location in Host	Method of Infection	Incidence in Nature	Remarks	Reference
Haemohormidium sp.	Europe	Greek tortoise	Blood	Bite of unknown bloodsucking arthropod	Uncommon	Pathologic effects unknown	Krasilnikov 1965
Tunetella emydis	Europe	Pond turtles	Blood	Bite of unknown bloodsucking arthropod	Uncommon	Pathologic effects unknown	Reichenbach-Klinke and Elkan 1965
Cytamoeba bacterifera	United States, Europe	Leopard frog, green frog, bullfrog, edible frog, mole frogs, mole salamanders, dusky salamanders, other salamanders, red-spotted newt, other newts, axolotl	Blood	Bite of unknown bloodsucking invertebrate	Common	Incidence of 35% in mole salamanders, 28 to 50% in dusky salamanders in eastern United States. Pathologic effects unknown	Rankin 1937 Reichenbach-Klinke and Elkan 1965 Walton 1964
Cytamoeba grassi	Europe	Treefrogs	Blood	Bite of unknown bloodsucking invertebrate	Uncommon	Pathologic effects unknown	Walton 1964
Leptotheca ohlmacheri	United States, Europe	Leopard frog, green frog, bullfrog, grass frog, edible frog, American toad, common toad, other toads	Kidneys	Unknown; probably ingestion of organism passed in urine	Common	Causes renal hypertrophy, congestion	Kudo 1930, 1966 Walton 1964 Wenyon 1926
Myxosoma ranae	Europe, Australia	Grass frog, treefrogs	Various tissues	Unknown; probably ingestion of spores released from tissue	Rare	Pathologic effects unknown	Reichenbach-Klinke and Elkan 1965 Walton 1964
Myxobolus conspicuus	United States	Red-spotted newt	Muscle	Unknown; probably ingestion of spores released from tissue	Uncommon	Incidence of 3% reported in eastern United States. Pathologic effects unknown	Rankin 1937 Reichenbach-Klinke and Elkan 1965 Walton 1964
Myxidium serotinum	United States	Leopard frog, green frog, other frogs, common toad	Gallbladder	Unknown; probably ingestion of organism passed in feces	Uncommon	Pathologic effects unknown	Kudo 1966 Kudo and Sprague 1940 Mitchell 1967 Walton 1964, 1966
Myxidium immersum	South America	Marine toad, other toads, frogs	Gallbladder	Unknown; probably ingestion of organism passed in feces	Common	Pathologic effects unknown	Kudo 1966 Kudo and Sprague 1940
Myxidium chelonarum	United States, Mexico	Painted turtle, map turtles, cooters, snapping turtle, other turtles	Bile duct, gallbladder	Unknown; probably ingestion of organism passed in feces	Common	Pathologic effects unknown	Johnson 1969

540

TABLE 17.4 *(continued)*

Parasite	Geographic Distribution	Reptilian or Amphibian Host	Location in Host	Method of Infection	Incidence in Nature	Remarks	Reference
Myxidium americanum	North central United States	Softshell turtles	Kidneys	Unknown; probably ingestion of organism passed in urine	Uncommon	Pathologic effects unknown	Hoffman 1967 Mitchell 1967
Pleistophora bufonis	United States, Europe	American toad, European toad	Bidder's organ	Unknown	Uncommon	Pathologic effects unknown	King 1907 Walton 1964
*Pleistophora myotrophica**	Europe	European toad	Muscle	Ingestion of invertebrate mechanical vector	Common in Great Britain	Causes anorexia, emaciation, death	Canning 1966 Canning et al. 1964 Reichenbach-Klinke and Elkan 1965
Glugea danilewskyi	Europe	Grass frog, European pond terrapin, water snakes	Muscle	Unknown	Uncommon	Causes intramuscular cysts	Kudo 1924 Reichenbach-Klinke and Elkan 1965 Walton 1964
Sarcocystis lacertae	Europe	Wall lizard	Muscle	Unknown	Uncommon	Pathologic effects unknown	Reichenbach-Klinke and Elkan 1965 Senaud and de Puytorac 1964–1965
*Dermocystidium ranae** (possibly a fungus)	Europe	Grass frog, edible frog, other frogs	Skin	Unknown	Uncommon	Causes dermal cysts	Reichenbach-Klinke and Elkan 1965
*Dermocystidium pusula** (possibly a fungus)	Europe	Newts	Skin	Unknown	Uncommon	Causes dermal cysts	Reichenbach-Klinke and Elkan 1965
*Dermosporidium granulosum** (possibly a fungus)	Europe	Grass frog	Skin	Unknown	Rare	Causes dermal cysts	Reichenbach-Klinke and Elkan 1965
*Dermosporidium multigranulosum** (possibly a fungus)	Europe	Edible frog	Skin	Unknown	Rare	Causes dermal cysts	Reichenbach-Klinke and Elkan 1965

*Discussed in text.

541

TABLE 17.5. Ciliates affecting laboratory reptiles and amphibians

Parasite	Geographic Distribution	Reptilian or Amphibian Host	Location in Host	Method of Infection	Incidence in Nature	Remarks	Reference
*Balantidium entozoon**	Europe	Grass frog, edible frog, other frogs, European toad, common newt, crested newt	Intestine	Ingestion of organism passed in feces	Common	Nonpathogenic	Reichenbach-Klinke and Elkan 1965 Walton 1964 Wenyon 1925
*Balantidium elongatum**	Europe, Asia	Grass frog, edible frog, other frogs, alpine newt, common newt, crested newt	Intestine	Ingestion of organism passed in feces	Common	Nonpathogenic	Reichenbach-Klinke and Elkan 1965 Walton 1964
*Balantidium duodeni**	Europe, Asia	Grass frog, edible frog, other frogs	Intestine	Ingestion of organism passed in feces	Common	Nonpathogenic	Kudo 1966 Reichenbach-Klinke and Elkan 1965 Walton 1964 Wenyon 1926
Balantidium helenae	Europe, Asia	Grass frog, edible frog, other frogs	Intestine	Ingestion of organism passed in feces	Common	Nonpathogenic	Walton 1964 Wenyon 1926
Balantidium nucleus	Europe	Grass frog, edible frog	Intestine	Ingestion of organism passed in feces	Common	Nonpathogenic	Walton 1964
Balantidium giganteum	Europe, Asia	Edible frog, other frogs	Intestine	Ingestion of organism passed in feces	Common	Nonpathogenic	Walton 1964 Wenyon 1926
Balantidium falciformis	United States	Pickerel frog	Intestine	Ingestion of organism passed in feces	Common	Nonpathogenic	Walton 1964
Balantidium sp.	North America	Green treefrog, wood frog, other frogs, American toad, other toads	Intestine	Ingestion of organism passed in feces	Unknown	Nonpathogenic	Walton 1964
Balantidium sp.	Africa	South African clawed toad	Intestine	Ingestion of organism passed in feces	Unknown	Nonpathogenic	Walton 1964
Balantidium amblystomatis	United States	Tiger salamander	Intestine	Ingestion of organism passed in feces	Common	Nonpathogenic	Reichenbach-Klinke and Elkan 1965 Walton 1964
Balantidium sp.	Asia	Newts	Intestine	Ingestion of organism passed in feces	Uncommon	Nonpathogenic	Matubayasi 1937c
Balantidium testudinis	South America, Asia, Africa	Greek tortoise, other tortoises	Intestine	Ingestion of organism passed in feces	Uncommon	Nonpathogenic	Geiman and Wichterman 1937 Wenyon 1926
Balantidium sp.	West Indies	Iguanas, other lizards	Intestine	Ingestion of organism passed in feces	Uncommon	Nonpathogenic	L. H. Saxe, personal communication
Glaucoma sp.	United States	Axolotl	Brain, spinal cord	Unknown	Unknown	Pathologic effects unknown	Reichenbach-Klinke and Elkan 1965 Walton 1964

*Discussed in text.

TABLE 17.5 (continued)

Parasite	Geographic Distribution	Reptilian or Amphibian Host	Location in Host	Method of Infection	Incidence in Nature	Remarks	Reference
Haptophrya michiganensis*	United States	Leopard frog, wood frog, American toad, Jefferson salamander, marbled salamanders, dusky salamanders, other salamanders, axolotl	Intestine	Ingestion of organism passed in feces	Common in salamanders, axolotl	Pathologic effects unknown	Kudo 1966, Rankin 1937, Reichenbach-Klinke and Elkan 1965, Walton 1964, Woodhead 1928
Haptophrya gigantea*	United States, Europe, Africa	Edible frog, other frogs, toads, salamanders	Intestine	Ingestion of organism passed in feces	Common in Europe, northern Africa	Pathologic effects unknown	Rankin 1937, Reichenbach-Klinke and Elkan 1965, Walton 1964
Haptophrya virginiensis	United States	Pickerel frog	Intestine	Ingestion of organism passed in feces	Uncommon	Pathologic effects unknown	Kudo 1966, Walton 1964
Haptophrya tritonis	Europe	Alpine newt	Intestine	Ingestion of organism passed in feces	Uncommon	Pathologic effects unknown	Reichenbach-Klinke and Elkan 1965, Walton 1964
Nyctotherus cordiformis*	Worldwide	Leopard frog, green frog, bullfrog, grass frog, wood frog, pickerel frog, edible frog, green treefrog, spring peeper, European treefrog, cricket frogs, other frogs, American toad, European toad, other toads, red-spotted newt, California newt, other newts	Intestine	Ingestion of organism passed in feces	Common	Nonpathogenic	Kudo 1966, Rankin 1937, Reichenbach-Klinke and Elkan 1965, Walton 1964, Wenyon 1926
Nyctotherus kyphodes	Asia	Tortoises	Intestine	Ingestion of organism passed in feces	Uncommon	Nonpathogenic	Geiman and Wichterman 1937
Nyctotherus teleascus	Asia	Tortoises	Intestine	Ingestion of organism passed in feces	Uncommon	Nonpathogenic	Geiman and Wichterman 1937
Nyctotherus sp.	West Indies	Iguanas, other lizards	Intestine	Ingestion of organism passed in feces	Uncommon	Nonpathogenic	L. H. Saxe, personal communication
Trichodina urinicola*	North America, Europe, Africa	Edible frog, toads, common newt, crested newt, palmate newt	Urinary bladder	Direct contact with organism in water	Uncommon	Pathologic effects unknown	Kudo 1966, Lom 1958, Reichenbach-Klinke and Elkan 1965, Walton 1964
Trichodina pediculus*	North America, Europe, Asia	Edible frog, other frogs	Skin	Direct contact with organism in water	Unknown	Pathologic effects unknown	Kudo 1966, Lom 1970, Reichenbach-Klinke and Elkan 1965, Walton 1964
Trichodina fultoni*	United States	Mudpuppy	Gills	Direct contact with organism in water	Uncommon	Pathologic effects unknown	Hoffman 1967, Lom 1970, Rankin 1937, Walton 1964

*Discussed in text.

REFERENCES

Acholonu, A. D. 1966. Occurrence of *Hae-mogregarina* (Protozoa) in Louisiana turtles. J. Protozool. 13:20.

Anderson, D. R., D. W. Duszynski, and W. C. Marquardt. 1968. Three new coccidia (Protozoa: Telosporea) from kingsnakes, *Lampropeltis* spp., in Illinois, with a redescription of *Eimeria zamenis* Phisalix, 1921. J. Parasitol. 54:577–81.

Anderson, J. R., and S. C. Ayala. 1968. Trypanosome transmitted by *Phlebotomus:* First report from the Americas. Science 161:1023–25.

Ayala, S. C. 1970. Lizard malaria in California; description of a strain of *Plasmodium mexicanum,* and biogeography of lizard malaria in western North America. J. Parasitol. 56:417–25.

Ayala, S. C., and D. Lee. 1970. Saurian malaria: Development of sporozoites in two species of phlebotomine sandflies. Science 167:891–92.

Barrow, J. H., Jr. 1958. The biology of *Trypanosoma diemyctyli,* Tobey: III. Factors influencing the cycle of *Trypanosoma diemyctyli* in the vertebrate host *Triturus* v. *viridescens.* J. Protozool. 5:161–70.

Barrow, J. H., Jr., and J. B. Hoy. 1960. Two new species of *Eimeria* from the common newt, *Notopthalmus viridescens.* J. Protozool. 7:217–21.

Bishop, Ann. 1931. A description of *Embadomonas* n. spp. from *Blatta orientalis, Rana temporaria, Bufo vulgaris, Salamandra maculosa;* with a note upon the "cyst" of *Trichomonas batrachorum.* Parasitology 23:286–300.

———. 1932. A note upon *Retortamonas rotunda* n. sp., an intestinal flagellate in *Bufo vulgaris.* Parasitology 24:233–37.

Bovee, E. C., and S. R. Telford, Jr. 1965. *Eimeria sceloporis* and *Eimeria molochis* spp. n. from lizards. J. Parasitol. 51:85–94.

Canning, E. U. 1966. The transmission of *Plistophora myotrophica,* a microsporidian infecting the voluntary muscles of the common toad, pp. 446–47. *In* A. Corradetti, ed. Proc. First Intern. Congr. Parasitol. Pergamon Press, New York.

Canning, E. U., E. Elkan, and P. I. Trigg. 1964. *Plistophora myotrophica* spec. nov., causing high mortality in the common toad *Bufo bufo* L., with notes on the maintenance of *Bufo* and *Xenopus* in the laboratory. J. Protozool. 11:157–66.

Carini, A. 1945. Consideracões sobre o *Plasmodium rhadinarum* [*sic*] (Thompson e Huff 1944) da iguana. Arquiv. Biol. (São Paulo) 29:147–49.

Cheng, T. C. 1964. The biology of animal parasites. W. B. Saunders, Philadelphia. 727 pp.

Corliss, J. O. 1959a. An illustrated key to the higher groups of the ciliated protozoa, with definition of terms. J. Protozool. 6:265–81.

———. 1959b. Comments on the systematics and phylogeny of the protozoa. Syst. Zool. 8:169–90.

Cowan, D. F. 1968. Diseases of captive reptiles. J. Am. Vet. Med. Assoc. 153:848–59.

Davis, H. S. 1947. Studies of the protozoan parasites of fresh-water fishes. U.S. Fish Wildlife Serv. Fishery Bull. 41. 29 pp.

DeGiusti, D. L. 1965. *Haemoproteus metchnikovi* of cheloneans, its tissue phases, peripheral parasitemia, host specificity, and geographical distribution, p. 176. *In* Ph. Vuysje, ed. Progress in protozoology. Excerpta Medica Foundation, New York.

Diamond, L. S. 1965. A study of the morphology, biology and taxonomy of the trypanosomes of anura. Wildlife Disease 44. 77 pp. (Microfiche).

Dobell, C. C. 1909. Researches on the intestinal protozoa of frogs and toads. Quart. J. Microscop. Sci. 53:201–77.

Doran, D. J. 1953. *Isospora jeffersoni* n. sp. from the blue spotted salamander *Ambystoma jeffersonianum* (Green), and *Eimeria grobbeni* Rudovsky, 1925 from California newt *Triturus torosus* (Rathke). Proc. Helminthol. Soc. Wash. D.C. 20:60–61.

Duszynski, D. W. 1969. Two new coccidia (Protozoa: Eimeriidae) from Costa Rican lizards with a review of the *Eimeria* from lizards. J. Protozool. 16:581–85.

Edney, J. M. 1949. *Haemogregarina stepanowi* Danilewsky (1885) in middle Tennessee turtles. J. Tenn. Acad. Sci. 24:220–23.

Ernst, J. V., T. B. Stewart, J. R. Sampson, and G. T. Fincher. 1969. *Eimeria chelydrae* n. sp. (Protozoa: Eimeriidae) from the snapping turtle, *Chelydra serpentina.* Bull. Wildlife Dis. Assoc. 5:410–11.

Fantham, H. B., and Annie Porter. 1953–1954. The endoparasites of some North American snakes and their effects on the Ophidia. Proc. Zool. Soc. London 123:867–98.

Garnham, P. C. C. 1966. Malaria parasites and other haemosporidia. Blackwell Scientific Publ., Oxford. 1114 pp.

Geiman, Q. M., and H. L. Ratcliffe. 1936. Morphology and life-cycle of an amoeba producing amoebiasis in reptiles. Parasitology 28:208–28.

Geiman, Q. M., and R. Wichterman. 1937. Intestinal protozoa from Galapagos tortoises (with descriptions of three new species). J. Parasitol. 23: 331–47.

Geus, A. 1960. Nachträgliche Bemerkungen zur Biologie des fischpathogenen Dinoflagellaten *Oodinium pillularis* Schäperclaus. Aquar. Terrar. Z. 13:305–6.

Golikova, M. N. 1963. Morphological and cytochemical study of the life cycle of *Nyctotherus cordiformis* Stein (in Russian). Acta Protozool. 1:31–42.

Grassé, P.-P. 1952. Traité de zoologie, anatomie, systémique, biologie. Vol. 1. Phylogénie, Protozoaires: generalités. Flagellés. Fasc. 1. 1064 pp. Masson, Paris.

Gutierrez-Ballesteros, E., and D. H. Wenrich. 1950. *Endolimax clevelandi*, n. sp., from turtles. J. Parasitol. 36:489–93.

Herban, Nancy L., and R. G. Yaeger. 1969. Blood parasites of certain Louisiana reptiles and amphibians. Am. Midland Naturalist 82:600–601.

Hoffman, G. L. 1967. Parasites of North American freshwater fishes. Univ. California Press, Berkeley. 486 pp.

Honigberg, B. M. 1950a. Intestinal flagellates of amphibians and reptiles. I. Survey of intestinal flagellates of reptiles. II. Structure and morphogenesis of the members of the genus *Trichomonas* Donné, 1836 from amphibians and reptiles. Doctoral dissertation, Univ. of California, Berkeley. 260 pp.

———. 1950b. On the structure of the parabasal body in *Tritrichomonas batrachorum* (Perty) and *Tritrichomonas augusta* (Alexeieff) of amphibians and reptiles. J. Parasitol. 36:89.

———. 1951. Structure and morphogenesis of *Trichomonas prowazeki* Alexeieff and *Trichomonas brumpti* Alexeieff. Univ. Calif. Publ. Zool. 55:337–94.

———. 1953. Structure, taxonomic status, and host list of *Tritrichomonas batrachorum* (Perty). J. Parasitol. 39:191–208.

———. 1955. Structure and morphogenesis of two new species of *Hexamastix* from lizards. J. Parasitol. 41:1–17.

———. 1963. Evolutionary and systematic relationships in the flagellate order Trichomonadida Kirby. J. Protozool. 10:20–63.

Honigberg, B. M., W. Balamuth, E. C. Bovee, J. O. Corliss, M. Gojdics, R. P. Hall, R. R. Kudo, N. D. Levine, A. R. Loeblich, Jr., J. Weiser, and D. H. Wenrich. 1964. A revised classification of the phylum Protozoa. J. Protozool. 11:7–20.

Honigberg, B. M., and H. H. Christian. 1952. Intestinal flagellates of *Ambystoma macu-*

latum (Shaw) and *Ambystoma trigrinum* (Green). J. Parasitol. 38:274.

———. 1954. Characteristics of *Hexamastix batrachorum* (Alexeieff). J. Parasitol. 40:508–14.

Hull, R. W., and J. H. Camin. 1960. Haemogregarines in snakes: The incidence and identity of the erythrocytic stages. J. Parasitol. 46:515–23.

Jacobs, D. L. 1946. A new parasitic dinoflagellate from fresh-water fish. Trans. Am. Microscop. Soc. 65:1–17.

Johnson, C. A., III. 1969. A redescription of *Myxidium chelonarum* Johnson, 1969 (Cnidospora: Myxidiidae) from various North American turtles. J. Protozool. 16:700–702.

Jordan, Helen B. 1964. Lizard malaria in Georgia. J. Protozool. 11:562–66.

King, Helen D. 1907. *Bertramia bufonis*, a new sporozoan parasite of *Bufo lentiginosus*. Proc. Acad. Nat. Sci. Phila. 59:273–78.

Krasilnikov, E. N. 1965. Blood parasites of turtles of southeast Georgia (in Russian). Zool. Zh. 44:1454–60.

Kudo, R. R. 1924. A biologic and taxonomic study of the Microsporidia. III. Biol. Monographs 9:79–346.

———. 1930. Myxosporidia, pp. 303–24. *In* R. Hegner and J. Andrews, eds. Problems and methods of research in protozoology. Macmillan, New York.

———. 1966. Protozoology. 5th ed. Charles C Thomas, Springfield, Ill. 1174 pp.

Kudo, R. R., and V. Sprague. 1940. On *Myxidium immersum* (Lutz) and *M. serotinum* n. sp., two myxosporidian parasites of Salientia of South and North America. Rev. Med. Trop. Parasitol. Bacteriol. Clin. Lab. 6:65–73.

Lainson, R. 1968. Parasitologic studies in British Honduras: IV. Some coccidial parasites of reptiles. Ann. Trop. Med. Parasitol. 62:260–66.

Laird, M., and W. L. Bullock. 1969. Marine fish haematozoa from New Brunswick and New England. J. Fisheries Res. Board Can. 26:1075–1102.

Lee, J. J. 1960. *Hypotrichomonas acosta* (Moskowitz) gen. nov. from reptiles: I. Structure and division. J. Protozool. 7:393–401.

Levine, N. D. 1961. Protozoan parasites of domestic animals and of man. Burgess, Minneapolis. 412 pp.

Lom, J. 1958. A contribution to the systematics and morphology of endoparasitic trichodinids from amphibians, with a proposal of uniform specific characteristics. J. Protozool. 5:251–63.

Lom, J. 1970. Observations on trichodinid ciliates from freshwater fishes. Arch. Protistenk. 112:153–77.

Mansour, N. S., and A. H. H. Mohammed. 1966a. Development of *Haemogregarina pestanae* in the toad *Bufo regularis*. J. Protozool. 13:265–69.

———. 1966b. *Haemogregarina faiyumensis* n. sp. in the toad *Bufo regularis* in Egypt. J. Protozool. 13:269–71.

Marcus, L. C. 1968. Diseases of snakes and turtles, pp. 435–42. *In* R. W. Kirk, ed. Current veterinary therapy III: Small animal practice. W. B. Saunders, Philadelphia.

Marquardt, W. C. 1966. Haemogregarines and *Haemoproteus* in some reptiles in southern Illinois. J. Parasitol. 52:823–24.

Marzinowsky, E. 1927. Du développement de l'*Haemogregarina stepanovi*. Ann. Parasitol. Humaine Comparee 5:140–42.

Matubayasi, H. 1937a. Studies on parasitic protozoa in Japan: I. On flagellates parasitic in snakes. Annot. Zool. Japon. 16:245–53.

———. 1937b. Studies on parasitic protozoa in Japan: II. Coccidia parasitic in snakes; with special remarks on *Tyzzeria (Koidzumiella) natrix*, parasitic in *Natrix tigrina*. Annot. Zool. Japon. 16:255–75.

———. 1937c. Studies on parasitic protozoa in Japan: III. On protozoa parasitic in the newt, *Triturus pyrrhogaster*. Annot. Zool. Japon. 16:277–91.

Meerovitch, E. 1957. On the relation of the biology of *Entamoeba invadens* to its pathogenicity in snakes. J. Parasitol. 43 (Supp.):41.

———. 1958. A new host of *Entamoeba invadens* Rodhain, 1934. Can. J. Zool. 36: 423–27.

Mitchell, L. G. 1967. *Myxidium macrocheili* n. sp. (Cnidospora: Myxidiidae) from the largescale sucker *Catostomus macrocheilus* Girard, and a synopsis of the *Myxidium* of North American freshwater vertebrates. J. Protozool. 14:415–24.

Mohammed, A. H. H., and N. S. Mansour. 1966. Development of *Haemogregarina boueti* in the toad *Bufo regularis*. J. Protozool. 13:259–64.

Moskowitz, N. 1951. Observations on some intestinal flagellates from reptilian host (Squamata). J. Morphol. 89:257–321.

Nigrelli, R. F. 1929a. *Dactylosoma jahni* sp. nov., a sporozoan parasite of the erythrocytes and erythroplastids of *Triturus viridescens*. Anat. Record 44:249.

———. 1929b. Atypical erythrocytes and erythroplastids in the blood of *Triturus viridescens*. Anat. Record 43:257–70.

Noble, G. K. 1931. The biology of the Amphibia. McGraw-Hill, New York, 577 pp.

O'Connor, Patricia. 1966. Diseases of snakes, pp. 582–85. *In* R. W. Kirk, ed. Current veterinary therapy 1966–1967: Small animal practice. W. B. Saunders, Philadelphia.

Page, L. A. 1966. Diseases and infections of snakes: A review. Bull. Wildlife Dis. Assoc. 2:111–26.

Pelaez, D., R. Perez-Reyes, and A. Barrera. 1948. Estudios sobre hematozoarios: I. *Plasmodium mexicanum* Thompson y Huff, 1944, en sus huéspedes naturales. Anales Escuela Nac. Cienc. Biol. Mex. 5:197–215.

Pellérdy, L. P. 1963. Catalogue of Eimeriidea (Protozoa: Sporozoa). Akadémiai Kiadó, Budapest. 160 pp.

Rankin, J. S. 1937. An ecological study of parasites of some North Carolina salamanders. Ecol. Monographs 7:169–269.

Ratcliffe, H. L. 1961. Report of the Penrose Research Laboratory of the Zoological Society of Philadelphia. 18 pp.

Ratcliffe, H. L., and Q. M. Geiman. 1934. Amebiasis in reptiles. Science 79:324–25.

———. 1938. Spontaneous and experimental amebic infection in reptiles. Arch. Pathol. 25:160–84.

Reichenbach-Klinke, H., and E. Elkan. 1965. The principal diseases of lower vertebrates. Academic Press, New York. 600 pp.

Roudabush, R. L. 1937. Some coccidia of reptiles found in North America. J. Parasitol. 23:354–59.

Roudabush, R. L., and G. R. Coatney. 1937. On some blood protozoa of reptiles and amphibians. Trans. Am. Micro. Soc. 56: 291–97.

Sampson, J. R., and J. V. Ernst. 1969. *Eimeria scriptae* n. sp. (Sporozoa: Eimeriidae) from the red-eared turtle *Pseudemys scripta elegans*. J. Protozool. 16:444–45.

Saxe, L. H. 1955. Observations on *Eimeria* from *Ambystoma tigrinum*, with descriptions of four new species. Proc. Iowa Acad. Sci. 62:663–73.

Schmittner, Stella M., and R. B. McGhee. 1961. The intra-erythrocytic development of *Babesiosoma stableri* n. sp. in *Rana pipiens pipiens*. J. Protozool. 8:381–86.

Senaud, J., and P. de Puytorac. 1964–1965. Observation de la Sarcosporidie du lézard (*Lacerta muralis*). Arch. Zool. Exp. Gen. 104:182–86.

Tanabe, M. 1933. The morphology and division of *Monocercomonas lacertae* n. sp.

from a lizard. Keijo J. Med. 4:367–77.

Vetterling, J. M., and E. A. Widmer. 1968. *Eimeria cascabeli* sp. n. (Eimeriidae: Sporozoa) from rattlesnakes, with a review of the species of *Eimeria* from snakes. J. Parasitol. 54:569–76.

Wallach, J. D. 1969. Medical care of reptiles. J. Am. Vet. Med. Assoc. 155:1017–34.

Walton, A. C. 1964. The parasites of Amphibia. Wildlife Disease 40. (Microcard and microfiche).

———. 1966. Supplemental catalog of the parasites of Amphibia. Wildlife Disease 48. 58 pp. (Microfiche).

———. 1967. Supplemental catalog of the parasites of Amphibia. Wildlife Disease 50. 38 pp. (Microfiche).

Wang, C. C., and S. H. Hopkins. 1965. *Haemogregarina* and *Haemoproteus* (Protozoa, Sporozoa) in blood of Texas freshwater turtles. J. Parasitol. 51:682–83.

Wenyon, C. M. 1926. Protozoology. 2 vol. Hafner, New York.

Woo, P. T. K. 1969a. Trypanosomes in amphibians and reptiles in southern Ontario. Can. J. Zool. 47:981–88.

———. 1969b. The life cycle of *Trypanosoma chrysemydis*. Can. J. Zool. 47:1139–51.

Woodhead, A. E. 1928. *Haptophrya michiganensis* sp. nov., a protozoan parasite of the four-toed salamander. J. Parasitol. 14:177–82.

Zwart, P. 1964. Studies on renal pathology in reptiles. Pathol. Vet. 1:542–56.

Chapter 18

HELMINTHS and LEECHES

HUNDREDS of helminths and many annelids have been reported in and on reptiles and amphibians, but the information concerning most of them is incomplete. Only those which are apparently common or likely to be encountered in reptiles and amphibians used in the laboratory are described in this chapter.

Most laboratory amphibians and reptiles are obtained from their natural habitat and only a few are raised in the laboratory (Nace 1968). Those obtained from nature are invariably parasitized (Nace 1968). Those raised in the laboratory have a lower incidence of infection because of the absence of intermediate hosts, but completely parasite-free colonies of reptiles and amphibians have not yet been developed.

MONOGENETIC, ASPIDOBOTHRETIC TREMATODES

Monogenetic trematodes have a direct life cycle involving a single host (Noble and Noble 1964; Reichenbach-Klinke and Elkan 1965). Most species that affect amphibians and reptiles are ectoparasites; however, some occur in the urinary bladder, nose, mouth, esophagus, and lungs.

Aspidobothretic trematodes also have a direct life cycle that usually involves a single host (a freshwater clam) (Olsen 1967). They have no asexual generations, but an alternation of hosts occurs in some species. Some of these parasites are occasionally found as accidental inhabitants of the digestive tract of turtles.

Few monogenetic and aspidobothretic trematodes appear to be important pathogens. Those likely to be found affecting laboratory reptiles and amphibians are listed in Table 18.1. The most important are discussed below.

Gyrodactylus

Gyrodactylus, an important pathogen of fishes throughout the world, is common on the skin of frogs or gills of frog tadpoles in North America and Europe (Cameron 1956; Hoffman and Putz 1964). There are many species of this genus, almost one for every species of fish (Hoffman 1967). Most are host-specific except possibly *G. elegans* (Hoffman 1967), and presumably it is this species that affects frogs, but even this is uncertain. The incidence of *Gyrodactylus* in laboratory frogs obtained from nature is unknown; it is probably common.

MORPHOLOGY

Adults (Fig. 18.1) are very small; those of *G. elegans* measure 0.5 to 0.8 mm in length (Cameron 1956; Dawes 1946). The

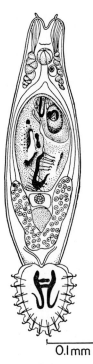

FIG. 18.1. *Gyrodactylus elegans* adult. (From Dogiel, Polyanski, and Kheisin 1964. Courtesy of Oliver and Boyd.)

anterior tip is bilobed; eye spots and an oral sucker are lacking (Hoffman 1967; Noble and Noble 1964). The posterior attachment organ (haptor) is fringed by 16 small hooks, each of which can be moved independently. A pair of large but apparently functionless hooks is located in the center of the haptor.

LIFE CYCLE

This trematode is viviparous and gives birth to a well-developed larva (Hoffman 1967). The life cycle is direct. The larva swims until it reaches a new host, attaches to the surface structures, and develops into an adult (Cameron 1956). It is extremely host-dependent and cannot survive more than 20 minutes unattached (Cameron 1956).

PATHOLOGIC EFFECTS

This fluke attaches to the gills, fins, and skin of tadpoles and the skin of adult frogs and ingests blood from the superficial capillaries (Cameron 1956; Cheng 1964). The affected surfaces become covered with a layer of mucus, and the fins of tadpoles are often frayed and torn. Large numbers of parasites on the gills sometimes cause death through asphyxiation. Fatal secondary mycotic infections also occur. Other clinical signs have not been reported in the frog, but affected fish rub themselves against a firm object in an attempt to dislodge the parasites (Davis 1953), and affected frogs are likely to respond similarly.

DIAGNOSIS

Diagnosis is based on demonstration and identification of the flukes in the mucus covering affected surfaces.

CONTROL

Control and treatment for frogs have not been described. Presumably treatments effective for fishes are equally satisfactory for frogs. These include formalin in the water at a level of 200 to 250 ppm for 1 hour; potassium permanganate in the water at a level of 0.1% for 30 to 40 seconds, 10 ppm for 5 to 30 minutes or 1 to 2 ppm for prolonged periods; acriflavine in the water at a level of 3 to 5 ppm for 1 to 4 hours; acetic acid in the water at a level of 0.2% for 1 to 2 minutes; and sodium chloride in the water at a level of 1 to 3% for several minutes to 1 hour (Snieszko and Hoffman 1963).

PUBLIC HEALTH CONSIDERATIONS

This trematode does not affect man.

Polystoma nearcticum, Polystoma integerrimum

These are the commonest monogenetic trematodes of amphibians (Reichenbach-Klinke and Elkan 1965; Savage 1962). They affect frogs, occurring on the gills of tadpoles and in the urinary bladder of both tadpoles and adults. *Polystoma nearcticum* is found in North America and affects treefrogs (Paul 1938). *Polystoma integerrimum* is found in Europe, Asia, and Africa and affects frogs, treefrogs, and toads (Walton 1964, 1966, 1967).

In a survey of grass frogs in Great Britain, 12.5% were found infected (Lees 1962). Young male frogs are most suscep-

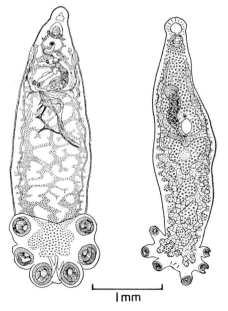

1mm

FIG. 18.2. *Polystoma nearcticum.* *(Left)* Adult from bladder. *(Right)* Adult from gills. (From Paul 1938.)

tible, and the rate of infection is highest in the autumn.

MORPHOLOGY

Adults vary in size and morphology, depending on whether they are located in the bladder or on the gills (Fig. 18.2) (Paul 1938). Those found in the bladder are 2.5 to 4.5 (avg 3.6) mm long by 0.9 to 1.5 (avg 1.2) mm wide; those found on the gills are 1.6 to 5.0 (avg 2.0) mm long by 0.3 to 0.8 (avg 0.5) mm wide. The bladder form has a cordiform caudal disc with six cup-shaped, muscular suckers and two large hooks. The gill form has a caudal disc with six pedunculated suckers and only rudimentary hooks, if any. The larva is just slightly smaller than the adult. It is partly covered with cilia and has four eye-spots and a posterior sucker with 16 hooks. Eggs produced by both forms of adults appear identical. They are ovoid and measure 300 by 150μ.

LIFE CYCLE

Adult flukes in the bladder lay eggs during the spawning period of the host

(Cameron 1956; Paul 1938). The eggs hatch in about 2 weeks and the larvae attach to the gills of a tadpole. They mature in about 3 weeks and begin to lay eggs. Larvae from these eggs apparently enter the bladder of a tadpole either by migrating down the digestive tract to the cloaca or entering it through the anus. They remain with the host through metamorphosis and mature at the same time as the host, at 3 years of age. Thus there is an alternation of generations, one requiring 3 weeks, one requiring 3 years.

PATHOLOGIC EFFECTS

These parasites feed on blood from the gills and urinary bladder (Paul 1938), but their effect is apparently slight.

DIAGNOSIS

Diagnosis is based on demonstration and identification of the parasites.

CONTROL

No treatment has been reported.

PUBLIC HEALTH CONSIDERATIONS

These parasites do not affect man.

Sphyranura

Sphyranura oligorchis, S. polyorchis, and *S. osleri* are common on the gills of the mudpuppy in North America (Rankin 1937; Reichenbach-Klinke and Elkan 1965; Walton 1964). Although there are no specific reports of these parasites in the laboratory, they are probably common on mudpuppies obtained from their natural habitat.

MORPHOLOGY

Adults are about 2.5 to 3.0 mm long (Fig. 18.3) (Olsen 1967; Rankin 1937). The haptor has two large muscular suckers, two large hooks, seven small hooks on each side, and one hook in each sucker. Five to 23 testes are usually arranged linearly between the intestinal branches. The ovary is ovoid and is located just anterior to the center of the body.

LIFE CYCLE

Adults living on the gills lay eggs which settle to the bottom of the water

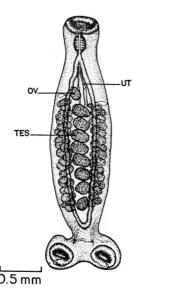

FIG. 18.3. *Sphyranura* adult. *OV*, ovary; *TES*, testes; *UT*, uterus. (From Cheng 1964. Courtesy of W. B. Saunders Co.)

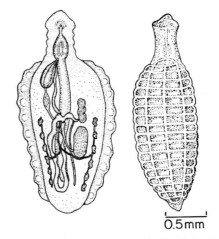

FIG. 18.4. *Aspidogaster conchicola* adult. *(Left)* Translucent view. *(Right)* Ventral view. *(Left* from Cheng 1964; courtesy of W. B. Saunders Co. *Right* from Cheng 1964; after Monticelli 1892; courtesy of W. B. Saunders Co.)

and hatch after 28 to 32 days (Olsen 1967). The larvae creep or use the caudal disc to swim. If a larva does not find a host within a few hours after hatching, it dies. Otherwise it attaches to the gills and develops to the adult stage in about 2 months. The complete cycle takes about 3 months.

PATHOLOGIC EFFECTS

Sphyranura sucks blood from the branchial circulation (Olsen 1967). The gills sometimes become frayed and asphyxiation occasionally occurs.

DIAGNOSIS

Diagnosis is based on demonstration and identification of the parasites on the gills.

CONTROL

Control and treatment have not been described.

PUBLIC HEALTH CONSIDERATIONS

This trematode does not affect man.

Aspidogaster conchicola

This fluke, a common parasite of freshwater clams throughout the world, is frequently found in the digestive tract of turtles (Olsen 1967). Although there are no specific reports of its occurrence in the laboratory, it is probably common in turtles obtained from their natural habitat.

MORPHOLOGY

The adult is 2.5 to 2.7 mm long by 1.1 to 1.2 mm wide (Fig. 18.4) (Olsen 1967). It is covered over most of its ventral surface by an alveolated sucker that contains four rows of sucking grooves. There is an ovary that is located toward the anterior end of the worm and one median testis.

LIFE CYCLE

The entire life cycle is passed in one invertebrate host, usually a freshwater clam (Olsen 1967). Adult worms in the pericardial or renal cavities of the clam lay eggs which presumably pass through the renopericardial pore, kidney, kidney pore, and suprabranchial gill chambers to the water, where the larvae hatch. A new host is apparently infected by drawing larvae into the suprabranchial gill chambers. These then enter the renal pore and pass through the kidney to the pericardium where they mature to adults. The turtle is not a necessary part of the life cycle and becomes infected only by eating clams containing the worms.

PATHOLOGIC EFFECTS

Nothing is known of the pathologic effects of this fluke for the turtle.

DIAGNOSIS

Diagnosis is based on demonstration and identification of the worm in the digestive tract.

CONTROL

No treatment has been reported.

PUBLIC HEALTH CONSIDERATIONS

This fluke does not affect man.

ADULT DIGENETIC TREMATODES

The adults of many digenetic trematodes are endoparasites of reptiles and amphibians (Noble and Noble 1964; Yamaguti 1958). The worms usually occur in the intestine, urinary bladder, and lungs. Although detrimental effects have been noted only when their numbers are large (Reichenbach-Klinke and Elkan 1965), it is probable that even in small numbers they cause wounding of the tissues, mechanical obstruction of ducts, hyperplasia of certain tissues, nutritional deprivation, and toxic effects (Noble and Noble 1964). For this reason, both known and probable pathogenic species are described in this section.

Those adult trematodes which are likely to be encountered in laboratory reptiles and amphibians are listed in Table 18.2. The most important are discussed below.

Gorgodera, Gorgoderina

These flukes are found in the kidneys and urinary bladder of amphibians throughout the world (Goodchild 1948, 1950; Walton 1964, 1967; Yamaguti 1958). The most important species and their hosts and geographic distribution are listed in Table 18.2. Many are common in nature. An incidence of 35.0% has been reported for *Gorgodera amplicava* in the bullfrog in southern United States (Harwood 1932). Incidences of 2.4 to 16.5% have been reported for *Gorgoderina bilobata* in dusky salamanders and 7.3% in the red-spotted newt in southeastern United States (Rankin 1937), and an incidence of 11.8% has been reported for *Gorgoderina vitelliloba*

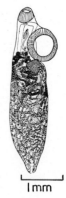

Fig. 18.5. *Gorgodera amplicava* adult. (From Goodchild 1948. Courtesy of American Society of Parasitologists.)

in the grass frog in Great Britain (Lees 1962).

MORPHOLOGY

All species of these genera are morphologically similar (Yamaguti 1958). *Gorgodera amplicava* is typical. Adults are about 4 mm long and have an oral sucker and a much larger ventral one (Fig. 18.5) (Goodchild 1948). A pharynx is absent; the esophagus is short, and the ceca are simple and terminate at the posterior end. Several testes are present. They are round or irregular in shape and usually arranged in two rows or one zigzag row. The genital pore is median or slightly submedian. The ovary is submedian, and the vitellaria are compact or lobed and paired. Eggs are nonoperculate and embryonated when passed.

LIFE CYCLE

The life cycle is similar for all species of these genera (Goodchild 1950; Olsen 1967). Eggs passed by adults hatch upon reaching water or within 24 hours. They are drawn into the mantle of a clam, enter through the gills, and develop into cercariae. These cercariae are ingested by frog tadpoles, salamander larvae, snails, or crayfish, and within 24 hours develop into metacercariae. The final host becomes infected by ingesting the second intermediate host. After excysting in the stomach or intestine, the larval flukes migrate down the alimentary tract to the cloaca and then up the reproductive and excretory ducts. They remain in the ducts for 2 weeks and then migrate to the urinary bladder and sometimes the kidneys, where they mature to adults in 3 weeks to 2 months.

PATHOLOGIC EFFECTS

Massive infections are harmful (Goodchild 1950). Adult worms in the kidneys occlude the tubules and ducts and cause listlessness, anorexia, uremia, and sometimes death.

DIAGNOSIS

Diagnosis is based on demonstration and identification of these parasites in the kidneys or urinary bladder at necropsy.

CONTROL

Because of the need for a mollusk intermediate host, it is unlikely that the life cycle of these trematodes would be completed in the laboratory. No treatment is known.

PUBLIC HEALTH CONSIDERATIONS

These flukes do not affect man.

Opisthioglyphe ranae, Dolichosaccus rastellus

These are the commonest intestinal trematodes of European anurans (Reichenbach-Klinke and Elkan 1965). *Opisthioglyphe ranae* (syn. *O. endoloba, Lecithopyge ranae*) occurs in the edible frog, grass frog, treefrog, European toad, clawed toad, European salamanders, and crested newt; it is the predominant species in continental Europe (Reichenbach-Klinke and Elkan 1965; Walton 1964; Yamaguti 1958). *Dolichosaccus rastellus* (syn. *Lecithopyge rastellum*) occurs in the edible frog, grass frog, European toad, European salamanders, and newts. It is the predominant species in Great Britain, where an 8% incidence has been observed in grass frogs obtained from their natural habitat (Lees 1962).

MORPHOLOGY

Adults of these species are oval and wide and measure 2 to 4 mm long and 0.8 to 1.2 mm wide (Fig. 18.6) (Dawes 1946). The testes are at the posterior end of the body and the uterus anterior to them; the vitellaria extend beyond the

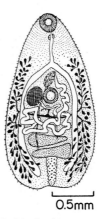

FIG. 18.6. *Opisthioglyphe ranae* adult. (From Dawes 1946. Courtesy of Cambridge University Press.)

level of the testes (Skrjabin 1964; Yamaguti 1958).

LIFE CYCLE

The life cycle of these species involves two intermediate hosts (Reichenbach-Klinke and Elkan 1965). The first is a snail; the second is usually an insect but sometimes a tadpole. The final host becomes infected by ingesting the insect or tadpole.

PATHOLOGIC EFFECTS

Nothing is known of the pathologic effects of these species.

DIAGNOSIS

Diagnosis is based on demonstration and identification of these parasites in the intestine at necropsy.

CONTROL

Because of the need for a mollusk and usually an insect as intermediate hosts, it is unlikely that the life cycle of these trematodes would be completed in the laboratory. No treatment is known.

PUBLIC HEALTH CONSIDERATIONS

These flukes do not affect man.

Lechriorchis, Zeugorchis, Dasymetra, Ochetosoma

These flukes, the so-called renifers, inhabit the lung, mouth, and digestive tract of snakes (Marcus 1968; Yamaguti 1958).

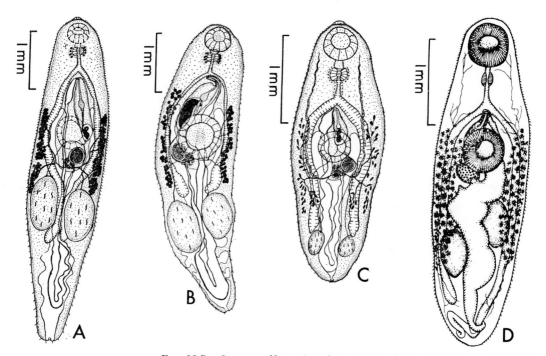

FIG. 18.7. Some renifers of snakes. *(A) Lechriorchis primus* adult. *(B)
L. tygarti* adult. *(C) Zeugorchis eurinus* adult. *(D) Dasymetra conferta*
adult. *(A, B, C* from Talbot 1933. *D* from Skrjabin 1964; courtesy of
University of Illinois Press.)

Although common throughout the world, little is known of their exact incidence (Reichenbach-Klinke and Elkan 1965; Stewart 1960; Walton 1964). A 25% incidence of *Lechriorchis primus* has been reported in the garter snake in north central United States (Talbot 1933).

MORPHOLOGY

Adults of all these species are similar (Fig. 18.7) (Olsen 1967). The ovary is anterior to the testes, the ascending and descending parts of the uterus pass between the testes, the genital pore is located between the suckers, and the excretory duct is Y-shaped. The adult of *L. primus* measures about 1.8 to 5.7 mm long and 0.6 to 1.3 mm wide; the egg is oval, has an operculum, and measures 48 to 50 μ by 23 to 25 μ (Talbot 1933). The adult of *L. tygarti* is 2.2 to 6.9 mm long by 0.6 to 1.6 mm wide; its eggs are also oval and operculate and measure 43 to 53 μ by 20 to 34 μ. The adult of *Zeugorchis eurinus* is

1.9 to 3.3 mm long and 0.6 to 0.8 mm wide. Its eggs are similar to those of *Lechriorchis* and measure 42 to 46 μ by 18 to 23 μ. The adult of *Dasymetra conferta* is 3.8 by 1.1 mm (Skrjabin 1964). The adult of *Ochetosoma aniarum* (syn. *Neorenifer aniarum*) is 1.8 to 3.5 mm long and 0.7 to 1.1 mm wide; the eggs are 32 to 42 μ by 20 to 25 μ (Harwood 1932).

LIFE CYCLE

The life cycles of all species of these genera are similar (Olsen 1967; Talbot 1933). Eggs deposited by the adults in the lung are swallowed and passed in the feces. They hatch when ingested by a snail and, after 4 to 5 weeks, leave the snail as cercariae. The cercariae are ingested by tadpoles and encyst in the muscles. The snake becomes infected by ingestion of the tadpole. The metacercariae excyst in the stomach and develop into young worms in the small intestine. After about 7 months, the young worms migrate through the stomach to the esophagus. Here they remain for another 3 months after which they pass through the mouth to the lung. Another year is required before the young worms in the lung become adults.

PATHOLOGIC EFFECTS

Weight loss and occasional dyspnea have been associated with heavy infections with these parasites (Marcus 1968; Nelson 1950). It has also been suggested that such infections cause nervousness and irritability, but this is disputed (Goodman 1951). Otherwise, nothing is known of the pathologic effects of these flukes (Page 1966).

DIAGNOSIS

Diagnosis is based on demonstration and identification of eggs in the feces or parasites in the mouth of living animals, or in the digestive tract or lung at necropsy.

CONTROL

Because of the need for a mollusk and tadpole intermediate host, it is unlikely that the life cycle of these flukes would be completed in the laboratory. The oral administration of tetrachlorethylene, 0.2 ml per kg of body weight by capsule, has been reported to be an effective treatment for the immature flukes in the intestine (Nelson 1950). The drug is given 4 days after feeding to avoid its absorption by residual fats in the stomach. No treatment is known for the adult flukes in the lungs.

PUBLIC HEALTH CONSIDERATIONS

These trematodes do not affect man.

Haplometra cylindracea

This fluke occurs in Europe in the lungs of the edible frog, grass frog, treefrogs, and European toad (Dawes 1946; Walton 1964; Yamaguti 1958). It is common and an incidence of 54.2% has been reported in the grass frog in Great Britain (Lees 1962). Usually about 5 and sometimes as many as 60 parasites occur in one host.

MORPHOLOGY

The adult is elongate, cylindrical, and usually about 10 mm long, but sometimes

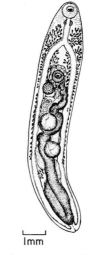

FIG. 18.8. *Haplometra cylindracea* adult. (From Skrjabin 1964. Courtesy of University of Illinois Press.)

as long as 20 mm (Fig. 18.8) (Dawes 1946; Yamaguti 1958). The ventral sucker is smaller than the oral sucker and posterior to it. The intestine bifurcates anterior to the ventral sucker. The testes are spherical, one behind the other, in the third quarter of the body; the ovary is anterior to the testes. The genital pore is median and near the ventral sucker. Eggs are dark brown and measure 220 by 40 μ.

LIFE CYCLE

The life cycle involves two intermediate hosts, a snail and a water beetle (Walton 1964). The frog or toad becomes infected by ingestion of the second intermediate host.

PATHOLOGIC EFFECTS

This parasite becomes fixed to the pulmonary epithelium and ingests blood (Arvy 1950). The pulmonary tissues undergo intensive changes but no inflammation is produced, and no apparent gross effects are seen even in heavy infections (Lees 1962).

DIAGNOSIS

Diagnosis is made at necropsy by demonstration and identification of parasites in the lungs.

CONTROL

Because of the need for two intermediate hosts, one of which is a water beetle, it is unlikely that the life cycle would be completed in the laboratory. Treatment is unknown.

PUBLIC HEALTH CONSIDERATIONS

This fluke does not affect man.

Glypthelmins pennsylvaniensis, Glypthelmins quieta

Glypthelmins pennsylvaniensis occurs in the intestine of the spring peeper and chorus frogs *(Pseudacris)* in the United States; *G. quieta* occurs in the intestine of the leopard frog, green frog, pickerel frog, bullfrog, chorus frogs, spring peeper, other frogs, and toads in the United States, Mexico, South America, and Asia (Rankin 1945; Ubelaker, Duszynski, and Beaver 1967; Walton 1964; Yamaguti 1958). A 10 to 15% incidence of infection with *G. pennsylvaniensis* has been reported in chorus frogs in western United States; a 30% incidence has been reported in the bullfrog and 18% in the spring peeper in northeastern United States.

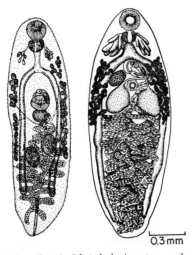

FIG. 18.9. *(Left) Glypthelmins pennsylvaniensis* adult. *(Right) G. quieta* adult. *(Left* from Cheng 1961; courtesy of American Society of Parasitologists. *Right* from Skrjabin 1964; courtesy of University of Illinois Press.)

MORPHOLOGY

The adult of *G. pennsylvaniensis* is about 1.8 mm long by 0.6 mm wide (Fig. 18.9) (Cheng 1961). Its ovary is located posterior to the acetabulum, and its testes are arranged obliquely in the posterior half of the body. The adult of *G. quieta* is similar in size and morphology. It is distinguished primarily by the position of its gonads. The ovary is anterior to the acetabulum, and the testes are more anterior and are situated side by side.

LIFE CYCLE

The life cycle is similar for both species and involves a snail as the intermediate host (Cheng 1961; Schell 1962). Free-swimming cercariae escape from the snail, penetrate the skin of the definitive host (a frog), encyst, and form metacercariae. The metacercariae are sloughed during molting, are ingested by the frog, and become adult flukes in the intestine.

PATHOLOGIC EFFECTS

Nothing is known of the pathologic effects of these flukes.

DIAGNOSIS

Diagnosis is based on demonstration and identification of the parasites in the skin or intestine at necropsy.

CONTROL

Because of the need for a snail intermediate host, it is unlikely that the life cycle would be completed in the laboratory. Treatment is unknown.

PUBLIC HEALTH CONSIDERATIONS

These flukes do not affect man.

Haematoloechus

Over 40 species of this genus occur in the lungs of frogs and toads throughout the world (Cheng 1964; Walton 1964; Yamaguti 1958). Although little is known of their exact incidence, many are common. Those most likely to be found in laboratory frogs and toads obtained from their natural habitat are listed together with their geographic distribution, hosts, and other information in Table 18.2.

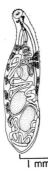

FIG. 18.10. *Haematoloechus* adult. (From Cheng 1964; redrawn after Ingles 1936. Courtesy of W. B. Saunders Co.)

MORPHOLOGY

The adult has a flattened body with a densely spined cuticle; it measures up to 8.0 mm long by 1.2 mm wide (Fig. 18.10) (Cheng 1964; Olsen 1967; Skrjabin 1964). The testes are oval and situated in the posterior one-third of the body. The ovary is elongate, smaller than the testes, and located in the middle third of the body. The genital pore is near the cecal bifurcation. Vitellaria are arranged in rosettelike configurations or clusters.

LIFE CYCLE

The life cycle requires both a snail and an insect host (Olsen 1967; Walton 1964). Embryonated eggs deposited by the adult in the lung cavity pass up the bronchioles to the mouth, are swallowed, and are voided in the feces. They do not hatch until ingested by a snail. Cercariae develop in the snail, are released, and are ingested by an insect. The frog or toad becomes infected by ingesting the insect.

PATHOLOGIC EFFECTS

Nothing is known of specific pathologic effects. Small numbers of flukes in the lungs are said to cause little harm and only a heavy infection is thought to cause serious effects (Reichenbach-Klinke and Elkan 1965). Presumably such effects do occur since up to 75 flukes have been observed in one frog (Olsen 1967).

DIAGNOSIS

Diagnosis is based on demonstration and identification of the flukes in the lungs at necropsy.

CONTROL

Because of the need for two intermediate hosts, it is unlikely that the life cycle would be completed in the laboratory. No treatment is known.

PUBLIC HEALTH CONSIDERATIONS

This trematode does not affect man.

Brachycoelium salamandrae

This trematode occurs throughout the world and is one of the commonest intestinal flukes of amphibians (Fischthal 1955a, b; Rankin 1937; Reichenbach-Klinke and Elkan 1965; Yamaguti 1958). It has also been reported in reptiles. It occurs in the wood frog, pickerel frog, cricket frog, chorus frogs *(Pseudacris)*, green treefrog, spring peeper, other frogs, toads, mole salamanders, dusky salamanders, woodland salamanders *(Plethodon)*, other salamanders, red-spotted newt, and amphiumas in North America, and in the grass frog, European toad, European salamander, and newts in Europe (Walton 1964, 1966; Yamaguti 1958). Terrestrial salamanders are more commonly infected than aquatic salamanders or frogs (Rankin 1945). In surveys of several amphibians obtained from their natural habitat in eastern United States, it was found in various terrestrial salamanders in incidences ranging up to 100%, with as many as 60 specimens in one animal, whereas incidences of 11 to 19% occurred in the aquatic red-spotted newt and 11% in the pickerel frog (Fischthal 1955a, b; Rankin 1937, 1945).

MORPHOLOGY

The adult is 3.0 to 5.0 mm in length and is characterized by short intestinal ceca which reach only to the ventral sucker (Fig. 18.11) (Dawes 1946; Skrjabin 1964). The testes are rounded and symmetrical; the ovary is anterior to the left testis; the uterus has long, folded, descending and ascending limbs and fills the posterior part of the body; the genital pore is anterior

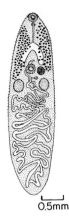

FIG. 18.11. *Brachycoelium salamandrae* adult. (From Dawes 1946. Courtesy of Cambridge University Press.)

to the ventral sucker. Vitellaria are confined to the anterior region. The eggs are light brown and measure 45 to 50 μ by 32 to 36 μ.

LIFE CYCLE

The life cycle involves a mollusk intermediate host (Cheng 1964; Walton 1964). Both the cercariae and metacercariae develop in snails. The amphibian host is infected by ingestion of an infected snail.

PATHOLOGIC EFFECTS

Nothing is known of the pathologic effects of this trematode.

DIAGNOSIS

Diagnosis is based on demonstration and identification of the parasite in the intestine at necropsy.

CONTROL

Because of the need for a mollusk intermediate host, it is unlikely that the life cycle would be completed in the laboratory. Treatment is unknown.

PUBLIC HEALTH CONSIDERATIONS

This fluke does not affect man.

Megalodiscus, Diplodiscus, Opisthodiscus

These flukes occur in the intestine, rectum, and sometimes in the bladder and cloaca of amphibians (Walton 1964; Yamaguti 1958). *Megalodiscus temporatus* is common in North America, Central America, and South America; it occurs in the large intestine of the leopard frog, green frog, bullfrog, green treefrog, spring peeper, chorus frogs *(Pseudacris)*, other frogs, common toad, mole salamanders, dusky salamanders, other salamanders, water newt, and amphiumas (Fischthal 1955a; Walton 1964; Yamaguti 1958). Incidences of 16 to 48% have been reported in the red-spotted newt in eastern United States (Fischthal 1955a; Rankin 1937, 1945). *Megalodiscus americanus* occurs in the intestine of the leopard frog, other frogs, mole salamanders, the dusky salamander, California newt, other salamanders, and amphiumas in North America and Central America. *Megalodiscus intermedius* occurs in the rectum of the bullfrog and dusky salamander; *M. microphagus* in the large intestine and urinary bladder of frogs, toads, and salamanders; and *M. rankini* in the intestine of the red-spotted newt in the United States (Efford and Tsumura 1969; Walton 1964; Yamaguti 1958).

Diplodiscus subclavatus (syn. *Opisthodiscus subclavatus*) is common in Europe, Africa, Asia, Australia, and New Zealand; it occurs in the large intestine of the grass frog, edible frog, treefrogs, other frogs, European toad, clawed toad, other toads, European salamander, and newts (Walton 1964; Yamaguti 1958). *Diplodiscus japonicus* occurs in the large intestine and cloaca of frogs in Asia; it is the commonest trematode of amphibians in Japan (Reichenbach-Klinke and Elkan 1965; Walton 1964; Yamaguti 1958). *Diplodiscus unguiculatus* occurs in the rectum of newts and *Opisthodiscus diplodiscoides* occurs in the large intestine of the edible frog in Europe (Walton 1964; Yamaguti 1958).

MORPHOLOGY

Adults are conical rather than flat; they measure up to 6.0 mm in length and about 2.0 to 2.2 mm in thickness (Fig. 18.12) (Cheng 1964; Olsen 1967; Reichenbach-Klinke and Elkan 1965). All species have a well-developed oral sucker (which has a pair of posterior diverticula) and a large, terminal posterior sucker. Mature forms of *Megalodiscus* and *Opisthodiscus* have two testes; mature forms of *Diplodiscus* have but one (Skrjabin 1964).

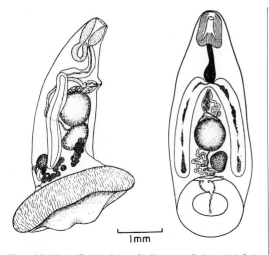

FIG. 18.12. *(Left) Megalodiscus* adult. *(Right) Diplodiscus* adult. (From Skrjabin 1964. Courtesy of University of Illinois Press.)

LIFE CYCLE

The life cycle involves two intermediate hosts, a snail and an amphibian (Cheng 1964; Efford and Tsumura 1969; Olsen 1967; Walton 1964). Adults deposit embryonated eggs which hatch, enter a snail, and develop into cercariae. This requires about 90 days. The cercariae escape from the snail and encyst as metacercariae in the skin of an amphibian or amphibian larva (tadpole). The adult amphibian is ordinarily infected by eating metacercariae in its own skin sloughed during molting. Tadpoles and possibly adults are sometimes infected directly by ingestion of cercariae. In this case the cercariae encyst in the mouth, pass to the intestine, excyst, and remain there through metamorphosis. The fluke usually matures in about 2 to 3 months after ingestion and remains in the host for about a year.

PATHOLOGIC EFFECTS

Nothing is known of the pathologic effects of these trematodes.

DIAGNOSIS

Diagnosis is based on demonstration and identification of the parasites at necropsy.

CONTROL

Because of the need for two intermediate hosts, completion of the life cycle in the laboratory is unlikely. No treatment has been reported.

PUBLIC HEALTH CONSIDERATIONS

These flukes do not affect man.

Halipegus

Flukes of this genus inhabit the mouth, ear canals, pharynx, stomach, and intestine of frogs, toads, and occasionally reptiles (Walton 1964; Yamaguti 1958). *Halipegus eccentricus, H. occidualis,* and *H. amherstensis* occur in North America. *Halipegus eccentricus* is found in the ear canals of the leopard frog, green frog, and bull frog; *H. occidualis* is found in the mouth, ear canals, and pharynx of the leopard frog, green frog, bullfrog, and other frogs; and *H. amherstensis* is found in the mouth and ear canals of the green frog, bullfrog, and other frogs. *Halipegus ovocaudatus* occurs in Europe and southern Africa; it is found in the mouth of the edible frog, grass frog, other frogs, and toads. Little is known of the incidence of these parasites. They are presumably common in certain localities.

MORPHOLOGY

Adults are fairly cylindrical and about 6.0 to 6.5 mm long by about 1.8 mm wide (Fig. 18.13) (Cheng 1964; Olsen 1967; Skrjabin 1964). The ventral sucker is near the middle of the body, the testes are in the posterior one-third, the ovary is posterior to the testes, and the two compact vitellaria are posterior to the ovary.

LIFE CYCLE

The life cycle involves two intermediate hosts, a snail and a copepod or insect (Olsen 1967; Rankin 1945; Reichenbach-Klinke and Elkan 1965; Walton 1964). Eggs deposited by the adult pass through the alimentary tract and are voided in the feces. When eaten by a snail they hatch and subsequently develop into cercariae. The cercariae are ingested by the copepod or insect and the final host becomes infected by ingestion of the arthropod.

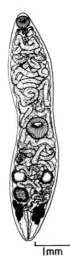

FIG. 18.13. *Halipegus* adult. (From Skrjabin 1964. Courtesy of University of Illinois Press.)

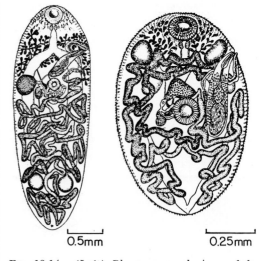

FIG. 18.14. *(Left) Pleurogenes claviger* adult. *(Right) Prosotocus confusus* adult. (From Skrjabin 1964. Courtesy of University of Illinois Press.)

PATHOLOGIC EFFECTS

Nothing is known of the pathologic effects.

DIAGNOSIS

Diagnosis is based on demonstration and identification of the parasite at necropsy.

CONTROL

Because of the need for two intermediate hosts, it is unlikely that the life cycle would be completed in the laboratory. Treatment is unknown.

PUBLIC HEALTH CONSIDERATIONS

Halipegus does not affect man.

Pleurogenes claviger, Pleurogenes medians, Prosotocus confusus

These flukes are common inhabitants of the small intestine of frogs, toads, and newts in Europe, Africa, and southwestern Asia (Reichenbach-Klinke and Elkan 1965; Walton 1964; Yamaguti 1958). *Pleurogenes claviger* occurs in the grass frog, edible frog, treefrogs, other frogs, European toad, other toads, common newt, crested newt, and other newts in Europe (Walton 1964). *Pleurogenes medians* occurs in the grass frog, edible frog, treefrogs, other frogs, European toad, other toads, common newt, and crested newt in Europe and Africa (Walton 1964). *Prosotocus confusus* occurs in the grass frog, edible frog, other frogs, European toad, and other toads in Europe and southwestern Asia (Walton 1964).

MORPHOLOGY

The adult of *P. claviger* is cylindrical and about 3.0 mm long; mature forms of *P. medians* and *P. confusus* are oval and about 1.0 mm long (Fig. 18.14) (Reichenbach-Klinke and Elkan 1965). In all three species the vitellaria are restricted to the anterior half of the body and the genital pore is located laterally, anterior to the ventral sucker (Skrjabin 1964). In *P. claviger* and *P. medians* the intestinal ceca are long, extending beyond the ventral sucker, and the testes are posterior to them; in *P. confusus* the intestinal ceca are short and the testes anterior to them.

LIFE CYCLE

The life cycle involves two intermediate hosts, a snail in which the cercariae develop and an arthropod in which the metacercariae develop (Reichenbach-Klinke and Elkan 1965; Walton 1964). A frog or toad is infected by ingestion of the infected arthropod.

PATHOLOGIC EFFECTS

Nothing is known of the pathologic effects of these flukes.

DIAGNOSIS

Diagnosis is based on demonstration and identification of the parasite in the intestine at necropsy.

CONTROL

Because of the need for two intermediate hosts, completion of the life cycle in the laboratory is unlikely. No treatment has been described.

PUBLIC HEATH CONSIDERATIONS

These flukes do not affect man.

Spirorchis

Species of this genus inhabit the vascular system of turtles in North America (Wall 1941; Yamaguti 1958). *Spirorchis parvus* and *S. elephantis* occur in painted turtles, *S. artericola* and *S. innominata* in pond turtles and other turtles, and *S. haematobium* in the snapping turtle (Thatcher 1954; Wall 1941; Williams 1953). All are common. An 18% incidence of *S. parvus* has been reported in painted turtles obtained from their natural habitat in north central United States (Wall 1941), and a 70% incidence of *S. haematobium* in snapping turtles in central United States (Williams 1953).

MORPHOLOGY

Adults are thin, transparent, and about 1 to 2 mm long, and do not have a ventral sucker (Fig. 18.15) (Olsen 1967; Skrjabin 1964; Wall 1941). The esophagus is long, and the two ceca extend almost to the posterior end of the body. The testes are arranged in a linear series anterior to the ovary; the ovary and the genital pore are located near the posterior end of the body. Vitellaria are follicular and usually occupy all available space in the body not occupied by reproductive organs from the esophagus to beyond the ends of the ceca. Eggs are large, about 55 by 40 μ, and with or without an operculum.

LIFE CYCLE

Adults of *S. parvus* occur in the mesenteric arterioles in the wall of the stomach and intestine (Wall 1941). Adults of other

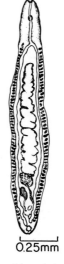

FIG. 18.15. *Spirorchis* adult. (From Skrjabin 1964. Courtesy of University of Illinois Press.)

species are found in the heart or in the arteries of the lungs and other organs. Eggs are deposited in the blood vessels, collect in the gut wall, pass into the lumen, and are voided in the feces. They hatch in water in 4 to 6 days and the miracidia penetrate a snail, where they develop into cercariae. The cercariae, when released from the snail, penetrate the thin epithelial membranes of a turtle, migrate through the tissues to the blood vessels, and circulate until they reach the heart or arteries, where they become adults. The development time in the snail is about 18 days, the time required to reach maturity in the turtle is about 3 months, and the time for eggs passed by the adult worm to reach the lumen of the gut is about 2 weeks.

PATHOLOGIC EFFECTS

Spirorchis parvus cercariae cause irritation when attempting to penetrate a turtle, and in massive infections the fluke eggs solidly coat large areas of the gut of small turtles, often causing death (Wall 1941). Otherwise, nothing is known of the pathologic effects of this or other species.

DIAGNOSIS

Diagnosis is based on demonstration and identification of the parasite in the blood vessels or heart.

Because of the need for a snail intermediate host, completion of the life cycle in the laboratory is unlikely. No treatment has been reported.

PUBLIC HEALTH CONSIDERATIONS

Spirorchis does not affect man.

LARVAL DIGENETIC TREMATODES

Amphibians are sometimes the second and rarely the third intermediate host of trematodes whose final hosts are certain mammals, birds, reptiles, or other amphibians (Reichenbach-Klinke and Elkan 1965; Walton 1964; Yamaguti 1958). The first intermediate host is a mollusk, usually a snail. Cercariae released from the mollusk enter an amphibian either by burrowing into the skin or by attaching themselves to a plant or transport host and being ingested. The cercariae invade and often encyst in the tissues of the amphibian, usually in the skin and muscles but sometimes in the eyes, central nervous system, heart, liver, lungs, or lateral line system. Their pathogenicity depends on the number present and the tissues affected.

Reptiles are not natural second intermediate hosts for trematodes, but rarely they are transport hosts for larvae (Reichenbach-Klinke and Elkan 1965; Walton 1964).

Larval digenetic trematodes which are likely to be encountered in laboratory reptiles and amphibians are listed in Table 18.3. The most important are discussed below.

Diplostomulum scheuringi

This larval diplostomulid fluke occurs in the brain and eyes of the red-spotted newt and greater siren *(Siren lacertina)* in the United States (Etges 1961; Walton 1964). It is common in the red-spotted newt, with incidences of 12 to 100% reported, and is likely to be encountered in laboratory specimens obtained from their natural habitat (Etges 1961; Lautenschlager 1959).

MORPHOLOGY

The larva as it occurs in amphibians (second intermediate host) is unencysted and measures about 1.0 mm long by 0.2

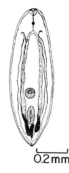

FIG. 18.16. *Diplostomulum scheuringi*. Fully developed, unencysted larva from brain of red-spotted newt. (From Etges 1961. Courtesy of American Society of Parasitologists.)

mm wide (Fig. 18.16) (Hughes 1929). It has a poorly differentiated hindbody and lateral suckers, and small, numerous calcareous corpuscles irregularly scattered throughout the parenchyma. Large, longitudinal muscle fibers give the body a striated appearance. The stage that occurs in the mollusk (first intermediate host), the cercaria, is typicaly strigeid (Etges 1961). An encysted form (third intermediate stage) has been experimentally produced in rodents (Etges 1961), but the adult and the egg are unknown (Walton 1964).

LIFE CYCLE

The life cycle is incompletely known (Etges 1961). Cercariae develop in a snail. These are shed by the snail and penetrate either the cornea of an adult newt or the cornea or skin of a larval newt. Cercariae that penetrate the skin of a larval newt usually migrate to the brain. It is also possible that those that enter the eye migrate through the optic stalk to the brain. They do not encyst. The experimental administration of unencysted larvae to rodents produces encysted larvae in the latter. This suggests a four-host life cycle. The definitive host and the time of the entire cycle are unknown.

PATHOLOGIC EFFECTS

The cercariae produce small hemorrhages at the point of penetration (Etges 1961). Those that enter the eye lodge chiefly in the vitreous body and possibly migrate along the optic stalk to the brain but apparently never invade the lens (Hughes 1929). Those that enter through the skin are carried by the circulatory system to the brain. They cause an increase in ventricular size, hyperplasia, and increased pigmentation of the meninges and either hyperplasia of the choroid plexus or, when located intraventricularly, an absence of the plexus (Lautenschlager 1959). A relationship between the presence of the parasite and brain tumor formation has been suggested.

DIAGNOSIS

Diagnosis is based on identification of the larva in affected tissues.

CONTROL

Because of the need for a snail intermediate host and an unknown definitive host, it is unlikely that the life cycle would be completed in the laboratory. No treatment is known.

PUBLIC HEALTH CONSIDERATIONS

This trematode is not known to affect man.

Diplostomulum xenopi

This larval diplostomulid fluke occurs in the pericardial cavity and causes pericarditis, respiratory distress, and death in the South African clawed toad (Nigrelli and Maraventano 1944; Southwell and Kirshner 1937). The larvae have been observed in imported South African clawed toads in the United States and in Great Britain and apparently occur wherever the toads are used. They are common, and an incidence of 78% has been reported in laboratory specimens imported into the United States (Nigrelli and Maraventano 1944).

MORPHOLOGY

The larva as it occurs in the clawed toad is unencysted and is about 0.5 mm long and 0.3 mm wide (Fig. 18.17) (Nigrelli and Maraventano 1944). The cuticle is thin and has no spines. The oral sucker is subterminal and has an auricular projection on either side. The lateral suckers are poorly developed and the acetabulum, which is located in the anterior part of the posterior half, is comparatively small and oval. Slightly posterior to the acetabulum

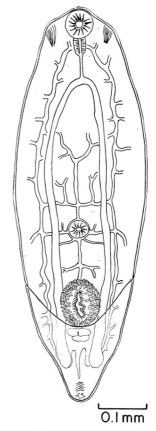

FIG. 18.17. *Diplostomulum xenopi.* Fully developed, unencysted larva from pericardial cavity of South African clawed toad. (From Nigrelli and Maraventano 1944. Courtesy of American Society of Parasitologists.)

is the tribocytic or holdfast organ. The latter is large, oval, and covered with proteolytic gland cells. Primordial gonads are immediately posterior to the tribocytic organ; the hindbody is poorly developed. Calcareous concretions are scattered throughout the body. Nothing is known of the morphology of the adult, egg, or cercarial forms.

LIFE CYCLE

The life cycle is unknown. It is presumed to involve a mollusk, probably a snail, as the first intermediate host and possibly a reptile as the definitive host (Nigrelli and Maraventano 1944; Walton 1964).

PATHOLOGIC EFFECTS

The larval flukes are readily observable in the pericardial cavity with the aid of a hand lens (Nigrelli and Maraventano 1944). They are motile and are often present in large numbers, 25 to 150 per toad. They never encyst and, consequently, remain in the pericardial sac as long as the toad lives. The larvae act as foreign bodies and cause an exudative response by the host. The pericardial sac distends, encroaches on the lungs, and causes a reduced respiratory capacity. Concurrently, the increased intrapericardial pressure interferes with venous input and results in decreased cardiac output. These combine to produce anoxemia, respiratory failure, and death.

DIAGNOSIS

Diagnosis is based on the signs and lesions and identification of the parasites in the pericardial cavity.

CONTROL

Because of the probable need for a mollusk intermediate host and an unknown definitive host, it unlikely that the life cycle would be completed in the laboratory. No treatment is known.

PUBLIC HEALTH CONSIDERATIONS

This trematode is not known to affect man.

Cercaria ranae

When experimentally placed in contact with tadpoles of unspecified species, cercariae of this strigeid trematode obtained from naturally infected snails in north central United States penetrate the skin, migrate to the body cavity and other tissues, and develop into diplostomula (Cort and Brackett 1937). Heavy infection causes abdominal distention and death ("bloat disease"). Natural infection of tadpoles has not been reported. The definitive host is unknown.

Neascus sp.

A diplostomatid metacercaria presumably of the larval genus *Neascus* has been reported once in Great Britain in a group of four imported South African clawed toads (Elkan and Murray 1952). The met-

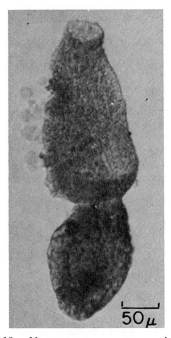

FIG. 18.18. *Neascus* sp. metacercaria from cyst in skin of South African clawed toad. (From Elkan and Murray 1952. Courtesy of Zoological Society of London.)

acercariae (Fig. 18.18) encyst in the skin below the lateral line system and cause a local proliferation of melanophores at the site of each neuromast (Fig. 18.19). Affected toads die shortly after the infection becomes apparent. Nothing is known of the life cycle, control, or public health importance of this parasite. The definitive host is also unknown.

ADULT CESTODES

The cestode life cycle usually involves two or more hosts (Wardle and McLeod 1952). Reptiles and amphibians are often intermediate hosts, but are only occasionally definitive hosts (Fischthal 1955a; Grünberg, Kutzer, and Otte 1963; Harwood 1932; Rankin 1937; Rausch 1947; Yamaguti 1959).

The effects of adult cestodes on reptiles and amphibians are generally unknown. Interference with nutrient absorption is likely, especially when there is massive infection (Reichenbach-Klinke and Elkan 1965).

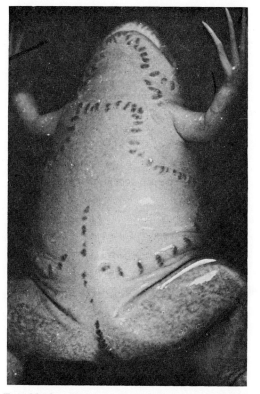

FIG. 18.19. *Neascus* sp. infection of South African clawed toad. Metacercariae encysted in the skin below the lateral line system cause a local proliferation of melanophores at the site of each neuromast. (From Elkan and Murray 1952. Courtesy of Zoological Society of London.)

Adult cestodes which are likely to be encountered in laboratory reptiles and amphibians are listed in Table 18.4. The most important are discussed below.

Bothriocephalus rarus

The adult of this pseudophyllid cestode is common in the small intestine of the red-spotted newt, California newt, and two-lined salamander *(Eurycea bislineata)* in the United States (Fischthal 1955a; Thomas 1937b; Walton 1964; Yamaguti 1959). Laboratory newts obtained from their natural habitat are likely to be infected. Incidences of 0.1, 12.3, 25.0, 26.0, and 29.6% have been reported in north central and eastern United States (Fischthal 1955a; Rankin 1945; Thomas 1937b).

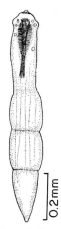

FIG. 18.20. *Bothriocephalus rarus,* young adult. (From Thomas 1937b).

MORPHOLOGY

The scolex of this tapeworm is small and has two shallow, longitudinal slits or bothria and a rectangular terminal disc (Fig. 18.20) (Thomas 1937a). Segmentation begins immediately posterior to the scolex; there is no neck. The mature worm has 60 to 250 segments and is 67 to 300 mm in length. The reproductive organs begin to appear in about the 30th segment. The genital apertures are nearly median, the ovary is compact and bilobed, and the uterine sac is ventral. The egg has a thick shell, is operculated, and is not embryonated when laid. It measures about 59 to 65 μ by 41 to 56 μ.

LIFE CYCLE

Eggs passed in the feces of the newt or salamander hatch in water in 3 to 8 days, depending on temperature, and release free-swimming larvae called coracidia (Thomas 1937b). The coracidia are ingested by a copepod and, within 8 to 12 days, develop into mature procercoids. When the copepod is ingested by a larval newt, the procercoid changes to a plerocercoid in the intestine. The adult worm matures after several months. Adult newts can be infected directly by ingestion of an infected copepod but are usually infected by ingestion of an infected larval newt.

PATHOLOGIC EFFECTS

Heavy infections cause weakness, debilitation, and death (Thomas 1937b).

DIAGNOSIS

Diagnosis is based on the clinical signs and demonstration of proglottids in the feces or the adult worms in the small intestine at necropsy.

CONTROL

Because the life cycle cannot be completed in the absence of copepods, routine sanitation will prevent the spread of the infection in the laboratory. No treatment is reported; however, abrupt changes in water temperature will cause newts in captivity to shed the tapeworms (Thomas 1937b).

PUBLIC HEALTH CONSIDERATIONS

This cestode is not known to affect man.

Cephalochlamys namaquensis
(SYN. *Chlamydocephalus xenopi*)

Adults of this pseudophyllid tapeworm are common in the small intestine of the South African clawed toad in its natural habitat, and they are frequently encountered in this toad in the laboratory (Elkan 1960; Reichenbach-Klinke and Elkan 1965; Yamaguti 1959). An incidence of 100% has been reported in one group of laboratory toads in Great Britain (Southwell and Kirshner 1937).

MORPHOLOGY

The scolex has two large, oval bothridia that stand away from the body and give an arrowhead appearance (Fig. 18.21) (Elkan 1960; Ortlepp 1926; Wardle and McLeod 1952). The total length of the worm is 16.0 to 36.0 mm, with a maximum breadth of 1.6 mm across the last segment. The segments, which throughout are wider than long, are at first very short, but their length increases toward the posterior end where they sometimes reach a length of almost 0.5 mm. Mature segments begin to appear at about 5 mm from the anterior end. The ovary is posterior, near the base of the segment; the uterus is narrow, coiled, and extends almost to the anterior border; the genital aperture is medial and in the anterior half of the segment. Eggs are oval, thin shelled, nonoperculated, and measure 37 μ long by 26 μ wide.

LIFE CYCLE

The life cycle is unknown (Elkan 1960).

PATHOLOGIC EFFECTS

Invasion of the jejunal mucosa by this parasite has been observed (Fig. 18.22), but although heavy infections (over 100 scolices in one toad) sometimes occur (Elkan 1960;

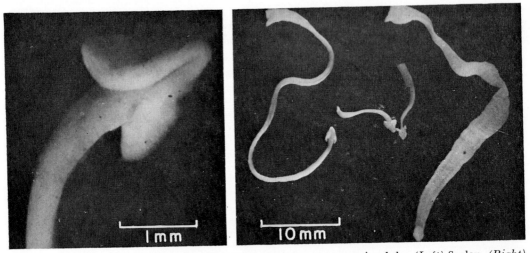

FIG. 18.21. *Cephalochlamys namaquensis* adult. *(Left)* Scolex. *(Right)* Entire worm. (From Elkan 1960. Courtesy of Zoological Society of London.)

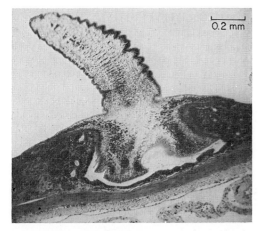

FIG. 18.22. *Cephalochlamys namaquensis* invading jejunal mucosa of South African clawed toad. (From Reichenbach-Klinke and Elkan 1965. Courtesy of Academic Press.)

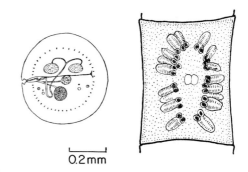

FIG. 18.23. *Nematotaenia dispar*, mature proglottid. *(Left)* Cross section. Note cylindrical shape. *(Right)* Longitudinal view. Note paruterine organs. *(Left* from Wardle and McLeod 1952; courtesy of University of Minnesota Press. *Right* from Cheng 1964; courtesy of W. B. Saunders Co.)

Reichenbach-Klinke and Elkan 1965), no other pathologic effects have been reported.

DIAGNOSIS

Diagnosis is based on demonstration and identification of the parasite in the small intestine.

CONTROL

Because of the lack of knowledge of the life cycle, recommendations for control cannot be made. Once freed of infection, toads in captivity do not appear to become reinfected, thus indicating that the life cycle is not likely to be completed in the laboratory (Elkan 1960). Bromphenol blue, in doses used as an internal indicator in pregnancy testing, is an effective treatment (Elkan 1960; Reichenbach-Klinke and Elkan 1965).

PUBLIC HEALTH CONSIDERATIONS

This cestode is not known to affect man.

Nematotaenia dispar

Adults of this cyclophyllid cestode have reported from the small intestine of the edible frog, grass frog, treefrogs, other frogs, European toad, other toads, fire salamander, other European salamanders, and the alpine newt in Europe, Africa, and Asia (Walton 1964, 1966; Yamaguti 1959).

It is common in southern Europe and northern Africa and is likely to be encountered in laboratory amphibians obtained from their natural habitat in these regions (Reichenbach-Klinke and Elkan 1965; Walton 1964). This cestode has also been reported from the leopard frog, cricket frog, American toad, common toad, and mudpuppy in North America, but these reports are of dubious validity (Walton 1964; Wardle and McLeod 1952).

MORPHOLOGY

Nematotaenia dispar (Fig. 18.23) is cylindrical, 5 to 22 cm long, and 0.5 to 0.6 mm wide (Reichenbach-Klinke and Elkan 1965; Wardle and McLeod 1952). It has an unarmed scolex with four suckers; a rostellum is either poorly developed or absent. Segmentation is inapparent except in the last few segments. The species is characterized by the presence in each segment of two testes and numerous so-called paruterine organs.

LIFE CYCLE

The life cycle is unknown.

PATHOLOGIC EFFECTS

In small numbers this cestode appears harmless, but in heavy infections, it causes intestinal obstruction and death (Elkan 1960).

Diagnosis is based on demonstration and identification of the parasite in the small intestine at necropsy.

CONTROL

Control and treatment are unknown.

PUBLIC HEALTH CONSIDERATIONS

This tapeworm is not known to affect man.

LARVAL CESTODES

Reptiles and amphibians are often intermediate hosts of cestodes (Reichenbach-Klinke and Elkan 1965). The pathologic effects of such infections are not well defined, but it is presumed that the migrating and rapidly growing larvae cause mechanical damage and interfere with the nutrition of the host.

Although larval cestodes are frequently observed in reptiles and amphibians, the parasites are usually not identified as to genus and species (Reichenbach-Klinke and Elkan 1965). Plerocercoid larvae of unidentified species are usually called spargana and probably belong to the genus *Diphyllobothrium* or *Spirometra;* tetrathyridium larvae of unidentified species are usually assigned to the genus *Mesocestoides* (Belding 1965; Wardle and McLeod 1952).

Larval cestodes which are likely to be encountered in laboratory reptiles and amphibians are listed in Table 18.5. The most important are discussed below.

Diphyllobothrium erinacei, Spirometra mansonoides

Larvae (spargana) of these pseudophyllid cestodes have been reported to be encysted in muscle and connective tissue of amphibians and reptiles throughout the world (Galliard and Ngu 1946; Noble and Noble 1961; Walton 1964, 1966, 1967; Witenberg 1964; Yamaguti 1959). Because of controversy about proper nomenclature and also because of the difficulty in precise identification of larval forms, disagreement exists concerning specific names of spargana in various geographic locations (Belding 1965; Burrows 1965; Witenberg 1964). *Diphyllobothrium erinacei* (syn. *Diphyllobothrium mansoni, D. ranarum, D. rep-*

tans, Spirometra erinacei) is commonly applied to larval forms reported from Europe, Asia, Indonesia, Australia, and South America, and *Spirometra mansonoides* (syn. *Diphyllobothrium mansonoides*) is applied to those reported from North America. *Diphyllobothrium erinacei* has been found in the grass frog, edible frog, treefrogs, other frogs, toads, fire salamander, common newt, other salamanders, snakes, and turtles (Galliard and Ngu 1946; Noble and Noble 1961; Walton 1964, 1966); *S. mansonoides* has been reported in the green frog, bullfrog, treefrogs, other frogs, toads, tiger salamander, red-spotted newt, kingsnakes, racers, water snakes, garter snakes, other snakes, and turtles (Corkum 1966; Noble and Noble 1961; Walton 1964, 1966). *Diphyllobothrium erinacei* is commonest in eastern Asia and Indonesia (Belding 1965), with an incidence of 82% reported in frogs *(Rana tigrina)* in southeastern Asia (Galliard 1948). In a survey of several species of tadpoles, adult frogs, and snakes in south central United States, *S. mansonoides* was found in 1% of the frogs and 18% of the snakes (Corkum 1966; Walton 1964, 1967).

Laboratory reptiles and amphibians obtained from their natural habitat in these regions are likely to be infected; the incidence in laboratory reptiles and amphibians in other parts of the world is unknown.

MORPHOLOGY

The plerocercoid larva is white, flattened, and transversely wrinkled, and has a longitudinal medial groove on the ventral surface (Fig. 18.24) (Belding 1965; Corkum 1966; Hoffman 1967). In amphibians it measures 10 to about 30 mm long by about 0.7 mm wide, whereas in reptiles it is 200 mm long or longer.

LIFE CYCLE

Eggs passed by the definitive host (dog, cat, other carnivores) hatch after reaching water and are ingested by a copepod in which they develop into procercoid larvae (Belding 1965; Corkum 1966; Galliard and Ngu 1946). Amphibians are usually infected in the immature stage (frog tadpole, newt larva) by ingesting the infected copepod. Adult amphibians and reptiles be-

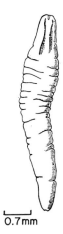

FIG. 18.24. *Diphyllobothrium,* plerocercoid larva. (From Lapage 1962. Courtesy of Ballière, Tindall and Cassell.)

come infected by ingesting an infected immature amphibian, and the definitive host becomes infected by ingesting an infected amphibian or reptile. Snakes are also infected by ingesting other snakes. The complete life cycle of *D. erinacei* requires about 54 days.

PATHOLOGIC EFFECTS

The migration of plerocercoid larvae through the intestinal wall and body cavity is known to cause mechanical damage and adhesions in fishes (Hoffman 1967) and, presumably, it is equally detrimental to reptiles and amphibians. Rapidly growing larvae also probably interfere with the nutrition of the host (Reichenbach-Klinke and Elkan 1965). Heavily infected frog tadpoles cease to grow (Galliard and Ngu 1946).

DIAGNOSIS

A tentative diagnosis is based on demonstration of the characteristic plerocercoid larva in the muscle (Belding 1965). A definitive diagnosis requires the experimental feeding of the immature parasite to a definitive host and the identification of the adult parasite.

CONTROL

Because the life cycle cannot be completed in the absence of copepods, routine sanitation will prevent the spread of the infection in the laboratory. No treatment is known.

PUBLIC HEALTH CONSIDERATIONS

Although these parasites cause sparganosis in man, infected laboratory reptiles and amphibians are unlikely to be a public health hazard as man is infected only by ingestion of uncooked flesh from infected animals (Belding 1965).

NEMATODES

Most nematodes have a life cycle involving only one host, but a few require an intermediate host (Belding 1965). Hundreds of species of nematodes have been reported from reptiles and amphibians (Walton 1964, 1966, 1967; Yamaguti 1961; Yorke and Maplestone 1926). In most cases the reptile or amphibian is the definitive host; in a few cases it is the intermediate host. Nematode larvae are frequently reported encysted in the stomach and intestinal wall of the green frog, water newt, and other aquatic amphibians in eastern United States (Fischthal 1955a, b; Rankin 1937, 1945). Although they are called spirurid larvae, their exact identity is unknown.

The nematodes affecting reptiles and amphibians are usually found in the alimentary tract or lungs, but some occur in the abdominal or thoracic cavity, liver, muscle, heart, blood vessels, and eyes (Walton 1964). The pathologic effects of these parasites are generally unknown. Most are probably harmless except in heavy infections (Reichenbach-Klinke and Elkan 1965).

Nematodes likely to be encountered in laboratory reptiles and amphibians are listed in Table 18.6. The most important are discussed below.

Rhabdias ranae, Rhabdias bufonis

These relatively nonpathogenic rhabditid nematodes are the common lungworms of frogs and toads (Reichenbach-Klinke and Elkan 1965). *Rhabdias ranae* occurs in North America in the lungs of the leopard frog, bullfrog, wood frog, pickerel frog, cricket frog, chorus frogs *(Pseudacris),* spring peeper, other frogs, common toad, other toads, kingsnakes, and garter snakes (Rankin 1945; Walton 1964;

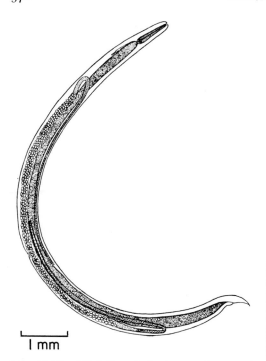

Fig. 18.25. *Rhabdias bufonis,* parthenogenic female. (From Yorke and Maplestone 1926.)

Yamaguti 1961). *Rhabdias bufonis* occurs in Europe and Asia in the lungs of the grass frog, edible frog, treefrogs, other frogs, European toad, and other toads (Walton 1964, 1966; Yamaguti 1961). A 31% incidence of *R. ranae* has been reported from several frog species in northeastern United States (Rankin 1945). A 48% incidence of *R. bufonis* has been observed in grass frogs in Great Britain (Lees 1962) and it is likely that most laboratory frogs and toads obtained from their natural habitat are infected (Reichenbach-Klinke and Elkan 1965).

MORPHOLOGY

The parthenogenic female, the stage of these species that occurs in the lungs of anurans, is about 11 to 13 mm long (Fig. 18.25) (Reichenbach-Klinke and Elkan 1965; Yorke and Maplestone 1926). It is characterized by a mouth that has six insignificant lips, a short esophagus, a vulva near the middle of the body, and a sharply tapered posterior extremity that ends in a finely conical point. The egg is thin shelled and embryonated. The larval stage that occurs in the intestine of the frog or toad is typically rhabditiform. The free-living male and female are similar to the parthenogenic female; the infective larva is filariform.

LIFE CYCLE

Eggs passed by the parthenogenic female are carried up the bronchus to the mouth and swallowed (Reichenbach-Klinke and Elkan 1965; Yorke and Maplestone 1926). They develop into rhabditiform larvae in the intestine and pass out in the feces. Outside the host they transform either directly into infective larvae or indirectly by first passing through a bisexual generation. The frog or toad is sometimes infected by ingestion of the infective larvae but usually by penetration of the skin. The larvae migrate through the body tissues to the lungs, where they develop to maturity.

PATHOLOGIC EFFECTS

Nothing is known of the pathologic effects of these nematodes. The adults are so ubiquitous in apparently healthy frogs that they are often regarded as symbionts (Elkan 1960; Reichenbach-Klinke and Elkan 1965). Migrating nematode larvae sometimes cause cysts or are associated with tumors in amphibians, and it has been suggested that the larvae of these worms can cause such effects (Reichenbach-Klinke and Elkan 1965).

DIAGNOSIS

Diagnosis is based on identification of the parthenogenic female in the lungs or the rhabditiform larvae in the intestine.

CONTROL

No attempts at control have been reported, but it would seem that the life cycle could be interrupted in the laboratory by frequent sanitation of cages. There is no treatment.

PUBLIC HEALTH CONSIDERATIONS

These nematodes are not known to affect man.

Cosmocerca, Cosmocercoides, Oxysomatium, Aplectana

These relatively nonpathogenic oxyurid nematodes are common in the intestine of frogs, toads, and salamanders in North America and Europe (Table 18.6) (Reichenbach-Klinke and Elkan 1965; Walton 1964; Yamaguti 1961). Incidences of 81% for *Cosmocerca ornata* and 23% for *Aplectana acuminata* have been reported in the grass frog in Great Britain (Lees 1962); incidences of 4 to 16% have been reported for *Cosmocercoides dukae* in the red-spotted newt (Rankin 1937, 1945) and 2 to 7% for *Oxysomatium americana* in salamanders (Fischthal 1955a) in northeastern United States. Laboratory amphibians obtained from their natural habitat are likely to be infected.

MORPHOLOGY

These are medium to small nematodes (about 2 to 7 mm in length), with a mouth that has three lips, an esophagus which terminates in a bulb, and a simple intestine that has no diverticulum (Fig. 18.26) (Yorke and Maplestone 1926). The males have two spicules of equal length; the females have a posterior extremity that is conical and pointed.

LIFE CYCLE

The life cycle is unknown but is probably direct, with infection by ingestion of an embryonated egg or infective larva (Cheng 1964; Yorke and Maplestone 1926).

PATHOLOGIC EFFECTS

Heavy infection of reptiles and amphibians with intestinal nematodes sometimes causes debilitation, intestinal obstruction, peritonitis, and death (Reichenbach-Klinke and Elkan 1965), but nothing is known of the specific pathologic effects of these nematodes.

DIAGNOSIS

Diagnosis is based on identification of the parasites in the intestine.

CONTROL

Control and treatment are unknown.

PUBLIC HEALTH CONSIDERATIONS

These nematodes are not known to affect man.

Falcaustra

(SYN. *Spironoura*)

This genus includes the commonest intestinal nematodes of turtles in the United States (Rausch 1947; Walton 1964; Williams 1953; Yamaguti 1961). *Falcaustra affinis* occurs in the box turtle, map turtle, spotted turtle, and Blanding's turtle; *F. procera* occurs in the painted turtle, cooters, and sliders; *F. wardi* occurs in the map turtle and snapping turtle; and *F. chely-*

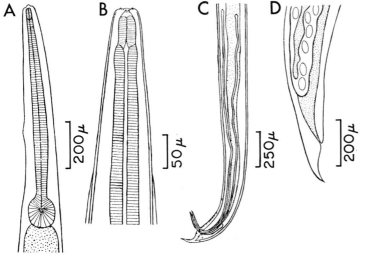

FIG. 18.26. *Aplectana.* (*A*) Anterior end, lateral view. (*B*) Anterior end, ventral view. (*C*) Posterior end of male. (*D*) Posterior end of female. (From Yorke and Maplestone 1926.)

drae occurs in the snapping turtle, red-eared turtle, and other turtles. Another species, *F. catesbianae,* is common in the bullfrog and also occurs in the leopard frog, chorus frogs *(Pseudacris),* treefrogs, and other frogs (Harwood 1932; Walton 1964; Yamaguti 1961). None is apparently pathogenic. Incidences of 19 to 97% have been reported in turtles and 50% in the bullfrog (Harwood 1932; Rausch 1947; Williams 1953). Laboratory turtles and bullfrogs obtained from their natural habitat are likely to be infected.

MORPHOLOGY

Adults of this genus are about 8 to 16 mm long and have an esophagus with a terminal bulb, a simple intestine without a diverticulum, and a pointed posterior extremity in both sexes (Fig. 18.27) (Harwood 1932; Yorke and Maplestone 1926). The male has spicules of equal length, a gubernaculum, but no caudal alae.

LIFE CYCLE

The life cycle is unknown but is probably direct, with infection by ingestion of

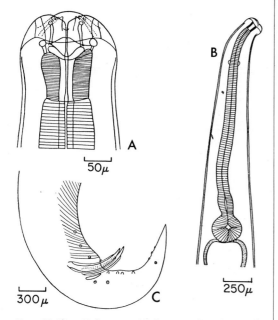

FIG. 18.27. *Falcaustra (Spironoura).* (A) Head, ventral view. (B) Anterior end, lateral view. (C) Posterior end of male, lateral view. (From Yorke and Maplestone 1926.)

an embryonated egg (Cheng 1964; Yorke and Maplestone 1926).

PATHOLOGIC EFFECTS

Nothing is known of the pathologic effects of nematodes of this genus.

DIAGNOSIS

Diagnosis is based on identification of the parasite in the intestine.

CONTROL

Piperazine, given orally 25 to 50 mg per kg of body weight daily for 3 days, is completely effective against intestinal nematodes of the Greek tortoise (Graham-Jones 1961) and is probably effective against *Falcaustra.* DDVP (dichlorvos), at a rate of 12.5 mg per kg of body weight daily for 2 days, is also effective for gastrointestinal nematodes in reptiles (Wallach 1969). The dose should be reduced for debilitated animals.

PUBLIC HEALTH CONSIDERATIONS

Falcaustra is not known to affect man.

Tachygonetria

This genus includes the commonest nematodes of the large intestine of the Greek tortoise in Europe and northern Africa (Reichenbach-Klinke and Elkan 1965; Schad 1963a; Yamaguti 1961). Laboratory tortoises are usually infected, often with several different species and hundreds of worms (Schad 1963a).

MORPHOLOGY

Adults are small worms, 1.5 to 4.6 mm in length (Fig. 18.28) (Forstner 1960; Yorke and Maplestone 1926). They have a mouth with six small lips, a long esophagus with a terminal bulb, and a simple intestine. The female has a short conical tail, and the vulva is posterior to the middle of the body. The male has a single, short spicule and a gubernaculum.

LIFE CYCLE

The life cycle is unknown but is probably direct, with infection by ingestion of an embryonated egg or infective larva (Cheng 1964; Yorke and Maplestone 1926).

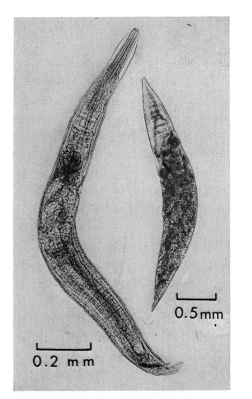

FIG. 18.28. *Tachygonetria longicollis. (Left)* Male. *(Right)* Female. (From Forstner 1960. Courtesy of Springer-Verlag, Berlin.)

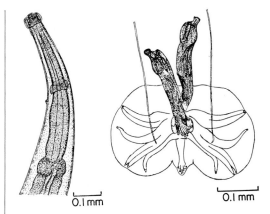

FIG. 18.29. *Oswaldocruzia. (Left)* Anterior end, lateral view. *(Right)* Posterior end of male, dorsal view. (From Yorke and Maplestone 1926.)

PATHOLOGIC EFFECTS

Although heavy infections are common and usually cause no apparent ill effects (Graham-Jones 1956; Schad 1963a), intestinal impaction and death have been reported (Graham-Jones 1961).

DIAGNOSIS

Diagnosis is based on identification of the parasite in the intestine.

CONTROL

Piperazine, given orally 25 to 50 mg per kg of body weight daily for 3 days, is completely effective in removing this parasite (Graham-Jones 1961). DDVP (dichlorvos), at a rate of 12.5 mg per kg of body weight daily for 2 days, is also effective for gastrointestinal nematodes in reptiles (Wallach 1969). The dose should be reduced for debilitated animals.

PUBLIC HEALTH CONSIDERATIONS

Tachygonetria is not known to affect man.

Oswaldocruzia

This relatively nonpathogenic trichostrongylid nematode occurs in the intestine of reptiles and amphibians throughout the world (Table 18.6) (Reichenbach-Klinke and Elkan 1965; Walton 1964; Yamaguti 1961). It is commonest in frogs, toads, salamanders, and turtles, occurring primarily in aquatic species (Rankin 1945). Typical reported incidences for *Oswaldocruzia pipiens* are 18% in the leopard frog in south central United States (Harwood 1932), and 70% in several species of frogs and 23% in the dusky salamander in northeastern United States (Rankin 1945). Incidences of 63% have been reported for *O. filiformis* in the grass frog in Great Britain (Lees 1962) and 53% for *O. leidyi* in the box turtle in north central United States (Rausch 1947). Laboratory frogs, toads, salamanders, and turtles obtained from their natural habitat are likely to be infected.

MORPHOLOGY

Adults of this genus are filiform worms about 6 to 14 mm long (Harwood 1932; Yorke and Maplestone 1926). The buccal cavity is rudimentary or absent, the vulva of the female is in the posterior half of the body, and the spicules of the male are short and stout and end in a number of processes (Fig. 18.29).

LIFE CYCLE

The life cycle is unknown but is probably direct, with infection by ingestion of an embryonated egg or infective larva (Cheng 1964; Yorke and Maplestone 1926).

PATHOLOGIC EFFECTS

Heavy infection of reptiles and amphibians with intestinal nematodes sometimes causes debilitation, intestinal obstruction, peritonitis, and death (Reichenbach-Klinke and Elkan 1965), but nothing is known of the specific pathologic effects of this nematode.

DIAGNOSIS

Diagnosis is based on demonstration and identification of the parasite in the intestine at necropsy.

CONTROL

Control is unknown and treatment has not been reported for amphibians. DDVP (dichlorvos), at a rate of 12.5 mg per kg of body weight daily for 2 days, is effective for gastrointestinal nematodes in reptiles (Wallach 1969). The dose should be reduced for debilitated animals.

PUBLIC HEALTH CONSIDERATIONS

Oswaldocruzia is not known to affect man.

Camallanus microcephalus, Camallanus trispinosus, Spiroxys contortus

These are common stomach and duodenal worms of turtles in the United States (Harwood 1932; Rausch 1947; Wieczorowski 1939; Williams 1953; Yamaguti 1961). *Camallanus microcephalus* is common in the painted turtle, map turtle, Blanding's turtle, and snapping turtle. Incidences of 54% have been reported in the painted turtle in north central United States and 83% in the snapping turtle in south central United States (Rausch 1947; Williams 1953). *Camallanus trispinosus* is common in the painted turtle, snapping turtle, and other turtles. Incidences of 87 to 100% have been reported in south central United States (Harwood 1932). *Spiroxys contortus* is common in the painted turtle, map turtle, snapping turtle, and other turtles and also occurs in the red-spotted newt. Incidences of 25% have been reported in the painted turtle and 38% in the snapping turtle in south central United States (Harwood 1932; Williams 1953). Laboratory turtles obtained from their natural habitat are usually heavily infected (Wieczorowski 1939).

MORPHOLOGY

Adults of *C. microcephalus* and *C. trispinosus* have a filiform body about 5 to 10 mm in length, a slitlike mouth with two lateral chitinous valves and an esophagus that has a short anterior muscular portion and a long posterior glandular portion (Fig. 18.30) (Yorke and Maplestone 1926). The posterior extremity of the male is rolled ventrally and has small caudal alae, dissimilar and unequal spicules, and no gubernaculum. The vulva of the female is near the middle of the body.

Adults of *S. contortus* have a filiform body that is about 15 to 30 mm in length, a mouth with two large, distinctly trilobed lips, and an esophagus that has a short anterior muscular portion and a longer posterior glandular portion (Fig. 18.31) (Yorke and Maplestone 1926). The male

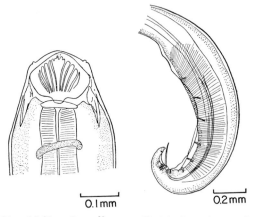

0.1mm   0.2mm

Fig. 18.30. *Camallanus.* *(Left)* Anterior end, lateral view. *(Right)* Posterior end of male, lateral view. (From Yorke and Maplestone 1926.)

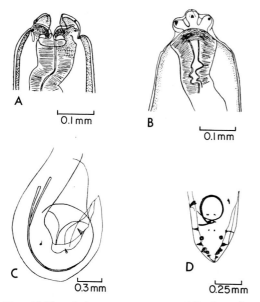

FIG. 18.31. *Spiroxys contortus*. *(A)* Anterior end, ventral view. *(B)* Anterior end, lateral view. *(C)* Posterior end of male, lateral view. *(D)* Posterior end of male, ventral view. (From Yorke and Maplestone 1926.)

has well-developed caudal alae, delicate and subequal spicules, and no gubernaculum. The vulva of the female is near the middle of the body.

LIFE CYCLE

The life cycle is indirect and involves a copepod as an intermediate host and sometimes an amphibian or fish as a transport host (Crites 1961; Hoffman 1967; Walton 1964). The definitive host is infected by ingestion of an infected copepod, amphibian, or fish.

PATHOLOGIC EFFECTS

These worms embed deeply in the stomach and duodenal wall and sometimes cause abscess formation (O'Connor 1966).

DIAGNOSIS

Diagnosis is based on identification of the parasite in the stomach or duodenum.

CONTROL

Because of the need for a copepod intermediate host, it is unlikely that the life cycle would be completed in the laboratory, and no special control procedures are needed. Piperazine, given orally 25 to 50 mg per kg of body weight daily for 3 days, is effective against the intestinal nematodes of the Greek tortoise (Graham-Jones 1961) and is probably effective for these species. DDVP (dichlorvos), at a rate of 12.5 mg per kg of body weight daily for 2 days, is also effective for gastrointestinal nematodes in reptiles (Wallach 1969). The dose should be reduced for debilitated animals.

PUBLIC HEALTH CONSIDERATIONS

These parasites are not known to affect man.

Foleyella, Icosiella

These filarial nematodes are common in frogs (Crans 1969; Kotcher 1941; Reichenbach-Klinke and Elkan 1965; Walton 1964; Yamaguti 1961). Adults are found in the abdominal cavity and mesentery and subcutaneous tissues; the microfilariae are found in the blood, lymph, and tissue fluids. *Foleyella brachyoptera* and *F. dolichoptera* occur in the leopard frog in southeastern United States; *F. americana* in the leopard frog and green frog in the United States and Canada; *F. ranae* in the leopard frog, green frog, and bullfrog in the United States and Canada; and *F. duboisi* in the edible frog in Israel. *Icosiella quadrituberculata* occurs in the leopard frog, bullfrog, and amphiumas in the United States and *I. neglecta* in the grass frog and edible frog in Europe, Asia, and Africa. These parasites are likely to be encountered in laboratory frogs obtained from endemic areas (Crans 1969; Kotcher 1941). Incidences as high as 100% have been reported (Reichenbach-Klinke and Elkan 1965).

MORPHOLOGY

Adults of these nematodes are white, fragile, filiform worms (Crans 1969; Kotcher 1941; Yorke and Maplestone 1926). Males are 15 to 25 mm in length; females are 60 to 72 mm long. The mouth of *Foleyella* is simple with no lips or teeth; the mouth of *Icosiella* is surrounded by four small spinous teeth. The esophagus of both genera is divided into two parts, a muscular and a glandular portion (Fig. 18.32); it is short in *Foleyella* and long in

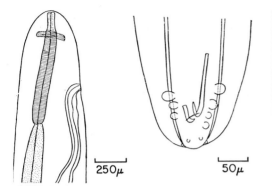

FIG. 18.32. *Foleyella.* *(Left)* Anterior end of female, lateral view. *(Right)* Posterior end of male, ventral view. (From Yorke and Maplestone 1926.)

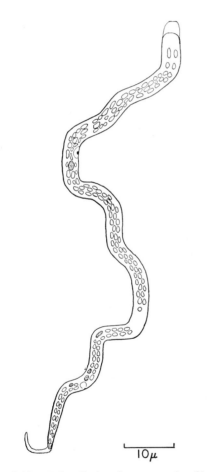

FIG. 18.33. *Foleyella brachyoptera* microfilaria. (From Kotcher 1941.)

Icosiella. The male of *Foleyella* has long caudal alae, anal papillae, and unequal spicules; the male of *Icosiella* has unequal spicules but no caudal alae or papillae. The vulva of the female in both genera is near the posterior end of the esophagus. The microfilariae (Fig. 18.33) are sheathed and vary in length with the genus and species. The microfilaria of *F. brachyoptera* is 120 to 168 μ long; that of *F. dolichoptera,* 263 to 295 μ; and that of *F. ranae,* 114 to 163 μ.

LIFE CYCLE

Adults occur in the body cavity of the frog, usually in the mesentery, but sometimes in the subcutis (Olsen 1967; Reichenbach-Klinke and Elkan 1965; Walton 1964). Fertilized eggs develop into sheathed microfilariae in the female, pass out into the tissues, and enter the lymph and blood vessels (Crans 1969; Kotcher 1941). Here they can survive about 2 years awaiting ingestion by a mosquito intermediate host. Once within a mosquito, the microfilariae migrate through the body, molt twice, and after about 18 days become infective larvae. The frog is infected when bitten by an infected mosquito.

PATHOLOGIC EFFECTS

Infected frogs are generally listless, but only in heavy infections does death occur (Reichenbach-Klinke and Elkan 1965). Adult worms cause either dermal, subcuticular, or mesenteric cysts, depending on the species, and microfilariae cause dermal tumors (Reichenbach-Klinke and Elkan 1965; Walton 1964).

DIAGNOSIS

Diagnosis is based on identification of the adult worm in the body cavity or the microfilariae in the blood (Reichenbach-Klinke and Elkan 1965).

CONTROL

Insect control will prevent infection of uninfected frogs. Treatment is unknown.

PUBLIC HEALTH CONSIDERATIONS

These nematodes are not known to affect man.

ACANTHOCEPHALANS

The life cycle of acanthocephalans involves an invertebrate intermediate host and one or two vertebrate hosts (Hyman 1951; Van Cleave 1948; Yamaguti 1963). Reptiles and amphibians serve as either definitive, intermediate, or transport hosts (Walton 1964). Only a few species of adult acanthocephalans are common in reptiles and amphibians, and larval acanthocephalans in these animals are rare (Harwood 1932; Rankin 1937; Van Cleave 1915, 1931; Walton 1964).

These parasites are characterized by a hook-bearing proboscis which is embedded in the tissues of the host for anchorage. All adult acanthocephalans of reptiles and amphibians occur in the stomach or intestine of their host. They cause local injury and inflammation at the point of attachment and sometimes death (Bullock 1961; Elkan 1960; Rankin 1937).

Acanthocephalans likely to be encountered in laboratory reptiles and amphibians are listed in Table 18.7. The most important are discussed below.

Neoechinorhynchus

Several species of this genus occur in the intestines of turtles in North America. *Neoechinorhynchus emydis* is found in the map turtle, false map turtle *(Graptemys pseudogeographica)*, Blanding's turtle, and red-eared turtle (Cable and Fisher 1961; Cable and Hopp 1954; Fisher 1960; Rausch 1947; Van Cleave and Bullock 1950); *N. pseudemydis* occurs in the painted turtle, Blanding's turtle, red-eared turtle, and other turtles (Acholonu 1967; Cable and Hopp 1954; Fisher 1960; Johnson 1968); *N. chrysemydis* is found in the painted turtle, red-eared turtle, and other cooters and sliders (Acholonu 1967; Cable and Hopp 1954; Fisher 1960; Johnson 1968); *N. emyditoides* occurs in the painted turtle, Blanding's turtle, and red-eared turtle (Acholonu 1967; Fisher 1960); and *N. stunkardi* occurs in the false map turtle (Cable and Fisher 1961). All are common and likely to be encountered in laboratory turtles obtained from their natural habitat.

Another species, *N. rutili*, which is common in fishes in North America, Europe, and Asia, occurs in turtles and the edible frog in Europe (Reichenbach-Klinke and Elkan 1965).

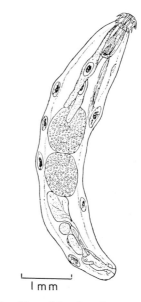

FIG. 18.34. *Neoechinorhynchus* male. (From Borradaile and Potts 1958. Courtesy of Cambridge University Press.)

MORPHOLOGY

Adults are small worms with a cylindrical, unspined, and usually curved body (Fig. 18.34) (Hoffman 1967). Males are 4.7 to 26.4 mm long by 0.4 to 1.0 mm wide, depending on the species; females are 7.0 to 39.2 mm long by 0.4 to 1.5 mm wide (Cable and Fisher 1961; Cable and Hopp 1954; Fisher 1960; Ward 1940). The proboscis is short and globular and contains three circles of six hooks each. Eggs are generally oval to elliptical but vary greatly in size and shape, depending on the species (Cable and Hopp 1954).

LIFE CYCLE

The life cycle of the North American species is not completely known. Eggs passed in the feces of a turtle hatch when ingested by an aquatic crustacean *(ostracod)* and unencysted immature worms develop (Lincicome 1948; Van Cleave and Bullock 1950). Snails become infected by ingestion of infected ostracods, and presumably a turtle is infected by ingesting an infected snail. It is uncertain, however, if the snail is a required intermediate host or if a turtle can become infected directly by ingestion of an infected ostracod. The life cycle of the species that affects turtles in Europe, *N. rutili,* does not require a second intermediate host (Reichenbach-Klinke and Elkan 1965). A turtle is infected with this species by ingesting an infected ostracod.

PATHOLOGIC EFFECTS

Heavy infections, 200 to 700 worms per turtle, are common (Rausch 1947; Van Cleave and Bullock 1950; Wieczorowski 1939). Often the worms are so numerous that they occlude the lumen of the intestine (Harwood 1932). The worms have a short proboscis and penetrate only the intestinal mucosa and a small amount of the lamina propria (Bullock 1961). Although they cause inflammation and thickening of the mucosa (Rausch 1947), tissue damage apparently is not extensive (Bullock 1961). They have also been associated with benign neoplastic lesions of the intestine (Rausch 1947) and benign granulomatous lesions of the pancreatic duct (Wieczorowski 1939).

DIAGNOSIS

Diagnosis is based on identification of the parasite in the intestine.

CONTROL

Because of the need for an ostracod and possibly a snail intermediate host, it is unlikely that the life cycle would be completed in the laboratory, and no special control procedures are required. There is no treatment.

PUBLIC HEALTH CONSIDERATIONS

Neoechinorhynchus is not known to affect man.

Acanthocephalus ranae

(SYN. *Acanthocephalus falcatus*)

This sometimes severely pathogenic acanthocephalan is common in the stomach and intestine of the grass frog, edible frog, and toad in Europe (Lees 1962; Reichenbach-Klinke and Elkan 1965). It also occurs in other European frogs, toads, salamanders, newts, and water snakes (Walton

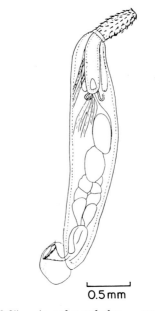

FIG. 18.35. *Acanthocephalus ranae* male. (From Van Cleave 1915.)

0.5 mm

1964). An incidence of 18% has been reported in the grass frog in Great Britain (Lees 1962), and 50% in the edible frog on the European continent (Van Cleave 1915). It is likely to be encountered in Europe in laboratory frogs obtained from their natural habitat.

MORPHOLOGY

The body of adults is cylindrical and the proboscis elongate, with 6 to 28 longitudinal rows of 4 to 15 hooks each (Fig. 18.35) (Hoffman 1967). The male is about 3.2 mm long and has two tandem, oval testes in the midregion of the body (Van Cleave 1915). The female is longer, about 6 mm in length.

LIFE CYCLE

The life cycle involves an aquatic crustacean (isopod) as an intermediate host (Walton 1964). Eggs passed in the feces of a definitive host are ingested by a crustacean, and the amphibian is infected by ingesting the crustacean. Snakes, which normally do not feed on isopods, become infected by ingesting an infected amphibian (Reichenbach-Klinke and Elkan 1965).

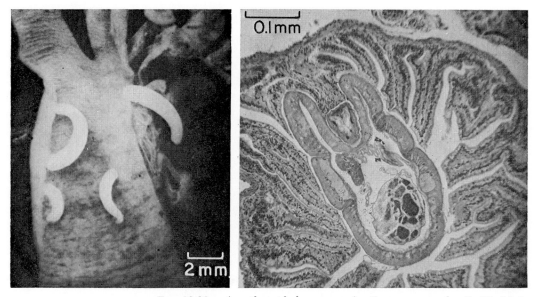

FIG. 18.36. *Acanthocephalus ranae* in European toad. *(Left)* Adult worms attached to intestinal mucosa. *(Right)* Section of small intestine containing a worm. (Courtesy of E. Elkan, London.)

PATHOLOGIC EFFECTS

The elongated proboscis of this worm penetrates deeply into the gastric or intestinal wall, causing severe tissue reaction and mechanical damage to the mucosa and submucosa at the point of attachment (Fig. 18.36) (Bullock 1961; Elkan 1960; Reichenbach-Klinke and Elkan 1965). Heavy infections accompanied by secondary bacterial infection result in death.

DIAGNOSIS

Diagnosis is based on recognition of the parasite in the stomach or intestine.

CONTROL

Because of the need for an isopod intermediate host, it is unlikely that the life cycle would be completed in the laboratory and no special control procedures are needed. There is no treatment.

PUBLIC HEALTH CONSIDERATIONS

This parasite does not affect man.

NEMATOMORPHS (GORDIACEAN WORMS)

Nematomorphs are long, slender, cylindrical worms that have a degenerate, nonfunctional alimentary tract (Cheng 1964). The adults are free-living, but the larvae are usually parasites of arthropods. There are a few reports of mole salamanders in the United States and the grass frog in Europe being infected with nematomorph larvae, but these are only accidental pseudoparasitic associations (Walton 1964).

LEECHES

Leeches are only temporary ectoparasites that leave the host when engorged (Cheng 1964). Those that have been reported to affect reptiles and amphibians used in the laboratory are listed in Table 18.8. All are rare or uncommon as ectoparasites of reptiles and amphibians and none is likely to be encountered in the laboratory.

TABLE 18.1. Monogenetic and aspidobothretic trematodes affecting laboratory reptiles and amphibians

Parasite	Geographic Distribution	Reptilian or Amphibian Host	Location in Host	Method of Infection	Incidence in Nature	Remarks	Reference
Gyrodactylus elegans[*]	North America, Europe	Frogs	Gills, skin	Direct contact	Unknown; probably common	Ingests blood; causes mucus coating on gills, skin; frayed fins; sometimes asphyxiation, death	Cameron 1956 Cheng 1964 Davis 1953 Dawes 1946 Hoffman 1967 Hoffman and Putz 1964 Noble and Noble 1964
Polystoma nearcticum[*]	North America	Treefrogs	Gills, urinary bladder	Direct contact	Common	Ingests blood; pathologic effects slight	Cameron 1956 Paul 1938 Walton 1964
Polystoma integerrimum[*]	Europe, Asia, Africa	Frogs, treefrogs, toads, clawed toads	Urinary bladder	Direct contact	Common	Ingests blood; pathologic effects slight	Cameron 1956 Lees 1962 Reichenbach-Klinke and Elkan 1965 Savage 1962 Walton 1964, 1966, 1967
Polystoma gallieni	Europe	Treefrogs	Urinary bladder	Direct contact	Unknown; apparently common	Pathologic effects unknown; probably causes slight effects	Reichenbach-Klinke and Elkan 1965 Walton 1964
Polystoma africanum	Africa	Toads	Urinary bladder	Direct contact	Unknown; apparently common	Pathologic effects unknown; probably causes slight effects	Reichenbach-Klinke and Elkan 1965 Walton 1964
Polystoma stellai	Cuba	Treefrogs	Urinary bladder	Direct contact	Unknown; apparently common	Pathologic effects unknown; probably causes slight effects	Reichenbach-Klinke and Elkan 1965 Walton 1964
Polystomoides terrapenis	North America	Box turtles	Urinary bladder	Direct contact	Common	Pathologic effects unknown	Harwood 1932 Reichenbach-Klinke and Elkan 1965
Polystomoides orbiculare	North America	Painted turtles, red-eared turtle, softshell turtles, snapping turtles, pond turtles	Urinary bladder	Direct contact	Common	Pathologic effects unknown	Harwood 1932 Rausch 1947 Reichenbach-Klinke and Elkan 1965 Thatcher 1954 Williams 1953
Polystomoides hassalli	North America	Snapping turtles, other turtles	Urinary bladder	Direct contact	Common	Pathologic effects unknown	Harwood 1932 Reichenbach-Klinke and Elkan 1965
Polystomoides oblongum	North America	Painted turtles, snapping turtles, other turtles	Urinary bladder	Direct contact	Common	Pathologic effects unknown	Reichenbach-Klinke and Elkan 1965 Williams 1953
Polystomoides multiflax	North America	Painted turtles	Mouth	Direct contact	Common	Pathologic effects unknown	Reichenbach-Klinke and Elkan 1965
Polystomoides coronatus	North America	Painted turtles, red-eared turtle, map turtles, softshell turtles, snapping turtles, pond turtles	Mouth	Direct contact	Common	Pathologic effects unknown	Reichenbach-Klinke and Elkan 1965 Thatcher 1954 Williams 1953

[*]Discussed in text.

580

TABLE 18.1 *(continued)*

Parasite	Geographic Distribution	Reptilian or Amphibian Host	Location in Host	Method of Infection	Incidence in Nature	Remarks	Reference
Polystomoides oris	North America	Painted turtles	Mouth	Direct contact	Common	Pathologic effects unknown	Paul 1938, Reichenbach-Klinke and Elkan 1965
Polystomoides megacotyle	North America	Painted turtles, red-eared turtle	Mouth	Direct contact	Common	Pathologic effects unknown	Harwood 1932
Polystomoides rugosum	North America	Softshell turtles	Nose	Direct contact	Common	Pathologic effects unknown	Reichenbach-Klinke and Elkan 1965
Polystomoides ocellatus	Europe, Asia	Semi-box turtles	Urinary bladder	Direct contact	Common	Pathologic effects unknown	Reichenbach-Klinke and Elkan 1965
Polystomoides japonicus	Japan	Pond turtles	Mouth	Direct contact	Common	Pathologic effects unknown	Reichenbach-Klinke and Elkan 1965
*Sphyranura oligorchis**	United States	Mudpuppy	Gills	Direct contact	Common	Ingests blood; causes frayed gills, sometimes asphyxiation	Olsen 1967, Rankin 1937, Reichenbach-Klinke and Elkan 1965, Walton 1964
*Sphyranura polyorchis**	United States	Mudpuppy	Gills	Direct contact	Common	Ingests blood; causes frayed gills, sometimes asphyxiation	Olsen 1967, Rankin 1937, Reichenbach-Klinke and Elkan 1965, Walton 1964
*Sphyranura osleri**	Canada	Mudpuppy	Gills	Direct contact	Common	Ingests blood; causes frayed gills, sometimes asphyxiation	Olsen 1967, Rankin 1937, Reichenbach-Klinke and Elkan 1965, Walton 1964
*Aspidogaster conchicola**	Worldwide	Various turtles	Stomach, intestine	Ingestion of infected clam	Unknown; probably common	Turtle is only accidental host. Pathologic effects unknown	Olsen 1967
Cotylaspis cokeri	North America	Map turtles, other turtles	Stomach, intestine	Ingestion of infected clam	Common	Turtle is probably only accidental host. Pathologic effects unknown	Rausch 1947, Reichenbach-Klinke and Elkan 1965
Cotylaspis stunkardi	North America	Snapping turtles	Stomach, intestine	Ingestion of infected clam	Unknown; probably common	Turtle is probably only accidental host. Pathologic effects unknown	Reichenbach-Klinke and Elkan 1965
Cotylaspis sinensis	China	Softshell turtles	Stomach, intestine	Ingestion of infected clam	Unknown; probably common	Turtle is probably only accidental host. Pathologic effects unknown	Reichenbach-Klinke and Elkan 1965
Lophotaspis orientalis	China	Softshell turtles	Stomach, intestine	Ingestion of infected clam	Unknown; probably common	Turtle is probably only accidental host. Pathologic effects unknown	Reichenbach-Klinke and Elkan 1965

*Discussed in text.

TABLE 18.2. Adult digenetic trematodes affecting laboratory reptiles and amphibians

Parasite	Geographic Distribution	Reptilian or Amphibian Host	Location in Host	Method of Infection	Incidence in Nature	Remarks	Reference
Gorgodera amplicava*	North America	Leopard frog, green frog, bullfrog, pickerel frog, toads, mole salamanders	Kidneys, urinary bladder	Ingestion of second intermediate host (frog tadpole, salamander larva, snail, crayfish)	Common	Incidence of 35% reported in bullfrog in southern United States. Heavy infections cause listlessness, anorexia, uremia, death	Goodchild 1948, 1950 Harwood 1932 Olsen 1967 Rankin 1937 Walton 1964 Yamaguti 1958
Gorgodera cygnoides	North America, Europe	Leopard frog, green frog, bullfrog, grass frog, pickerel frog, edible frog, treefrogs, toads, spotted salamander	Urinary bladder	Ingestion of second intermediate host (frog tadpole, salamander larva, snail, crayfish)	Common	Syn. Gorgodera pagenstecheri. Heavy infections cause listlessness, anorexia, uremia, death	Dawes 1946 Walton 1964 Yamaguti 1958
Gorgodera varsoviensis	Europe, Africa	Edible frog, grass frog	Urinary bladder	Ingestion of second intermediate host (frog tadpole, salamander larva, snail, crayfish)	Common	Heavy infections cause listlessness, anorexia, uremia, death	Dawes 1946 Walton 1964 Yamaguti 1958
Gorgoderina attenuata	North America, Central America	Leopard frog, green frog, bullfrog, wood frog, pickerel frog, other frogs, red-spotted newt, other newts, garter snakes	Kidneys, urinary bladder	Ingestion of second intermediate host (frog tadpole, salamander larva, snail, crayfish)	Common	Incidences of 22 to 100% reported in frogs, 29% in red-spotted newt in eastern United States. Heavy infections cause listlessness, anorexia, uremia, death	Caballero 1946 Fischthal 1955a Goodchild 1950 Olsen 1967 Rankin 1945 Yamaguti 1958
Gorgoderina bilobata*	Southeastern United States	Leopard frog, bullfrog, toads, marbled salamander, dusky salamanders, red-spotted newt	Urinary bladder	Ingestion of second intermediate host (frog tadpole, salamander larva, snail, crayfish)	Common	Incidences of 2 to 16% reported in salamanders. Pathologic effects unknown; heavy infections probably cause listlessness, anorexia, uremia, death	Rankin 1937 Walton 1964 Yamaguti 1958
Gorgoderina intermedia	North America	Red-spotted newt	Urinary bladder	Ingestion of second intermediate host (frog tadpole, salamander larva, snail, crayfish)	Common	Pathologic effects unknown; heavy infections probably cause listlessness, anorexia, uremia, death	Rankin 1937 Walton 1964 Yamaguti 1958
Gorgoderina parvicava	Mexico, Central America, South America	Frogs, toads	Urinary bladder	Ingestion of second intermediate host (frog tadpole, salamander larva, snail, crayfish)	Common	Pathologic effects unknown; heavy infections probably cause listlessness, anorexia, uremia, death	Caballero 1946 Walton 1964, 1967 Yamaguti 1958
Gorgoderina vitelliloba*	Europe, southwestern Asia, Africa	Grass frog, other frogs, toads	Urinary bladder	Ingestion of second intermediate host (frog tadpole, salamander larva, snail, crayfish)	Common	Incidence of 12% reported in grass frog in Great Britain. Pathologic effects unknown; heavy infections probably cause listlessness, anorexia, uremia, death	Lees 1962 Walton 1964, 1967 Yamaguti 1958

* Discussed in text.

TABLE 18.2 *(continued)*

Parasite	Geographic Distribution	Reptilian or Amphibian Host	Location in Host	Method of Infection	Incidence in Nature	Remarks	Reference
Phyllodistomum solidum	Eastern United States	Dusky salamanders	Urinary bladder	Ingestion of second intermediate host (arthropod)	Common	Incidences of 5 to 18% reported. Pathologic effects unknown	Fischthal 1955a, b Goodchild 1948 Rankin 1937 Walton 1964 Yamaguti 1958
Phyllodistomum americanum	North America	Toads, spotted salamander, tiger salamander, other salamanders	Urinary bladder	Ingestion of second intermediate host (arthropod)	Unknown; probably common	Pathologic effects unknown	Rankin 1937 Walton 1964 Yamaguti 1958
Crepidostomum cooperi	North America, Europe	Mudpuppies, snapping turtles, softshell turtles	Intestine	Ingestion of second intermediate host (arthropod)	Unknown; probably common	Pathologic effects unknown	Hoffman 1967 Rankin 1937 Reichenbach-Klinke and Elkan 1965 Walton 1964 Yamaguti 1958
Crepidostomum cornutum	North America	Frogs, salamanders, mudpuppies, amphiumas	Intestine	Ingestion of second intermediate host (arthropod)	Unknown; probably common	Pathologic effects unknown	Hoffman 1967 Walton 1964 Yamaguti 1958
Crepidostomum farionis	North America, Europe	Mudpuppies	Intestine	Ingestion of second intermediate host (arthropod)	Unknown; probably common	Pathologic effects unknown	Hoffman 1967 Rankin 1937 Walton 1964 Yamaguti 1958
Auridistomum chelydrae	North America	Painted turtles, snapping turtles	Intestine	Ingestion of second intermediate host (arthropod)	Unknown; probably common	Pathologic effects unknown	Harwood 1932 Rausch 1947 Walton 1964 Williams 1953 Yamaguti 1958
Telorchis necturi	North America	Mudpuppies	Intestine	Ingestion of second intermediate host (arthropod)	Common	Pathologic effects unknown	Rankin 1937 Reichenbach-Klinke and Elkan 1965 Yamaguti 1958
Telorchis stunkardi	Southern United States	Amphiumas	Intestine	Ingestion of second intermediate host (arthropod)	Unknown; probably common	Pathologic effects unknown	Rankin 1937 Walton 1964 Yamaguti 1958
Telorchis ercolani	North America, Europe	Painted turtles, red-eared turtle, water snakes	Intestine	Ingestion of second intermediate host (arthropod)	Common	Syn. *Telorchis nematoides*. Sometimes causes pancreatitis, pancreatic necrosis	Dawes 1946 Wieczorowski 1939 Yamaguti 1958
Telorchis attenuatus	North America	Painted turtles	Intestine	Ingestion of second intermediate host (arthropod)	Common	Pathologic effects unknown	Rausch 1947 Yamaguti 1958
Telorchis corti	North America	Painted turtles, map turtles, pond turtles, snapping turtles	Intestine	Ingestion of second intermediate host (arthropod)	Common	Pathologic effects unknown	Rausch 1947 Williams 1953 Yamaguti 1958
Telorchis medius	North America	Blanding's turtle, cooters, sliders, box turtle, garter snakes	Intestine	Ingestion of second intermediate host (arthropod)	Common	Pathologic effects unknown	Rausch 1947 Yamaguti 1958

TABLE 18.2 (continued)

Parasite	Geographic Distribution	Reptilian or Amphibian Host	Location in Host	Method of Infection	Incidence in Nature	Remarks	Reference
Telorchis robustus	United States, Mexico	Pond turtles, spotted turtle, red-eared turtle, other cooters	Intestine	Ingestion of second intermediate host (arthropod)	Common	Pathologic effects unknown	Harwood 1932 Rausch 1947 Yamaguti 1958
Telorchis thamnophidis	North America	Garter snakes	Intestine	Ingestion of second intermediate host (arthropod)	Unknown; probably common	Pathologic effects unknown	Bravo 1943 Yamaguti 1958
Telorchis bonnerensis	Western United States	Garter snakes	Intestine	Ingestion of second intermediate host (arthropod)	Unknown; probably common	Pathologic effects unknown	Waitz 1961
Protenes chapmani	North America	Red-eared turtle	Intestine	Ingestion of second intermediate host (arthropod)	Common	Pathologic effects unknown	Harwood 1932
Protenes angustus	North America	Painted turtles, red-eared turtle	Intestine	Ingestion of second intermediate host (arthropod)	Common	Pathologic effects unknown	Yamaguti 1958
*Opisthioglyphe ranae**	Europe, Africa	Edible frog, grass frog, treefrogs, European toad, clawed toads, European salamanders, crested newt	Intestine	Ingestion of second intermediate host (insect, tadpole)	Common	Syn. *Opisthioglyphe endoloba, Lecithopyge ranae.* Pathologic effects unknown	Dawes 1946 Reichenbach-Klinke and Elkan 1965 Walton 1964 Yamaguti 1958
*Dolichosaccus rastellus**	Europe	Edible frog, grass frog, European toad, European salamanders, newts	Intestine	Ingestion of second intermediate host (insect, tadpole)	Common	Syn. *Lecithopyge rastellum.* Incidence of 8% reported in grass frog in Great Britain. Pathologic effects unknown	Dawes 1946 Lees 1962 Reichenbach-Klinke and Elkan 1965 Walton 1964 Yamaguti 1958
*Lechriorchis primus**	North America	Water snakes, garter snakes	Lung, mouth, esophagus, intestine	Ingestion of second intermediate host (frog tadpole)	Common	Incidence of 25% reported in garter snakes in north central United States. Heavy infections cause dyspnea, weight loss; other pathologic effects unknown	Olsen 1967 Talbot 1933 Walton 1964 Yamaguti 1958
*Lechriorchis tygarti**	United States	Garter snakes	Lung, mouth, esophagus, intestine	Ingestion of second intermediate host (frog tadpole)	Common	Heavy infections cause dyspnea, weight loss; other pathologic effects unknown	Nelson 1950 Olsen 1967 Talbot 1933 Walton 1964 Yamaguti 1958
Lechriorchis plesientera	Western United States	Garter snakes	Lung, mouth, esophagus, intestine	Ingestion of second intermediate host (frog tadpole)	Common	Pathologic effects unknown; heavy infections probably cause dyspnea, weight loss	Waitz 1961 Yamaguti 1958

*Discussed in text.

584

TABLE 18.2 (continued)

Parasite	Geographic Distribution	Reptilian or Amphibian Host	Location in Host	Method of Infection	Incidence in Nature	Remarks	Reference
*Zeugorchis eurinus**	United States	Garter snakes	Lung, mouth, esophagus, intestine	Ingestion of second intermediate host (frog tadpole)	Common	Heavy infections cause dyspnea, weight loss; other pathologic effects unknown	Olsen 1967, Talbot 1933, Walton 1964, Yamaguti 1958
Zeugorchis megacystis	Central United States	Garter snakes	Lung, mouth, esophagus, intestine	Presumably by ingestion of frog tadpole	Unknown	Pathologic effects unknown; heavy infections probably cause dyspnea, weight loss	Stewart 1960
Zeugorchis signatus	Europe	Water snakes	Lung, mouth, esophagus, intestine	Ingestion of second intermediate host (frog tadpole)	Common	Heavy infections cause dyspnea, weight loss; other pathologic effects unknown	Walton 1964
*Dasymetra conferta**	North America	Water snakes	Lung, mouth, esophagus, intestine	Ingestion of second intermediate host (frog tadpole)	Common	Heavy infections cause dyspnea, weight loss; other pathologic effects unknown	Byrd and Maples 1969, Harwood 1932, Walton 1964, Yamaguti 1958
Dasymetra villicaeca	United States	Water snakes	Lung, mouth, esophagus, intestine	Ingestion of second intermediate host (frog tadpole)	Common	Heavy infections cause dyspnea, weight loss; other pathologic effects unknown	Olsen 1967, Walton 1964, Yamaguti 1958
*Ochetosoma aniarum**	United States	Water snakes, hognose snakes, kingsnakes	Lung, mouth, esophagus, intestine	Ingestion of second intermediate host (frog tadpole)	Common	Syn. *Neorenifer aniarum*. Heavy infections cause dyspnea, weight loss; other pathologic effects unknown	Harwood 1932, Marcus 1968, Olsen 1967, Walton 1964, Yamaguti 1958
Ochetosoma kansensis	United States	Racers, common kingsnake, other snakes	Lung, mouth, esophagus, intestine	Ingestion of second intermediate host (frog tadpole)	Common	Syn. *Neorenifer kansensis*. Heavy infections cause dyspnea, weight loss; other pathologic effects unknown	Harwood 1932, Marcus 1968, Walton 1964, Yamaguti 1958
Ochetosoma lateriporus	Central United States	Racers	Lung, mouth, esophagus, intestine	Presumably by ingestion of frog tadpole	Unknown	Syn. *Neorenifer batereporus*. Pathologic effects unknown; heavy infections probably cause dyspnea, weight loss	Stewart 1960
Encyclometra colabrimurorum	Europe, Asia	Racers, water snakes	Intestine	Presumably by ingestion of frog tadpole	Unknown	Pathologic effects unknown	Dawes 1946, Walton 1964, Yamaguti 1958
Plagitura parva	Eastern United States	Red-spotted newt	Small intestine	Ingestion of metacercaria in tissue of second intermediate host (snail, insect)	Common	Syn. *Manodistomum parvum*. Incidences of 5 to 7% reported. Pathologic effects unknown	Fischthal 1955a, b, Rankin 1937, 1945, Russell 1951, Walton 1964, Yamaguti 1958

*Discussed in text.

TABLE 18.2 (continued)

Parasite	Geographic Distribution	Reptilian or Amphibian Host	Location in Host	Method of Infection	Incidence in Nature	Remarks	Reference
Plagitura salamandra	Eastern United States	Marbled salamander, dusky salamanders, other salamanders, red-spotted newt	Small intestine	Ingestion of metacercaria in tissue of second intermediate host (snail, insect)	Common in water newt; rare in other salamanders	Syn. *Manodistomum salamandra*. Incidence of 57% reported in red-spotted newt. Pathologic effects unknown	Fischthal 1955a, b; Rankin 1937; Russell 1951; Walton 1964; Yamaguti 1958
*Haplometra cylindracea**	Europe	Grass frog, edible frog, treefrogs, European toad	Lungs	Ingestion of second intermediate host (water beetle)	Common	Incidence of 54% reported in grass frog in Great Britain. Ingests blood; causes pulmonary tissue alteration, no inflammation; heavy infections cause no apparent gross effects	Arvy 1950; Dawes 1946; Lees 1962; Reichenbach-Klinke and Elkan 1965; Walton 1964; Yamaguti 1958
Haplometrana intestinalis	Western United States	Frogs, toads	Intestine	Ingestion of metacercaria formed in skin of frog after penetration by free-swimming cercaria	Common	Pathologic effects unknown	Olsen 1967; Walton 1964; Yamaguti 1958
*Glypthelmins pennsylvaniensis**	United States	Spring peeper, chorus frogs (*Pseudacris*)	Intestine	Ingestion of metacercaria formed in skin of frog after penetration by free-swimming cercaria	Common	Pathologic effects unknown	Cheng 1961; Ubelaker et al. 1967; Walton 1964
*Glypthelmins quieta**	United States, Mexico, South America, Asia	Leopard frog, green frog, bullfrog, pickerel frog, spring peeper, other frogs, toads	Intestine	Ingestion of metacercaria formed in skin of frog after penetration by free-swimming cercaria	Common	Incidence of 30% reported in bullfrog, 18% in spring peeper in northeastern United States. Pathologic effects unknown	Rankin 1945; Schell 1962; Walton 1964; Yamaguti 1958
Glypthelmins californiensis	United States, Mexico	Leopard frog, other frogs	Intestine	Ingestion of metacercaria formed in skin of frog after penetration by free-swimming cercaria	Common	Syn. *Margeana californiensis*. Pathologic effects unknown	Walton 1964; Yamaguti 1958
Glypthelmins linguatula	South America, Asia	Frogs, toads	Intestine	Ingestion of metacercaria formed in skin of frog after penetration by free-swimming cercaria	Common	Syn. *Margeana linguatula*. Pathologic effects unknown	Cheng 1964; Walton 1964; Yamaguti 1958
Haematoloechus variegatus	Worldwide	Leopard frog, bullfrog, grass frog, edible frog, American toad, European toad	Lungs	Ingestion of second intermediate host (arthropod)	Common	Pathologic effects unknown; heavy infections occur	Dawes 1946; Reichenbach-Klinke and Elkan 1965; Walton 1964; Yamaguti 1958
Haematoloechus medioplexus	North America, South America	Leopard frog, green frog, bullfrog, pickerel frog, toads	Lungs	Ingestion of second intermediate host (arthropod)	Common	Incidence of 18% reported in frogs in northeastern United States. Pathologic effects unknown; heavy infections occur	Olsen 1967; Rankin 1945; Walton 1964; Yamaguti 1958
Haematoloechus breviplexus	North America	Leopard frog, green frog, bullfrog, toads	Lungs	Ingestion of second intermediate host (arthropod)	Common	Pathologic effects unknown; heavy infections occur	Walton 1964; Yamaguti 1958

*Discussed in text.

TABLE 18.2 *(continued)*

Parasite	Geographic Distribution	Reptilian or Amphibian Host	Location in Host	Method of Infection	Incidence in Nature	Remarks	Reference
Haematoloechus varioplexus	North America	Leopard frog, bullfrog, wood frog,	Lungs	Ingestion of second intermediate host (arthropod)	Common	Pathologic effects unknown; heavy infections occur	Walton 1964 Yamaguti 1958
Haematoloechus similiplexus	United States, Canada	Leopard frog, green frog, American toad	Lungs	Ingestion of second intermediate host (arthropod)	Common	Pathologic effects unknown; heavy infectons occur	Walton 1964 Yamaguti 1958
Haematoloechus complexus	United States, Mexico	Leopard frog, green frog, bullfrog	Lungs	Ingestion of second intermediate host (arthropod)	Common	Pathologic effects unknown; heavy infections occur	Olsen 1967 Reichenbach-Klinke and Elkan 1965 Walton 1964 Yamaguti 1958
Haematoloechus longiplexus	United States, Mexico	Leopard frog, green frog, bullfrog, other frogs	Lungs	Ingestion of second intermediate host (arthropod)	Common	Pathologic effects unknown; heavy infections occur	Olsen 1967 Walton 1964 Yamaguti 1958
Haematoloechus parviplexus	United States	Green frog, bullfrog, other frogs	Lungs	Ingestion of second intermediate host (arthropod)	Common	Pathologic effects unknown; heavy infections occur	Olsen 1967 Walton 1964 Yamaguti 1958
Haematoloechus asper	Europe, Africa	Edible frog, grass frog, European toad	Lungs	Ingestion of second intermediate host (arthropod)	Common	Pathologic effects unknown; heavy infections occur	Dawes 1946 Walton 1964 Yamaguti 1958
Haematoloechus similis	Europe, Africa	Edible frog, grass frog	Lungs	Ingestion of second intermediate host (arthropod)	Common	Pathologic effects unknown; heavy infections occur	Dawes 1946 Walton 1964 Yamaguti 1958
*Brachycoelium salamandrae**	Worldwide	Grass frogs, wood frog, pickerel frog, green treefrog, spring peeper, cricket frogs, other frogs, European toad, other toads, mole salamanders, dusky salamanders, European salamanders, other salamanders, red-spotted newt, amphiumas, various reptiles	Intestine	Ingestion of metacercaria in tissues of intermediate host (snail)	Common	Incidences of 3 to 100% reported in salamanders, 11% in pickerel frog in eastern United States. Pathologic effects unknown	Dawes 1946 Fischthal 1955a, b Rankin 1937, 1945 Rausch 1947 Reichenbach-Klinke and Elkan 1965 Russell 1951 Walton 1964, 1966 Yamaguti 1958
Brachycoelium stablefordi	Eastern United States	Dusky salamanders	Small intestine	Presumably by ingestion of snail	Unknown	Pathologic effects unknown	Cheng and Chase 1961
Brachycoelium ambystomae	Southeastern United States	Marbled salamander	Small intestine	Presumably by ingestion of snail	Common	Incidence of 100% reported. Pathologic effects unknown	Couch 1966
Leptophallus nigrovenosus	Europe, Africa	Water snakes, other snakes	Esophagus, intestine	Ingestion of second intermediate host (arthropod)	Common	Pathologic effects unknown; heavy infections occur	Dawes 1946 Walton 1964 Yamaguti 1958

*Discussed in text.

TABLE 18.2 (continued)

Parasite	Geographic Distribution	Reptilian or Amphibian Host	Location in Host	Method of Infection	Incidence in Nature	Remarks	Reference
Paradistomum mutabile	Europe, Asia	Sand lizard, other lizards	Gallbladder	Ingestion of second intermediate host (arthropod)	Common	Pathologic effects unknown; heavy infections occur	Dawes 1946 Yamaguti 1958
Megalodiscus temporatus*	North America, Central America, South America	Leopard frog, green frog, bullfrog, green treefrog, spring peeper, other frogs, common toad, mole salamanders, other salamanders, dusky salamanders, red-spotted newt, amphiumas	Large intestine	Ingestion of metacercaria in skin of amphibian	Common	Incidences of 16 to 48% reported in red-spotted newt in eastern United States. Pathologic effects unknown	Cheng 1964 Fischthal 1955a Olsen 1967 Rankin 1937, 1945 Reichenbach-Klinke and Elkan 1965 Skrjabin 1965 Walton 1964 Yamaguti 1958
Megalodiscus americanus*	North America, Central America	Leopard frog, other frogs, mole salamanders, dusky salamanders, other salamanders, California newt, amphiumas	Intestine	Ingestion of metacercaria in skin of amphibian	Common	Pathologic effects unknown	Skrjabin 1964 Walton 1964 Yamaguti 1958
Megalodiscus intermedius*	United States	Bullfrog, dusky salamanders	Rectum	Ingestion of metacercaria in skin of amphibian	Common	Pathologic effects unknown	Skrjabin 1964 Walton 1964 Yamaguti 1958
Megalodiscus microphagus*	United States	Frogs, toads, salamanders	Large intestine, urinary bladder	Ingestion of metacercaria in skin of amphibian	Common	Pathologic effects unknown	Efford and Tsumura 1969 Skrjabin 1964 Walton 1964 Yamaguti 1958
Megalodiscus rankini*	United States	Red-spotted newt	Intestine	Ingestion of metacercaria in skin of amphibian	Common	Pathologic effects unknown	Russell 1951 Walton 1964 Yamaguti 1958
Diplodiscus subclavatus*	Europe, Africa, Asia, Australia, New Zealand	Grass frog, edible frog, treefrogs, other frogs, European toad, clawed toads, other toads, European salamanders, newts	Large intestine	Ingestion of metacercaria in skin of amphibian	Common	Syn. Opisthodiscus subclavatus. Pathologic effects unknown	Cheng 1964 Reichenbach-Klinke and Elkan 1965 Skrjabin 1964 Walton 1964 Yamaguti 1958
Diplodiscus japonicus*	Asia	Frogs	Large intestine, cloaca	Ingestion of metacercaria in skin of amphibian	Common	Pathologic effects unknown	Reichenbach-Klinke and Elkan 1965 Skrjabin 1964 Walton 1964 Yamaguti 1958
Diplodiscus amphichrus*	Asia	Frogs	Large intestine, cloaca	Ingestion of metacercaria in skin of amphibian	Common	Pathologic effects unknown	Skrjabin 1964 Walton 1964 Yamaguti 1958

*Discussed in text.

TABLE 18.2 (*continued*)

Parasite	Geographic Distribution	Reptilian or Amphibian Host	Location in Host	Method of Infection	Incidence in Nature	Remarks	Reference
Diplodiscus unguiculatus[*]	Europe	Newts	Rectum	Ingestion of metacercaria in skin of amphibian	Unknown; probably common in certain localities	Pathologic effects unknown	Walton 1964 Yamaguti 1958
Opisthodiscus diplodiscoides[*]	Europe	Edible frog	Large intestine	Ingestion of metacercaria in skin of amphibian	Unknown; probably common in certain localities	Pathologic effects unknown	Walton 1964 Yamaguti 1958
Allassostoma magnum	North America	Red-eared turtle, other cooters	Large intestine	Unknown; possibly by ingestion of metacercaria in crustacean, tadpole, on aquatic plant	Common	Pathologic effects unknown	Johnson 1968 Yamaguti 1958
Allassostomoides parvum	North America	Leopard frog, bullfrog, cooters, snapping turtle	Colon, urinary bladder, cloaca	Unknown; possibly by ingestion of metacercaria in crustacean, tadpole, on aquatic plant	Common in turtle, uncommon in frogs	Syn. *Allassostoma parvum*. Incidence of 37% reported in snapping turtle in central United States. Pathologic effects unknown	Walton 1964 Williams 1953 Yamaguti 1958
Heronimus chelydrae	North America	Painted turtles, red-eared turtle, snapping turtle, Blanding's turtle, map turtle, other turtles	Lungs	Ingestion of intermediate host (snail)	Common	Incidence of 43% reported in snapping turtle in central United States. Pathologic effects unknown	Crandell 1960 Harwood 1932 Rausch 1947 Reichenbach-Klinke and Elkan 1965 Skrjabin 1964 Williams 1953 Yamaguti 1958
Halipegus eccentricus[*]	United States	Leopard frog, green frog, bullfrog	Ear canals	Ingestion of second intermediate host (arthropod)	Unknown; probably common in certain localities	Pathologic effects unknown	Olsen 1967 Skrjabin 1964 Walton 1964 Yamaguti 1958
Halipegus occidualis[*]	North America	Leopard frog, green frog, bullfrog, other frogs	Mouth, ear canals, pharynx	Ingestion of second intermediate host (arthropod)	Unknown; probably common in certain localities	Pathologic effects unknown	Olsen 1967 Skrjabin 1964 Walton 1964 Yamaguti 1958
Halipegus amherstensis[*]	United States, Mexico	Green frog, bullfrog, other frogs	Mouth, ear canals	Ingestion of second intermediate host (arthropod)	Unknown; probably common in certain localities	Pathologic effects unknown	Olsen 1967 Rankin 1945 Skrjabin 1964 Walton 1964 Yamaguti 1958
Halipegus ovocaudatus[*]	Europe, southern Africa	Edible frog, grass frog, other frogs, toads	Mouth	Ingestion of second intermediate host (arthropod)	Unknown; probably common in certain localities	Pathologic effects unknown	Cheng 1964 Dawes 1946 Olsen 1967 Rankin 1945 Reichenbach-Klinke and Elkan 1965 Skrjabin 1964 Walton 1964 Yamaguti 1958

[*]Discussed in text.

TABLE 18.2 (continued)

Parasite	Geographic Distribution	Reptilian or Amphibian Host	Location in Host	Method of Infection	Incidence in Nature	Remarks	Reference
Microphallus opacus	Central United States	Painted turtles, snapping turtles, map turtles	Intestine	Ingestion of second intermediate host (crustacean)	Common	Syn. *Microphallus ovatus*. Pathologic effects unknown	Hoffman 1967, Rausch 1946, 1947, Yamaguti 1958
Microphallus eversum	Central United States	Map turtles	Intestine	Ingestion of second intermediate host (crustacean)	Common	Pathologic effects unknown	Rausch 1947
*Pleurogenes claviger**	Europe	Grass frog, edible frog, treefrogs, other frogs, European toad, other toads, common newt, other newts	Small intestine	Ingestion of second intermediate host (arthropod)	Common	Pathologic effects unknown	Reichenbach-Klinke and Elkan 1965, Skrjabin 1964, Walton 1964, Yamaguti 1958
*Pleurogenes medians**	Europe, Africa	Grass frog, edible frog, other frogs, European toad, other toads, common newt, crested newt	Small intestine	Ingestion of metacercaria encysted in second intermediate host (insect) or in skin of tadpole	Common	Syn. *Pleurogenoides medians*. Pathologic effects unknown	Dawes 1946, Walton 1964, Yamaguti 1958
*Prosotocus confusus**	Europe, southwestern Asia	Grass frog, edible frog, other frogs, European toad, other toads	Small intestine	Ingestion of second intermediate host (arthropod)	Common	Pathologic effects unknown	Reichenbach-Klinke and Elkan 1965, Skrjabin 1964, Walton 1964, Yamaguti 1958
Loxogenes arcanum	United States, Canada	Leopard frog, green frog, bullfrog	Intestine, viscera	Ingestion of metacercaria encysted in second intermediate host (insect)	Common	Causes cysts in viscera	Walton 1964, Yamaguti 1958
Cephalogonimus retusus	North America, Europe	Leopard frog, green frog, bullfrog, grass frog, edible frog	Intestine	Ingestion of metacercaria in skin of amphibian, possibly by ingestion of arthropod	Common	Syn. *Cephalogonimus americanus, C. europaeus*. Pathologic effects unknown	Dawes 1946, Lang 1969, Rankin 1945, Walton 1964, Yamaguti 1958
Cephalogonimus amphiumae	United States	Amphiumas	Intestine	Unknown; probably by ingestion of metacercaria in arthropod or skin of amphibian	Common	Pathologic effects unknown	Rankin 1937, Walton 1964, Yamaguti 1958
*Spirorchis parvus**	United States	Painted turtles	Heart, blood vessels	Penetration of skin by free-swimming cercaria released from snail	Common	Incidence of 18% reported in central United States. Penetrating cercaria causes irritation; egg masses sometimes cause death by coating gastrointestinal mucosa	Olsen 1967, Rausch 1947, Skrjabin 1964, Wall 1941, Yamaguti 1958

*Discussed in text.

TABLE 18.2 (continued)

Parasite	Geographic Distribution	Reptilian or Amphibian Host	Location in Host	Method of Infection	Incidence in Nature	Remarks	Reference
*Spirorchis elephantis**	United States	Painted turtles	Heart, blood vessels	Penetration of skin by free-swimming cercaria released from snail	Common	Pathologic effects unknown; massive infections probably cause death	Olsen 1967 Skrjabin 1964 Yamaguti 1958
*Spirorchis artericola**	United States	Painted turtles, pond turtles, map turtles, cooters	Heart, blood vessels	Penetration of skin by free-swimming cercaria released from snail	Common	Pathologic effects unknown; massive infections probably cause death	Rausch 1947 Skrjabin 1964 Thatcher 1954 Wall 1941 Yamaguti 1958
Spirorchis blandigioides	United States	Red-eared turtle, other cooters	Heart, blood vessels	Penetration of skin by free-swimming cercaria released from snail	Unknown; probably common	Pathologic effects unknown; massive infections probably cause death	Yamaguti 1958
Spirorchis elegans	North America	Painted turtles, cooters	Heart, blood vessels	Penetration of skin by free-swimming cercaria released from snail	Unknown; probably common	Pathologic effects unknown; massive infections probably cause death	Yamaguti 1958
Spirorchis scripta	North America	Red-eared turtle, cooters, map turtles	Heart, blood vessels	Penetration of skin by free-swimming cercaria released from snail	Unknown; probably common	Pathologic effects unknown; massive infections probably cause death	Yamaguti 1958
*Spirorchis innominata**	North America	Map turtles, pond turtles	Heart, blood vessels	Penetration of skin by free-swimming cercaria released from snail	Common	Pathologic effects unknown; massive infections probably cause death	Rausch 1947 Skrjabin 1964 Wall 1941 Yamaguti 1958
*Spirorchis haematobium**	United States	Snapping turtles	Heart, blood vessels	Penetration of skin by free-swimming cercaria released from snail	Common	Incidence of 70% reported in central United States. Pathologic effects unknown; massive infections probably cause death	Rausch 1947 Skrjabin 1964 Williams 1953 Yamaguti 1958

*Discussed in text.

591

TABLE 18.3. Larval digenetic trematodes affecting laboratory reptiles and amphibians

Parasite	Geographic Distribution	Reptilian or Amphibian Host	Location in Host	Method of Infection	Incidence in Nature	Remarks	Reference
Diplostomum flexicaudum	United States	Tadpoles of leopard frog, green frog, American toad	Eye lens	Penetration by cercaria released from snail	Uncommon	Possible syn. *Diplostomum spathaceum*. Pathologic effects unknown	Ferguson 1943, Hoffman 1967, Southwell and Kirshner 1937, Walton 1964, Yamaguti 1958
*Diplostomulum scheuringi**	United States	Red-spotted newt, greater siren (*Siren lacertina*)	Eyes, brain	Penetration by cercaria released from snail	Common	Incidences of 12 to 100% reported in water newt. Adult stage unknown. Larva causes small hemorrhages in eyes, brain; lesions in brain; possibly brain tumors	Erges 1961, Hughes 1929, Lautenschlager 1959, Reichenbach-Klinke and Elkan 1965, Walton 1964
*Diplostomulum xenopi**	United States, Great Britain, southern Africa	South African clawed toad	Pericardial cavity	Presumably by penetration by cercaria released from snail	Common	Incidence of 78% reported. Adult stage unknown. Causes pericarditis, decreased respiratory capacity, death	Nigrelli and Maraventano 1944, Reichenbach-Klinke and Elkan 1965, Walton 1964
Diplostomulum ambystomae	United States	Spotted salamander, marbled salamander	Body cavity	Unknown	Common	Incidences of 11 to 70% reported in southeastern United States. Adult stage unknown. Pathologic effects unknown	Rankin 1937, Walton 1964, Yamaguti 1958
Diplostomulum desmognathi	United States	Dusky salamanders, other salamanders	Body cavity	Unknown	Common	Incidences of 9 to 31% reported in southeastern United States. Adult stage unknown. Pathologic effects unknown	Rankin 1937, Walton 1964, Yamaguti 1958
Diplostomulum vegrandis	United States	Tadpole of leopard frog; snakes	Muscle	Presumably by penetration by cercaria released from snail	Unknown	Adult stage unknown. Pathologic effects unknown	Walton 1964
*Cercaria ranae**	North central United States	Tadpole of unspecified species	Body cavity, other tissues	Penetration by cercaria released from snail	Unknown	Natural infection of tadpole not reported; experimental infection causes abdominal distention, death ("bloat disease")	Cort and Brackett 1937, Walton 1964
Cercaria elodes	United States	Tadpole of leopard frog	Notochord	Unknown	Unknown	Adult stage unknown. Pathologic effects unknown	Walton 1964

*Discussed in text.

592

TABLE 18.3 *(continued)*

Parasite	Geographic Distribution	Reptilian or Amphibian Host	Location in Host	Method of Infection	Incidence in Nature	Remarks	Reference
Cercaria vesculosa	Canada	Leopard frog, bullfrog	Throat muscle	Unknown	Unknown; probably common	Adult stage unknown. Pathologic effects unknown	Walton 1964
Neascus sp.*	Great Britain, southern Africa	South African clawed toad	Lateral line system	Unknown	Unknown	Adult stage unknown. Causes local proliferation of melanophores, death	Elkan and Murray 1952 Walton 1964
Tetracotyle crystallina	United States	Leopard frog	Muscle	Unknown	Uncommon	Adult stage unknown. Pathologic effects unknown	Walton 1964
Cotylurus variegatus	Europe	Frogs	Liver	Unknown	Common	Adult stage unknown. Pathologic effects unknown	Reichenbach-Klinke and Elkan 1965 Walton 1967
Strigea elegans	United States	Tadpoles of leopard frog, green frog, bullfrog, wood frog, American toad; larva of marbled salamander; snakes	Various tissues	Penetration by cercaria released from snail or ingestion of tadpole	Unknown; probably common	Pathologic effects unknown	Pearson 1959 Walton 1964, 1967 Yamaguti 1958
Fibricola cratera	United States	Leopard frog, green frog, green treefrog, other frogs	Skin, muscle, body cavity	Penetration by cercaria released from snail	Unknown; probably common	Pathologic effects unknown	Reichenbach-Klinke and Elkan 1965 Walton 1964 Yamaguti 1958
Alaria canis	United States, Canada	Tadpoles, occasionally adults of leopard frog, green frog, other frogs, toads; larvae of Jefferson salamander, spotted salamander, other salamanders	Skin, subcutis, muscle	Penetration by cercaria released from snail	Uncommon	Apparently non-pathogenic	Olsen 1967 Pearson 1956 Walton 1966 Yamaguti 1958
Alaria arisaemoides	United States	Tadpoles, occasionally adults of leopard frog, green frog, bullfrog, spring peeper, other frogs; larvae of Jefferson salamander, spotted salamander, other salamanders	Skin, subcutis, muscle	Penetration by cercaria released from snail	Uncommon	Apparently non-pathogenic	Pearson 1956 Walton 1966 Yamaguti 1958
Alaria mustelae	United States	Leopard frog, green frog, bullfrog, pickerel frog, other frogs	Various tissues	Penetration by cercaria released from snail	Unknown; probably common	Pathologic effects unknown	Dawes 1946 Southwell and Kirshner 1937 Walton 1964 Yamaguti 1958
Alaria intermedia	United States	Leopard frog, garter snakes	Muscle, kidneys, pericardium	Penetration by cercaria released from snail	Uncommon	Pathologic effects unknown	Nigrelli and Maraventano 1944 Walton 1964 Yamaguti 1958

*Discussed in text.

593

TABLE 18.3 *(continued)*

Parasite	Geographic Distribution	Reptilian or Amphibian Host	Location in Host	Method of Infection	Incidence in Nature	Remarks	Reference
Alaria marcianae	United States	Tadpoles of leopard frog, green frog; snakes	Various tissues	Penetration by cercaria released from snail	Uncommon	Syn. *Cercaria marcianae.* Pathologic effects unknown	Walton 1964 Yamaguti 1958
Alaria micradena	United States	Tadpoles of leopard frog, American toad	Various tissues	Penetration by cercaria released from snail	Uncommon	Syn. *Cercaria micradena.* Pathologic effects unknown	Walton 1964 Yamaguti 1958
Alaria alata	Europe	Grass frog, edible frog, European toad, European viper, other snakes	Skin, subcutis, muscle	Penetration by cercaria released from snail	Uncommon	Apparently non-pathogenic	Reichenbach-Klinke and Elkan 1965 Walton 1966 Yamaguti 1958
Apharyngostrigea pipientis	United States	Tadpoles of leopard frog, treefrogs	Various tissues	Penetration by cercaria released from snail	Unknown; probably common	Syn. *Tetracotyle pipientis.* Pathologic effects unknown	Dawes 1946 Southwell and Kirshner 1937 Walton 1964 Yamaguti 1958
Codonocephalus urnigerus	Europe	Grass frog, edible frog, snakes	Skin, subcutis, muscle	Penetration by cercaria released from snail	Common	Pathologic effects unknown	Dawes 1946 Niewiadomska 1964 Reichenbach-Klinke and Elkan 1965 Southwell and Kirshner 1937 Walton 1964 Yamaguti 1958
Gorgodera amplicava	North America	Tadpoles of green frog, bullfrog, pickerel frog, treefrogs; larva of spotted salamander	Intestinal wall	Ingestion of cercaria released from clam	Common	Pathologic effects unknown	Goodchild 1950 Olsen 1967 Walton 1964 Yamaguti 1958
Gorgodera cygnoides	North America, Europe	Edible frog, other frogs, toads	Urinary bladder	Penetration by cercaria released from clam	Uncommon	Syn. *Gorgodera pagenstecheri.* Pathologic effects unknown	Dawes 1946 Walton 1964 Yamaguti 1958
Gorgoderina capensis	Europe, northern Africa	Edible frog	Muscle	Unknown	Uncommon	Pathologic effects unknown	Dawes 1946 Walton 1964 Yamaguti 1958
Allocreadium angusticolle	Europe	Grass frog	Various tissues	Penetration by cercaria released from snail	Uncommon	Pathologic effects unknown	Dawes 1946 Walton 1964
Sphaerostoma bramae	Europe	Treefrogs	Various tissues	Penetration by cercaria released from snail	Uncommon	Pathologic effects unknown	Dawes 1946 Walton 1964 Yamaguti 1958

TABLE 18.3 (continued)

Parasite	Geographic Distribution	Reptilian or Amphibian Host	Location in Host	Method of Infection	Incidence in Nature	Remarks	Reference
Clinostomum complanatum	Eastern Europe, southern Asia	Leopard frog, green frog, bullfrog, pickerel frog, other frogs	Muscle	Penetration by cercaria released from snail	Common	Pathologic effects unknown	Dawes 1946, Olsen 1967, Reichenbach-Klinke and Elkan 1965, Walton 1964, Yamaguti 1958
Clinostomum attenuatum	North America	Frogs, salamanders, snakes	Muscle	Penetration by cercaria released from snail	Uncommon	Pathologic effects unknown	Dawes 1946, Walton 1964, Yamaguti 1958
Lechriorchis primus	North America	Leopard frog, green frog	Muscle	Ingestion of cercaria released from snail	Uncommon	Pathologic effects unknown	Olsen 1967, Walton 1964, Yamaguti 1958
Lechriorchis tygarti	United States	Leopard frog, green frog	Muscle	Ingestion of cercaria released from snail	Uncommon	Pathologic effects unknown	Walton 1964, Yamaguti 1958
Zeugorchis eurinus	United States	Tadpoles of leopard frog, green frog	Muscle	Ingestion of cercaria released from snail	Uncommon	Pathologic effects unknown	Walton 1964, Yamaguti 1958
Zeugorchis signatus	Europe	Tadpoles of frogs	Muscle	Ingestion of cercaria released from snail	Uncommon	Pathologic effects unknown	Walton 1964
Dasymetra conferta	North America	Tadpoles of green frog, bullfrog	Muscle	Ingestion of cercaria released from snail	Uncommon	Pathologic effects unknown	Walton 1964, Yamaguti 1958
Dasymetra villicaeca	United States	Tadpoles of green frog, bullfrog, other frogs	Muscle	Ingestion of cercaria released from snail	Uncommon	Pathologic effects unknown	Walton 1964, Yamaguti 1958
Ochetosoma aniarum	United States	Tadpoles of green frog, bullfrog, treefrogs, other frogs	Muscle	Ingestion of cercaria released from snail	Uncommon	Syn. *Neorenifer aniarum.* Pathologic effects unknown	Walton 1964, Yamaguti 1958
Ochetosoma kansensis	United States	Tadpoles of frogs	Muscle	Ingestion of cercaria released from snail	Uncommon	Syn. *Neorenifer kansensis.* Pathologic effects unknown	Walton 1964, Yamaguti 1958
Encyclometra colubrimurorum	Europe, Asia	Edible frog, other frogs	Muscle	Ingestion of cercaria released from snail	Uncommon	Pathologic effects unknown	Walton 1964, Yamaguti 1958
Glypthelmins pennsylvaniensis	United States	Spring peeper	Skin	Penetration by cercaria released from snail	Uncommon	Pathologic effects unknown	Walton 1964
Glypthelmins quieta	United States, Mexico, South America, Asia	Leopard frog, green frog, bullfrog, pickerel frog, spring peeper, other frogs	Skin, intestine	Penetration by cercaria released from snail	Common	Pathologic effects unknown	Walton 1964, Yamaguti 1958

TABLE 18.3 (continued)

Parasite	Geographic Distribution	Reptilian or Amphibian Host	Location in Host	Method of Infection	Incidence in Nature	Remarks	Reference
Opisthioglyphe xenopi	Southern Africa	South African clawed toad	Skin	Ingestion of cercaria released from snail	Uncommon	Pathologic effects unknown	Walton 1964 Yamaguti 1958
Platynosomum fastosum	North America, South America	Anoles	Bile duct	Ingestion of isopod	Common	Pathologic effects unknown	Maldonado 1945 Walton 1964 Yamaguti 1958
Leptophallus nigrovenosus	Europe, Africa	Tadpoles of frogs, toads, newts	Various tissues	Penetration by cercaria released from snail	Uncommon	Pathologic effects unknown	Walton 1964 Yamaguti 1958
Echinoparyphium flexum	North America	Leopard frog, green frog, wood frog, treefrogs, other frogs	Kidneys	Penetration by cercaria released from snail	Common	Pathologic effects unknown	Walton 1964 Yamaguti 1958
Echinoparyphium recurvatum	Worldwide	Grass frog, edible frog, other frogs, treefrogs, European toad, newts	Liver, kidneys	Penetration by cercaria released from snail	Common	Pathologic effects unknown	Walton 1964 Yamaguti 1958
Echinoparyphium spinigerum	Europe	Edible frog	Various tissues	Penetration by cercaria released from snail	Uncommon	Possible syn. Pegosomum spiniferum. Pathologic effects unknown	Walton 1964 Yamaguti 1958
Echinostoma revolutum	Worldwide	Leopard frog, bullfrog, edible frog, other frogs, American toad, other toads, other amphibians	Various tissues	Penetration by cercaria released from snail	Common	Pathologic effects unknown	Walton 1964, 1966 Yamaguti 1958
Echinostoma xenopi	Southern Africa	South African clawed toad	Brain, subcutis	Penetration by cercaria released from snail	Uncommon	Adult stage unknown. Pathologic effects unknown	Walton 1964
Euparyphium melis	North America, Europe, Asia	Tadpoles of green frog, other frogs	Tail	Penetration by cercaria released from snail	Common	Syn. Isthmiophora melis. Pathologic effects unknown	Dawes 1946 Walton 1964 Yamaguti 1958
Hypoderaeum conoideum	United States, Europe, Asia	Edible frog	Various tissues	Penetration by cercaria released from snail	Common	Pathologic effects unknown	Dawes 1946 Walton 1964 Yamaguti 1958
Euryhelmis monorchis	United States	Leopard frog, green frog, pickerel frog	Skin, subcutis	Penetration by cercaria released from snail	Common	Incidence of 67% reported. Causes skin vesicles, cysts	Dawes 1946 Walton 1964 Yamaguti 1958
Euryhelmis squamula	Europe	Grass frog, edible frog, toads, newts	Skin	Penetration by cercaria released from snail	Common	Pathologic effects unknown	Dawes 1946 Reichenbach-Klinke and Elkan 1965 Walton 1964 Yamaguti 1958

TABLE 18.3 *(continued)*

Parasite	Geographic Distribution	Reptilian or Amphibian Host	Location in Host	Method of Infection	Incidence in Nature	Remarks	Reference
Pleurogenes medians	Europe, Africa	Grass frog, treefrogs	Skin	Penetration by cercaria released from snail	Uncommon	Pathologic effects unknown	Dawes 1946 Walton 1964 Yamaguti 1958
Ratzia parva	Europe, Africa	Edible frog	Muscle	Unknown	Uncommon	Pathologic effects unknown	Dawes 1946 Walton 1964 Yamaguti 1958
Allassostomoides parvum	North America	Tadpole of leopard frog	Skin	Penetration by cercaria released from snail	Uncommon	Syn. *Allassostoma parvum.* Pathologic effects unknown	Dawes 1946 Walton 1964 Yamaguti 1958
Megalodiscus temporatus	North America, Central America, South America	Leopard frog, green frog, spring peeper	Skin	Penetration by cercaria released from snail	Uncommon	Pathologic effects unknown	Walton 1964 Yamaguti 1958

TABLE 18.4. Adult cestodes affecting laboratory reptiles and amphibians

Parasite	Geographic Distribution	Reptilian or Amphibian Host	Location in Host	Method of Infection	Incidence in Nature	Remarks	Reference
*Bothriocephalus rarus**	United States	Red-spotted newt, California newt, two-lined salamander (*Eurycea bislineata*)	Small intestine	Ingestion of intermediate host (copepod) or newt larva	Common	Incidences of 0.1 to 30.0% reported. Heavy infections cause weakness, debilitation, death	Fischthal 1955a Rankin 1937, 1945 Reichenbach-Klinke and Elkan 1965 Thomas 1937a, b Walton 1964 Wardle and McLeod 1952 Yamaguti 1959
*Cephalochlamys namaquensis**	Great Britain, southern Africa	South African clawed toad	Small intestine	Unknown	Common	Syn. *Chlamydocephalus xenopi*. Incidence of 100% reported. Pathologic effects unknown	Elkan 1960 Ortlepp 1926 Reichenbach-Klinke and Elkan 1965 Southwell and Kirshner 1937 Thomas 1937a Walton 1964, 1966, 1967 Wardle and McLeod 1952 Yamaguti 1959
*Nematotaenia dispar**	Europe, Africa, Asia	Grass frog, edible frog, treefrogs, other frogs, European toad, other toads, fire salamander, other European salamanders, alpine newt	Small intestine	Unknown	Common in southern Europe, northern Africa	Heavy infections cause intestinal obstruction, death	Elkan 1960 Reichenbach-Klinke and Elkan 1965 Walton 1964, 1966 Wardle and McLeod 1952 Yamaguti 1959
Cylindrotaenia americana	North America, South America	Leopard frog, bullfrog, treefrogs, cricket frogs, other frogs, common toad, other toads, dusky salamanders, softshell turtles, snakes, lizards	Small intestine	Unknown	Common	Pathologic effects unknown	Acholonu 1970 Fischthal 1955a Harwood 1932 Rankin 1945 Reichenbach-Klinke and Elkan 1965 Walton 1964 Wardle and McLeod 1952 Yamaguti 1959
Cylindrotaenia quadrijugosa	North central United States	Leopard frog	Small intestine	Unknown	Uncommon	Pathologic effects unknown	Lawler 1939 Reichenbach-Klinke and Elkan 1965 Walton 1964 Wardle and McLeod 1952
Distoichometra bufonis	Southeastern United States	American toad, common toad, other toads	Small intestine	Unknown	Uncommon	Pathologic effects unknown	Reichenbach-Klinke and Elkan 1965 Walton 1964 Wardle and McLeod 1952 Yamaguti 1959

*Discussed in text.

TABLE 18.4 *(continued)*

Parasite	Geographic Distribution	Reptilian or Amphibian Host	Location in Host	Method of Infection	Incidence in Nature	Remarks	Reference
Oochoristica anolis	Southern United States	Green anole	Intestine	Ingestion of intermediate host (tick)	Unknown; probably common in some localities	Pathologic effects unknown	Harwood 1932 Wardle and McLeod 1952 Yamaguti 1959
Oochoristica natricis	North America, southern Africa	Water snakes, other snakes, collared lizards	Intestine	Ingestion of intermediate host (tick)	Unknown; probably common in some localities	Pathologic effects unknown	Harwood 1932 Waitz 1961 Wardle and McLeod 1952 Yamaguti 1959
Oochoristica elaphis	Southern United States	Rat snakes	Intestine	Ingestion of intermediate host (tick)	Unknown; probably common in some localities	Pathologic effects unknown	Harwood 1932 Wardle and McLeod 1952 Yamaguti 1959
Oochoristica fibrata	Western United States, Asia	Racers, other snakes	Intestine	Ingestion of intermediate host (tick)	Unknown; probably common in some localities	Pathologic effects unknown	Waitz 1961 Yamaguti 1959
Oochoristica scelopori	Western United States	Spiny lizards	Intestine	Ingestion of intermediate host (tick)	Unknown; probably common in some localities	Pathologic effects unknown	Waitz 1961 Yamaguti 1959
Oochoristica whitentoni	North America	Box turtles	Intestine	Ingestion of intermediate host (tick)	Unknown; probably common in some localities	Pathologic effects unknown	Reichenbach-Klinke and Elkan 1965 Wardle and McLeod 1952 Yamaguti 1959
Oochoristica rostellata	Europe, Africa	Racers, other snakes	Intestine	Ingestion of intermediate host (tick)	Unknown; probably common in some localities	Pathologic effects unknown	Yamaguti 1959
Oochoristica tuberculata	Europe, Africa	European lizards, other lizards, snakes	Intestine	Ingestion of intermediate host (tick)	Unknown; probably common in some localities	Pathologic effects unknown	Yamaguti 1959
Ophiotaenia perspicua	North America, Central America	Leopard frog, water snakes, garter snakes	Intestine	Ingestion of intermediate host (copepod) or frog tadpole or fish	Unknown; probably common in some localities	Pathologic effects unknown	Reichenbach-Klinke and Elkan 1965 Waitz 1961 Walton 1964 Wardle and McLeod 1952 Yamaguti 1959
Ophiotaenia saphena	North central United States	Green frog, bullfrog	Small intestine	Ingestion of intermediate host (copepod)	Unknown	Pathologic effects unknown	Osler 1931 Reichenbach-Klinke and Elkan 1965 Thomas 1931 Walton 1964 Wardle and McLeod 1952 Yamaguti 1959

599

TABLE 18.4 *(continued)*

Parasite	Geographic Distribution	Reptilian or Amphibian Host	Location in Host	Method of Infection	Incidence in Nature	Remarks	Reference
Ophiotaenia magna	North America	Cricket frogs, green frog, bullfrog, other frogs, toads	Intestine	Unknown	Unknown; probably common in some localities	Pathologic effects unknown	Harwood 1932; Reichenbach-Klinke and Elkan 1965; Walton 1964; Wardle and McLeod 1952; Yamaguti 1959
Ophiotaenia gracilis	United States	Bullfrog	Intestine	Unknown	Unknown; probably common in some localities	Pathologic effects unknown	Walton 1964; Yamaguti 1959
Ophiotaenia cryptobranchi	United States	Dusky salamanders, red-spotted newt, other salamanders	Intestine	Unknown	Common	Syn. *Crepidobothrium cryptobranchi.* Incidences of 6 to 17% reported in salamanders. Pathologic effects unknown	Rankin 1937; Walton 1964; Wardle and McLeod 1952; Yamaguti 1959
Ophiotaenia filaroides	Central United States	Tiger salamander	Intestine	Unknown	Unknown; probably common in some localities	Pathologic effects unknown	Rankin 1937; Reichenbach-Klinke and Elkan 1965; Walton 1964; Wardle and McLeod 1952; Yamaguti 1959
Ophiotaenia loennbergii	Central United States	Mudpuppies	Intestine	Unknown	Unknown; probably common in some localities	Pathologic effects unknown	Rankin 1937; Reichenbach-Klinke and Elkan 1965; Walton, 1964; Wardle and McLeod 1952; Yamaguti 1959
Ophiotaenia amphiumae	Southern United States	Amphiumas, dusky salamanders	Intestine	Unknown	Unknown; probably common in some localities	Syn. *Crepidobothrium amphiumae.* Pathologic effects unknown	Rankin 1937; Walton 1964; Wardle and McLeod 1952; Yamaguti 1959
Ophiotaenia alternans	Central United States	Amphiumas	Small intestine	Unknown	Unknown; probably common in some localities	Pathologic effects unknown	Walton 1964; Wardle and McLeod 1952; Yamaguti 1959
Proteocephalus testudo	United States	Softshell turtles	Intestine	Unknown	Common in some localities	Pathologic effects unknown	Acholonu 1970
Proteocephalus trionychinum	United States	Softshell turtles	Intestine	Unknown	Unknown; probably common in some localities	Pathologic effects unknown	Acholonu 1970

TABLE 18.5. Larval cestodes affecting laboratory reptiles and amphibians

Parasite	Geographic Distribution	Reptilian or Amphibian Host	Location in Host	Method of Infection	Incidence in Nature	Remarks	Reference
Diphyllobothrium erinacei *	Europe, Asia, Indonesia, Australia, South America	Grass frog, edible frog, treefrogs, other frogs, toads, common newt, fire salamander, other salamanders, turtles, snakes	Muscle, connective tissue	Ingestion of first intermediate host (copepod) or immature amphibian	Common in southeastern Asia, Indonesia	Syn. *Diphyllobothrium mansoni, D. ranarum, D. reptans, Spirometra erinacei.* Incidence of 82% reported in treefrogs in southeastern Asia. Larval migration presumably causes mechanical damage, adhesions; rapidly growing larvae presumably interfere with nutrition of host, cause cessation of growth of tadpoles. A cause of sparganosis in man	Belding 1965 Galliard 1948 Galliard and Ngu 1946 Noble and Noble 1961 Reichenbach-Klinke and Elkan 1965 Walton 1964, 1966 Wardle and McLeod 1952 Witenberg 1964 Yamaguti 1959
Diphyllobothrium latum	North America, southern South America, Europe, Japan	Edible frog, other frogs	Various tissues	Ingestion of first intermediate host (copepod)	Uncommon	Pathologic effects in amphibians unknown. Adults occur in man	Reichenbach-Klinke and Elkan 1965 Walton 1964, 1967 Yamaguti 1959
Spirometra mansonoides *	United States	Green frog, bullfrog, treefrogs, other frogs, toads, tiger salamander, red-spotted newt, turtles, racers, kingsnakes, water snakes, garter snakes, other snakes	Muscle	Ingestion of first intermediate host (copepod) or amphibian or reptile	Common	Syn. *Diphyllobothrium mansonoides.* Incidences of 1% in frogs, 18% in snakes in south central United States. Pathologic effects in amphibians and reptiles unknown. A cause of sparganosis in man	Belding 1965 Burrows 1965 Corkum 1966 Noble and Noble 1961 Walton 1964, 1967 Wardle and McLeod 1952 Witenberg 1964 Yamaguti 1959
Schistocephalus solidus	Europe	Edible frog	Body cavity	Ingestion of first intermediate host (copepod)	Uncommon	Pathologic effects unknown	Walton 1964 Wardle and McLeod 1952 Yamaguti 1959
Ligula intestinalis	North America, Europe, Asia	Tiger salamander	Intestine	Ingestion of first intermediate host (copepod)	Uncommon	Pathologic effects unknown	Rankin 1937 Walton 1964 Wardle and McLeod 1952 Yamaguti 1959
Mesocestoides sp.	United States	Leopard frog, American toad, other toads, garter snakes, other snakes, lizards	Kidneys, intestinal wall, mesentery, other tissues	Ingestion of unknown first intermediate host	Uncommon	Pathologic effects unknown	James and Ulmer 1967 Reichenbach-Klinke and Elkan 1965 Voge 1953 Wardle and McLeod 1952
Ophiotaenia perspicua	United States	Leopard frog, other frogs	Liver	Ingestion of first intermediate host (copepod)	Uncommon	Pathologic effects unknown	Walton 1964 Wardle and McLeod 1952 Yamaguti 1959

*Discussed in text.

TABLE 18.6. Nematodes affecting laboratory reptiles and amphibians

Parasite	Geographic Distribution	Reptilian or Amphibian Host	Location in Host	Method of Infection	Incidence in Nature	Remarks	Reference
*Rhabdias ranae**	North America	Leopard frog, bullfrog, wood frog, pickerel frog, spring peeper, cricket frogs, other frogs, common toad, other toads, kingsnakes, garter snakes	Lungs	Ingestion of infective larva or penetration of skin by larva	Common	Incidence of 31% reported in frogs in northeastern United States. Pathologic effects unknown	Rankin 1945, Walton 1964, Yamaguti 1961
Rhabdias entomelas	United States	Pickerel frog, other frogs	Lungs	Ingestion of infective larva or penetration of skin by larva	Uncommon	Pathologic effects unknown	Walton 1964, Yamaguti 1961
Rhabdias vellardi	North America	Hognose snakes, garter snakes	Lung	Ingestion of infective larva or penetration of skin by larva	Common	Pathologic effects unknown	Harwood 1932, Yamaguti 1961
Rhabdias fuscovenosa	United States, Europe, Asia, Africa	Racers, rat snakes, kingsnakes, water snakes, garter snakes, other snakes	Lung	Ingestion of infective larva or penetration of skin by larva	Unknown; probably common	Pathologic effects unknown	Reichenbach-Klinke and Elkan 1965, Yamaguti 1961
*Rhabdias bufonis**	Europe, Asia	Grass frog, edible frog, treefrogs, other frogs, European toad, other toads	Lungs	Ingestion of infective larva or penetration of skin by larva	Common	Incidence of 48% reported in grass frog in Great Britain. Pathologic effects unknown	Elkan 1960, Lees 1962, Reichenbach-Klinke and Elkan 1965, Walton 1964, 1966, Yamaguti 1961, Yorke and Maplestone 1926
Rhabdias rubrovenosa	Europe	Grass frog, edible frog, European toad, other toads	Lungs	Ingestion of infective larva or penetration of skin by larva	Common	Pathologic effects unknown	Walton 1964, Yamaguti 1961
Rhabdias sphaerocephala	Europe, Central America	European toad, other toads	Lungs	Ingestion of infective larva or penetration of skin by larva	Common	Pathologic effects unknown	Reichenbach-Klinke and Elkan 1965, Walton 1964, Yamaguti 1961
Strongyloides serpentis	South central United States	Racers, hognose snakes, kingsnakes, water snakes	Small intestine	Unknown; probably by ingestion of infective larva or penetration of skin by larva	Common	Pathologic effects unknown	Little 1966
Strongyloides gulae	South central United States	Racers, hognose snakes, kingsnakes, water snakes	Esophagus	Unknown; probably by ingestion of infective larva or penetration of skin by larva	Common	Pathologic effects unknown	Little 1966

*Discussed in text.

TABLE 18.6 (continued)

Parasite	Geographic Distribution	Reptilian or Amphibian Host	Location in Host	Method of Infection	Incidence in Nature	Remarks	Reference
Ophidascaris labiatopapillosa	United States	Definitive: racers, eastern hognose snake, common kingsnake, water snakes; Intermediate: leopard frog, green frog, bullfrog, other frogs, amphiumas	Adult: stomach wall; Larva: muscle, mesentery	Definitive: ingestion of intermediate host (amphibian); Intermediate: ingestion of embryonated egg	Locally common (south-western Louisiana; Michigan in summer)	Larva causes cyst in muscle, mesentery; adult sometimes causes necrosis of stomach wall	Ash and Beaver 1963 Kutzer and Grünberg 1965 Walton 1964, 1966
Cosmocerca ornata*	Europe	Grass frog, edible frog, other frogs, European toad, other toads, alpine newt, crested newt	Intestine	Unknown; probably by ingestion of infective larva	Common	Incidence of 81% reported in grass frog in Great Britain. Pathologic effects unknown; possibly causes debilitation, intestinal obstruction, peritonitis, death	Lees 1962 Reichenbach-Klinke and Elkan 1965 Walton 1964 Yamaguti 1961 Yorke and Maplestone 1926
Cosmocerca commutata	Europe, South America	Grass frog, edible frog, treefrogs, other frogs, European toad, other toads, European salamanders, crested newt	Intestine	Unknown; probably by ingestion of infective larva	Common	Pathologic effects unknown; possibly causes debilitation, intestinal obstruction, peritonitis, death	Walton 1964 Yamaguti 1961 Yorke and Maplestone 1926
Cosmocercoides dukae*	North America	Leopard frog, green frog, bullfrog, wood frog, pickerel frog, green treefrog, spring peeper, cricket frogs, other frogs, common toad, other toads, mole salamanders, dusky salamanders, red-spotted newt, California newt, other newts, box turtle, western box turtle, hognose snakes	Intestine	Unknown; probably by ingestion of infective larva	Common	Incidences of 4 to 29% reported in salamanders, 4 to 16% in red-spotted newt in eastern United States. Pathologic effects unknown; possibly causes debilitation, intestinal obstruction, peritonitis, death	Fischthal 1955a, b Harwood 1932 Rankin 1937, 1945 Walton 1964 Yamaguti 1961
Oxysomatium americana*	United States	Leopard frog, bullfrog, wood frog, pickerel frog, treefrogs, other frogs, common toad, dusky salamanders	Large intestine	Unknown; probably by ingestion of embryonated egg or infective larva	Common	Incidences of 2 to 7% reported in salamanders in north-eastern United States. Pathologic effects unknown; possibly causes debilitation, intestinal obstruction, peritonitis, death	Fischthal 1955a Walton 1964 Yamaguti 1961
Oxysomatium brevicaudatum	Europe	Grass frog, edible frog, treefrogs, other frogs, European toad, other toads, European salamanders, common newt, alpine newt	Large intestine	Unknown; probably by ingestion of embryonated egg or infective larva	Common	Pathologic effects unknown; possibly causes debilitation, intestinal obstruction, peritonitis, death	Rankin 1937 Walton 1964, 1967 Yamaguti 1961

*Discussed in text.

TABLE 18.6 *(continued)*

Parasite	Geographic Distribution	Reptilian or Amphibian Host	Location in Host	Method of Infection	Incidence in Nature	Remarks	Reference
*Aplectana acuminata**	Europe, Africa, South America	Grass frog, edible frog, treefrogs, other frogs, European toad, other toads, European salamanders, common newt, crested newt	Intestine	Unknown; probably by ingestion of embryonated egg or infective larva	Common	Syn. *Oxysomatium acuminata.* Incidence of 23% reported in grass frog in Great Britain. Pathologic effects unknown; possibly causes debilitation, intestinal obstruction, peritonitis, death	Lees 1962 Reichenbach-Klinke and Elkan 1965 Walton 1964, 1966 Yamaguti 1961 Yorke and Maplestone 1926
*Falcaustra affinis**	United States	Spotted turtle, Blanding's turtle, map turtles, box turtles	Large intestine	Unknown; probably by ingestion of embryonated egg	Common	Syn. *Spironoura affinis.* Incidences of 23 to 91% reported in north central United States. Pathologic effects unknown	Harwood 1932 Rausch 1947 Yamaguti 1961 Yorke and Maplestone 1926
*Falcaustra procera**	United States	Painted turtle, cooters	Large intestine	Unknown; probably by ingestion of embryonated egg	Common	Syn. *Spironoura procera.* Incidence of 19% reported in south central United States. Pathologic effects unknown	Harwood 1932 Yamaguti 1961
*Falcaustra wardi**	United States	Map turtle, snapping turtle	Large intestine	Unknown; probably by ingestion of embryonated egg	Common	Syn. *Spironoura wardi.* Incidence of 45% reported in snapping turtle in south central United States. Pathologic effects unknown	Rausch 1947 Williams 1953 Yamaguti 1961
*Falcaustra chelydrae**	South central United States	Snapping turtle, red-eared turtle, other turtles	Large intestine	Unknown; probably by ingestion of embryonated egg	Common	Syn. *Spironoura chelydrae.* Incidence of 97% reported in south central United States. Pathologic effects unknown	Harwood 1932 Williams 1953 Yamaguti 1961
*Falcaustra catesbianae**	United States	Leopard frog, bullfrog, treefrogs, other frogs	Large intestine	Unknown; probably by ingestion of embryonated egg	Common in bullfrog	Syn. *Spironoura catesbianae.* Incidence of 50% reported in bullfrog in south central United States. Pathologic effects unknown	Harwood 1932 Walton 1964 Yamaguti 1961
Tachygonetria longicollis	Europe, northern Africa	Greek tortoise	Large intestine	Unknown; probably by ingestion of embryonated egg	Common	Syn. *Tachygonetria pusilla, T. testudinis.* Sometimes causes intestinal obstruction, death	Forstner 1960 Graham-Jones 1961 Petter 1962 Yamaguti 1961 Yorke and Maplestone 1926
Tachygonetria dentata	Europe, northern Africa	Greek tortoise, other tortoises	Large intestine	Unknown; probably by ingestion of embryonated egg	Common	Incidence of 100% reported. Sometimes causes intestinal obstruction, death	Forstner 1960 Graham-Jones 1961 Reichenbach-Klinke and Elkan 1965 Schad 1963a Yamaguti 1961 Yorke and Maplestone 1926

*Discussed in text.

604

TABLE 18.6 *(continued)*

Parasite	Geographic Distribution	Reptilian or Amphibian Host	Location in Host	Method of Infection	Incidence in Nature	Remarks	Reference
Tachygonetria macrolaimus	Europe, northern Africa	Greek tortoise, other tortoises	Large intestine	Unknown; probably by ingestion of embryonated egg	Common	Incidence of 100% reported. Sometimes causes intestinal obstruction, death	Graham-Jones 1961; Reichenbach-Klinke and Elkan 1965; Schad 1963a; Yamaguti 1961; Yorke and Maplestone 1926
Tachygonetria conica	Europe, northern Africa	Greek tortoise, other tortoises	Large intestine	Unknown; probably by ingestion of embryonated egg	Common	Incidence of 100% reported. Soemtimes causes intestinal obstruction, death	Graham-Jones 1961; Reichenbach-Klinke and Elkan 1965; Schad 1963a; Yamaguti 1961; Yorke and Maplestone 1926
Tachygonetria microstoma	Europe, northern Africa	Greek tortoise, other tortoises	Large intestine	Unknown; probably by ingestion of embryonated egg	Common	Syn. *Mehdiella microstoma.* Incidence of 100% reported. Sometimes causes intestinal obstruction, death	Dyk and Dykova 1956; Forstner 1960; Graham-Jones 1961; Reichenbach-Klinke and Elkan 1965; Schad 1963a; Yamaguti 1961; Yorke and Maplestone 1926
Tachygonetria robusta	Europe, northern Africa	Greek tortoise, other tortoises	Large intestine	Unknown; probably by ingestion of embryonated egg	Common	Syn. *Mehdiella robusta.* Incidence of 100% reported. Sometimes causes intestinal obstruction, death	Forstner 1960; Graham-Jones 1961; Petter 1962; Reichenbach-Klinke and Elkan 1965; Schad 1963a; Yamaguti 1961
Tachygonetria uncinata	Europe, northern Africa	Greek tortoise, other tortoises	Large intestine	Unknown; probably by ingestion of embryonated egg	Common	Syn. *Mehdiella uncinata.* Incidence of 90% reported. Sometimes causes intestinal obstruction, death	Graham-Jones 1961; Reichenbach-Klinke and Elkan 1965; Schad 1963a; Yamaguti 1961; Yorke and Maplestone 1926
Tachygonetria stylosa	Europe, northern Africa	Greek tortoise, other tortoises	Large intestine	Unknown; probably by ingestion of embryonated egg	Common	Syn. *Mehdiella stylosa.* Incidence of 70% reported. Sometimes causes intestinal obstruction, death	Graham-Jones 1961; Petter 1962; Reichenbach-Klinke and Elkan 1965; Schad 1963a; Yamaguti 1961; Yorke and Maplestone 1926

TABLE 18.6 (continued)

Parasite	Geographic Distribution	Reptilian or Amphibian Host	Location in Host	Method of Infection	Incidence in Nature	Remarks	Reference
Tachygonetria numidica	Europe, northern Africa	Greek tortoise, other tortoises	Large intestine	Unknown; probably by ingestion of embryonated egg	Common	Incidence of 60% reported. Sometimes causes intestinal obstruction, death	Graham-Jones 1961 Reichenbach-Klinke and Elkan 1965 Schad 1963a Yamaguti 1961 Yorke and Maplestone 1925
Tachygonetria microlamus	Northern Africa	Greek tortoise	Large intestine	Unknown; probably by ingestion of embryonated egg	Unknown	Pathologic effects unknown	Petter 1962
Atractis dactyluris	Europe, northern Africa	Greek tortoise	Intestine	Unknown; probably by ingestion of infective larva	Common	Pathologic effects unknown	Dyk and Dykova 1956 Forstner 1960 Yamaguti 1961 Yorke and Maplestone 1926
Atractis carolinea	United States, Bermuda	Box turtles, anoles	Intestine	Unknown; probably by ingestion of infective larva	Unknown; probably common	Pathologic effects unknown	Harwood 1932 Williams 1959 Yamaguti 1961
Thelandros magnavulvaris	United States	Dusky salamander, red-spotted newt, other salamanders	Intestine	Unknown; probably by ingestion of embryonated egg	Common	Incidences of 10 to 48% reported in dusky salamander in eastern United States. Pathologic effects unknown	Fischthal 1955a Rankin 1937 Schad 1960, 1963b Walton 1964
Pharyngodon spinicauda	Europe, northern Africa	Salamanders, newts, European lizards	Intestine	Unknown; probably by ingestion of embryonated egg	Common	Pathologic effects unknown	Yamaguti 1961
*Oswaldocruzia pipiens**	North America	Leopard frog, green frog, wood frog, pickerel frog, green treefrog, spring peeper, other frogs, American toad, common toad, other toads, dusky salamanders, box turtle, western box turtle, eastern fence lizard	Small intestine	Unknown; probably by ingestion of infective larva	Common	Incidences of 18 to 70% reported in amphibians. Pathologic effects unknown; possibly causes debilitation, intestinal obstruction, peritonitis, death	Fischthal 1955b Harwood 1932 Rankin 1937, 1945 Walton 1964 Yamaguti 1961
*Oswaldocruzia leidyi**	North America	Green frog, bullfrog, pickerel frog, cricket frogs, green treefrog, American toad, common toad, dusky salamanders, box turtle	Small intestine	Unknown; probably by ingestion of infective larva	Common	Incidence of 53% reported in box turtle in north central United States. Pathologic effects unknown; possibly causes debilitation, intestinal obstruction, peritonitis, death	Rausch 1947 Reichenbach-Klinke and Elkan 1965 Walton 1964 Yamaguti 1961 Yorke and Maplestone 1926
Oswaldocruzia subauricularis	United States, Central America, South America	Leopard frog, treefrogs, other frogs, toads, mudpuppies	Small intestine	Unknown; probably by ingestion of infective larva	Common	Pathologic effects unknown; possibly causes debilitation, intestinal obstruction, peritonitis, death	Rankin 1937 Reichenbach-Klinke and Elkan 1965 Walton 1964 Yamaguti 1961

*Discussed in text.

TABLE 18.6 (continued)

Parasite	Geographic Distribution	Reptilian or Amphibian Host	Location in Host	Method of Infection	Incidence in Nature	Remarks	Reference
Oswaldocruzia filiformis*	Europe, Asia	Grass frog, edible frog, treefrogs, other frogs, European toad, other toads, European salamanders, common newt, crested newt, European lizards	Small intestine	Unknown; probably by ingestion of infective larva	Common	Incidence of 63% reported in grass frog in Great Britain. Pathologic effects unknown; possibly causes debilitation, intestinal obstruction, peritonitis, death	Lees 1962, Reichenbach-Klinke and Elkan 1965, Walton 1964, Yamaguti 1961, Yorke and Maplestone 1926
Oswaldocruzia goezi	Europe, Asia	Grass frog, edible frog, treefrogs, other frogs, European toad, other toads, European salamanders, common newt	Small intestine	Unknown; probably by ingestion of infective larva	Common	Pathologic effects unknown. Possibly causes debilitation, intestinal obstruction, peritonitis, death	Walton 1964, Yamaguti 1961
Oswaldocruzia bialata	Europe, Asia, Africa	Grass frog, edible frog, other frogs, European toad, other toads	Small intestine	Unknown; probably by ingestion of infective larva	Common	Pathologic effects unknown. Possibly causes debilitation, intestinal obstruction, peritonitis, death	Walton 1964, Yamaguti 1961, Yorke and Maplestone 1926
Kalicephalus agkistrodontis	United States	Racers, hognose snakes, common kingsnake, water snakes, garter snakes	Stomach, intestine	Unknown; probably by ingestion of arthropod	Common	Pathologic effects unknown	Harwood 1932, Rankin 1945, Yamaguti 1961
Camallanus microcephalus*	United States	Leopard frog, painted turtle, Blanding's turtle, map turtle, snapping turtle	Stomach, duodenum	Ingestion of copepod	Common in turtles	Incidences of 54 to 83% reported in turtles in central United States. Penetrates mucosa, causes abscesses in stomach, duodenal wall	Hoffman 1967, O'Connor 1966, Rausch 1947, Walton 1964, Williams 1953, Yamaguti 1961
Camallanus trispinosus*	United States	Painted turtle, snapping turtle, other turtles	Stomach, duodenum	Ingestion of copepod	Common	Syn. Camallanus americanus. Incidences of 87 to 100% reported in turtles in south central United States. Penetrates mucosa, causes abscesses in stomach, duodenal wall	Harwood 1932, Hoffman 1967, O'Connor 1966, Wieczorowski 1939, Yamaguti 1961
Procamallanus slomei	Southern Africa	South African clawed toad	Stomach	Unknown; probably by ingestion of copepod	Common	Embeds head deeply in stomach wall; apparently ingests blood, causes trauma	Southwell and Kirshner 1937, Walton 1964, Yamaguti 1961
Spiroxys contortus*	United States	Red-spotted newt, painted turtle, map turtle, snapping turtle, other turtles	Stomach	Ingestion of copepod or transport host (fish, amphibian)	Common	Syn. Spiroxys constricta. Incidences of 25 to 38% reported in turtles in south central United States. Penetrates mucosa, causes abscess formation in stomach, duodenal wall	Crites 1961, Harwood 1932, O'Connor 1966, Rankin 1937, Rausch 1947, Walton 1964, Wieczorowski 1939, Williams 1953, Yamaguti 1961

*Discussed in text.

TABLE 18.6 (continued)

Parasite	Geographic Distribution	Reptilian or Amphibian Host	Location in Host	Method of Infection	Incidence in Nature	Remarks	Reference
Foleyella brachyoptera*	Southeastern United States	Leopard frog	Adult: body cavity, mesentery Larva: blood, lymph, tissue fluids	Bite of mosquito	Common	Causes mesenteric cysts, listlessness, sometimes death	Crans 1969 Kotcher 1941 Reichenbach-Klinke and Elkan 1965 Walton 1964 Yamaguti 1961
Foleyella dolichoptera*	Southeastern United States	Leopard frog	Adult: body cavity, mesentery Larva: blood, lymph, tissue fluids	Bite of mosquito	Common	Causes mesenteric cysts, listlessness, sometimes death	Crans 1969 Kotcher 1941 Reichenbach-Klinke and Elkan 1965 Walton 1964 Yamaguti 1961
Foleyella americana*	United States, Canada	Leopard frog, green frog	Adult: body cavity, mesentery Larva: blood, lymph, tissue fluids	Bite of mosquito	Common	Causes mesenteric cysts, listlessness, sometimes death	Crans 1969 Reichenbach-Klinke and Elkan 1965 Walton 1964 Yamaguti 1961
Foleyella ranae*	United States, Canada	Leopard frog, green frog, bullfrog	Adult: body cavity, mesentery Larva: blood, lymph, tissue fluids	Bite of mosquito	Common	Causes mesenteric cysts, listlessness, sometimes death	Crans 1969 Kotcher 1941 Reichenbach-Klinke and Elkan 1965 Walton 1964
Foleyella duboisi*	Israel	Edible frog	Adult: body cavity, mesentery Larva: blood, lymph, tissue fluids	Bite of mosquito	Common	Causes mesenteric cysts, listlessness, sometimes death	Reichenbach-Klinke and Elkan 1965 Walton 1964 Yamaguti 1961
Icosiella quadrituberculata*	United States	Leopard frog, bullfrog, amphiumas	Adult: body cavity, mesentery Larva: blood, lymph, tissue fluids	Unknown; probably by bite of mosquito	Common	Causes mesenteric cysts, listlessness, sometimes death	Rankin 1937 Reichenbach-Klinke and Elkan 1965 Walton 1964, 1966 Yamaguti 1961
Icosiella neglecta*	Europe, Asia, Africa	Grass frog, edible frog	Adult: subcutis Larva: blood, lymph, tissue fluids	Bite of mosquito or midge	Common	Causes subcuticular cysts, listlessness, sometimes death	Reichenbach-Klinke and Elkan 1965 Walton 1964 Yamaguti 1961
Ophiodracunculus ophidensis	United States	Garter snakes	Subcutis	Ingestion of copepod or tadpole	Common	Syn. Dracunculus ophidensis. Pathologic effects unknown	Walton 1964 Yamaguti 1961
Chelonidracunculus globocephalus	United States	Snapping turtles	Pelvic fasciae	Unknown; probably by ingestion of copepod or tadpole	Common	Syn. Dracunculus globocephalus. Incidence of 70% reported in south central United States. Pathologic effects unknown	Williams 1953 Yamaguti 1961

*Discussed in text.

TABLE 18.6 *(continued)*

Parasite	Geographic Distribution	Reptilian or Amphibian Host	Location in Host	Method of Infection	Incidence in Nature	Remarks	Reference
Capillaria temua	Eastern United States	Green frog, pickerel frog, red-spotted newt	Intestine	Unknown; probably by ingestion of embryonated egg or earthworm	Common	Incidences of 21 to 49% reported in red-spotted newt. Pathologic effects unknown	Fischthal 1955a, b Rankin 1937, 1945 Walton 1964 Yamaguti 1961
Capillaria inequalis	Eastern United States	Marbled salamander, dusky salamanders, red-spotted newt	Intestine	Unknown; probably by ingestion of embryonated egg or earthworm	Common	Incidences of 2 to 57% reported in salamanders, 8 to 86% in red-spotted newt. Pathologic effects unknown	Rankin 1937 Walton 1964 Yamaguti 1961
Capillaria serpentina	South central United States	Snapping turtles	Intestine	Unknown; probably by ingestion of embryonated egg or earthworm	Common	Incidence of 30% reported. Pathologic effects unknown	Harwood 1932 Williams 1953 Yamaguti 1961
Capillaria sp.	Northeastern United States	Racers, kingsnakes	Intestine	Unknown; probably by ingestion of embryonated egg or earthworm	Unknown	Possibly *Capillaria serpentina*. Pathologic effects unknown	Rankin 1945

TABLE 18.7. Acanthocephalans affecting laboratory reptiles and amphibians

Parasite	Geographic Distribution	Reptilian or Amphibian Host	Location in Host	Method of Infection	Incidence in Nature	Remarks	Reference
Neoechinorhynchus emydis*	Eastern United States	Map turtles, Blanding's turtle, red-eared turtle	Intestine	Ingestion of first intermediate host (ostracod) or second intermediate host (snail)	Common	Causes intestinal occlusion, enteritis, thickening of mucosa; associated with neoplastic, granulomatous lesions	Cable and Fisher 1961 Cable and Hopp 1954 Fisher 1960 Harwood 1932 Rausch 1947 Van Cleave and Bullock 1950 Wieczorowski 1939
Neoechinorhynchus pseudemydis*	Eastern United States	Painted turtle, Blanding's turtle, red-eared turtle, other turtles	Intestine	Ingestion of first intermediate host (ostracod) or second intermediate host (snail)	Common	Causes intestinal occlusion, enteritis, thickening of mucosa; associated with neoplastic, granulomatous lesions	Acholonu 1967 Cable and Hopp 1954 Fisher 1960 Johnson 1968
Neoechinorhynchus chrysemydis*	Eastern United States	Painted turtle, red-eared turtle, other cooters	Intestine	Ingestion of first intermediate host (ostracod) or second intermediate host (snail)	Common	Causes intestinal occlusion, enteritis, thickening of mucosa; associated with neoplastic, granulomatous lesions	Acholonu 1967 Cable and Hopp 1954 Fisher 1960 Johnson 1968
Neoechinorhynchus emyditoides*	United States, Mexico	Painted turtle, Blanding's turtle, red-eared turtle	Intestine	Ingestion of first intermediate host (ostracod) or second intermediate host (snail)	Common	Causes intestinal occlusion, enteritis, thickening of mucosa; associated with neoplastic, granulomatous lesions	Acholonu 1967 Fisher 1960
Neoechinorhynchus stunkardi*	North central United States	Map turtles	Intestine	Ingestion of first intermediate host (ostracod) or second intermediate host (snail)	Common	Unknown; probably causes intestinal occlusion, enteritis, thickening of mucosa	Cable and Fisher 1961
Neoechinorhynchus rutili*	Europe	Edible frog, turtles	Stomach, intestine	Ingestion of intermediate host (ostracod)	Uncommon	Unknown; probably causes intestinal occlusion, gastritis, enteritis, thickening of mucosa	Reichenbach-Klinke and Elkan 1965
Acanthocephalus ranae*	Europe	Grass frog, edible frog, treefrogs, other frogs, European toad, other toads, European salamanders, alpine newt, common newt, crested newt, palmate newt, water snakes	Stomach, intestine	Amphibians: ingestion of intermediate host (isopod) Snakes: ingestion of amphibian	Common in amphibians; uncommon in snakes	Syn. *Acanthocephalus falcatus*. Incidence of 18% reported in grass frog in Great Britain, 50% in edible frog in Europe. Causes traumatic gastritis, enteritis, sometimes death	Bullock 1961 Elkan 1960 Lees 1962 Reichenbach-Klinke and Elkan 1965 Van Cleave 1915 Walton 1964
Acanthocephalus bufonicola	Eastern Europe	European toad	Intestine	Unknown; probably by ingestion of isopod or amphipod	Uncommon	Pathologic effects unknown; probably causes traumatic enteritis	Bullock 1961 Walton 1964

*Discussed in text.

TABLE 18.7 *(continued)*

Parasite	Geographic Distribution	Reptilian or Amphibian Host	Location in Host	Method of Infection	Incidence in Nature	Remarks	Reference
Acanthocephalus bufonis	Asia	Edible frog, other frogs, toads	Intestine	Unknown; probably by ingestion of isopod or amphipod	Common	Pathologic effects unknown; probably causes traumatic enteritis	Bullock 1961 Walton 1964
Acanthocephalus lucidus	Southeastern Asia	Edible frog, other frogs, toads	Intestine	Unknown; probably by ingestion of isopod or amphipod	Common	Pathologic effects unknown; probably causes traumatic enteritis	Bullock 1961 Walton 1964
Acanthocephalus acutulus	Eastern United States	Marbled salamander, dusky salamander, red-spotted newt, other salamanders	Intestine	Unknown; probably by ingestion of isopod or amphipod	Common	Incidences of 3 to 31% reported. Pathologic effects unknown; probably causes traumatic enteritis	Bullock 1961 Rankin 1937 Van Cleave 1931 Walton 1964
Acanthocephalus anthuris	Europe	Common newt, crested newt, palmate newt, turtles	Intestine	Unknown; probably by ingestion of isopod or amphipod	Uncommon	Pathologic effects unknown; probably causes traumatic enteritis	Bullock 1961 Reichenbach-Klinke and Elkan 1965 Walton 1964
Leptorhynchoides thecatus	United States	Amphiumas, mudpuppies	Intestine	Unknown; probably by ingestion of amphipod	Uncommon	Pathologic effects unknown	Hoffman 1967 Walton 1964
Pomphorhynchus bulbocolli	Eastern United States	Red-spotted newt	Intestine	Unknown; probably by ingestion of amphipod	Rare	Penetrates deeply into intestinal wall; causes traumatic enteritis	Bullock 1961 Hoffman 1967 Rankin 1937 Walton 1964
Corynosoma semerme	Europe	Edible frog	Intestine	Ingestion of aquatic crustacean (amphipod)	Uncommon	Pathologic effects unknown	Walton 1964
Centrorhynchus aluconis	Europe, Asia	Edible frog, treefrogs, other frogs, toads, water snakes, other snakes, lizards	Intestine	Amphibians: ingestion of insect larva; Snakes, lizards: ingestion of amphibian	Uncommon	Pathologic effects unknown	Reichenbach-Klinke and Elkan 1965 Walton 1964

TABLE 18.8. Leeches affecting laboratory reptiles and amphibians

Parasite	Geographic Distribution	Reptilian or Amphibian Host	Location in Host	Method of Infection	Incidence in Nature	Remarks	Reference
Haementeria montifera	North central United States	Frogs, toads	Skin	Direct contact	Rare	Syn. *Placobdella montifera.* Pathologic effects unknown	Hoffman 1967; Walton 1964
Haementeria costata	Europe, Asia	Edible frog, European pond terrapin	Skin	Direct contact	Rare	Syn. *Placobdella costata.* Vector of *Haemogregarina*; otherwise, pathologic effects unknown	Reichenbach-Klinke and Elkan 1965; Walton 1964
Hemiclepsis marginata	Europe, Asia	Frogs, turtles	Skin	Direct contact	Rare	Syn. *Placobdella marginata.* Pathologic effects unknown	Reichenbach-Klinke and Elkan 1965; Walton 1964
Protoclepsis occidentalis	Europe	Frogs	Skin	Direct contact	Rare	Pathologic effects unknown	Walton 1964
Glossiphonia swampina	Europe	Frogs	Skin	Direct contact	Rare	Pathologic effects unknown	Walton 1964
Limnatis nilotica	Africa	Edible frog	Skin	Direct contact	Rare	Pathologic effects unknown	Walton 1964
Macrobdella decora	United States	Frogs	Skin	Direct contact	Rare	Pathologic effects unknown	Walton 1964
Macrobdella ditetra	United States	Bullfrog	Skin	Direct contact	Rare	Pathologic effects unknown	Walton 1964
Batrachobdella picta	United States	Bullfrog	Dorsal lymph sac	Direct contact	Rare	Accidental invasion. Pathologic effects unknown	Reichenbach-Klinke and Elkan 1965; Walton 1964
Batrachobdella algira	Eastern Europe	Edible frog, other frogs	Skin	Direct contact	Rare	Vector of unidentified rickettsialike organism; otherwise, pathologic effects unknown	Walton 1964
Oligobdella biannulata	United States	Dusky salamanders	Skin	Direct contact	Rare	Pathologic effects unknown	Walton 1964
Actinobdella annectens	United States	Snapping turtles	Skin	Direct contact	Rare	Pathologic effects unknown	Reichenbach-Klinke and Elkan 1965
Ozobranchus branchiatus	Southern United States	Green turtle	Skin of neck, eyelids	Direct contact	Uncommon	Associated with skin tumors	Nigrelli and Smith 1943; Reichenbach-Klinke and Elkan 1965

REFERENCES

Acholonu, A. D. 1967. Studies on the acanthocephalan parasites of Louisiana turtles. Bull. Wildlife Dis. Assoc. 3:40.

———. 1970. On *Proteocephalus testudo* (Magath, 1924) (Cestoda: Proteocephalidae) from *Trionyx spinifer* (Chelonia) in Louisiana. J. Wildlife Diseases 6:171–72.

Arvey, L. 1950. Donées cytologiques et histochimiques sur l'hématophagie chez *Haplometra cylindracea* Zeder 1800. Ann. Parasitol. Humaine Comparee 25:27–36.

Ash, L. R., and P. C. Beaver. 1963. Redescription of *Ophidascaris labiatopapillosa* Walton, 1927, an ascarid parasite of North American snakes. J. Parasitol. 49:765–70.

Belding, D. L. 1965. Textbook of parasitology. 3rd ed. Appleton-Century-Crofts, New York. 1374 pp.

Borradaile, L. A., and F. A. Potts. 1958. The invertebrata: A manual for the use of students. 3d ed. Cambridge Univ. Press, Cambridge, England. 795 pp.

Bravo, H. Margarita. 1943. Tremátodos parásitos de las culebras *Thamnophis angustirostris melanogaster* de agua dulce. Ann. Inst. Biol. Univ. Nacion. Mexico 14:491–97.

Bullock, W. L. 1961. A preliminary study of the histopathology of Acanthocephala in the vertebrate intestine. J. Parasitol. 47 (Supp.):31.

Burrows, R. B. 1965. Microscopic diagnosis of the parasites of man. Yale Univ. Press, New Haven. 328 pp.

Byrd, E. E., and W. P. Maples. 1969. Intramolluscan stages of *Dasymetra conferta* Nicoll, 1911 (Trematoda: Plagiorchiidae). J. Parasitol. 55:509–26.

Caballero, E. 1946. Estudios helmintológicos de la región oncocercosa de Mexico y de la República de Guatemala: Trematoda II. Presencia de Paragonimus en reservorios naturales y descripción de un nuevo género. Ann. Inst. Biol. Univ. Nacion. Mexico 17:137–65.

Cable, R. M., and F. M. Fisher, Jr. 1961. A fifth species of *Neoechinorhynchus* (Acanthocephala) in turtles. J. Parasitol. 47:666–67.

Cable, R. M., and W. B. Hopp. 1954. Acanthocephalan parasites of the genus *Neoechinorhynchus* in North American turtles with the description of two new species. J. Parasitol. 40:674–80.

Cameron, T. W. M. 1956. Parasites and parasitism. John Wiley, New York. 322 pp.

Cheng, T. C. 1961. Description, life history, and developmental pattern of *Glypthelmins pennsylvaniensis* n. sp. (Trematoda: Brachycoeliidae), new parasite of frogs. J. Parasitol. 47:469–77.

———. 1964. The biology of animal parasites. W. B. Saunders, Philadelphia. 727 pp.

Cheng, T. C., and R. S. Chase, Jr. 1961. *Brachycoelium stablefordi*, a new parasite of salamanders; and a case of abnormal polylobation of the testes of *Brachycoelium storerliae* Harwood, 1932 (Trematoda: Brachycoeliidae). Trans. Am. Microscop. Soc. 80:33–38.

Corkum, K. C. 1966. Sparganosis in some vertebrates of Louisiana and observations on a human infection. J. Parasitol. 52:444–48.

Cort, W. W., and S. Brackett. 1937. A new strigeid cercaria which produces a bloat disease in tadpoles. J. Parasitol. 23:263–71.

Couch, J. A. 1966. *Brachycoelium ambystomae* sp. n. (Trematoda: Brachycoeliidae) from *Ambystoma opacum*. J. Parasitol. 52: 46–49.

Crandall, R. B. 1960. The life history and affinities of the turtle lung fluke, *Heronimus chelydrae* MacCallum, 1902. J. Parasitol. 46:289–307.

Crans, W. J. 1969. Preliminary observations of frog filariasis in New Jersey. Bull. Wildlife Dis. Assoc. 5:342–47.

Crites, J. L. 1961. Observations on *Spiroxys contortus* (Rudolphi, 1819) a parasite of turtles, with a summary of Ohio records (Trematoda: Gnathosomatidae). Biobriefs 2:1–4.

Davis, H. S. 1953. Culture and diseases of game fishes. Univ. California Press, Berkeley. 332 pp.

Dawes, B. 1946. The Trematoda, with special reference to British and other European forms. Cambridge Univ. Press, Cambridge, England. 644 pp.

Dogiel, V. A., Yu. I. Polyanski, and E. M. Kheisin. 1964. General parasitology (translated edition). Oliver and Boyd, Edinburgh and London. 516 pp.

Dyk, V., and S. Dykova. 1956. Hlistice nalezené v dovezených zelvách řeckých *(Testudo graeca* L.). Cesk. Parasitol. 3:43–48.

Efford, I. E., and K. Tsumura. 1969. Observations on the biology of the trematode *Megalodiscus microphagus* in amphibians from Marion Lake, British Columbia. Am. Midland Naturalist 82:197–203.

Elkan, E. 1960. Some interesting pathological cases in amphibians. Proc. Zool. Soc. London 134:275–96.

Elkan, E., and R. W. Murray. 1952. A larval trematode infection of the lateral line system of the toad, *Xenopus laevis* (Daudin). Proc. Zool. Soc. London 122:121–26.

Etges, F. J. 1961. Contributions to the life history of the brain fluke of newts and fish, *Diplostomulum scheuringi* Hughes, 1929 (Trematoda: Diplostomatidae). J. Parasitol. 47:453–58.

Ferguson, M. S. 1943. Development of eye flukes of fishes in the lenses of frogs, turtles, birds, and mammals. J. Parasitol. 29: 136–42.

Fischthal, J. H. 1955a. Ecology of worm parasites in south-central New York salamanders. Am. Midland Naturalist 53: 176–83.

———. 1955b. Helminths of salamanders from Promised Land State Forest Park, Pennsylvania. Proc. Helminthol. Soc. Wash. D.C. 22:46–48.

Fisher, F. M., Jr. 1960. On Acanthocephala of turtles, with the description of *Neoechinorhynchus emyditoides*, n. sp. J. Parasitol. 46:257–66.

Forstner, M. J. 1960. Ein Beitrag zur Kenntnis parasitischer Nematoden aus griechischen Landschildkröten. Z. Parasitenk. 20:1–22.

Galliard, H. 1948. Infestation naturelle des batraciens et reptiles par les larves plérocercoides de *Diphyllobothrium mansoni* au Tonkin. Ann. Parasitol. Humaine Comparee 23:23–26.

Galliard, H., and D. V. Ngu. 1946. Particularités du cycle évolutif de *Diphyllobothrium mansoni* au Tonkin. Ann. Parasitol. Humaine Comparee 21:246–53.

Goodchild, C. G. 1948. Additional observations on the bionomics and life history of *Gorgodera amplicava* Looss, 1899 (Trematoda: Gorgoderidae). J. Parasitol. 34:407–27.

———. 1950. Establishment and pathology of gorgoderid infections in anuran kidneys. J. Parasitol. 36:439–46.

Goodman, J. D. 1951. Some aspects of the role of parasitology in herpetology. Herpetologica 7:65–67.

Graham-Jones, O. 1956. Common diseases of cage birds and other less usual pets. Vet. record 68:918–33.

———. 1961. Some clinical conditions affecting the North African tortoise ("Greek" tortoise), *Testudo graeca*. Vet. Record 73: 317–21.

Grünberg, W., E. Kutzer, and E. Otte. 1963. Abszessähnliche Nekrosen bei Schlangen aus zoologischen Gärten. Berlin. Muench. Tieraerztl. Wochschr. 76:90–95.

Harwood, P. D. 1932. The helminths parasitic in the Amphibia and Reptilia of Houston. Texas, and vicinity. Proc. U.S. Natl. Museum 81:1–71.

Hoffman, G. L. 1967. Parasites of North American fishes. Univ. California Press, Berkeley. 486 pp.

Hoffman, G. L., and R. E. Putz. 1964. Studies on *Gyrodactylus macrochiri* n. sp. (Trematoda: Monogenea) from *Lepomis macrochirus*. Proc. Helminthol. Soc. Wash. D.C. 31:76–82.

Hughes, R. C. 1929. Studies on the trematode family Strigeidae (Holostomidae) No. XIX: *Diplostomulum scheuringi* sp. nov. and *D. vegrandis* (La Rue). J. Parasitol. 15:267–71.

Hyman, Libbie H. 1951. The invertebrates: Acanthocephala, Aschelminthes, and Entoprocta: The pseudocoelomate bilateria. Vol. III. McGraw-Hill, New York. 572 pp.

James, H. A., and M. J. Ulmer. 1967. New amphibian host records for *Mesocestoides* sp. (Cestoda: Cyclophyllidea). J. Parasitol. 53:59.

Johnson, C. A. III. 1968. New host for *Allassostoma* (Trematoda: Digenea) and *Neoechinorhynchus* (Acanthocephala) from *Pseudemys concinna* (Le Conte) (Chelonia). Bull. Wildlife Dis. Assoc. 4:129.

Kotcher, E. 1941. Studies on the development of frog filariae. Am. J. Hyg. 34:36–65.

Kutzer, E., and W. Grünberg. 1965. Parasitologie und Pathologie der Spulwurmkrankheit der Schlangen. Zentr. Veterinaermed. 12:155–75.

Lang, B. Z. 1969. Modes of infection of *Rana clamitans* with *Cephalogonimus americanus* (Trematoda). J. Parasitol. 55:832.

Lautenschlager, E. W. 1959. Meningeal tumors of the newt associated with trematode infection of the brain. Proc. Helminthol. Soc. Wash. D.C. 26:11–14.

Lawler, H. J. 1939. A new cestode, *Cylindrotaenia quadrijugosa* n. sp. from *Rana pipiens*, with a key to the nematotaeniidae. Trans. Am. Microscop. Soc. 58:73–77.

Lees, E. 1962. The incidence of helminth parasites in a particular frog population. Parasitology 52:95–102.

Lincicome, D. R. 1948. Observations on *Neoechinorhynchus emydis* (Leidy), an acanthocephalan parasite of turtles. J. Parasitol. 34:51–54.

Little, M. D. 1966. Seven new species of *Strongyloides* (Nematoda) from Louisiana. J. Parasitol. 52:85–97.

Maldonado, J. F. 1945. The life history and biology of *Platynosomum fastosum* Kossak, 1910 (Trematoda: Dicrocoeliidae). Puerto Rico J. Publ. Health Trop. Med. 21:17–39.

Marcus, L. C. 1968. Diseases of snakes and turtles, pp. 435–42. *In* R. W. Kirk, ed. Current veterinary therapy III: Small animal practice. W. B. Saunders, Philadelphia.

Nace, G. W. 1968. The amphibian facility of

the University of Michigan. Bioscience 18: 767–75.

Nelson, D. J. 1950. A treatment for helminthiasis in Ophidia. Herpetologica 6:57–59.

Niewiadomska, Katarzyna. 1964. The life cycle of *Codonocephalus urnigerus* (Rudolphi, 1819): Strigeidae. Acta Parasit. Pol. 12: 283–96.

Nigrelli, R. F., and L. W. Maraventano. 1944. Pericarditis in *Xenopus laevis* caused by *Diplostomulum xenopi* sp. nov., a larval strigeid. J. Parasitol. 30:184–90.

Nigrelli, R. F., and G. M. Smith. 1943. The occurrence of leeches, *Ozobranchus branchiatus* (Menzies), on fibro-epithelial tumors of marine turtles, *Chelonia mydas* (Linnaeus). Zoologica 28:107–8.

Noble, E. R., and G. A. Noble. 1961. Parasitology: The biology of animal parasites. Lea and Febiger, Philadelphia. 767 pp.

———. 1964. Parasitology. 2d ed. Lea and Febiger, Philadelphia. 724 pp.

O'Connor, Patricia. 1966. Diseases of snakes, pp. 582–85. *In* R. W. Kirk, ed. Current veterinary therapy 1966–1967: Small animal practice. W. B. Saunders, Philadelphia.

Olsen, O. W. 1967. Animal parasites: Their biology and life cycles. 2d ed. Burgess, Minneapolis. 431 pp.

Ortlepp, R. J. 1926. On a collection of helminths from a South African farm. J. Helminthol. 4:127–42.

Osler, Carmen P. 1931. A new cestode from *Rana clamitans* Latr. J. Parasitol. 17:183–86.

Page, L. A. 1966. Diseases and infections of snakes: A review. Bull. Wildlife Dis. Assoc. 2:11–26.

Paul, A. A. 1938. Life history studies of North American fresh-water polystomes. J. Parasitol. 24:489–510.

Pearson, J. C. 1956. Studies on the life cycles and morphology of the larval stages of *Alaria arisaemoides* Augustine and Uribe, 1927 and *Alaria canis* LaRue and Fallis, 1936 (Trematoda: Diplostomidae). Can. J. Zool. 34:295–387.

———. 1959. Observations on the morphology and life cycle of *Strigea elegans* Chandler and Rausch, 1947 (Trematoda: Strigeidae). J. Parasitol. 45:155–74.

Petter, Annie-J. 1962. Redescription et analyse critique de quelques especès d'oxyures de la tortue grecque *(Testudo graeca* L.): Diversité des structures cephaliques (II). Ann. Parasitol. 37:140–52.

Rankin, J. S., Jr. 1937. An ecological study of parasites of some North Carolina salamanders. Ecol. Monographs 7:170–269.

———. 1945. An ecological study of the helminth parasites of amphibians and reptiles of western Massachusetts and vicinity. J. Parasitol. 31:142–50.

Rausch, R. 1946. New host records for *Microphallus ovatus* Osborn, 1919. J. Parasitol. 32:93–94.

———. 1947. Observations on some helminths parasitic in Ohio turtles. Am. Midland Naturalist 38:434–42.

Reichenbach-Klinke, H., and E. Elkan. 1965. The principal diseases of lower vertebrates. Academic Press, New York. 600 pp.

Russell, Catherine M. 1951. Survey of the intestinal helminths of *Triturus v. viridescens* in the vicinity of Charlottesville, Va. Virginia J. Sci. 2:215–19.

Savage, R. M. 1962. The ecology and life history of the common frog *(Rana temporaria temporaria).* Hafner, New York. 221 pp.

Schad, G. A. 1960. The genus *Thelandros* (Nematoda: Oxyuroidea) in North American salamanders, including a description of *Thelandros salamandrae* n. sp. Can. J. Zool. 38:115–20.

———. 1963a. Niche diversification in a parasitic species flock. Nature 196:404–6.

———. 1963b. *Thelandros magnavulvaris* (Rankin, 1937) Schad, 1960 (Nematoda: Oxyuroidea) from the green salamander, *Aneides aeneus.* Can. J. Zool. 41:943–46.

Schell, S. C. 1962. Development of the sporocyst generations of *Glypthelmins quieta* (Stafford, 1900) (Trematoda: Plagiorchioidea), a parasite of frogs. J. Parasitol. 48: 387–94.

Skrjabin, K. I. 1964. Keys to the trematodes of animals and man (English translation). H. P. Arai, ed. Univ. Illinois Press, Urbana. 351 pp.

Snieszko, S. F., and G. L. Hoffman. 1963. Control of fish diseases. Lab. Animal Care 13: 197–206.

Southwell, T., and A. Kirshner. 1937. On some parasitic worms found in *Xenopus laevis,* the South African clawed toad. Ann. Trop. Med. Parasitol. 31:245–65.

Stewart, Peggy L. 1960. Lung-flukes of snakes, genera *Thamnophis* and *Coluber,* in Kansas. Univ. Kansas Sci. Bull. 41:877–90.

Talbot, S. B. 1933. Life history studies on trematodes of the subfamily Reniferinae. Parasitology 25:518–45.

Thatcher, V. E. 1954. Some helminths parasitic in *Clemmys marmorata.* J. Parasitol. 40:481–82.

Thomas, L. J. 1931. Notes on the life history of *Ophiotaenia saphena* from *Rana clamitans* Latr. J. Parasitol. 17:187–95.

———. 1937a. *Bothriocephalus rarus* n. sp.: A

cestode from the newt, *Triturus viridescens* Raf. J. Parasitol. 23:119–32.

Thomas, L. J. 1937b. Environmental relations and life history of the tapeworm *Bothriocephalus rarus* Thomas. J. Parasitol. 23:133–52.

Ubelaker, J. E., D. W. Duszynski, and D. L. Beaver. 1967. Occurrence of the trematode, *Glypthelmins pennsylvaniensis* Cheng, 1961, in chorus frogs, *Pseudacris triseriata,* in Colorado. Bull. Wildlife Dis. Assoc. 3:177.

Van Cleave, H. J. 1915. Acanthocephala in North American Amphibia. J. Parasitol. 1:175–78.

———. 1931. Acanthocephala in North American Amphibia: II. A new species of the genus *Acanthocephalus.* Trans. Am. Microscop. Soc. 50:46–47.

———. 1948. Expanding horizons in the recognition of a phylum. J. Parasitol. 34:1–20.

Van Cleave, H. J., and W. L. Bullock. 1950. Morphology of *Neoechinorhynchus emydis,* a typical representative of the Eoacanthocephala: I. The praesoma. Trans. Am. Microscop. Soc. 69:288–308.

Voge, Marietta. 1953. New host records for Mesocestoides (Cestoda: Cyclophyllidea) in California. Am. Midland Naturalist 49:249–51.

Waitz, J. A. 1961. Parasites of Idaho reptiles. J. Parasitol. 47:51.

Wall, L. D. 1941. *Spirorchis parvus* (Stunkard) its life history and the development of its excretory system (Trematoda: Spirorchiidae). Trans. Am. Microscop. Soc. 60:221–60.

Wallach, J. D. 1969. Medical care of reptiles. J. Am. Vet. Med. Assoc. 155:1017–34.

Walton, A. C. 1964. The parasites of Amphibia. Wildlife Disease 40. (Microcard and microfiche).

———. 1966. Supplemental catalog of the parasites of Amphibia. Wildlife Disease 48. 58 pp. (Microfiche).

———. 1967. Supplemental catalog of the parasites of Amphibia. Wildlife Disease 50. 38 pp. (Microfiche).

Ward, Helen L. 1940. Studies on the life history of *Neoechinorhynchus cylindratus* (Van Cleave, 1913) (Acanthocephala). Trans. Am. Microscop. Soc. 59:327–47.

Wardle, R. A., and J. A. McLeod. 1952. The zoology of tapeworms. Univ. Minnesota Press, Minneapolis. 780 pp.

Wieczorowski, Elsie. 1939. Parasitic lesions in turtles. J. Parasitol. 25:395–99.

Williams, R. W. 1953. Helminths of the snapping turtle, *Chelydra serpentina,* from Oklahoma, including the first report and description of the male of *Capillaria serpentina* Harwood, 1932. Trans. Am. Microscop. Soc. 72:175–78.

———. 1959. Some nematode parasites of tree frogs, toads, lizards and land crabs of the Bermuda Islands. J. Parasitol. 49:239.

Witenberg, G. G. 1964. Zooparasitic diseases: A. Helminthozoonoses, pp. 529–719. *In* J. van der Hoeden, ed. Zoonoses. Elsevier, New York.

Yamaguti, S. 1958. The digenetic trematodes of vertebrates. Vol. I. 2 Parts. *In* S. Yamaguti. *Systema helminthum.* Interscience, New York.

———. 1959. The cestodes of vertebrates. Vol. II. *In* S. Yamaguti. *Systema helminthum.* Interscience, New York.

———. 1961. The nematodes of vertebrates. Vol. III. 2 Parts. *In* S. Yamaguti. *Systema helminthum.* Interscience, New York.

———. 1963. Acanthocephala. Vol. V. *In* S. Yamaguti. *Systema helminthum.* Interscience, New York.

Yorke, W., and P. A. Maplestone. 1926. The nematode parasites of vertebrates. Blakiston, Philadelphia. 536 pp.

Chapter 19

MOLLUSKS

LARVAE of freshwater clams (Table 19.1) sometimes spend part of their life cycle embedded in the gills of amphibian larvae (Howard 1951; Reichenbach-Klinke and Elkan 1965; Walton 1964a, b, 1966, 1967). Larvae of *Simpsoniconcha ambigua* and *Megalonaeas gigantea* have been found on the mudpuppy in the United States (Harris 1954; Howard 1951), and larvae of *Anodonta cygnaea* on the axolotl in Europe (Reichenbach-Klinke and Elkan 1965). There are no specific reports of these parasites on laboratory amphibians, but they could be introduced into a colony on newly acquired specimens or in pond water.

TABLE 19.1. Mollusks affecting laboratory amphibians

Parasite	Geographic Distribution	Amphibian Host	Usual Habitat	Incidence in Nature	Remarks	Reference
Simpsoniconcha ambigua	United States	Mudpuppy	Larva: gills	Rare	Causes cysts in gills	Howard 1951
Megalonaeas gigantea	United States	Mudpuppy	Larva: gills	Rare	Causes cysts in gills	Harris 1954
Anodonta cygnaea	Europe	Axolotl	Larva: gills	Rare	Causes cysts in gills	Reichenbach-Klinke and Elkan 1965

REFERENCES

Harris, J. P., Jr. 1954. The parasites of Amphibia. Field Lab. 22:52–58.
Howard, A. D. 1951. A river mussel parasitic on a salamander. Chicago Acad. Sci. Nat. Hist. Misc. 77:1–6.
Reichenbach-Klinke, H., and E. Elkan. 1965. The principal diseases of lower vertebrates. Academic Press, New York. 600 pp.
Walton, A. C. 1964a. The parasites of Amphibia. Wildlife Disease 39. 28 pp. (Microcard and microfiche).
———. 1964b. The parasites of Amphibia, continued. Wildlife Disease 40. (Microcard and microfiche).
———. 1966. Supplemental catalog of the parasites of Amphibia. Wildlife Disease 48. 58 pp. (Microfiche).
———. 1967. Supplemental catalog of the parasites of Amphibia. Wildlife Disease 50. 38 pp. (Microfiche).

Chapter 20

ARTHROPODS

WITH the exception of certain mites, arthropods are not important pathogens of reptiles and amphibians maintained in the laboratory. Some mites are common, but most mites and crustaceans, insect larvae, ticks, and pentastomids are rare and are encountered only in reptiles and amphibians obtained from their natural habitat.

CRUSTACEANS

A few branchiurans and copepods have been reported on adult amphibians and their larvae (Walton 1964, 1966, 1967). Although these parasitic crustaceans are important fish pathogens, they are of little importance in amphibians (Reichenbach-Klinke and Elkan 1965). The species which have been encountered on amphibians used in the laboratory are listed in Table 20.1. None is common.

Crustaceans sometimes occur on reptiles, for example, barnacles on marine turtles (Wells 1966), but descriptions are rare and information is meager. No crustaceans have been reported affecting reptiles used in the laboratory.

FLIES

Several members of the order Diptera cause myiasis in laboratory reptiles and amphibians, and a few are vectors of blood-borne pathogens. Those likely to affect laboratory reptiles and amphibians are listed in Table 20.2. The most important are discussed below.

Bufolucilia bufonivora, Bufolucilia silvarum

(Toad Flies)

The larvae of these calliphorid flies cause a severe and often fatal myiasis of toads and frogs (Bleakney 1963; Zumpt 1965). *Bufolucilia bufonivora* (syn. *Lucilia bufonivora*) occurs in Europe, Asia, northern Africa, and possibly North America (Zumpt 1965). It is common in the European toad and sometimes affects other toads, the grass frog, edible frog, treefrogs, other frogs, European salamanders, crested newt, palmate newt, and other newts (Walton 1964, 1966, 1967; Zumpt 1965). *Bufolucilia silvarum* (syn. *L. silvarum*) occurs in North America and possibly Europe and northern Africa (Stone et al. 1965). In North America it has been reported from the bullfrog and American toad (Bleakney 1963); it is rare. Infection with larvae of these flies would not be expected in laboratories with proper fly control, but it could be present in specimens recently obtained from their natural environment.

MORPHOLOGY

Mature larvae are typically calliphorid (Fig. 20.1) (Zumpt 1965). They are white, measure 10 to 18 mm in length, and have

618

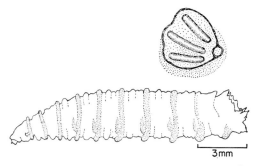

FIG. 20.1. Calliphorid larva. *(Inset)* Posterior spiracles. (From Peterson 1951. Courtesy of A. Peterson.)

several bands of microspines around the body. The head is retractile and has paired mouth hooks. Adults resemble the housefly but are larger, 6 to 11 mm in length. The body is metallic green, the legs are black, and the arista of the antenna is plumose.

LIFE CYCLE

Bufolucilia bufonivora is an obligate parasite of amphibians; *B. silvarum* is a facultative parasite (Zumpt 1965). Eggs usually hatch in 1 to 3 days, but sometimes remain unhatched for many days. Larvae pupate in 2 to 7 days and metamorphose to adults in 10 to 21 days. The entire life cycle requires 2 to 4 weeks.

PATHOLOGIC EFFECTS

Eggs laid on the skin of the host hatch and the larvae enter the nasal passages (Zumpt 1965). They cause erosion of the mucous membrane and occasionally penetrate the underlying bone and enter the orbit or brain (Fig. 20.2) (Sandner 1955; Stadler 1930). Infected toads usually die.

DIAGNOSIS

Diagnosis is based on the clinical signs and the presence of the larvae in the lesions.

CONTROL

Newly acquired specimens should be examined and, if infected, discarded. Proper fly control will prevent infection.

PUBLIC HEALTH CONSIDERATIONS

These flies have not been reported to affect man.

Cistudinomyia cistudinis

(SYN. *Sarcophaga cistudinis*)

Larvae of this sarcophagid fly cause a serious and sometimes fatal myiasis of turtles and tortoises in eastern and southern United States (Dodge 1955; Jackson, Jackson, and Davis 1969; Knipling 1937). The parasite affects several species of land turtles, including the box turtle, western box turtle, painted turtle, and gopher tortoise (*Gopherus polyphemus*). Infection with larvae of this fly is particularly common in southeastern United States. An incidence of approximately 25% was observed in 136 turtles collected in Georgia. It would not be expected in laboratories with proper fly

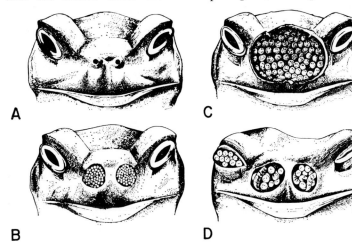

A

B

C

D

FIG. 20.2. *Bufolucilia bufonivora* infection in a toad. *(A)* Healthy toad. *(B)* Infected toad after 24 to 36 hours. *(C)* Infected toad after 48 to 72 hours. Note destruction of nasal septum and formation of a single cavity. *(D)* Infected toad after 48 to 72 hours; nasal cavities and right orbit infected. (From Zumpt 1965. Courtesy of Butterworth and Co.)

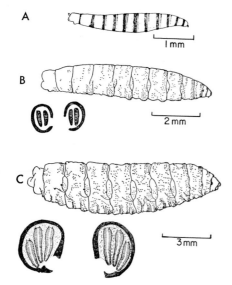

FIG. 20.3. *Cistudinomyia cistudinis* larvae. *(A)* First instar larva. *(B)* Second instar larva and posterior spiracles. *(C)* Third instar larva and posterior spiracles. (From Knipling 1937.)

control, but it could be encountered in specimens recently obtained from their natural habitat.

MORPHOLOGY

All larvae are heavily spined (Fig. 20.3) (Knipling 1937). The first instar larva measures about 2 mm in length when newly deposited and about 4 mm at the time of molting; the second instar larva is 4 to 10 mm long, and the third instar larva about 10 to 15 mm long. Adults are typically sarcophagid and resemble the housefly.

LIFE CYCLE

A gravid female deposits first instar larvae in an open wound, often in lesions produced by the gopher-tortoise tick, *Amblyomma tuberculatum* (Knipling 1937). Larval development requires about 50 to 60 days, pupation takes 14 to 21 days, and the entire life cycle requires 69 to 81 days.

PATHOLOGIC EFFECTS

Feeding larvae congregate in closely packed groups with their posterior ends toward the wound opening (Knipling 1937). They destroy considerable tissue and

produce a fetid odor and a dark discharge from the wound. The larval invasion is usually contained by the formation of a cyst wall. Only occasionally is the infection heavy enough to cause death (King and Griffo 1958; Knipling 1937; Peters 1948; Rainey 1953).

DIAGNOSIS

Diagnosis is based on demonstration of the larvae in the wounds.

CONTROL

Newly acquired specimens should be examined and, if infected, treated or discarded. Proper fly control will prevent infection. Treatment consists of removing the parasites mechanically, washing the affected area, and applying a mild antiseptic (Graham-Jones 1961; Kaplan 1957).

PUBLIC HEALTH CONSIDERATIONS

This fly is not known to affect man.

Culicids, Ceratopogonids, Psychodids

Several species of bloodsucking insects including mosquitoes *(Aedes, Culex)*, biting midges *(Forcipomyia)*, and sand flies *(Phlebotomus)* feed on reptiles and amphibians throughout the world (Pechuman and Wirth 1961; Stone et al. 1965; Walton 1964). They are important only because they are vectors of blood-borne viruses, bacteria, protozoans, and particularly the filariid nematodes, *Foleyella* and *Icosiella* (Gebhardt, Stanton, and de St. Jeor 1966; O'Connor 1966).

TICKS

Ticks frequently occur on reptiles but rarely on amphibians (Reichenbach-Klinke and Elkan 1965; Walton 1964). They are commonest on turtles, snakes, and lizards native to tropical and subtropical regions and are usually encountered in temperate regions only on imported specimens (Bishopp and Trembley 1945; Cooley and Kohls 1944a, b; Graham-Jones 1961; Worms 1967; W. H. Summerville, personal communication). Those likely to be encountered on laboratory reptiles and amphibians are listed in Table 20.3. The most important species are discussed below.

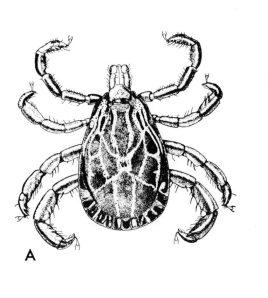

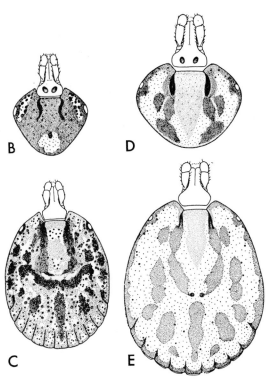

2mm

FIG. 20.4. *(A) Amblyomma* male, dorsal view. *(B)* Scutum of *A. dissimile* female. *(C)* Scutum of *A. dissimile* male. *(D)* Scutum of *A. tuberculatum* female. *(E)* Scutum of *A. tuberculatum* male. *(A* courtesy of U.S. Department of Agriculture. *B, C, D, E* from Cooley and Kohls 1944a; courtesy of Journal of Parasitology.)

Amblyomma dissimile

(Iguana Tick)

The iguana tick (Fig. 20.4), which is native to southeastern United States, Mexico, West Indies, Central America, and South America, is common on reptiles and amphibians obtained from these areas (Bishopp and Trembley 1945; Walton 1964, 1966). It attacks only ectothermal animals. The principal host is the iguana, but the toad, gopher snake, rattlesnake *(Crotalus)*, eastern fence lizard, and several other amphibians and reptiles are occasionally affected (Bishopp and Trembley 1945; Cooley and Kohls 1944a). It is likely to be encountered on laboratory amphibians and reptiles obtained from endemic regions.

Although no specific pathologic effects of this parasite have been reported, it is presumed that its presence is detrimental, especially to reptiles in captivity (Bishopp and Trembley 1945; O'Connor 1966). Treatment consists of removing the tick manually with a blunt forceps, taking care not to leave the mouth parts embedded (O'Connor 1966). The use of insecticides is not recommended.

Amblyomma tuberculatum

(Gopher-tortoise Tick)

This tick (Fig. 20.4D, E) is one of the largest known (Bishopp and Trembley 1945). The male measures 6.2 mm long by 5.5 mm wide; the female is 7.0 to 7.5 mm by 5.5 to 6.0 mm (Cooley and Kohls 1944a). Engorged females attain a length of 18 to 24 mm. The larva of *Amblyomma tuberculatum* occurs on mammals and birds. The adults and nymph occur almost exclusively on the gopher tortoise *(Gopherus poly-*

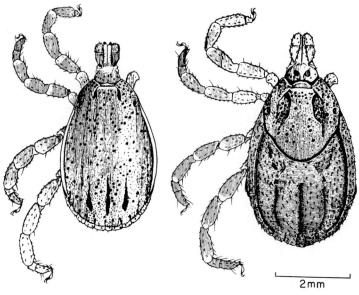

FIG. 20.5. *Hyalomma aegyptium.* *(Left)* Adult male, dorsal view. *(Right)* Adult female, dorsal view. (Courtesy of Harry Hoogstraal, U.S. Naval Medical Research Unit. No. 3.)

2mm

phemus), and the geographic distribution of this parasite (southeastern United States) is identical with that of its primary host (Bishopp and Trembley 1945; Cooley and Kohls 1944a). It is likely to occur in the laboratory only on gopher tortoises obtained from their natural habitat.

Hyalomma aegyptium
(Tortoise *Hyalomma*)

This tick (Fig. 20.5) is the commonest ectoparasite of the Greek tortoise and European pond terrapin (Graham-Jones 1961; Worms 1967). It occurs in southern Europe and southwestern Asia and, although originally described from a tortoise in Egypt, it now appears to be extinct in Africa (Hoogstraal 1956). It is a vector of *Haemogregarina* in the tortoise (Hoogstraal 1956; Marzinowsky 1927); otherwise, its pathologic effects have not been described. Treatment consists of applying ether or chloroform to the tick until it releases its grip and then removing it with a forceps (Graham-Jones 1961).

Ornithodoros turicata
(Relapsing Fever Tick)

This tick (Fig. 20.6) is native to the United States and Mexico (Cooley and Kohls 1944b). It is common on endothermal hosts and usually uncommon on ectotherms.

However, heavy infections occur occasionally on the box turtle in its natural habitat, and it was reported once as having become established in captive reptiles in the United States (Cooley and Kohls 1944b). The pathologic effects of *Ornithodoros turicata* for reptiles are unknown, but it transmits the agent of relapsing fever in man and may be a vector of *Leptospira pomona* (Cooley and Kohls 1944b; Philip and Burgdorfer 1961). All stages readily attack man.

MITES

Several species of mites affect reptiles and amphibians. Those likely to be encountered in laboratory specimens are listed in Table 20.4. The most important are discussed below.

Ophionyssus natricis
(SYN. *Ophionyssus serpentium,* *Serpenticola serpentium*)

This bloodsucking, debilitating, dermanyssid mite, the most serious ectoparasite of snakes, occurs on the skin or under the scales of several species of captive snakes and lizards throughout the world (Baker et al. 1956; Fain 1962b; Page 1966; Reichenbach-Klinke and Elkan 1965). Although common on most snakes in captivity, including racers, rat snakes, hognose snakes, king snakes, water snakes, and garter

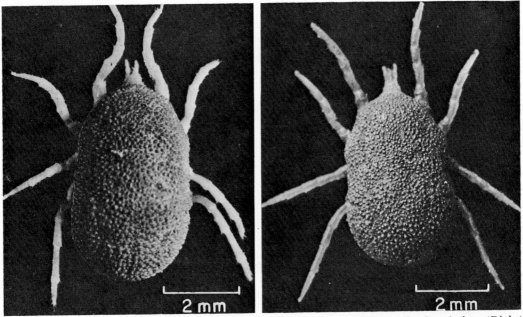

FIG. 20.6. *Ornithodoros turicata (Left)* Adult male, dorsal view. *(Right)* Nymph, dorsal view. (Courtesy of U.S. Department of Agriculture.)

snakes, it is seldom found on wild specimens and then only in Africa (Fain 1962b; Yunker 1956). Laboratory snakes are frequently infected (Pope 1950; Steward 1969). The source of infection is usually other laboratories or zoos (Klauber 1956).

MORPHOLOGY

Adults are 0.6 to 1.3 mm long (Fig. 20.7) (Camin 1953). Unfed females are

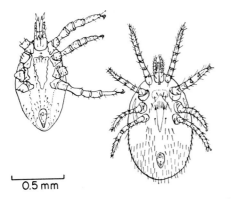

0.5 mm

FIG. 20.7. *Ophionyssus natricis. (Left)* Male, ventral view. *(Right)* Female, ventral view. (From Reichenbach-Klinke and Elkan 1965. Courtesy of Academic Press.)

yellow-brown; engorged females are dark red or black.

LIFE CYCLE

The engorged female leaves the host and deposits eggs in cage crevices or in debris (Camin 1953). The eggs hatch in 1 to 4 days, and the parasite goes through larval, protonymphal, and deutonymphal stages before reaching the adult stage. The larva does not feed; nymphs must feed before molting to the next stage. The entire life cycle requires 13 to 19 days. Some individuals live as long as 40 days.

PATHOLOGIC EFFECTS

The number of mites present on captive snakes is frequently large (Steward 1969). They suck blood and actively feed at several locations, usually on the rim of the eye or beneath the scales anterior to the neck (Camin 1948; Yunker 1956). Heavy infestations are characterized by irritation, listlessness, debilitation, severe anemia, and death (Baker et al. 1956; Klauber 1956; O'Connor 1966; Schroeder 1934).

Ophionyssus natricis is a mechanical vector of *Aeromonas hydrophila (A. lique-*

faciens), an important pathogen of snakes (Camin 1948; Heywood 1968).

DIAGNOSIS

Infestation with *O. natricis* is often first recognized by the appearance of small white deposits of mite feces on the body; clinical signs are also an aid (Page 1966). Final diagnosis is based on recognition and identification of the mite.

CONTROL

Newly acquired snakes should be carefully inspected and, if infected, isolated, treated, and placed in clean, sterilized cages. Malathion applied topically as a 4% dust (Page 1966), pyrethrins applied topically as a dust (concentration, vehicle, and method of application not given) (Page 1966; Pope 1950), and p-chlorophenyl phenyl sulfone (Sulphenone, Hazleton Laboratories) applied topically as a 10% dust or 1% suspension (Baker et al. 1956) are effective treatments, but they are sometimes toxic for reptiles (Camin et al. 1964; Page 1966; Tarshis 1960, 1962). The topical application of a sorptive silica dust (Dri-Die

67, FMC Corporation) is reportedly effective and generally nontoxic (Tarshis 1960, 1962), but it may be injurious to small reptiles (Camin et al. 1964). Spraying with an aqueous mixture of 500 to 1,000 ppm of a 64.5% emulsion of naled (Dibrom, Chevron Chemical Co.) or 2,000 to 4,000 ppm of a 25% emulsion of Diazinon (Geigy Chemical) is effective and apparently nontoxic (Camin et al. 1964). If the cage and cage contents become infested, thorough cleaning and treatment with insecticides or sterilization with steam or an open flame are necessary (Baker et al. 1956; Klauber 1956; Pope 1950).

PUBLIC HEALTH CONSIDERATIONS

Infection of laboratory personnel has been reported (Reichenbach-Klinke and Elkan 1965). The mite causes intense irritation and small pustules.

Entonyssus, Entophionyssus

Entonyssid mites are common parasites of the trachea and lungs of snakes (Fain 1961b). The genera most likely to be encountered in laboratory snakes are *Ento-*

FIG. 20.8. Entonyssid mites. *(Left) Entonyssus colubri* female, ventral view. *(Right) Entophionyssus glasmacheri* female, ventral view. (From Fain 1961b. Courtesy of Institut royal des Sciences naturelles de Belgique.)

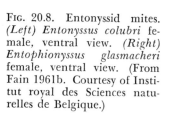
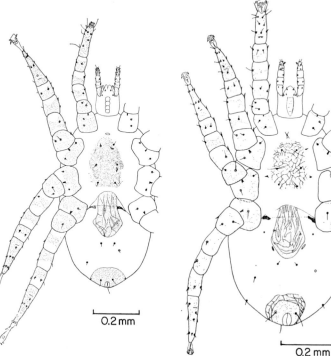

0.2 mm

0.2 mm

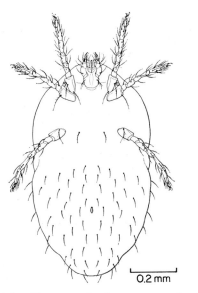

FIG. 20.9. *Hannemania* larva, ventral view. (From Sambon 1928.)

nyssus and *Entophionyssus* (Fig. 20.8). Although these parasites are frequently found in snakes that have died of pulmonary disease, no evidence exists of a causal relationship or the production of any harmful effects by the mites (Turk 1947).

Hannemania

The larva of this trombiculid genus embeds beneath the skin of various amphibians in North and South America (Hyland 1956; Sambon 1928; Walton 1964). The commonest species, *Hannemania dunni,* is prevalent in eastern United States (Hyland 1950; Murphy 1965; Sambon 1928). It has been reported from the pickerel frog, spotted salamander, marbled salamander, dusky salamander, and other amphibians (Murphy 1965; Walton 1964). Incidences of 60 to 90% have been observed in the pickerel frog (Murphy 1965), 7% in the marbled salamander, and 17 to 33% in other salamanders (Rankin 1937). Another common species is *H. penetrans,* which occurs in eastern United States and affects the leopard frog, green frog, bullfrog, toads, and other amphibians (Sambon 1928; Walton 1964). Laboratory specimens obtained from their natural habitat are likely to be infected.

MORPHOLOGY

The larva has six legs and an ovoid body, 0.6 to 1.0 mm in length and 0.3 to 0.6 mm in width (Fig. 20.9) (Sambon 1928). As it approaches the nymphal stage, rudiments of the fourth pair of legs become apparent. The nymph and adults have eight legs.

LIFE CYCLE

The life cycle involves an egg, larva, nymph, and adults (Hyland 1950). Although most trombiculid mites are ecto-

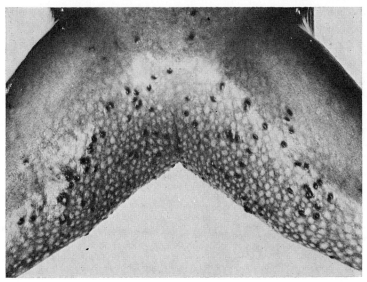

FIG. 20.10. *Hannemania* infection in a frog. Note vesicles produced by mites embedded in skin. (From Worms 1967. Courtesy of Institute of Animal Technicians.)

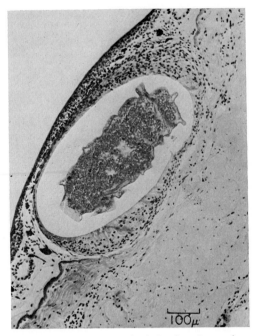

FIG. 20.11. *Hannemania* infection in a frog. Note mite in section of vesicle. (From Worms 1967. Courtesy of Institute of Animal Technicians.)

parasites, the larva of this genus is usually found beneath the skin of the host. Unengorged larvae penetrate the skin and become completely embedded in about 2 hours. The length of time spent under the skin varies, sometimes lasting 6 months. The nymph and adults are free-living and feed on small arthropods or arthropod eggs.

PATHOLOGIC EFFECTS

The embedded larvae cause the formation of orange-to-red vesicles less than 1 mm in diameter on the ventral surface of the rear legs and in the cloacal region (Fig. 20.10) (Sambon 1928; Worms 1967). In microscopic sections, encysted mites are seen in the vesicles (Fig. 20.11).

DIAGNOSIS

Diagnosis is based on the typical lesions and the identification of the mite.

CONTROL

Newly acquired amphibians should be carefully examined and, if infected, discarded. No treatment has been reported.

PUBLIC HEALTH CONSIDERATIONS

Mites of this genus have not been reported to affect man.

Eutrombicula, Neotrombicula

Larvae of these trombiculid mites are often found on reptiles and sometimes on amphibians obtained from their natural habitat (Feider 1958; Reichenbach-Klinke and Elkan 1965; Sambon 1928; Walton 1964). The commonest species in North America is *Eutrombicula alfreddugesi*, the common chigger (Fig. 20.12). It is prevalent throughout the Western Hemisphere and has been reported to affect toads, the box turtle, other turtles, racers, hognose snakes, kingsnakes, garter snakes, other snakes, and lizards (Ewing 1926; Sambon 1928; Walton

FIG. 20.12. *Eutrombicula alfreddugesi.* (*Left*) Adult female, dorsal view. (*Right*) Larva, dorsal view. (From Ewing 1929.)

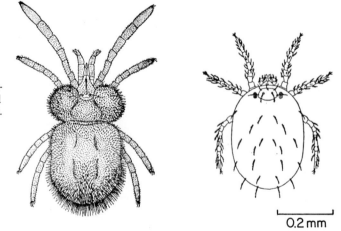

0.2 mm

1964). Another common species which occurs in southeastern United States is *E. splendens*, which affects treefrogs, snakes, and lizards (Chandler and Read 1961; Walton 1964). The common harvest mite of Europe, *Neotrombicula autumnalis*, also parasitizes reptiles; it has been found on the viviparous lizard and possibly occurs on snakes (Sambon 1928).

Only the larvae of these genera are parasitic; the nymphs and adults are free-living (Faust, Beaver, and Jung 1968). The larvae feed on tissue fluids from a single host until engorged. They are often so abundant on reptiles that they form red patches on the skin (Marcus 1968). Control is similar to that described for *Ophionyssus natricis*. The life cycle cannot be completed in the laboratory.

These mites cause a severe dermatitis in man (Faust, Beaver, and Jung 1968). Infested laboratory animals are not a hazard, however, because the larvae feed but once, and a host can become infested only by contact with unfed, unattached larvae.

PENTASTOMIDS

These vermiform arthropods are common in tropical snakes and lizards but rare in amphibians (Fain 1966; Walton 1964, 1966). Since laboratory snakes and lizards are usually obtained from temperate regions, most of these parasites are of little importance.

The morphology of pentastomids has been carefully described (Heymons 1935), but little is known of their life cycle or pathologic effects (Fain 1966; Self and Kuntz 1966). All pentastomids are endoparasites. The adults usually live in the lungs, bronchi, trachea, pharynx, or oral cavity; larvae and nymphs occur in the lungs or other organs and tissues. Infection of the definitive host is usually by ingestion of immature stages in tissues of the intermediate host, which may be a fish, amphibian, reptile, or endothermal animal. Sometimes the entire life cycle is completed in one host (Fain and Mortelmans 1960). Neither adults nor immature forms seem to cause any detrimental effects (Fain 1966; Self and Kuntz 1966). Inflammation is not produced, even in heavy infections, and no pathology has been reported.

Pentastomids that could be encoun-

tered in the laboratory are listed in Table 20.5. The most important are discussed below.

Kiricephalus coarctatus
Kiricephalus pattoni

Kiricephalus coarctatus (Fig. 20.13) is common in North, Central, and South American colubrid snakes (Fain 1961a, 1966; Heymons 1935; Self and Cosgrove 1968). Immature stages are found in the subcutaneous muscles of racers, rat snakes, garter snakes, and other snakes. Adults occur in the lung of rat snakes, garter snakes, and other snakes.

Kiricephalus pattoni occurs in colubrid and boid snakes in Asia, Indonesia, Australia, and Madagascar (Fain 1961a, 1966; Heymons 1935). Immature stages have been found in the subcutaneous tissues of toads and frogs and in subcutaneous tissues or the stomach wall of snakes (Fain 1966; Sambon 1928; Walton 1964, 1966). Adults occur in the lung of racers and other snakes.

Although these parasites have not been specifically reported in laboratory amphibians and snakes, both species are common and could be encountered in hosts obtained from their natural habitat in endemic areas.

Raillietiella

Several species of this cosmopolitan genus (Fig. 20.14) affect reptiles that are used in the laboratory (Fain 1961a, 1964a, 1966; Heymons 1935). Only one species, *Raillietiella bicaudata*, occurs in North America. It is found in the lung of rat snakes and other snakes (Fain 1966). The commonest species in Europe, *R. orientalis*, occurs in the lung of racers, rat snakes, and other snakes (Fain 1966). *Raillietiella boulengeri* is the commonest species in Africa (Fain 1966). Immature stages of this species are found in various tissues of snakes and lizards, and adults occur in colubrid, boid, viperid, and other snakes (Fain 1964a). Only one species, *R. furcocerca*, occurs in South America (Fain 1966). Larvae and nymphs of this species are found in various tissues of racers and rat snakes, and adults occur in the lung of colubrid, boid, crotalid, and other snakes. Although not specifically reported in lab-

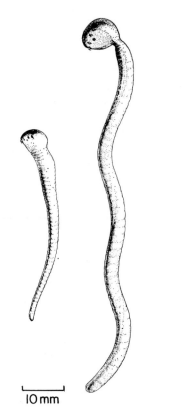

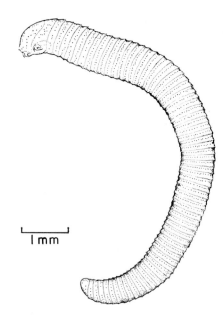

Fig. 20.15. *Sebekia oxycephala* larva. (From Heymons 1935.)

Fig. 20.13. *Kiricephalus coarctatus.* *(Left)* Male. *(Right)* Female. (From Heymons 1935.)

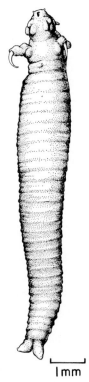

Fig. 20.14. *Raillietiella.* (From Heymons 1935.)

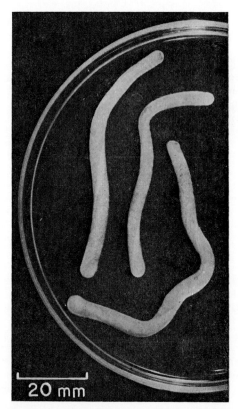

Fig. 20.16. *Porocephalus* females. (From Fain 1961a. Courtesy of Musée royal de l'Afrique Centrale.)

oratory reptiles, *Raillietiella* is likely to be encountered in certain snakes obtained from their natural habitat in endemic areas.

Sebekia oxycephala

Adults of this species occur in the lungs, trachea, and pharynx of the crocodile, alligator, and spectacled caiman in North and South America (Fain 1961a, 1966; Heymons 1935). Immature stages (Fig. 20.15) are frequently encountered in hognose snakes and other snakes and occasionally in lizards. They also occur in fishes (Hoffman 1967). Although no specific reports have been made of this parasite in laboratory animals, adults are likely to be encountered in crocodilians, and larvae and nymphs in snakes obtained from their natural habitat in endemic areas.

Porocephalus

Adults of this genus (Fig. 20.16) occur in the lung of crotalid, boid, and some colubrid snakes in North and South America and Africa (Fain 1961a, 1966). *Porocephalus crotali* is particularly common in rattlesnakes *(Crotalus)* in the United States with an incidence of over 50% reported in some areas (Self and McMurry 1948). Although *Porocephalus* does not occur in species of snakes usually used in the laboratory, members of this genus are important because immature stages occur in certain laboratory rodents (Esslinger 1962a, b; da Fonseca 1939; Layne 1967; Penn 1942; Self and McMurry 1948) and primates (Cosgrove, Nelson, and Gengozian 1968; Heymons 1935; Nelson, Cosgrove, and Gengozian 1966; Self and Cosgrove 1968).

TABLE 20.1. Crustaceans affecting laboratory amphibians

Parasite	Geographic Distribution	Reptilian or Amphibian Host	Location in Host	Incidence in Nature	Remarks	Reference
Argulus americanus	United States	Leopard frog, salamanders	Skin	Unknown; probably uncommon	Fish louse. Ingests blood, causes irritation, sometimes death; possible vector of pathogens	Hoffman 1967 Reichenbach-Klinke and Elkan 1965 Walton 1966
Argulus japonicus	Worldwide	Tadpole of leopard frog	Skin	Unknown; probably uncommon	Fish louse. Ingests blood, causes irritation, sometimes death; possible vector of pathogens	Hoffman 1967 Reichenbach-Klinke and Elkan 1965 Walton 1967
Lernaea cyprinacea	United States, Europe, Asia, Africa	Leopard frog, bullfrog, wood frog, common newt, salamanders	Gills, skin	Unknown; probably uncommon	Syn. *L. carassii*, *L. elegans*; probable syn. *L. ranae*; anchor worm. Vermiform female embeds in tissues of host. Causes trauma of gills, skin	Baldauf 1961 Hoffman 1967 Reichenbach-Klinke and Elkan 1965 Tidd and Shields 1963 Walton 1964, 1966
Lernaea ranae	United States	Tadpole of green frog	Gills	Unknown; probably uncommon	Probable syn. *L. cyprinacea*; anchor worm. Vermiform female embeds in tissues of host. Causes trauma of gills	Hoffman 1967 Walton 1964

630

TABLE 20.2. Flies affecting laboratory reptiles and amphibians

Parasite	Geographic Distribution	Reptilian or Amphibian Host	Location in Host	Incidence in Nature	Remarks	Reference
Bufolucilia bufonivora*	Europe, Asia, northern Africa, possibly North America	Grass frog, edible frog, tree-frogs, other frogs, European toad, European salamanders, crested newt, palmate newt, other newts	Larva: nasal passages, orbit, brain	Common in European toad; uncommon in other species	Syn. Lucilia bufonivora. Causes severe myiasis, death	Sandner 1955 Stadler 1930 Walton 1964, 1966, 1967 Zumpt 1965
Bufolucilia silvarum*	North America, possibly Europe, northern Africa	Bullfrog, American toad	Larva: nasal passages, orbit, brain	Rare	Syn. Lucilia silvarum. Causes myiasis, death	Bleakney 1963 Stone et al. 1965
Lucilia porphyrina	India	Toads	Larva: skin, orbit	Uncommon	Causes myiasis, death	Dasgupta 1962 Zumpt 1965
Blowfly (calliphorid of undetermined species)	Europe	Greek tortoise, other turtles	Larva: skin of tail, skin of cloacal region, under carapace	Common	Causes myiasis	Graham-Jones 1961 Reichenbach-Klinke and Elkan 1965
Batrachomyia mertensi	Australia	Treefrogs, toads	Larva: skin	Uncommon	Causes myiasis	Reichenbach-Klinke and Elkan 1965 Walton 1964, 1967
Cistudinomyia cistudinis*	Eastern United States, southern United States	Painted turtle, box turtle, western box turtle, gopher tortoise (Gopherus polyphemus)	Larva: skin	Common	Syn. Sarcophaga cistudinis. Causes myiasis, sometimes death	Dodge 1955 Jackson et al. 1969 King and Griffo 1958 Knipling 1937 Peters 1948 Rainey 1953
Sarcophaga ruralis	Europe	European toad	Larva: skin	Uncommon	Causes myiasis	Walton 1964
Anolisimyia blakeae	Eastern United States	Green anole	Larva: skin	Uncommon	Causes myiasis	Dodge 1955 Gunter 1958
Aedes	Worldwide	Leopard frog, green frog, other frogs	Skin	Common	Ingests blood; transmits filarial nematodes, other blood-borne pathogens	Walton 1964
Culex	Worldwide	Leopard frog, green frog, other frogs, snakes	Skin	Common	Ingests blood; transmits viruses of western and eastern equine encephalitis, filarial nematodes, other blood-borne pathogens	Gebhardt et al. 1966 O'Connor 1966 Walton 1964
Forcipomyia fairfaxensis	Eastern Canada	Leopard frog	Skin	Common	Ingests blood; probably transmits blood-borne pathogens	Pechuman and Wirth 1961 Stone et al. 1965
Forcipomyia pilosipennis	Europe	Edible frog	Skin	Common	Syn. F. velox. Ingests blood; transmits blood-borne pathogens	Stone et al. 1965 Walton 1964
Phlebotomus sp.	United States	Frogs, toads	Skin	Common	Ingests blood; transmits blood-borne pathogens	Walton 1964
Phlebotomus squamirostris	China	Toads	Skin	Common	Ingests blood; transmits trypanosomes	Walton 1964

*Discussed in text.

TABLE 20.3. Ticks affecting laboratory reptiles and amphibians

Parasite	Geographic Distribution	Reptilian or Amphibian Host	Location in Host	Incidence in Nature	Remarks	Reference
Amblyomma dissimile*	Southeastern United States, Mexico, West Indies, Central America, South America	Toads, gopher snake, other snakes, iguanas, eastern fence lizard, other lizards	Skin	Common	Iguana tick. Pathologic effects unknown; probably causes irritation, trauma	Bishopp and Trembley 1945; Cooley and Kohls 1944a; O'Connor 1966; Walton 1964, 1966
Amblyomma tuberculatum*	Southeastern United States	Gopher tortoise (Gopherus polyphemus), box turtle, eastern fence lizard	Skin	Common	Gopher-tortoise tick. Pathologic effects unknown; probably causes irritation	Bishopp and Trembley 1945; Cooley and Kohls 1944a
Amblyomma humerale	Southern United States, South America	Box turtle	Skin	Uncommon	Pathologic effects unknown; probably causes irritation	Bilsing and Eads 1947; Robinson 1926
Amblyomma testudinis	South America	Various reptiles	Skin	Uncommon	Pathologic effects unknown; probably causes irritation	Becklund 1968; Robinson 1926
Amblyomma rotundatum	Mexico, West Indies, South America	Toads, various reptiles	Skin	Uncommon	Pathologic effects unknown; probably causes irritation	Becklund 1968; Walton 1964, 1966
Amblyomma marmoreum	Africa	Tortoises, warrener lizards (Varanus)	Skin	Uncommon	Large reptile Amblyomma. Pathologic effects unknown; probably causes irritation	Hoogstraal 1956
Amblyomma nuttalli	Africa	Tortoises	Skin	Uncommon	Small reptile Amblyomma. Pathologic effects unknown; probably causes irritation	Hoogstraal 1956
Aponomma elaphensis	Southwestern United States, Mexico	Rat snake	Skin	Uncommon	Pathologic effects unknown; probably causes irritation	Degenhardt and Degenhardt 1965
Aponomma gervaisi	Southern Asia	Snakes	Skin	Common	Pathologic effects unknown; probably causes irritation	Hughes 1959
Aponomma exornatum	Africa	Tortoises, crocodiles, snakes, warrener lizards (Varanus)	Skin	Common on warrener lizard; otherwise uncommon	Monitor lizard tick. Pathologic effects unknown; probably causes irritation	Hoogstraal 1956
Aponomma latum	Africa	Large snakes (Python, Naja, Dasypeltis, Bitis)	Skin	Common	Snake tick. Pathologic effects unknown; probably causes irritation	Hoogstraal 1956
Hyalomma aegyptium*	Southern Europe, southwestern Asia	European pond terrapin, Greek tortoise	Skin	Common	Tortoise Hyalomma. Pathologic effects unknown; probably causes irritation; vector of Haemogregarina	Graham-Jones 1961; Hoogstraal 1956; Marzinowsky 1927; Worms 1967
Haemaphysalis punctata	Europe, northwestern Africa, southwestern Asia	Lizards, European viper	Skin	Uncommon on reptiles	Only immature stages occur on reptiles. Pathologic effects unknown; probably causes irritation. Transmits agent of Siberian tick typhus	Hoogstraal 1967; Lapage 1968

*Discussed in text.

TABLE 20.3 *(continued)*

Parasite	Geographic Distribution	Reptilian or Amphibian Host	Location in Host	Incidence in Nature	Remarks	Reference
Haemaphysalis concinna	Europe, northern Asia	Various reptiles	Skin	Uncommon on reptiles	Only immature stages occur on reptiles. Pathologic effects unknown; probably causes irritation. Transmits agents of Russian spring-summer encephalitis, Siberian tick typhus	Hoogstraal 1966, 1967
Ixodes pacificus	Pacific coastal region of North America	Garter snakes, spiny lizards, other lizards	Skin	Common on lizards	California black-legged tick. Only immature stages occur on reptiles. Pathologic effects in reptiles unknown; probably causes irritation, trauma. Bite causes irritation, trauma in man; possibly transmits agent of tularemia	Arthur and Snow 1968 Bishopp and Trembley 1945 Cooley and Kohls 1945 Philip and Burgdorfer 1961 U.S. Dept. Agr. 1965
Ixodes ricinus	Europe	Green lizard, other lizards	Skin	Uncommon on reptiles	Only immature stages occur on reptiles. Pathologic effects in reptiles unknown; probably causes irritation, trauma. Bite causes irritation, severe trauma, paralysis in man; transmits agent of central European tick-borne encephalitis; possible vector of agents of boutonneuse fever, Bukhovian hemorrhagic fever	Hoogstraal 1966, 1967 Lapage 1962, 1968 Reichenbach-Klinke and Elkan 1965
*Ornithodoros turicata****	United States, Mexico	Box turtle, gopher tortoise *(Gopherus polyphemus)*, rattlesnakes *(Crotalus)*	Skin	Common on box turtle in some regions	Relapsing fever tick. Pathologic effects in reptiles unknown; probably causes irritation, trauma. Causes painful bite, inflammation, edema, subcutaneous nodules, itching in man; transmits agents of relapsing fever and possibly leptospirosis	Cooley and Kohls 1944b Philip and Burgdorfer 1961
Ornithodoros erraticus	Southern Europe, southwestern Asia, northern Africa	Toads, various reptiles	Skin	Uncommon	Pathologic effects in reptiles unknown; probably causes irritation, trauma	Hoogstraal 1956 Walton 1964, 1966
Ornithodoros moubata complex	Southern Africa	Tortoises	Skin	Uncommon on tortoises	Pathologic effects in reptiles unknown; probably causes irritation, trauma	Hoogstraal 1956

*Discussed in text.

TABLE 20.4. Mites affecting laboratory reptiles and amphibians

Parasite	Geographic Distribution	Reptilian or Amphibian Host	Location in Host	Incidence in Nature	Remarks	Reference
Ophionyssus natricis*	Africa; worldwide in snakes in captivity	Racers, rat snakes, hognose snakes, kingsnakes, water snakes, garter snakes, other snakes, lizards	Skin	Uncommon	Syn. O. serpentium, Serpenticola serpentium. Common on laboratory snakes. Serious blood-sucking ectoparasite of captive snakes; causes loss of blood, irritation, debilitation, anemia, sometimes death; mechanical vector of Aeromonas hydrophila (A. liquefaciens)	Baker et al. 1956 Camin 1948, 1953 Fain 1962b Heywood 1968 Klauber 1956 O'Connor 1966 Page 1966 Pope 1950 Reichenbach-Klinke and Elkan 1965 Schroeder 1934 Steward 1969 Yunker 1956
Neoliponyssus lacertarum	Europe, western Asia	Green lizard, other lizards	Skin	Uncommon	Syn. N. lacertinus, Liponyssus lacertarum. Apparently nonpathogenic	Hughes 1959 Till 1957
Neoliponyssus saurarum	Europe	Sand lizard	Skin	Uncommon	Syn. Liponyssus saurarum. Apparently nonpathogenic	Till 1957
Entonyssus colubri	United States	Racers	Trachea, lungs	Common	Apparently nonpathogenic	Fain 1961b Turk 1947
Entonyssus halli	United States	Pine snake, other snakes	Trachea, lungs	Common	Apparently nonpathogenic	Fain 1961b Turk 1947
Entonyssus asiaticus	Indonesia	Water snakes	Trachea, lungs	Common	Apparently nonpathogenic	Fain 1961b
Entonyssus javanicus	Indonesia	Water snakes	Trachea, lungs	Common	Apparently nonpathogenic	Fain 1961b Turk 1947
Entophionyssus hamertoni	North America	Garter snakes	Trachea, lungs	Common	Apparently nonpathogenic	Fain 1961b Turk 1947
Entophionyssus glasmacheri	North America	Rat snakes, common king-snake, bullsnakes	Trachea, lungs	Common	Apparently nonpathogenic	Fain 1961b Turk 1947
Entophionyssus heterodontos	United States	Hognose snakes, kingsnakes	Trachea, lungs	Common	Apparently nonpathogenic	Fain 1961b Turk 1947
Entophionyssus natricis	Southeastern United States	Water snakes	Trachea, lungs	Common	Apparently nonpathogenic	Fain 1961b Turk 1947
Entophionyssus fragilis	North America	Common kingsnake	Trachea, lungs	Common	Apparently nonpathogenic	Fain 1961b Keegan 1946
Viperacarus europaeus	Europe	European viper	Trachea, lungs	Common	Apparently nonpathogenic	Fain 1961b
Haemolaelaps natricis	Eastern Europe	Water snakes	Skin	Uncommon	Pathologic effects unknown	Fain 1962b
Ixodorhynchus liponyssoides	North America	Garter snakes, other colubrid snakes	Skin	Uncommon	Pathologic effects unknown	Fain 1962b Turk 1947

*Discussed in text.

634

TABLE 20.4 (continued)

Parasite	Geographic Distribution	Reptilian or Amphibian Host	Location in Host	Incidence in Nature	Remarks	Reference
Ixodorhynchus johnstoni	Southeastern United States	Eastern hognose snake	Skin	Uncommon	Pathologic effects unknown	Fain 1962b
Ixobioides butantanensis	South America	Colubrid snakes	Skin	Uncommon	Pathologic effects unknown	Fain 1962b Hughes 1959 Turk 1947
Hemilaelaps triangulus	Eastern United States	Rat snake, kingsnakes, other colubrid snakes	Skin	Uncommon	Syn. *Liponyssus triangulus*, *Hemilaelaps distinctus*. Pathologic effects unknown	Fain 1962b Hughes 1959 Turk 1947
Hemilaelaps feideri	Southern Europe	Water snakes	Skin	Uncommon	Pathologic effects unknown	Fain 1962b
Hemilaelaps radfordi	Eastern Europe	Water snakes, other colubrid snakes	Skin	Uncommon	Pathologic effects unknown	Fain 1962b
Hemilaelaps piger	Southern Europe	Colubrid snakes	Skin	Uncommon	Pathologic effects unknown	Fain 1962b
Hemilaelaps farrieri	Africa	Colubrid snakes	Skin	Uncommon	Pathologic effects unknown	Fain 1962b
Hemilaelaps imphialensis	Southern Asia	Colubrid snakes	Skin	Uncommon	Pathologic effects unknown	Fain 1962b
Asiatolaelaps tanneri	Eastern Asia	Water snakes	Skin	Uncommon	Pathologic effects unknown	Fain 1962b
Asiatolaelaps evansi	Southern Asia	Rat snakes	Skin	Uncommon	Pathologic effects unknown	Fain 1962b
Strandtibbettsia gordoni	Eastern Asia, Indonesia	Water snakes	Skin	Uncommon	Pathologic effects unknown	Fain 1962b
*Hannemania dunni**	Eastern United States	Pickerel frog, spotted salamander, marbled salamander, dusky salamander, other amphibians	Skin	Common	Encysted larvae cause orange-red dermal vesicles	Hyland 1950, 1956 Murphy 1965 Rankin 1937 Sambon 1928 Walton 1964 Worms 1967
*Hannemania penetrans**	Eastern United States	Leopard frog, green frog, bullfrog, other frogs, toads, other amphibians	Skin	Common	Encysted larvae cause orange-red dermal vesicles	Hyland 1956 Sambon 1928 Walton 1964
Hannemania eltoni	South central United States	Leopard frog	Skin	Uncommon	Encysted larvae cause orange-red dermal vesicles	Hyland 1956 Walton 1964
Hannemania hegeneri	Southeastern United States	Leopard frog	Skin	Uncommon	Encysted larvae cause orange-red dermal vesicles	Hyland 1956, 1961 Walton 1964
Hannemania hylae	Southwestern United States	Treefrogs	Skin	Uncommon	Encysted larvae cause orange-red dermal vesicles	Hughes 1959 Hyland 1956 Sambon 1928 Walton 1964

*Discussed in text.

635

TABLE 20.4 (continued)

Parasite	Geographic Distribution	Reptilian or Amphibian Host	Location in Host	Incidence in Nature	Remarks	Reference
Hannemania mexicana	Mexico	Leopard frog, other frogs	Skin	Uncommon	Encysted larvae cause orange-red dermal vesicles	Hyland 1956, 1961 Walton 1964
Hannemania pelaesi	Mexico	Leopard frog	Skin	Uncommon	Encysted larvae cause orange-red dermal vesicles	Walton 1967 Worms 1967
Hannemania newsteadi	South America	Treefrogs	Skin	Uncommon	Encysted larvae cause orange-red dermal vesicles	Hughes 1959 Sambon 1928 Walton 1964
Hannemania edwardsi	South America	Toads	Skin	Uncommon	Encysted larvae cause orange-red dermal vesicles	Sambon 1928 Walton 1964
Eutrombicula alfreddugesi*	North America, West Indies, South America	Toads, box turtle, other turtles, racers, hognose snakes, kingsnakes, garter snakes, other snakes, lizards	Skin	Common	Syn. Trombicula irritans; common chigger. Only larva parasitic. Feeds on tissue fluids; pathologic effects unknown. Causes dermatitis in man	Ewing 1926 Sambon 1928 Walton 1964
Eutrombicula splendens*	Southeastern United States	Treefrogs, snakes, lizards	Skin	Common	Syn. Trombicula splendens. Only larva parasitic. Feeds on tissue fluids; pathologic effects unknown.	Chandler and Read 1961 Walton 1964
Eutrombicula insularis	West Indies	Anoles	Skin	Uncommon	Only larva parasitic. Pathologic effects unknown	Reichenbach-Klinke and Elkan 1965
Eutrombicula vorkei	South America	Treefrogs	Skin	Uncommon	Only immature stages occur on frogs. Pathologic effects unknown	Sambon 1928 Walton 1964
Eutrombicula hirsti	Southeastern Asia	Racers	Skin	Uncommon	Syn. Trombicula hakei. Only larva parasitic. Pathologic effects unknown	Reichenbach-Klinke and Elkan 1965
Neotrombicula autumnalis*	Europe	Viviparous lizard, possibly snakes	Skin	Uncommon	Syn. Trombicula autumnalis. Common harvest mite. Only larva parasitic. Pathologic effects unknown. Causes dermatitis in man	Sambon 1928
Neotrombicula trogardhiana	Europe	Sand lizard	Skin	Uncommon	Pathologic effects unknown	Feider 1958
Trombicula hasei	Europe	European lizards	Skin	Uncommon	Only larva parasitic. Pathologic effects unknown	Feider 1958
Trombicula agamae	Near East	Starred lizard (Agamo stellio)	Skin	Uncommon	Only larva parasitic. Pathologic effects unknown	Reichenbach-Klinke and Elkan 1965
Neoschoengastia scelopori	Southern United States	Spiny lizards	Skin	Uncommon	Pathologic effects unknown	Hughes 1959

* Discussed in text.

636

TABLE 20.4 (continued)

Parasite	Geographic Distribution	Reptilian or Amphibian Host	Location in Host	Incidence in Nature	Remarks	Reference
Ophioptes parkeri	South America	Colubrid snakes	Skin	Uncommon	Pathologic effects unknown	Fain 1964b Sambon 1928
Ophioptes tropicalis	Northern South America	Colubrid snakes	Skin	Uncommon	Pathologic effects unknown	Fain 1964b
Ophioptes dromicus	West Indies	Colubrid snakes	Skin	Uncommon	Pathologic effects unknown	Fain 1964b
Geckobiella texana	Western United States	Western fence lizard, other lizards	Skin	Uncommon	Pathologic effects unknown	Lawrence 1953
Hirstiella bakeri	North America	Iguanas	Skin	Uncommon	Pathologic effects unknown	Hughes 1959
Hirstiella pelaezi	North America	Spiny lizards	Skin	Uncommon	Pathologic effects unknown	Hughes 1959
Lawrencarus hylae	North America, South America, Africa, Asia, Australia	Treefrogs, other amphibians	Nasal passages	Uncommon	Pathologic effects unknown	Fain 1962a Walton 1967
Lawrencarus americanus	Southeastern United States	Treefrogs	Skin	Uncommon	Pathologic effects unknown	Fain 1962a
Lawrencarus eweri	Southern Europe, Africa, southeastern Asia	Toads	Nasal passages	Uncommon	Pathologic effects unknown	Fain 1962a Walton 1967
Xenopacarus africanus	Southern Africa	South African clawed toad	Nasal passages	Unknown	Pathologic effects unknown	Fain et al. 1969
Cloacarus beeri	North central United States	Painted turtle	Rectum	Unknown	Pathologic effects unknown	Fain 1968
Cloacarus faini	Central United States	Snapping turtle	Rectum	Unknown	Pathologic effects unknown	Fain 1968
Theodoracarus testudinis	Israel	Greek tortoise	Rectum, muscle	Unknown	Pathologic effects unknown	Fain 1968
Caminacarus theodori	Israel	Pond turtles	Rectum	Unknown	Pathologic effects unknown	Fain 1968
Caminacarus costai	Israel	Pond turtles	Rectum	Unknown	Pathologic effects unknown	Fain 1968
Caminacarus sinensis	China	Softshell turtles	Rectum	Unknown	Pathologic effects unknown	Fain 1968

637

TABLE 20.5. Pentastomids affecting laboratory reptiles and amphibians

Parasite	Geographic Distribution	Reptilian or Amphibian Host	Location in Host	Incidence in Nature	Remarks	Reference
*Kiricephalus coarctatus**	North America, Central America, South America	Definitive: rat snakes, garter snakes, other snakes. Intermediate: racers, rat snakes, garter snakes, other snakes	Adult: lung. Larva, nymph: subcutaneous muscles	Common	Apparently nonpathogenic	Fain 1961a, 1966; Heymons 1935; Self and Cosgrove 1968
*Kiricephalus pattoni**	Asia, Indonesia, Australia, Madagascar	Definitive: racers, other snakes. Intermediate: toads, frogs, snakes	Adult: lung. Larva, nymph: subcutaneous tissues, stomach wall	Common	Apparently nonpathogenic	Fain 1961a, 1966; Heymons 1935; Sambon 1928; Walton 1964, 1966
*Raillietiella bicaudata**	North America	Rat snakes, other snakes	Lung	Common	Apparently nonpathogenic	Fain 1961a, 1966; Heymons 1935
*Raillietiella orientalis**	Southern Europe, southwestern Asia, Africa	Racers, rat snakes, other snakes	Lung	Common	Apparently nonpathogenic	Fain 1961a, 1966; Heymons 1935
Raillietiella mediterranea	Europe, northern Africa	Racers	Lung	Uncommon	Apparently nonpathogenic	Fain 1961a, 1966; Heymons 1935; Walton 1964
*Raillietiella boulengeri**	Africa, Asia	Definitive: colubrid, boid, viperid, other snakes. Intermediate: snakes, lizards	Adult: lung. Larva, nymph: many tissues	Common	Apparently nonpathogenic	Fain 1961a, 1964a; Heymons 1935
*Raillietiella furcocerca**	South America	Definitive: colubrid, boid, crotalid, other snakes. Intermediate: racers, rat snakes	Adult: lung. Larva, nymph: many tissues	Common	Apparently nonpathogenic	Fain 1961a, 1966; Heymons 1935
*Sebekia oxycephala**	North America, South America	Definitive: American alligator, spectacled caiman, American crocodile. Intermediate: hognose snakes, other snakes, lizards	Adult: lung, trachea, pharynx. Larva, nymph: viscera	Common	Apparently nonpathogenic	Fain 1961a, 1966; Heymons 1935; Hoffman 1967
Sebekia divestei	North America	American crocodile	Lungs	Uncommon	Apparently nonpathogenic	Fain 1961a, 1966; Heymons 1935
Sebekia acuminata	South America	Caimans	Lungs	Uncommon	Apparently nonpathogenic	Fain 1961a; Heymons 1935
Sebekia samboni	South America	Caimans	Lungs	Uncommon	Apparently nonpathogenic	Fain 1961a; Heymons 1935
Sebekia wedli	Africa	Nile crocodile	Lungs	Uncommon	Apparently nonpathogenic	Fain 1961a; Heymons 1935
Sebekia cesarisi	Africa	Nile crocodile	Lungs	Uncommon	Apparently nonpathogenic	Fain 1961a; Heymons 1935
Sebekia jubini	Southeastern Asia	Crocodiles	Nasal pit	Uncommon	Apparently nonpathogenic	Fain 1961a; Heymons 1935

*Discussed in text.

TABLE 20.5 (continued)

Parasite	Geographic Distribution	Reptilian or Amphibian Host	Location in Host	Incidence in Nature	Remarks	Reference
Porocephalus crotali*	North America, South America	Definitive: crotalid snakes; Intermediate: snakes, amphibians	Adult: lung; Larva, nymph: subcutaneous tissues	Common	Apparently nonpathogenic. Immature stages occur in rodents	Fain 1961a, 1966; Heymons 1935
Porocephalus clavatus	South America	Boid snakes	Lung	Common	Apparently nonpathogenic. Immature stages occur in simian primates	Fain 1961a, 1966; Heymons 1935
Porocephalus stilesi	South America	Crotalid, colubrid snakes	Lung	Common	Apparently nonpathogenic	Fain 1961a, 1966; Heymons 1935
Porocephalus subulifer	Tropical Africa	File snakes (Mehelya)	Lung	Common	Apparently nonpathogenic. Immature stages occur in simian primates	Fain 1961a, 1966; Heymons 1935
Armillifer armillatus	Tropical Africa	Boid, viperid snakes	Lung	Common	Apparently nonpathogenic. Immature stages occur in mammals, including man; rarely in birds	Fain 1961a, 1966; Heymons 1935
Armillifer moniliformis	Asia, Africa, Australia	Boid snakes	Lung	Common	Apparently nonpathogenic. Immature stages occur in mammals, including man	Fain 1966; Heymons 1935
Alofia platycephala	South America	American alligator, spectacled caiman	Lungs	Uncommon	Apparently nonpathogenic	Fain 1961a; Heymons 1935
Alofia indica	India	Crocodiles	Lungs, trachea	Uncommon	Apparently nonpathogenic	Fain 1961a; Heymons 1935
Subtriquetra subtriquetra	South America	Spectacled caiman, other caimans	Mouth, pharynx	Uncommon	Apparently nonpathogenic	Fain 1961a; Heymons 1935
Subtriquetra shipleyi	India	Crocodiles	Pharynx	Uncommon	Apparently nonpathogenic	Fain 1961a; Heymons 1935
Subtriquetra megacephala	Africa	Crocodiles	Cephalic tissues	Uncommon	Apparently nonpathogenic	Fain 1961a
Leiperia gracilis	South America	Spectacled caiman, American crocodile	Lungs	Uncommon	Apparently nonpathogenic	Fain 1961a, 1966; Heymons 1935
Leiperia cincinnalis	Africa	Nile crocodile	Lungs, heart, aorta	Uncommon	Apparently nonpathogenic	Fain 1961; Heymons 1935
Waddycephalus teretiusculus	Asia, Australia	Rat snakes, other snakes	Lung	Uncommon	Apparently nonpathogenic	Fain 1961a, 1966; Heymons 1935

*Discussed in text.

REFERENCES

Arthur, D. R., and K. R. Snow. 1968. *Ixodes pacificus* Cooley and Kohls, 1943: Its life-history and occurrence. Parasitology 58: 893–906.

Baker, E. W., T. M. Evans, D. J. Gould, W. B. Hull, and H. L. Keegan. 1956. A manual of parasitic mites of medical or economic importance. Natl. Pest Control Assoc., New York. 170 pp.

Baldauf, R. J. 1961. Another case of parasitic copepods on amphibians. J. Parasitol. 47: 195.

Becklund, W. W. 1968. Ticks of veterinary significance found on imports in the United States. J. Parasitol. 54:622–28.

Bilsing, S. W., and R. B. Eads. 1947. An addition to the tick fauna of the United States. J. Parasitol. 33:85–86.

Bishopp, F. C., and Helen L. Trembley. 1945. Distribution and hosts of certain North American ticks. J. Parasitol. 31:1–54.

Bleakney, J. S. 1963. First North American record of *Bufolucilia silvarum* (Meigen) (Diptera: Calliphoridae) parasitizing *Bufo terrestris americanus* Holbrook. Can. Entomol. 95:107.

Camin, J. H. 1948. Mite transmission of a hemorrhagic septicemia in snakes. J. Parasitol. 34:345–54.

———. 1953. Observations on the life-history and sensory behavior of the snake mite, *Ophionyssus natricis* (Gervais). Chicago Acad. Sci. Spec. Publ. 10. 75 pp.

Camin, J. H., G. K. Clarke, L. H. Goodson, and H. R. Shuyler. 1964. Control of the snake mite, *Ophionyssus natricis* (Gervais), in captive reptile collections. Zoologica 49: 65–79.

Chandler, A. C., and C. P. Read. 1961. Introduction to parasitology. 10th ed. John Wiley, New York. 822 pp.

Cooley, R. A., and G. M. Kohls. 1944a. The genus *Amblyomma* (Ixodidae) in the United States. J. Parasitol. 30:77–111.

———. 1944b. The Argasidae of North America, Central America, and Cuba. Am. Midland Naturalist Monograph 1. 152 pp.

———. 1945. The genus *Ixodes* in North America. Natl. Inst. Health Bull. 184. U.S. Public Health Serv. 246 pp.

Cosgrove, G. E., B. Nelson, and N. Gengozian. 1968. Helminth parasites of the tamarin, *Saguinus fuscicollis*. Lab. Animal Care 18:654–56.

Dasgupta, B. 1962. On the myiasis of the Indian toad *Bufo melanostictus*. Parasitology 52: 63–66.

Degenhardt, W. G., and Paula B. Degenhardt. 1965. The host-parasite relationship between *Elaphe subocularis* (Reptilia: Colubridae) and *Aponomma elaphensis* (Acarina: Ixodidae). Southwestern Naturalist 10:167–78.

Dodge, H. R. 1955. Sarcophagid flies parasitic on reptiles (Diptera: Sarcophagidae). Proc. Entomol. Soc. Wash. D.C. 57:183–87.

Esslinger, J. H. 1962a. Development of *Porocephalus crotali* (Humboldt, 1808) (Pentastomida) in experimental intermediate hosts. J. Parasitol. 48:452–56.

———. 1962b. Hepatic lesions in rats experimentally infected with *Porocephalus crotali* (Pentastomida). J. Parasitol. 48:631–38.

Ewing, H. E. 1926. The common box-turtle, a natural host for chiggers. Proc. Biol. Soc., Wash. D.C. 39:19–20.

———. 1929. A manual of external parasites. Charles C Thomas, Springfield, Ill. 225 pp.

Fain, A. 1961a. Les pentastomidés de l'Afrique Centrale. Ann. Musee Roy. Afrique Centrale, Ser. 8, Sci. Zool. 92:1–115.

———. 1961b. Les acariens parasites endopulmonaires des serpents (Entonyssidae: Mesostigmata). Inst. Roy. Sci. Nat. Belg. Bull. 37:1–135.

———. 1962a. Les acariens parasites nasicoles des batriciens. Revision des Lawrencarinae Fain 1957 (Ereynetidae: Trombidiformes). Inst. Roy. Sci. Nat. Belg. Bull. 38:1–69.

———. 1962b. Les acariens mesostigmatiques ectoparasites des serpents. Inst. Roy. Sci. Nat. Belg. Bull. 38:1–149.

———. 1964a. Observations sur le cycle évolutif du genre *Raillietiella* (Pentastomida). Bull. Acad. Roy. Belg. 50:1036–60.

———. 1964b. Les Ophioptidae, acariens parasites des ecailles des serpents (Trombidiformes). Inst. Roy. Sci. Nat. Belg. Bull. 40:1–57.

———. 1966. Pentastomida of snakes—their parasitological role in man and animals. Mem. Inst. Butantan (São Paulo) 33:167–74.

———. 1968. Notes sur les acariens de la famille Cloacaridae Camin et al. Parasites du cloaque et des tissus profonds des tortues (Cheyletoidea: Trombidiformes). Inst. Roy. Sci. Natl. Belg. Bull. 44:1–33.

Fain, A., R. A. Baker, and R. C. Tinsley. 1969. Notes on a mite *Xenopacarus africanus* n.g., n.sp. parasitic in the nasal cavities of the African clawed frog *Xenopus laevis* (Ereynetidae: Trombidiformes). Rev. Zool. Bot. Afr. 80:340–45.

Fain, A., and J. Mortelmans. 1960. Observations sur le cycle évolutif de Sambonia lohrmanni chez le varan. Preuve d'un développement direct chez les Pentastomida. Bull. Acad. Roy. Sci. Belg. 46:518–31.

Faust, E. C., P. C. Beaver, and R. C. Jung. 1968. Animal agents and vectors of human disease. 3d ed. Lea and Febiger, Philadelphia. 461 pp.

Feider, Z. 1958. Sur une larve du genre *Trombicula* (Acari) parasite sur les lézards de la roumanie. Z. Parasitenk. 18:441–56.

Fonseca, F. da. 1939. Observacoes sobre o ciclo evolutivo de *Porocephalus clavatus*, especialmente sobre o seu orquidotropismo em cobaias. Mem. Inst. Butantan (São Paulo) 12:185–90.

Gebhardt, L. P., G. J. Stanton, and S. de St. Jeor. 1966. Transmission of WEE virus to snakes by infected *Culex tarsalis* mosquitoes. Proc. Soc. Expt. Biol. Med. 123:233–35.

Graham-Jones, O. 1961. IV. Some clinical conditions affecting the North African tortoise ("Greek" tortoise) *Testudo graeca*. Vet. Record 73:317–21.

Gunter, G. 1958. A sarcophagid fly larva parasitic in *Anolis carolinensis*. Copeia 1958 (4):336.

Heymons, R. 1935. Pentastomida, pp. 1–268. *In* H. G. Bronn's Klassen und Ordnungen des Tierreichs. Vol. 5, Sect. 4, Bk. 1. Akademische Verlagsgesellschaft, M.B.H., Leipzig.

Heywood, R. 1968. *Aeromonas* infection in snakes. Cornell Vet. 236–41.

Hoffman, G. L. 1967. Parasites of North American freshwater fishes. Univ. California Press, Berkeley. 486 pp.

Hoogstraal, H. 1956. African Ixodoidea: I. Ticks of the Sudan (with special reference to Equatoria Province and with preliminary reviews of the genera *Boophilus*, *Margaropus*, and *Hyalomma*). U. S. Navy Dept., Wash. D.C. Res. Rept. NM 005 050.29.07. 1101 pp.

———. 1966. Ticks in relation to human diseases caused by viruses, pp. 261–308. *In* R. F. Smith and T. E. Mittler, eds. Ann. Rev. Entomol. Annual Reviews, Palo Alto, Calif.

———. 1967. Ticks in relation to human diseases caused by Rickettsia species, pp. 377–420. *In* R. F. Smith and T. E. Mittler, eds. Ann. Rev. Entomol. Annual Reviews, Palo Alto, Calif.

Hughes, T. E. 1959. Mites or the Acari. Athlone Press, London. 225 pp.

Hyland, K. E., Jr. 1950. The life cycle and parasitic habit of the chigger mite *Hannemania dunni* Sambon, 1928, a parasite of amphibians. J. Parasitol. 36(Supp.):32–33.

———. 1956. A new species of chigger mite, *Hannemania hegeneri* (Acarina: Trombiculidae). J. Parasitol. 42:176–79.

———. 1961. Parasitic phase of the chigger mite, *Hannemania hegeneri*, on experimentally infested amphibians. Exp. Parasitol. 2:212–25.

Jackson, C. G., Jr., M. M. Jackson, and J. D. Davis. 1969. Cutaneous myiasis in the three-toed box turtle, *Terrapene carolina triunguis*. Bull. Wildlife Dis. Assoc. 5:114.

Kaplan, H. M. 1957. The care and diseases of laboratory turtles. Proc. Animal Care Panel 7:259–72.

Keegan, H. L. 1946. Six new mites of the superfamily Parasitoidea. Trans. Am. Microscop. Soc. 65:69–77.

King, W., and J. V. Griffo, Jr. 1958. A box turtle fatality apparently caused by *Sarcophaga cistudinis* larvae. Florida Entomologist 41:44.

Klauber, L. M. 1956. Rattlesnakes: Their habits, life histories, and influence on mankind. 2 vol. Univ. Calif. Press, Berkeley.

Knipling, E. F. 1937. The biology of *Sarcophaga cistudinis* Aldrich (Diptera), a species of Sarcophagidae parasitic on turtles and tortoises. Proc. Entomol. Soc. Wash. D.C. 39:91–101.

Lapage, G. 1962. Mönnig's veterinary helminthology and entomology. 5th ed. Williams and Wilkins, Baltimore. 600 pp.

———. 1968. Veterinary parasitology. 2d ed. Oliver and Boyd, Edinburgh and London. 1182 pp.

Lawrence, R. F. 1953. Two new scale-mite parasites of lizards. Proc. U.S. Natl. Museum 103:9–18.

Layne, J. N. 1967. Incidence of *Porocephalus crotali* (Pentastomida) in Florida mammals. Bull. Wildlife Dis. Assoc. 3:105–9.

Marcus, L. C. 1968. Diseases of snakes and turtles, pp. 435–42. *In* R. W. Kirk, ed. Current veterinary therapy III: Small animal practice. W. B. Saunders, Philadelphia.

Marzinowsky, E. 1927. Du développement de l'*Haemogregarina stepanovi*. Ann. Parasitol. Humaine Comparee 5:140–42.

Murphy, T. D. 1965. High incidence of two parasitic infestations and two morphological abnormalities in a population of the frog, *Rana pulustris* Le Conte. Am. Midland Naturalist 74:233–39.

Nelson, B., G. E. Cosgrove, and N. Gengozian. 1966. Diseases of an imported primate *Tamarinus nigricollis*. Lab. Animal Care 16:255–75.

O'Connor, Patricia. 1966. Diseases of snakes, pp. 582–84. *In* R. W. Kirk, ed. Current veterinary therapy 1966–1967: Small animal practice. W. B. Saunders, Philadelphia.

Page, L. A. 1966. Diseases and infections of snakes: A review. Bull. Wildlife Dis. Assoc. 2:111–26.

Pechuman, L. L., and W. W. Wirth. 1961. A new record of Ceratopogonidae (Diptera) feeding on frogs. J. Parasitol. 47:600.

Penn, G. H., Jr. 1942. The life history of *Porocephalus crotali,* a parasite of the Louisiana muskrat. J. Parasitol. 28:277–83.

Peters, J. A. 1948. The box turtle as a host for dipterous parasites. Am. Midland Naturalist 40:472–74.

Peterson, A. 1951. Larvae of insects: An introduction to nearctic species. II. Coleoptera, Diptera, Neuroptera, Siphonaptera, Mecoptera, Trichoptera. J. W. Edwards, Ann Arbor, Mich. 416 pp.

Philip, C. B., and W. Burgdorfer. 1961. Arthropod vectors as reservoirs of microbial disease agents, pp. 391–412. *In* E. A. Steinhaus and R. F. Smith, eds. Ann. Rev. Entomol. Annual Reviews, Palo Alto, Calif.

Pope, C. H. 1950. Snakes, pp. 309–23. *In* E. J. Farris, ed. The care and breeding of laboratory animals. John Wiley, New York.

Rainey, D. G. 1953. Death of an ornate box turtle parasitized by dipterous larvae. Herpetologica 9:109–110.

Rankin, J. S. 1937. An ecological study of parasites of some North Carolina salamanders. Ecol. Monographs 7:169–269.

Reichenbach-Klinke, H., and E. Elkan. 1965. The principal diseases of lower vertebrates. Academic Press, New York. 600 pp.

Robinson, L. E. 1926. The genus *Amblyomma:* Part IV. Ticks, a monograph of the Ixodoidea, pp. 1–285.

Sambon, L. W. 1928. The parasitic acarians of animals and the part they play in the causation of the eruptive fevers and other diseases of man: Preliminary considerations based upon an ecological study of typhus fever. Ann. Trop. Med. 22:67–132.

Sandner, H. 1955. *Lucilia bufonivora* Moniez, 1876 *(Diptera)* w Polsce. Acta Parasitol. Pol. 2:319–29.

Schroeder, C. R. 1934. The snake mite *(Ophionyssus serpentium,* Hirst.). J. Econ. Entomol. 27:1004–14.

Self, J. T., and G. E. Cosgrove. 1968. Pentastome larvae in laboratory primates. J. Parasitol. 54:969.

Self, J. T., and R. E. Kuntz. 1966. The Pentastomida: A review, pp. 620–21. *In* A. Corradetti, ed. Proc. First Intern. Congr. Parasitol. Pergamon Press, New York.

Self, J. T., and F. B. McMurry. 1948. *Poro-*

cephalus crotali Humboldt (Pentastomida) in Oklahoma. J. Parasitol. 34:21–23.

Stadler, H. 1930. Über den Befall einer Kröte *(Bufo vulgaris* Laur.) durch die Larven von *Lucilia sylvarum* Meig.; Krankheitsgeschiche und Sektionsbefund. Z. Parasitenk. 2:360–67.

Steward, J. W. 1969. Care and management of amphibians, reptiles, and fish in the laboratory: Amphibians and reptiles, pp. 285–309. *In* D. J. Short and Dorothy P. Woodnott, eds. The I.A.T. manual of laboratory animal practice and techniques. 2d ed. Charles C Thomas, Springfield, Ill.

Stone, A., C. W. Sabrosky, W. W. Wirth, R. H. Foote, and J. R. Coulson. 1965. A catalog of the Diptera of America north of Mexico. U.S. Dept. Agr. Handbook 276. 1696 pp.

Tarshis, I. B. 1960. Control of the snake mite *(Ophionyssus natricis),* other mites and certain insects with the sorptive dust, SG 67. J. Econ. Entomol. 53:903.

———. 1962. The use of silica aerogel compounds for the control of ectoparasites. Proc. Animal Care Panel 12:217–54.

Tidd, W. M., and R. J. Shields. 1963. Tissue damage inflicted by *Lernaea cyprinacea* Linnaeus, a copepod parasitic on tadpoles. J. Parasitol. 49:693–96.

Till, W. M. 1957. Mesostigmatic mites living as parasites of reptiles in the Ethiopian region (Acarina: Laelaptidae). J. Entomol. Soc. S. Afr. 20:120–43.

Turk, F. A. 1947. Studies of Acari: IV. A review of the lung mite of snakes. Parasitology 38:17–26.

U.S. Department of Agriculture. 1965. Manual on livestock ticks. U.S. Dept. Agr. ARS 91–49. 142 pp.

Walton, A. C. 1964. The parasites of Amphibia. Wildlife Disease 40. (Microcard and microfiche).

———. 1966. Supplemental catalog of the parasites of Amphibia. Wildlife Disease 48. 58 pp. (Microfiche).

———. 1967. Supplemental catalog of the parasites of Amphibia. Wildlife Disease 50. 38 pp. (Microfiche).

Wells, H. W. 1966. Barnacles of the northeastern Gulf of Mexico. Quart. J. Fla. Acad. Sci. 28:81–95.

Worms, M. J. 1967. Parasites in newly imported animals. J. Inst. Animal Tech. 18: 39–47.

Yunker, C. E. 1956. Studies on the snake mite, *Ophionyssus natricis,* in nature. Science 124:979–80.

Zumpt, F. 1965. Myiasis in man and animals in the Old World: A textbook for physicians, veterinarians and zoologists. Butterworth, London. 267pp.

Parasites of Laboratory Fishes

Chapter 21

PROTOZOANS

MANY protozoans occur in and on fishes. Their significance as pathogens in nature is not well known, but several are important in fishes in captivity (Hoffman 1967a). Of those which attach externally, some affect the fish by feeding on cells and mucus while others cause hypersecretion of mucus or injury by covering the gill epithelium and interfering with respiration. Little is known of the pathogenicity of those which occur internally. In small numbers, they probably cause little harm, but in heavy infections, resulting from crowding, malnutrition, or sudden changes in temperature or other environmental factors, they often cause extensive damage (Lom 1969).

FLAGELLATES

The flagellates that affect laboratory fishes are listed in Table 21.1. Several occur in the blood or on the skin or gills of fishes used in the laboratory, but only one genus occurs in the intestine (Hoffman 1967a). *Cryptobia*, the commonest hemoflagellate; *Costia* and *Oodinium,* the commonest ectoparasitic flagellates; and *Hexamita,* the sole enteric flagellate, are described below.

Cryptobia

(Syn. *Trypanoplasma*)

Many species of this pathogenic flagellate have been described from fishes some-times used in the laboratory (Table 21.1) (Hoffman 1967a). *Cryptobia salmositica* is the commonest species in North America; it occurs in the blood of the rainbow trout, brown trout, Pacific salmons, sticklebacks, and other fishes in northwestern United States and southwestern Canada (Becker and Katz 1965). *Cryptobia cyprini* and *C. borreli* are the species most likely to be encountered in Europe; they occur in the blood of the goldfish, carp, European minnow, and other fishes (van Duijn 1967; Kraneveld and Keidel 1969; Wenyon 1926). *Cryptobia* is likely to be encountered only in laboratory fishes obtained from their natural habitat or from hatcheries infested with leeches (van Duijn 1967; Wales and Wolf 1955).

MORPHOLOGY

This protozoan is trypanosomelike except that it has two flagella, one that forms the outer margin of an undulating membrane and one that is free (Fig. 21.1) (Hoffman 1967a). The body is 10 to 30 μ long, curved and blunt at the anterior end, and pointed posteriorly (Kudo 1966; Olsen 1967).

LIFE CYCLE

The life cycle of species affecting fishes requires a leech as an intermediate host (Hoffman 1967a; Olsen 1967). Flagellates ingested by a feeding leech develop and

645

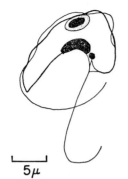

FIG. 21.1. *Cryptobia salmositica* trophozoite. (From Hoffman 1967a. Courtesy of University of California Press.)

---

multiply in the leech and infect another fish the next time the leech feeds. Multiplication in the fish is by binary fission.

PATHOLOGIC EFFECTS

Infection is sometimes inapparent (Kraneveld and Keidel 1969). Signs reported in heavily infected fish include lethargy; anorexia; weight loss; enophthalmos or exophthalmos; reduced blood-clotting time; anemia; pale skin and gills; excess mucus on the skin; white, translucent, gelatinous exudate on the gills; protrusion of the scales; a distended abdomen; darkened external appearance; lateral recumbency; and death (van Duijn 1967; Wales and Wolf 1955). Internal lesions include ascites and a slight paleness of the liver. The causative organisms are seen on microscopic examination of the blood and ascitic fluid and in sections of the muscle and kidneys.

DIAGNOSIS

Diagnosis is based on the clinical signs and on identification of the organism in the blood, ascitic fluid, or tissue sections (van Duijn 1967; Wales and Wolf 1955).

CONTROL

Because of the need for a leech intermediate host, the life cycle is not likely to be completed in the laboratory, and no special control procedures are needed (van Duijn 1967). There is no treatment.

PUBLIC HEALTH CONSIDERATIONS

This flagellate does not affect man.

Costia necatrix, Costia pyriformis

These ectoparasitic flagellates occur on many species of fishes sometimes used in the laboratory (Davis 1953; Hoffman 1967a; Tavolga and Nigrelli 1947). *Costia necatrix* is the commonest species; it is found on the skin and gills of the guppy, platyfish, swordtail, tropical mouthbreeders, other aquarium fishes, salmonids, and other fishes in North America, Europe, and Asia. *Costia pyriformis* (possibly a synonym of *C. necatrix*) occurs on the skin and gills of the rainbow trout, brook trout, and other fishes in the United States. Aquarium and hatchery fishes are frequently parasitized, and laboratory fishes obtained from such sources are likely to be infected.

MORPHOLOGY

These flagellates have two long and two short flagella (Fig. 21.2) (Hoffman 1967a; Tavolga and Nigrelli 1947). The long flagella are about 18 μ long and easily seen; the short flagella are about 9 μ long and difficult to see. The body varies in size from 5 to 18 μ in length and 2.5 to 7.7 μ in width. It also varies in shape; attached forms are pyriform while free-swimming

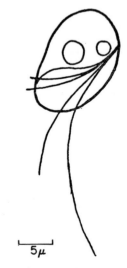

FIG. 21.2. *Costia necatrix* trophozoite. (From Hoffman 1967a. Courtesy of University of California Press.)

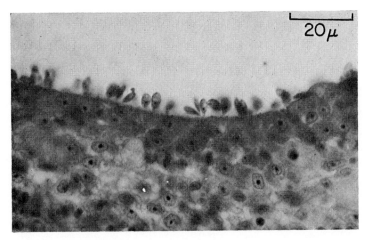

Fig. 21.3. *Costia necatrix* trophozoites attached to skin of channel catfish. (From Davis 1947a. Courtesy of Bureau of Sport Fisheries and Wildlife, U.S. Department of the Interior.)

forms are ovoid, flattened, and concave ventrally.

LIFE CYCLE

The life cycle is direct (Tavolga and Nigrelli 1947). Individual parasites readily leave a host and swim about. When ready to attach to a new host they make contact and fasten to the skin by means of a flat, posterior disc (Fig. 21.3) (Schubert 1968). Reproduction is by binary fission. It occurs on the host, or off the host in accumulations of sloughed scales and debris.

PATHOLOGIC EFFECTS

The parasites attach to the epidermis, insert fingerlike processes, and ingest portions of the epidermal cells (Lom 1969; Schubert 1968). In light infections, they occur on the cells between overlapping scales (Davis 1953; Tavolga and Nigrelli 1947). In heavy infections, they attach to the external surface of the scales, especially near the base of the tail and fins, and sometimes to the gills. Affected fish appear coated with a gray mucus. If untreated, they cease eating, become debilitated, and die.

DIAGNOSIS

Because the signs are nonspecific, microscopic identification of the parasites in scrapings of the skin or gills is essential for diagnosis (Davis 1953; Tavolga and Nigrelli 1947; Walliker 1966).

CONTROL

These parasites have a free-swimming form, therefore it is important that both infected fish and their holding tanks be treated at the same time. Effective treatments include formalin, 200 to 250 ppm for 1 hour; pyridylmercuric acetate, 2 ppm for 1 hour (toxic for some trouts); potassium permanganate, 1,000 ppm for 30 to 40 seconds; and acetic acid, 2,000 ppm for 1 to 2 minutes (Hoffman 1970; Snieszko and Hoffman 1963).

PUBLIC HEALTH CONSIDERATIONS

These flagellates do not affect man.

Oodinium

This dinoflagellate, a common ectoparasite of marine fishes, frequently causes a high mortality in freshwater aquarium fishes (van Duijn 1967; Hoffman 1967a; Jacobs 1946; Reichenbach-Klinke and Elkan 1965). *Oodinium limneticum* has been reported from the skin and gills of the Siamese fighting fish, guppy, mollies, platyfish, swordtail, and other aquarium fishes in the United States (Jacobs 1946). *Oodinium pillularis* has been reported from the skin and gills of the goldfish, Siamese fighting fish, tetras, guppy, swordtail, other aquarium fishes, carp, and brown trout in Europe (van Duijn 1967; Reichenbach-Klinke and Elkan 1965; Walliker 1966). Although this parasite is frequently reported on aquarium fishes, its incidence in laboratory fishes is unknown; it is probably uncommon.

MORPHOLOGY

The parasitic stage is spherical or piriform, measures 12 to 150 μ at the greatest diameter, and has a short stalk, yellow-

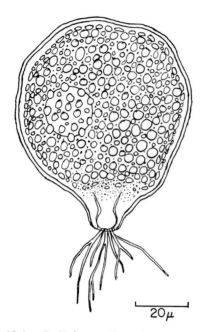

FIG. 21.4. *Oodinium limneticum,* parasitic stage. (From Jacobs 1946. Courtesy of American Microscopical Society.)

green chromoplasts, and pseudopodia, but no flagella (Fig. 21.4) (Hoffman 1967a; Jacobs 1946). The free-swimming stage, or gymnodinium, is oval to round, measures 10 to 19 μ in diameter, and has one posterior and one transverse flagellum, but no pseudopodia.

LIFE CYCLE

The mature parasitic stage drops off the fish and becomes a spherical cyst (Jacobs 1946). It divides by binary fission for 3 to 4 days to produce 64 to 256 free-swimming gymnodinia. When a gymnodinium contacts a suitable host it attaches, changes to the parasitic form, and matures in about a week. Gymnodinia, which do not reach a host in 12 to 48 hours, encyst. Their subsequent development and ultimate fate are unknown.

PATHOLOGIC EFFECTS

Affected fish appear covered with a dull, yellow-brown coating (van Duijn 1967; Jacobs 1946; Reichenbach-Klinke and Elkan 1965). The parasite apparently feeds by withdrawing organic material from the cells of the host through its pseudopodia. Mortality is highest in young fish, and death is probably the result of the direct effects of the feeding parasite. In older and large fish, light infection causes no apparent discomfort or loss of vigor, but heavy infection involving the gills causes impaired respiration, debility, and death.

DIAGNOSIS

Diagnosis is based on the signs and confirmed by microscopic identification of the parasite in scrapings of the skin or gills (van Duijn 1967).

CONTROL

Because the incidence of the parasite in the laboratory is unknown, specific routine prophylactic treatment is probably not indicated. Effective therapeutic treatments include methylene blue, 2.6 ppm (Jacobs 1946); copper sulfate, 2 ppm (Dempster 1955; Reichenbach-Klinke and Elkan 1965); and acriflavine, 10 ppm (Patterson 1950), in the water for about 3 days.

PUBLIC HEALTH CONSIDERATIONS

Oodinium does not affect man.

Hexamita

This is the only intestinal flagellate of fishes (Hoffman 1967a). *Hexamita salmonis* has been encountered in the goldfish and is common in salmonids and other fishes in North America (Davis 1926b, 1953; Hoffman 1967a), and *H. intestinalis* (a possible synonym of *H. salmonis*) has been reported from the goldfish and other aquarium fishes and is common in salmonids in Europe (Bykhovskaya-Pavlovskaya et al. 1962; van Duijn 1967; Hoffman 1967a; Reichenbach-Klinke and Elkan 1965). This flagellate is generally considered to be a pathogen (Davis 1926b, 1947a, 1953; McElwain and Post 1968; Yasutake, Buhler, and Shanks 1961), but it is not certain if the large numbers recovered from diseased fish are the cause or the result of the illness (Uzmann and Jesse 1963). The incidence in laboratory fishes is unknown; it is probably common in laboratory salmonids.

MORPHOLOGY

Trophozoites are piriform and have two nuclei near the anterior end, two axo-

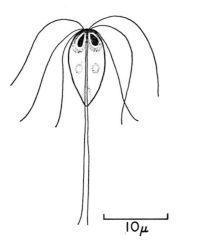

Fig. 21.5. *Hexamita salmonis* trophozoite. (From Hoffman 1967a. Courtesy of University of California Press.)

styles, and six anterior and two posterior flagella (Fig. 21.5) (Hoffman 1967a). *Hexamita salmonis* is 10 to 12 μ long by 6 to 8 μ wide; *H. intestinalis* is 10 to 16 μ long and 6 to 7 μ wide (Davis 1926b; van Duijn 1967; Kudo 1966).

LIFE CYCLE

Reproduction is by binary fission (Davis 1926b, 1947a, 1953). Cysts, which can live for a long time outside the host, are formed and excreted in the feces. A fish is infected by ingesting a cyst or, possibly, a trophozoite.

PATHOLOGIC EFFECTS

The pathologic effects of *Hexamita* are uncertain. It is generally thought to cause either an acute disease, characterized by a catarrhal enteritis and death, or a chronic disease, characterized by anorexia, listlessness, emaciation, decreased growth rate, and increased mortality (Davis 1926b, 1947a, 1953; van Duijn 1967; Reichenbach-Klinke and Elkan 1965). It is also thought that heavy infections interfere with the usefulness of infected fish for research, especially for nutritional studies (Yasutake, Buhler, and Shanks 1961). However, although mortality often decreases and growth improves after infected fish are treated (McElwain and Post 1968), this is possibly because the drug used is effective

against a concurrent infection with some other unrecognized agent (Uzmann and Jesse 1963). In a series of controlled studies using naturally infected Pacific salmon and rainbow trout, untreated fishes gained more weight and converted food better than treated controls (Uzmann and Jesse 1963).

DIAGNOSIS

Diagnosis is made by microscopic examination of intestinal contents; however, the presence of the flagellate in debilitated fishes is not conclusive evidence that the parasite is the cause of the illness (Davis 1947a).

CONTROL

Because of the widespread distribution of this flagellate, especially in salmonid fishes, attempts to eliminate the infection from laboratory fishes by sanitation and restocking are impractical, and control is based on treatment (Davis 1947a, 1953). Effective treatments include 2-acetamido-5-nitrothiazole (Enheptin-A, American Cyanamid Co.), given in the food at a rate of 20 ppm for 3 days (McElwain and Post 1968); and 2-amino-5-nitrothiazole (Enheptin, American Cyanamid Co.), p-carbamido-benzene arsonic acid (Carbarsone, Eli Lilly and Co.), or p-carbamidophenyl arsenoxide (Carbarsone oxide, Eli Lilly and Co.), given in the food at a rate of 2,000 ppm for 5 to 7 days (Davis 1953; Yasutake, Buhler, and Shanks 1961).

PUBLIC HEALTH CONSIDERATIONS

Hexamita salmonis and *H. intestinalis* are not known to affect man.

SARCODINES

Only one sarcodine, *Schizamoeba salmonis*, has been identified from freshwater fishes sometimes used in the laboratory (Table 21.2), and it is apparently nonpathogenic (Davis 1926a, 1947a; Hoffman 1967a).

SPOROZOANS

These protozoans lack flagella, cilia, and typical pseudopodia and are characterized by spore formation (Hoffman 1967a). All are parasitic and many affect fishes. Several species have been associated with increased mortality in fishes in captivity, but the specific pathology they cause is often unknown. Most sporozoans affecting fishes belong to the order Myxosporida. These undergo considerable development and multiplication in the host's tissues and frequently form visible cysts containing huge masses of spores. Damage to the fish from such cysts ranges from negligible to fatal.

Sporozoans likely to be encountered in laboratory fishes are listed in Table 21.3. The most important are described below.

Eimeria

Several species of this genus occur in laboratory fishes (Table 21.3) (van Duijn 1967; Hoffman 1965, 1967a; Marinček 1965; Wenyon 1926). *Eimeria aurati* occurs in the goldfish (Hoffman 1965) and *Eimeria* sp. in the brook trout and other fishes (Davis 1947a) in eastern United States; both are uncommon and, although *E. aurati* is thought to cause enteritis, their specific pathogenicity is uncertain. *Eimeria carpelli* and *E. subepithelialis* are the commonest species in Europe (Marinček 1965; Reichenbach-Klinke and Elkan 1965; Wenyon 1926); both affect carp, causing a mild enteritis and sometimes debility and death.

MORPHOLOGY

Eimeria is characterized by an oocyst that produces four sporocysts, each with two sporozoites (Kudo 1966). Oocysts of *E. aurati* (Fig. 21.6) measure 16 to 24 μ by 14 to 17 μ (Hoffman 1965). Those of *E. carpelli* are 6 to 12 μ in diameter (Marinček 1965), and those of *E. subepithelialis* are 18 to 21 μ in diameter (Reichenbach-Klinke and Elkan 1965).

LIFE CYCLE

The life cycle is direct (Kudo 1966; Levine 1961). Unsporulated oocysts passed in the feces sporulate in 2 to 5 days (Hoffman 1965). Infection is by ingestion of a sporulated oocyst. Schizogony and gametogony occur in the same host.

PATHOLOGIC EFFECTS

The pathologic effects of most species of *Eimeria* that affect laboratory fishes are unknown. *Eimeria aurati* has been associated with enteritis and lethargy in the goldfish, but a causal relationship has not been established (Hoffman 1965). *Eimeria carpelli* and *E. subepithelialis* cause a mild enteritis in the carp (Marinček 1965; Rei-

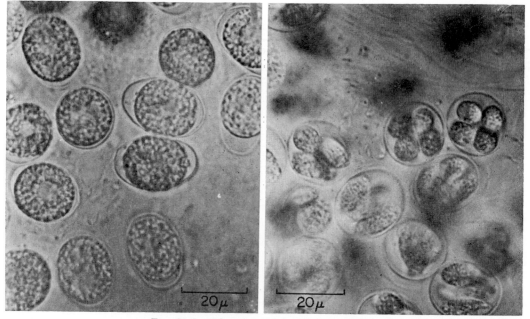

FIG. 21.6. *Eimeria aurati.* *(Left)* Freshly voided, nonsporulated oocysts. *(Right)* Sporulated oocysts. (From Hoffman 1965. Courtesy of Society of Protozoologists.)

chenbach-Klinke and Elkan 1965). Infection is usually mild and only heavy infections cause debility and death.

DIAGNOSIS

Diagnosis is based on recognition of lesions and identification of the oocyst in feces or intestinal contents.

CONTROL

Control is based on sanitation and elimination of infected fish. Furazolidone in the food (dose not given) has been used for treatment (Musselius and Strelkov 1968).

PUBLIC HEALTH CONSIDERATIONS

None of the species of *Eimeria* that occur in fishes is known to affect man.

Myxosoma

Several species of *Myxosoma* occur in laboratory fishes (Table 21.3) (van Duijn 1967; Hoffman 1967a; Hoffman, Putz, and Dunbar 1965). *Myxosoma cerebralis* is common in North America, Europe, and Asia. It localizes in the cartilage of the head and spine of brook trout, rainbow trout, brown trout, and other salmonids, causing destruction of the parasitized parts, deformation, and impaired movement ("whirling disease"). *Myxosoma cartilaginis,* which is common in eastern United States, localizes in the cartilaginous parts of the head of the bluegill, sunfishes, and black bass but does not cause deformation or impaired movement. *Myxosoma dujardini* is common in carp and other fishes in Europe and Asia; it localizes in the gills and causes cysts, dyspnea, and death. Other species of *Myxosoma* are less common and most cause cysts in the tissues they affect. The incidence of *Myxosoma* in laboratory fishes is unknown; it is probably uncommon.

MORPHOLOGY

Spores are ovoid in front view, lenticular in profile, and have two piriform polar capsules at the anterior end (Fig. 21.7) (Hoffman, Putz, and Dunbar 1965; Kudo 1966). They measure about 6 to 13 μ in diameter and 5 to 7 μ in thickness.

LIFE CYCLE

The life cycle is not completely known but is presumed to be direct (Bogdanova

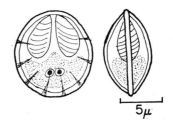

FIG. 21.7. *Myxosoma* spore. *(Left)* Front view. *(Right)* Side view. (From Hoffman, Putz, and Dunbar 1965. Courtesy of Society of Protozoologists.)

1968; Elson 1969; Hoffman, Putz, and Dunbar 1965). Infection is apparently by ingestion of a spore released from disintegrated infected tissue; the spore of *M. cerebralis* must age for 4 months before it is infective. The sporoplasm, which is released from the spore in the intestine, migrates to the tissue for which it has specificity, develops into a multinucleate trophozoite, and produces pansporoblasts and spores. Infection usually occurs during the first year of life; species which affect cartilage infect the host in the first few weeks of life, prior to bone formation.

PATHOLOGIC EFFECTS

Various stages of the organism are found in the skin, cartilage, eyes, and other body tissue, depending on the species involved. Typically, *Myxosoma* causes cyst formation; it also occurs free in the tissue and necrosis is seen in heavy infection (Elson 1969; Hoffman, Putz, and Dunbar 1965; Lom 1969; Roberts and Elson 1970). Clinical signs depend on the location of the organism. *Myxosoma cerebralis* causes destruction of the cartilaginous parts of the head and vertebral column, resulting in skeletal deformation (Fig. 21.8). Damage to the nerves that control the melanophores of the posterior part of the body causes a blackening of the tail, and damage to the auditory organ combined with the skeletal deformities causes the affected fish to swim in circles. *Myxosoma cartilaginis* causes the formation of 0.4 to 1.5 mm cysts in the cartilaginous parts of the head (Fig. 21.9) of affected fishes but does not produce whirling, darkening of the body, or other signs. *Myxosoma dujardini* causes the for-

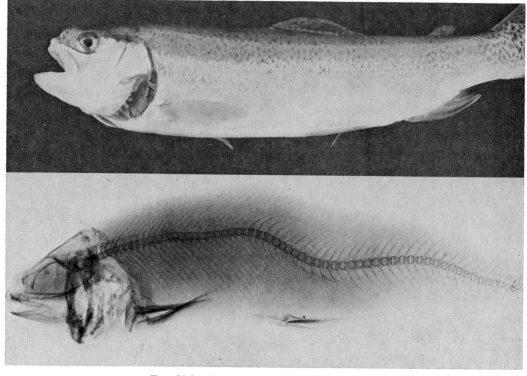

FIG. 21.8. *Myxosoma cerebralis* infection (whirling disease). *(Top)* Two-year-old rainbow trout; note misshapen head. *(Bottom)* Radiograph of yearling rainbow trout; note spinal curvature and "sunken" head. (Courtesy of G. L. Hoffman, Eastern Fish Disease Laboratory.)

mation of irregular, yellow-to-white, 1.0 to 1.5 mm cysts in the gills of affected fishes. Signs of infection with this species are dyspnea and death.

DIAGNOSIS

Diagnosis is based on the signs, if present, recognition of the lesions, and identification of the spores (Hoffman, Putz, and Dunbar 1965).

CONTROL

No effective treatment is known, and control is based on sanitation and elimination of affected fish (van Duijn 1967; Hoffman, Dunbar, and Bradford 1962; Snieszko and Hoffman 1963). Agents presumed to be effective against *Myxosoma* spores include benzalkonium chloride, 200 to 800 ppm for 24 hours; calcium hydroxide, 0.5 to 2.0% for 24 hours; chlorine, 1,600 ppm

for 24 hours; and hot water, 60 to 100 C for 10 minutes (Hoffman and Putz 1969).

PUBLIC HEALTH CONSIDERATIONS

Myxosoma does not affect man.

Myxobolus, Henneguya, Unicauda, Hoferellus

Many species of these closely related myxosporidan genera affect laboratory fishes and produce cysts in the tissues for which each has an affinity (Table 21.3) (van Duijn 1967; Hoffman 1967a; Reichenbach-Klinke and Elkan 1965). Most are uncommon.

MORPHOLOGY

Spores are subspherical, ovoid, ellipsoid, or pyriform in front view and flattened in side view (Hoffman 1967a; Kudo 1966). Those of *Myxobolus* (Fig. 21.10*A*) are

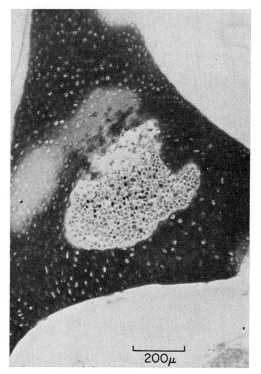

FIG. 21.9. *Myxosoma cartilaginis* infection in cartilage of bluegill. (Courtesy of **G. L. Hoff-man, Eastern Fish Disease Laboratory.**)

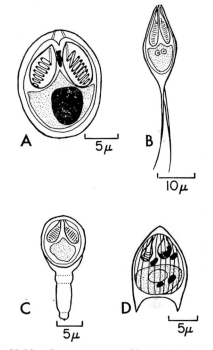

FIG. 21.10. Some myxosporidans of laboratory fishes (spores). *(A) Myxobolus. (B) Henneguya. (C) Unicauda. (D) Hoferellus.* (From Hoffman 1967a. Courtesy of University of California Press.)

about 8 to 13 μ in diameter and have two anterior polar capsules and a sporoplasm containing an iodinophilous vacuole. Spores of *Henneguya* (Fig. 21.10B) are similar but differ in that the posterior end of each shell valve is prolonged into a long process. Those of *Unicauda* (Fig. 21.10C) are also similar except that they have a single posterior appendage which is not an extension of the shell valves. *Hoferellus* spores (Fig. 21.10D) are pyramidal, measure about 10 to 12 μ in diameter, and have 9 to 10 longitudinal striae on each shell valve and two posterior spinous processes.

LIFE CYCLE

The life cycle is similar to that of *Myxosoma* (Kudo 1966).

PATHOLOGIC EFFECTS

These sporozoans produce cysts of varying size in the tissues for which each has a specific affinity (Table 21.3) (Hoffman 1967a; Kudo 1920). Those most frequently

recognized in fishes used in the laboratory are the cysts which occur in the skin and gills (Figs. 21.11, 21.12).

DIAGNOSIS

Diagnosis is based on identification of spores in typical cysts. Care must be taken to differentiate cutaneous cysts produced by these organisms from the granulomatous lesions caused by *Ichthyophthirius multifiliis* (van Duijn 1967).

CONTROL

No effective treatment is known, and control is based on sanitation and elimination of affected fish (van Duijn 1967; Snieszko and Hoffman 1963).

PUBLIC HEALTH CONSIDERATIONS

These sporozoans do not affect man.

Pleistophora, Glugea

Some species of these microsporidan genera occasionally affect fishes used in the

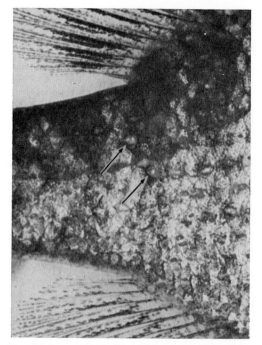

FIG. 21.11. *Myxobolus* infection in a bluegill. Note dermal cysts. (Courtesy of G. L. Hoffman, Eastern Fish Disease Laboratory.)

laboratory (Hoffman 1967a; Putz, Hoffman, and Dunbar 1965). The most important are *Pleistophora hyphessobryconis,* which causes muscular necrosis, emaciation, and death (neon tetra disease) in tetras, swordtails, and other fishes in Europe (van Duijn 1967); *P. salmonae,* which causes gill cysts and increased mortality in rainbow trout, Pacific salmons, and other salmonids in western United States (Putz, Hoffman, and Dunbar 1965; Wales and Wolf 1955); and *Glugea anomala,* which causes subcutaneous cysts in sticklebacks in Alaska and Europe (van Duijn 1967; Putz, Hoffman, and Dunbar 1965; Reichenbach-Klinke and Elkan 1965).

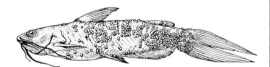

FIG. 21.12. *Henneguya exilis* infection in a channel catfish. Note dermal cysts. (From Kudo 1966. Courtesy of Charles C Thomas, Publisher.)

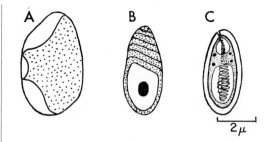

FIG. 21.13. Some microsporidans of laboratory fishes (spores). *(A) Pleistophora hyphessobryconis. (B) P. salmonae. (C) Glugea anomala.* (From Putz, Hoffman, and Dunbar 1965. Courtesy of Society of Protozoologists.)

The incidence in laboratory fishes is unknown.

MORPHOLOGY

The morphology of the vegetative forms varies widely, depending on the stage of the life cycle (Kudo 1966; Putz, Hoffman, and Dunbar 1965). Spores are small, usually 3 to 6 μ long, and simple in appearance (Fig. 21.13) (Hoffman 1967a). Each has a single, but not readily apparent, polar filament.

LIFE CYCLE

The life cycle involves both asexual division and sporogony within the host cell (Hoffman 1967a; Wenyon 1926). Each *Pleistophora* sporont (pansporoblast) develops into 16 or more spores while each *Glugea* sporont develops into only 2 spores. The method of transmission is unknown, but it is presumed to be by ingestion of spores carried in water (Reichenbach-Klinke and Elkan 1965).

PATHOLOGIC EFFECTS

Pleistophora hyphessobryconis primarily affects the subcutaneous muscles in which it produces widespread necrosis and parasite-filled cysts (Fig. 21.14) (van Duijn 1967; Reichenbach-Klinke and Elkan 1965). The muscles become pale and transparent and cause the external surface of the fish to appear spotted and patchy. Emaciation and death are common. *Pleistophora salmonae* affects the gill filaments (Putz, Hoffman, and Dunbar 1965; Wales and Wolf 1955). Various stages occur throughout the

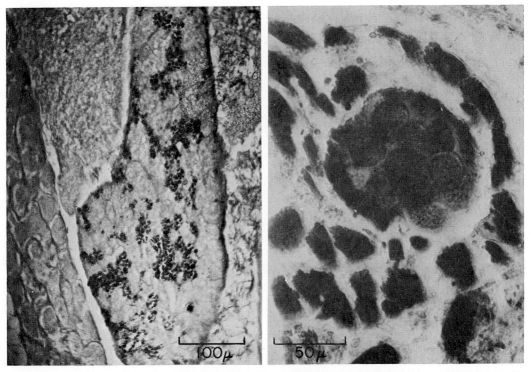

FIG. 21.14. *Pleistophora hyphessobryconis* infection (neon tetra disease) in fish muscle. *(Left)* Numerous pansporoblasts in necrotic muscle tissue. *(Right)* Cyst containing pansporoblasts. *(Left* courtesy of C. van Duijn, Zeist, Netherlands. *Right* from Reichenbach-Klinke and Elkan 1965; courtesy of Academic Press.)

gill tissue, and cysts varying in size up to 180 μ in diameter and containing numerous mature spores are sometimes seen (Fig. 21.15). Heavy infections cause anemia, inflammation, and moderate to extensive epithelial proliferation of the gill lamellae, and rapid death without pronounced weight loss. *Glugea anomala* affects both visceral and subcutaneous connective tissue, resulting in hypertrophy of infected cells and the development of thick-walled cysts up to 4 mm in diameter (Fig. 21.16) (van Duijn 1967; Reichenbach-Klinke and Elkan 1965; Sindermann 1966). Heavy infections cause extensive body deformation and a high mortality.

DIAGNOSIS

Because the lesions produced by these microsporidans are similar to those produced by other agents, a definitive diagnosis requires the identification of the caus-

ative agent in histologic sections or smears of cyst contents (van Duijn 1967; Wales and Wolf 1955).

CONTROL

There is no known treatment (van Duijn 1967; Snieszko and Hoffman 1963). Control is based on sanitation and elimination of affected fish.

PUBLIC HEALTH CONSIDERATIONS

These microsporidans are not known to affect man.

Dermocystidium

Parasites of this genus have some characteristics of a fungus and some of a sporozoan (Davis 1947b; Hoffman 1967a; Reichenbach-Klinke and Elkan 1965). *Dermocystidium salmonis* occurs in the gills of the chinook salmon in western United States (Davis 1947b) and *D. branchialis* in the

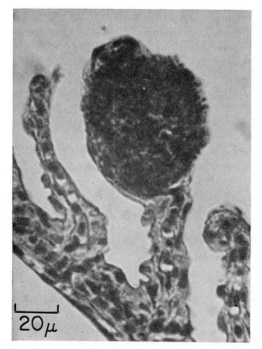

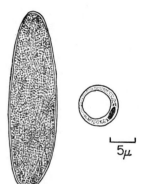

FIG. 21.17. *Dermocystidium.* *(Left)* Cyst. *(Right)* Spore. (From Hoffman 1967a. Courtesy of University of California Press.)

FIG. 21.15. *Pleistophora salmonae* infection in a salmonid. Note cyst in gill filament. (Courtesy of G. L. Hoffman, Eastern Fish Disease Laboratory.)

gills of the brown trout in Europe (van Duijn 1967; Reichenbach-Klinke and Elkan 1965). *Dermocystidium gasterostei* occurs in the skin of sticklebacks in Europe (Elkan 1962), *D. koi* in the skin and muscle of the carp in Japan, and an unnamed species in the skin of the goldfish, bluegill, and

brook trout in the United States (Hoffman 1967a). None is common; they are important only because they produce cysts in the affected tissues.

MORPHOLOGY

The immature stage appears as a cyst consisting of a hyaline wall of varying thickness, filled with an amorphous protoplasmic mass (Fig. 21.17) (Hoffman 1967a). Spores are round, 3 to 12 μ in diameter, and contain a nucleus and a conspicuous, large, eccentric vacuole.

LIFE CYCLE

The complete life cycle is unknown (Davis 1947b; Hoffman 1967a; Reichenbach-Klinke and Elkan 1965). Chromatin granules in the immature stage coalesce to

FIG. 21.16. *Glugea anomala* infection in a stickleback. Note subcutaneous cysts. (From Reichenbach-Klinke and Elkan 1965. Courtesy of Academic Press.)

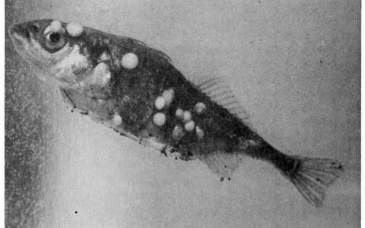

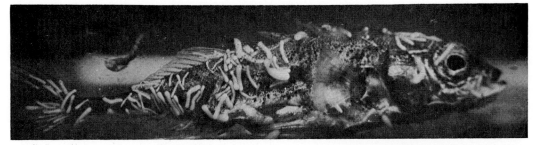

FIG. 21.18. *Dermocystidium gasterostei* infection in a stickleback. Note dermal cysts. (From Elkan 1962. Courtesy of Macmillan Journals, Ltd.)

form nuclei, and the protoplasmic mass reforms into spores. The method of transmission is unknown.

PATHOLOGIC EFFECTS

Dermocystidium salmonis and *D. branchialis* cause the formation of small, rounded cysts in the gill filaments, *D. koi* causes similar cysts in skin and muscle, and the unnamed species found in eastern United States causes similar cysts in the skin (Davis 1947b; van Duijn 1967; Hoffman 1967a; Reichenbach-Klinke and Elkan 1965). In contrast, *D. gasterostei* produces wormlike, cylindrical dermal cysts that are 2 to 3 mm long and about 0.2 to 0.3 mm wide (Fig. 21.18) (Elkan 1962). None of these species, including *D. gasterostei,* appears to have any significant pathologic effects on affected fish.

DIAGNOSIS

Diagnosis is based on the appearance of the cysts and identification of the causative agent in tissue sections.

CONTROL

Nothing is known of control (Snieszko and Hoffman 1963).

PUBLIC HEALTH CONSIDERATIONS

Dermocystidium is not known to affect man.

CILIATES

The ciliates likely to be encountered in laboratory fishes are listed in Table 21.4. All are ectoparasites and many are serious pathogens (Davis 1947a, b; van Duijn 1967; Hoffman 1967a; Reichenbach-Klinke and Elkan 1965). The most important are discussed below.

Ichthyophthirius multifiliis

This ciliate, the cause of ichthyophthiriasis ("ich") or white spot disease, affects the skin and gills of all freshwater fishes throughout the world (Bauer 1958; van Duijn 1967; Hoffman 1967a; Reichenbach-Klinke and Elkan 1965). Although uncommon in fishes in their natural habitat, it is the commonest ectoparasite of captive fishes. It is a serious pathogen and often causes extensive skin damage and death. Laboratory fishes obtained from hatcheries or aquariums are likely to be infected (Anthony 1969). The parasite can also be introduced into a laboratory colony with water plants or live food (van Duijn 1967; Reichenbach-Klinke and Elkan 1965).

MORPHOLOGY

Ichthyophthirius multifiliis is the largest parasitic protozoan affecting fishes (Hoffman and Sindermann 1962). Trophozoites are oval to round, 50 μ to 1 mm in length, and uniformly ciliated with a characteristic crescent-shaped macronucleus (Fig. 21.19) (Davis 1947a; Hoffman 1967a). The cytostome, which is at or near the anterior end, is not readily visible in large individuals. Young forms, called tomites, are oval, 30 to 45 μ long and uniformly ciliated, and have an anterior knob or perforatorium.

LIFE CYCLE

A mature trophozoite leaves the fish, swims feebly about for a short time, and comes to rest on a plant or other object in the water or on the bottom of the tank

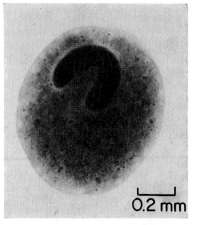

FIG. 21.19. *Ichthyophthirius multifiliis* trophozoite. (Courtesy of Bureau of Sport Fisheries
and Wildlife, U.S. Department of the Interior.)

(Davis 1947a; Wenyon 1926). It encloses
itself in a gelatinous sheath or cyst and
multiplies by simple transverse division until the cyst contains hundreds or thousands
of tomites (Fig. 21.20). The cyst wall breaks
and the tomites leave, attach to a fish, penetrate the skin, and grow to adults. Multiplication does not occur in the skin of the
fish. The time required for the complete
life cycle depends on the temperature (Hoffman 1967a). At the optimum temperature,
24 to 26 C, multiplication within the cyst is
completed in about 7 to 8 hours. Unattached tomites live about 48 hours, and
the entire cycle is completed in about 4
days. Infection of a fish is by direct contact
with the parasite in water. Cysts can be
transferred into a tank on plants or other
objects.

PATHOLOGIC EFFECTS

Penetration of the skin by a tomite
causes irritation (Davis 1947a). Affected
fish often scratch or rub themselves against
the sides of the tank or other objects. The
epidermis of the fish reacts to the irritation by overgrowing and enclosing the parasite, producing the typical gray-white
granulomatous lesions (Fig. 21.21). In severe infections, the whole body surface, including the gills, is affected. Damage to the
epithelium is extensive. The fish becomes

FIG. 21.20. Life cycle of
Ichthyophthirius multifiliis.
(A) Adult parasite on catfish.
(B) Mature trophozoite after
leaving fish. *(C)* Division of
adult into many tomites after
cyst formation. *(D)* Rupture
of cyst releasing tomites which
reinfect fish. (From Davis
1947a.)

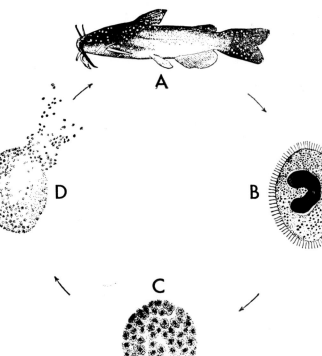

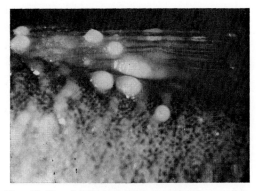

FIG. 21.21. Ichthyophthiriasis ("ich") or white spot disease in a fish. Note typical white foci on skin. (Courtesy of E. Elkan, London.)

lethargic and death is common (Anthony 1969). Decreased hemoglobin, increased sedimentation rate, anemia, neutrophilia, and monocytemia also occur in heavy infection (Lom 1969).

DIAGNOSIS

Diagnosis is based on the typical lesions and identification of the parasite (Davis 1947a; Walliker 1966). Living trophozoites are easily recognized by their large size, their constantly beating cilia, and their rotating motion (van Duijn 1967; Hoffman and Sindermann 1962). Fixed specimens or those in tissue sections are identified by the large, crescent-shaped macronucleus (Mawdesley-Thomas and Jolly 1967). Care must be taken to differentiate ichthyophthiriasis lesions from cutaneous myxosporidian cysts (Hoffman and Sindermann 1962). The scratching or rubbing resulting from the epidermal irritation is not sufficiently specific to be diagnostic (Davis 1947a).

CONTROL

Prevention is based on interruption of the life cycle and on quarantine. Because the free-living tomites survive only about 48 hours at 24 to 26 C, removing all fish from a tank for 3 days will free the tank of this parasite (Bauer 1959; van Duijn 1967). New fish, before being introduced into a clean colony, should be held in isolation at 20 to 25 C for 1 week (van Duijn 1967; Walliker 1966). If no evidence of infection is apparent after this period of quar-

antine, it is probable that the fish are not infected; however, a holding period of 2 to 8 weeks is safer.

There is no treatment that will kill the parasites in the skin of the fish without killing the fish (Bauer 1958; van Duijn 1967). Thus control based on treatment is aimed at destroying the mature parasite, after it leaves the host, along with immature free-swimming forms, and preventing reinfection until all trophozoites have left the host. For this reason, treatment must be continued for an extended period: 10 days at 24 C and 30 days at 10 C (Clemens 1958). Effective agents given in the water daily include formalin, 200 to 250 ppm for 1 hour; malachite green, 2 ppm for 1/2 hour; pyridylmercuric acetate, 2 ppm for 1 hour (toxic for some trouts); acriflavine, 2 to 5 ppm for 1 to 4 hours; and methylene blue, 3 to 4 ppm, or potassium permanganate, 1 to 2 ppm, for a prolonged period (Hoffman 1970; Meyer 1966, 1969; Snieszko and Hoffman 1963; Walliker 1966).

PUBLIC HEALTH CONSIDERATIONS

Ichthyophthirius multifiliis does not affect man.

Chilodonella cyprini

(SYN. *Chilodon cyprini*)

Chilodonella cyprini is frequently encountered on the skin and gills of cyprinids and other freshwater fishes in North America, Europe, and Asia (Davis 1947a; Hoffman 1967a). It is usually pathogenic only at temperatures below 10 C (Bauer and Nikolskaya 1957) and is therefore unlikely to be a problem in fishes in the laboratory.

MORPHOLOGY

This ciliate is ovoid and dorsoventrally flattened (Fig. 21.22) (Hoffman 1967a). It measures 50 to 70 μ long by 30 to 40 μ wide (Kudo 1966). Ciliation is incomplete. The ventral surface has 8 to 15 rows of cilia; the dorsal surface has a cross-row of bristles. The cytostome is rounded, the oral basket is conspicuous, and the macronucleus is oval.

LIFE CYCLE

Reproduction by simple division occurs on the host (Bauer and Nikolskaya

FIG. 21.22. *Chilodonella* trophozoites. *(Left* from Hoffman 1967a; courtesy of University of California Press.
Right courtesy of Bureau of
Sport Fisheries and Wildlife,
U.S. Department of the Interior.)

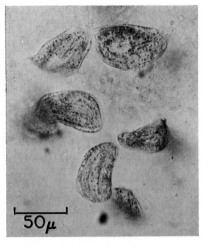

20μ   50μ

1957). Transmission is by direct contact
with the organism in water. The optimum
temperature for division is 5 to 10 C; it
ceases at 20 C.

PATHOLOGIC EFFECTS

Chilodonella cyprini is a strict ectoparasite; it occurs on the skin and gills but
does not penetrate the epidermis (Wenyon
1926). This ciliate usually causes inapparent infection and is an important pathogen
only in debilitated fish at 5 to 10 C (van
Duijn 1967; Reichenbach-Klinke and
Elkan 1965). It causes irritation, epithelial
hyperplasia, and excessive mucus production (van Duijn 1967; Mawdesley-Thomas
and Jolly 1967). The gills are usually
more severely damaged than the rest of the
body; heavy infections cause impaired respiration and death (Davis 1947a; Reichenbach-Klinke and Elkan 1965; Wenyon
1956).

DIAGNOSIS

Because the signs and lesions are nonspecific, microscopic identification of the
parasite in scrapings of the skin and gills
is essential for diagnosis (Walliker 1966).

CONTROL

Agents effective against *Costia necatrix, C. pyriformis,* and *Ichthyophthirius
multifiliis* are effective against this parasite
(van Duijn 1967; Reichenbach-Klinke and
Elkan 1965; Snieszko and Hoffman 1963).

PUBLIC HEALTH CONSIDERATIONS

This ciliate does not affect man.

Ambiphrya ameiuri

(SYN. *Scyphidia macropodia*)

This peritrichid ciliate occurs on the
gills of the channel catfish and other ictalurids in the United States (Hoffman
1967a). Although uncommon on ictalurids
in their natural habitat, it is common on
such fishes reared in hatcheries (Clemens
1958; Davis 1947b; Geibel and Murray
1961), and it is likely to be encountered on
laboratory ictalurids obtained from these
sources. It is usually nonpathogenic, but
sometimes causes a high mortality in young
fish (Davis 1947b; Reichenbach-Klinke and
Elkan 1965).

MORPHOLOGY

The body is generally cylindrical but
usually somewhat constricted anterior to
the base (Fig. 21.23) (Davis 1947b). The
peristome, which is at the anterior or adoral end, has a slightly greater diameter than
the body proper. At the base or posterior
end is a large, flexible holdfast organ called
the scopula. At about one-third of the distance toward the posterior end is a collar
of cilia. When fully extended, the organism is about 35 to 45 μ long and 20 to 25
μ in diameter.

LIFE CYCLE

Asexual reproduction is by binary fission and sexual reproduction by conjugation (Davis 1947b; Hoffman 1967a). No
cysts are formed. Transmission is by direct

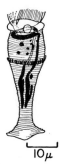

FIG. 21.23. *Ambiphrya ameiuri (Scyphidia macropodia)* trophozoite. (From Hoffman 1967a. Courtesy of University of California Press.)

contact with young, free-swimming forms in water.

PATHOLOGIC EFFECTS

Heavy infection in young fish causes a high mortality (Davis 1947b). Otherwise, this organism is not pathogenic.

DIAGNOSIS

Because the pathologic effects are non-specific, diagnosis is based on the microscopic identification of massive numbers of the organism on the gills of affected fish.

CONTROL

Control is based on chemical treatment (Clemens 1958; Geibel and Murray 1961;

Snieszko and Hoffman 1963). Agents effective against *Costia necatrix, C. pyriformis,* and *Ichthyophthirius multifiliis* are also effective against this parasite.

PUBLIC HEALTH CONSIDERATIONS

This ciliate does not affect man.

Epistylis sp.

Epistylis sp. is common on the skin of the bluegill, black bass, rainbow trout, brook trout, and other fishes in the United States (Hoffman 1967a). Although usually considered to be nonpathogenic (van Duijn 1967), heavy infections sometimes cause dermal lesions (W. A. Rogers, personal communication). Its incidence on laboratory fishes is unknown.

MORPHOLOGY

The body is cone shaped and has a zone of cilia at the adoral end (Fig. 21.24) (Wenyon 1926). Young, free-swimming forms have an additional circle of cilia around the posterior end of the body. *Epistylis* sp. characteristically forms colonies in which the individual organisms are united on noncontractile, branched filaments with a common stem.

LIFE CYCLE

Asexual reproduction is by binary fission and sexual reproduction by conjugation (Wenyon 1926). Transmission is by

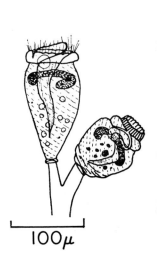

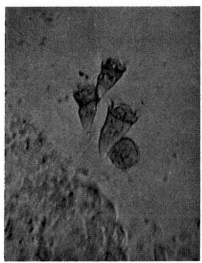

FIG. 21.24. *Epistylis* sp. *(Left)* Drawing of attached forms. *(Right)* Photomicrograph of organisms on skin of bluegill. *(Left* from Hoffman 1967a; courtesy of University of California Press. *Right* courtesy of G. L. Hoffman, Eastern Fish Disease Laboratory.)

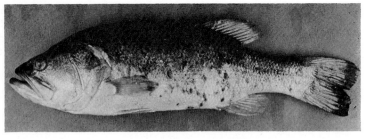

FIG. 21.25. *Epistylis* sp. infection in a black bass. Note dermal lesions. (Courtesy of W. A. Rogers and Southern Cooperative Fish Disease Project, Auburn University.)

direct contact with young, free-swimming forms in water.

PATHOLOGIC EFFECTS

Heavy infections sometimes cause erosion of scales and dermal ulcers (Fig. 21.25) (W. A. Rogers, personal communication). Otherwise, the organism is not pathogenic (van Duijn 1967).

DIAGNOSIS

Diagnosis is based on the microscopic identification of the organism in the lesions.

CONTROL

Control is based on chemical treatment. Agents effective against *Costia necatrix*, *C. pyriformis*, and *Ichthyophthirius multifiliis* are usually effective against this organism (Snieszko and Hoffman 1963).

PUBLIC HEALTH CONSIDERATIONS

Epistylis sp. is not pathogenic for man.

Trichodina, Trichodinella, Tripartiella

These closely related peritrichid ciliates occur on many species of laboratory fishes (Table 20.4) (Davis 1947b; Hoffman 1967a; Lom 1970; Wellborn 1967). *Trichodina fultoni* is the most important species in North America; it occurs on the skin and gills of chubs, shiners, the bluegill, sunfishes, black bass, brook trout, channel catfish, and other fishes. Its incidence in nature is unknown, but it is common on hatchery-reared fishes (Davis 1947a). Several species of *Trichodina*, many often erroneously called *Trichodina domerguei*, are common on the skin and gills of the goldfish and other aquarium fishes in Europe and Asia (van Duijn 1967; Reichenbach-Klinke and Elkan 1965). Laboratory fishes are frequently infected with tricho-

dinids (Anthony 1969). When the infections are heavy, they cause dermal lesions or dyspnea and death (Davis 1947b).

MORPHOLOGY

These ciliates have a saucer- to bell-shaped body with a highly developed basal adhesive disc and an adoral zone of cilia arranged in a spiral (Davis 1947b; Kudo 1966). When viewed dorsoventrally, they are seen to contain a skeletal ring, with radially arranged denticles (Fig. 21.26). The genera are differentiated by the extent of the ciliary spiral and by the shape of the denticles (Fig. 21.27) (Hoffman 1967a). *Trichodina* has a ciliary spiral that makes more than one but less than two complete turns, and denticles that have a flat outer blade, a central cone, and an inner ray or thorn; *Trichodinella* has a ciliary spiral that makes less than one complete turn, and denticles that have an outer flat blade, a central cone, and a poorly developed inner ray. *Tripartiella* has a ciliary spiral

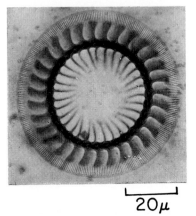

FIG. 21.26. *Trichodina* skeletal ring. Note radially arranged denticle. (From Davis 1947b. Courtesy of Bureau of Sport Fisheries and Wildlife, U.S. Department of the Interior.)

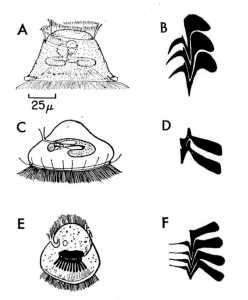

FIG. 21.27. Some peritrichids of laboratory fishes. *(A) Trichodina.* *(B)* Denticles of *Trichodina.* *(C) Trichodinella.* (D) Denticles of *Trichodinella.* *(E) Tripartiella.* *(F)* Denticles of *Tripartiella.* *(A* from Lom 1958; courtesy of Society of Protozoologists. *B, F* from Davis 1947b. *C, D, E* from Hoffman 1967a; courtesy of University of California Press.)

similar to that of *Trichodinella* and denticles that have an outer flat blade and a central cone but a highly developed inner ray. The size varies with the species. *Trichodina fultoni* is about 75 to 90 μ in diameter (Wellborn 1967); common European species of *Trichodina* are about 40 to 105 μ in diameter (Lom 1970).

LIFE CYCLE

Asexual reproduction is by binary fission and sexual reproduction by conjuga-

tion; cysts are not formed (Davis 1947a, b). Transmission is by direct contact with the organism in water.

PATHOLOGIC EFFECTS

Light infections probably have little pathologic effect, but heavy infections cause severe damage (Anthony 1969; Davis 1947a, b; van Duijn 1967). Species that occur principally on the skin cause extensive dermal lesions, including excess mucus production, irregular white blotches on the head and dorsal surface of the body, loosened scales, frayed fins, epithelial hyperplasia, cutaneous hemorrhage, and sloughing of the epidermis; anorexia, listlessness, and death also occur. Species that occur principally on the gills cause hyperplasia of the gill epithelium, dyspnea, and death.

DIAGNOSIS

A tentative diagnosis of trichodinosis is based on identification of the organism associated with the lesions; however, since other protozoan parasites are usually concurrently present, it is sometimes impossible to make a definitive diagnosis (Davis 1947b).

CONTROL

Control is based on chemical treatment. Agents effective against *Costia necatrix, C. pyriformis,* and *Ichthyophthirius multifiliis* are usually effective against these organisms (van Duijn 1967; Reichenbach-Klinke and Elkan 1965; Snieszko and Hoffman 1963).

PUBLIC HEALTH CONSIDERATIONS

These ciliates are not pathogenic for man.

TABLE 21.1. Flagellates affecting laboratory fishes

Parasite	Geographic Distribution	Fish Host	Location in Host	Method of Infection	Incidence in Nature	Remarks	Reference
*Cryptobia salmositica**	Northwestern United States, south-western Canada	Rainbow trout, brown trout, Pacific salmons, stickle-backs, other fishes	Blood	Bite of intermediate host (leech)	Common	Syn. *Trypanoplasma salmositica*. Heavy infections cause lethargy, anorexia, weight loss, anemia, death	Becker and Katz 1965 Hoffman 1967a Wales and Wolf 1955
Cryptobia sp.	Western United States	Salmonids, other fishes	Blood	Bite of intermediate host (leech)	Unknown	Syn. *Trypanoplasma* sp. Pathologic effects unknown	Hoffman 1967a Wolf 1960
Cryptobia carassii	Western United States	Goldfish	Skin, gills	Unknown	Unknown; probably rare	Syn. *Trypanoplasma carassii*. Pathologic effects unknown; apparently a commensal	Becker and Katz 1965 Hoffman 1967a Swezy 1919
Cryptobia sp.	Eastern United States	Carp	Gills	Unknown	Unknown; probably rare	Syn. *Trypanoplasma* sp. Pathologic effects unknown	Becker and Katz 1965 Hoffman 1967a Wenrich 1931
Cryptobia sp.	Eastern United States	Chubs, other fishes	Blood	Bite of intermediate host (leech)	Unknown	Syn. *Trypanoplasma* sp. Pathologic effects unknown	Hoffman 1967a
Cryptobia gurneyorum	Northeastern Canada, Europe	Lake trout, other fishes	Blood	Bite of intermediate host (leech)	Unknown; probably uncommon	Syn. *Trypanoplasma gurneyorum*. Pathologic effects unknown	Becker and Katz 1965 Hoffman 1967a
*Cryptobia cyprini**	Europe	Goldfish, carp	Blood	Bite of intermediate host (leech)	Uncommon	Syn. *Trypanoplasma cyprini*. Heavy infection cause lethargy, anorexia, weight loss, anemia, death	van Duijn 1967 Kraneveld and Keidel 1969 Kudo 1966 Reichenbach-Klinke and Elkan 1965
*Cryptobia borreli**	Europe	European minnow, other fishes	Blood	Bite of intermediate host (leech)	Uncommon	Syn. *Trypanoplasma borreli*. Heavy infections cause lethargy, anorexia, weight loss, anemia, death	Becker and Katz 1965 van Duijn 1967 Hoffman 1967a Wales and Wolf 1955
Trypanosoma sp.	Northeastern United States, Canada	Brook trout, other fishes	Blood	Bite of intermediate host (leech)	Unknown; probably uncommon	Pathologic effects unknown	Hoffman 1967a
Trypanosoma danilewski	Europe	Carp	Blood	Bite of intermediate host (leech)	Uncommon	Heavy infections cause anemia, debilitation, death	van Duijn 1967 Wenyon 1926
Trypanosoma phoxini	Europe	European minnow	Blood	Bite of intermediate host (leech)	Uncommon	Heavy infections cause anemia, debilitation, death	van Duijn 1967 Wenyon 1926
Trypanosoma granulosum	Europe	Eels	Blood	Bite of intermediate host (leech)	Uncommon	Heavy infections cause anemia, debilitation, death	van Duijn 1967 Wenyon 1926

*Discussed in text.

664

TABLE 21.1 (continued)

Parasite	Geographic Distribution	Fish Host	Location in Host	Method of Infection	Incidence in Nature	Remarks	Reference
Costia necatrix*	North America, Europe, Asia	Guppy, platyfish, swordtail, tropical mouthbreeders, other aquarium fishes, salmonids, other fishes	Skin, gills	Direct contact with free-swimming stage	Common	Causes gray coating on skin, anorexia, debilitation, death	Davis 1953, Hoffman 1967a, Schubert 1968, Tavolga and Nigrelli 1947, Walliker 1966
Costia pyriformis*	United States	Brook trout, rainbow trout, other fishes	Skin, gills	Direct contact with free-swimming stage	Uncommon	Possible syn. Costia necatrix. Causes gray coating on skin, anorexia, debilitation, death	Davis 1953, Hoffman 1967a, Tavolga and Nigrelli 1947
Colponema agitans	Eastern United States	Bluegill, other fishes	Gills	Direct contact with free-swimming stage	Unknown	Pathologic effects unknown	Hoffman 1967a
Colponema sp.	South central United States	Channel catfish	Gills	Direct contact with free-swimming stage	Unknown	Pathologic effects unknown	Hoffman 1967a
Bodomonas concava	United States	Bluegill, other fishes	Gills	Direct contact with free-swimming stage	Unknown	Pathologic effects unknown	Hoffman 1967a
Oodinium limneticum*	United States	Guppy, mollies, platyfish, swordtail, Siamese fighting fish, other aquarium fishes	Skin, gills	Direct contact with free-swimming stage	Common	Causes yellow-brown coating on skin, gills; debilitation; impaired respiration; sometimes death	van Duijn 1967, Hoffman 1967a, Jacobs 1946, Reichenbach-Klinke and Elkan 1965, Walliker 1966
Oodinium pillularis*	Europe	Goldfish, carp, guppy, swordtail, Siamese fighting fish, paradise fish, tetras, other aquarium fishes, brown trout	Skin, gills	Direct contact with free-swimming stage	Common	Causes yellow-brown coating on skin, gills; debilitation; impaired respiration; sometimes death	Hoffman 1967a, Reichenbach-Klinke and Elkan 1965, Walliker 1966
Hexamita salmonis*	North America	Goldfish, salmonids, other fishes	Intestine	Ingestion of cyst passed in feces	Common in salmonids	Possible syn. Hexamita intestinalis. Pathologic effects unknown; generally thought to cause catarrhal enteritis, anorexia, listlessness, emaciation, retarded growth, death; also reported as nonpathogenic	Davis 1926b, 1947a, 1953, Hoffman 1967a, McElwain and Post 1968, Uzmann and Jesse 1963, Yasutake et al. 1961
Hexamita intestinalis*	Europe	Goldfish, other aquarium fishes, salmonids, other fishes	Intestine	Ingestion of cyst passed in feces	Common in salmonids	Syn. Hexamita truttae; possible syn. Hexamita salmonis. Pathologic effects unknown; generally thought to cause catarrhal enteritis, anorexia, listlessness, emaciation, retarded growth, death; also reported as nonpathogenic	Bykhovskaya-Pavlovskaya et al. 1962, van Duijn 1967, Hoffman 1967a, Reichenbach-Klinke and Elkan 1965

*Discussed in text.

TABLE 21.2. Sarcodines affecting laboratory fishes

Parasite	Geographic Distribution	Fish Host	Location in Host	Method of Infection	Incidence in Nature	Remarks	Reference
Schizamoeba salmonis	United States	Brook trout, rainbow trout, brown trout, Pacific salmons	Stomach, intestine	Ingestion of organism passed in feces	Common	Apparently nonpathogenic	Davis 1926a, 1947a Hoffman 1967a

TABLE 21.3. Sporozoans affecting laboratory fishes

Parasite	Geographic Distribution	Fish Host	Location in Host	Method of Infection	Incidence in Nature	Remarks	Reference
Eimeria aurati*	Eastern United States	Goldfish	Intestine	Ingestion of oocyst passed in feces	Uncommon	Pathologic effects unknown; possibly causes enteritis	Hoffman 1965, 1967a
Eimeria carassii	Europe	Goldfish	Intestine	Ingestion of oocyst passed in feces	Uncommon	Pathologic effects unknown	Hoffman 1965
Eimeria nicollei	Europe	Goldfish	Intestine	Ingestion of oocyst passed in feces	Uncommon	Pathologic effects unknown	Hoffman 1965
Eimeria carpelli*	Europe	Carp	Intestine	Ingestion of oocyst passed in feces	Common	Syn. Eimeria cyprini, E. wierzejskii, E. cyprinorum. Causes mild enteritis, sometimes debilitation, death	Marinček 1965, Walliker 1966, Wenyon 1926
Eimeria subepithelialis*	Europe	Carp	Intestine	Ingestion of oocyst passed in feces	Common	Causes mild enteritis, sometimes debilitation, death	Marinček 1965, Reichenbach-Klinke and Elkan 1965, Wenyon 1926
Eimeria cyprinorum	Europe	European minnows, other fishes	Intestine	Ingestion of oocyst passed in feces	Uncommon	Pathologic effects unknown	van Duijn 1967
Eimeria sp.*	Northeastern United States	Brook trout, other fishes	Intestine	Ingestion of oocyst passed in feces	Uncommon	Pathologic effects unknown	Davis 1947a, Hoffman 1967a
Eimeria truttae	Europe	Brown trout	Intestine	Ingestion of oocyst passed in feces	Uncommon	Pathologic effects unknown	van Duijn 1967, Wenyon 1926
Eimeria gasterostei	Europe	Sticklebacks	Liver	Ingestion of oocyst passed in feces	Uncommon	Pathologic effects unknown	van Duijn 1967, Wenyon 1926
Eimeria anguillae	Europe	Eels	Intestine	Ingestion of oocyst passed in feces	Uncommon	Pathologic effects unknown	van Duijn 1967, Wenyon 1926
Dactylosoma salvelini	Eastern Canada	Brook trout	Blood	Bite of unknown blood-sucking invertebrate	Uncommon	Pathologic effects unknown	Hoffman 1967a
Ceratomyxa shasta	Western United States	Rainbow trout	Intestine, liver, gallbladder, spleen, gonads, kidneys, heart, gills, skin	Unknown	Uncommon	One report of high mortality in a hatchery	Hoffman 1967a, Wales and Wolf 1955
Wardia ovinocua	North central United States	Bluegill, sunfishes	Ovaries	Unknown	Uncommon	Pathologic effects unknown	Hoffman 1967a, Kudo 1966

*Discussed in text.

TABLE 21.3 (continued)

Parasite	Geographic Distribution	Fish Host	Location in Host	Method of Infection	Incidence in Nature	Remarks	Reference
Sinuolinea gilsoni	Europe	Eels	Urinary bladder	Unknown; probably by ingestion of spores passed in urine	Uncommon	Pathologic effects unknown	van Duijn 1967
Sphaerospora elegans	Europe	European minnow, sticklebacks, other fishes	Kidneys, ovaries	Unknown; probably by ingestion of spores released from tissue or passed in urine	Uncommon	Pathologic effects unknown	van Duijn 1967
Sphaerospora reichnowi	Europe	Eels	Intestine	Unknown; probably by ingestion of spores passed in feces	Uncommon	Causes white cysts in intestine	van Duijn 1967
Myxosoma cerebralis*	North America, Europe, Asia	Brook trout, rainbow trout, brown trout, other salmonids	Cartilage of head, spine	Ingestion of spores released from tissue	Common	Syn. Lentospora cerebralis. Causes destruction of cartilage of head, spine; deformation of head, spine; blackened tail; impaired locomotion (whirling disease)	Bogdanova 1968 van Duijn 1967 Elson 1969 Hoffman 1967a Hoffman and Putz 1969 Hoffman et al. 1962, 1965 Kudo 1930, 1966 Olsen 1967 Reichenbach-Klinke and Elkan 1965 Roberts and Elson 1970
Myxosoma cartilaginis*	Eastern United States	Bluegill, sunfishes, black bass	Cartilage of head, spine	Unknown; probably by ingestion of spores released from tissue	Common	Causes cysts in cartilage of head	Hoffman 1967a Hoffman et al. 1965 Olsen 1967
Myxosoma squamalis	Northwestern United States	Rainbow trout, Pacific salmons	Skin	Unknown; probably by ingestion of spores released from tissue	Uncommon	Causes cysts in skin between scales, increased mortality	Hoffman 1967a Hoffman et al. 1965
Myxosoma hoffmani	North central United States	Fathead minnow	Eyes	Unknown; probably by ingestion of spores released from tissue	Uncommon	Causes cysts in sclera of eye	Hoffman 1967a Hoffman et al. 1965
Myxosoma grandis	Northeastern United States	Shiners, other fishes	Liver	Unknown; probably by ingestion of spores released from tissue	Uncommon	Causes enlarged liver	Hoffman 1967a Hoffman et al. 1965
Myxosoma robustrum	North central United States	Shiners	Skin	Unknown; probably by ingestion of spores released from tissue	Uncommon	Causes cysts in skin	Hoffman 1967a Hoffman et al. 1965
Myxosoma orbitalis	Eastern Canada	Shiners	Eyes	Unknown; probably by ingestion of spores released from tissue	Uncommon	Causes cysts in eyes	Hoffman 1967a Hoffman et al. 1965

*Discussed in text.

TABLE 21.3 *(continued)*

Parasite	Geographic Distribution	Fish Host	Location in Host	Method of Infection	Incidence in Nature	Remarks	Reference
Myxosoma notropis	Eastern Canada	Shiners	Abdominal cavity	Unknown; probably by ingestion of spores released from tissue	Uncommon	Causes cysts in abdominal cavity, destruction of liver	Hoffman 1967a, Hoffman et al. 1965
Myxosoma media	Eastern Canada	Shiners	Abdominal cavity	Unknown; probably by ingestion of spores released from tissue	Uncommon	Causes cysts in abdominal cavity	Hoffman 1967a, Hoffman et al. 1965
Myxosoma subtecalis	Eastern United States	Topminnows	Skin, viscera, fat of cranial cavity, kidneys	Unknown; probably by ingestion of spores released from tissue	Uncommon	Causes cysts in skin, cranial cavity, kidneys	Hoffman 1967a, Hoffman et al. 1965
Myxosoma hudsonis	Northeastern United States	Topminnows	Skin	Unknown; probably by ingestion of spores released from tissue	Uncommon	Causes cysts in skin between scales	Hoffman 1967a, Hoffman et al. 1965
Myxosoma funduli	Eastern United States	Topminnows, killifishes	Gills	Unknown; probably by ingestion of spores released from tissue	Uncommon	Causes cysts in gills	Hoffman 1967a, Hoffman et al. 1965
Myxosoma diaphana	Eastern Canada, Europe	Killifishes	Ovaries, testes	Unknown; probably by ingestion of spores released from tissue	Uncommon	Syn. *Lentospora diaphana.* Causes cysts in ovaries, testes; destruction of ovaries, testes	van Duijn 1967, Hoffman 1967a, Hoffman et al. 1965
Myxosoma eucalii	North central United States	Sticklebacks	Bone	Unknown; probably by ingestion of spores released from tissue	Uncommon	Pathologic effects unknown	Hoffman 1967a
Myxosoma dujardini*	Europe, Asia	Carp, other fishes	Gills	Unknown; probably by ingestion of spores released from tissue	Common	Syn. *Lentospora dujardini.* Causes yellow-white cysts in gills, dyspnea, death	van Duijn 1967, Kudo 1920, Reichenbach-Klinke and Elkan 1965
Myxosoma encephalina	Europe	Carp	Blood vessels of brain	Unknown; probably by ingestion of spores released from tissue	Uncommon	Syn. *Lentospora encephalina.* Pathologic effects unknown	van Duijn 1967, Kudo 1920, Reichenbach-Klinke and Elkan 1965
Myxobolus bellus	North central United States	Carp	Skin	Unknown; probably by ingestion of spores released from tissue	Uncommon	Causes cysts in skin	Hoffman 1967a
Myxobolus dispar	Europe	Carp, other fishes	Skin, gills, muscle, spleen, intestine	Unknown; probably by ingestion of spores released from tissue or passed in feces	Common	Causes cysts in skin, gills, muscle, spleen, intestine	van Duijn 1967, Kudo 1920, Reichenbach-Klinke and Elkan 1965

*Discussed in text.

TABLE 21.3 (continued)

Parasite	Geographic Distribution	Fish Host	Location in Host	Method of Infection	Incidence in Nature	Remarks	Reference
Myxobolus exiguus	Europe	Carp, other fishes	Skin, gills, kidneys, stomach, intestine	Unknown; probably by ingestion of spores released from tissue or passed in feces	Common	Causes cysts in skin, gills	van Duijn 1967 Reichenbach-Klinke and Elkan 1965
Myxobolus cyprini	Europe	Carp, other fishes	Liver, spleen, kidneys	Unknown; probably by ingestion of spores released from tissue	Common	Causes cysts in liver, spleen	van Duijn 1967 Reichenbach-Klinke and Elkan 1965
Myxobolus mülleri	Europe	Carp, European minnow, other fishes	Skin, ovaries, kidneys	Unknown; probably by ingestion of spores released from tissue	Common	Causes cysts in skin, ovaries	van Duijn 1967 Kudo 1920 Reichenbach-Klinke and Elkan 1965
Myxobolus koi	Japan	Carp	Gills	Unknown; probably by ingestion of spores released from tissue	Uncommon	Causes cysts in gills	Hoffman 1967a
Myxobolus aureatus	Northeastern United States	Bluntnose minnow	Fins	Unknown; probably by ingestion of spores released from tissue	Uncommon	Causes cysts in fins	Hoffman 1967a
Myxobolus mutabilis	North central United States	Bluntnose minnow	Skin	Unknown; probably by ingestion of spores released from tissue	Uncommon	Causes cysts in skin	Hoffman 1967a
Myxobolus nodosus	North central United States	Bluntnose minnow	Skin	Unknown; probably by ingestion of spores released from tissue	Uncommon	Causes cysts in skin	Hoffman 1967a
Myxobolus notatus	Canada	Bluntnose minnow	Muscle	Unknown; probably by ingestion of spores released from tissue	Uncommon	Causes cysts in muscle	Hoffman 1967a Kudo 1920
Myxobolus compressus	North central United States	Shiners	Skin	Unknown; probably by ingestion of spores released from tissue	Uncommon	Causes cysts in skin	Hoffman 1967a
Myxobolus orbiculatus	North central United States	Shiners	Muscle	Unknown; probably by ingestion of spores released from tissue	Uncommon	Causes cysts in muscle	Hoffman 1967a
Myxobolus teres	North central United States	Shiners	Muscle	Unknown; probably by ingestion of spores released from tissue	Uncommon	Causes cysts in muscle	Hoffman 1967a
Myxobolus notropis	Canada	Shiners	Skin	Unknown; probably by ingestion of spores released from tissue	Uncommon	Causes cysts in skin	Hoffman 1967a
Myxobolus transversalis	Canada	Shiners	Muscle	Unknown; probaby by ingestion of spores released from tissue	Uncommon	Causes cysts in muscle	Hoffman 1967a

TABLE 21.3 *(continued)*

Parasite	Geographic Distribution	Fish Host	Location in Host	Method of Infection	Incidence in Nature	Remarks	Reference
Myxobolus grandis	Canada	Shiners	Abdominal cavity	Unknown; probably by ingestion of spores released from tissue	Uncommon	Causes cysts in abdominal cavity	Hoffman 1967a
Myxobolus notemigoni	South central United States	Golden shiner	Skin	Unknown; probably by ingestion of spores released from tissue	Uncommon	Causes cysts in skin	Hoffman 1967a
Myxobolus musculi	Eastern United States	Topminnows	Skin	Unknown; probably by ingestion of spores released from tissue	Uncommon	Causes cysts in skin	Hoffman 1967a
Myxobolus bilineatum	Eastern United States	Topminnows	Brain, viscera	Unknown; probably by ingestion of spores released from tissue	Uncommon	Causes cysts in brain, viscera	Hoffman 1967a
Myxobolus lintoni	Northeastern United States	Topminnows	Subcutis	Unknown; probably by ingestion of spores released from tissue	Uncommon	Causes cysts in subcutis	Hoffman 1967a
Myxobolus capsulatus	Southern United States	Topminnows	Viscera	Unknown; probably by ingestion of spores released from tissue	Uncommon	Causes cysts in viscera	Hoffman 1967a
Myxobolus funduli	Northeastern United States	Topminnows, killifishes	Muscle	Unknown; probably by ingestion of spores released from tissue	Uncommon	Causes cysts in muscle	Hoffman 1967a
Myxobolus osburni	North central United States	Bluegill, sunfishes, black bass, other fishes	Mesentery, peritoneum, gallbladder	Unknown; probably by ingestion of spores released from tissue	Uncommon	Causes cysts in mesentery, peritoneum	Hoffman 1967a
Myxobolus gibbosus	Northeastern United States	Sunfishes	Connective tissue of gills	Unknown; probably by ingestion of spores released from tissue	Uncommon	Causes cysts in gills	Hoffman 1967a
Myxobolus mesentericus	North central United States	Sunfishes	Mesentery, liver, spleen, stomach, intestine, gallbladder	Unknown; probably by ingestion of spores released from tissue or passed in feces	Uncommon	Causes cysts in viscera	Hoffman 1967a Kudo 1920
Myxobolus kostiri	Northeastern United States	Black bass	Subcutis	Unknown; probably by ingestion of spores released from tissue	Uncommon	Causes cysts in subcutis	Hoffman 1967a
Myxobolus inornatus	United States	Black bass	Muscle	Unknown; probably by ingestion of spores released from tissue	Uncommon	Causes cysts in muscle	Hoffman 1967a
Myxobolus ovoidalis	Canada	Brook trout	Skin	Unknown; probably by ingestion of spores released from tissue	Uncommon	Causes cysts in skin	Hoffman 1967a

TABLE 21.3 (continued)

Parasite	Geographic Distribution	Fish Host	Location in Host	Method of Infection	Incidence in Nature	Remarks	Reference
Myxobolus neurobius	Europe	Brown trout	Spinal cord, nerves	Unknown; probably by ingestion of spores released from tissue	Uncommon	Causes cysts in nerves, spinal cord	van Duijn 1967 Hoffman 1967a
Myxobolus insidiosus	Northwestern United States	Chinook salmon	Muscle	Unknown; probably by ingestion of spores released from tissue	Uncommon	Causes cysts in muscle	Hoffman 1967a
Myxobolus kisutchi	Northwestern United States	Pacific salmons	Spinal cord	Unknown; probably by ingestion of spores released from tissue	Uncommon	Causes cysts in spinal cord	Hoffman 1967a Yasutake and Wood 1957
Myxobolus squamae	Northwestern United States	Pacific salmons, other fishes	Skin	Unknown; probably by ingestion of spores released from tissue	Uncommon	Causes cysts in skin	Hoffman 1967a
Henneguya zikaweiensis	Europe	Goldfish	Eyes	Unknown; probably by ingestion of spores released from tissue	Uncommon	Causes cysts in cornea	van Duijn 1967
Henneguya fontinalis var. *notropis*	Eastern Canada	Shiners	Skin	Unknown; probably by ingestion of spores released from tissue	Uncommon	Causes cysts in skin	Hoffman 1967a
Henneguya salminicola	Alaska, Siberia	Pacific salmons	Muscle, subcutis	Unknown; probably by ingestion of spores released from tissue	Uncommon	Causes cysts in muscle, subcutis (tapioca disease)	Hoffman 1967a Kudo 1920 Sindermann 1966
Henneguya salmonis	Canada	Atlantic salmon	Subcutis	Unknown; probably by ingestion of spores released from tissue	Uncommon	Causes cysts in subcutis	Hoffman 1967a
Henneguya exilis	North central United States	Channel catfish, other fishes	Skin, gills	Unknown; probably by ingestion of spores released from tissue	Uncommon	Causes cysts in skin, gills	Hoffman 1967a Kudo 1966
Henneguya media	Europe	Sticklebacks	Kidneys, ovaries	Unknown; probably by ingestion of spores released from tissues or passed in urine	Uncommon	Causes cysts in ovaries	van Duijn 1967
Henneguya brevis	Europe	Sticklebacks	Kidneys, ovaries	Unknown; probably by ingestion of spores released from tissue or passed in urine	Uncommon	Causes cysts in ovaries	van Duijn 1967
Unicauda clavicauda	North central United States	Shiners	Skin	Unknown; probably by ingestion of spores released from tissue	Uncommon	Causes cysts in skin	Hoffman 1967a Kudo 1966
Unicauda brachyura	Eastern United States	Shiners	Fins	Unknown; probably by ingestion of spores released from tissue	Uncommon	Causes cysts in fins	Hoffman 1967a

TABLE 21.3 *(continued)*

Parasite	Geographic Distribution	Fish Host	Location in Host	Method of Infection	Incidence in Nature	Remarks	Reference
Unicauda fontinalis	Eastern Canada	Brook trout	Skin	Unknown; probably by ingestion of spores released from tissue	Uncommon	Syn. *Henneguya fontinalis.* Causes cysts in skin	Hoffman 1967a
Unicauda plasmodia	United States	Channel catfish	Gills	Unknown; probably by ingestion of spores released from tissue	Uncommon	Syn. *Henneguya plasmodia.* Causes cysts in gills	Hoffman 1967a
Thelohanellus notatus	North central United States, eastern Canada	Bluntnose minnow, shiners	Skin	Unknown; probably by ingestion of spores released from tissue	Uncommon	Causes cysts in skin	Hoffman 1967a
Hoferellus cyprini	Europe	Carp	Kidneys	Unknown; probably by ingestion of spores passed in urine	Uncommon	Sometimes causes obstruction of renal tubules, ascites	van Duijn 1967 Hoffman 1967a Reichenbach-Klinke and Elkan 1965
Mitraspora elongata	Eastern United States	Bluegill, sunfishes, black bass	Kidneys	Unknown; probably by ingestion of spores passed in urine	Uncommon	Pathologic effects unknown	Hoffman 1967a
Mitraspora cyprini	Japan	Carp	Kidneys	Unknown; probably by ingestion of spores passed in urine	Uncommon	Pathologic effects unknown	van Duijn 1967
Myxobilatus mictospora	North central United States	Sunfishes, black bass	Urinary bladder	Unknown; probably by ingestion of spores passed in urine	Uncommon	Syn. *Henneguya mictospora.* Pathologic effects unknown	Hoffman 1967a Kudo 1966
Myxobilatus ohioensis	North central United States	Sunfishes	Urinary bladder	Unknown; probably by ingestion of spores passed in urine	Uncommon	Pathologic effects unknown	Hoffman 1967a
Chloromyxum legeri	Europe	Carp	Gallbladder	Unknown; probably by ingestion of spores passed in feces	Uncommon	Pathologic effects unknown	van Duijn 1967
Chloromyxum cyprini	Japan	Carp	Gallbladder	Unknown; probably by ingestion of spores passed in feces	Common in some areas	Incidence of 20% reported. Pathologic effects unknown	van Duijn 1967
Chloromyxum koi	Japan	Carp	Gallbladder	Unknown; probably by ingestion of spores passed in feces	Uncommon	Pathologic effects unknown	van Duijn 1967
Chloromyxum externum	Southern United States	Chubs, other fishes	Gills	Unknown; probably by ingestion of spores released from tissue	Uncommon	Pathologic effects unknown	Davis 1947b Hoffman 1967a
Chloromyxum renalis	Southern United States	Killifishes	Kidneys	Unknown; probably by ingestion of spores passed in urine	Uncommon	Pathologic effects unknown	Hoffman 1967a

673

TABLE 21.3 *(continued)*

Parasite	Geographic Distribution	Fish Host	Location in Host	Method of Infection	Incidence in Nature	Remarks	Reference
Chloromyxum gibbosum	Eastern United States	Bluegill, sunfishes	Gallbladder	Unknown; probably by ingestion of spores passed in feces	Uncommon	Pathologic effects unknown	Hoffman 1967a
Chloromyxum truttae	Eastern United States, Europe	Brook trout, brown trout	Gallbladder	Unknown; probably by ingestion of spores passed in feces	Uncommon	Sometimes causes hypertrophy of gallbladder, anorexia, debilitation, diarrhea, anemia, death	Davis 1947a van Duijn 1967 Hoffman 1967a Kudo 1930
Chloromyxum majori	Northwestern United States	Rainbow trout, chinook salmon	Kidneys	Unknown; probably by ingestion of spores passed in urine	Uncommon	Causes damage to renal glomeruli	Hoffman 1967a Yasutake and Wood 1957
Chloromyxum wardi	Northwestern United States	Salmonids	Gallbladder, intestine	Unknown; probably by ingestion of spores passed in feces	Uncommon	Pathologic effects unknown	Hoffman 1967a
Kudoa sp.	Eastern United States	Topminnows, other fishes	Blood	Unknown	Uncommon	Pathologic effects unknown	Hoffman 1967a
Myxidium histophilum	Europe	European minnow	Kidneys, ovaries	Unknown; probably by ingestion of spores released from tissue or passed in urine	Uncommon	Pathologic effects unknown	van Duijn 1967
Myxidium folium	Eastern United States	Topminnows	Liver, gallbladder	Unknown; probably by ingestion of spores passed in feces	Uncommon	Pathologic effects unknown	Hoffman 1967a Mitchell 1967
Myxidium incurvatum	Eastern United States, Europe	Killifishes, mosquito-fish	Gallbladder	Unknown; probably by ingestion of spores passed in feces	Uncommon	Pathologic effects unknown	Mitchell 1967
Myxidium phyllium	Eastern United States	Mosquitofish	Gallbladder	Unknown; probably by ingestion of spores passed in feces	Uncommon	Pathologic effects unknown	Mitchell 1967
Myxidium minteri	Northwestern United States	Brook trout, rainbow trout, chinook salmon, other salmonids	Kidneys, gallbladder, liver	Unknown; probably by ingestion of spores passed in urine or feces	Common in some salmonids	Heavy infections cause degeneration of renal tubules	Hoffman 1967a Mitchell 1967 Sanders and Fryer 1970 Yasutake and Wood 1957
Myxidium oviforme	Western United States, Europe	Rainbow trout, Atlantic salmon	Gallbladder	Unknown; probably by ingestion of spores passed in feces	Uncommon	Pathologic effects unknown	Hoffman 1967a Mitchell 1967
Myxidium sp.	United States	Black bass, rainbow trout, other salmonids	Gallbladder, kidneys	Unknown; probably by ingestion of spores passed in feces or urine	Uncommon	Pathologic effects unknown	Hoffman 1967a Mitchell 1967 Yasutake and Wood 1957

TABLE 21.3 (continued)

Parasite	Geographic Distribution	Fish Host	Location in Host	Method of Infection	Incidence in Nature	Remarks	Reference
Myxidium truttae	Europe	Brown trout	Gallbladder	Unknown; probably by ingestion of spores passed in feces	Uncommon	Pathologic effects unknown	van Duijn 1967
Myxidium oviforme	Europe	Atlantic salmon, other fishes	Gallbladder	Unknown; probably by ingestion of spores passed in feces	Uncommon	Pathologic effects unknown	van Duijn 1967
Myxidium bellum	North central United States	Channel catfish	Gallbladder	Unknown; probably by ingestion of spores passed in feces	Uncommon	Pathologic effects unknown	Hoffman 1967a Mitchell 1967
Myxidium gasterostei	Western United States	Sticklebacks	Gallbladder	Unknown; probably by ingestion of spores passed in feces	Uncommon	Pathologic effects unknown	Hoffman 1967a Mitchell 1967
Myxidium illinoisense	North central United States	Eels	Kidneys	Unknown; probably by ingestion of spores passed in urine	Uncommon	Pathologic effects unknown	Hoffman 1967a Mitchell 1967
Myxidium girardi	Europe	Eels	Kidneys	Unknown; probably by ingestion of spores passed in urine	Uncommon	Causes cysts in kidneys	van Duijn 1967
Zschokkella salvelini	Canada	Brook trout	Kidneys	Unknown; probably by ingestion of spores passed in urine	Uncommon	Pathologic effects unknown	Hoffman 1967a
Pleistophora ovariae	Central United States	Golden shiner	Ovaries, liver, kidneys	Unknown	Uncommon	Causes sterility in female	van Duijn 1967 Hoffman 1967a Putz et al. 1965
Pleistophora sp.	Eastern United States	Topminnows	Muscle	Unknown	Uncommon	Pathologic effects unknown	Bond 1937 Putz et al. 1965
Pleistophora hyphessobryconis*	Europe	Swordtail, tetras, other fishes	Muscle	Unknown; probably by ingestion of spores released from tissue	Uncommon	Causes cysts in muscle, muscular necrosis, emaciation, death (neon tetra disease)	van Duijn 1967 Putz et al. 1965 Reichenbach-Klinke and Elkan 1965
Pleistophora salmonae*	Western United States	Rainbow trout, Pacific salmons, other salmonids	Gills	Unknown; probably by ingestion of spores released from tissue	Uncommon	Causes cysts in gills, anemia, inflammation of gills, proliferation of gill lamellae, death	Hoffman 1967a Putz et al. 1965 Wales and Wolf 1955

*Discussed in text.

675

TABLE 21.3 *(continued)*

Parasite	Geographic Distribution	Fish Host	Location in Host	Method of Infection	Incidence in Nature	Remarks	Reference
Pleistophora typicalis	Europe	Sticklebacks, other fishes	Muscle	Unknown; probably by ingestion of spores released from tissue	Uncommon	Pathologic effects unknown	Putz et al. 1965 Reichenbach-Klinke and Elkan 1965
*Glugea anomala**	Alaska, Europe	Sticklebacks	Subcutaneous tissues, peritoneum, stomach, intestine, ovaries, cornea	Unknown; probably by ingestion of spores released from tissue	Uncommon	Causes large, thick-walled cysts in subcutaneous tissues; body deformation; death	van Duijn 1967 Kudo 1966 Putz et al. 1965 Reichenbach-Klinke and Elkan 1965 Sindermann 1966 Wenyon 1926
Sarcocystis salvelini	Canada	Brook trout	Muscle	Unknown	Uncommon	Pathologic effects unknown	Hoffman 1967a
*Dermocystidium salmonis** (possibly a fungus)	Western United States	Chinook salmon	Gills	Unknown	Uncommon	Causes cysts in gills	Davis 1947b Hoffman 1967a
*Dermocystidium branchialis** (possibly a fungus)	Europe	Brown trout	Gills	Unknown	Uncommon	Causes cysts in gills	van Duijn 1967 Hoffman 1967a Reichenbach-Klinke and Elkan 1965
*Dermocystidium gasterostei** (possibly a fungus)	Europe	Sticklebacks	Skin	Unknown	Uncommon	Causes wormlike cysts in skin	van Duijn 1967 Elkan 1962 Reichenbach-Klinke and Elkan 1965
*Dermocystidium koi** (possibly a fungus)	Japan	Carp	Skin, muscle	Unknown	Uncommon	Causes cysts in skin, muscle	Hoffman 1967a
*Dermocystidium sp.** (possibly a fungus)	Eastern United States	Goldfish, bluegill, brook trout	Skin	Unknown	Uncommon	Causes cysts in skin	Hoffman 1967a

*Discussed in text.

TABLE 21.4. Ciliates affecting laboratory fishes

Parasite	Geographic Distribution	Fish Host	Location in Host	Method of Infection	Incidence in Nature	Remarks	Reference
Ichthyophthirius multifiliis*	Worldwide	All freshwater fishes	Skin, gills	Direct contact with organism in water	Uncommon	Common on fishes in captivity. Causes irritation of skin, gray-white granulomatous dermal lesions, decreased hemoglobin, anemia, neutrophilia, monocytemia, lethargy, death (ichthyophthiriasis, "ich," white spot disease)	Anthony 1969 Davis 1947a van Duijn 1967 Hoffman 1967a Hoffman and Sindermann 1962 Lom 1969 Mawdesley-Thomas and Jolly 1967 Reichenbach-Klinke and Elkan 1965 Walliker 1966
Ophryoglena sp.	Eastern United States	Chubs, bluegill, black bass, other fishes	Skin	Direct contact with organism in water	Rare	Causes epithelial sloughing, lethargy, sometimes death	Hoffman 1967b
Chilodonella cyprini*	North America, Europe, Asia	Cyprinids, other fishes	Skin, gills	Direct contact with organism in water	Common	Syn. Chilodon cyprini. Usually pathogenic only at temperatures below 10 C; causes irritation of skin, epithelial hyperplasia, excessive mucus production, damage to gills, impaired respiration, death	Bauer and Nikolskaya 1957 Davis 1947a van Duijn 1967 Hoffman 1967a Kudo 1966 Reichenbach-Klinke and Elkan 1965 Walliker 1966 Wenyon 1926
Chilodonella dentatus	Eastern Canada	Black bass	Gills	Direct contact with organism in water	Uncommon	Pathologic effects unknown	Hoffman 1967a
Amphileptus voracus	United States	Channel catfish, other fishes	Gills	Direct contact with organism in water	Uncommon	Probably beneficial to host; ingests pathogenic protozoans	Davis 1947b Hoffman 1967a
Ambiphrya ameiuri*	United States	Channel catfish, other ictalurids	Gills	Direct contact with organism in water	Uncommon	Syn. Scyphidia macropodia. Common on hatchery-reared ictalurids. Heavy infections sometimes cause death	Clemens 1958 Davis 1947b Geibel and Murray 1961 Hoffman 1967a Reichenbach-Klinke and Elkan 1965
Ambiphrya tholiformis	Eastern United States	Black bass	Gills	Direct contact with organism in water	Uncommon	Pathologic effects unknown; heavy infections in young fish probably cause death	Hoffman 1967a

*Discussed in text.

677

TABLE 21.4 *(continued)*

Parasite	Geographic Distribution	Fish Host	Location in Host	Method of Infection	Incidence in Nature	Remarks	Reference
Apiosoma micropteri	Eastern United States	Black bass	Gills	Direct contact with organism in water	Uncommon	Syn. *Scyphidia micropteri*. Pathologic effects unknown; heavy infections in young fish probably cause death	Hoffman 1967a
Apiosoma piscicola	Europe	Goldfish, sticklebacks, other fishes	Gills	Direct contact with organism in water	Uncommon	Syn *Glossatella piscicola*. Pathologic effects unknown	van Duijn 1967 Reichenbach-Klinke and Elkan 1965
Epistylis sp.*	United States	Bluegill, black bass, brook trout, rainbow trout, other fishes	Skin	Direct contact with organism in water	Common	Heavy infections sometimes cause erosion of scales, dermal ulcers	van Duijn 1967 Hoffman 1967a W. A. Rogers, personal communication Wenyon 1926
Trichodina fultoni*	North America, Europe	Chubs, shiners, bluegill, sunfishes, black bass, brook trout, channel catfish, other fishes	Skin, gills	Direct contact with organism in water	Unknown	Syn. *T. domerguei* in part. Common in hatchery-reared fishes. Causes excess mucus production, skin blotches, loosened scales, frayed fins, epithelial hyperplasia, listlessness, dyspnea, death	Davis 1947a, b Lom 1970 Hoffman 1967a Wellborn 1967
Trichodina acuta	North America, Europe, Asia	Goldfish, carp, topminnows, sunfishes, other fishes	Skin, gills	Direct contact with organism in water	Common in Europe, Asia	Syn. *T. domerguei* in part. Pathologic effects unknown; heavy infections probably cause dermal lesions, dyspnea, death	Lom 1970
Trichodina reticulata	North America, Europe, Asia	Goldfish	Skin, gills	Direct contact with organism in water	Common in Europe, Asia	Syn. *T. domerguei* in part. Pathologic effects unknown; heavy infections probably cause dermal lesions, dyspnea, death	Hoffman 1967a Lom 1970
Trichodina pediculus	North America, Europe, Asia	Goldfish, carp, other fishes	Skin, gills	Direct contact with organism in water	Common in Europe, Asia	Pathologic effects unknown; heavy infections probably cause dermal lesions, dyspnea, death	Davis 1947b Hoffman 1967a Lom 1970 Wellborn 1967
Trichodina mutabilis	Europe, Asia	Goldfish, carp, other fishes	Skin, gills	Direct contact with organism in water	Common	Pathologic effects unknown; heavy infections probably cause dermal lesions, dyspnea, death	Lom 1970
Trichodina nigra	Europe, Asia	Carp, brown trout, Atlantic salmon, other fishes	Skin, gills	Direct contact with organism in water	Common	Pathologic effects unknown; heavy infections probably cause dermal lesions, dyspnea, death	Lom 1970
Trichodina nobilis	Asia	Goldfish, carp, other fishes	Skin, gills	Direct contact with organism in water	Common	Pathologic effects unknown; heavy infections probably cause dermal lesions, dyspnea, death	Lom 1970

*Discussed in text.

678

TABLE 21.4 *(continued)*

Parasite	Geographic Distribution	Fish Host	Location in Host	Method of Infection	Incidence in Nature	Remarks	Reference
Trichodina intermedia	Europe	European minnow	Skin	Direct contact with organism in water	Uncommon	Pathologic effects unknown; heavy infections probably cause dermal lesions, death	Lom 1970
Trichodina janovice	Europe	European minnow	Skin	Direct contact with organism in water	Uncommon	Pathologic effects unknown; heavy infections probably cause dermal lesions, death	Lom 1970
Trichodina hypsilepis	Southeastern United States	Shiners	Skin	Direct contact with organism in water	Uncommon	Pathologic effects unknown; heavy infections probably cause dermal lesions, death	Lom 1970 Wellborn 1967
Trichodina funduli	Southeastern United States	Topminnows	Skin	Direct contact with organism in water	Uncommon	Pathologic effects unknown; heavy infections probably cause dermal lesions, death	Lom 1970 Wellborn 1967
Trichodina uellborni	Southeastern United States	Black bass	Gills	Direct contact with organism in water	Uncommon	Pathologic effects unknown; heavy infections probably cause dyspnea, death	Lom 1970
Trichodina salmincola	Eastern United States	Brook trout, rainbow trout	Skin	Direct contact with organism in water	Uncommon	Pathologic effects unknown; heavy infections probably cause dermal lesions, death	Lom 1970 Wellborn 1967
Trichodina truttae	Western United States, Siberia	Pacific salmons, other salmonids	Skin, gills	Direct contact with organism in water	Uncommon	Pathologic effects unknown; heavy infections probably cause dermal lesions, dyspnea, death	Lom 1970
Trichodina sp.	Western United States, Siberia	Chinook salmon, other salmonids	Skin, gills	Direct contact with organism in water	Uncommon	Pathologic effects unknown; heavy infections probably cause dermal lesions, dyspnea, death	Davis 1947b Hoffman 1967a Lom 1970 Wellborn 1967
Trichodina tenuidens	North America, Europe, Asia	Sticklebacks, other fishes	Skin	Direct contact with organism in water	Uncommon	Pathologic effects unknown; heavy infections probably cause dermal lesions, death	Lom 1970 Wellborn 1967
Trichodina domerguei	Europe, Asia	Sticklebacks, other fishes	Skin, gills	Direct contact with organism in water	Uncommon	Pathologic effects unknown; heavy infections probably cause dermal lesions, dyspnea, death	Lom 1970
Trichodina gasterostei	Asia	Sticklebacks	Skin	Direct contact with organism in water	Uncommon	Pathologic effects unknown; heavy infections probably cause dermal lesions, death	Lom 1970
Trichodina anguilli	Europe	Eel	Gills	Direct contact with organism in water	Uncommon	Pathologic effects unknown; heavy infections probably cause dyspnea, death	Lom 1970

TABLE 21.4 (continued)

Parasite	Geographic Distribution	Fish Host	Location in Host	Method of Infection	Incidence in Nature	Remarks	Reference
Trichodinella myakkae	United States	Carp, black bass, brook trout, other fishes	Gills	Direct contact with organism in water	Uncommon	Syn. *Trichodina myakkae*. Heavy infections cause hyperplasia of gill epithelium, dypsnea, death	Davis 1947b, Hoffman 1967a
Trichodinella subtilis	Eastern United States, Europe	Goldfish, carp, European minnow	Gills	Direct contact with organism in water	Uncommon	Syn. *Foliella subtilis*. Pathologic effects unknown; heavy infections probably cause hyperplasia of gill epithelium, dyspnea, death	Hoffman 1967a, Lom 1970
Tripartiella symmetricus	United States	Chubs, channel catfish, other fishes	Gills	Direct contact with organism in water	Uncommon	Syn. *Trichodina symmetricus*. Pathologic effects unknown; heavy infections probably cause dyspnea, death	Davis 1947b, Hoffman 1967a
Tripartiella bulbosa	Eastern United States	Chubs	Gills	Direct contact with organism in water	Uncommon	Syn. *Trichodina bulbosa*. Pathologic effects unknown; heavy infections probably cause dyspnea, death	Davis 1947b, Hoffman 1967a
Tripartiella incisa	Europe	European minnow	Gills	Direct contact with organism in water	Uncommon	Pathologic effects unknown; heavy infections probably cause dyspnea, death	Lom 1970
Trichophrya piscium	United States, Canada	Black bass, brook trout, rainbow trout, Pacific salmons, channel catfish	Gills	Direct contact with organism in water	Common	Pathologic effects unknown	Davis 1947b
Trichophrya micropteri	Eastern United States	Black bass	Gills	Direct contact with organism in water	Rare	Possible syn. *Trichophrya piscium*. Pathologic effects unknown	Davis 1947b
Trichophrya ictaluri	Central United States	Channel catfish	Gills	Direct contact with organism in water	Rare	Possible syn. *Trichophrya piscium*. Pathologic effects unknown	Davis 1947b, Hoffman 1967a
Trichophrya sp.	United States	Brook trout	Gills	Direct contact with organism in water	Rare	Possible syn. *Trichophrya piscium*. Pathologic effects unknown	Davis 1947b, Hoffman 1967a

REFERENCES

Anthony, J. D. 1969. Temperature effect on the distribution of *Gyrodactylus elegans* on goldfish. Bull. Wildlife Dis. Assoc. 5: 44–47.

Bauer, O. N. 1958. Biologie und Bekämpfung von *Ichthyophthirius multifiliis* Fouquet. Z. Fischerei 7:575–81.

———. 1959. The ecology of parasites of freshwater fish (in Russian). Izv. Gos. Nauchn. Issled. Inst. Ozern. i Rechn. Rybn. Khoz. 49:5–206. (Translated edition: 1962. U.S. Dept. Commerce, Office Tech. Serv. TT61-31056. 236 pp.)

Bauer, O. N., and N. P. Nikolskaya. 1957. *Chilodonella cyprini* (Moroff, 1902), its biology and epizootiologic importance (in Russian) Izv. Vses. Nauchn. Issled. Inst. Ozern. i Rechn. Rybn. Khoz. 42:53–66.

Becker, C. D., and M. Katz. 1965. Infections of the hemoflagellate, *Cryptobia salmositica* Katz, 1951, in freshwater teleosts of the Pacific Coast. Trans. Am. Fisheries Soc. 94:327–33.

Bogdanova, E. A. 1968. Modern data on the distribution and biology of *Myxosoma cerebralis* (Protozoa, Cnidosporidia) as agent of whirling disease of salmonids. Bull. Office Intern. Epizootiol. 69:1499–1506.

Bond, F. F. 1937. A microsporidian infection of *Fundulus heteroclitis* (Linn.). J. Parasitol. 23:229–30.

Bykhovskaya–Pavlovskaya, Irina E., A. V. Gusev, M. N. Dubinina, N. A. Izyumova, T. S. Smirnova, I. L. Sokolovskaya, G. A. Shtein, S. S. Shul'man, and V. M. Epshtein. 1962. Key to parasites of freshwater fish of the U.S.S.R. (in Russian). Zool. Inst. Akad. Nauk SSSR, Moscow-Leningrad. (Translated edition: 1964. U.S. Dept. Commerce, Office Tech. Serv. TT64-11040. 919 pp.)

Clemens, H. P. 1958. The chemical control of some diseases and parasites of channel catfish. Progressive Fish-Culturist 20:8–15.

Davis, H. S. 1926a. *Schizamoeba salmonis*, a new ameba parasitic in salmonid fishes. Bull. Bur. Fish. 42:1–8.

———. 1926b. *Octomitus salmonis,* a parasitic flagellate of trout. Bull. Bur. Fish. 42: 9–26.

———. 1947a. Care and diseases of trout. U.S. Fish Wildlife Serv. Res. Rept. 12. 98 pp.

———. 1947b. Studies of the protozoan parasites of fresh-water fishes. U.S. Fish Wildlife Serv. Fishery Bull. 41. 29 pp.

———. 1953. Culture and diseases of game fishes. Univ. California Press, Berkeley. 332 pp.

Dempster, R. P. 1955. The use of copper sulfate as a cure for fish diseases caused by parasitic dinoflagellates of the genus *Oodinium*. Zoologica 40:133–38.

Duijn, C. van, Jr. 1967. Diseases of fishes. 2d ed. Iliffe Books, London. 309 pp.

Elkan, E. 1962. *Dermocystidium gasterostei* n. sp., a parasite of *Gasterosteus aculeatus* L. and *Gasterosteus pungitus* L. Nature 196: 958–60.

Elson, K. G. R. 1969. Whirling disease in trout. Nature 223:968.

Geibel, G. E., and P. J. Murray. 1961. Channel catfish culture in California. Progressive Fish-Culturist 23:99–105.

Hoffman, G. L. 1965. *Eimeria aurati* n. sp. (Protozoa: Eimeriidae) from goldfish *(Carassius auratus)* in North America. J. Protozool. 12:273–75.

———. 1967a. Parasites of North American freshwater fishes. Univ. California Press, Berkeley. 486 pp.

———. 1967b. An unusual case of fish disease caused by *Ophryoglena* sp. (Protozoa: Hymenostomatida). Bull. Wildlife Dis. Assoc. 3:111–12.

———. 1970. Control and treatment of parasitic diseases of freshwater fishes. U.S. Bureau Sport Fish. Wildlife. Fish Disease Leaflet 28. 7 pp.

Hoffman, G. L., C. E. Dunbar, and A. Bradford. 1962. Whirling disease of trouts caused by *Myxosoma cerebralis* in the United States. U.S. Fish. Wildlife Serv. Spec. Sci. Rept. Fisheries 427.

Hoffman, G. L., and R. E. Putz. 1969. Host susceptibility and the effect of aging, freezing, heat, and chemicals on spores of *Myxosoma cerebralis*. Progressive Fish-Culturist 31:35–37.

Hoffman, G. L., R. E. Putz, and C. E. Dunbar. 1965. Studies on *Myxosoma cartilaginis* n. sp. (Protozoa: Myxosporidea) of centrarchid fish and a synopsis of the *Myxosoma* of North American freshwater fishes. J. Protozool. 12:319–32.

Hoffman, G. L., and C. J. Sindermann. 1962. Common parasites of fishes. U.S. Fish Wildlife Serv. Circ. 144. 17 pp.

Jacobs, D. L. 1946. A new parasitic dinoflagellate from fresh-water fish. Trans. Am. Microscop. Soc. 65:1–17.

Kraneveld, F. C., and H. J. W. Keidel. 1969. Bloedparasieten bij vissen in Nederland: II. Cryptobia/Trypanoplasma-infecties bij karpersoorten. Tijdschr. Diergeneesk. 94: 297–307.

Kudo, R. R. 1920. Studies on Myxosporidia:

A synopsis of genera and species of Myxosporidia. Illinois Biol. Monographs 5:239–503.

———. 1930. Myxosporidia, pp. 303–24. *In* R. Hegner and J. Andrews, eds. Problems and methods of research in protozoology. Macmillan, New York.

———. 1966. Protozoology. 5th ed. Charles C Thomas, Springfield, Ill. 1174 pp.

Levine, N. D. 1961. Protozoan parasites of domestic animals and of man. Burgess, Minneapolis. 412 pp.

Lom, J. 1958. A contribution to the systematics and morphology of endoparasitic trichodinids from Amphibians, with a proposal of uniform specific characteristics. J. Protozool. 5:251–63.

———. 1969. Cold-blooded vertebrate immunity to protozoa, pp. 249–65. *In* G. J. Jackson, R. Herman, and I. Singer, eds. Immunity to parasitic animals. Appleton-Century-Crofts, New York.

———. 1970. Observations on trichodinid ciliates from freshwater fishes. Arch. Protistenk. 112:153–77.

Marinček, Magdalena. 1965. Coccidial infection in carp. Arch. Biol. Sci. 17:57–64.

Mawdesley-Thomas, L. E., and D. W. Jolly. 1967. Diseases of fish: II. The goldfish *(Carassius auratus)*. J. Small Animal Pract. 8:533–41.

McElwain, I. V., and G. Post. 1968. Efficacy of cyzine for trout hexamitiasis. Progressive Fish-Culturist 30:84–91.

Meyer, F. P. 1966. Parasites of freshwater fishes: IV. Miscellaneous. 6. Parasites of catfishes. U.S. Bureau Sport Fish. Wildlife. Fish Disease Leaflet 5. 7 pp.

———. 1969. Parasites of freshwater fishes: II. Protozoa. 3. *Ichthyophthirius multifilis*. U.S. Bureau Sport Fish. Wildlife. Fish Disease Leaflet 2. 4 pp.

Mitchell, L. G. 1967. *Myxidium macrocheili* n. sp. (Cnidospora: Myxidiidae) from the largescale sucker *Catostomus macrocheilus* Girard, and a synopsis of the *Myxidium* of North American freshwater vertebrates. J. Protozool. 14:415–24.

Musselius, V. A., and J. A. Strelkov. 1968. Diseases and control measures for fishes of Far-East Complex in farms of the U.S.S.R. Bull. Office Intern. Epizootiol. 69:1603–11.

Olsen, O. W. 1967. Animal parasites: Their biology and life cycles. 2d ed. Burgess, Minneapolis. 431 pp.

Patterson, E. E. 1950. Effects of acriflavine on birth rate. Aquarium J. 21 (2):36.

Putz, R. E., G. L. Hoffman, and C. E. Dunbar. 1965. Two new species of *Plistophora* (Microsporidea) from North American fish with a synopsis of Microsporidea of freshwater and euryhaline fishes. J. Protozool. 12:228–36.

Reichenbach–Klinke, H., and E. Elkan. 1965. The principal diseases of lower vertebrates. Academic Press, New York. 600 pp.

Roberts, R. J., and K. G. R. Elson. 1970. An outbreak of whirling disease in rainbow trout. Vet. Record 86:258–59.

Sanders, J. E., and J. L. Fryer. 1970. Occurrence of the myxosporidan parasite *Myxidium minteri* in salmonid fish. J. Protozool. 17:354–57.

Schubert, G. 1968. The injurious effects of *Costia necatrix*. Bull. Office Intern. Epizootiol. 69:1171–78.

Sindermann, C. J. 1966. Diseases of marine fishes. Advan. Marine Biol. 4:1-89.

Snieszko, S. F., and G. L. Hoffman. 1963. Control of fish diseases. Lab. Animal Care 13: 197–206.

Swezy, Olive. 1919. The occurrence of *Trypanoplasma* as an ectoparasite. Trans. Am. Microscop. Soc. 38:20–24.

Tavolga, W. N., and R. F. Nigrelli. 1947. Studies on *Costia necatrix* (Henneguy). Trans. Am. Microscop. Soc. 66:366–78.

Uzmann, J. R., and J. W. Jesse. 1963. The *Hexamita* (=*Octomitus*) problem: A preliminary report. Progressive Fish-Culturist 25:141–43.

Wales, J. H., and H. Wolf. 1955. Three protozoan diseases of trout in California. Calif. Fish Game 41:183–87.

Walliker, D. 1966. The management and diseases of fish: III. Protozoal diseases of fish with special reference to those encountered in aquaria. J. Small Animal Pract. 7:799–807.

Wellborn, T. L., Jr. 1967. *Trichodina* (Ciliata: Urceolariidae) of freshwater fishes of the Southeastern United States. J. Protozool. 14:399–412.

Wenrich, D. H. 1931. A trypanoplasm on the gills of carp from the Schuylkill River. J. Parasitol. 18:133.

Wenyon, C. M. 1926. Protozoology: A manual for medical men, veterinarians and zoologists. 2 vol. Hafner, New York.

Yasutake, W. T., D. R. Buhler, and W. E. Shanks. 1961. Chemotherapy of hexamitiasis in fish. J. Parasitol. 47:81–86.

Yasutake, W. T., and E. M. Wood. 1957. Some myxosporidia found in Pacific Northwest salmonids. J. Parasitol. 43:633–42.

Chapter 22

HELMINTHS and LEECHES

NUMEROUS helminths and several leeches are parasitic to fishes in nature (Amlacher 1961; Bykhovskaya-Pavlovskaya et al. 1962; Dogiel, Petrushevski, and Polyanski 1958; van Duijn 1967; Hoffman 1967; Reichenbach-Klinke 1966; Reichenbach-Klinke and Elkan 1965; Schäperclaus 1954; Sindermann 1970). Many have complicated life cycles with two or more intermediate hosts. Under aquarium or hatchery conditions, these life cycles are readily broken by elimination of the intermediate host. Nevertheless, certain helminths are a problem in cultured fishes, and all of these parasites must be considered when fishes are acquired from their natural environment.

Although helminths are often numerous in fishes in their natural environment, serious pathologic effects are uncommon. In the laboratory, however, crowding, inadequate oxygen, malnutrition, or other adverse conditions sometimes occur. When this happens, the pathologic effects are increased and a high mortality often results.

MONOGENETIC TREMATODES

Monogenetic trematodes are small parasites which have a direct life cycle involving a single host (Bykhovskaya-Pavlovskaya et al. 1962; Hoffman 1967; Sproston 1946; Yamaguti 1963). Species identification is

sometimes difficult, but it is aided by the fact that many monogenetic trematodes are host-specific. Identification is generally based on the morphology of the haptor, which is the primary organ of attachment. Immature forms usually resemble adults.

Except for one genus which occurs in the urinary tract, the monogenetic trematodes affecting fishes occur as ectoparasites on the gills, body, and fins. They feed on mucus, epithelium, and sometimes blood. Some species are important pathogens in hatchery- or aquarium-raised fishes, extensively damaging the gill filaments and skin and sometimes causing death.

Monogenetic trematodes that affect laboratory fishes are listed in Table 22.1. The most important are discussed below.

Gyrodactylus

Gyrodactylus, which occurs on the skin and gills of fishes throughout the world, is one of the commonest and most pathogenic parasites of laboratory fishes (Anthony 1969; van Duijn 1967; Hoffman and Putz 1964; Malmberg 1970; Reichenbach-Klinke and Elkan 1965). Most species are host-specific, there being a species of Gyrodactylus for almost every species of fish. This trematode is not only common on laboratory fishes obtained from their natural habitat but it is

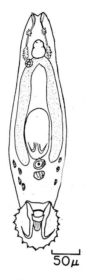

FIG. 22.1. *Gyrodactylus* adult. Note absence of eye spots and presence of embryo or larva. (From Hoffman 1967. Courtesy of University of California Press.)

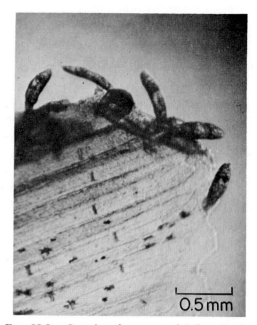

FIG. 22.2. *Gyrodactylus* on caudal fin of rainbow trout. (Courtesy of G. Hoffman, Eastern Fish Disease Laboratory.)

also likely to be encountered on fishes obtained from hatcheries (Hoffman and Putz 1964). Some species do not survive under laboratory conditions while others reproduce rapidly and cause severe pathologic effects.

MORPHOLOGY

The adult (Fig. 22.1) is a small, elongated parasite, measuring about 250 to 600 μ by 40 to 115 μ (Bykhovskaya-Pavlovskaya et al. 1962; Hoffman 1967). The posterior organ of attachment (haptor) is well developed and bears one pair of large anchors and 16 marginal hooklets. Eye spots are absent; a larva is usually present within the adult.

LIFE CYCLE

All species are viviparous, and the larva is born complete with anchors (Bykhovski 1957). The life cycle is direct, and the larva often attaches to the same host as the parent. The total time required for a complete life cycle is unknown for most species; for *G. bullatarudis* it is 60 hours (Turnbull 1956).

PATHOLOGIC EFFECTS

Gyrodactylus often occurs on the fins, body, and gills in large numbers (Fig. 22.2) (Hoffman and Putz 1964) and ingests mucus and epithelium from the body surface and sometimes blood from the superficial capillaries (Cheng 1964; Hoffman 1967). It apparently causes severe irritation since affected fish scrape their sides on the bottom of the aquarium (Davis 1953). Other signs of infestation include paleness, frayed fins, listlessness, emaciation, superficial petechial hemorrhages, a blue, slimy mucus covering the skin and gills, increased respiratory rate, asphyxiation, and death (Cheng 1964; van Duijn 1967).

DIAGNOSIS

Diagnosis is based on the clinical signs and is confirmed by demonstration and identification of the parasite.

CONTROL

Changing the water daily or providing a rapid, continuous flow will help to reduce or eliminate this parasite (Snieszko and Hoffman 1963). Effective chemical treatments include formalin in the water at a rate of 200 to 250 ppm for 1 hour; potassium permanganate in the water at a rate of 0.1% for 30 to 40 seconds, 10 ppm for 5 to 30 minutes, or 1 to 2 ppm for prolonged periods; pyridylmercuric acetate in the water at a rate of 2 ppm for 1 hour (not recommended for rainbow and cutthroat trout); acriflavine in the water at a rate of 3 to 5 ppm for 1 to 4 hours; acetic acid in the water at a rate of 0.2% for 1 to 2 minutes (but not for more than 2.5 minutes); sodium chloride in the water at a rate of 1 to 3% for several minutes to 1 hour; and trichlorfon in the water at a rate of 2.0 to 3.5% for 2 to 3 minutes or 0.25 ppm for prolonged periods (van Duijn 1967; F. Meyer 1968; Snieszko and Hoffman 1963).

PUBLIC HEALTH CONSIDERATIONS

This parasite does not affect man.

Dactylogyrus

Dactylogyrus occurs on the gills of goldfish, carp, and other fishes (Hoffman 1967). It is common throughout the world and is likely to be encountered not only on laboratory fishes obtained from their natural habitat but also on those obtained from hatcheries. Infestation of laboratory fishes with this parasite is even more dangerous than infestation with *Gyrodactylus* (van Duijn 1955).

MORPHOLOGY

The morphology is similar to that of *Gyrodactylus* except that the adult *Dactylogyrus* has eye spots and does not contain a larva (Fig. 22.3) (Hoffman 1967). It measures about 400 to 1,000 μ by 85 to 180 μ, depending on species.

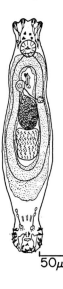

FIG. 22.3. *Dactylogyrus* adult. Note eye spots. (From Hoffman 1967. Courtesy of University of California Press.)

50μ

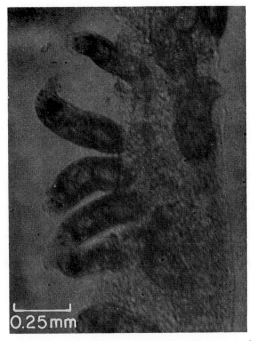

0.25mm

FIG. 22.4. *Dactylogyrus* on gill filament of minnow. (Courtesy of W. Rogers, Southeastern Cooperative Fish Disease Project, Auburn University.)

LIFE CYCLE

Dactylogyrus is oviparous. Its life cycle is direct and requires 1 to 5 days. Transmission is by direct contact with an infested fish or free-swimming larva.

PATHOLOGIC EFFECTS

The parasite attaches to the gills (Fig. 22.4). The number present and their effects increase with the age of the host (Noble and Noble 1961). Signs of infestation include increased respiratory rate, stretching of the gill covers, protrusion of gill filaments outside the covers, and an opaque mucus covering the gills (van Duijn 1967). Heavy infestations cause a high mortality (Bauer 1958; G. L. Hoffman, unpublished data). Microscopically, hypertrophy of the tips of the filaments is seen.

DIAGNOSIS

Diagnosis is based on the clinical signs and is confirmed by demonstration and identification of the parasite (van Duijn 1967).

CONTROL

Control is similar to that for *Gyrodactylus* (van Duijn 1967; F. Meyer 1968; Snieszko and Hoffman 1963). The formalin and trichlorfon treatments are particularly effective.

PUBLIC HEALTH CONSIDERATIONS

This trematode does not affect man.

ADULT DIGENETIC TREMATODES

The adults of many digenetic trematodes are endoparasites of fishes (Dawes 1946; Hoffman 1967; Van Cleave and Mueller 1934; Yamaguti 1958). The majority occur in the gastrointestinal tract and most, apparently, are not serious pathogens. A few species parasitize the body cavity but these do not occur in the usual laboratory fishes. One genus, *Sanguinicola*, which is found in the blood vessels, is an important pathogen in hatchery-raised fishes.

Adult digenetic trematodes that affect laboratory fishes are listed in Table 22.2. The most important are described below.

Sanguinicola

Members of this genus occur in the blood vessels of several species of fishes. *Sanguinicola davisi* is common in the rainbow trout in western United States, *S. huronis* is common in black bass in central United States, and *S. inermis* and *S. armata* are common in the carp in Europe (Dawes 1946; van Duijn 1967; Hoffman 1967; Reichenbach-Klinke and Elkan 1965; Wales 1958; Yamaguti 1958). Although these flukes are not likely to occur in laboratory fishes raised in aquariums, they could be encountered in fishes obtained from their natural habitat and from some hatcheries.

MORPHOLOGY

The adult is lanceolate and has a finely striated or denticulated margin and a variable size, up to 1.0 mm in length by 0.3 mm in width (Fig. 22.5) (Dawes 1946; Hoffman 1967). Suckers are absent. The intestine is short, X-shaped, and consists of four to six lobes. The testes are arranged medially in two rows between the ovary and intestine. The ovary is divided into two lobes and is

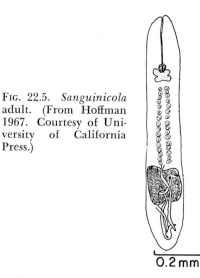

Fig. 22.5. *Sanguinicola* adult. (From Hoffman 1967. Courtesy of University of California Press.)

0.2 mm

situated in the posterior one-third of the body. The egg measures 30 to 70 μ in length and usually contains a ciliated miracidium that possesses an eyespot.

LIFE CYCLE

The adult occurs in the cardiovascular system, primarily in the main gill arteries, heart, and renal veins (Dawes 1946; van Duijn 1967; Hoffman 1967; Wales 1958). Eggs are carried in the bloodstream and lodge in capillaries of the gills and other organs, where they hatch. Miracidia pass out of the fish through the gills and invade the intermediate host, a snail. Cercariae develop in the snail, are released, penetrate a fish, and develop into adults. The longevity of adults in the fish is at least 4 months.

PATHOLOGIC EFFECTS

Eggs and migrating miracidia produce hemorrhages and embolisms, particularly in the gills (van Duijn 1967; Hoffman 1967; Wales 1958). In heavy infections the gill filaments are pale, flaccid, and sometimes so filled with eggs that the total gill volume appears to consist of fluke eggs. When such large numbers of eggs hatch at one time, it is probable that the trauma and blood loss cause death.

DIAGNOSIS

Diagnosis is usually based on recognition of the eggs and miracidia in the branchial blood vessels. Demonstration of the adult fluke is more difficult and is accomplished by stripping possibly infected veins in a physiologic saline solution under a dissecting microscope.

CONTROL

Because of the need for a snail intermediate host, completion of the life cycle in the laboratory is unlikely, and no specific control measures are necessary. Treatment is unknown (van Duijn 1967).

PUBLIC HEALTH CONSIDERATIONS

Sanguinicola does not affect man.

Crepidostomum

Species of *Crepidostomum* are common in the intestine of the carp, other cyprinids, bluegill, sunfishes, lake trout, rainbow trout, brown trout, Atlantic salmon, other salmonids, channel catfish, eels, and other fishes in North America and Europe (Dawes 1946; Dogiel, Polyanski, and Kheisin 1962; Hoffman 1967; Yamaguti 1958). Although these flukes are not likely to be encountered in laboratory fishes raised in aquariums, they could be encountered in fishes obtained from their natural habitat or from some hatcheries. A 100% incidence of *C. farionis* has been reported in hatchery-raised golden trout *(Salmo aquabonita)* in western United States (Mitchum and Moore 1969).

MORPHOLOGY

The adult is oval, usually elongated, measures about 1 to 2 mm in length and has two to six papillae located anterodorsally on the head (Fig. 22.6) (Hoffman 1967; Noble and Noble 1961; Olsen 1967). The oral sucker is terminal and the ventral sucker is in the anterior half of the body. The pharynx is well developed, the esophagus is short to moderate, and the ceca terminate at the posterior end. Usually two, but sometimes four, testes arranged in tandem are in the posterior half of the body. The ovary is anterior to the testes. Eggs are oval and unembryonated.

LIFE CYCLE

The life cycle requires a clam as the first intermediate host and either a mayfly

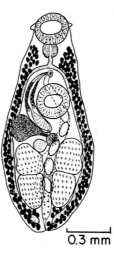

FIG. 22.6. *Crepidostomum* adult. (From Hoffman 1967. Courtesy of University of California Press.)

0.3 mm

or other aquatic insect or a crayfish or other crustacean as the second intermediate host (Hoffman 1967; Olsen 1967). The adult in the fish's intestine deposits unembryonated eggs which begin development in water when passed in the feces. The eggs hatch, releasing miracidia which enter a clam and develop into cercariae. The cercariae escape, penetrate an insect nymph or crustacean, and encyst. Fishes are infected by ingesting metacercariae encysted in the second intermediate host.

PATHOLOGIC EFFECTS

Heavy infection sometimes causes severe intestinal inflammation and death (Mitchum and Moore 1969). Otherwise, the pathologic effects are unknown.

DIAGNOSIS

Diagnosis is based on identification of the eggs in the feces or the adult worm in the intestine at necropsy.

CONTROL

Because a clam is necessary as the first intermediate host and an arthropod as the second intermediate host, completion of the life cycle is unlikely in the laboratory, and no specific control measures are necessary. Oral administration of dibutyltin oxide, at a rate of 150 mg per kg of body weight daily for 3 days, is an effective treatment (Mitchum and Moore 1969).

Crepidostomum does not affect man.

LARVAL DIGENETIC TREMATODES

Fishes are the second intermediate host of certain trematodes which infect mammals, birds, reptiles, and other fishes (Dawes 1946; Hoffman 1960, 1967; Van Cleave and Mueller 1934; Yamaguti 1958). The first intermediate host is a mollusk, usually a snail, in which cercariae are produced. These cercariae are free-swimming and actively penetrate the fish epidermis. They migrate through the tissues, encyst, and develop into metacercariae. Their pathologic effects depend on their number and the tissues they invade. Extensive mechanical damage and hemorrhage are often produced during the migrating phase, but once encysted, they usually produce little effect unless present in such large numbers that they interfere with physiologic functions (Burton 1956; Hoffman 1958a, 1967; G. L. Hoffman, unpublished data).

Laboratory fishes obtained from their natural habitat or from hatcheries with snails present are often infected; fishes obtained from hatcheries free of snails are not infected (Hoffman 1967).

Larval digenetic trematodes that affect laboratory fishes are listed in Table 22.3. The most important are discussed below.

Diplostomum spathaceum

(PROBABLE SYN. *Diplostomum flexicaudum,
Diplostomum huronense*)

The larva of this diplostomatid trematode localizes in the lens or vitreous body of the eye of many fishes, often causing blindness (Ashton, Brown, and Easty 1969; van Duijn 1967; Hoffman 1960, 1967; Reichenbach-Klinke and Elkan 1965). The European form, *Diplostomum spathaceum*, is common in the goldfish, carp, European minnow, black bass, rainbow trout, brown trout, Atlantic salmon, sticklebacks, and eels. In the United States, *D. flexicaudum*, which is thought to be identical with *D. spathaceum*, is common in black bass and other fishes. *Diplostomum huronense*, which occurs in the bluegill, sunfishes, and other fishes in north central United States, is also thought to be a synonym of *D. spathaceum*. Laboratory fishes obtained from

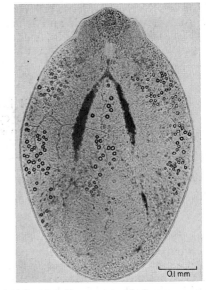

FIG. 22.7. *Diplostomum spathaceum* metacercaria. Note calcareous corpuscles in reserve excretory system. (From Ashton, Brown, and Easty 1969. Courtesy of Pergamon Press.)

their natural habitat or from hatcheries with snails present are likely to be infected. Fishes obtained from hatcheries free of snails or from those in which birds are prevented access are not infected (Bregnballe 1963).

MORPHOLOGY

The metacercaria, the form found in fishes, is about 0.5 to 0.9 mm long by 0.4 mm wide (Fig. 22.7) (Hoffman 1960, 1967). It has a concave foliaceous forebody, a small concave hindbody, a reserve excretory system containing calcareous corpuscles at the ends of the small branches, and two lateral pseudosuckers near the oral sucker.

LIFE CYCLE

Eggs are passed in the feces of a definitive host (gull or pelican) (Skrjabin 1964); those that enter water hatch in about 3 weeks, releasing free-swimming miracidia which invade the first intermediate host, a snail. Sporocysts and daughter sporocysts are formed and, after about 6 weeks, thousands of free-swimming cercariae are released. The cercariae penetrate the epider-

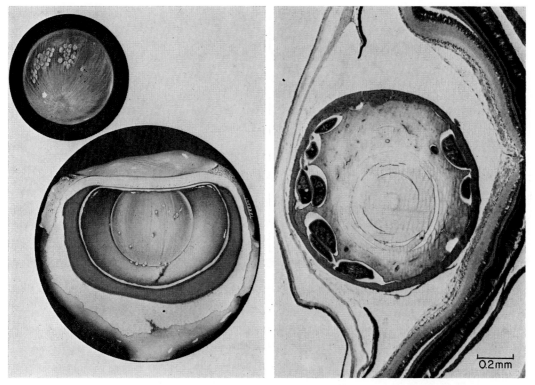

FIG. 22.8. *Diplostomum spathaceum* metacercariae in lens. *(Left)* Painting of open eye of a trout showing metacercariae entering lens capsule; *inset* shows metacercariae in lens cortex. *(Right)* Section of eye of guppy showing metacercariae in lens cortex. (From Ashton, Brown, and Easty 1969. Courtesy of Pergamon Press.)

mis of the fish and migrate to the eye. The definitive host is infected by ingesting an infected fish; the entire life cycle takes about 3 months.

PATHOLOGIC EFFECTS

Heavy infections cause blindness (Reichenbach-Klinke and Elkan 1965). Initially the metacercariae are visible as small white dots against the dark background of the pupil (Fig. 22.8) (van Duijn 1967). Later as the pathologic effects progress, the eye becomes completely white, the lens becomes opaque and flaccid, and the cortical substance liquefies (Ferguson 1943). Fluid accumulates in the eye, intraocular pressure increases, and eventually the cornea ruptures. Secondary bacterial or mycotic infection and death are common.

Microscopic lesions of the lens include larvae in the cortex (Fig. 22.8) and disruptions in the posterior capsule with herniation of lenticular material (Ashton, Brown, and Easty 1969; Larson 1965). A neoplastic-like proliferation of lens epithelium occurs adjacent to larvae after 2 to 3 weeks.

DIAGNOSIS

Diagnosis is based on the clinical signs and is confirmed by the demonstration and identification of the parasite.

CONTROL

Because a fish-eating bird is needed as a definitive host and a mollusk as a first intermediate host, it is unlikely that the life cycle would be completed in the laboratory, and no specific control measures are necessary.

Surgical treatment of individual fish by

lancing the eye and applying a disinfectant has been described (van Duijn 1967).

PUBLIC HEALTH CONSIDERATIONS

Although there is a remote possibility that the cercaria of this parasite can affect man (Ferguson 1943), the metacercaria (the stage found in fishes) is not infectious for man.

Uvulifer ambloplitis,
Crassiphiala bulboglossa,
Posthodiplostomum cuticola

(Blackspot *Neascus*)

Larvae of these diplostomatid flukes cause pigmented cysts in the skin and sometimes in the gills and muscle (Hoffman 1960; Yamaguti 1958). *Uvulifer ambloplitis* is common in the United States and Canada in the fathead minnow, bluntnose minnow, chubs, shiners, golden shiner, other cyprinids, sunfishes, and other centrarchids. *Crassiphiala bulboglossa* is common in northern United States in the fathead minnow, chubs, shiners, golden shiner, other cyprinids, killifishes, and other fishes. *Posthodiplostomum cuticola* is common in Eu-

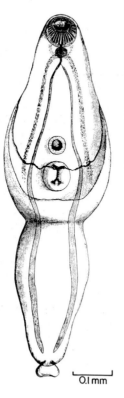

FIG. 22.9. *Uvulifer ambloplitis* metacercaria. (From Hughes 1927.)

0.1 mm

rope and occurs in the goldfish, sticklebacks, and other fishes (Hoffman 1960; Reichenbach-Klinke and Elkan 1965). These larvae are likely to be encountered in laboratory fishes obtained from their natural habitat or from hatcheries with snails present, but they do not occur in fishes obtained from hatcheries free of snails.

MORPHOLOGY

The metacercariae of these trematodes are of the *Neascus* type (Fig. 22.9) (Hoffman 1960, 1967). They have a concave, foliaceous forebody, a well-developed hindbody, a reserve excretory system with calcareous granules not confined to the ends of the small branches, and no lateral pseudosuckers. The forebody of *U. ambloplitis* is 0.22 to 0.67 mm long by 0.15 to 0.23 mm wide; the hindbody is 0.19 to 0.68 mm long by 0.07 to 0.19 mm wide. The metacercaria of *C. bulboglossa* is 0.31 to 0.40 mm long by 0.13 to 0.17 mm wide and that of *P. cuticola*, 0.73 to 1.98 mm long by 0.39 to 0.66 mm wide.

LIFE CYCLE

The life cycle of these species involves a fish-eating bird (kingfisher or heron) as a definitive host and a snail as a first intermediate host (Hoffman 1960). Cercariae released from the snail penetrate the epidermis of the fish, where they develop into metacercariae. The definitive host becomes infected by ingesting an infected fish.

PATHOLOGIC EFFECTS

Infection with larvae of these trematodes causes a host response that results in the formation of small brown or black spots, 0.8 to 3.8 mm in diameter, on the body and fins (Fig. 22.10) (van Duijn 1967; Hoffman and Sindermann 1962). In microscopic section, these cysts are seen to contain larval trematodes. In small numbers, the parasites apparently cause little discomfort, but massive infections cause death (Hoffman 1956, 1958b; Krull 1934).

DIAGNOSIS

Diagnosis is based on the characteristic lesions and on demonstration and identification of the parasite. The living, slowly

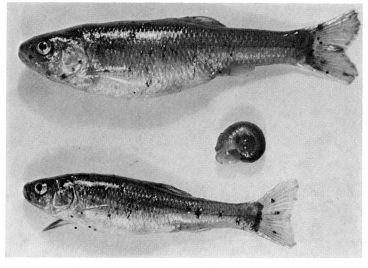

FIG. 22.10. *Crassiphiala bulboglossa* metacercariae (blackspot *Neascus*) in skin of bluntnose minnow. (Courtesy of G. Hoffman, Eastern Fish Disease Laboratory.)

moving larva is readily seen with the aid of a dissecting microscope.

CONTROL

Because a fish-eating bird is necessary as a definitive host and a mollusk as a first intermediate host, it is unlikely that the life cycle would be completed in the laboratory, and isolation of affected fish and similar control measures are unnecessary.

PUBLIC HEALTH CONSIDERATIONS

These trematodes are not known to affect man.

Posthodiplostomum minimum

(White Grub)

The larva of this diplostomatid trematode causes the formation of a nonpigmented cyst in the mesentery, kidneys, liver, pericardium, and spleen (Hoffman 1960; Spall and Summerfelt 1969). It is very common throughout the United States and Canada and frequently occurs in large numbers in the fathead minnow, bluntnose minnow, chubs, shiners, golden shiner, topminnows, mollies, mosquitofish, bluegill, sunfishes, black bass, brook trout, channel catfish, sticklebacks, and other fishes (Hoffman 1960, 1967; Lewis and Nickum 1964; Spall and Summerfelt 1969; Yamaguti 1958). It is likely to be encountered in laboratory fishes obtained from their natural habitat or from hatcheries with snails present; it is

not found in fishes obtained from hatcheries free of snails.

MORPHOLOGY

The metacercaria is of the *Neascus* type (Fig. 22.11) (Hoffman 1960, 1967). It measures 0.91 to 2.24 mm in length, has a distinct forebody which is 0.52 to 0.89 mm in length by 0.30 to 0.42 mm in width, and has a conical to spheroidal hindbody.

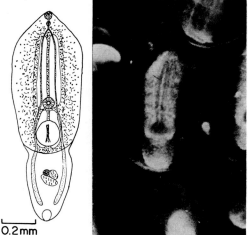

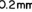
0.2mm

FIG. 22.11. *Posthodiplostomum minimum* metacercaria. (*Left* from Hoffman 1967; courtesy of University of California Press. *Right* courtesy of G. Hoffman, Eastern Fish Disease Laboratory.)

LIFE CYCLE

Eggs are passed in the feces of a definitive host (heron); those that reach water hatch into free-swimming miracidia in about 10 days and must penetrate an appropriate snail to continue their development (Hoffman 1958b). In the snail they grow into sporocysts which produce daughter sporocysts. After about 45 days, thousands of free-swimming cercariae are released. These penetrate the fish, migrate through the tissues, and after about 1 month, develop into the typical cysts. The definitive host is infected by ingesting an affected fish. The entire life cycle takes about 3 months.

PATHOLOGIC EFFECTS

The cysts produced by larvae of this trematode are white and about 1 mm in diameter (Hoffman 1958b; Lewis and Nickum 1964; Spall and Summerfelt 1969). Their pathologic effects are uncertain but depend to a large extent on the number involved and the rate of infection. Although heavy experimental infections cause death (Hoffman 1958b), the slower accumulation of the cysts in natural infections is not usually fatal.

DIAGNOSIS

Diagnosis is based on the lesions and on demonstration and identification of the parasite.

CONTROL

Because of the need for a fish-eating bird as the definitive host and a mollusk as the first intermediate host, it is unlikely that the life cycle would be completed in the laboratory. No specific control measures are necessary, and no treatment has been reported.

PUBLIC HEALTH CONSIDERATIONS

This trematode does not affect man.

Clinostomum marginatum, *Clinostomum complanatum*

(Yellow Grub)

The larvae of these trematodes cause the formation of large, unsightly yellow cysts in the muscle, connective tissue, and

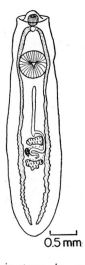

FIG. 22.12.   *Clinostomum marginatum* metacercaria. (From Hoffman 1967. Courtesy of University of California Press.)

gills. *Clinostomum marginatum* is common in North America; it affects the bluntnose minnow, chubs, shiners, killifishes, bluegill, sunfishes, black bass, brook trout, rainbow trout, and other fishes (Hoffman 1967; Yamaguti 1958). *Clinostomum complanatum* is less common; it occurs in the goldfish and other fishes in eastern Europe and southern Asia (van Duijn 1967; Reichenbach-Klinke and Elkan 1965). Laboratory fishes obtained from their natural habitat are likely to be infected. Infection is also common in North American laboratory fishes obtained from hatcheries with snails present, but it does not occur in fishes obtained from hatcheries free of snails.

MORPHOLOGY

The metacercariae of these species are 1.5 to 6.5 mm in length and 1.0 to 2.0 mm in width (Fig. 22.12) (van Duijn 1967; Reichenbach-Klinke and Elkan 1965). They have a stout body, an oral sucker surrounded by a collarlike fold, and a large ventral sucker in the anterior one-third of the body, but lack a typical pharynx (Hoffman 1967).

LIFE CYCLE

The life cycle involves a fish-eating bird (heron) as a definitive host and a snail as a first intermediate host (van Duijn 1967; Hoffman 1967; Reichenbach-Klinke and Elkan 1965). Cercariae released from the snail penetrate the epidermis of the fish, migrate through the tissues, and devel-

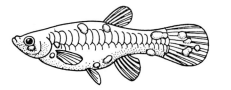

FIG. 22.13. Fish infected with *Clinostomum complanatum* metacercariae (yellow grub). (From van Duijn 1967. Courtesy of C. van Duijn, Jr. and Iliffe Books.)

op into metacercariae. The definitive host is infected by ingesting an infected fish.

PATHOLOGIC EFFECTS

Infection with larvae of these trematodes causes the formation of typical cysts (Fig. 22.13) (van Duijn 1967; Hoffman 1967; Hoffman and Sindermann 1962; Reichenbach-Klinke and Elkan 1965). The cysts are usually round or oval and vary in size from 1.0 to 2.5 mm, depending on their age. They require about 7 weeks to reach maximum size. Although usually yellow, white cysts sometimes occur. In light infections in large fishes, the presence of the parasite causes no apparent disability; however, in small fishes, in which the size of the parasite is large in relation to the size of the host (Fig. 22.14), the tissue displacement affects both the metabolism and mobility of the host.

DIAGNOSIS

Diagnosis is based on demonstration and identification of the parasite in the typical lesion.

CONTROL

Because of the complex life cycle involving a fish-eating bird as the definitive host and a mollusk as the first intermediate host, it is unlikely that the life cycle would be completed in the laboratory; consequently, affected fish need not be isolated, and no specific control measures are required.

Treatment of individual fish by incising the cysts, removing the parasites, and disinfecting the wound with merbromin (Mercurochrome, Hynson, Wescott, and Dunning) has been described (van Duijn 1967).

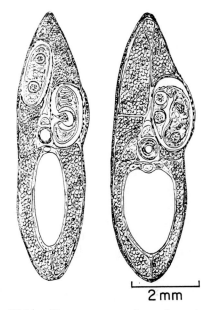

2 mm

FIG. 22.14. Transverse section through two fish affected with *Clinostomum* metacercariae (yellow grub). (From Reichenbach-Klinke and Elkan 1965. Courtesy of Academic Press.)

PUBLIC HEALTH CONSIDERATIONS

Although human infection with an unidentified species of *Clinostomum* has been reported in India and Japan (Cameron 1945), *C. marginatum* and *C. complanatum* are not known to affect man.

ADULT CESTODES

Cestodes have complicated life cycles which involve an arthropod intermediate host and sometimes a secondary vertebrate intermediate host (Hoffman 1967; Wardle and McLeod 1952; Yamaguti 1959). Fishes are often secondary intermediate hosts and also definitive hosts, sometimes for the same parasite. Although adult cestodes are common in fishes obtained from their natural habitat and are sometimes found in hatchery- or aquarium-raised fishes, little is known of their pathologic effects. Most are thought to cause little harm (van Duijn 1967).

Adult cestodes that affect laboratory fishes are listed in Table 22.4. The most important are described below.

Corallobothrium fimbriatum,
Corallobothrium giganteum

Adults of these proteocephalids are common in the intestine of the channel catfish and other ictalurids in the United States and other parts of North America (Essex 1927; Hoffman 1967; Spall and Summerfelt 1969; Yamaguti 1959). They are often numerous and are likely to be encountered in laboratory catfishes obtained from their natural habitat or from hatcheries that have stream or lake water sources.

MORPHOLOGY

The scolex (Fig. 22.15) is unarmed and has four suckers on the flat, anterior face (Essex 1927; Hoffman 1967). Body folds, sometimes called lappets, cover the suckers. The testes are in one layer between two ventral excretory stems, the ovary is posterior and intervitellarian and the genital

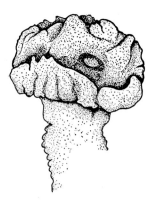

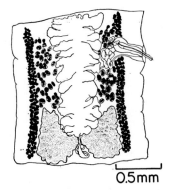

0.5mm

FIG. 22.15. *Corallobothrium.* (*Top*) Scolex. (*Bottom*) Mature proglottid. (From Essex 1927.)

pores are irregularly alternating. *Corallobothrium fimbriatum* reaches a maximum length of 80 mm; *C. giganteum* attains a length of 440 mm.

LIFE CYCLE

The life cycle involves a copepod and sometimes a small fish (Essex 1927; Hoffman 1967). Eggs passed in the feces of a catfish, when ingested by a copepod, develop into procercoid larvae. In *C. fimbriatum* and possibly in *C. giganteum,* a shiner or other small fish sometimes ingests an infected copepod. When this happens, the parasite migrates into the body cavity, ovaries, or muscle and develops to the plerocercoid larval stage but not to the adult. The catfish is infected by ingesting either an infected copepod or small fish.

PATHOLOGIC EFFECTS

Although the specific pathologic effects are unknown, the presence of these proteocephalids is probably harmful to the health of infected fish.

DIAGNOSIS

Diagnosis is based on identification of the eggs in the feces or the adult worms in the intestine at necropsy.

CONTROL

Because a copepod and sometimes a small fish are required as intermediate hosts, it is unlikely that the life cycle would be completed in the laboratory, and no specific control procedures are needed. Dibutyltin oxide, given orally at a rate of 250 mg per kg of body weight or 0.3% in the food for 1 day, is an effective treatment (Hoffman 1970; Mitchum and Moore 1969).

PUBLIC HEALTH CONSIDERATIONS

These cestodes are not known to affect man.

Proteocephalus

The adults of many species of this proteocephalid occur in the intestine of fishes sometimes used in the laboratory (Hoffman 1967; Spall and Summerfelt 1969; Wardle and McLeod 1952; Yamaguti 1959). Several species (Table 22.4) are common in North America and Europe and are likely to be encountered in laboratory fishes

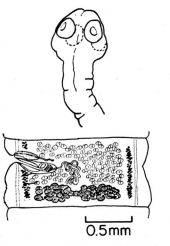

FIG. 22.16. *Proteocephalus ambloplitis.* *(Top)* Scolex. *(Bottom)* Mature proglottid. (From Hoffman 1967. Courtesy of University of California Press.)

obtained from their natural habitat in these regions.

MORPHOLOGY

The scolex is unarmed and has four and sometimes five suckers (Fig. 22.16) (Hoffman 1967; Wardle and McLeod 1952). Body folds do not cover the suckers. The testes are characteristically in a single, continuous field, but the size and other morphologic features vary widely with the species. *Proteocephalus ambloplitis* measures about 100 by 2 mm.

LIFE CYCLE

In some species, eggs passed in the feces of the definitive host develop into procercoid and plerocercoid larvae in copepods; in other species, the plerocercoid larvae develop in the body cavity of small fishes; but in most species the life cycle is unknown (Hoffman 1967). Presumably the definitive host becomes infected by ingesting either an infected copepod or small fish. In *P. ambloplitis,* plerocercoid larvae in the celom of a fish can penetrate the intestinal wall, enter the lumen, attach to the mucosa, and become adults (Fischer and Freeman 1969.)

PATHOLOGIC EFFECTS

The pathologic effects of the adults of this genus are unknown.

DIAGNOSIS

Diagnosis is based on identification of the eggs in the feces or the adult worms in the intestine at necropsy.

CONTROL

Because of the need for one or two intermediate hosts, it is unlikely that the life cycle would be completed in the laboratory, and no special control procedures are needed. Dibutyltin oxide, given orally at the rate of 0.3% in the food for 1 day, or kamala, given orally at the rate of 1.5 to 2.0% in the food for 2 weeks, is an effective treatment (van Duijn 1967; Snieszko and Hoffman 1963).

PUBLIC HEALTH CONSIDERATIONS

Proteocephalus is not known to affect man.

Eubothrium crassum, Eubothrium salvelini

Adults of these pseudophyllid cestodes are common in the pyloric ceca of salmonid fishes of North America and Europe (Hoffman 1967; Wardle and McLeod 1952; Yamaguti 1959). *Eubothrium crassum* occurs in the brook, rainbow, and brown trouts, Atlantic and Pacific salmons, and other fishes; *E. salvelini* occurs in the brook, rainbow, and lake trouts, Pacific salmons, and other fishes. Laboratory fishes obtained from their natural habitat or from hatcheries having stream or lake water supplies are likely to be infected.

MORPHOLOGY

The scolex has two simple bothria and no chitinoid hooks (Fig. 22.17) (Hoffman 1967; Wardle and McLeod 1952). The body is usually distinctly segmented and has dorsal and ventral median furrows. The cirrovaginal pore is marginal. *Eubothrium crassum* attains a maximum length of 120 to 600 mm and a width of 2.5 to 5.6 mm; *E. salvelini* reaches a length of 280 mm and a width of 2.25 mm. The eggs are nonoperculated.

LIFE CYCLE

Embryonated eggs passed in the feces of infected fishes develop into procercoid larvae in copepods (Hoffman 1967). No

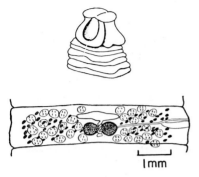

FIG. 22.17. *Eubothrium crassum.* *(Top)* Scolex. *(Bottom)* Mature proglottid. *(Top* from Wardle and McLeod 1952; courtesy of University of Minnesota Press. *Bottom* from Hoffman 1967; courtesy of University of California Press.)

second intermediate host is necessary, and the definitive host becomes infected by ingesting an infected copepod. Adult worms live for several years.

PATHOLOGIC EFFECTS

The pathologic effects are uncertain. Intestinal obstruction and decreased growth rate have been reported (Dogiel, Polyanski, and Kheisin 1962; Richardson 1936). It is also stated that fishes harboring worms up to 600 mm in length seemed as healthy as uninfected fishes (Wardle and McLeod 1952).

DIAGNOSIS

Diagnosis is based on identification of the eggs in the feces or the adult worms in the pyloric cecum at necropsy.

CONTROL

Because a copepod is needed as an intermediate host, it is unlikely that the life cycle would be completed in the laboratory, and no specific control measures are required. Dibutyltin oxide, given orally at a rate of 500 mg per kg of body weight in the food over a period of 3 days, is an effective treatment (Hnath 1970).

PUBLIC HEALTH CONSIDERATIONS

These cestodes are not known to affect man.

LARVAL CESTODES

Fishes are secondary intermediate hosts for some cestodes (Hoffman 1967; Wardle and McLeod 1952; Yamaguti 1959). Plerocercoid larvae of these cestodes occur in the muscles and viscera of the fish. The migration of these larvae, which range in size from less than a millimeter to several centimeters in length, sometimes causes extensive mechanical damage and adhesions and results in impaired metabolism, decreased reproductive capacity, and death (Hoffman 1967).

Larval cestodes that affect laboratory fishes are listed in Table 22.5. The most important are described below.

Proteocephalus ambloplitis
(Bass Tapeworm)

The plerocercoid larva of this proteocephalid cestode is frequently encountered in the viscera (especially gonads) of shiners, chubs, topminnows, killifishes, bluegill, sunfishes, black bass, rainbow trout, channel catfish, and other fishes of North America (Hoffman 1967; Yamaguti 1959). It is extremely pathogenic and often causes extensive tissue damage and sexual sterility. Laboratory fishes obtained from their natural habitat or from hatcheries having stream or lake water supplies are likely to be infected.

MORPHOLOGY

The plerocercoid larva (Fig. 22.18) is typically proteocephalid and is distinguished only by the presence of an apical, fifth, vestigial sucker (Wardle and McLeod 1952).

LIFE CYCLE

Eggs passed in the feces of the definitive host, usually a black bass, develop to the procercoid stage in copepods (Hoffman 1967; Wardle and McLeod 1952). The second intermediate host, a small fish in which the plerocercoid larva develops, is infected by ingestion of the infected copepod. The definitive host is usually infected by ingesting an infected small fish, but in the black bass the plerocercoid larva sometimes migrates from the viscera into the gut and matures (Fischer and Freeman 1969). Adults live in the intestine for about a year.

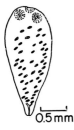

FIG. 22.18. *Proteocephalus ambloplitis,* plerocercoid larva. (From Hoffman 1967. Courtesy of University of California Press.)

0.5mm

PATHOLOGIC EFFECTS

The plerocercoid larva does not encyst but continues to migrate through the tissues, producing much damage (Hoffman 1967; Hoffman and Sindermann 1962; Wardle and McLeod 1952). Sometimes as many as 400 larvae are found in one fish. Extensive fibrosis and adhesions result, often causing gross distortions of the body (Fig. 22.19). The gonads, the organs most heavily affected, frequently become nonfunctional.

DIAGNOSIS

Diagnosis is based on identification of the parasite in the viscera of affected fish.

CONTROL

Because a copepod is necessary as an intermediate host, it is unlikely that the life cycle would be completed in the laboratory, and no special control procedures are needed. There is no treatment (van Duijn 1967; Snieszko and Hoffman 1963).

PUBLIC HEALTH CONSIDERATIONS

Proteocephalus ambloplitis does not affect man.

Diphyllobothrium cordiceps,
Diphyllobothrium sebago

The migration of the plerocercoid larvae of these diphyllobothriid cestodes often causes extensive tissue damage to salmonid fishes of North America (Hoffman 1967; Yamaguti 1959). *Diphyllobothrium cordiceps* is frequently encountered in the muscle, connective tissue, mesentery, liver, and spleen of the brook trout, rainbow trout, Pacific salmons, and other salmonids of western United States; *D. sebago* is frequently found in the viscera of the brook trout and other fishes in northeastern United States. Laboratory fishes obtained from their natural habitat or from hatcheries having stream or lake water supplies are likely to be infected.

MORPHOLOGY

The plerocercoid larvae, the stage of these cestodes found in fishes, are about 10 to 20 mm in length and 2 to 3 mm in width and have a wrinkled but nonsegmented strobila and an elongated scolex with two bothria but no hooks or tentacles (Fig. 22.20) (Hoffman 1967).

LIFE CYCLE

Eggs passed in the feces of the definitive host (fish-eating birds for *D. cordiceps* and fish-eating birds and mammals for *D. sebago*) develop into procercoid larvae in copepods (Hoffman 1967). The second intermediate host, a salmonid fish, becomes infected by ingesting an infected copepod, and the definitive host becomes infected by ingesting the infected fish. Eggs of *D. se-*

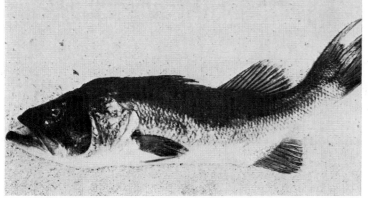

FIG. 22.19. *Proteocephalus ambloplitis* larval infection in black bass. Note gross distortion of body resulting from adhesions caused by migrating larvae. (Courtesy of G. Hoffman, Eastern Fish Disease Laboratory, and C. Johnson, North Carolina State University.)

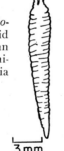

Fig. 22.20. *Diphyllobothrium,* plerocercoid larva. (From Hoffman 1967. Courtesy of University of California Press.)

3 mm

bago hatch in about 10 days and develop into procercoid larvae in about 13 days, into plerocercoid larvae in 3 to 5 months, depending on the temperature, and into adults in about 7 days (M. Meyer and Vik 1963). Presumably the time required for *D. cordiceps* is similar.

PATHOLOGIC EFFECTS

The plerocercoid larvae of these cestodes do not encyst but continue to migrate, causing hemorrhage, fibrosis, adhesions, emaciation, reduced fertility, and often death (Hoffman 1967).

DIAGNOSIS

Diagnosis is based on identification of the parasites in the viscera of affected fish.

CONTROL

Because a copepod is necessary as intermediate host, it is unlikely that the life cycles would be completed in the laboratory, and no special control procedures are needed. There is no treatment (van Duijn 1967; Snieszko and Hoffman 1963).

PUBLIC HEALTH CONSIDERATIONS

These diphyllobothriid cestodes do not affect man (Hoffman 1967).

Ligula intestinalis

The large and often highly pathogenic plerocercoid larva of this diphyllobothriid cestode is frequently encountered in the abdominal cavity of the goldfish, carp, European minnow, bluntnose minnow, fathead minnow, shiners, black bass, brook trout, rainbow trout, and other fishes in North America, Europe, and Asia (van Duijn 1967; Hoffman 1967; Reichenbach-Klinke

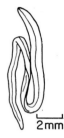

Fig. 22.21. *Ligula intestinalis,* plerocercoid larva. (From Hoffman 1967. Courtesy of University of California Press.)

2 mm

and Elkan 1965; Yamaguti 1959). Laboratory fishes obtained from their natural habitat or from hatcheries having stream or lake water supplies are likely to be infected.

MORPHOLOGY

The stage found in fishes, the plerocercoid larva, is 20 to 600 mm long (Fig. 22.21) (Wardle and McLeod 1952). It has a smooth, nonsegmented strobila with dorsoventral grooves and a blunt scolex with two indistinct bothria and no hooks.

LIFE CYCLE

Eggs passed in the feces of the definitive host, a fish-eating bird, develop to the procercoid stage in copepods (Hoffman 1967; Wardle and McLeod 1952). The second intermediate host, a fish, is infected by ingesting an infected copepod, and the definitive host is infected by ingesting an infected fish.

PATHOLOGIC EFFECTS

Signs of infection are abdominal distention and infertility (van Duijn 1967). The extent of the distention is dependent on the number of worms present and their size. In small, heavily parasitized fish the intraabdominal pressure often becomes so great that the body wall ruptures (Hoffman and Sindermann 1962). Short of this, the parasites cause compression of the abdominal organs, extensive proliferation of fibrous connective tissue, and almost complete obliteration of the gonads (Owen and Arme 1966; Reichenbach-Klinke and Elkan 1965). Death is common.

DIAGNOSIS

Diagnosis is based on the clinical signs and is confirmed by demonstration and identification of the parasite in the abdominal cavity.

CONTROL

Because of the need for a copepod intermediate host, it is unlikely that the life cycle would be completed in the laboratory, and no special control procedures are needed. There is no treatment (van Duijn 1967; Snieszko and Hoffman 1963).

PUBLIC HEALTH CONSIDERATIONS

Although two cases of accidental infection have been reported, man is not considered to be a natural host for this parasite (Belding 1965).

Schistocephalus solidus

The plerocercoid larva of this diphyllobothriid cestode is common in the abdominal cavity of sticklebacks and occurs occasionally in other fishes in North America, Europe, and Asia (Bykhovskaya-Pavlovskaya et al. 1962; Hoffman 1967; Yamaguti 1959). It is pathogenic in heavy infections (Arme and Owen 1967; van Duijn 1967; Reichenbach-Klinke and Elkan 1965) and is likely to be encountered in laboratory sticklebacks obtained from their natural habitat or in those raised in hatcheries that have a lake or stream water supply.

MORPHOLOGY

The plerocercoid larva, the stage found in fishes, is white and 20 to 76 mm long by about 6 mm wide (Bykhovskaya-Pavlovskaya et al. 1962; Hoffman 1967; Wardle and McLeod 1952). The scolex is triangular with an anterior longitudinal bothrium; the strobila is distinctly segmented (Fig. 22.22).

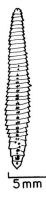

FIG. 22.22. *Schistocephalus solidus*, plerocercoid larva. (From Hoffman 1967. Courtesy of University of California Press.)

5mm

LIFE CYCLE

Eggs passed in the feces of the definitive host, a fish-eating bird, develop into procercoid larvae in copepods (Hoffman 1967; Wardle and McLeod 1952). The second intermediate host, a stickleback, is infected by ingesting an infected copepod, and the definitive host is infected by ingesting the fish.

PATHOLOGIC EFFECTS

Heavy infections cause abdominal distention and decreased reproduction (Arme and Owen 1967; van Duijn 1967; Reichenbach-Klinke and Elkan 1965). The plerocercoid larvae fill the abdominal cavity, causing compression of the visceral organs and obliteration of the gonads (Fig. 22.23).

DIAGNOSIS

Diagnosis is based on the clinical signs and is confirmed by demonstration and identification of the parasite in the abdominal cavity.

CONTROL

Because a copepod is needed as intermediate host, it is unlikely that the life cycle would be completed in the laboratory, and no special control procedures are needed. There is no treatment (van Duijn 1967; Snieszko and Hoffman 1963).

PUBLIC HEALTH CONSIDERATIONS

This cestode does not affect man.

Triaenophorus nodulosus
Triaenophorus crassus

The plerocercoid larvae of these triaenophoriid cestodes are common in those parts of North America and Europe where the definitive host, usually the northern pike *(Esox)* and occasionally other predatory fishes, is common (Hoffman 1967; Wardle and McLeod 1952; Yamaguti 1959). The highly pathogenic plerocercoid larva of *Triaenophorus nodulosus* (syn. *T. lucii*) occurs in the liver of the goldfish, other cyprinids, bluegill, sunfishes, black bass, other centrarchids, Atlantic salmon, other salmonids, channel catfish, sticklebacks, and other fishes. The somewhat less pathogenic larva of *T. crassus* occurs in the muscle and connective tissues of the Atlantic salmon,

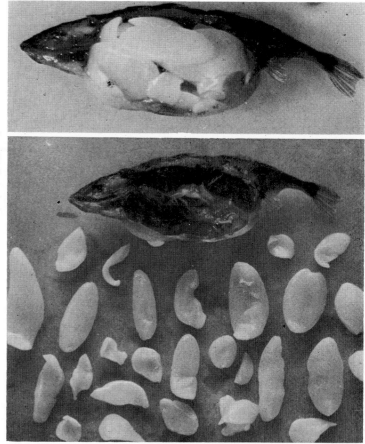

FIG. 22.23. *Schistocephalus solidus.* *(Top)* Plerocercoid larvae in abdominal cavity of stickleback. *(Bottom)* Larvae removed from abdominal cavity. (From Reichenbach-Klinke and Elkan 1965. Courtesy of Academic Press.)

Pacific salmons, other salmonids, and other fishes. These larval cestodes are likely to occur in laboratory fishes obtained from their natural habitat or from hatcheries that use lake or stream water in endemic areas. Incidences of 7 to 33% have been reported (Dogiel, Polyanski, and Kheisin 1962).

MORPHOLOGY

The plerocercoid larvae of these cestodes are long (up to 130 mm), white, and about 1 mm in width (Fig. 22.24) (Hoffman 1967). They are differentiated from all other cestode larvae of freshwater fishes by the presence of chitinoid hooks on the scolex (Fig. 22.25).

LIFE CYCLE

Eggs passed in the feces of the definitive host (predatory fish) develop into procercoid larvae in copepods (Hoffman 1967; Wardle and McLeod 1952). The sec-

ond intermediate host (small fish) is infected by ingesting an infected copepod, and the definitive host, by ingesting an infected small fish.

PATHOLOGIC EFFECTS

The plerocercoid larva of *T. nodulosus* produces cysts in the liver (van Duijn 1967).

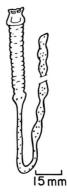

FIG. 22.24. *Triaenophorus,* plerocercoid larva. (From Hoffman 1967. Courtesy of University of California Press.)

15 mm

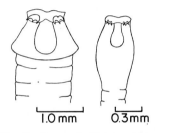

FIG. 22.25. Scolices of *Triaenophorus* plerocercoid larvae. *(Left)* T. *nodulosus. (Right)* T. *crassus.* (From Wardle and McLeod 1952. Courtesy of University of Minnesota Press.)

If the infection is heavy, most of the liver tissue is destroyed and death results (Reichenbach-Klinke and Elkan 1965). Massive mortalities have been reported (Matthey 1963). The less pathogenic plerocercoid larva of T. *crassus* produces yellow cysts in the muscle and connective tissue and rarely causes death (Hoffman 1967).

DIAGNOSIS

Diagnosis is based on demonstration and identification of the plerocercoid larvae coiled in cysts.

CONTROL

Because a copepod is required as an intermediate host, it is unlikely that the life cycles of these tapeworms would be completed in the laboratory, and no special control procedures are needed. There is no treatment (van Duijn 1967; Snieszko and Hoffman 1963).

PUBLIC HEALTH CONSIDERATIONS

These cestodes do not affect man.

NEMATODES

Many species of nematodes have been reported from fishes (Hoffman 1967; Reichenbach-Klinke and Elkan 1965; Van Cleave and Mueller 1934; Yorke and Maplestone 1926). Although nematodes usually have a life cycle involving only one host, those that affect fishes almost always require an invertebrate intermediate host, such as a copepod or insect. Sometimes the fish is a second intermediate host; sometimes it is the definitive host.

Adult nematodes affecting fishes are usually found in the stomach or intestine, but some occur in the body cavity or caudal fin. Larval nematodes occur in the muscle or body cavity. Adult nematodes that occur in the stomach and intestine usually cause little apparent effect, but adults and larvae that occur in the muscle and body cavity often produce severe damage (Hoffman 1967; M. Meyer 1960).

Nematodes that affect laboratory fishes are listed in Tables 22.6 and 22.7. The most important are discussed below.

Philonema agubernaculum,
Philonema oncorhynchi

Adults of these filarial nematodes occur in the body cavity of salmonid fishes where they sometimes cause extensive pathology (Hoffman 1967; Yamaguti 1961). *Philonema agubernaculum* is common in the brook trout, lake trout, rainbow trout, brown trout, and other salmonids in the United States and Canada. *Philonema oncorhynchi* is common in the brook trout, rainbow trout, Pacific salmons, and other salmonids in the United States, Canada, and the USSR. An incidence of about 20% has been reported in the Pacific salmons in southwestern Canada (Northcote 1957). Laboratory fishes obtained from their natural habitat or from hatcheries having stream or lake water supplies are likely to be infected.

MORPHOLOGY

Adults are long, thin, filiform, and glistening white worms that have a rounded anterior end and a sharply pointed posterior extremity (Fig. 22.26) (Hoffman 1967; Northcote 1957). The esophagus is cylindrical and is divided into a short anterior portion and longer posterior portion. The female measures up to 300 mm in length by 0.8 mm in diameter and has two small ovaries and a large uterus that occupies most of the body. The male is much shorter, ranging up to 35 mm in length. It has a spirally coiled posterior extremity with two slender, equal spicules and no gubernaculum.

LIFE CYCLE

These nematodes are viviparous (Hoffman 1967). Larvae pass out of the fish during spawning and are eaten by a copepod. Small salmonid fishes are infected by ingesting an infected copepod and larger salmo-

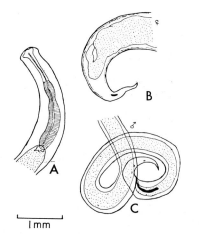

FIG. 22.26. *Philonema.* *(A)* Anterior end. *(B)* Posterior end of female. *(C)* Posterior end of male. (From Hoffman 1967. Courtesy of University of California Press.)

nid fishes by ingesting a small fish which has recently ingested an infected copepod.

PATHOLOGIC EFFECTS

Infection with these worms is usually inapparent (Northcote 1957), but sometimes it results in severe visceral adhesions (M. Meyer 1960; Richardson 1936). In extreme cases all the abdominal organs are bound together in a solid mass of adhesions, and normal functions, including reproduction, are precluded.

DIAGNOSIS

Diagnosis is based on identification of the parasite in the abdominal cavity.

CONTROL

Because a copepod is necessary as the intermediate host, it is unlikely that the life cycle would be completed in the laboratory, and no special control procedures are necessary. There is no treatment.

PUBLIC HEALTH CONSIDERATIONS

These nematodes do not affect man.

Capillaria catenata,
Capillaria eupomotis

Capillaria catenata occurs in the intestine of the bluegill, sunfishes, black bass, channel catfish, and other fishes in North America and sometimes causes enteritis (Hoffman 1967). *Capillaria eupomotis* (possible syn. *Hepaticola petruschewskii*) is common in the liver of the European minnow, sunfishes, rainbow trout, and other fishes in Europe and often causes extensive tissue damage (Ghittino 1961; Hoffman 1967; Reichenbach-Klinke and Elkan 1965). Both species are common in fishes obtained from their natural habitat and in those raised in hatcheries, and they are likely to be encountered in laboratory fishes.

MORPHOLOGY

Adults of these species have a capillary body with a long, narrow esophagus (Fig. 22.27) (Hoffman 1967; Yorke and Maplestone 1926). The females are about 21 to 28 mm long. Males are about 11 to 13 mm long and are characterized by a long, slender spicule with a spinose sheath. The eggs

FIG. 22.27. *Capillaria.* *(A)* Female. *(B)* Male. *(C)* Anterior end of *C. catenata* showing narrowing of esophagus. *(D)* *C. catenata* female, posterior end. *(E)* *C. catenata* male, posterior end. *(A, B* from Yorke and Maplestone 1926. *C, D, E* from Hoffman 1967; courtesy of University of California Press.)

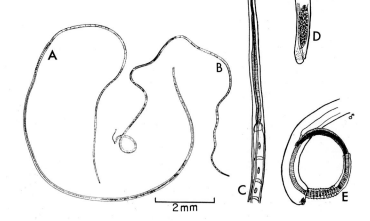

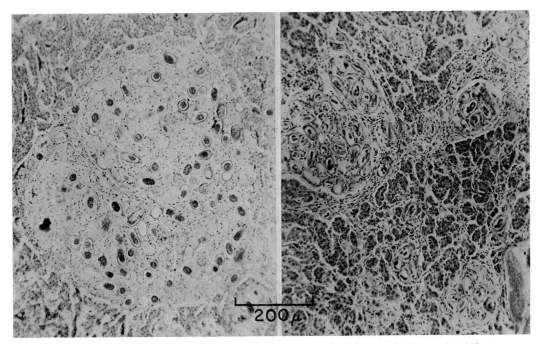

FIG. 22.28. *Capillaria eupomotis* infection in liver of rainbow trout. Note mass of eggs *(left)* and extensive damage *(right)*. (From Ghittino 1961. Courtesy of Rivista di Parassitologia.)

are elliptical and have opercular plugs at the poles.

LIFE CYCLE

The life cycle is unknown (Hoffman 1967).

PATHOLOGIC EFFECTS

Heavy infection with *C. catenata* sometimes causes a severe enteritis (Hoffman 1967), and infection with *C. eupomotis* often causes extensive liver damage (Fig. 22.28) (Ghittino 1961).

DIAGNOSIS

Diagnosis is based on identification of the parasite in the intestine or liver.

CONTROL

Nothing is known of control or treatment.

PUBLIC HEALTH CONSIDERATIONS

It is not known if these nematodes affect man.

Contracaecum spiculigerum

The larva of this nematode occurs in the body cavity of fishes, where it often causes extensive visceral damage (Hoffman 1967). *Contracaecum spiculigerum* is common in many species of fishes, including the golden shiner, topminnows, bluegill, sunfishes, black bass, rainbow trout, channel catfish, and eels, and it is likely to be encountered in laboratory fishes obtained from their natural habitat. An incidence of 28.4% has been reported in the channel catfish in south central United States (Spall and Summerfelt 1969).

MORPHOLOGY

This nematode is characterized by three indistinct lips, an esophagus that has a solid posterior appendix, and a cecum that projects anteriorly (Fig. 22.29) (Hoffman 1967; Yorke and Maplestone 1926). Adults are 30 to 44 mm in length. The larva, the stage that occurs in fishes, is similar to the adults except that it is smaller, and

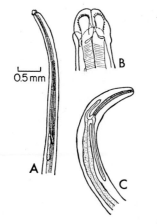

FIG. 22.29. *Contracaecum.* *(A)* Anterior end of adult showing cecum and appendix. *(B)* Anterior end of adult showing lips. *(C)* Anterior end of larva. (From Hoffman 1967. Courtesy of University of California Press.)

it is often encysted in the viscera in cysts up to 5 mm in diameter.

LIFE CYCLE

Adult worms occur in fish-eating birds (Hoffman 1967). The first intermediate host is unknown, but it is probably a copepod or amphipod. The fish is the second intermediate host.

PATHOLOGIC EFFECTS

The larva causes extensive damage to the viscera as it migrates through the body cavity (Hoffman 1967). Larvae that fail to encyst are the most injurious.

DIAGNOSIS

Diagnosis is based on recognition and identification of the parasite in affected tissues.

CONTROL

Nothing is known of control or treatment.

PUBLIC HEALTH CONSIDERATIONS

This nematode is not known to affect man.

Spiroxys

Larvae of unidentified species of this genus are commonly encountered in the body cavity of carp, shiners, other cyprinids, sunfishes, black bass, other centrarchids, channel catfish, sticklebacks, and other fishes in North America (Hoffman 1967). Their pathogenicity is uncertain. Laboratory fishes obtained from their natural habitat or from hatcheries that have lake or stream water supplies are likely to be infected.

MORPHOLOGY

Adults of this genus have a filiform body, about 15 to 30 mm long, a mouth that has two large, distinctly trilobed lips, and an esophagus that has a short anterior muscular portion and a longer posterior glandular portion (Hoffman 1967; Yorke and Maplestone 1926). There is no intestinal cecum or esophageal appendix. The larva, the stage found in fishes, is similar only much smaller (Fig. 22.30).

LIFE CYCLE

The life cycle is indirect and involves a copepod intermediate host (Hoffman 1967; Walton 1964). Adults occur in the stomach of turtles or in the intestine of the red-spotted newt. Fishes are second intermediate or transport hosts and are infected by ingesting an infected copepod.

PATHOLOGIC EFFECTS

Little is known of the pathologic effects of these larvae. They usually encyst in the mesentery and probably cause little damage unless present in large numbers.

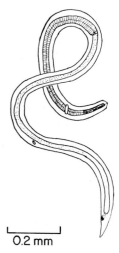

FIG. 22.30. *Spiroxys* larva. (From Hoffman 1967. Courtesy of University of California Press.)

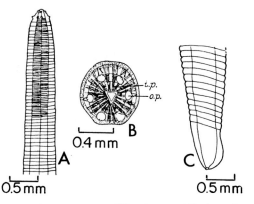

FIG. 22.31. *Eustrongylides* larva. *(A)* Anterior end. *(B)* Head-on view of anterior end showing inner circle of papillae *(i.p.)* and outer circle *(o.p.)*. *(C)* Posterior end. *(A, C* from Hoffman 1967; courtesy of University of California Press. *B* from Yorke and Maplestone 1926.)

DIAGNOSIS

Diagnosis is based on identification of the parasite encysted in the mesentery.

CONTROL

Because of the need for a copepod intermediate host, completion of the life cycle in the laboratory is unlikely, and no special control procedures are required. There is no treatment.

PUBLIC HEALTH CONSIDERATIONS

This nematode is not known to affect man.

Eustrongylides

(Red Roundworm)

Larvae of this genus are frequently found encysted in the muscle and viscera of fishes (Hoffman and Sindermann 1962; Northcote 1957; Yamaguti 1961). The larva of an unidentified species of *Eustrongylides* is common in killifishes, the bluegill, sunfishes, lake trout, rainbow trout, and sticklebacks in the United States and Canada (Hoffman 1967). In Europe, the larva of *E. escisus* is common in the muscle and viscera of the carp, ictalurids, and other fishes (Bykhovskaya-Pavlovskaya et al. 1962). Laboratory fishes obtained from their natural habitat are likely to be infected.

MORPHOLOGY

The larva, the stage found in fishes, is characteristically bright red (Hoffman 1967). It has a simple mouth and a head that has 12 or 18 small papillae arranged in two circles (Fig. 22.31) (Yorke and Maplestone 1926). In the North American species, it reaches a maximum length of 100 mm. In the European species, it is shorter, about 27 mm long (Bykhovskaya-Pavlovskaya et al. 1962).

LIFE CYCLE

The adult is found in fish-eating birds (Hoffman 1967). The first intermediate host is unknown or unnecessary, and it is not known how fishes become infected.

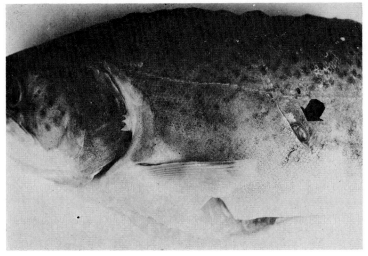

FIG. 22.32. *Eustrongylides* larva encysted in muscle of fish. (Courtesy of G. Hoffman, Eastern Fish Disease Laboratory.)

The larvae cause the formation of large red cysts, up to 10 mm in diameter, in the muscle and viscera (Fig. 22.32) (Hoffman 1967). Often the cysts become purulent and ulcerate (Bykhovskaya-Pavlovskaya et al. 1962).

DIAGNOSIS

Diagnosis is based on identification of the larva in a cyst.

CONTROL

Control and treatment are unknown.

PUBLIC HEALTH CONSIDERATIONS

This nematode is not known to affect man.

ACANTHOCEPHALANS

Acanthocephalans, which are easily recognized by their typical hook-bearing proboscis, are frequently encountered in the intestine of fishes (Hoffman 1967). The life cycle of these helminths always involves an invertebrate intermediate host and a vertebrate definitive host, and sometimes a vertebrate second intermediate host. Fishes serve as either definitive or second intermediate hosts. Adult acanthocephalans affecting fishes often cause extensive damage to the intestinal mucosa (Bullock 1961, 1963; Bykhovskaya-Pavlovskaya et al. 1962; Venard and Warfel 1953). The pathologic effects of larval acanthocephalans on fishes are unknown.

Acanthocephalans that affect laboratory fishes are listed in Table 22.8. The most important are discussed below.

Neoechinorhynchus cylindratus, Neoechinorhynchus rutili

Adults of *Neoechinorhynchus cylindratus* are common in the intestine of shiners, golden shiners, topminnows, killifishes, the bluegill, sunfishes, black bass, other centrarchids, brook trout, Atlantic salmon, other salmonids, eels, and other fishes in the United States and Canada (Hoffman 1967). The larva of this species is common in the liver of the bluegill, sunfishes, black bass, other centrarchids, mosquitofish, and other fishes in the same geographic region. Adults of *N. rutili* are common in the in-

testine of the goldfish, carp, shiners, other cyprinids, black bass, other centrarchids, brook trout, rainbow trout, brown trout, Atlantic salmon, Pacific salmons, other salmonids, sticklebacks, eels, and other fishes in North America, Europe, and Asia (Hoffman 1967; Van Cleave and Lynch 1950). The larva of this species does not occur in fishes. Laboratory fishes obtained from their natural environment or from hatcheries that have lake or stream water sup-

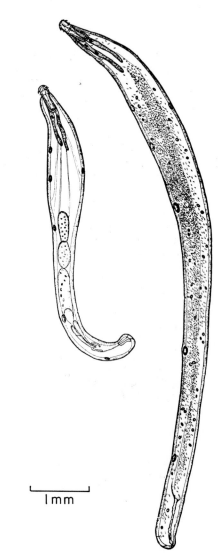

FIG. 22.33. *Neoechinorhynchus cylindratus*. *(Left)* Adult male. *(Right)* Adult female. (From Ward 1940.)

plies are likely to be infected. A 9% incidence of *N. rutili* has been reported in sticklebacks obtained from their natural habitat in Great Britain (Chappell 1969).

MORPHOLOGY

Adults of these species are small, cylindrical worms with an unspined body (Fig. 22.33) (Hoffman 1967; Ward 1940). The males are 4.7 to 6.3 mm long and 0.36 to 0.63 mm wide. The females are 7.0 to 11.2 mm long and 0.35 to 0.70 mm wide. The proboscis is globular and contains three circles of six hooks each. The encysted larval stage of *N. cylindratus* that occurs in fishes (Fig. 22.34) is similar to the adult except in size and degree of development of the reproductive organs. The larval male is about 1.3 to 2.7 mm long and the larval female about 1.5 to 3.6 mm long. The eggs are oval, 57 μ in length by 28 μ in width, and contain an ensheathed embryo when discharged from the adult female worm.

LIFE CYCLE

The life cycle of both species requires an aquatic crustacean (ostracod) as an intermediate host (Hoffman 1967; Olsen 1967; Ward 1940). Fishes are infected with *N. rutili* by ingesting an infected ostracod. *Neoechinorhynchus cylindratus* requires a second intermediate host. When a small fish ingests an infected ostracod, the immature acanthocephalan escapes from the crustacean and encysts in the liver of the fish. The definitive host, a large, predatory fish, is infected by ingesting an infected small fish.

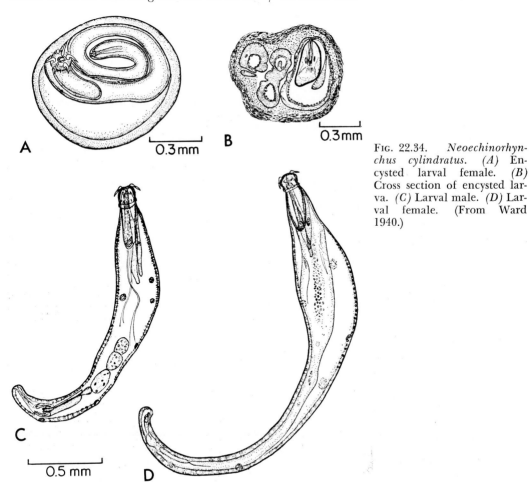

FIG. 22.34. *Neoechinorhynchus cylindratus.* *(A)* Encysted larval female. *(B)* Cross section of encysted larva. *(C)* Larval male. *(D)* Larval female. (From Ward 1940.)

PATHOLOGIC EFFECTS

Adults of these species have a relatively short proboscis and penetrate only the intestinal mucosa and a small portion of the submucosa (Venard and Warfel 1953). Individual worms do not cause extensive damage or tissue reaction, but heavy infections produce severe injury.

The larval stage of *N. cylindratus* apparently causes local inflammation in the liver of the host and cyst formation (Bogitsh 1961). Otherwise, nothing is known of its pathologic effects.

DIAGNOSIS

Diagnosis is based on identification of the adult worms in the intestine or the larva in the liver.

CONTROL

Because an ostracod is required as an intermediate host, it is unlikely that the life cycle would be completed in the laboratory, and no special control procedures are needed. There is no treatment (Snieszko and Hoffman 1963).

PUBLIC HEALTH CONSIDERATIONS

These helminths do not affect man.

Echinorhynchus

Adults of this genus are found in the intestine of many species of fishes and are often associated with severe enteric pathology (Bykhovskaya-Pavlovskaya et al. 1962; Dogiel, Polyanski, and Kheisin 1962; Hoffman 1967). *Echinorhynchus salmonis* occurs in shiners, the bluegill, sunfishes, black bass, other centrarchids, lake trout, rainbow trout, brown trout, Atlantic salmon, other salmonids, eels, and other fishes in North America, Europe, and Siberia. *Echinorhynchus leidyi* occurs in black bass, rainbow trout, lake trout, other salmonids, and other fishes in northern United States and Canada. *Echinorhynchus truttae* is found in the rainbow trout, brown trout, Atlantic salmon, and other fishes in Europe and Siberia. All are common and likely to be encountered in laboratory fishes obtained from their natural habitat or from hatcheries that have lake or stream water supplies.

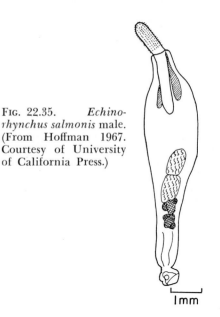

FIG. 22.35. *Echinorhynchus salmonis* male. (From Hoffman 1967. Courtesy of University of California Press.)

1mm

MORPHOLOGY

Adults of this genus have a small to medium unspined body (Fig. 22.35) (Hoffman 1967). *Echinorhynchus salmonis* attains a length of 7 mm and *E. truttae* a length of 20 mm. The proboscis is long and cylindrical and contains 9 to 26 longitudinal rows of 5 to 16 hooks each. The testes are oval to elliptical and are arranged in tandem in the middle one-third of the body. Posterior to the testes are five to seven oval cement glands. The egg is oval and fusiform and has prominent polar prolongations of the middle shell.

LIFE CYCLE

The life cycle requires an amphipod as an intermediate host but no second intermediate host (Hoffman 1967). A fish is infected by ingesting an infected amphipod.

PATHOLOGIC EFFECTS

Heavy infection with *E. truttae* causes intestinal obstruction, and *E. salmonis* causes the formation in the intestinal wall of many deep pits (Dogiel, Polyanski, and Kheisin 1962). Both species cause traumatic, ulcerative enteritis (Bykhovskaya-Pavlovskaya et al. 1962). The pathologic effects of *E. leidyi* are unknown but are probably similar.

Diagnosis is based on identification of the parasite in the intestine.

CONTROL

The need for an amphipod intermediate host makes the completion of the life cycle in the laboratory unlikely, and no special control procedures are required. There is no treatment (Snieszko and Hoffman 1963).

PUBLIC HEALTH CONSIDERATIONS

Echinorhynchus does not affect man.

Acanthocephalus

Adults of this genus occur in the intestine of several species of fishes, often causing extensive intestinal pathology (Bullock 1961, 1962, 1963; Bykhovskaya-Pavlovskaya et al. 1962; Hoffman 1967). *Acanthocephalus anguillae* occurs in the goldfish, carp, brook trout, rainbow trout, brown trout, Atlantic salmon, eels, and other fishes in the United States and Europe. *Acanthocephalus dirus* occurs in the bluegill, sunfishes, black bass, channel catfish, and other fishes in southern United States. *Acanthocephalus jacksoni* occurs in sunfishes, the brook trout, rainbow trout, and other fishes in northeastern United States. *Acanthocephalus lateralis* occurs in the brook trout, Pacific salmons, other salmonids, and other fishes in the United States and Canada. *Acanthocephalus lucii* occurs in the brown trout, Atlantic salmon, sticklebacks, eels, and other fishes in Europe. All are common and likely to be found in laboratory fishes obtained from their natural environment or from hatcheries with stream or lake water supplies.

MORPHOLOGY

Adults of this genus have a small to medium unspined body (Fig. 22.36) (Bullock 1962; Hoffman 1967). The male of *A. jacksoni* measures 2.9 to 5.5 mm long by 0.5 to 1.5 mm wide; the female measures 7.0 to 14.3 mm long by 0.7 to 0.9 mm wide. The proboscis is long and contains 6 to 28 longitudinal rows of 4 to 15 hooks each. The testes are oval and arranged in tandem in the middle one-third of the body. Posterior to the testes are six cement glands. The egg is elongated and fusiform.

LIFE CYCLE

The life cycle requires an aquatic crustacean (amphipod or isopod) as an intermediate host, but no second intermediate host (Hoffman 1967). A fish is infected by ingesting an infected crustacean.

PATHOLOGIC EFFECTS

Adults of *A. jacksoni* firmly embed in the intestinal mucosa and cause extensive mechanical damage by the insertion, withdrawal, and reinsertion of the proboscis as they change locations in the intestine (Fig. 22.37) (Bullock 1961, 1963). Their long-term effect is to cause a chronic fibrinous enteritis. Adults of *A. anguillae* not only damage the mucosa but usually penetrate into or through the muscularis and sometimes cause death (Bullock 1963; Nigrelli 1943). Although no specific pathology has been associated with the other species of *Acanthocephalus* affecting fishes, they probably cause similar effects.

DIAGNOSIS

Diagnosis is based on identification of the parasite in the intestine.

CONTROL

Because an aquatic crustacean intermediate host is needed, it is unlikely that the life cycle would be completed in the laboratory, and no special control procedures are needed. There is no treatment (Snieszko and Hoffman 1963).

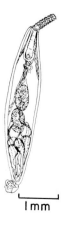

FIG. 22.36. *Acanthocephalus jacksoni* male. (From Bullock 1962. Courtesy of American Society of Parasitologists.)

1mm

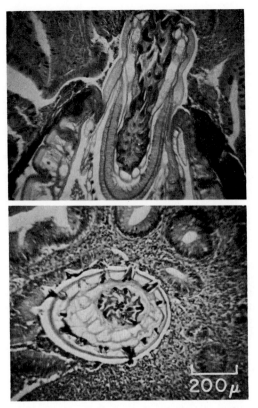

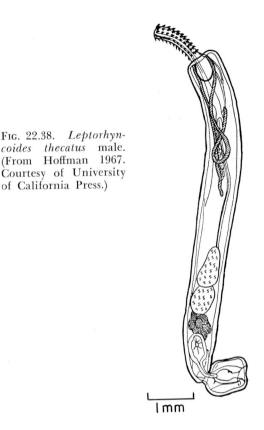

FIG. 22.38. *Leptorhyncoides thecatus* male. (From Hoffman 1967. Courtesy of University of California Press.)

FIG. 22.37. *Acanthocephalus jacksoni* proboscis in intestine of brook trout. *(Top)* Longitudinal section. *(Bottom)* Cross section. Note marked destruction of intestinal epithelium at site of attachment. (From Bullock 1963. Courtesy of the Wistar Institute Press.)

PUBLIC HEALTH CONSIDERATIONS

Acanthocephalus does not affect man.

Leptorhynchoides thecatus

Adults of this acanthocephalan occur in the pyloric ceca of the carp, shiners, other cyprinids, topminnows, sunfishes, bluegill, black bass, other centrarchids, brook trout, lake trout, other salmonids, channel catfish, sticklebacks, eels, and other fishes in the United States and Canada (Hoffman 1967; Spall and Summerfelt 1969). The larvae encyst in the mesentery and liver of chubs, topminnows, killifishes, mosquitofish, bluegill, sunfishes, black bass, brook trout, channel catfish, eels, and other fishes in the same geographic region. Both the adults and larvae are common and are likely to be encountered in laboratory fishes obtained from their natural habitat or from hatcheries that have lake or stream water supplies.

MORPHOLOGY

Adults are 7 to 26 mm long and have an elongated, unspined, cylindrical body (Fig. 22.38) (Hoffman 1967). The proboscis is subcylindrical and has 12 to 14 longitudinal rows of 8 to 24 hooks each. The testes are contiguous and in the posterior half of the body. Massed together immediately posterior to the testes are eight compact cement glands. The larvae are similar to the adults except in size and degree of development of the reproductive organs. The egg is elongate and has polar prolongations of the middle shell.

LIFE CYCLE

The life cycle requires an amphipod intermediate host (Hoffman 1967). It does not require a second intermediate host, but when larvae that have been in an amphipod less than 30 days are ingested by a fish, they do not develop into adults but encyst in the mesentery and liver. The definitive host is infected either by ingestion of an amphipod that has been infected for more than 30 days, or by ingestion of a small fish.

PATHOLOGIC EFFECTS

Adults in the cecum penetrate the mucosa and submucosa, causing extensive mechanical damage, tissue reaction, and cellular infiltration (Venard and Warfel 1953). The worms change their location frequently, leaving open wounds in the mucosa at previous sites of penetration. Secondary bacterial infection is common.

Nothing is known of the pathologic effects of the encysted larvae.

DIAGNOSIS

Diagnosis is based on identification of the adults in the pyloric ceca or the larva in the mesentery or liver.

CONTROL

Because of the requirement for an amphipod intermediate host, the life cycle is not likely to be completed in the laboratory, and no special control procedures are necessary. There is no treatment (Snieszko and Hoffman 1963).

PUBLIC HEALTH CONSIDERATIONS

This acanthocephalan does not affect man.

Pomphorhynchus bulbocolli, Pomphorhynchus laevis

The adults of these species are often extremely pathogenic (Saidov 1953). Those of *Pomphorhynchus bulbocolli* occur in the intestine of the goldfish, carp, bluntnose minnow, chubs, shiners, golden shiner, other cyprinids, topminnows, bluegill, sunfishes, black bass, other centrarchids, rainbow trout, and other salmonids in the United States and Canada (Hoffman 1967). The larvae of this species occur in the mesentery, liver, and spleen of shiners, other cyprinids, and other fishes in the same geographic region. Adults of *P. laevis* occur in the goldfish, carp, salmonids, sticklebacks, eels, and other fishes in Europe (Bykhovskaya-Pavlovskaya et al. 1962). Both

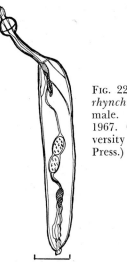

FIG. 22.39. *Pomphorhynchus bulbocolli* male. (From Hoffman 1967. Courtesy of University of California Press.)

species are common and are likely to be encountered in laboratory fishes obtained from their natural habitat or from hatcheries that have lake or stream water supplies.

MORPHOLOGY

Adults of these species are small, about 4 to 5 mm in length, and have an aspinose trunk and a characteristic long neck with a globular expansion immediately posterior to the proboscis (Fig. 22.39) (Hoffman 1967). The proboscis is long and almost cylindrical and contains 12 to 20 longitudinal rows of 10 to 14 hooks each. The testes are arranged in tandem near the middle of the trunk. There are six oval cement glands. The genital pore in both the male and the female is terminal and not surrounded by spines. The larvae are similar to the adults except in size and degree of development. The eggs are fusiform and have prominent polar prolongations of the middle shell.

LIFE CYCLE

The life cycle of both species requires an aquatic crustacean (amphipod) as an intermediate host (Hoffman 1967). *Pomphorhynchus bulbocolli* requires a second intermediate host, a small fish, but *P. laevis* does not. Fishes are infected with *P. laevis* by ingesting an infected amphipod. Small fishes are infected with *P. bulbocolli* in the same manner, but the parasite fails to mature and encysts in the mesentery, liver, or spleen. Adults develop when a large, predatory fish is infected by ingesting an infected small fish.

PATHOLOGIC EFFECTS

Adults penetrate through the submucosa of the intestinal wall and into the muscularis (Bullock 1961; Northcote 1957). Tissue reaction is marked and a thick, fibrous capsule, which appears as a macroscopic nodule on the serosal surface, develops around the proboscis. Sometimes the intestine is perforated and the liver traumatized (Saidov 1953). The larvae encyst in the viscera but otherwise nothing is known of their pathologic effects.

DIAGNOSIS

Diagnosis is based on identification of the adult worms in the intestine or the larvae in the mesentery, liver, or spleen.

CONTROL

The need for an aquatic crustacean as an intermediate host makes it unlikely that the life cycles of these species would be completed in the laboratory, and no special control procedures are required. There is no treatment (Snieszko and Hoffman 1963).

PUBLIC HEALTH CONSIDERATIONS

These acanthocephalans do not affect man.

NEMATOMORPHS (GORDIACEAN WORMS)

Nematomorphs resemble nematodes except that they are extremely long and blunt at both ends (Hoffman 1967). Larvae of these helminths are usually parasites of insects. Adults are free-living. Nematomorphs have been observed in the stomach and body cavity of fishes Nigrelli 1943), but these occurrences are rare and only accidental.

LEECHES

The leeches that affect fishes sometimes used in the laboratory are listed in Table 22.9 and illustrated in Figure 22.40. Although many are common on fishes in their natural environment, they are seldom encountered in hatcheries and are absent in aquariums (van Duijn 1967; Hoffman

1967). Some might rarely be encountered on fishes recently obtained from their natural environment, but none is likely to be an important pathogen in the laboratory.

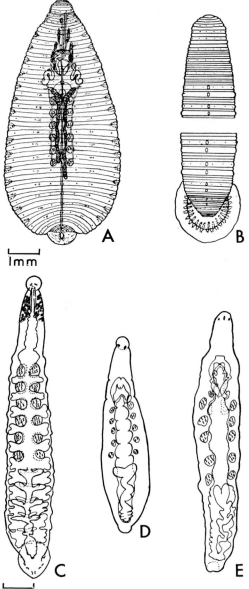

FIG. 22.40. Leeches. *(A) Haementeria (Placobdella). (B) Cystobranchus. (C) Piscicola. (D) Piscicolaria. (E) Illinobdella.* (From Hoffman 1967. Courtesy of University of California Press.)

TABLE 22.1. Monogenetic trematodes affecting laboratory fishes

Parasite	Geographic Distribution	Fish Host	Location in Host	Method of Infection	Incidence in Nature	Remarks	Reference
Gyrodactylus elegans	North America, Europe, Japan	Goldfish, carp, bluegill, brook trout, lake trout, rainbow trout, brown trout, sticklebacks, other fishes	Skin, gills	Direct contact	Common	Possible syn. *G. katherineri*. Ingests blood; causes mucus coating on skin, gills; frayed fins; sometimes death	van Duijn 1967 Hoffman 1967 Hoffman and Putz 1964 Malmberg 1970 Reichenbach-Klinke and Elkan 1965
Gyrodactylus medius	North America, Europe	Goldfish, carp, tropical mouth-breeders, black bass, brook trout	Skin, gills	Direct contact	Common	Ingests blood; causes mucus coating on skin, gills; frayed fins; sometimes death	Dawes 1946 van Duijn 1967 Hoffman 1967 Reichenbach-Klinke and Elkan 1965
Gyrodactylus gurleyi	South central United States	Goldfish	Skin, gills	Direct contact	Unknown; probably common	Pathologic effects unknown; probably causes mucus coating on skin, gills; frayed fins; sometimes death	Hoffman 1967
Gyrodactylus mutabilitas	Europe	Goldfish	Skin, gills	Direct contact	Unknown; probably common	Pathologic effects unknown; probably causes mucus coating on skin, gills; frayed fins; sometimes death	Hoffman 1967
Gyrodactylus sprostonae	Europe	Goldfish, carp	Skin, gills	Direct contact	Unknown; probably common	Pathologic effects unknown; probably causes mucus coating on skin, gills; frayed fins; sometimes death	Hoffman 1967
Gyrodactylus carassii	Northern Europe	Goldfish	Skin, gills	Direct contact	Common	Pathologic effects unknown; probably causes mucus coating on skin, gills; frayed fins; sometimes death	Hoffman 1967
Gyrodactylus chinensis	Asia	Goldfish	Skin, gills	Direct contact	Unknown; probably common	Pathologic effects unknown; probably causes mucus coating on skin, gills; frayed fins; sometimes death	Hoffman 1967
Gyrodactylus fairporti	United States	Carp, other fishes	Skin, gills	Direct contact	Unknown; probably common	Pathologic effects unknown; probably causes mucus coating on skin, gills; frayed fins; sometimes death	Hoffman 1967 Rogers 1968b
Gyrodactylus cyprini	United States, Europe	Carp	Skin, gills	Direct contact	Unknown; probably common	Pathologic effects unknown; probably causes mucus coating on skin, gills; frayed fins; sometimes death	Rogers 1968b
Gyrodactylus gracilis	Europe	Carp, other cyprinids	Skin, gills	Direct contact	Unknown; probably common	Pathologic effects unknown; probably causes mucus coating on skin, gills; frayed fins; sometimes death	Dawes 1946 van Duijn 1967 Hoffman 1967

TABLE 22.1 (continued)

Parasite	Geographic Distribution	Fish Host	Location in Host	Method of Infection	Incidence in Nature	Remarks	Reference
Gyrodactylus nagtibinae	Europe	Carp	Skin, gills	Direct contact	Unknown; probably common	Ingests blood; causes mucus coating on skin, gills; frayed fins; sometimes death	Hoffman 1967
Gyrodactylus hoffmani	Southeastern United States	Bluntnose minnow	Skin, gills	Direct contact	Unknown; probably common	Pathologic effects unknown; probably causes mucus coating on skin, gills; frayed fins; sometimes death	Wellborn and Rogers 1967
Gyrodactylus atratuli	Eastern United States	Chubs	Skin, gills	Direct contact	Unknown; probably common	Pathologic effects unknown; probably causes mucus coating on skin, gills; frayed fins; sometimes death	Hoffman 1967
Gyrodactylus protuberus	Southeastern United States	Shiners	Skin, gills	Direct contact	Unknown; probably common	Pathologic effects unknown; probably causes mucus coating on skin, gills; frayed fins; sometimes death	Hoffman 1967 Rogers and Wellborn 1965
Gyrodactylus albeoli	Southeastern United States	Shiners	Skin, gills	Direct contact	Unknown; probably common	Pathologic effects unknown; probably causes mucus coating on skin, gills; frayed fins; sometimes death	Rogers 1968b
Gyrodactylus asperus	Southeastern United States	Shiners	Skin, gills	Direct contact	Unknown; probably common	Pathologic effects unknown; probably causes mucus coating on skin, gills; frayed fins; sometimes death	Rogers 1967c
Gyrodactylus baeacanthus	Southeastern United States	Shiners	Skin, gills	Direct contact	Unknown; probably common	Pathologic effects unknown; probably causes mucus coating on skin, gills; frayed fins; sometimes death	Wellborn and Rogers 1967
Gyrodactylus illigatus	Southeastern United States	Shiners	Skin, gills	Direct contact	Unknown; probably common	Pathologic effects unknown; probably causes mucus coating on skin, gills; frayed fins; sometimes death	Rogers 1968b
Gyrodactylus lambanus	Southeastern United States	Shiners	Skin, gills	Direct contact	Unknown; probably common	Pathologic effects unknown; probably causes mucus coating on skin, gills; frayed fins; sometimes death	Rogers 1967c
Gyrodactylus stephanus	United States	Killifishes	Skin, gills	Direct contact	Unknown; probably common	Pathologic effects unknown; probably causes mucus coating on skin, gills; frayed fins; sometimes death	Hoffman 1967 Hoffman and Putz 1964
Gyrodactylus stegurus	Eastern United States	Killifishes, other fishes	Skin, gills	Direct contact	Unknown; probably common	Pathologic effects unknown; probably causes mucus coating on skin, gills; frayed fins; sometimes death	Hoffman 1967

TABLE 22.1 (continued)

Parasite	Geographic Distribution	Fish Host	Location in Host	Method of Infection	Incidence in Nature	Remarks	Reference
Gyrodactylus prolongis	Southern United States	Killifishes, other fishes	Skin, gills	Direct contact	Unknown; probably common	Pathologic effects unknown; probably causes mucus coating on skin, gills; frayed fins; sometimes death	Hoffman 1967 Hoffman and Putz 1964
Gyrodactylus funduli	Southern United States	Killifishes	Skin, gills	Direct contact	Unknown; probably common	Pathologic effects unknown; probably causes mucus coating on skin, gills; frayed fins; sometimes death	Hoffman 1967 Hoffman and Putz 1964
Gyrodactylus megacanthus	Southeastern United States	Killifishes	Skin, gills	Direct contact	Unknown; probably common	Pathologic effects unknown; probably causes mucus coating on skin, gills; frayed fins; sometimes death	Wellborn and Rogers 1967
Gyrodactylus bullatarudis	North America	Guppy	Skin, gills	Direct contact	Common	Pathologic effects unknown; probably causes mucus coating on skin, gills; frayed fins; sometimes death	Hoffman 1967 Hoffman and Putz 1964 Reichenbach-Klinke and Elkan 1965
Gyrodactylus gambusiae	Southeastern United States	Mosquitofish	Skin, gills	Direct contact	Unknown; probably common	Pathologic effects unknown; probably causes mucus coating on skin, gills; frayed fins; sometimes death	Hoffman 1967 Rogers and Wellborn 1965
Gyrodactylus macrochiri	Eastern United States	Bluegill, sunfishes, other fishes	Skin, gills	Direct contact	Common	Pathologic effects unknown; probably causes mucus coating on skin, gills; frayed fins; sometimes death	Hoffman 1967 Hoffman and Putz 1964 Rogers and Wellborn 1965
Gyrodactylus salaris	Europe	Brown trout, Atlantic salmon	Skin, gills	Direct contact	Unknown; probably common	Pathologic effects unknown; probably causes mucus coating on skin, gills; frayed fins; sometimes death	Hoffman 1967
Gyrodactylus ictaluri	Southeastern United States	Channel catfish	Skin, gills	Direct contact	Unknown; probably common	Pathologic effects unknown; probably causes mucus coating on skin, gills; frayed fins; sometimes death	Rogers 1967c
Gyrodactylus aculeati	Europe	Sticklebacks	Skin, gills	Direct contact	Unknown; probably common	Pathologic effects unknown; probably causes mucus coating on skin, gills; frayed fins; sometimes death	Hoffman 1967
Gyrodactylus rarus	Europe	Sticklebacks	Skin, gills	Direct contact	Unknown; probably common	Pathologic effects unknown; probably causes mucus coating on skin, gills; frayed fins; sometimes death	Dawes 1946 Hoffman 1967

TABLE 22.1 (continued)

Parasite	Geographic Distribution	Fish Host	Location in Host	Method of Infection	Incidence in Nature	Remarks	Reference
Gyrodactylus bychowskii	Europe, Asia	Sticklebacks	Skin, gills	Direct contact	Common	Pathologic effects unknown; probably causes mucus coating on skin, gills; frayed fins; sometimes death	Hoffman 1967
Gyrodactylus arcuatus	Europe	Sticklebacks	Skin, gills	Direct contact	Unknown; probably common	Pathologic effects unknown; probably causes mucus coating on skin, gills; frayed fins; sometimes death	Hoffman 1967
Gyrodactylus anguillae	Europe	Eels	Skin, gills	Direct contact	Common	Pathologic effects unknown; probably causes mucus coating on skin, gills; frayed fins; sometimes death	Hoffman 1967
Dactylogyrus vastator	United States, Europe, Israel, Japan	Goldfish, carp	Gills	Direct contact	Unknown; probably common	Causes hypertrophy of gill filaments, sometimes death	Dawes 1946 Dogiel et al. 1958 Hoffman 1967 Rogers 1967b
Dactylogyrus anchoratus	United States, Europe, Israel	Goldfish, carp	Gills	Direct contact	Common	Pathologic effects unknown; probably causes hypertrophy of gill filaments, sometimes death	Dawes 1946 Dogiel et al. 1962 Hoffman 1967 Rogers 1967b
Dactylogyrus extensus	North America, Europe, Israel	Goldfish, carp, black bass	Gills	Direct contact	Common	Probable syn. *Dactylogyrus solidus*. Pathologic effects unknown; probably causes hypertrophy of gill filaments, sometimes death	Hoffman 1967 Rogers 1967b
Dactylogyrus wegeneri	United States, Europe	Goldfish, carp	Gills	Direct contact	Unknown; probably common	Pathologic effects unknown; probably causes hypertrophy of gill filaments, sometimes death	Dawes 1946 Hoffman 1967
Dactylogyrus auriculatus	Europe	Goldfish, carp	Gills	Direct contact	Unknown; probably common	Pathologic effects unknown; probably causes hypertrophy of gill filaments, sometimes death	Dawes 1946 van Duijn 1967 Hoffman 1967
Dactylogyrus crassus	Europe	Goldfish, carp	Gills	Direct contact	Unknown; probably common	Pathologic effects unknown; probably causes hypertrophy of gill filaments, sometimes death	Dawes 1946 Hoffman 1967
Dactylogyrus dujardinianus	Europe	Goldfish, carp	Gills	Direct contact	Unknown; probably common	Pathologic effects unknown; probably causes hypertrophy of gill filaments, sometimes death	Dawes 1946 Hoffman 1967
Dactylogyrus fallax	Europe	Goldfish, carp, other cyprinids	Gills	Direct contact	Unknown; probably common	Pathologic effects unknown; probably causes hypertrophy of gill filaments, sometimes death	van Duijn 1967 Hoffman 1967

TABLE 22.1 (continued)

Parasite	Geographic Distribution	Fish Host	Location in Host	Method of Infection	Incidence in Nature	Remarks	Reference
Dactylogyrus arquatus	Europe	Goldfish	Gills	Direct contact	Unknown; probably common	Pathologic effects unknown; probably causes hypertrophy of gill filaments, sometimes death	Hoffman 1967
Dactylogyrus baueri	United States, Europe	Goldfish	Gills	Direct contact	Unknown; probably common	Pathologic effects unknown; probably causes hypertrophy of gill filaments, sometimes death	Hoffman 1967 Rogers 1967b
Dactylogyrus dogieli	Europe	Goldfish	Gills	Direct contact	Unknown; probably common	Pathologic effects unknown; probably causes hypertrophy of gill filaments, sometimes death	Hoffman 1967
Dactylogyrus dulkeiti	Europe	Goldfish	Gills	Direct contact	Unknown; probably common	Pathologic effects unknown; probably causes hypertrophy of gill filaments, sometimes death	Hoffman 1967
Dactylogyrus formosus	United States, Europe	Goldfish	Gills	Direct contact	Unknown; probably common	Pathologic effects unknown; probably causes hypertrophy of gill filaments, sometimes death	Bykhovskaya-Pavlovskaya et al. 1962 Dawes 1946 Rogers 1967b
Dactylogyrus inexpectatus	Europe	Goldfish	Gills	Direct contact	Unknown; probably common	Pathologic effects unknown; probably causes hypertrophy of gill filaments, sometimes death	Bykhovskaya-Pavlovskaya et al. 1962
Dactylogyrus intermedius	Europe	Goldfish	Gills	Direct contact	Unknown; probably common	Pathologic effects unknown; probably causes hypertrophy of gill filaments, sometimes death	Bykhovskaya-Pavlovskaya et al. 1962
Dactylogyrus minutus	United States, Europe, Israel	Carp	Gills	Direct contact	Unknown; probably common	Pathologic effects unknown; probably causes hypertrophy of gill filaments, sometimes death	Dawes 1946 Hoffman 1967 Rogers 1967b
Dactylogyrus solidus	Europe	Carp	Gills	Direct contact	Unknown; probably common	Probable syn. Dactylogyrus extensus. Causes hypertrophy of gill filaments, sometimes death	Dogiel et al. 1958 Hoffman 1967
Dactylogyrus falcatus	Europe	Carp	Gills	Direct contact	Unknown; probably common	Pathologic effects unknown; probably causes hypertrophy of gill filaments, sometimes death	Dawes 1946 Hoffman 1967
Dactylogyrus mollis	Europe	Carp	Gills	Direct contact	Unknown; probably common	Pathologic effects unknown; probably causes hypertrophy of gill filaments, sometimes death	Bykhovskaya-Pavlovskaya et al. 1962 Dawes 1946

TABLE 22.1 (continued)

Parasite	Geographic Distribution	Fish Host	Location in Host	Method of Infection	Incidence in Nature	Remarks	Reference
Dactylogyrus achmerovi	Europe	Carp	Gills	Direct contact	Unknown; probably common	Pathologic effects unknown; probably causes hypertrophy of gill filaments, sometimes death	Hoffman 1967
Dactylogyrus falciformis	Europe	Carp	Gills	Direct contact	Unknown, probably common	Pathologic effects unknown; probably causes hypertrophy of gill filaments, sometimes death	Hoffman 1967
Dactylogyrus cyprini	Java	Carp	Gills	Direct contact	Unknown; probably common	Pathologic effects unknown; probably causes hypertrophy of gill filaments, sometimes death	Hoffman 1967
Dactylogyrus bifurcatus	United States	Bluntnose minnow	Gills	Direct contact	Unknown; probably common	Pathologic effects unknown; probably causes hypertrophy of gill filaments, sometimes death	Hoffman 1967 Rogers 1967b
Dactylogyrus bychowskyi	United States	Bluntnose minnow	Gills	Direct contact	Unknown; probably common	Pathologic effects unknown; probably causes hypertrophy of gill filaments, sometimes death	Hoffman 1967 Rogers 1967b
Dactylogyrus simplex	United States	Bluntnose minnow	Gills	Direct contact	Unknown; probably common	Syn. *Neodactylogyrus simplex.* Pathologic effects unknown; probably causes hypertrophy of gill filaments, sometimes death	Hoffman 1967
Dactylogyrus attenuatus	United States	Chubs	Gills	Direct contact	Unknown; probably common	Syn. *Neodactylogyrus attenuatus.* Pathologic effects unknown; probably causes hypertophy of gill filaments, sometimes death	Hoffman 1967 Rogers 1967b
Dactylogyrus atromaculatus	North central United States	Chubs	Gills	Direct contact	Unknown; probably common	Pathologic effects unknown; probably causes hypertrophy of gill filaments, sometimes death	Hoffman 1967
Dactylogyrus claviformis	North central United States	Chubs, other cyprinids	Gills	Direct contact	Unknown; probably common	Pathologic effects unknown; probably causes hypertrophy of gill filaments, sometimes death	Hoffman 1967
Dactylogyrus corporalis	Eastern United States	Chubs, other cyprinids	Gills	Direct contact	Unknown; probably common	Pathologic effects unknown; probably causes hypertrophy of gill filaments, sometimes death	Hoffman 1967
Dactylogyrus lineatus	United States	Chubs, other cyprinids	Gills	Direct contact	Unknown; probably common	Pathologic effects unknown; probably causes hypertrophy of gill filaments, sometimes death	Hoffman 1967 Rogers 1967b

TABLE 22.1 (continued)

Parasite	Geographic Distribution	Fish Host	Location in Host	Method of Infection	Incidence in Nature	Remarks	Reference
Dactylogyrus microphallus	United States	Chubs, other cyprinids	Gills	Direct contact	Unknown; probably common	Pathologic effects unknown; probably causes hypertrophy of gill filaments, sometimes death	Hoffman 1967 Rogers 1967b
Dactylogyrus semotilus	North central United States	Chubs, other cyprinids	Gills	Direct contact	Unknown; probably common	Pathologic effects unknown; probably causes hypertrophy of gill filaments, sometimes death	Hoffman 1967
Dactylogyrus tenax	Northeastern United States	Chubs, other cyprinids	Gills	Direct contact	Unknown; probably common	Pathologic effects unknown; probably causes hypertrophy of gill filaments, sometimes death	Hoffman 1967
Dactylogyrus banghami	North America	Shiners, other cyprinids	Gills	Direct contact	Common	Pathologic effects unknown; probably causes hypertrophy of gill filaments, sometimes death	Hoffman 1967 Rogers 1967b
Dactylogyrus bulbus	North America	Shiners	Gills	Direct contact	Unknown; probably common	Syn. Neodactylogyrus bulbus. Pathologic effects unknown; probably causes hypertrophy of gill filaments, sometimes death	Hoffman 1967 Rogers 1967b
Dactylogyrus cornutus	North America	Shiners	Gills	Direct contact	Unknown; probably common	Syn. Neodactylogyrus cornutus. Pathologic effects unknown; probably causes hypertrophy of gill filaments, sometimes death	Hoffman 1967 Rogers 1967b
Dactylogyrus perlus	Northeastern United States, Canada	Shiners	Gills	Direct contact	Unknown; probably common	Syn. Neodactylogyrus perlus. Pathologic effects unknown; probably causes hypertrophy of gill filaments, sometimes death	Hoffman 1967
Dactylogyrus acus	Northeastern United States	Shiners, other fishes	Gills	Direct contact	Unknown; probably common	Syn. Neodactylogyrus acus. Pathologic effects unknown; probably causes hypertrophy of gill filaments, sometimes death	Hoffman 1967
Dactylogyrus fulcrum	Northeastern United States	Shiners	Gills	Direct contact	Unknown; probably common	Syn. Neodactylogyrus fulcrum. Pathologic effects unknown; probably causes hypertrophy of gill filaments, sometimes death	Hoffman 1967
Dactylogyrus orchis	Northeastern United States	Shiners	Gills	Direct contact	Unknown; probably common	Syn. Neodactylogyrus orchis. Pathologic effects unknown; probably causes hypertrophy of gill filaments, sometimes death	Hoffman 1967

TABLE 22.1 (continued)

Parasite	Geographic Distribution	Fish Host	Location in Host	Method of Infection	Incidence in Nature	Remarks	Reference
Dactylogyrus photogenis	Northeastern United States	Shiners	Gills	Direct contact	Unknown; probably common	Syn. *Neodactylogyrus photogenis*. Pathologic effects unknown; probably causes hypertrophy of gill filaments, sometimes death	Hoffman 1967
Dactylogyrus rubellus	Northeastern United States	Shiners	Gills	Direct contact	Unknown; probably common	Syn. *Neodactylogyrus rubellus*. Pathologic effects unknown; probably causes hypertrophy of gill filaments, sometimes death	Hoffman 1967
Dactylogyrus distinctus	North central United States	Shiners	Gills	Direct contact	Unknown; probably common	Syn. *Neodactylogyrus distinctus*. Pathologic effects unknown; probably causes hypertrophy of gill filaments, sometimes death	Hoffman 1967
Dactylogyrus dubius	North central United States	Shiners	Gills	Direct contact	Unknown; probably common	Pathologic effects unknown; probably causes hypertrophy of gill filaments, sometimes death	Hoffman 1967
Dactylogyrus pyriformis	North central United States	Shiners	Gills	Direct contact	Unknown; probably common	Syn. *Neodactylogyrus pyriformis*. Pathologic effects unknown; probably causes hypertrophy of gill filaments, sometimes death	Hoffman 1967
Dactylogyrus vannus	North central United States	Shiners	Gills	Direct contact	Unknown; probably common	Syn. *Neodactylogyrus vannus*. Pathologic effects unknown; probably causes hypertrophy of gill filaments, sometimes death	Hoffman 1967
Dactylogyrus moorei	Southern United States	Shiners	Gills	Direct contact	Unknown; probably common	Pathologic effects unknown; probably causes hypertrophy of gill filaments, sometimes death	Hoffman 1967 Rogers 1967b
Dactylogyrus arcus	Southeastern United States	Shiners	Gills	Direct contact	Unknown; probably common	Pathologic effects unknown; probably causes hypertrophy of gill filaments, sometimes death	Rogers 1967b
Dactylogyrus argenteus	Southeastern United States	Shiners	Gills	Direct contact	Unknown; probably common	Pathologic effects unknown; probably causes hypertrophy of gill filaments, sometimes death	Rogers 1967b
Dactylogyrus caudoluminis	Southeastern United States	Shiners	Gills	Direct contact	Unknown; probably common	Pathologic effects unknown; probably causes hypertrophy of gill filaments, sometimes death	Rogers 1967b

TABLE 22.1 *(continued)*

Parasite	Geographic Distribution	Fish Host	Location in Host	Method of Infection	Incidence in Nature	Remarks	Reference
Dactylogyrus cursitans	Southeastern United States	Shiners	Gills	Direct contact	Unknown; probably common	Pathologic effects unknown; probably causes hypertrophy of gill filaments, sometimes death	Rogers 1967b
Dactylogyrus lepidus	Southeastern United States	Shiners	Gills	Direct contact	Unknown; probably common	Pathologic effects unknown; probably causes hypertrophy of gill filaments, sometimes death	Rogers 1967b
Dactylogyrus luxili	Southeastern United States	Shiners	Gills	Direct contact	Unknown; probably common	Pathologic effects unknown; probably causes hypertrophy of gill filaments, sometimes death	Rogers 1967b
Dactylogyrus manicatus	Southeastern United States	Shiners	Gills	Direct contact	Unknown; probably common	Pathologic effects unknown; probably causes hypertrophy of gill filaments, sometimes death	Rogers 1967b
Dactylogyrus crucis	Southeastern United States	Shiners	Gills	Direct contact	Unknown; probably common	Pathologic effects unknown; probably causes hypertrophy of gill filaments, sometimes death	Rogers 1967b
Dactylogyrus fungulus	Southeastern United States	Shiners	Gills	Direct contact	Unknown; probably common	Pathologic effects unknown; probably causes hypertrophy of gill filaments, sometimes death	Rogers 1967b
Dactylogyrus ornatus	Southeastern United States	Shiners	Gills	Direct contact	Unknown; probably common	Pathologic effects unknown; probably causes hypertrophy of gill filaments, sometimes death	Rogers 1967b
Dactylogyrus pronatus	Southeastern United States	Shiners	Gills	Direct contact	Unknown; probably common	Pathologic effects unknown; probably causes hypertrophy of gill filaments, sometimes death	Rogers 1967b
Dactylogyrus venusti	Southeastern United States	Shiners	Gills	Direct contact	Unknown; probably common	Pathologic effects unknown; probably causes hypertrophy of gill filaments, sometimes death	Rogers 1967b
Dactylogyrus welakae	Southeastern United States	Shiners	Gills	Direct contact	Unknown; probably common	Pathologic effects unknown; probably causes hypertrophy of gill filaments, sometimes death	Rogers 1967b
Dactylogyrus percobromus	South central United States	Shiners	Gills	Direct contact	Unknown; probably common	Pathologic effects unknown; probably causes hypertrophy of gill filaments, sometimes death	Rogers 1967b

TABLE 22.1 (continued)

Parasite	Geographic Distribution	Fish Host	Location in Host	Method of Infection	Incidence in Nature	Remarks	Reference
Dactylogyrus pollex	Eastern Canada	Shiners	Gills	Direct contact	Unknown; probably common	Pathologic effects unknown; probably causes hypertrophy of gill filaments, sometimes death	Hoffman 1967
Dactylogyrus aureus	United States	Golden shiner, bluegill, sunfishes, other centrarchids	Gills	Direct contact	Common	Pathologic effects unknown; probably causes hypertrophy of gill filaments, sometimes death	Hoffman 1967 Rogers 1967b
Dactylogyrus parvicirrus	Southern United States	Golden shiner	Gills	Direct contact	Unknown; probably common	Pathologic effects unknown; probably causes hypertrophy of gill filaments, sometimes death	Hoffman 1967 Rogers 1967b
Pseudacolpenteron pavlovskyi	United States, Europe, Asia	Carp, other cyprinids	Gills, fins	Direct contact	Unknown; probably common	Pathologic effects unknown; probably causes hypertrophy of gill filaments, sometimes death	Rogers 1968a
Lyrodiscus seminolensis	Southeastern United States	Bluegill	Skin, gills	Direct contact	Unknown; probably common	Pathologic effects unknown; probably causes hypertrophy of gill filaments, sometimes death	Rogers 1967a
Lyrodiscus muricatus	Southeastern United States	Sunfishes	Skin, gills	Direct contact	Unknown; probably common	Pathologic effects unknown; probably causes hypertrophy of gill filaments, sometimes death	Rogers 1967a
Anchoradiscoides serpentinus	Southeastern United States	Sunfishes	Skin, gills	Direct contact	Unknown; probably common	Pathologic effects unknown	Rogers 1967a
Cleidodiscus bedardi	United States	Sunfishes	Gills	Direct contact	Common	Heavy infections probably cause dyspnea, death	Hoffman 1967
Cleidodiscus diversus	United States	Bluegill, sunfishes	Gills	Direct contact	Common	Heavy infections probably cause dyspnea, death	Hoffman 1967
Cleidodiscus nematocirrus	Southern United States	Bluegill, sunfishes	Gills	Direct contact	Common	Heavy infections probably cause dyspnea, death	Hoffman 1967
Cleidodiscus robustus	United States	Bluegill, sunfishes	Gills	Direct contact	Common	Heavy infections probably cause dyspnea, death	Hoffman 1967
Cleidodiscus floridanus	United States	Channel catfish, other ictalurids	Gills	Direct contact	Common	Heavy infections probably cause dyspnea, death	Hoffman 1967
Cleidodiscus pricei	United States	Channel catfish, other ictalurids	Gills	Direct contact	Common	Heavy infections probably cause dyspnea, death	Hoffman 1967
Cleidodiscus longus	United States	Ictalurids	Gills	Direct contact	Common	Heavy infections probably cause dyspnea, death	Hoffman 1967

TABLE 22.1 (continued)

Parasite	Geographic Distribution	Fish Host	Location in Host	Method of Infection	Incidence in Nature	Remarks	Reference
Urocleidoides reticulatus	United States, West Indies	Guppy	Gills	Direct contact	Common	Heavy infections probably cause dypsnea, death	Mizelle and Price 1964
Urocleidus acer	United States	Bluegill, sunfishes	Gills	Direct contact	Common	Heavy infections probably cause dypsnea, death	Hoffman 1967
Urocleidus terox	United States	Bluegill, sunfishes	Gills	Direct contact	Common	Heavy infections probably cause dypsnea, death	Hoffman 1967
Urocleidus furcatus	United States	Bluegill, sunfishes, black bass	Gills	Direct contact	Common	Heavy infections probably cause dypsnea, death	Hoffman 1967
Urocleidus attenuatus	Southern United States	Bluegill, sunfishes	Gills	Direct contact	Common	Heavy infections probably cause dypsnea, death	Hoffman 1967
Urocleidus dispar	Northern United States, Canada	Bluegill, sunfishes	Gills	Direct contact	Common	Heavy infections probably cause dypsnea, death	Hoffman 1967
Urocleidus principalis	United States, Great Britain	Black bass	Gills	Direct contact	Common	Heavy infections probably cause dypsnea, death	Hoffman 1967 Maitland and Price 1969
Clavunculus bursatus	United States	Bluegill, black bass	Gills	Direct contact	Common	Heavy infections probably cause dypsnea, death	Hoffman 1967
Actinocleidus fergusoni	United States	Bluegill, sunfishes	Gills	Direct contact	Common	Heavy infections probably cause dypsnea, death	Hoffman 1967
Actinocleidus fusiformis	United States	Black bass	Gills	Direct contact	Common	Heavy infections probably cause dypsnea, death	Hoffman 1967
Discocotyle sagittata	North America, Europe	Brook trout, rainbow trout, brown trout, Atlantic salmon	Gills	Direct contact	Common	Syn. *Discocotyle salmonis*. Heavy infections probably cause dyspnea, death	Hoffman 1967 Hoffman and Sinder-mann 1962 Reichenbach-Klinke and Elkan 1965
Diplozoon paradoxum	Europe	Carp, European minnow, other cyprinids, sticklebacks	Gills	Direct contact	Common	Causes adhesions, edema of gills; dyspnea; death	Dawes 1946 van Duijn 1967 Reichenbach-Klinke and Elkan 1965
Diplozoon nipponicum	Japan	Carp, other cyprinids	Gills	Direct contact	Unknown; probably common	Pathologic effects unknown; probably causes adhesions, edema of gills; dyspnea; death	Dawes 1946 Reichenbach-Klinke and Elkan 1965

TABLE 22.2. Adult digenetic trematodes affecting laboratory fishes

Parasite	Geographic Distribution	Fish Host	Location in Host	Method of Infection	Incidence in Nature	Remarks	Reference
*Sanguinicola davis**	Western United States	Rainbow trout	Blood vessels	Penetration of skin by cercaria released from snail	Common	Ova and miracidia cause extensive gill damage, death	Hoffman 1967 Wales 1958
*Sanguinicola huronis**	Central United States	Black bass	Blood vessels	Penetration of skin by cercaria released from snail	Common	Ova and miracidia cause extensive gill damage, death	Hoffman 1967 Yamaguti 1958
Sanguinicola intermedius	Europe	Goldfish, carp, other fishes	Blood vessels	Penetration of skin by cercaria released from snail	Unknown; probably common	Ova and miracidia cause extensive gill damage, death	Bykhovskaya-Pavlovskaya et al. 1962 Yamaguti 1958
*Sanguinicola inermis**	Europe	Carp	Blood vessels	Penetration of skin by cercaria released from snail	Common	Ova and miracidia cause extensive gill damage, death	Dawes 1946 Hoffman 1967 Reichenbach-Klinke and Elkan 1965 Yamaguti 1958
*Sanguinicola armata**	Europe	Carp, other fishes	Blood vessels	Penetration of skin by cercaria released from snail	Common	Ova and miracidia cause extensive gill damage, death	Hoffman 1967 Yamaguti 1958
Bucephalus elegans	United States	Bluegill, sunfishes, other fishes	Intestine	Ingestion of metacercaria in muscle or skin of fish	Common	Pathologic effects unknown	Hoffman 1967 Yamaguti 1958
Bucephalus polymorphus	Europe	Goldfish, carp, Atlantic salmon, eels, other fishes	Intestine	Ingestion of metacercaria in gills or skin of fish	Common	Pathologic effects unknown	Dawes 1946 Hoffman 1967 Yamaguti 1958
Rhipidocotyle septpapillata	United States	Sunfishes, other fishes	Intestine	Ingestion of metacercaria in gills or skin of fish	Common	Pathologic effects unknown	Hoffman 1967 Yamaguti 1958
Cryptogonimus chyli	United States, Canada	Bluegill, sunfishes, other fishes	Stomach, intestine	Ingestion of metacercaria in muscle of fish	Common	Pathologic effects unknown	Hoffman 1967 Yamaguti 1958
Acetodextra amiuri	United States, Canada	Channel catfish, other ictalurids	Ovaries	Probably by ingestion of metacercaria in liver of fish	Common	Pathologic effects unknown	Hoffman 1967 Yamaguti 1958
Centrovarium lobotes	North America	Black bass, other centrarchids, channel catfish, eels, other fishes	Stomach, intestine	Ingestion of metacercaria in muscle of fish	Common	Pathologic effects unknown	Hoffman 1967 Yamaguti 1958
Phyllodistomum superbum	United States, Canada	Sunfishes, brook trout, other fishes	Ureters, urinary bladder	Ingestion of cercaria released from mollusk	Common	Pathologic effects unknown	Hoffman 1967
Phyllodistomum lohrenzi	United States	Bluegill, sunfishes, other fishes	Ureters, urinary bladder	Ingestion of cercaria released from clams or metacercaria in arthropod	Common	Pathologic effects unknown	Hoffman 1967 Yamaguti 1958

* Discussed in text.

724

TABLE 22.2 (continued)

Parasite	Geographic Distribution	Fish Host	Location in Host	Method of Infection	Incidence in Nature	Remarks	Reference
Phyllodistomum pearsii	United States	Sunfishes, other fishes	Ureters, urinary bladder	Ingestion of cercaria released from clam	Common	Pathologic effects unknown	Hoffman 1967 Yamaguti 1958
Phyllodistomum lachancei	United States, Canada	Brook trout, rainbow trout	Ureters, urinary bladder	Ingestion of cercaria released from mollusk	Common	Pathologic effects unknown	Hoffman 1967 Yamaguti 1958
Phyllodistomum lacustri	United States	Channel catfish, other ictalurids	Ureters, urinary bladder	Unknown; presumably ingestion of cercaria encysted in arthropod	Common	Pathologic effects unknown	Hoffman 1967 Spall and Summerfelt 1969 Yamaguti 1958
Phyllodistomum folium	Europe	Goldfish, sticklebacks, other fishes	Urinary bladder	Ingestion of cercaria released from mollusk	Common	Pathologic effects unknown	Bykhovskaya-Pavlovskaya et al. 1962 Dawes 1946 Yamaguti 1958
Phyllodistomum elongatum	Europe	Goldfish, carp, other cyprinids	Urinary bladder	Ingestion of cercaria released from mollusk	Common	Pathologic effects unknown	Bykhovskaya-Pavlovskaya et al. 1962 Dawes 1946 Yamaguti 1958
Phyllodistomum simile	Europe	Brown trout, other fishes	Urinary bladder	Ingestion of cercaria released from mollusk	Common	Syn. *Phyllodistomum megalorchis.* Pathologic effects unknown	Dawes 1946 Hoffman 1967 Yamaguti 1958
Phyllodistomum macrocotyle	Europe	Carp, other fishes	Ureters, urinary bladder	Ingestion of cercaria released from mollusk	Common	Pathologic effects unknown	Dawes 1946 Yamaguti 1958
Proterometra macrostoma	United States	Bluegill, sunfishes, other fishes	Esophagus	Ingestion of metacercaria in snail	Unknown; probably common	Pathologic effects unknown	Hoffman 1967 Yamaguti 1958
Proterometra dickermani	North central United States	Bluegill, sunfishes	Intestine	Ingestion of metacercaria in snail	Unknown; probably common	Pathologic effects unknown	Hoffman 1967
Proterometra catenaria	Southeastern United States	Sunfishes	Intestine	Ingestion of metacercaria in snail	Unknown; probably common	Pathologic effects unknown	Hoffman 1967 Yamaguti 1958
Proterometra hodgesiana	Southeastern United States	Sunfishes	Intestine	Ingestion of metacercaria in snail	Unknown; probably common	Pathologic effects unknown	Hoffman 1967
Azygia angusticauda	North America	Bluegill, sunfishes, channel catfish, other fishes	Intestine	Ingestion of cercaria in snail	Common	Pathologic effects unknown	Hoffman 1967 Yamaguti 1958
Azygia longa	United States, Canada	Sunfishes, lake trout, other salmonids, other fishes	Stomach, intestine	Ingestion of cercaria in snail or encysted in fish	Common	Pathologic effects unknown	Hoffman 1967

TABLE 22.2 (continued)

Parasite	Geographic Distribution	Fish Host	Location in Host	Method of Infection	Incidence in Nature	Remarks	Reference
Azygia acuminata	United States	Bluegill, other fishes	Stomach	Ingestion of cercaria in snail	Common	Pathologic effects unknown	Hoffman 1967
Azygia lucii	Europe	Salmonids, eels, other fishes	Stomach, intestine	Ingestion of cercaria in snail	Common	Pathologic effects unknown	Yamaguti 1958
Microphallus opacus	North America	Black bass, channel catfish, eels, other fishes	Stomach, intestine	Ingestion of metacercaria in crustacean	Common	Syn. *Microphallus ovatus*. Pathologic effects unknown	Hoffman 1967 Yamaguti 1958
Alloglossidium corti	United States, Canada	Channel catfish, other fishes	Intestine	Ingestion of intermediate host (dragonfly, mayfly nymph)	Common	Pathologic effects unknown	Hoffman 1967 Yamaguti 1958
Creptotrema funduli	United States	Topminnows, sticklebacks, other fishes	Intestine	Ingestion of metacercaria in insect	Common	Pathologic effects unknown	Hoffman 1967 Yamaguti 1958
Crepidostomum cooperi	North America, Europe	Carp, topminnows, bluegill, sunfishes, black bass, rainbow trout, brown trout, other fishes	Intestine	Ingestion of intermediate host (mayfly)	Common	Pathologic effects unknown	Hoffman 1967 Olsen 1967 Yamaguti 1958
Crepidostomum farionis	North America, Europe	Sunfishes, lake trout, rainbow trout, brown trout, Atlantic salmon, other fishes	Intestine	Ingestion of intermediate host (mayfly, crustacean)	Common	Heavy infections sometimes cause severe enteritis, death	Dawes 1946 Dogiel et al. 1962 Hoffman 1967 Mitchum and Moore 1969 Olsen 1967 Yamaguti 1958
Crepidostomum cornutum	North America	Bluegill, sunfishes, black bass, brook trout, Atlantic salmon, eels, other fishes	Intestine	Ingestion of intermediate host (crayfish)	Common	Pathologic effects unknown	Hoffman 1967 Olsen 1967 Yamaguti 1958
Crepidostomum laureatium	United States	Sunfishes, rainbow trout	Intestine	Ingestion of intermediate host (arthropod)	Common	Pathologic effects unknown	Hoffman 1967
Crepidostomum metoecus	United States Europe	Brown trout, Atlantic salmon	Intestine	Ingestion of intermediate host (arthropod)	Common	Pathologic effects unknown	Hoffman 1967 Yamaguti 1958
Crepidostomum ictaluri	United States, Canada	Channel catfish, other ictalurids	Intestine	Ingestion of intermediate host (mayfly nymph)	Common	Syn. *Megalogonia ictaluri*. Pathologic effects unknown	Hoffman 1967 Olsen 1967 Spall and Summerfelt 1969
Crepidostomum breviviteIlum	Northeastern United States, Canada	Eels	Intestine	Ingestion of intermediate host (arthropod)	Common	Pathologic effects unknown	Hoffman 1967 Yamaguti 1958

TABLE 22.2 (continued)

Parasite	Geographic Distribution	Fish Host	Location in Host	Method of Infection	Incidence in Nature	Remarks	Reference
Bunodera lucioþercae	United States, Europe	Carp, black bass, brown trout, other fishes	Intestine	Ingestion of intermediate host (arthropod)	Common	Pathologic effects unknown	Bykhovskaya-Pavlovskaya et al. 1962 Hoffman 1967 Yamaguti 1958
Bunodera sacculata	United States, Canada	Shiners, sunfishes, black bass, other fishes	Intestine	Ingestion of intermediate host (arthropod)	Common	Syn. *Bunoderina sacculata.* Pathologic effects unknown	Bykhovskaya-Pavlovskaya et al. 1962 Hoffman 1967 Yamaguti 1958
Bunoderina eucaliae	United States, Canada, England	Sticklebacks	Intestine	Ingestion of intermediate host (arthropod)	Common	Pathologic effects unknown	Bykhovskaya-Pavlovskaya et al. 1962 Hoffman 1967 Yamaguti 1958
Vietosoma parvum	Eastern United States	Channel catfish	Stomach, intestine	Ingestion of intermediate host (arthropod)	Common	Pathologic effects unknown	Bykhovskaya-Pavlovskaya et al. 1962 Hoffman 1967 Yamaguti 1958
Allocreadium lobatum	United States	Shiners, brook trout, rainbow trout, other fishes	Stomach, intestine	Ingestion of metacercaria in arthropod, clam	Common	Pathologic effects unknown	Hoffman 1967 Yamaguti 1958
Allocreadium ictaluri	United States, Canada	Channel catfish, other ictalurids	Intestine	Ingestion of metacercaria in arthropod, clam	Common	Pathologic effects unknown	Hoffman 1967 Olsen 1967
Allocreadium isoporum	Europe	Goldfish, carp, other cyprinids	Intestine	Ingestion of metacercaria in arthropod, clam	Unknown; probably common	Pathologic effects unknown	Dawes 1946 Hoffman 1967 Reichenbach-Klinke and Elkan 1965 Yamaguti 1958
Allocreadium transversale	Europe	Goldfish	Intestine	Ingestion of metacercaria in arthropod, clam	Unknown; probably common	Pathologic effects unknown	Dawes 1946 Hoffman 1967 Yamaguti 1958
Homalometron armatum	Southern United States	Sunfishes, other fishes	Intestine	Ingestion of metacercaria in clam	Common	Pathologic effects unknown	Hoffman 1967 Yamaguti 1958
Podocotyle shawi	Northwestern United States	Rainbow trout, Pacific salmons	Intestine	Unknown	Common	Pathologic effects unknown	Hoffman 1967
Podocotyle simplex	Canada	Atlantic salmon, other fishes	Intestine	Unknown	Common	Pathologic effects unknown	Hoffman 1967 Yamaguti 1958
Podocotyle atomon	Canada, Europe	Atlantic salmon, sticklebacks, eels	Intestine	Unknown; probably by ingestion of infected amphipod	Common	Pathologic effects unknown	Hanek and Threlfall 1969 Hoffman 1967 Yamaguti 1958
Plagioporus lepomis	United States	Sunfishes, other centrarchids	Intestine	Ingestion of metacercaria in intermediate host (arthropod)	Common	Syn. *Podocotyle letpomis.* Pathologic effects unknown	Hoffman 1967 Yamaguti 1958

TABLE 22.2 *(continued)*

Parasite	Geographic Distribution	Fish Host	Location in Host	Method of Infection	Incidence in Nature	Remarks	Reference
Plagioporus angusticollis	United States, Europe	Rainbow trout, eels, other fishes	Intestine	Ingestion of metacercaria in intermediate host (arthropod)	Common	Pathologic effects unknown	Hoffman 1967 Yamaguti 1958
Plagioporus cooperi	United States	Shiners, other fishes	Intestine	Ingestion of metacercaria in intermediate host (arthropod)	Common	Pathologic effects unknown	Hoffman 1967 Yamaguti 1958
Plagioporus sinitsini	United States	Chubs, shiners, eels	Intestine	Ingestion of metacercaria in intermediate host (arthropod)	Common	Pathologic effects unknown	Hoffman 1967 Yamaguti 1958
Plagioporus bilaris	Israel	Tropical mouthbreeders	Intestine	Ingestion of metacercaria in intermediate host (arthropod)	Common	Pathologic effects unknown	Hoffman 1967
Plagioporus angulatus	USSR	Eels	Intestine	Ingestion of metacercaria in intermediate host (arthropod)	Common	Pathologic effects unknown	Hoffman 1967 Yamaguti 1958
Sphaerostoma bramae	Europe	Carp, European minnow, chubs, eels, other fishes	Intestine	Ingestion of cercaria released from mollusk	Common	Pathologic effects unknown	Dawes 1946 Hoffman 1967 Reichenbach-Klinke and Elkan 1965 Yamaguti 1958
Sphaerostoma globiporum	Europe	Brown trout	Intestine	Ingestion of cercaria released from mollusk	Unknown; probably common	Syn. *Sphaerostoma bramae*. Pathologic effects unknown	Hoffman 1967 Yamaguti 1958
Sphaerostoma majus	Europe	Brown trout	Intestine	Ingestion of cercaria released from mollusk	Unknown; probably common	Pathologic effects unknown	Hoffman 1967
Sphaerostoma salmonis	Europe	Brown trout	Intestine	Ingestion of cercaria released from mollusk	Unknown; probably common	Pathologic effects unknown	Hoffman 1967
Holostephanus ictaluri	United States	Channel catfish	Intestine	Ingestion of cercaria released from mollusk	Unknown; probably common	Fish possibly accidental host. Pathologic effects unknown	Hoffman 1967 Yamaguti 1958
Holostephanus lukei	Great Britain	Sticklebacks	Intestine	Ingestion of cercaria released from mollusk	Unknown; probably common	Fish possibly accidental host. Pathologic effects unknown	Hoffman 1967 Yamaguti 1958
Peracreadium gasterostei	Europe	Sticklebacks	Intestine	Ingestion of cercaria released from mollusk	Unknown; probably common	Pathologic effects unknown	Hoffman 1967 Yamaguti 1958

TABLE 22.3 Larval digenetic trematodes affecting laboratory fishes

	Geographic Distribution	Fish Host	Location in Host	Method of Infection	Incidence in Nature	Remarks	Reference
*Diplostomum spathaceum**	Europe	Goldfish, carp, European minnow, black bass, rainbow trout, brown trout, Atlantic salmon, sticklebacks, eels, other fishes	Eye lens, vitreous body	Penetration by cercaria released from snail	Common	Possible syn. *Diplostomum flexicaudum, D. huronense*. Causes opacity of lens, blindness, increased intraocular pressure, rupture of cornea, death	Ashton et al. 1969 Bykhovskaya-Pavlovskaya et al. 1962 van Duijn 1967 Ferguson 1943 Hoffman 1960, 1967 Larson 1965 Reichenbach-Klinke and Elkan 1965 Yamaguti 1958
*Diplostomum flexicaudum**	United States	Black bass, other fishes	Eye lens	Penetration by cercaria released from snail	Common	Possible syn. *Diplostomum spathaceum*. Causes opacity of lens, blindness	Hoffman 1960, 1967 Yamaguti 1958
*Diplostomum huronense**	North central United States	Bluegill, sunfishes, other fishes	Eye lens, vitreous body	Penetration by cercaria released from snail	Uncommon	Possible syn. *Diplostomum spathaceum*. Pathologic effects unknown; probably causes opacity of lens, blindness	Hoffman 1960, 1967 Yamaguti 1958
Diplostomum phoxini	Europe	European minnow	Brain	Penetration by cercaria released from snail	Common	Unencysted in brain; pathologic effects unknown	Hoffman 1960
Diplostomum baeri eucaliae	Northern United States	Sticklebacks	Brain	Penetration by cercaria released from snail	Uncommon	Unencysted in brain; sometimes causes death	Hoffman 1960, 1967 Yamaguti 1958
Diplostomulum scheuringi	United States	Carp, bluntnose minnow, shiners, other cyprinids, mosquitofish, bluegill, sunfishes, black bass, other centrarchids, brown trout, other salmonids	Vitreous body	Penetration by cercaria released from snail	Common	Adults unknown. Pathologic effects unknown; probably causes blindness	Hoffman 1960, 1967
Diplostomulum clavatum	Europe	Goldfish, carp, other fishes	Vitreous body	Penetration by cercaria released from snail	Common	Adults unknown. Pathologic effects unknown; probably causes blindness	Bykhovskaya-Pavlovskaya et al. 1962 Hoffman 1960, 1967 Reichenbach-Klinke and Elkan 1965
Diplostomulum truttae	Great Britain	Brown trout	Eye	Penetration by cercaria released from snail	Uncommon	Adults unknown. Pathologic effects unknown; probably causes blindness	Hoffman 1960, 1967
Bolbophorus confusus	Northwestern United States, Europe, Africa	Rainbow trout, brown trout, other fishes	Muscle	Penetration by cercaria released from snail	Common in Europe, uncommon in United States	Causes cysts in muscle; new cysts are unpigmented, old cysts are black	Hoffman 1960, 1967 Yamaguti 1958

*Discussed in text.

TABLE 22.3 (continued)

Parasite	Geographic Distribution	Fish Host	Location in Host	Method of Infection	Incidence in Nature	Remarks	Reference
Hysteromorpha triloba	North America, South America, Europe, Japan, Australia	Golden shiner, other fishes	Muscle	Penetration by cercaria released from snail	Common	Causes cysts in muscle	Hoffman 1960, 1967; Yamaguti 1958
Tetracotyle lepomensis	United States	Shiners, bluegill	Vitreous body, mesentery	Penetration by cercaria released from snail	Common in some areas	Probably causes blindness; cysts in mesentery	Hoffman 1967; G. L. Hoffman, unpublished data
Tetracotyle intermedia	North central United States, USSR	Brown trout, other fishes	Pericardium	Penetration by cercaria released from snail	Uncommon	Causes cysts in pericardium	Bykhovskaya-Pavlovskaya et al. 1962; Hoffman 1960, 1967
Tetracotyle echinata	Europe	Carp, other cyprinids	Peritoneum	Penetration by cercaria released from snail	Uncommon	Causes cysts in peritoneum	Bykhovskaya-Pavlovskaya et al. 1962; Hoffman 1960, 1967
Tetracotyle sogdiana	USSR	Carp, other cyprinids, salmonids	Peritoneum	Penetration by cercaria released from snail	Uncommon	Causes peritonitis, adhesions	Bykhovskaya-Pavlovskaya et al. 1962; Hoffman 1960, 1967
Uvulifer ambloplitis*	United States, Canada	Fathead minnow, bluntnose minnow, chubs, shiners, golden shiner, other cyprinids, sunfishes, other centrarchids	Skin, muscle	Penetration by cercaria released from snail	Common	Causes black cysts in skin, muscle (blackspot Neascus); heavy infections cause death	Hoffman 1960, 1967; Krull 1934; Yamaguti 1958
Crassiphiala bulboglossa*	Northern United States	Fathead minnow, chubs, shiners, golden shiner, other cyprinids, killifishes, other fishes	Skin, gills, muscle	Penetration by cercaria released from snail	Common	Causes black cysts in skin, branchial arches, muscle (blackspot Neascus); heavy infections cause death	Hoffman 1956, 1960, 1967; Yamaguti 1958
Posthodiplostomum cuticola*	Europe	Goldfish, sticklebacks, other fishes	Skin, gills, muscle, mouth	Unknown; probably penetration by cercaria released from snail	Common	Causes black cysts in skin (blackspot Neascus); heavy infections probably cause death	Bykhovskaya-Pavlovskaya et al. 1962; van Duijn 1967; Hoffman 1960; Reichenbach-Klinke and Elkan 1965; Yamaguti 1958
Posthodiplostomum minimum*	United States, Canada	Fathead minnow, bluntnose minnow, chubs, shiners, golden shiner, topminnows, mollies, mosquitofish, bluegill, sunfishes, black bass, brook trout, channel catfish, sticklebacks, other fishes	Mesentery, kidneys, liver, spleen, pericardium	Penetration by cercaria released from snail	Common	Causes cysts in mesentery, kidneys, liver, spleen, pericardium (white grub); heavy infections cause death	Hoffman 1958b, 1960, 1967; Lewis and Nickum 1964; Yamaguti 1958

* Discussed in text.

TABLE 22.3 *(continued)*

Parasite	Geographic Distribution	Fish Host	Location in Host	Method of Infection	Incidence in Nature	Remarks	Reference
Ornithodiplostomum ptychocheilus	Northern United States	Fathead minnow, chubs, shiners	Peritoneum, viscera, brain	Penetration by cercaria released from snail	Uncommon	Causes cysts in peritoneum, viscera, brain	Hoffman 1958a, 1960, 1967 Yamaguti 1958
Neodiplostomum perlatum	Eastern Europe	Carp	Skin, muscle	Unknown; probably penetration by cercaria released from snail	Uncommon	Causes cysts in skin, muscle	van Duijn 1967 Hoffman 1960 Yamaguti 1958
Prohemistomum ovatus	Europe	Carp, other cyprinids	Muscle	Penetration by cercaria released from snail	Uncommon	Probable syn. *Prohemistomum circulare*. Causes cysts in muscle	Hoffman 1960
*Clinostomum marginatum**	North America	Bluntnose minnow, chubs, shiners, killifishes, bluegill, sunfishes, black bass, brook trout, rainbow trout, other fishes	Muscle, connective tissue, gills	Penetration by cercaria released from snail	Common	Causes light yellow cysts in muscle, connective tissue, gills (yellow grub); serious pathogen in some hatcheries	van Duijn 1967 Hoffman 1967 Reichenbach-Klinke and Elkan 1965 Yamaguti 1958
*Clinostomum complanatum**	Eastern Europe, southern Asia	Goldfish, other fishes	Muscle, connective tissue	Penetration by cercaria released from snail	Uncommon	Causes light yellow cysts in muscle, connective tissue (yellow grub)	Bykhovskaya-Pavlovskaya et al. 1962 van Duijn 1967 Reichenbach-Klinke and Elkan 1965 Yamaguti 1958
Bucephalus elegans	United States	Shiners, other fishes	Muscle, skin	Penetration by cercaria released from snail	Uncommon	Causes cysts in muscle, skin	Hoffman 1967 Yamaguti 1958
Bucephalus polymorphus	Europe	Cyprinids, eels, other fishes	Gills, skin, fins	Penetration by cercaria released from snail	Common	Causes cysts in gills, skin, fins; hemorrhagic necrosis in fins, eyes, mouth; sometimes death	Bykhovskaya-Pavlovskaya et al. 1962 van Duijn 1967 de Kinkelin et al. 1968 Yamaguti 1958
Petasiger nitidus	North America	Shiners, guppy, bluegill, other fishes	Esophagus	Ingestion of cercaria released from snail	Uncommon	Causes cysts in esophagus	Hoffman 1967 Yamaguti 1958
Echinochasmus donaldsoni	North central United States	Sticklebacks	Gills	Penetration by cercaria released from snail	Uncommon	Causes cysts in gills	Hoffman 1967 Yamaguti 1958
Echinochasmus schwartzi	United States	Killifishes	Gills	Penetration by cercaria released from snail	Uncommon	Causes cysts in gills	Hoffman 1967 Yamaguti 1958
Euparyphium melis	United States, Europe, Asia	Bluegill, other fishes	Nares, cloaca	Penetration by cercaria released from snail	Uncommon	Syn. *Isthmiophora melis*. Pathologic effects unknown	Dawes 1946 Hoffman 1967 Walton 1964 Yamaguti 1958

*Discussed in text.

TABLE 22.3 *(continued)*

Parasite	Geographic Distribution	Fish Host	Location in Host	Method of Infection	Incidence in Nature	Remarks	Reference
Itibeiroia ondatrae	North America	Bluegill, sunfishes, black bass, other fishes	Subcutis	Penetration by cercaria released from snail	Uncommon	Causes cysts in lateral line system	Hoffman 1967 Yamaguti 1958
Macroderoides spinifera	North America	Killifishes, mollies, mosquito-fish	Muscle	Penetration by cercaria released from snail	Uncommon	Causes cysts in muscle	Hoffman 1967 Yamaguti 1958
Paramacroderoides echinus	United States	Killifishes, mollies, mosquito-fish	Muscle	Penetration by cercaria released from snail	Uncommon	Causes cysts in muscle	Hoffman 1967 Yamaguti 1958
Nanophyetus salmincola	Pacific coast of North America, Siberia	Goldfish, other cyprinids, mosquitofish, sunfishes, brook trout, lake trout, rainbow trout, brown trout, Atlantic salmon, other salmonids, sticklebacks	Gills, eyes, tongue, muscle, heart, kidneys, liver, gall-bladder, pancreas, intestine	Penetration by cercaria released from snail	Common	Syn. *Troglotrema salmincola.* Transmits *Neorickettsia helminthoeca* to canids. Causes cysts which produce mechanical damage; heavy infections cause death; serious pathogen in some hatcheries. Reported in man in Siberia	Belding 1965 Hoffman 1967 Wood and Yasutake 1956 Yamaguti 1958
Sellacotyle mustelae	North America	Fathead minnow, chubs, shiners, other fishes	Muscle, mesentery	Penetration by cercaria released from snail	Uncommon	Causes small cysts in muscle, mesentery	Hoffman 1967 Yamaguti 1958
Apophallus brevis	United States, Canada	Brook trout, brown trout	Skin	Penetration by cercaria released from snail	Uncommon	Causes black cysts in skin	Hoffman 1967 Yamaguti 1958
Apophallus venustus	North America, Europe	Carp, shiners, sunfishes, black bass, other fishes	Skin	Penetration by cercaria released from snail	Uncommon	Syn. *Apophallus donicus.* Causes unpigmented cysts in skin	Hoffman 1967 Yamaguti 1958
Apophallus muelingi	Europe	Cyprinids	Muscle, gills	Penetration by cercaria released from snail	Common	Causes cysts in muscle, gills	Yamaguti 1958
Ascocotyle angrense	United States	Topminnows, killifishes, mollies, other fishes	Gills	Penetration by cercaria released from snail	Common	Causes cysts in gills	Hoffman 1967
Ascocotyle chandleri	Southern United States	Topminnows, mollies	Liver	Penetration by cercaria released from snail	Uncommon	Causes cysts in liver	Hoffman 1967
Ascocotyle leighi	Southern United States	Topminnows, killifishes, mollies	Beneath endothelium in conus arteriosus	Penetration by cercaria released from snail	Uncommon	Causes cysts in conus arteriosus which sometimes block flow of blood	Hoffman 1967
Ascocotyle tenuicollis	Southern United States	Mollies, mosquitofish, other fishes	Conus arteriosus	Penetration by cercaria released from snail	Uncommon	Causes cysts in conus arteriosus	Hoffman 1967 Yamaguti 1958
Ascocotyle mcintoshi	Southern United States	Mollies, mosquitofish	Mesentery, viscera	Penetration by cercaria released from snail	Uncommon	Causes cysts in mesentery, viscera	Hoffman 1967 Yamaguti 1958
Ascocotyle moliensicola	Southern United States	Mollies	Intestinal wall, muscle, gills	Penetration by cercaria released from snail	Uncommon	Causes cysts in intestinal wall, muscle, gills	Hoffman 1967

TABLE 22.3 *(continued)*

Parasite	Geographic Distribution	Fish Host	Location in Host	Method of Infection	Incidence in Nature	Remarks	Reference
Ascocotyle coleostoma	Europe	Carp, other fishes	Gills	Penetration by cercaria released from snail	Uncommon	Causes cysts in gills	Bykhovskaya-Pavlovskaya et al. 1962 Hoffman 1967 Yamaguti 1958
Centrovarium lobotes	North America	Bluntnose minnow, shiners, other fishes	Muscle	Penetration by cercaria released from snail	Common	Causes unpigmented cysts in muscle	Hoffman 1967 Yamaguti 1958
Opisthorchis tenuicollis	North America, Europe, Asia	Carp, other cyprinids	Muscle, connective tissue	Penetration by cercaria released from snail	Common	Syn. *Opisthorchis felineus.* Causes cysts in muscle, connective tissue. Sometimes affects man	Belding 1965 Bykhovskaya-Pavlovskaya et al. 1962 Reichenbach-Klinke and Elkan 1965 Yamaguti 1958
Opisthorchis tonkae	United States	Sunfishes, other fishes	Muscle	Penetration by cercaria released from snail	Common	Causes cysts in muscle	Yamaguti 1958

TABLE 22.4. Adult cestodes affecting laboratory fishes

Parasite	Geographic Distribution	Fish Host	Location in Host	Method of Infection	Incidence in Nature	Remarks	Reference
*Corallobothrium fimbriatum**	North America	Channel catfish, other ictalurids	Intestine	Ingestion of intermediate host (copepod, small fish)	Common	Pathologic effects unknown; probably harmful to host	Essex 1927 Hoffman 1967 Mitchum and Moore 1969 Wardle and McLeod 1952 Yamaguti 1959
*Corallobothrium giganteum**	United States	Channel catfish, other ictalurids	Intestine	Ingestion of intermediate host (copepod, small fish)	Common	Pathologic effects unknown; probably harmful to host	Essex 1927 Hoffman 1967 Wardle and McLeod 1952 Yamaguti 1959
Corallobothrium thompsoni	United States	Channel catfish	Intestine	Ingestion of intermediate host (copepod, small fish)	Rare	Pathologic effects unknown	Hoffman 1967 Yamaguti 1959
Ophotaenia fragilis	North central United States	Channel catfish	Intestine	Unknown	Rare	Pathologic effects unknown	Hoffman 1967 Wardle and McLeod 1952 Yamaguti 1959
Proteocephalus perplexus	Northern United States	Bluntnose minnow, other fishes	Intestine	Ingestion of intermediate host (small fish)	Uncommon	Pathologic effects unknown	Hoffman 1967 Wardle and McLeod 1952 Yamaguti 1959
Proteocephalus pearsei	Northern United States	Shiners, sunfishes, black bass, other fishes	Intestine, pyloric ceca	Ingestion of intermediate host (small fish)	Uncommon in sunfishes	Pathologic effects unknown	Hoffman 1967 Wardle and McLeod 1952 Yamaguti 1959
Proteocephalus ambloplitis	North America	Shiners, sunfishes, black bass, salmonids, ictalurids, other fishes	Intestine	Ingestion of intermediate host (copepod, small fish)	Common in black bass	Bass tapeworm. Pathologic effects unknown	Fischer and Freeman 1969 Hoffman 1967 Mitchum and Moore 1969 Wardle and McLeod 1952 Yamaguti 1959
Proteocephalus stizostethi	North America	Black bass, sunfishes, other fishes	Intestine	Unknown	Uncommon	Pathologic effects unknown	Hoffman 1967 Wardle and McLeod 1952 Yamaguti 1959
Proteocephalus microcephalus	United States	Black bass	Intestine	Unknown	Rare	Pathologic effects unknown	Hoffman 1967 Yamaguti 1959
Proteocephalus fluviatilis	North central United States	Black bass, lake trout	Intestine	Unknown	Uncommon	Pathologic effects unknown	Hoffman 1967 Wardle and McLeod 1952 Yamaguti 1959
Proteocephalus pinguis	North America	Brook trout, brown trout, other fishes	Intestine	Ingestion of intermediate host (small fish)	Common	Pathologic effects unknown	Hoffman 1967 Wardle and McLeod 1952 Yamaguti 1959
Proteocephalus pusillus	Eastern North America	Brook trout, lake trout, Atlantic salmon	Intestine	Unknown	Uncommon	Pathologic effects unknown	Hoffman 1967 Wardle and McLeod 1952 Yamaguti 1959

*Discussed in text.

734

TABLE 22.4 *(continued)*

Parasite	Geographic Distribution	Fish Host	Location in Host	Method of Infection	Incidence in Nature	Remarks	Reference
Proteocephalus parallacticus	Northeastern North America	Brook trout, lake trout, brown trout	Intestine	Ingestion of intermediate host (copepod)	Uncommon	Pathologic effects unknown	Hoffman 1967 Wardle and McLeod 1952 Yamaguti 1959
Proteocephalus tumidicollis	Western United States	Brook trout, rainbow trout	Intestine	Ingestion of intermediate host (copepod)	Uncommon	Pathologic effects unknown	Hoffman 1967 Yamaguti 1959
Proteocephalus arcticus	Canada	Brook trout, Pacific salmons, other salmonids	Intestine	Unknown	Uncommon	Pathologic effects unknown	Hoffman 1967 Wardle and McLeod 1952 Yamaguti 1959
Proteocephalus salmonidicola	Western North America	Rainbow trout, other salmonids	Intestine	Unknown	Uncommon	Pathologic effects unknown	Hoffman 1967 Yamaguti 1959
Proteocephalus laruei	North America	Pacific salmons, other salmonids	Intestine	Unknown	Uncommon	Pathologic effects unknown	Hoffman 1967 Wardle and McLeod 1952 Yamaguti 1959
Proteocephalus exiguus	North America, USSR	Pacific salmons, other salmonids	Intestine	Unknown	Common	Length: 9 to 38 mm. Pathologic effects unknown	Bykhovskaya-Pavlovskaya et al. 1962 Hoffman 1967 Wardle and McLeod 1952 Yamaguti 1959
Proteocephalus pugetensis	Western North America	Sticklebacks	Intestine	Ingestion of intermediate host (copepod)	Uncommon	Pathologic effects unknown	Hoffman 1967 Wardle and McLeod 1952 Yamaguti 1959
Proteocephalus macrocephalus	United States, Europe	Eels	Intestine	Unknown	Uncommon	Length: 400 mm. Pathologic effects unknown	Bykhovskaya-Pavlovskaya et al. 1962 Hoffman 1967 Wardle and McLeod 1952 Yamaguti 1959
Proteocephalus longicollis	Europe	Rainbow trout, brown trout, other fishes	Intestine	Unknown	Uncommon	Length: 20 to 50 mm. Pathologic effects unknown	Bykhovskaya-Pavlovskaya et al. 1962 Wardle and McLeod 1952 Yamaguti 1959
Proteocephalus neglectus	Europe	Brown trout	Intestine	Unknown	Uncommon	Pathologic effects unknown	Bykhovskaya-Pavlovskaya et al. 1962 Yamaguti 1959
Proteocephalus cernuae	Europe	Sticklebacks, other fishes	Intestine	Unknown	Common	Pathologic effects unknown	Bykhovskaya-Pavlovskaya et al. 1962 Wardle and McLeod 1952 Yamaguti 1959
Proteocephalus filicollis	Europe	Sticklebacks	Intestine	Unknown	Common	Incidence of 17% reported in Great Britain. Pathologic effects unknown	Chappell 1969 Wardle and McLeod 1952 Yamaguti 1959

735

TABLE 22.4 (continued)

Parasite	Geographic Distribution	Fish Host	Location in Host	Method of Infection	Incidence in Nature	Remarks	Reference
*Eubothrium crassum**	North America, Europe	Brook trout, rainbow trout, brown trout, Atlantic salmons, Pacific salmons, other fishes	Pyloric ceca	Ingestion of intermediate host (copepod)	Common	Pathologic effects unknown	Bykhovskaya-Pavlovskaya et al. 1962; Dogiel et al. 1962; Hoffman 1967; Wardle and McLeod 1952; Yamaguti 1959
*Eubothrium salvelini**	North America, Europe	Brook trout, rainbow trout, lake trout, Pacific salmons, other fishes	Pyloric ceca	Ingestion of intermediate host (copepod)	Common	Pathologic effects unknown	Hoffman 1967; Richardson 1936; Wardle and McLeod 1952; Yamaguti 1959
Bothriocephalus claviceps	United States, Europe	Bluegill, sunfishes, black bass, sticklebacks, eels, other fishes	Intestine	Ingestion of intermediate host (copepod, small fish)	Common	Pathologic effects unknown	Hoffman 1967; Wardle and McLeod 1952; Yamaguti 1959
Bothriocephalus cuspidatus	North America	Bluegill, sunfishes, other fishes	Pyloric ceca, intestine	Ingestion of intermediate host (copepod, small fish)	Common	Pathologic effects unknown	Hoffman 1967; Wardle and McLeod 1952; Yamaguti 1959
Bothriocephalus gowkongensis	Europe, Asia	Carp	Intestine	Ingestion of intermediate host (copepod, small fish)	Common	Heavy infections cause death	Bykhovskaya-Pavlovskaya et al. 1962
Cyathocephalus truncatus	North America, Europe	Brown trout, other fishes	Intestine	Ingestion of intermediate host (small fish)	Common	Pathologic effects unknown	Hoffman 1967; Reichenbach-Klinke and Elkan 1965; Wardle and McLeod 1952; Yamaguti 1959
Triaenophorus nodulosus	North America, Europe	Carp, sunfishes, black bass, rainbow trout, eels, other fishes	Intestine	Ingestion of intermediate host (small fish)	Common	Syn. *Triaenophorus lucii.* Pathologic effects unknown	Hoffman 1967; Reichenbach-Klinke and Elkan 1965; Yamaguti 1959
Triaenophorus crassus	North America, Europe	Shiners, black bass, salmonids, sticklebacks, other fishes	Intestine	Ingestion of intermediate host (small fish)	Common	Pathologic effects unknown	Yamaguti 1959
Khawia iowensis	Central United States	Carp, other cyprinids	Intestine	Unknown	Uncommon	Pathologic effects unknown	Hoffman 1967
Atractolytocestus huronensis	United States	Carp	Intestine	Unknown	Uncommon	Pathologic effects unknown	Hoffman 1967
Caryophyllaeus terebrans	North America	Carp, other fishes	Intestine	Ingestion of intermediate host (oligochete)	Common	Pathologic effects unknown	Hoffman 1967; Wardle and McLeod 1952; Yamaguti 1959

*Discussed in text.

TABLE 22.4 *(continued)*

Parasite	Geographic Distribution	Fish Host	Location in Host	Method of Infection	Incidence in Nature	Remarks	Reference
Caryophyllaeus fimbriceps	Europe	Carp, other fishes	Intestine	Ingestion of intermediate host (oligochete)	Common	Causes acute enteritis, death	Dogiel et al. 1958 van Duijn 1967 Wardle and McLeod 1952 Yamaguti 1959
Caryophyllaeus laticeps	Europe	Carp, other fishes	Intestine	Ingestion of intermediate host (oligochete)	Common	Pathologic effects unknown	Dogiel et al. 1962 van Duijn 1967 Reichenbach-Klinke and Elkan 1965 Wardle and McLeod 1952 Yamaguti 1959

TABLE 22.5. Larval cestodes affecting laboratory fishes

Parasite	Geographic Distribution	Fish Host	Location in Host	Method of Infection	Incidence in Nature	Remarks	Reference
*Corallobothrium fimbriatum**	North America	Shiners	Viscera	Ingestion of intermediate host (copepod)	Common	Pathologic effects unknown	Essex 1927 Hoffman 1967 Wardle and McLeod 1952 Yamaguti 1959
*Proteocephalus ambloplitis**	North America	Chubs, shiners, topminnows killifishes, bluegill, sunfishes, black bass, rainbow trout, channel catfish, other fishes	Viscera, gonads	Ingestion of intermediate host (copepod)	Common	Bass tapeworm. Migrating plerocercoids cause extensive damage to viscera, fibrosis, adhesions, distortion of body, sterility	Fischer and Freeman 1969 Hoffman 1967 Wardle and McLeod 1952 Yamaguti 1959
Proteocephalus pearsei	Northern United States	Fathead minnow, bluegill, other fishes	Viscera, muscle	Ingestion of intermediate host (copepod)	Common	Pathologic effects unknown	Hoffman 1967 Wardle and McLeod 1952 Yamaguti 1959
Proteocephalus pinguis	North America	Brook trout, rainbow trout	Viscera	Ingestion of intermediate host (copepod)	Common	Pathologic effects unknown	Hoffman 1967 Wardle and McLeod 1952 Yamaguti 1959
*Diphyllobothrium cordiceps**	Western United States	Brook trout, rainbow trout, Pacific salmons, other salmonids	Muscle, connective tissue, mesentery, liver, spleen	Ingestion of intermediate host (copepod)	Common	Causes hemorrhage, fibrosis, adhesions, emaciation, reduced fertility, death	Hoffman 1967 Yamaguti 1959
*Diphyllobothrium sebago**	Northeastern United States	Brook trout	Viscera	Ingestion of intermediate host (copepod)	Common	Causes hemorrhage, fibrosis, adhesions, emaciation, reduced fertility, death	Hoffman 1967
Diphyllobothrium latum	North America, southern South America, Europe, Japan	Lake trout, brown trout, eels, other fishes	Muscle, viscera	Ingestion of intermediate host (copepod)	Common in northern United States, Canada, east central Europe; uncommon in western Europe	Broad fish tapeworm. Pathologic effects of larva unknown. Adult occurs in man	van Duijn 1967 Hoffman 1967 Reichenbach-Klinke and Elkan 1965 Yamaguti 1959
Diphyllobothrium ursi	Alaska	Pacific salmons	Viscera	Ingestion of intermediate host (copepod)	Uncommon	Pathologic effects unknown	Hoffman 1967 Yamaguti 1959
Diphyllobothrium osmeri	Alaska, Europe	Atlantic salmon, other fishes	Viscera	Ingestion of intermediate host (copepod)	Uncommon	Pathologic effects unknown	Hoffman 1967 Reichenbach-Klinke and Elkan 1965 Yamaguti 1959
Diphyllobothrium dendriticum	North America, Europe	Brown trout, sticklebacks, other fishes	Viscera	Ingestion of intermediate host (copepod)	Uncommon	Pathologic effects unknown	Bykhovskaya-Pavlovskaya et al. 1962 Reichenbach-Klinke and Elkan 1965 Threlfall 1969 Yamaguti 1959

*Discussed in text.

738

TABLE 22.5 *(continued)*

Parasite	Geographic Distribution	Fish Host	Location in Host	Method of Infection	Incidence in Nature	Remarks	Reference
Diphyllobothrium ditremum	Europe	Brown trout, other fishes	Viscera	Ingestion of intermediate host (copepod)	Uncommon	Pathologic effects unknown	Hoffman 1967 Reichenbach-Klinke and Elkan 1965 Yamaguti 1959
Diphyllobothrium norvegicum	Europe	Brown trout, Atlantic salmon, sticklebacks	Viscera	Ingestion of intermediate host (copepod)	Uncommon	Pathologic effects unknown. Adult occurs in man	Hoffman 1967 Yamaguti 1959
Ligula intestinalis*	North America, Europe, Asia	Goldfish, carp, European minnow, fathead minnow, bluntnose minnow, shiners, black bass, brook trout, rainbow trout, other fishes	Abdominal cavity	Ingestion of intermediate host (copepod)	Common	Causes abdominal distention, compression of viscera, excessive proliferation of connective tissue, obliteration of gonads, sterility, rupture of body wall, death	Belding 1965 van Duijn 1967 Hoffman 1967 Hoffman and Sindermann 1962 Owen and Arme 1966 Reichenbach-Klinke and Elkan 1965 Wardle and McLeod 1952 Yamaguti 1959
Schistocephalus solidus*	North America, Europe, Asia	Sticklebacks, other fishes	Abdominal cavity	Ingestion of intermediate host (copepod)	Common in sticklebacks	Heavy infections cause abdominal distention, compression of viscera, obliteration of gonads, decreased fertility	Arme and Owen 1967 Bykhovskaya-Pavlovskaya et al. 1962 van Duijn 1967 Hoffman 1967 Reichenbach-Klinke and Elkan 1965 Yamaguti 1959
Schistocephalus thomasi	North central United States	Sticklebacks	Abdominal cavity	Ingestion of intermediate host (copepod)	Rare	Pathologic effects unknown	Hoffman 1967
Haplobothrium globuliforme	North America	Guppy, sunfishes	Liver	Ingestion of intermediate host (copepod)	Common	Pathologic effects unknown	Hoffman 1967 Yamaguti 1959
Triaenophorus nodulosus*	North America, Europe	Goldfish, other cyprinids, bluegill, sunfishes, black bass, other centrarchids, Atlantic salmon, other salmonids, ictalurids, sticklebacks, eels, other fishes	Liver	Ingestion of intermediate host (copepod)	Common	Syn. *Triaenophorus lucii.* Causes cysts in liver; massive infections cause destruction of liver, death	Dogiel et al. 1962 van Duijn 1967 Hoffman 1967 Reichenbach-Klinke and Elkan 1965 Wardle and McLeod 1952 Yamaguti 1959
Triaenophorus crassus*	North America, Europe	Atlantic salmon, Pacific salmons, other salmonids, other fishes	Muscle, connective tissue	Ingestion of intermediate host (copepod)	Common	Causes yellow cysts in muscle, connective tissue	Hoffman 1967 Reichenbach-Klinke and Elkan 1965 Wardle and McLeod 1952 Yamaguti 1959

*Discussed in text.

TABLE 22.6. Adult nematodes affecting laboratory fishes

Parasite	Geographic Distribution	Fish Host	Location in Host	Method of Infection	Incidence in Nature	Remarks	Reference
Philonema agubernaculum*	United States, Canada	Brook trout, lake trout, rainbow trout, brown trout, other salmonids	Abdominal cavity	Ingestion of intermediate host (copepod)	Common	Sometimes causes massive adhesions, sterility	Hoffman 1967 Hoffman and Sindermann 1962 M. Meyer 1960 Northcote 1957 Richardson 1936 Yamaguti 1961
Philonema oncorhynchi*	United States, Canada, USSR	Brook trout, rainbow trout, Pacific salmons, other salmonids	Abdominal cavity	Ingestion of intermediate host (copepod)	Common	Sometimes causes massive adhesions, sterility	Hoffman 1967 Richardson 1936 Yamaguti 1961
Philometra carassii	North central United States	Goldfish	Caudal fin	Ingestion of intermediate host (copepod)	Uncommon	Pathologic effects unknown	Hoffman 1967
Philometra cylindracea	North America	Black bass, other fishes	Abdominal cavity	Ingestion of intermediate host (copepod)	Common	Pathologic effects unknown	Hoffman 1967 Yamaguti 1961
Philometra sanguinea	Canada, Europe	Goldfish, other fishes	Caudal fin	Ingestion of intermediate host (copepod)	Common	Pathologic effects unknown	Hoffman 1967 Reichenbach-Klinke and Elkan 1965 Yamaguti 1961 Yorke and Maplestone 1926
Philometra abdominalis	Europe	Cyprinids	Abdominal cavity	Ingestion of intermediate host (copepod)	Common	Length: 40 to 60 mm. Pathologic effects unknown	van Duijn 1967 Reichenbach-Klinke and Elkan 1965 Yamaguti 1961
Capillaria catenata*	North America	Bluegill, sunfishes, black bass, channel catfish, other fishes	Intestine	Unknown; probably by accidental ingestion of egg	Common	Heavy infections cause enteritis	Hoffman 1967 Yamaguti 1961
Capillaria eupomotis*	Europe	European minnow, sunfishes, rainbow trout, other fishes	Liver	Unknown; probably by accidental ingestion of egg	Common	Possible syn. Hepaticola petruschewskii. Causes extensive liver damage	Ghittino 1961 Hoffman 1967 Reichenbach-Klinke and Elkan 1965
Hepaticola bakeri	United States, Canada	Salmonids	Intestine	Unknown	Common	Pathologic effects unknown	Hoffman 1967
Camallanus lacustris	Northeastern United States, Europe	Carp, other cyprinids, Atlantic salmon, sticklebacks, eels, other fishes	Intestine	Ingestion of intermediate host (copepod)	Common	Possible syn. Camallanus truncatus. Length: 5 to 18 mm. Pathologic effects unknown	van Duijn 1967 Hoffman 1367 Reichenbach-Klinke and Elkan 1965 Yamaguti 1961 Yorke and Maplestone 1926

*Discussed in text.

740

TABLE 22.6 *(continued)*

Parasite	Geographic Distribution	Fish Host	Location in Host	Method of Infection	Incidence in Nature	Remarks	Reference
Camallanus truncatus	Northeastern United States, Europe	Black bass, other fishes	Intestine	Ingestion of intermediate host (copepod)	Common	Possible syn. *Camallanus lacustris*. Pathologic effects unknown	Hoffman 1967; Reichenbach-Klinke and Elkan 1965
Camallanus oxycephalus	United States	Shiners, sunfishes, black bass, salmonids, channel catfish, other fishes	Intestine	Ingestion of intermediate host (copepod)	Common	Incidence of 17.4% reported in channel catfish in south central United States. Pathologic effects unknown	Hoffman 1967; Spall and Summerfelt 1969; Yamaguti 1961; Yorke and Maplestone 1926
Camallanus ancylodirus	Central United States	Carp, other cyprinids	Stomach, intestine	Ingestion of intermediate host (copepod)	Common	Pathologic effects unknown	Hoffman 1967; Yamaguti 1961; Yorke and Maplestone 1926
Cucullanus truttae	North America, Europe	Brook trout, rainbow trout, brown trout, Pacific salmons, other salmonids, eels	Intestine	Unknown; probably by ingestion of copepod	Common	Syn. *Cucullanus occidentalis, C. globosus, Bulbodacnitis occidentalis*. Pathologic effects unknown	Hoffman 1967; Spall and Summerfelt 1969; Yamaguti 1961; Yorke and Maplestone 1926
Dacnitoides cotylophora	United States, Canada	Chubs, sunfishes, black bass, ictalurids, other fishes	Intestine	Unknown; probably by ingestion of copepod	Common	Pathologic effects unknown	Hoffman 1967; Yamaguti 1961; Yorke and Maplestone 1926
Dacnitoides robusta	United States	Channel catfish, other ictalurids	Intestine	Unknown; probably by ingestion of copepod	Common	Pathologic effects unknown	Hoffman 1967; Spall and Summerfelt 1969; Yamaguti 1961
Haplonema aditum	United States	Eels	Intestine	Unknown; probably by ingestion of copepod	Uncommon	Pathologic effects unknown	Hoffman 1967; Yamaguti 1961
Cystidicola stigmatura	North America	Brook trout, lake trout, rainbow trout, other salmonids	Swim bladder	Ingestion of intermediate host (shrimp)	Common	Pathologic effects unknown	van Duijn 1967; Hoffman 1967; Margolis 1966; Northcote 1957; Reichenbach-Klinke and Elkan 1965; Yamaguti 1961; Yorke and Maplestone 1926
Cystidicola farionis	Europe	Salmonids, sticklebacks	Swim bladder	Ingestion of intermediate host (amphipod)	Common	Pathologic effects unknown	Hoffman 1967; Yamaguti 1961
Rhabdochona cascadilla	North America, South America	Carp, chubs, shiners, black bass, Pacific salmons, other salmonids, sticklebacks, other fishes	Swim bladder, intestine	Ingestion of intermediate host (mayfly)	Common	Pathologic effects unknown	Hoffman 1967; Yamaguti 1961

TABLE 22.6 (continued)

Parasite	Geographic Distribution	Fish Host	Location in Host	Method of Infection	Incidence in Nature	Remarks	Reference
Rhabdochona decaturensis	United States	Channel catfish, other fishes	Swim bladder, intestine	Ingestion of intermediate host (mayfly)	Common	Incidence of 52% reported in channel catfish in south central United States. Pathologic effects unknown	Hoffman 1967 Spall and Summerfelt 1969 Yamaguti 1961
Rhabdochona denudata	Europe, Asia	Salmonids, other fishes	Intestine	Ingestion of intermediate host (mayfly)	Common	Pathologic effects unknown	Yamaguti 1961
Spinitectus carolini	United States	Bluegill, sunfishes, black bass, channel catfish, other fishes	Stomach, intestine	Ingestion of intermediate host (mayfly)	Common	Incidence of 17% reported in channel catfish in south central United States. Pathologic effects unknown	Hoffman 1967 Spall and Summerfelt 1969 Yamaguti 1961
Spinitectus gracilis	United States	Carp, shiners, sunfishes, black bass, ictalurids, sticklebacks, other fishes	Stomach, intestine	Ingestion of intermediate host (mayfly)	Common	Pathologic effects unknown	Hoffman 1967 Spall and Summerfelt 1969 Yamaguti 1961
Spinitectus inermis	Europe	Eels	Intestine	Ingestion of intermediate host (mayfly)	Common	Causes severe enteritis, death	Reichenbach-Klinke and Elkan 1965 Yamaguti 1961
Metabronema salvelini	Northern United States, Canada	Brook trout, lake trout, rainbow trout, brown trout, Pacific salmons, other salmonids, other fishes	Intestine	Ingestion of intermediate host (mayfly)	Common	Pathologic effects unknown	Hoffman 1967 Reichenbach-Klinke and Elkan 1965 Yamaguti 1961
Contracaecum brachyurum	North America	Bluegill, sunfishes, black bass, other centrarchids, other fishes	Stomach, intestine	Ingestion of second intermediate host (small fish)	Common	Length: up to 90 mm. Pathologic effects unknown	Hoffman 1967 Yamaguti 1961
Contracaecum aduncum	Europe	Brown trout, Atlantic salmon, Pacific salmons, other salmonids, eels, other fishes	Stomach	Ingestion of second intermediate host (small fish)	Common	Length: 18 to 36 mm. Pathologic effects unknown	Bykhovskaya-Pavlovskaya et al. 1962 Reichenbach-Klinke and Elkan 1965 Yamaguti 1961 Yorke and Maplestone 1926

TABLE 22.7. Larval nematodes affecting laboratory fishes

Parasite	Geographic Distribution	Fish Host	Location in Host	Method of Infection	Incidence in Nature	Remarks	Reference
*Contracaecum spiculigerum**	United States, Canada	Golden shiner, topminnows, bluegill, sunfishes, black bass, rainbow trout, channel catfish, eels	Viscera	Unknown; probably by ingestion of copepod, amphipod	Common	Incidence of 28% reported in channel catfish in south central United States. Migrating larvae cause extensive visceral damage	Hoffman 1967 Reichenbach-Klinke and Elkan 1965 Spall and Summerfelt 1969
Spiroxys sp.*	North America	Carp, shiners, other cyprinids, sunfishes, black bass, other centrarchids, channel catfish, sticklebacks, other fishes	Viscera, mesentery	Ingestion of first intermediate host (copepod)	Common	Causes cysts in mesentery; otherwise pathologic effects unknown; probably causes little damage except in heavy infections	Hoffman 1967 Spall and Summerfelt 1969
Eustrongylides sp.*	United States, Canada	Killifishes, bluegill, sunfishes, lake trout, rainbow trout, sticklebacks	Muscle, viscera	Unknown	Common	Causes large red cysts up to 10 mm in diameter in muscle, viscera	Hoffman 1967 Hoffman and Sindermann 1962 Northcote 1957 Yamaguti 1961
*Eustrongylides escius**	Europe	Carp, ictalurids, other fishes	Muscle, viscera	Unknown	Common	Causes large red cysts in muscle, viscera	Bykhovskaya-Pavlovskaya et al. 1962

*Discussed in text.

TABLE 22.8. Acanthocephalans affecting laboratory fishes

Parasite	Geographic Distribution	Fish Host	Location in Host	Method of Infection	Incidence in Nature	Remarks	Reference
Neoechinorhynchus cylindratus*	United States, Canada	Definitive: shiners, golden shiner, topminnows, killifishes, bluegill, sunfishes, black bass, other centrarchids, brook trout, Atlantic salmon, other salmonids, eels, other fishes. Intermediate: mosquitofish, bluegill, sunfishes, black bass, other centrarchids, other fishes	Adult: intestine. Larva: liver	Definitive: ingestion of second intermediate host (small fish). Intermediate: ingestion of first intermediate host (ostracod)	Common	Adult: causes local damage to intestinal mucosa. Larva: causes cysts in liver	Bogitsh 1961, Hoffman 1967, Olsen 1967, Venard and Warfel 1953, Ward 1940
Neoechinorhynchus rutili*	North America, Europe, Asia	Goldfish, carp, shiners, other cyprinids, black bass, other centrarchids, brook trout, rainbow trout, brown trout, Atlantic salmon, Pacific salmons, other salmonids, sticklebacks, eels, other fishes	Intestine	Ingestion of intermediate host (ostracod)	Common	Incidence of 9% reported in sticklebacks in Great Britain. Causes damage to intestinal mucosa	Chappell 1969, Hoffman 1967, Olsen 1967, Van Cleave and Lynch 1950
Neoechinorhynchus saginatus	Northern United States	Chubs, other cyprinids	Intestine	Unknown	Uncommon	Pathologic effects unknown	Hoffman 1967
Octospiniferoides chandleri	Southern United States	Killifishes, mosquitofish	Intestine	Ingestion of intermediate host (probably ostracod)	Common	Pathologic effects unknown	Hoffman 1967
Echinorhynchus salmonis*	North America, Europe, Siberia	Shiners, bluegill, sunfishes, black bass, other centrarchids, lake trout, rainbow trout, brown trout, Atlantic salmon, other salmonids, eels, other fishes	Intestine	Ingestion of intermediate host (amphipod)	Common	Causes deep pits in intestinal wall, ulcerative enteritis	Bykhovskaya-Pavlovskaya et al. 1962, Dogiel et al. 1962, Hoffman 1967
Echinorhynchus leidyi*	Northern United States, Canada	Black bass, lake trout, rainbow trout, other salmonids, other fishes	Intestine	Ingestion of intermediate host (amphipod)	Common	Pathologic effects unknown; probably causes ulcerative enteritis	Hoffman 1967
Echinorhynchus truttae*	Europe, Siberia	Rainbow trout, brown trout, Atlantic salmon, other fishes	Intestine	Ingestion of intermediate host (amphipod)	Common	Causes intestinal obstruction, ulcerative enteritis	Bykhovskaya-Pavlovskaya et al. 1962, Dogiel et al. 1962
Acanthocephalus anguillae*	United States, Europe	Goldfish, carp, brook trout, rainbow trout, brown trout, Atlantic salmon, eels, other fishes	Intestine	Ingestion of intermediate host (amphipod)	Common	Causes damage to intestinal mucosa, muscularis; sometimes death	Bullock 1963, Hoffman 1967, Nigrelli 1943
Acanthocephalus dirus*	Southern United States	Bluegill, sunfishes, black bass, channel catfish, other fishes	Intestine	Ingestion of intermediate host (amphipod)	Common	Unknown; probably causes damage to intestinal mucosa	Hoffman 1967

*Discussed in text.

TABLE 22.8 (continued)

Parasite	Geographic Distribution	Fish Host	Location in Host	Method of Infection	Incidence in Nature	Remarks	Reference
*Acanthocephalus jacksoni**	Northeastern United States	Sunfishes, brook trout, rainbow trout, other fishes	Intestine	Ingestion of intermediate host (amphipod)	Common	Causes damage to intestinal mucosa, chronic fibrinous enteritis	Bullock 1961, 1962, 1963 Hoffman 1967
*Acanthocephalus lateralis**	United States, Canada	Brook trout, Pacific salmons, other salmonids, other fishes	Intestine	Ingestion of intermediate host (amphipod)	Common	Unknown; probably causes damage to intestinal mucosa	Hoffman 1967
*Acanthocephalus lucii**	Europe	Brown trout, Atlantic salmon, sticklebacks, eels, other fishes	Intestine	Ingestion of intermediate host (amphipod)	Common	Unknown; probably causes damage to intestinal mucosa	Bykhovskaya-Pavlovskaya et al. 1962 Hoffman 1967
*Leptorhynchoides thecatus**	United States, Canada	Definitive: carp, shiners, other cyprinids, topminnows, bluegill, sunfishes, black bass, other centrarchids, brook trout, lake trout, other salmonids, channel catfish, sticklebacks, eels, other fishes Intermediate: chubs, topminnows, killifishes, mosquitofish, bluegill, sunfishes, black bass, brook trout, channel catfish, eels, other fishes	Adult: pyloric ceca Larva: mesentery, liver	Definitive: ingestion of intermediate host (amphipod, small fish); Intermediate: ingestion of intermediate host (amphipod)	Common	Adult: causes extensive damage to cecal mucosa Larva: causes cysts in mesentery, liver; otherwise pathologic effects unknown	Hoffman 1967 Spall and Summerfelt 1969 Venard and Warfel 1953
*Pomphorhynchus bulbocolli**	United States, Canada	Definitive: goldfish, carp, bluntnose minnow, chubs, shiners, golden shiner, other cyprinids, topminnows, bluegill, sunfishes, black bass, other centrarchids, rainbow trout, other salmonids Intermediate: shiners, other cyprinids, other fishes	Adult: intestine Larva: mesentery, liver, spleen	Definitive: ingestion of second intermediate host (small fish) Intermediate: ingestion of first intermediate host (amphipod)	Common	Adult: causes extensive damage to intestinal mucosa; sometimes perforation of intestine, trauma to liver Larva: causes cysts in mesentery, liver, spleen; otherwise pathologic effects unknown	Bullock 1961 Hoffman 1967 Northcote 1957
*Pomphorhynchus laevis**	Europe	Goldfish, carp, salmonids, sticklebacks, eels, other fishes	Intestine	Ingestion of intermediate host (amphipod)	Common	Causes extensive damage to intestinal mucosa; sometimes perforation of intestine, trauma to liver	Bykhovskaya-Pavlovskaya et al. 1962 Hoffman 1967 Saidov 1953

*Discussed in text.

TABLE 22.9. Leeches affecting laboratory fishes

Parasite	Geographic Distribution	Fish Host	Location in Host	Method of Infection	Incidence in Nature	Remarks	Reference
Haementeria montifera	North central United States	Carp, black bass, other fishes	Skin	Direct contact	Common	Syn. *Placobdella montifera.* Ingests blood	Hoffman 1967
Haementeria parasitica	North central United States	Killifishes, bluegill, other fishes	Skin	Direct contact	Rare	Syn. *Placobdella parasitica.* Ingests blood	Hoffman 1967 F. Meyer 1969
Cystobranchus verrilli	North central United States	Bluegill, black bass, channel catfish, other fishes	Gills	Direct contact	Common	Ingests blood; otherwise pathologic effects unknown	Hoffman 1967
Cystobranchus respirans	Europe	Atlantic salmon, other salmonids, other fishes	Skin	Direct contact	Uncommon	Ingests blood; otherwise pathologic effects unknown	Bykhovskaya-Pavlovskaya et al. 1962 van Duijn 1967 Hoffman 1967 Reichenbach-Klinke and Elkan 1965
Piscicola geometra	North central United States, Europe	Goldfish, carp, rainbow trout, brown trout, Atlantic salmon, sticklebacks, other fishes	Skin	Direct contact	Common	Ingests blood; causes weight loss; vector of *Crytobia*	Bykhovskaya-Pavlovskaya et al. 1962 van Duijn 1967 Hoffman 1967 F. Meyer 1969 Reichenbach-Klinke and Elkan 1965
Piscicola punctata	Northern United States, Canada	Sunfishes, black bass, brook trout, rainbow trout, other salmonids, other fishes	Skin	Direct contact	Common	Ingests blood; otherwise pathologic effects unknown	Hoffman 1967
Piscicola milneri	Northern United States, Canada	Lake trout, other salmonids, other fishes	Skin	Direct contact	Uncommon	Ingests blood; otherwise pathologic effects unknown	Hoffman 1967
Piscicola salmositica	Western North America	Rainbow trout, Pacific salmons, other salmonids	Skin	Direct contact	Common	Ingests blood; causes death; vector of *Crytobia*	Becker and Katz 1965 F. Meyer 1969 Thomas 1969
Piscicolaria reducta	United States	Golden shiner, bluegill, channel catfish, other fishes	Skin	Direct contact	Uncommon	Ingests blood; otherwise pathologic effects unknown	Hoffman 1967
Piscicolaria sp.	Northern United States	Black bass, channel catfish, other fishes	Skin	Direct contact	Uncommon	Ingests blood; otherwise pathologic effects unknown	Hoffman 1967
Illinobdella alba	United States, Canada	Golden shiner, bluegill, sunfishes, black bass, channel catfish, other fishes	Skin	Direct contact	Common	Ingests blood; otherwise pathologic effects unknown	Hoffman 1967
Illinobdella moorei	United States, Canada	Golden shiner, bluegill, sunfishes, black bass, other centrarchids, channel catfish, other fishes	Skin	Direct contact	Common	Ingests blood; otherwise pathologic effects unknown	Hoffman 1967 F. Meyer 1969
Illinobdella richardsoni	United States	Sunfishes, black bass, other fishes	Skin	Direct contact	Uncommon	Ingests blood; otherwise pathologic effects unknown	Hoffman 1967
Illinobdella elongata	Northern United States, Canada	Black bass, other fishes	Skin	Direct contact	Uncommon	Ingests blood; otherwise pathologic effects unknown	Hoffman 1967

REFERENCES

Amlacher, E. 1961. Taschenbuch der Fischkrankheiten für Fischereibiologen, Tierärzte, Fischzüchter und Aquarianer. Fischer Verlag, Jena. 286 pp.

Anthony, J. D. 1969. Temperature effect on the distribution of Gyrodactylus elegans on goldfish. Bull. Wildlife Dis. Assoc. 5:44–47.

Arme, C., and R. Wynne Owen. 1967. Infections of the three-spined stickleback, Gasterosteus aculeatus L., with the plerocercoid larvae of Schistocephalus solidus (Müller, 1776), with special reference to pathologic effects. Parasitology 57:301–14.

Ashton, N., N. Brown, and E. Easty. 1969. Trematode cataract in fresh water fish. J. Small Animal Practice 10:471–78.

Bauer, O. N. 1958. Interrelationships between parasites and host fishes, pp. 90–108. In V. A. Dogiel, G. K. Petrushevski, and Yu. I. Polyanski, eds. Parasitology of fishes (in Russian). Leningrad Univ. Press, Leningrad. (Translated edition: 1961. Oliver and Boyd, Edinburgh. 384 pp.)

Becker, C. D., and M. Katz. 1965. Distribution, ecology, and biology of the salmonid leech, Piscicola salmositica (Rhynchobdellae: Piscicolidae). J. Fish. Res. Board Can. 22:1175–95.

Belding, D. L. 1965. Textbook of parasitology. 3d ed. Appleton-Century-Crofts, New York. 1374 pp.

Bogitsh, B. J. 1961. Histological and histochemical observations on the nature of the cyst of Neoechinorhynchus cylindratus in Lepomis sp. Proc. Helminthol. Soc. Wash. D.C. 28:75–81.

Bregnballe, F. 1963. Trout cultures in Denmark. Progressive Fish-Culturist 25:115–20.

Bullock, W. L. 1961. A preliminary study of the histopathology of Acanthocephala in the vertebrate intestine. J. Parasitol. 47(Supp. 4):31.

———. 1962. A new species of Acanthocephalus from New England fishes, with observations on variability. J. Parasitol. 48:442–51.

———. 1963. Intestinal histology of some salmonid fishes with particular reference to the histopathology of acanthocephalan infections. J. Morphol. 112:23–44.

Burton, P. R. 1956. Morphology of Ascocotyle leighi, n. sp. (Heterophyidae), an avian trematode with metacercaria restricted to the conus arteriosus of the fish, Mollienesia latipinna LeSueur. J. Parasitol. 42:540–43.

Bykhovski, B. E. 1957. Monogenetic trematodes, their systematics and phylogeny (in Russian). Izd-vo Akad. Nauk SSSR, Moscow. 509 pp. (Translated edition: 1961. Am. Inst. Biol. Sci., Wash. D.C. 627 pp.)

Bykhovskaya-Pavlovskaya, Irina E., A. V. Gusev, M. N. Dubinina, N. A. Izyumova, T. S. Smirnova, I. L. Sokolovskaya, G. S. Shtein, S. S. Shul'man, and V. M. Epshtein. 1962. Key to parasites of freshwater fish of the USSR (in Russian). Zool. Inst. Akad. Nauk SSSR, Moscow-Leningrad. (Translated edition: 1964. U.S. Dept. Commerce, Office Tech. Serv. TT64-11040. 919 pp.)

Cameron, T. W. M. 1945. Fish-carried parasites in Canada: I. Parasites carried by freshwater fish. Can. J. Comp. Med. 9:245–54, 283–86, 302–11.

Chappell, L. H. 1969. Competitive exclusion between two intestinal parasites of the three-spined stickleback, Gasterosteus aculeatus L. J. Parasitol. 55:775–78.

Cheng, T. C. 1964. The biology of animal parasites. W. B. Saunders, Philadelphia. 727 pp.

Davis, H. S. 1953. Culture and diseases of game fishes. Univ. California Press, Berkeley. 332 pp.

Dawes, B. 1946. The Trematoda, with special reference to British and other forms. Cambridge Univ. Press, Cambridge. 644 pp.

Dogiel, V. A., G. K. Petrushevski, and Yu. I. Polyanski, eds. 1958. Parasitology of fishes (in Russian). Leningrad Univ. Press, Leningrad. (Translated edition: 1964. Oliver and Boyd, Edinburgh. 384 pp.)

Dogiel, V. A., Yu. I. Polyanski, and E. M. Kheisin. 1962. General parasitology (in Russian). Leningrad Univ. Press, Leningrad. (Translated edition: 1964. Oliver and Boyd, Edinburgh. 516 pp.)

Duijn, C. van, Jr. 1955. Diseases of fishes and their cure, pp. 125–53. In H. R. Axelrod and L. P. Schultz, eds. Handbook of tropical aquarium fishes. McGraw-Hill, New York.

———. 1967. Diseases of fishes. 2d ed. Iliffe Books, London. 309 pp.

Essex, H. E. 1927. The structure and development of Corallobothrium. Illinois Biol. Monographs. Univ. Illinois Press, Urbana. 11(3):7–74.

Ferguson, M. S. 1943. Development of eye flukes of fishes in the lenses of frogs, turtles, birds and mammals. J. Parasitol. 29:136–42.

Fischer, H., and R. S. Freeman. 1969. Penetration of parenteral plerocercoids of Proteocephalus ambloplitis (Leidy) into the gut of smallmouth bass. J. Parasitol. 55:766–74.

Ghittino, P. 1961. Su una capillariosi epatica

in trote di allevamento e in altri teleostei delle acque libere del bacino del Po in Piemonte, con descrizione di una nuova specie *(Capillaria eupomotis)*. Riv. Parassitol. 22:193–204.

Hanek, G., and W. Threlfall. 1969. Digenetic trematodes from Newfoundland, Canada. I. Three species from *Gasterosteus aculeatus* Linnaeus, 1758. Can. J. Zool. 47: 793–94.

Hoffman, G. L. 1956. The life cycle of *Crassiphiala bulboglossa* (Trematoda: Strigeida): Development of the metacercaria and cyst, and effect on the fish hosts. J. Parasitol. 42:435–44.

———. 1958a. Studies on the life-cycle of *Ornithodiplostomum ptychocheilus* (Faust) (Trematoda: Strigeoidea) and the "self cure" of infected fish. J. Parasitol. 44:416–21.

———. 1958b. Experimental studies on the cercaria and metacercaria of strigeoid trematode, *Posthodiplostomum minimum*. Exp. Parasitol. 7:23–50.

———. 1960. Synopsis of Strigeoidea (Trematoda) of fishes and their life cycles. U.S. Fish Wildlife Serv. Fishery Bull. 175. 60: 439–69.

———. 1967. Parasites of North American freshwater fishes. Univ. California Press, Berkeley. 486 pp.

———. 1970. Control and treatment of parasitic diseases of freshwater fishes. U.S. Bureau Sport Fish. Wildlife. Fish Disease Leaflet 28. 7pp.

Hoffman, G. L., and R. E. Putz. 1964. Studies on *Gyrodactylus macrochiri* n. sp. (Trematoda: Monogenea) from *Lepomis macrochirus*. Proc. Helminthol. Soc. Wash. D.C. 31:76–82.

Hoffman, G. L., and C. J. Sindermann. 1962. Common parasites of fishes. U.S. Fish Wildlife Serv. Circ. 144. 17 pp.

Hnath, J. G. 1970. Di-n-butyl tin oxide as a vermifuge on *Eubothrium crassum* (Bloch, 1779) in rainbow trout. Progressive Fish-Culturist 32:47–50.

Hughes, R. C. 1927. Studies on the trematode family Strigeidae (Holostomidae): VI. A new metacercaria, *Neascus ambloplitis* sp. nov. representing a new larval group. Trans. Am. Microscop. Soc. 46:248–67.

Kinkelin, P. de, P. Besse, and G. Tuffery. 1968. Une nouvelle affection nécrosante des téguments et des nageoires: La Bucéphalose larvaire à *Bucephalus polymorphus* (Baer, 1827). Bull. Office Intern. Epiz. 69: 1207–30.

Krull, W. H. 1934. *Cercaria bessiae* Cort and

Brooks, 1928, an injurious parasite of fish. Copeia 1934:69–73.

Larson, O. R. 1965. *Diplostomulum* (Trematoda: Strigeoidea) associated with herniations of bullhead lenses. J. Parasitol. 51: 224–29.

Lewis, W. M., and J. Nickum. 1964. The effect of *Posthodiplostomum minimum* upon the body weight of the bluegill. Progressive Fish-Culturist 26:121–23.

Maitland, P. S., and C. E. Price. 1969. *Urocleidus principalis* (Mizelle, 1936): A North American monogenetic trematode new to the British Isles, probably introduced with the largemouth bass *Micropterus salmonoides* Lacépède, 1802). J. Fish Biol. 1:17–18.

Malmberg, G. 1970. The excretory systems and the marginal hooks as a basis for the systematics of *Gyrodactylus* (Trematoda: Monogenea). Arkiv. Zool. Ser. 2. 23:1–192.

Margolis, L. 1966. The swim bladder nematodes of Pacific salmons (genus *Oncorhynchus*), pp. 559–60. *In* A. Corradetti, ed. Proc. First Intern. Congr. Parasitol. Pergamon Press, New York.

Matthey, R. 1963. Rapport sur les maladies des poissons en Suisse. Bull. Office Intern. Epiz. 59:121–26.

Meyer, F. P. 1968. Dylox as a control for ectoparasites of fish. Proc. 22nd Ann. Conf. S.E. Assoc. Game and Fish Comm. 12 pp. (Mimeo).

———. 1969. A potential control for leeches. Progressive Fish-Culturist 31:160–63.

Meyer, M. C. 1960. Notes on *Philonema agubernaculum* and other related dracunculoids infecting salmonids. Libro Hom. Caballero y Caballero Jubileo 1930-1960. Sec. Educ. Publ., Mexico, D.F.

Meyer, M. C., and R. Vik. 1963. The life cycle of *Diphyllobothrium sebago* (Ward, 1910). J. Parasitol. 49:962–68.

Mitchum, D. L., and T. D. Moore. 1969. Efficacy of di-n-butyl tin oxide on an intestinal fluke, *Crepidostomum farionis*, in golden trout. Progressive Fish-Culturist 31: 143–48.

Mizelle, J. D., and C. E. Price. 1964. Studies on monogenetic trematodes: XXVII. Dactylogyrid species with the proposal of *Urocleidoides* gen. n. J. Parasitol. 50:579–84.

Nigrelli, R. F. 1943. Causes of diseases and death of fishes in captivity. Zoologica 28: 203–16.

Noble, E. R., and G. A. Noble. 1961. Parasitology: The biology of animal parasites. Lea and Febiger, Philadelphia. 767 pp.

Northcote, T. G. 1957. Common diseases and parasites of fresh-water fishes in British

Columbia. Brit. Columbia Game Comm. Management Publ. 6. 25 pp.

Olsen, O. W. 1967. Animal parasites: Their biology and life cycles. 2d ed. Burgess, Minneapolis. 431 pp.

Owen, R. Wynne, and C. Arme. 1966. Some pathological effects produced in freshwater fishes by the plerocercoid larvae of the pseudophyllidean cestode, *Ligula intestinalis* (L.), pp. 553–54. *In* A. Corradetti, ed. Proc. First Intern. Congr. Parasitol. Pergamon Press, New York.

Reichenbach-Klinke, H. 1966. Krankheiten und Schädigungen der Fische. Fischer, Stuttgart. 388 pp.

Reichenbach-Klinke, H., and E. Elkan. 1965. The principal diseases of lower vertebrates. Academic Press, New York. 600 pp.

Richardson, L. R. 1936. Observations on the parasites of the speckled trout in Lake Edward, Quebec. Trans. Am. Fisheries Soc. 66:343–56.

Rogers, W. A. 1967a. New genera and species of Ancyrocephalinae (Trematoda: Monogenea) from centrarchid fishes of the Southeastern U.S. J. Parasitol. 53:15–20.

———. 1967b. Studies on Dactylogyrinae (Monogenea) with descriptions of 24 new species of *Dactylogyrus,* 5 new species of *Pellucidhaptor,* and the proposal of *Aplodiscus* gen. n. J. Parasitol. 53:501–24.

———. 1967c. Six new species of *Gyrodactylus* (Monogenea) from the Southeastern U.S. J. Parasitol. 53:747–51.

———. 1968a. *Pseudacolpenteron pavlovskyi* Bychowsky and Gussev, 1955 (Monogenea), from North America, with notes on its taxonomic status. J. Parasitol. 54:339.

———. 1968b. Eight new species of *Gyrodactylus* (Monogenea) from the Southeastern U.S. with redescriptions of *G. fairporti* Van Cleave, 1921, and *G. cyprini* Diarova, 1964. J. Parasitol. 54:490–95.

Rogers, W. A., and T. L. Wellborn, Jr. 1965. Studies on *Gyrodactylus* (Trematoda: Monogenea) with descriptions of five new species from the Southeastern U.S. J. Parasitol. 51:977–82.

Saidov, Hu. S. 1953. Helminth fauna of Dagestan fish and piscivorous birds (in Russian). Avtoreferat Dissertatsii (Moscow):1–16.

Schäperclaus, W. 1954. Fischkrankheiten. 3d ed. Akademie-Verlag, Berlin. 708 pp.

Sindermann, C. J. 1970. The principal diseases of marine fish and shellfish. Academic Press, New York. 369 pp.

Skrjabin, K. I. 1964. Keys to the trematodes of animals and man (English translation). H. P. Arai, ed. Univ. Illinois Press, Urbana. 351 pp.

Snieszko, S. F., and G. L. Hoffman. 1963. Control of fish diseases. Lab. Animal Care 13: 197–206.

Spall, R. D., and R. C. Summerfelt. 1969. Host-parasite relations of certain endoparasitic helminths of the channel catfish and white crappie in an Oklahoma reservoir. Bull. Wildlife Dis. Assoc. 5:48–67.

Sproston, Nora G. 1946. A synopsis of monogenetic trematodes. Trans. Zool. Soc. London 25:185–600.

Thomas, A. E. 1969. Mortality due to leech infestation in an incubation channel. Progressive Fish-Culturist 31:164–65.

Threlfall, W. 1969. Further records of helminths from Newfoundland mammals. Can. J. Zool. 47:197–201.

Turnbull, Eleanor R. 1956. *Gyrodactylus bullatarudis* n. sp. from *Lebistes reticulatus* Peters with a study of its life cycle. Can. J. Zool. 34:583–94.

Van Cleave, H. J., and J. E. Lynch. 1950. The circumpolar distribution of *Neoechinorhynchus rutili,* an acanthocephalan parasite of fresh-water fishes. Trans. Am. Microscop. Soc. 69:156–71.

Van Cleave, H. J., and J. F. Mueller. 1934. Parasites of Oneida Lake fishes: Part III. A biological and ecological survey of the worm parasites. Roosevelt Wild Life Ann. 3. Bull. N.Y. State Coll. Forestry 7:161–334.

Venard, C. E., and J. H. Warfel. 1953. Some effects of two species of Acanthocephala on the alimentary canal of the largemouth bass. J. Parasitol. 39:187–90.

Wales, J. H. 1958. Two new blood fluke parasites of trout. Calif. Fish Game 44:125–36.

Walton, A. C. 1964. The parasites of Amphibia. Wildlife Disease 40. (Microcard and microfiche).

Ward, Helen L. 1940. Studies on the life history of *Neoechinorhynchus cylindratus* (Van Cleave, 1913) (Acanthocephala). Trans. Am. Microscop. Soc. 59:327–47.

Wardle, R. A., and J. A. McLeod. 1952. The zoology of tapeworms. Univ. Minnesota Press, Minneapolis. 780 pp.

Wellborn, T. L., Jr., and W. A. Rogers. 1967. Five new species of *Gyrodactylus* (Trematoda: Monogenea) from the Southeastern U.S. J. Parasitol. 53:10–14.

Wood, E. M., and W. T. Yasutake. 1956. Histopathology of fish: II. The salmon-poisoning fluke. Progressive Fish-Culturist 18: 22–25.

Yamaguti, S. 1958. The digenetic trematodes of vertebrates. Vol. I. 2 Parts. *In* S. Yamaguti. *Systema helminthum.* Interscience, New York.

———. 1959. The cestodes of vertebrates. Vol. II. *In* S. Yamaguti. *Systema helminthum.* Interscience, New York.

———. 1961. The nematodes of vertebrates. Vol. III. 2 Parts. *In* S. Yamaguti. *Systema helminthum.* Interscience, New York.

———. 1963. Monogenea and Aspidocotylea. Vol. IV. *In* S. Yamaguti. *Systema helminthum.* Interscience, New York.

Yorke, W., and P. A. Maplestone. 1926. The nematode parasites of vertebrates. Blakiston, Philadelphia. 536 pp.

Chapter 23

MOLLUSKS

LARVAE, or glochidia, of freshwater clams and adult sphaerid clams sometimes affect fishes used in the laboratory (Table 23.1).

LARVAL MOLLUSKS

The larvae of most freshwater clams spend part of their life cycle embedded in the gills, skin, or fins of fishes (Davis 1953). Glochidia of several species of clams, many of them unidentified, have been reported to affect the goldfish, carp, shiners, minnows, sunfishes, bluegill, black bass, brook trout, rainbow trout, brown trout, sticklebacks, and other fishes throughout the world (Hoffman 1967; Reichenbach-Klinke and Elkan 1965). There are no specific reports of these parasites on laboratory fishes, but they could be introduced into a colony on newly acquired specimens or in pond water.

The glochidium has a thin bivalve shell with small anchoring hooks on the inner edges and is about 50 μ in diameter when first released by the female clam (Fig. 23.1) (Hoffman 1967; Northcote 1957; Reichenbach-Klinke and Elkan 1965). It is nonmotile and is carried by the current or settles to the bottom. When the glochidium comes in contact with a host, it attaches to the gills, skin, or fins and compresses the epidermis between the two halves of its shell. This stimulates the epidermis to pro-

liferate around the larval clam and to form a cyst which measures up to 3 mm in diameter (Hoffman and Sindermann 1962). The larva remains encysted for 9 to 80, usually 10 to 20, days. Grossly, it resembles a metacercarial cyst but is easily differentiated by the presence of a shell. Heavy gill infections are sometimes fatal.

There is no known treatment. The use of pond water for laboratory aquariums should be avoided during late spring and early summer when glochidia are present (Davis 1947). A filter or settling basin can be used to remove larvae from the water supply.

ADULT MOLLUSKS

Adults of the sphaerid clam, *Pisidium variable,* sometimes attach to the mouths of young rainbow trout and other fishes (Hoffman 1967).

REFERENCES

Davis, H. S. 1947. Care and diseases of trout. U.S. Fish Wildlife Serv. Res. Rept. 12. 98 pp.

———. 1953. Culture and diseases of game fishes. Univ. California Press, Berkeley. 332 pp.

Hoffman, G. L. 1967. Parasites of North American freshwater fishes. Univ. California Press, Berkeley. 486 pp.

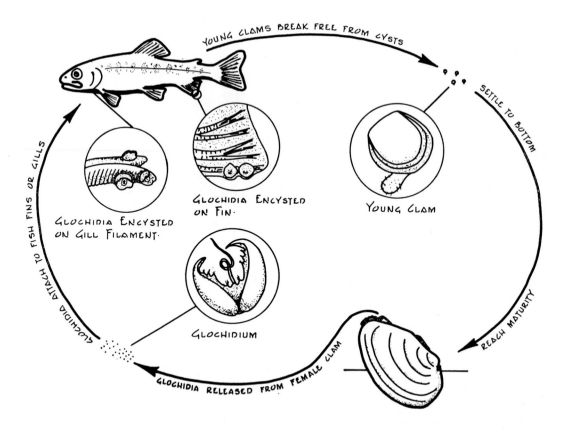

FIG. 23.1.   Life cycle of a freshwater clam. (Courtesy of T. G. Northcote, Fish and Wildlife Branch, Department of Recreation and Conser-
vation, Province of British Columbia.)

Hoffman, G. L., and C. J. Sindermann. 1962.
    Common parasites of fishes. U.S. Fish
    Wildlife Serv. Circ. 144. 17 pp.
Northcote, T. G. 1957. Common diseases and
    parasites of fresh-water fishes in British
    Columbia. Brit. Columbia Game Comm.
    Management Publ. 6. 25 pp.
Reichenbach-Klinke, H., and E. Elkan. 1965.
    The principal diseases of lower vertebrates.
    Academic Press, New York. 600 pp.

TABLE 23.1. Mollusks affecting laboratory fishes

Parasite	Geographic Distribution	Fish Host	Usual Habitat	Incidence in Nature	Remarks	Reference
Freshwater clams of unknown species	Worldwide	Goldfish, carp, bluntnose minnow, shiners, bluegill, sunfishes, black bass, brook trout, rainbow trout, brown trout, sticklebacks, other fishes	Larva: gills, skin, fins	Common	Causes cysts in gills; heavy infections sometimes cause death	Davis 1946, 1953 Hoffman 1967 Hoffman and Sindermann 1962 Northcote 1957 Reichenbach-Klinke and Elkan 1965
Margaritifera margaritifera	Western North America	Brook trout, rainbow trout, brown trout, other salmonids	Larva: gills	Common	Causes cysts in gills; heavy infections sometimes cause death	Davis 1946 Hoffman 1967
Pisidium variabile	North America	Rainbow trout, other fishes	Adult: mouth	Rare	Attaches to mouth of young fish; causes irritation	Hoffman 1967

Chapter 24

ARTHROPODS

HE most important arthropods affecting laboratory fishes are the crustaceans. Pentastomid larvae are sometimes seen, but they are much less common in fishes than in reptiles. Mite infections are rare. Some arthropods serve as intermediate hosts for fish parasites, but these are not likely to be encountered in fishes in the laboratory.

CRUSTACEANS

Branchiurans and copepods are the subgroups of crustaceans that parasitize freshwater fishes (Hoffman 1967; Schäperclaus 1954; Yamaguti 1963). The parasitic stages of these crustaceans are specialized morphologically and are often unrecognizable as arthropods. The free-swimming stages are more characteristic, and classification is based on them.

Crustaceans that affect laboratory fishes are listed in Table 24.1. The most important are discussed below.

Argulus

(Fish Louse)

This branchiuran is a common and serious bloodsucking ectoparasite of fishes (van Duijn 1967; Hoffman 1967; Reichenbach-Klinke and Elkan 1965; Wilson 1959). The genus contains about 110 species (Yamaguti 1963). They occur throughout the world and are frequently found on the skin of aquarium fishes.

Argulus japonicus and *A. foliaceus* are the commonest species. They are cosmopolitan and occur on the goldfish, carp, brown trout, sticklebacks, eel, and other fishes. *Argulus americanus* is common in North America on the bluegill and other fishes, and *A. coregoni* is common in North America and Europe on the brown trout, other salmonids, and the European minnow.

Other species that occur on laboratory fishes are listed in Table 24.1. Many are common in nature and are likely to be encountered on fishes obtained from their natural habitat. They can also be introduced into laboratory aquariums with live fish foods, such as *Daphnia,* obtained from waters in which infected fishes are present (van Duijn 1967).

MORPHOLOGY

Adults are light green to brown and flattened dorsoventrally. They have a leaf-like carapace that covers most of the dorsal surface and two prominent suction discs, a retractable preoral stinger, a proboscis, two pairs of antennae, and four pairs of thoracic legs on the ventral surface (van Duijn 1967; Hoffman 1967; Wilson 1959) (Fig. 24.1). The female is usually 6 to 7 mm long, and the male 4 to 5 mm long, but some species reach a length of 25 mm.

LIFE CYCLE

After copulation, the female lays eggs in batches on any object in the water (Bau-

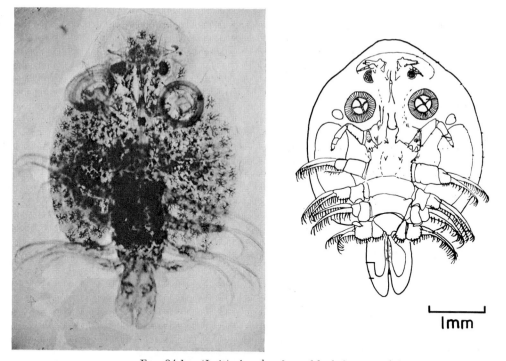

FIG. 24.1. *(Left) Argulus* from black bass. *(Right) Argulus japonicus* male, ventral view. *(Left* courtesy of W. A. Rogers, Southeastern Cooperative Fish Disease Project, Auburn University. *Right* from Hoffman, 1967; courtesy of University of California Press.)

er 1959; van Duijn 1967; Hoffman 1967). Eggs hatch in 15 to 55 days, and free-swimming larvae must attach to a suitable host in 2 to 3 days or die. After attachment, the larval stage grows, molts several times, and becomes sexually mature in 30 to 35 days. Adults can survive up to 15 days off a host.

PATHOLOGIC EFFECTS

The parasite moves freely over the surface of the fish, punctures the skin with its preoral stinger, inserts its proboscis, and sucks plasma (Bauer 1959; van Duijn 1967; Reichenbach-Klinke and Elkan 1965). Irritation, inflammation, and edema occur at the site of the puncture, and affected fish become restless and rub against objects in the water in an attempt to scratch the parasite loose. Small fishes attacked by large numbers of parasites sometimes die, apparently from the effects of a toxic substance believed to be secreted by the proboscis. *Argulus* also serves as a vector of

bacterial and probably of viral and protozoan pathogens.

DIAGNOSIS

Diagnosis is based on the presence of the localized areas of inflammation and edema and on identification of the parasite (Bowen and Putz 1966).

CONTROL

Newly acquired fishes should be carefully examined and, if infected, isolated and treated. Larval stages can be removed by placing the fishes in an aquarium with continuously flowing water. Adults are easily removed with a forceps or by gently rubbing the infected fish, always from head to tail (van Duijn 1967). Other effective treatments include the addition of 0.25 to 0.5 ppm trichlorfon (Dylox, Chemagro Corporation; Neguvon, Bayer) or 0.12 ppm naled (Dibrom, Chevron Chemical Co.) to the tank water, or the removal of infected fishes to a solution containing either 100 ppm trichlorfon for 1 hour, 2.0 to 3.5% trichlorfon for 2 to 3 minutes, or 10 ppm potassium permanganate for 5 to 60 minutes (van Duijn 1967; Hoffman 1970; Schäperclaus 1954; Snieszko and Hoffman 1963).

PUBLIC HEALTH CONSIDERATIONS

Argulus laticauda has been reported once as a fortuitous parasite of the eye of man; it caused no permanent damage (Hoffman 1967). Otherwise, the fish louse is of no known public health importance.

Lernaea cyprinacea
(Anchor Worm)
(SYN. *Lernaea carassii, Lernaea elegans;* probable syn. *Lernaea ranae*)

This copepod is a common and serious ectoparasite of freshwater fishes in North America, Europe, Africa, and Asia. It occurs on the gills, fins, and skin of the goldfish, carp, minnows, shiners, mosquitofish, tropical mouthbreeders, bluegill, sunfishes, black bass, trout, Pacific salmons, channel catfish, other fishes, and occasionally on amphibians (Harding 1950; Hoffman 1967; Putz and Bowen 1968; Reichenbach-Klinke

and Elkan 1965; Yamaguti 1963). Although usually uncommon on aquarium-raised laboratory fishes, it is sometimes introduced on plants, in pond water, on newly acquired specimens, or with live fish foods, such as *Daphnia* (Fletcher 1961; Reichenbach-Klinke and Elkan 1965).

MORPHOLOGY

The free-living copepodid male (Fig. 24.2*A*) and female (Fig. 24.2*B*) are recognizable as crustaceans, but the mature female (Fig. 24.2*C*) has a light green to dark brown, vermiform body, 7.5 to 22.5 mm long, with a large anchoring appendage at the anterior end and two egg sacs at the posterior end (Harding 1950; Hoffman 1967; Yamaguti 1963).

LIFE CYCLE

The eggs hatch in the egg sacs in 1 to 3 days, releasing six-legged, free-living larvae or nauplii (Grabda 1963; Hoffman 1967; Sarig 1968; Tidd 1938). Two more brief, free-living stages (nauplii) and parasitic larval stages follow until the sexual copepodid stage is reached. The time required from the hatching of the eggs to the

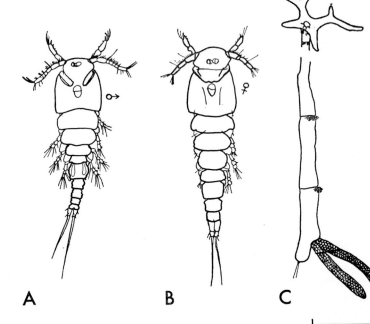

FIG. 24.2. *Lernaea cyprinacea.* (*A*) Copepodid male. (*B*) Copepodid female. (*C*) Mature female. (From Hoffman 1967. Courtesy of University of California Press.)

A   B   C

2mm

sexual copepodid stage, at 20 to 25 C, is about 14 days. Fertilization occurs on the host during the last free-swimming larval stage, after which the female embeds its head in the flesh of the fish, and the male dies. The head of the female becomes modified to form the large anchoring structure, and the body becomes elongated and vermiform. Although the life cycle is seasonal in nature in the temperate zones, it is continuous in aquariums (Fletcher 1961). The time required for the entire cycle at 20 to 25 C is about 20 to 25 days.

PATHOLOGIC EFFECTS

Heavy infection with fifth-stage copepodids sometimes causes serious gill damage and death, but the usual and most important pathologic effects of this parasite are those produced by the embedded female (Bauer 1959; van Duijn 1967; McNeil 1961; Reichenbach-Klinke and Elkan 1965). The adult female attaches to the gills, fins, and skin, usually at the base of the fins, and penetrates to the musculature, causing extensive tissue damage. Sometimes a protective connective tissue sheath encapsulates the embedded part of the parasite, but the usual lesion is a large hole in the skin and subcutaneous tissues that heals slowly, if at all. Secondary infection with bacteria and fungi is common. Debilitation and death occur in heavy infections, and small fishes are sometimes killed by perforation of the abdominal wall. Dermal tumors on fish have been associated with anchorworm infection, but a causal relationship has not been established (Schlumberger 1952).

DIAGNOSIS

Diagnosis is based on recognition of the parasite in association with the typical lesions.

CONTROL

Newly acquired fishes should be examined and, if infected, isolated and treated. Treatments effective against larvae include trichlorfon added to the water at a rate of 0.25 to 0.5 ppm, weekly for 4 to 5 weeks (Hoffman 1970; Meyer 1966); malathion in the water at a rate of 0.5 ppm for one application (P. Osborn, personal communication); and potassium permanganate in the water at a rate of 25 ppm for 90 minutes plus 50 ppm for an additional 60 min-

utes (Shilo, Sarig, and Rosenberger 1960). Benzene hexachloride has been used to control this parasite (Hindle 1949; McNeil 1961; Lewis 1961; Saha and Sen 1958), but it is not as effective as trichlorfon. Treatment of individual fish with 0.1% potassium permanganate solution has been described (van Duijn 1967). Only the parasite is brushed with the solution, not the fish. The parasite shrivels and drops off, and the wound is treated with merbromin (Mercurochrome, Hynson, Wescott, and Dunning).

PUBLIC HEALTH CONSIDERATIONS

Lernaea cyprinacea is of no known public health importance.

Ergasilus

This copepod is a common parasite of the gills of fishes in North America, Europe, and Asia (Yamaguti 1963). *Ergasilus caeruleus, E. centrarchidarum,* and *E. versicolor,* the commonest species of North America, are found on chubs, shiners, bluegill, sunfishes, black bass, rainbow trout, channel catfish, eels, and other fishes (Hoffman 1967; Roberts 1970). *Ergasilus sieboldi,* the common species of Europe, is found on many fishes, including the goldfish, carp, rainbow trout, and brown trout (Bykhovskaya-Pavlovskaya et al. 1962; Reichenbach-Klinke and Elkan 1965). *Ergasilus* is common in nature and is likely to be encountered on laboratory fishes obtained from their natural habitat. It appears only occasionally on aquarium-raised specimens (van Duijn 1967). This parasite can, however, be introduced into laboratory aquariums with live fish foods, such as *Daphnia,* obtained from waters in which infected fish are present.

MORPHOLOGY

Adults have a white, cyclopslike body which is flattened dorsoventrally (Hoffman 1967; Wilson 1959). The mature female, the only parasitic stage, is 1 to 2 mm long and has two long egg sacs with a pair of pointed, curved cephalic claspers (Fig. 24.3).

LIFE CYCLE

The eggs hatch in the egg sacs in 2 to 4 days and release the first-stage larvae or nauplii (Hoffman 1967). Another brief

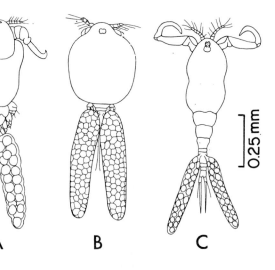

FIG. 24.3. *Ergasilus* females. *(A) E. caeruleus.* *(B) E. centrarchidarum.* *(C) E. versicolor.* (From Wilson 1959. Courtesy of John Wiley & Sons.)

larval stage (metanauplius) and four, free-swimming copepodid stages follow. Development to sexual maturity takes 10 to 70 days. Copulation occurs and the male dies. The female attaches to the gills of a suitable host and produces eggs at intervals of 3 to 12 days, depending on the species and temperature (Bowen 1966).

PATHOLOGIC EFFECTS

Ergasilus infection is characterized by the appearance of small white nodules (parasites) on the gills (Reichenbach-Klinke and Elkan 1965). Other signs are anorexia, weight loss, and debilitation. Gill damage is often extensive and consists of proliferation of the gill epithelium, with subsequent fusion of the lamellae (Fig. 24.4) and impaired respiration (Bauer 1958; Rogers 1969). Hemorrhage, lymphocytic infiltration, local epithelial degeneration, necrosis of lamellar stroma, and secondary bacterial or mycotic infection also occur. Heavy infections are sometimes fatal.

DIAGNOSIS

Diagnosis is based on identification of the parasite on the gills.

CONTROL

Newly acquired fishes should be carefully examined and, if infected, isolated and treated. Very little is known of specific control measures, but agents effective

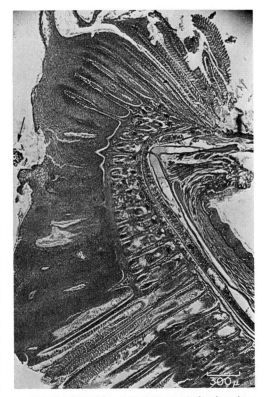

FIG. 24.4. *Ergasilus cyprinaceus* infection in a shiner. Note parasite *(arrow)* and proliferation of gill epithelium and fusion of lamellae. (Courtesy of W. A. Rogers, Southeastern Cooperative Fish Disease Project, Auburn University.)

against *Lernaea cyprinacea* are probably effective against this copepod. Individual fish can be treated by mechanically removing the parasites with forceps (van Duijn 1967). Care should be taken to avoid injuring the delicate gill epithelium.

Ergasilus is of no known public health importance.

Achtheres

This copepod occurs on the inner surface of the gill arches of several freshwater fishes sometimes used in the laboratory (Table 24.1) (Hoffman 1967). Most species are common and are likely to be encountered on specimens brought into the laboratory from their natural habitat. Morphology and the life cycle are generally similar to those of other copepods. The parasitic stage, the adult female (Fig. 24.5), causes gill damage. Otherwise, little is known of the pathologic effects of this parasite or of its treatment.

Salmincola

This copepod is found on the gills and occasionally on the skin of several salmonid fishes sometimes used in the laboratory (Hoffman 1967; Kabata 1969). *Salmincola edwardsii* and *S. californiensis* are the commonest species. They occur on the brook trout, rainbow trout, and other salmonids and are likely to be encountered on laboratory specimens of these fishes obtained from their natural habitat. Morphology and the

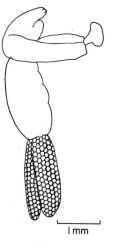

FIG. 24.6. *Salmincola edwardsii* female. (From Hoffman 1967. Courtesy of University of California Press.)

life cycle are generally similar to those of other copepods. The larva attaches to the gills and, after about 17 to 21 days, becomes sexually mature. Copulation occurs, the male dies, and the female degenerates into a grublike parasite (Fig. 24.6). While attached to the gills, the parasite sucks blood and causes local tissue damage and sometimes debilitation and death. Adults are difficult to kill, but it is likely that agents used against *Lernaea cyprinacea* are effective against the larvae of this parasite.

INSECTS

When ingested by salmonid fishes, larvae (caterpillars) of the silver-spotted tiger moth, *Halisidota argentata* (Fig. 24.7), cause lesions in various internal organs, usually in the viscera (Wood and Yasutake

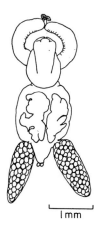

FIG. 24.5. *Achtheres ambloplitis* female. (From Hoffman 1967. Courtesy of University of California Press.)

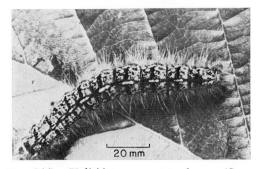

FIG. 24.7. *Halisidota argentata* larva. (Courtesy of W. T. Yasutake, Western Fish Disease Laboratory.)

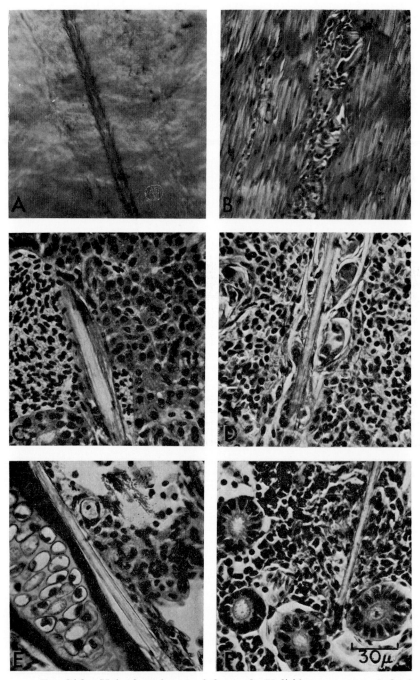

Fig. 24.8. Hairs from larvae of the moth, *Halisidota argentata*, lodged in several visceral organs and the vertebral column of a salmonid fish. (A) Mesentery. (B) Stomach wall. (C) Liver. (D) Spleen. (E) Adjacent to vertebra. (F) Kidney. (From Wood and Yasutake 1956. Courtesy of American Society of Parasitologists.)

1956). The lesions have been observed in the brook trout, rainbow trout, brown trout, Pacific salmons, and other salmonid fishes in northwestern United States. Ten of 75 samples of wild salmonid fishes were found affected, but only 1 of 75 samples of hatchery-reared fishes was affected. The condition is not likely to be encountered in laboratory-reared fishes, but it could be encountered in salmonid fishes obtained from their natural habitat in endemic areas.

The lesions are observable only microscopically and consist of focal inflammation caused by a central foreign body, a spine-covered hair (Fig. 24.8). The hairs, which remain in the stomach of the fish after the rest of the caterpillar is digested, penetrate the stomach wall and apparently migrate through the viscera, producing the foreign-body reaction.

No treatment is reported; control consists of preventing the ingestion of the caterpillars.

MITES

The larvae of some mites have been reported from the skin, gills, and esophagus of fishes, but they are rare. An unidentified mite encysted in the esophagus of the blue-gill has been reported in eastern United States (Hoffman 1967).

PENTASTOMIDS

Pentastomid larvae are sometimes found in fishes (Hoffman 1967). *Sebekia oxycephala* (Fig. 24.9) occurs in viscera of the mosquitofish, sunfishes, and other fishes in southern United States; *Leiperia cincinnalis* occurs in the muscle tissue of tropical mouthbreeders. Adults of these parasites occur in the respiratory tract of crocodiles, alligators, and caimans (Heymons 1935).

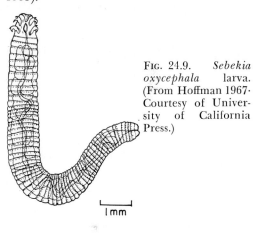

FIG. 24.9. *Sebekia oxycephala* larva. (From Hoffman 1967. Courtesy of University of California Press.)

1 mm

TABLE 24.1. Crustaceans affecting laboratory fishes

Parasite	Geographic Distribution	Fish Host	Usual Habitat	Incidence in Nature	Remarks	Reference
*Argulus japonicus**	Worldwide	Goldfish, carp, brown trout, stickle-backs, eels, other fishes	Skin	Common	Possible syn. *Argulus foliaceus, A. trilineatus.* Causes irritation of skin, loss of blood, sometimes death; possible vector of pathogens	Bauer 1958 van Duijn 1967 Hoffman 1967 Reichenbach-Klinke and Elkan 1965 Wilson 1959
*Argulus foliaceus**	Worldwide	Goldfish, carp, brown trout, stickle-backs, eels, other fishes	Skin	Common	Possible syn. *Argulus japonicus.* Causes irritation of skin, loss of blood, sometimes death; possible vector of pathogens	Bauer 1958 van Duijn 1967 Hoffman 1967 Reichenbach-Klinke and Elkan 1965 Wilson 1959
Argulus trilineatus	Western United States	Goldfish	Skin	Unknown; probably common	Possible syn. *Argulus japonicus.* Causes irritation of skin, loss of blood, sometimes death; possible vector of pathogens	Hoffman 1967 Reichenbach-Klinke and Elkan 1965 Wilson 1959
Argulus lunatus	Eastern United States	Goldfish	Skin	Unknown; probably common	Causes irritation of skin, loss of blood, sometimes death; possible vector of pathogens	Hoffman 1967 Reichenbach-Klinke and Elkan 1965
Argulus biramosus	United States, Europe, Israel	Carp, other fishes	Skin	Common	Possible syn. *Argulus appendiculosus.* Causes irritation of skin, loss of blood, sometimes death; possible vector of pathogens	Hoffman 1967
Argulus flavescens	North America	Carp, sunfishes, black bass, other fishes	Skin	Common	Causes irritation of skin, loss of blood, sometimes death; possible vector of pathogens	Hoffman 1967
Argulus catostomi	Northern United States	Carp, other fishes	Skin	Common	Causes irritation of skin, loss of blood, sometimes death; possible vector of pathogens	Hoffman 1967
*Argulus americanus**	North America	Bluegill, other fishes	Skin	Common	Causes irritation of skin, loss of blood, sometimes death; possible vector of pathogens	Hoffman 1967
Argulus versicolor	United States	Sunfishes, other fishes	Skin	Common	Causes irritation of skin, loss of blood, sometimes death; possible vector of pathogens	Hoffman 1967
Argulus appendiculosus	United States	Black bass, channel catfish, other ictalurids	Skin	Common	Possible syn. *Argulus biramosus.* Causes irritation of skin, loss of blood, sometimes death; possible vector of pathogens	Hoffman 1967
*Argulus coregoni**	North America, Europe	European minnow, brown trout, other salmonids	Skin	Common	Causes irritation of skin, loss of blood, sometimes death; possible vector of pathogens	van Duijn 1967 Hoffman 1967 Reichenbach-Klinke and Elkan 1965

*Discussed in text.

TABLE 24.1 *(continued)*

Parasite	Geographic Distribution	Fish Host	Usual Habitat	Incidence in Nature	Remarks	Reference
Argulus canadensis	Eastern United States, Canada	Brook trout, lake trout, sticklebacks, other fishes	Skin	Common	Possible syn. *Argulus stizostethi*. Causes irritation of skin, loss of blood, sometimes death; possible vector of pathogens	Hoffman 1967
Argulus stizostethi	Northern United States, Canada	Brook trout, Atlantic salmon, sticklebacks, other fishes	Skin	Common	Possible syn. *Argulus canadensis*. Causes irritation of skin, loss of blood, sometimes death; possible vector of pathogens	Hoffman 1967
Argulus pugettensis	Western United States	Rainbow trout, Pacific salmons, other fishes	Skin	Common	Causes irritation of skin, loss of blood, sometimes death; possible vector of pathogens	Hoffman 1967
Argulus funduli	Southern United States	Topminnows, killifishes	Skin	Common	Causes irritation of skin, loss of blood, sometimes death; possible vector of pathogens	Hoffman 1967 Reichenbach-Klinke and Elkan 1965
Argulus laticauda	United States	Eels, other fishes	Skin	Unknown	Causes irritation of skin, loss of blood, sometimes death; possible vector of pathogens. Reported once in eye of man	Hoffman 1967
*Lernaea cyprinacea****	North America, Europe, Asia, Africa	Goldfish, carp, fathead minnow, bluntnose minnow, shiners, golden shiner, other cyprinids, mosquito-fish, tropical mouthbreeders, bluegill, sunfishes, black bass, rainbow trout, Pacific salmons, channel cat-fish, other fishes	Gills, fins, skin	Common	Syn. *Lernaea carassii, L. elegans*; probable syn. *L. ranae*. Causes extensive damage to gills, fins, skin; debilitation; sometimes death	Bauer 1959 van Duijn 1967 Fletcher 1961 Harding 1950 Hoffman 1967 McNeil 1961 Putz and Bowen 1968 Reichenbach-Klinke and Elkan 1965 Yamaguti 1963
Lernaea esocina	Europe	Carp, rainbow trout, brown trout, sticklebacks, other fishes	Skin, gills	Common	Syn. *Lernaeocera branchialis*. Pathologic effects unknown; probably causes extensive damage to skin, gills	van Duijn 1967 Hoffman 1967 Reichenbach-Klinke and Elkan 1965
Lernaea phoxinacea	Europe	European minnow	Skin, gills	Common	Pathologic effects unknown; probably causes extensive damage to skin, gills	van Duijn 1967 Reichenbach-Klinke and Elkan 1965
Lernaea catostomi	United States	Shiners, mosquitofish, bluegill, sunfishes, other fishes	Skin, gills	Unknown; probably confused with *Lernaea cyprinacea*	Syn. *Lernaea tortua*. Pathologic effects unknown; probably causes extensive damage to skin, gills	Hoffman 1967
Lernaea pectoralis	Central United States	Shiners	Skin, gills	Rare	Syn. *Lernaeocera pectoralis*. Pathologic effects unknown; probably causes extensive damage to skin, gills	Hoffman 1967
Lernaea variabilis	Central United States	Bluegill, other fishes	Skin, gills	Unknown	Pathologic effects unknown; probably causes extensive damage to skin, gills	Hoffman 1967

*Discussed in text.

TABLE 24.1 *(continued)*

Parasite	Geographic Distribution	Fish Host	Usual Habitat	Incidence in Nature	Remarks	Reference
Lernaea dolabrodes	Central United States	Bluegill	Skin, gills	Unknown	Pathologic effects unknown; probably causes extensive damage to skin, gills	Hoffman 1967
Lernaea pomotidis	Central United States	Bluegill	Skin, gills	Unknown	Syn. *Lernaeocera pomotidis*. Pathologic effects unknown; probably causes extensive damage to skin, gills	Hoffman 1967
Lernaea cruciata	United States	Sunfishes, black bass, other centrarchids, brown trout, other fishes	Skin, gills	Unknown; probably common	Syn. *Lernaeocera cruciata*. Pathologic effects unknown; probably causes extensive damage to skin, gills	Hoffman 1967
Lernaea anomala	Southern United States	Black bass	Skin, gills	Unknown	Syn. *Lernaea insolens*. Pathologic effects unknown; probably causes extensive damage to skin, gills	Hoffman 1967
Lernaea lophiara	Africa	Tropical mouthbreeders, other fishes	Skin, gills	Unknown; probably common	Pathologic effects unknown; probably causes extensive damage to skin, gills	Hoffman 1967
Lernaea laterobranchialis	Africa	Tropical mouthbreeders	Skin, gills	Unknown	Pathologic effects unknown; probably causes extensive damage to skin, gills	Hoffman 1967
Lernaea tilapiae	Africa	Tropical mouthbreeders	Skin, gills	Unknown	Pathologic effects unknown; probably causes extensive damage to skin, gills	Hoffman 1967
Ergasilus caeruleus*	North America	Chubs, other cyprinids, bluegill, sunfishes, black bass, other centrarchids, rainbow trout, other salmonids, ictalurids, eels, other fishes	Gills	Common	Causes nodules on gills, anorexia, loss of weight, debilitation, fusion of gill lamellae, impaired respiration, death	Hoffman 1967 Roberts 1970
Ergasilus centrarchidarum*	North America	Bluegill, sunfishes, black bass, other centrarchids, other fishes	Gills	Common	Causes damage to gills, impaired respiration, death	Hoffman 1967 Roberts 1970
Ergasilus versicolor*	United States	Shiners, bluegill, sunfishes, black bass, other centrarchids, channel catfish, other ictalurids, other fishes	Gills	Common	Causes damage to gills, impaired respiration, death	Hoffman 1967 Roberts 1970
Ergasilus megaceros	United States	Chubs, golden shiner, other cyprinids, ictalurids	Gills, nasal fossae of ictalurids	Unknown; probably uncommon	Pathologic effects unknown; probably causes damage to gills, impaired respiration, death	Hoffman 1967 Roberts 1970
Ergasilus cyprinaceus	Southeastern United States	Chubs, shiners, other fishes	Gills	Uncommon	Causes damage to gills, impaired respiration, death	Roberts 1970 Rogers 1969
Ergasilus funduli	Southern United States	Killifishes	Gills	Unknown	Pathologic effects unknown; probably causes damage to gills, impaired respiration, death	Hoffman 1967 Roberts 1970
Ergasilus manicatus	Eastern United States	Mosquitofish, sticklebacks	Gills	Unknown; probably uncommon	Pathologic effects unknown; probably causes damage to gills, impaired respiration, death	Hoffman 1967 Roberts 1970

*Discussed in text.

TABLE 24.1 *(continued)*

Parasite	Geographic Distribution	Fish Host	Usual Habitat	Incidence in Nature	Remarks	Reference
Ergasilus lizae	Eastern United States, southern South America, Israel	Topminnows, killifishes, bluegill, sunfishes, other fishes	Gills	Unknown; probably uncommon	Causes severe damage to gills, impaired respiration, death	Hoffman 1967 Roberts 1970
Ergasilus arthrosis	United States	Bluegill, sunfishes, channel catfish, other ictalurids	Gills	Common on ictalurids; uncommon on other fishes	Pathologic effects unknown; probably causes damage to gills, impaired respiration, death	Roberts 1970
Ergasilus turgidus	Alaska, western Canada	Black bass, Pacific salmons, sticklebacks, other fishes	Gills	Unknown	Pathologic effects unknown; probably causes damage to gills, impaired respiration, death	Hoffman 1967 Roberts 1970
Ergasilus nerkae	United States, southwestern Canada	Rainbow trout, Pacific salmons, other fishes	Gills	Unknown	Pathologic effects unknown; probably causes damage to gills, impaired respiration, death	Hoffman 1967 Roberts 1970
Ergasilus auritus	Canada, USSR	Pacific salmons, sticklebacks	Gills	Uncommon	Pathologic effects unknown; probably causes damage to gills impaired respiration, death	Hanek and Threlfall 1970 Hoffman 1967 Roberts 1970
*Ergasilus sieboldi**	Europe	Goldfish, Pacific salmons, other fishes trout, other fishes	Gills	Common	Causes damage to gills, anorexia, debilitation, impaired respiration, death	Hoffman 1967 Reichenbach-Klinke and Elkan 1965
Ergasilus briani	USSR, China	Goldfish, Pacific salmons, other fishes	Gills	Common	Pathologic effects unknown; probably causes damage to gills, impaired respiration, death	Hoffman 1967
Ergasilus boettgeri	Europe	Mollies	Gills	Unknown	Pathologic effects unknown; probably causes damage to gills, impaired respiration, death	Hoffman 1967 Reichenbach-Klinke and Elkan 1965
Ergasilus gibbus	Europe	Eels, other fishes	Gills	Common	Causes damage to gills, impaired respiration, death	van Duijn 1967 Hoffman 1967
Ergasilus magnicornis	China	Goldfish	Gills	Unknown	Pathologic effects unknown; probably causes damage to gills, impaired respiration, death	Hoffman 1967
Ergasilus fryeri	Israel	Tropical mouthbreeders, eels, other fishes	Gills	Unknown; probably uncommon	Pathologic effects unknown; probably causes damage to gills, impaired respiration, death	Hoffman 1967
Achtheres ambloplitis	North America	Black bass, other centrarchids, salmonids, ictalurids	Gills	Common	Causes damage to gills, impaired respiration, death	Hoffman 1967 Kabata 1969
Achtheres micropteri	North America	Bluegill, black bass, other centrarchids, channel catfish, other fishes	Gills	Common	Causes damage to gills, impaired respiration, death	Hoffman 1967 Kabata 1969
Achtheres pimelodi	North America	Channel catfish, other ictalurids	Gills	Common	Causes damage to gills, impaired respiration, death	Hoffman 1967 Kabata 1969

*Discussed in text.

765

TABLE 24.1 *(continued)*

Parasite	Geographic Distribution	Fish Host	Usual Habitat	Incidence in Nature	Remarks	Reference
*Salmincola edwardsii**	United States, Canada, USSR	Brook trout, rainbow trout, other salmonids	Gills	Common	Syn. *Lernaeopoda edwardsii, L. fontinalis, Basanistes salmonea.* Causes loss of blood, damage to gills, debilitation, death	Hoffman 1967 Kabata 1969
*Salmincola californiensis**	Western United States, western Canada, Japan	Rainbow trout, Atlantic salmon, Pacific salmons, other salmonids, other fishes	Gills	Common	Syn. *S. falculata, S. beani, S. carpenteri, S. lata.* Causes loss of blood, damage to gills, debilitation, death	Hoffman 1967 Kabata 1969
Salmincola carpionis	Alaska, Canada, Greenland, Iceland, Siberia	Brook trout, other salmonids	Gills	Unknown	Pathologic effects unknown; probably causes loss of blood, damage to gills, debilitation, death	Hoffman 1967 Kabata 1969
Salmincola siscowet	Northern United States, Canada, Greenland	Lake trout	Gills	Unknown	Pathologic effects unknown; probably causes loss of blood, damage to gills, debilitation, death	Hoffman 1967 Kabata 1969
Salmincola salmoneus	Eastern Canada, Europe	Brown trout, Atlantic salmon, other salmonids	Gills	Unknown	Pathologic effects unknown; probably causes loss of blood, damage to gills, debilitation, death	Hoffman 1967 Kabata 1969
Lepeophtheirus salmonis	North America, USSR	Brook trout, brown trout, Atlantic salmon, other salmonids	Perianal skin	Common	Salmon louse. Causes damage to skin	Hoffman 1967 Reichenbach-Klinke and Elkan 1965
Lepeophtheirus strömii	Europe	Atlantic salmon	Perianal skin	Unknown	Salmon louse. Causes damage to skin	Hoffman 1967
Lepeophtheirus pollachii	USSR	Atlantic salmon, other fishes	Perianal skin	Unknown	Salmon louse. Causes damage to skin	Hoffman 1967

* Discussed in text.

REFERENCES

Bauer, O. N. 1958. Interrelationships between parasites and host fishes, pp. 90–108. *In* V. A. Dogiel, G. K. Petrushevski, and Yu. I. Polyanski, eds. Parasitology of fishes (in Russian). Leningrad Univ. Press, Leningrad. (Translated edition: 1961. Oliver and Boyd, Edinburgh. 384 pp.)

———. 1959. The ecology of parasites of freshwater fish (in Russian). Izv. Gos. Nauchn. Issled. Inst. Ozern. i Rechn. Rybn. Khoz. 49:5–206. (Translated edition: 1962. U.S. Dept. Commerce, Office Tech. Serv. TT61-31056. 236 pp.)

Bowen, J. T. 1966. Parasites of freshwater fish: IV. Miscellaneous. 4. Parasitic copepods *Ergasilus, Actheres,* and *Salmincola.* U.S. Bureau Sport Fish. Wildlife. Fish Disease Leaflet 4. 4 pp.

Bowen, J. T., and R. E. Putz. 1966. Parasites of freshwater fish: IV. Miscellaneous. 3. Parasitic copepod *Argulus.* U.S. Bureau Sport Fish. Wildlife. Fish Disease Leaflet 3. 4 pp.

Bykhovskaya-Pavlovskaya, Irina E., A. V. Gusev, M. N. Dubinina, N. A. Izyumova, T. S. Smirnova, I. L. Sokolovskaya, G. A. Shtein, S. S. Shul'man, and V. M. Epshtein. 1962. Key to parasites of freshwater fish of the USSR (in Russian). Zool. Inst. Akad. Nauk SSSR, Moscow-Leningrad. (Translated edition: 1964. U.S. Dept. Commerce, Office Tech. Serv. TT64-11040. 919 pp.)

Duijn, C. van, Jr. 1967. Diseases of fishes. 2d ed. Iliffe Books, London. 309 pp.

Fletcher, A. 1961. Anchor worm: Aquarium pest. All-Pets Magazine 32:27–28.

Grabda, Jadwiga. 1963. Life cycle and morphogenesis of *Lernaea cyprinacea* L. Acta Parasitol. Polon. 11:169–98.

Hanek, G., and W. Threlfall. 1970. *Ergasilus auritus* Markewitsch, 1940 (Copepoda: Ergasilidae) from *Gasterosteus aculeatus* Linnaeus, 1758 in Newfoundland. Can. J. Zool. 48:185–87.

Harding, J. P. 1950. On some species of *Lernaea* (Crustacea; Copepoda: parasites of freshwater fish). Bull. Brit. Museum Zool. 1:1–27.

Heymons, R. 1935. Pentastomida, pp. 1–268. *In* H. G. Bronn's Klassen and Ordnungen des Tierreichs. Vol. 5, Sect. 4, Bk. 1. Akademische Verlagsgesellschaft M.B.H., Leipzig.

Hindle, E. 1949. Notes on the treatment of fish infected with *Argulus.* Proc. Zool. Soc. London 119:79–81.

Hoffman, G. L. 1967. Parasites of North American freshwater fishes. Univ. California Press, Berkeley. 486 pp.

———. 1970. Control and treatment of parasitic diseases of freshwater fishes. U.S. Bureau Sport Fish. Wildlife. Fish Disease Leaflet 28. 7 pp.

Kabata, Z. 1969. Revision of the genus *Salmincola* Wilson, 1915 (Copepoda: Lernaeopodidae). J. Fisheries Res. Board Can. 26: 2987–3041.

Lewis, W. M. 1961. Benzene hexachloride vs. lindane in the control of anchor worm. Progressive Fish-Culturist 23:69.

McNeil, P. L. 1961. The use of benzene hexachloride as a copepodicide and some observations on lernaean parasites in trout rearing units. Progressive Fish-Culturist 23: 127–33.

Meyer, F. P. 1966. A new control for the anchor parasite, *Lernaea cyprinacea.* Progressive Fish-Culturist 28:33–39.

Putz, R. E., and J. T. Bowen. 1968. Parasites of freshwater fishes: IV. Miscellaneous. The anchor worm *(Lernaea cyprinacea)* and related species. U.S. Bureau Sport Fish. Wildlife. Fish Disease Leaflet 12. 4 pp.

Reichenbach-Klinke, H., and E. Elkan. 1965. The principal diseases of lower vertebrates. Academic Press, New York. 600 pp.

Roberts, L. S. 1970. *Ergasilus* (Copepoda: Cyclopoida): Revision and key to species in North America. Trans. Am. Microscop. Soc. 89:134–61.

Rogers, W. A. 1969. *Ergasilus cyprinaceus* sp. n. (Copepoda: Cyclopoida) from cyprinid fishes of Alabama, with notes on its biology and pathology. J. Parasitol. 55: 443–46.

Saha, K. C., and D. P. Sen. 1958. Gammexane in the treatment of *Argulus* and fish leech infection in fish. Ann. Biochem. Exp. Med. 15:71–72.

Sarig, S. 1968. Possibilities of prophylaxis and control of ectoparasites under conditions of intensive warm-water pondfish culture in Israel. Bull. Off. Int. Epiz. 69:1577–90.

Schäperclaus, W. 1954. Fischkrankheiten. 3d ed. Akademie-Verlag, Berlin. 708 pp.

Schlumberger, H. G. 1952. Nerve sheath tumours in an isolated goldfish population. Cancer Res. 12:890–99.

Shilo, M., S. Sarig, and R. Rosenberger. 1960. Ton scale treatment of *Lernaea* infected carps. Bamidgeh. Bull. Fish-Culturist 12: 37–42.

Snieszko, S. F., and G. L. Hoffman. 1963. Control of fish diseases. Lab. Animal Care 13: 197–206.

Tidd, W. M. 1938. Studies on the life history

of a parasitic copepod, *Lernaea carassii* Tidd. Doctoral Diss. Abstr. Ohio State Univ. 26:59–62.

Wilson, Mildred S. 1959. Branchiura and parasitic copepoda, pp. 862–68. *In* W. T. Edmondson, ed. Fresh-water biology. 2d ed. John Wiley, New York.

Wood, E. M., and W. T. Yasutake. 1956. Tissue damage in salmonids caused by *Halisidota argentata* Packard. J. Parasitol. 42: 544–46.

Yamaguti, S. 1963. Parasitic copepoda and branchiura of fishes. Interscience, New York. 1104 pp.

APPENDIX

LIST OF COMMON and PROPER NAMES

THIS LIST, based on the references given, is not meant to be authoritative, as some entries are arbitrary. The reader should bear in mind also that the identity of an animal mentioned in the text is that given in the supporting reference, and its correctness depends to a large extent on the accuracy of the original report.

MAMMALS
RODENTS

MURIDS

Mouse, laboratory mouse, house mouse	*Mus musculus*
Rat, laboratory rat, Norway rat	*Rattus norvegicus*
Black rat, roof rat	*Rattus rattus*
Multimammate mouse	*Praomys natalensis* (syn. *Rattus natalensis, Mastomys natalensis*)
European field mice, Old World field mice	*Apodemus*

CRICETIDS

Hamster, golden hamster, Syrian hamster	*Mesocricetus auratus*
Chinese hamster	*Cricetulus barabensis*
Deer mice, whitefooted mice	*Peromyscus*
Grasshopper mice	*Onychomys*
Cotton rat	*Sigmodon hispidus*
Wood rats, pack rats	*Neotoma*
Meadow mice, common meadow mice, voles	*Microtus*
Red-backed mice, bank voles	*Clethrionomys*
Rice rat	*Oryzomys palustris*
Gerbils	*Gerbillus*
Mongolian gerbil, clawed jird, tamarisk gerbil	*Meriones unguiculatus*
Muskrat	*Ondatra zibethica*

CAVIIDS
Guinea pig   *Cavia porcellus*

CHINCHILLIDS
Chinchilla   *Chinchilla laniger*

CAPROMYIDS
Nutria, coypu   *Myocaster coypus*

HETEROMYIDS
Pocket mice   *Perognathus*
Kangaroo rats   *Dipodomys*

SCIURIDS
Ground squirrels, gophers   *Citellus* (syn. *Spermophilus*)
Squirrels   *Sciurus*
Prairie dogs   *Cynomys*
Eastern chipmunk   *Tamias striatus*
Western chipmunks   *Eutamias*

LAGOMORPHS

LEPORIDS
Rabbit, laboratory rabbit, domestic   *Oryctolagus cuniculus*
   rabbit, European rabbit
Cottontail rabbits   *Sylvilagus*
Hares, jack rabbits   *Lepus*

CARNIVORES

CANIDS
Dog   *Canis familiaris*
Coyote   *Canis latrans*
Wolf, gray wolf, timber wolf   *Canis lupus*
Red foxes   *Vulpes*
Gray fox   *Urocyon cinereoargenteus*

FELIDS
Cat   *Felis catus*

MUSTELIDS
Mink   *Mustela vison*
Skunk, striped skunk   *Mephitis mephitis*

PRIMATES

LEMURIDS
Lemurs   *Lemur*

LORISIDS
Lorises   *Loris*
Slow lorises   *Nycticebus*
Galagos, bush babies   *Galago*

CALLITHRICIDS, CEBIDS (NEW WORLD MONKEYS, PLATYRRHINES)

Marmosets, tamarins	*Callithrix* (syn. *Hapale*)
	Saguinus (syn. *Leontocebus, Marikina, Oedipomidas, Tamarin, Tamarinus*)
	Leontideus (syn. *Leontocebus*)
	Callimico
	Cebuella
Common marmoset	*Callithrix jacchus*
Capuchins	*Cebus*
Howler monkeys	*Alouatta*
Spider monkeys	*Ateles*
Squirrel monkeys	*Saimiri*
Night monkey, owl monkey	*Aotus trivirgatus*
Titi monkeys, titis	*Callicebus*
Uakarises	*Cacajao*
Woolly monkeys	*Lagothrix*

CERCOPITHECIDS (OLD WORLD MONKEYS, CATARRHINES)

Rhesus monkey, monkey	*Macaca mulatta*
Cynomolgus monkey, crab-eating monkey, Java monkey	*Macaca irus* (syn. *M. cynomolgus, M. fascicularis, M. philippinensis*)
Pigtail macaque, pigtail monkey	*Macaca nemestrina*
Stumptailed macaque	*Macaca speciosa* (syn. *M. arctoides*)
Bonnet monkey, bonnet macaque	*Macaca radiata*
Japanese macaque	*Macaca fuscata*
Formosan macaque, Taiwan macaque	*Macaca cyclopis*
Macaques	*Macaca*
Green monkey, grivet, vervet	*Cercopithecus aethiops*
Guenons	*Cercopithecus*
Mangabeys	*Cercocebus*
Baboons	*Papio* (syn. *Chaeropithecus*)
Mandrills	*Mandrillus*
Gelada, gelada baboon	*Theropithecus gelada*
Patas monkey	*Erythrocebus patas*
Langurs, leaf monkeys	*Presbytis* (syn. *Semnopithecus, Kasi, Trachypithecus*)
Colobus monkeys, leaf monkeys	*Colobus*

PONGIDS

Gibbons	*Hylobates*
Orangutan	*Pongo pygmaeus*
Chimpanzee	*Pan troglodytes*
Gorilla	*Gorilla gorilla*

INSECTIVORES

ERINACEIDS

Hedgehog, European hedgehog	*Erinaceus europaeus*

MARSUPIALS

DIDELPHIDS

Opossum, common opossum	*Didelphis marsupialis*

EDENTATES

DASYPODIDS
  Armadillo, nine-banded armadillo   *Dasypus novemcintus*

BATS (CHIROPTERANS)

VESPERTILIONIDS
  Little brown bats   *Myotis*
  Big brown bats   *Eptesicus*

ARTIODACTYLIDS

BOVIDS
  Ox, cattle   *Bos taurus*
  Sheep   *Ovis aries*
  Goat   *Capra hircus*

SUIDS
  Pig   *Sus scrofa*

PERISSODACTYLIDS

EQUIDS
  Horse   *Equus caballus*

B I R D S
GALLIFORMS

PHASIANIDS
  Chicken   *Gallus domesticus*
  Coturnix quail   *Coturnix coturnix*

MELEAGRIDIDS
  Turkey   *Meleagris gallopavo*

COLUMBIFORMS

COLUMBIDS
  Pigeon   *Columba livia*

ANSERIFORMS

ANATIDS
  Duck   *Anas domesticus* (syn. *A. platyrhynchos*)

PASSERIFORMS

FRINGILLIDS
  Canary   *Serinus canarius*

PSITTACIFORMS

PSITTACIDS
  Parakeet, budgerigar   *Melopsittacus undulatus*

A M P H I B I A N S
FROGS AND TOADS (SALIENTIANS, ANURANS)

RANIDS

Frogs, true frogs	*Rana*
Leopard frog	*Rana pipiens*
Green frog	*Rana clamitans*
Bullfrog	*Rana catesbeiana*
Grass frog, common European frog	*Rana temporaria* (syn. *R. fusca*)
Wood frog	*Rana sylvatica*
Pickerel frog	*Rana palustris*
Edible frog	*Rana esculenta*

HYLIDS

Treefrogs	*Hyla*
Green treefrog	*Hyla cinerea*
Spring peeper	*Hyla crucifer*
European treefrog	*Hyla arborea*
Cricket frogs	*Acris*
Cricket frog	*Acris gryllus*

BUFONIDS

Toads	*Bufo*
American toad	*Bufo americanus*
Common toad	*Bufo terrestris*
European toad, common European toad	*Bufo bufo*
Marine toad	*Bufo marinus*

PIPIDS

Clawed toads	*Xenopus*
South African clawed toad	*Xenopus laevis*

SALAMANDERS AND NEWTS (CAUDATES, URODELES)

AMBYSTOMIDS

Mole salamanders	*Ambystoma*
Jefferson salamander	*Ambystoma jeffersonianum*
Spotted salamander	*Ambystoma maculatum*
Marbled salamander	*Ambystoma opacum*
Tiger salamander	*Ambystoma tigrinum*
Mexican axolotl, axolotl	*Ambystoma mexicanum* (syn. *Siredon mexicanum*)

PLETHODONTIDS

Dusky salamanders	*Desmognathus*
Dusky salamander	*Desmognathus fuscus*

SALAMANDRIDS

Newts	*Diemictylus* (syn. *Triturus, Notophthalmus*) *Triturus* (syn. *Triton, Taricha*)
Red-spotted newt, water newt, red eft	*Diemictylus viridescens* (syn. *Triturus viridescens, Notophthalmus viridescens*)
Alpine newt	*Triturus alpestris*

Common newt, smooth newt	*Triturus vulgaris*
Crested newt	*Triturus cristatus*
Palmate newt	*Triturus helveticus* (syn. *T. palmatus*)
Pacific newt, California newt, Western American newt	*Triturus torosus*
European salamanders	*Salamandra*
Fire salamander	*Salamandra salamandra*

PROTEIDS
| Waterdogs, mudpuppies | *Necturus* |
| Waterdog, mudpuppy | *Necturus maculosus* |

AMPHIUMIDS
| Amphiumas | *Amphiuma* |
| Amphiuma | *Amphiuma means* |

R E P T I L E S
TURTLES, TORTOISES, TERRAPINS (CHELONIANS)

TESTUDINIDS
Painted turtles	*Chrysemys*
Painted turtle	*Chrysemys picta*
Pond turtles	*Clemmys*
Spotted turtle	*Clemmys guttata*
Semi-box turtles	*Emydoidea* (syn. *Emys*)
Blanding's turtle	*Emydoidea blandingi* (syn. *Emys blandingi*)
European pond terrapin	*Emydoidea orbicularis* (syn. *Emys orbicularis*)
Map turtles, sawbacks	*Graptemys*
Map turtle	*Graptemys geographica*
Cooters, sliders	*Pseudemys*
Cooter	*Pseudemys floridana*
Florida red-bellied turtle	*Pseudemys nelsoni*
Pond slider, red-eared turtle	*Pseudemys scripta*
Box turtles	*Terrapene*
Box turtle, Eastern box turtle	*Terrapene carolina*
Western box turtle, ornate box turtle	*Terrapene ornata*
Tortoises, land tortoises	*Testudo*
South American tortoise	*Testudo denticulata*
Greek tortoise	*Testudo graeca*
Mediterranean tortoise	*Testudo hermanni*

CHELONIIDS
| Green turtles | *Chelonia* |
| Green turtle | *Chelonia mydas* |

CHELYDRIDS
| Snapping turtles | *Chelydra* |
| Snapping turtle | *Chelydra serpentina* |

TRIONYCHIDS
| Softshell turtles | *Trionyx* |
| Spiny softshell turtle | *Trionyx ferox* |

CROCODILIANS

ALLIGATORIDS

Alligators   *Alligator*
American alligator   *Alligator mississippiensis*
Caimans   *Caiman*
Broad-fronted caiman   *Caiman latirostris*
Spectacled caiman   *Caiman sclerops*

CROCODYLIDS

Crocodiles   *Crocodylus*
American crocodile   *Crocodylus acutus*
Nile crocodile   *Crocodylus niloticus*

SNAKES (SERPENTENS, OPHIDIANS)

COLUBRIDS

Racers   *Coluber*
Racer   *Coluber constrictor*
Rat snakes   *Elaphe*
Rat snake   *Elaphe obsoleta*
Corn snake   *Elaphe guttata*
Hognose snakes   *Heterodon*
Eastern hognose snake   *Heterodon platyrhinos*
Southern hognose snake   *Heterodon simus*
Western hognose snake   *Heterodon nasicus*
Kingsnakes   *Lampropeltis*
Common kingsnake   *Lampropeltis getulus*
Milk snake   *Lampropeltis doliata* (syn. *L. triangulum*)

Water snakes   *Natrix*
Common water snake   *Natrix sipedon*
Green water snake   *Natrix cyclopion*
Green snakes   *Opheodrys*
Rough green snake   *Opheodrys aestivus*
Bullsnakes   *Pituophis*
Gopher snake   *Pituophis catenifer*
Pine snake   *Pituophis melanoleucus*
Garter snakes   *Thamnophis*
Garter snake, ribbon snake   *Thamnophis sauritus*
Butler's garter snake   *Thamnophis butleri*

VIPERIDS

True vipers, Old World vipers   *Vipera*
Common European viper, adder   *Vipera berus*

LIZARDS (SAURIANS, LACERTILIANS)

IGUANIDS

Anoles   *Anolis*
Green anole, American chameleon   *Anolis carolinensis*
Basilisks   *Basiliscus*
Basilisk lizard   *Basiliscus basiliscus*
Collared lizards, leopard lizards   *Crotaphytus*
Collared lizard   *Crotaphytus collaris*
Iguanas   *Iguana*

Green iguana, common iguana — *Iguana iguana*
Horned lizards, horned toads — *Phrynosoma*
Texas horned lizard, Texas horned toad — *Phrynosoma cornutum*
Spiny lizards — *Sceloporus*
Eastern fence lizard, fence lizard — *Sceloporus undulatus*
Western fence lizard — *Sceloporus occidentalis*

LACERTIDS
European lizards — *Lacerta*
Sand lizard — *Lacerta agilis*
Wall lizard — *Lacerta muralis*
Viviparous lizard — *Lacerta vivipara*
Green lizard — *Lacerta viridis*

CHAMAELEONTIDS
Chameleons — *Chamaeleo*
European chameleon — *Chamaeleo chamaeleon*

XANTUSIIDS
Night lizards — *Xantusia*
Desert night lizard — *Xantusia vigilis*

HELODERMATIDS
Beaded lizard — *Heloderma horridum*
Gila monster — *Heloderma suspectum*

FISHES
BONY FISHES (TELEOSTS)

CYPRINIDS
Goldfish — *Carassius auratus*
Carp — *Cyprinus carpio*
European minnow — *Phoxinus phoxinus*
Fathead minnow — *Pimephales promelas*
Bluntnose minnow — *Pimephales notatus*
Chubs — *Semotilus*
Shiners — *Notropis*
Golden shiner — *Notemigonus crysoleucas*

CYPRINODONTIDS
Topminnows, killifishes — *Cyprinodon, Fundulus*
Medaka — *Oryzias latipes*

POECILIIDS
Guppy — *Lebistes reticulatus*
Mollies — *Mollienesia*
Platyfish, platy — *Xiphophorus maculatus* (syn. *Platypoecilus maculatus*)
Swordtail — *Xiphophorus helleri*
Mosquitofish — *Gambusia affinis*

ANABANTIDS
Siamese fighting fish — *Betta splendens*
Paradise fish — *Macropodus opercularis*

CHARACIDS
    Tetras   *Hyphessobrycon, Hemigrammus*

CICHLIDS
    Tropical mouthbreeders   *Tilapia*

CENTRARCHIDS
    Sunfishes   *Lepomis*
    Bluegill   *Lepomis macrochirus*
    Black bass   *Micropterus*

SALMONIDS
    Brook trout   *Salvelinus fontinalis*
    Lake trout   *Salvelinus namaycush*
    Rainbow trout   *Salmo gairdneri*
    Brown trout   *Salmo trutta*
    Atlantic salmon   *Salmo salar*
    Pacific salmons   *Oncorhynchus*
    Chinook salmon   *Oncorhynchus tshawytscha*

ICTALURIDS
    Channel catfish   *Ictalurus punctatus*

GASTEROSTEIDS
    Sticklebacks   *Gasterosteus*

ANGUILLIDS
    Eels   *Anguilla*

REFERENCES

Blair, W. F., A. P. Blair, P. Brodkorb, F. R. Cagle, and G. A. Moore. 1957. Vertebrates of the United States. McGraw-Hill, New York. 819 pp.

Conant, R., F. R. Cagle, C. J. Goin, C. H. Lowe, Jr., W. T. Neill, M. G. Netting, K. P. Schmidt, C. E. Shaw, R. C. Stebbins, and C. M. Bodert. 1956. Common names for North American amphibians and reptiles. Copeia 1956:172–85.

Davis, D. H. S. 1965. Classification problems of African Muridae. Zoologica Africana 1:121–45.

Ellerman, J. R. 1940. The families and genera of living rodents. Vol. I. Rodents other than Muridae. Wheldon and Wesley, Codicote, England. 689 pp.

Ellerman, J. R. 1941. The families and genera of living rodents. Vol. II. Family Muridae. Wheldon and Wesley, Codicote, England. 690 pp.

Gray, P. 1967. The dictionary of the biological sciences. Reinhold, New York. 602 pp.

Hoffman, G. L. 1967. Parasites of North American freshwater fishes. Univ. of Calif. Press, Berkeley. 486 pp.

Hoffstetter, R., and J-P. Gasc. 1969. Vertebrae and ribs of modern reptiles, pp. 201–310. *In* C. Gans, A. d'A. Bellairs, and T. S. Parsons, eds. Biology of the Reptilia: Vol. I. Morphology A. Academic Press, New York.

Jordan, D. S. 1963. The genera of fishes and a classification of fishes. Stanford Univ. Press, Stanford, Calif. 800 pp.

Napier, J. R., and P. H. Napier. 1967. A handbook of living primates. Academic Press, New York. 456 pp.

Noble, G. K. 1931. The biology of the Amphibia. McGraw-Hill, New York. 577 pp.

Pope, C. H. 1956. The reptile world. Alfred A. Knopf, New York. 325 pp.

Simpson, G. G. 1945. The principles of classification and a classification of mammals. Bull. Am. Mus. Natl. Hist., Vol. 85. 350 pp.

Thomson, A. L. 1964. A new dictionary of birds. McGraw-Hill, New York. 928 pp.

Walker, E. P., Florence Warnick, S. E. Hamlet, K. I. Lange, Mary A. Davis, Howard E. Uible, and Patricia F. Wright. 1968. Mammals of the world. 2d ed. 2 vols. Johns Hopkins Press, Baltimore.

INDEX